Dear Colleague:

UnitedHealth Foundation is pleased to provide you with a complimentary copy of *Clinical Evidence,* Issue 4, an international resource that provides easy access to the most up-to-date information on what works in medicine. *Clinical Evidence* was developed by the BMJ Publishing Group, publisher of the 160-year old *British Medical Journal,* in conjunction with internationally recognized medical experts.

Today, the sheer volume of information on medical care that is available through the popular media and elsewhere is overwhelming — and much of it is biased, fragmentary and confusing. We recognize how difficult it can be for the practicing physician to discern what information is based on the latest scientific evidence. UnitedHealth Foundation is committed to helping physicians access objective, evidence-based information they can use to improve health care delivery.

This past summer, UnitedHealth Foundation distributed copies of *Clinical Evidence,* Issue 3 to approximately 400,000 physicians throughout the United States. The response to this initial distribution was so overwhelmingly positive that the Foundation now is distributing *Clinical Evidence,* Issue 4 and has expanded the recipients to include many academic teaching programs. This book has proven particularly timely given the increasing attention to, and support for, evidence-based decision-making as a standard for medical care.

Given the clear value and importance of this volume, coupled with the universally positive response to its distribution, UnitedHealth Foundation already has committed to provide complimentary copies of the next issue of *Clinical Evidence* to physicians and academic teaching programs. If you would like to receive a copy of ***Clinical Evidence,*** Issue 5, please e-mail us at uhfce@uhc.com, phone us at **1-877-485-8074**, or mail us at the address above with your name, specialty and the address where you would like the book sent.

The BMJ Publishing Group is solely responsible for the content of all issues of *Clinical Evidence* and is continually revising *Clinical Evidence* based on feedback from physicians. I encourage you to provide them with comments via CEfeedback@bmjgroup.com.

We hope that you continue to find *Clinical Evidence* a resource that can assist you and your patients in making the best decisions possible, and thus advance optimum medical care to all people.

Sincerely,

William W. McGuire, M.D.
Chairman
UnitedHealth Foundation

4 ISSUE

DECEMBER 2000

clinical
evidence

The international source of the
best available evidence for
effective health care

BMJ
Publishing
Group

Editorial Office
BMJ Publishing Group, BMA House, Tavistock Square, London, WC1H 9JR, United Kingdom Tel: +44 (0)20 7387 4499 Fax: +44 (0)20 7383 6242 www.bmjpg.com

Subscription prices
Clinical Evidence is published six monthly (June/December) by BMJ Publishing Group. The annual subscription rates for Issues 4 and 5 (December 2000 and June 2001) are:

Individual: £75 • US$110 • Can$160
Institutional: £160 • US$240 • Can$345
Student: £55 • US$80 • Can$120

The above rates include print and online formats for individuals and students. The institutional rate is for print only. Institutions may purchase online site licenses separately. For further information, visit the subscription pages of our website www.clinicalevidence.org or contact Miranda Lonsdale, Sales Manager mlonsdale@bmjgroup.com

All subscriptions from countries outside the Americas to be directed to BMJ Publishing Group, PO Box 299, London WC1H 9TD.
Tel: +44 (0)20 7383 6270 • Fax: +44 (0)20 7383 6402• Email: subscriptions@bmjgroup.com

All subscriptions from countries in the Americas to BMJ-Clinical Evidence, PO Box 512, Annapolis Jct, MD 20701-0512, USA.
Tel: 1-800-373-2897/1-240-646-700 • Fax: 1-240-646-7005 • Email: clinevide@pmds.com
Alternatively, you can visit the BMJ Publishing Group website to order online www.bmjpg.com

Bulk subscriptions for societies and organisations
The Publishers offer discounts for any society or organisation buying bulk quantities for their members/ specific groups. Please contact Miranda Lonsdale, Sales Manager mlonsdale@bmjgroup.com

Feedback
We are always looking to improve *Clinical Evidence* to make it as useful, accurate, and up to date as possible. Please give us your views, comments, and suggestions. You can email us on CEfeedback@bmjgroup.com

Contributors
If you are interested in becoming a contributor to *Clinical Evidence* please contact us on clinicalevidence@bmjgroup.com

Clinical Evidence Online
Individual subscribers to *Clinical Evidence* will receive full text internet access as part of their annual subscription: go to www.clinicalevidence.org to sign up. For information about electronic products, including access through Ovid and a standalone intranet version, please contact Diane Harris on clinicalevidence@bmjgroup.com

Rights
For information on translation rights, please contact Daniel Raymond-Barker on clinicalevidence@bmjgroup.com

British Library Cataloguing in Publication Data. A catalogue record for this book is available from the British Library. ISBN 0-7279-14987 ISSN 1462-3846

Permission to reproduce
Please write to Josephine Woodcock, BMJ *Clinical Evidence* at the address above when requesting permission to reprint all or part of any contribution in *Clinical Evidence*.

Legal Disclaimer
Care has been taken to confirm the accuracy of the information presented and to describe generally accepted practices. However, the authors, editors, and publishers are not responsible for errors or omissions or for any consequences from application of the information in this book and make no warranty, express or implied, with respect to the contents of the publication.

Printed by Quebecor Printing, Hawkins, Tennessee
Designed by Pete Wilder, The Designers Collective Limited, London UK

Acknowledgements

We especially acknowledge the continuing support and guidance of Fiona Godlee, Founding Editor of *Clinical Evidence*, whose vision, leadership and energy led to the production of issues 1 to 3.

We thank Anna Donald and Vivek Muthu for their unceasing enthusiasm and encouragement. We also thank the following people and organisations for their advice and support: The Cochrane Collaboration, and especially Iain Chalmers, Mike Clarke, Phil Alderson and Carol Lefebvre; the NHS Centre for Reviews and Dissemination, and especially Jos Kleijnen and Julie Glanville; the NHS Executive, and especially Andrew

Burnett, Chris Henshall, and Tom Mann; the British National Formulary, and especially Dinesh Mehta; the Health Information Research Unit at McMaster University and especially Brian Haynes and Ann McKibbon; the Sowerby Centre for Health Informatics at Newcastle especially Nick Booth, Peter Johnson and Neill Jones; and the clinicians, epidemiologists, and members of patient support groups who have acted as peer reviewers. We also thank the following people for their help as freelance advisors and editors during our early development: Martin Duerden, José García, Richard Hardern, Harry Hemingway, Per Hjortdahl, Denise Kendrick, Tim Lancaster, Richard LeBlond, Helen Manson, Linda McIntyre, Edward Merrens, Sarah Purdy, Liam Smeeth, Nick Summerton, and Kieran Sweeney. Finally, we are grateful to the clinicians and patients who spare time to take part in focus groups, which are crucial to the development of *Clinical Evidence*.

Contents

Welcome to Issue 4

Welcome to Issue 4 of *Clinical Evidence*. *Clinical Evidence* is a six monthly, updated compendium of evidence on the effects of clinical interventions. It summarises the current state of knowledge, ignorance, and uncertainty about the prevention and treatment of clinical conditions, based on thorough searches and appraisal of the literature. It is not a textbook of medicine nor a book of guidelines. It describes the best available evidence, and where there is no good evidence, it says so.

RESPONSE TO ISSUE 3

Since the publication of Issue 3, around 400,000 people, mainly in the UK and USA, have received a printed copy of *Clinical Evidence*. Each month, a thousand more people register online and, in September 2000, a German translation of *Clinical Evidence* was published.[1]

We are delighted with the huge amount of feedback from physicians, pharmacists, nurses, and members of the general public. It is overwhelmingly positive, and we are encouraged that straight evidence about important clinical questions is useful in so many areas of clinical practice, policy formulation, education and life.

Here are some examples of feedback from readers that have led to changes in *Clinical Evidence:*

- **Evidence relevant to hospitals and to community**
  Many readers have commented that we should provide more evidence that is relevant to clinical care outside hospitals. They have argued strongly that clinical problems in community settings are often less defined because they present early in their natural history before diagnostic features are apparent. Also, for conditions that usually resolve spontaneously, routine diagnostic testing may add few benefits to justify their risks and costs. Some topics in *Clinical Evidence* already address undifferentiated problems (e.g. low back pain and sciatica, p 614). Others, mainly from within hospitals, feel that these topics would be improved by focusing on specific conditions established by modern advanced diagnostic methods. Neither view is right or wrong — the evidence of benefits and harms will vary from setting to setting. This dilemma spurs us on to do better by considering questions in a variety of settings (as in the topic on croup, p 206), and to ask the question whether evidence is available about comparisons of care in different settings (as in the topic on stroke management, p 114).

- **Discarding old issues of Clinical Evidence**
  If you want to be sure that you are using the latest available evidence, then discard old issues of *Clinical Evidence* as soon as the new issue arrives. From now, we will use a distinct colour on the cover to help you to identify the latest issue at a glance.

- **New topics**
  Many of you have suggested topics for future coverage. A list of suggested and commissioned topics and questions can be found on our web site www.clinicalevidence.org. Soon you will be able to indicate your preferences on the web site so that we can prioritise the commissioning of topics.

- **Evaluation of Clinical Evidence**
  We have embarked on a number of simple evaluations of *Clinical Evidence*. So far these have been simple qualitative studies of existing users, but we hope to commission more studies of the impact of *Clinical Evidence* as part of a specified intervention. If you are interested in the organisation of such an evaluation, then please contact us.

The content has been updated and expanded. Firstly, there is one new section on Poisoning and 17 new topics, including Paracetamol poisoning, Obesity, Hip fracture, Wax in ear, Chronic tension-type headache, and Opportunistic infections in HIV. All the new topics are labelled on the contents page. Secondly, several topics have been expanded, including Changing behaviour, Alzheimer's disease, Depressive disorders, and Schizophrenia. The newly included interventions are labelled on the summary page for each topic. Thirdly, 99 of the 103 topics from Issue 3 have been updated and re-edited. This has involved performing a *Clinical Evidence* search from the date of the previous search, appraising any new studies that were identified, and incorporating the new evidence into the *Clinical Evidence* review (e.g. one new systematic review found that progesterone is likely to be inneffective or harmful for premenstrual syndrome — causing no improvement of symptoms but numerous minor adverse effects). The topics have also been re-edited to make them, we hope, even clearer, and to make good any instances where we felt that we had misrepresented the evidence in Issue 3. In some cases this has meant promoting or demoting an intervention from one summary category to another.

QUALITY ASSURANCE

We have appointed a Quality Assurance editor to help guarantee that we present the best available evidence. We will make all the results of our quality processes available on our web site. Our existing quality assurance methods include overt search, critical appraisal, peer review, and editing processes. As a result of quality considerations, we have made two small adjustments to the way we produce *Clinical Evidence*.

- **Categorising interventions**
  We have refined the criteria for categorising interventions to make interpretation easier. It is impossible to avoid a subjective element in the categorisations because different issues need to be combined within the interventions table. Opinions differ from person to person on the relative importance of each issue. For example, it is difficult to weigh a frequent but small benefit versus a rare but severe harm. Another difficulty arises from strong evidence of a small benefit versus weaker evidence of a much larger benefit). Now interventions categorised as "beneficial" have (a) evidence of significant benefits derived from RCTs and (b) expectation of harms that is small compared with the benefits. These changes do not remove the subjective element, and we recognise the importance of applying the value judgements of those involved in medical decisions to the evidence. In a few instances, where RCTs would be regarded as unethical or impractical, we have categorised interventions as beneficial if there is sufficient evidence from non-RCT sources (e.g. oxygen versus no oxygen in severe acute asthma; treatment of generalised epilepsy). These exceptions have been clearly identified within the tables. Preliminary tests to assess the agreement in categorisation between raters have found encouarging agreement at least among our editors; more about this in future issues.

- **Systematic reviews**
  We now use a tighter definition of systematic reviews to mean those reviews which provide operationally explicit descriptions of their search and selection criteria so that the systematic review could be replicated by others. When we count how many systematic reviews found for a clinical question, then recent systematic reviews replace earlier reviews that used the same analytical methods.

UPDATING

The biggest challenge facing *Clinical Evidence* is that of producing high quality updates for a large number of topics at regular intervals. From early 2001, we will post new updates immediately to our web site, and an e-mail alert system will be developed to inform subscribers of updates in selected areas. We aim to update all topics on a regular cycle. The paper version will continue to be published every six months, and will contain all the updates available at that time.

THE FUTURE

We will expand *Clinical Evidence* as fast as we reasonably can (currently around 40 new topics per year). However, many people have written asking for a book that fits in a pocket. One way to achieve both of these objectives is to produce a summary version that can be used in conjunction with a larger book, CD-ROM, or online version of *Clinical Evidence*.

We are piloting an option for subscribers to address particular "snippets" of information within *Clinical Evidence*, so that they can be electronically linked to guidelines and other documents owned by the subscriber. The web version of *Clinical Evidence* is itself already linked to the National Library of Medicine's PubMed database. These links lead to abstracts of references and, where possible, to full text versions.[3] We aim to provide additional links from each reference to critical appraisal information and extracts of results from that reference.

We have started projects aimed at developing specialty versions of *Clinical Evidence* (for paediatrics, cardiology and mental health), and aimed at creating topics about questions on diagnostic strategies.

Today, most of our subscribers and authors are from Western countries. We hope that before long *Clinical Evidence* becomes a global resource with international contributors and readers. We are keen to work with agencies around the world to overcome the technical, financial, language, and other barriers which impede access.[4]

We look forward to hearing your views on what we are doing, how we could do it better, and what we should include in future issues.

REFERENCES

1. Godlee F, ed. *Clinical Evidence*. Bern, Verlag Hans Huber, August/September 2000.
2. Murray Enkin, et al, eds. *A guide to effective care in pregnacy and childbirth*. Oxford, Oxford University Press, 1995.
3. http://www.ncbi.nlm.nih.gov/entrez/query.fcgi
4. Godlee F, Horton R, Smith R. Global information flow. Publishers should provide information free to resource poor countries. *BMJ* 2000 Sep 30;321(7264):776–777.

About Clinical Evidence

The inspiration for *Clinical Evidence* came in a phone call in 1995. Tom Mann and his colleagues at the NHS Executive asked the BMJ Publishing Group to explore the possibility of developing an evidence "formulary" along the lines of the *British National Formulary*. They recognised that clinicians were under increasing pressure to keep up to date and to base their practice more firmly on evidence, but that few had the necessary time or skills to do this. Their idea was to provide a pocket book containing concise and regularly updated summaries of the best available evidence on clinical interventions. However, they didn't think that the NHS could develop such a formulary itself. "It would be marvellous," said Tom Mann, "if somebody would just do it." A small team at the BMJ set to work to produce a pilot version of what was then called the *Clinical Effectiveness Directory*.

Since that pilot, a great deal has changed. In collaboration with the American College of Physicians–American Society of Internal Medicine, we convened an international advisory board, held focus groups of clinicians, talked to patient support groups, and adopted countless good ideas from early drafts by our contributors. Throughout we have kept in mind an equation set out by Slawson et al.[1] This states that the usefulness of any source of information is equal to its relevance, multiplied by its validity, divided by the work required to extract the information. In order to be as useful as possible, we aimed for high relevance, high validity, and low work in terms of the reader's time and effort. We also kept in mind principles of transparency and explicitness. Readers needed to understand where our information came from and how it was assembled.

A UNIQUE RESOURCE

Clinical Evidence joins a growing number of sources of evidence based information for clinicians. But it has several features that, we think, make it unique.

- Its contents are driven by questions rather than by the availability of research evidence. Rather than start with the evidence and summarise what is there, we have tried to identify important clinical questions, and then to search for and summarise the best available evidence to answer them.

- It identifies but does not try to fill important gaps in the evidence. In a phrase used by Jerry Osheroff, who has led much of the recent research on clinicians' information needs,[2] *Clinical Evidence* presents the dark as well as the light side of the moon. We feel that it will be helpful for clinicians to know when their uncertainty stems from gaps in the evidence rather than gaps in their own knowledge.

- It is updated every six months. This means that you can rely on it to keep you up to date in the areas that are covered.

- It specifically aims not to make recommendations. This is because we feel that simply summarising the evidence will make it more widely useful. The experience of the clinical practice guideline movement has shown that it is nearly impossible to make recommendations that are appropriate in every situation. Differences in individual patients' baseline risks and preferences, and in the local availability of interventions, will always mean that the evidence must be individually interpreted rather than applied across the board. *Clinical Evidence* provides the raw material for developing locally applicable clinical practice guidelines, and for clinicians and patients to make up their own minds on the best course of action. We supply the evidence, you make the decisions.

COMPLEMENTARY BUT DIFFERENT

We are often asked how *Clinical Evidence* differs from two other high quality sources of evidence based information: the Cochrane Library; and the evidence based journals *ACP Journal Club*, *Evidence Based Medicine*, *Evidence Based Mental Health*, and *Evidence Based Nursing*.

Clinical Evidence is complementary to but different from the work of the Cochrane Collaboration, which produces and publishes high quality systematic reviews of controlled trials.[3] Clinical Evidence has been called the friendly front end of the Cochrane Library, since it takes this, and other, high quality information and pulls it together in one place in a concise format. Many of our advisors and contributors are active members of the Cochrane Collaboration, and we are exploring closer ties between Clinical Evidence and the Collaboration in the way the evidence is searched for, summarised, and accessed by users.

Clinical Evidence is also complementary to but different from the evidence based journals, which select and abstract the best and most clinically relevant articles as they appear in the world's medical literature. Together these journals form a growing archive of high quality abstracts of individual articles, many of which are now pooled on the Best Evidence CD. Clinical Evidence takes a different approach. It begins not with the journals but with clinical questions. It is able to answer some. For others it simply reports that no good evidence was found.

A WORK IN PROGRESS
Clinical Evidence is an evolving project. We knew before we started that we were undertaking an enormous task, but the more we worked the more we realised its enormity. We recognise that there is some mismatch between what we aim eventually to achieve and what we have achieved so far. While we have made every effort to ensure that the searches were thorough and that the appraisals of studies were objective (see p xv), we will inevitably have missed some important studies. In order not to make unjustified claims about the accuracy of the information, we use phrases such as "we found no systematic review" rather than "there is no systematic review". In addition, some contributors helped us out by performing their own searches and appraisals in line with our guidance notes. In order to be as explicit as possible about the methods used for each contribution, we have asked each set of contributors to provide a brief methods section, describing the searches that were performed and how individual studies were selected.

UPDATING AND EXPANDING CLINICAL EVIDENCE
Our expectation is that Clinical Evidence will evolve rapidly in its early years. Indeed, it may well become a family of products, appearing in different formats and languages for different audiences: German, French, Italian, and Japanese language versions are already in development. In particular, Clinical Evidence will evolve in response to the needs of clinicians. We have tried hard to anticipate those needs (not least by involving clinicians at every stage), but it is only when people begin to use Clinical Evidence in daily practice that we can know how best to develop it. That's why your feedback is so important to us, and we are arranging for various ways to evaluate the product.

Clinical Evidence is updated every six months, and expanded to include summaries of the evidence on additional diseases, syndromes, and clinical questions. We also intend to develop versions of Clinical Evidence to cover questions about screening, diagnosis, and prognosis.

CLINICAL EVIDENCE ONLINE
Clinical Evidence Online is available to all individual subscribers as part of their annual subscription www.clinicalevidence.org. This provides full text of the current issue plus updates and new topics as they are finalised. Clinical Evidence is also available via Ovid www.ovid.com and we are developing versions for intranets and handheld computers.

REFERENCES
1. Slawson DC, Shaughnessy AF, Bennett JH. Becoming a medical information master: feeling good about not knowing everything. J Fam Pract 1994;38:505–513.
2. Ely JW, Osheroff JA, Ebell MJ, et al. Analysis of questions asked by family doctors regarding patient care. BMJ 1999; 319:358–361.
3. http://hiru.mcmaster.ca/cochrane/default.htm

SUMMARY PAGE

The summary page for each topic presents the questions addressed, some key messages, and a list of the interventions covered, categorised according to whether they have been found to be effective or not. We have borrowed the categories of effectiveness from one of the Cochrane Collaboration's first and most popular products, *A guide to effective care in pregnancy and childbirth*.[1] These categories are:

Beneficial: Interventions whose effectiveness has been demonstrated by clear evidence from randomised controlled trials, and expectation of harms that is small compared with the benefits.

Likely to be beneficial: Interventions for which effectiveness is less well established than for those listed under "beneficial".

Trade off between benefits and harms: Interventions for which clinicians and patients should weigh up the beneficial and harmful effects according to individual circumstances and priorities.

Unknown effectiveness: Interventions for which there are currently insufficient data or data of inadequate quality (includes interventions that are widely accepted as beneficial but have never been formally tested in RCTs, often because RCTs would be considered unethical).

Unlikely to be beneficial: Interventions for which lack of effectiveness is less well established than for those listed under "likely to be ineffective or harmful".

Likely to be ineffective or harmful: Interventions whose ineffectiveness or harmfulness has been demonstrated by clear evidence.

Fitting interventions into these categories is not always straightforward. For one thing, the categories represent a mix of several hierarchies: the level of benefit (or harm), the level of evidence (RCT or observational data), and the level of certainty around the finding (represented by the confidence interval). Another problem is that much of the evidence that is most relevant to clinical decisions relates to comparisons between different interventions rather than to comparison with placebo or no intervention. Where necessary, we have indicated the comparisons in brackets. A third problem is that interventions may have been tested, or found to be effective, in only one group of people, such as those at high risk of an outcome. Again, we have indicated this where possible. But perhaps most difficult of all has been to trying to maintain consistency across different topics. We are working on refining the criteria for putting interventions under each category.

NEGATIVE FINDINGS

A surprisingly hard aspect to get right has been the reporting of negative findings. As we have had to keep reminding ourselves, saying that there is no good evidence that a treatment works is not the same as saying that the treatment doesn't work. In trying to get this right, we may have erred too much on the side of caution; when in doubt we have changed summary phrases from, for example, "the review found no difference," to "the review found no evidence of a difference." We recognise that to get this right, we need a better handle on the power of individual systematic reviews and trials to demonstrate statistically significant differences between groups, and better information on what constitute clinically important differences in the major outcomes for each intervention. In the meantime, we hope that the text makes a clear distinction between lack of benefit and lack of evidence of benefit.

OUTCOMES
Clinical Evidence focuses on outcomes that matter to patients, meaning those that patients themselves are aware of, such as symptom severity, quality of life, survival, disability, walking distance, and live birth rate. We are less interested in proxy outcomes such as blood lipid concentrations, blood pressure, or ovulation rates. Each topic includes a list of the main patient oriented outcomes, and where possible describes how these are measured. We have for the moment decided not to address the vexed question of what constitutes a clinically important change in an outcome, but we would welcome any suggestions.

EFFECTS, NOT EFFECTIVENESS
A key aim of *Clinical Evidence* is to emphasise the important trade offs between the benefits and harms, advantages and disadvantages, of different treatment options. We therefore talk about the effects of interventions, both positive and negative, rather than the effectiveness, and for each question or intervention option we present data on benefits and harms under separate headings.

HARMS
"Harms" include adverse effects of treatment and inconvenience to the patient. Finding good data on harms of treatments is not easy. Ideally these would come from RCTs, but many trials are not sufficiently large or long term to capture rarer or more distant evnts, and many do not adequately report adverse effects. We have asked contributors to keep the negative effects of interventions in mind at all times. Where possible, from good data, we indicate the frequency of adverse effects, and to highlight which adverse effects have not been adequately studied or reported.

DRUG INFORMATION
We make no attempt to provide information on drug dosages, formulations, indications, and contraindications. For this information, we refer readers to their national drug formularies. Drug dosages are included when a question explores the relative effects of different doses.

INFORMATION ON COST
We have decided not to include information on the cost or cost effectiveness of interventions, for the first few issues of *Clinical Evidence* at least. This is not because we believe cost to be unimportant, but because the question of what constitutes good evidence on cost is much disputed and because costs vary greatly both within and between countries. However, we believe that it will become increasingly untenable for clinicians to act without paying attention to resources, and future issues of *Clinical Evidence* may provide relevant information on costs.

NUMERICAL DATA
Whenever possible, data are presented in the same form as in the original studies. However, sometimes we have changed the units or type of information used to allow comparison with results from other studies. This has mainly involved converting odds ratios into relative risks. For many situations (when the absolute risk of an outcome is low and the 95% confidence interval is not too wide) the relative risk and odds ratio are comparable. Where this was not the case, relative risks and their confidence intervals have been calculated from baseline event rates and odds ratios cited in studies or, where appropriate, from pooled results.[2, 3]

AN INTERNATIONAL APPROACH TO THE EVIDENCE
Clinical Evidence takes an international approach to the evidence. This means including drugs despite the fact that they are not licensed in some countries. It also means keeping in mind the practicalities of treating patients in rich as well as poorer countries, by covering

interventions even if they have been superceded (for example, single drug treatment for HIV infection as opposed to three drug treatment).

COMPETING INTERESTS
In line with the *BMJ*'s policy,[4] our aim is not to try to eliminate conflicts of interest but to make them explicit, so that readers can judge for themselves what influence if any these may have had on the contributors' interpretation of the evidence. We therefore ask all contributors to let us know about any potential conflicts or, as we now call them, competing interests, and we append any that are declared to the end of the contribution. Where the contributor gives no competing interests, we record "none declared".

CHANGES SINCE THE LAST ISSUE
The text has been edited and updated. Substantive changes since the last issue are listed at the end of each topic. These are defined as:
- Presentation of additional evidence that either confirms or alters the conclusions
- Re-evaluation of the evidence
- Correction of an important error

HOW TO USE THE INFORMATION IN CLINICAL EVIDENCE
The type of information contained in *Clinical Evidence* is necessary but not sufficient for the provision of effective, high quality health care. It is intended as an aid to clinical decision making, to be used in conjunction with other important sources of information. These other sources include estimates of patients' baseline risk of a condition or outcome based on history, physical examination, and clinical investigations; patients' preferences; economic arguments; availability of treatments; and local expertise.

Some guidance on how to apply research evidence in practice is available on our website www.clinicalevidence.org and in appendix 3 in this issue.

How Clinical Evidence is put together

The summaries in *Clinical Evidence* result from a rigorous process aimed at ensuring that the information they contain is both reliable and relevant to clinical practice.

SELECTING TOPICS
Clinical Evidence aims to cover common or important clinical conditions seen in primary and hospital care. To decide which conditions to cover in the first few issues, we reviewed national data on consultation rates, morbidity, and mortality, and took advice from generalist clinicians and patient groups. See our website www.clinicalevidence.org for a list of conditions that we are planning to cover in future issues. Further suggestions are welcome.

SELECTING THE QUESTIONS
The questions in *Clinical Evidence* concern the benefits and harms of preventative and therapeutic interventions, with emphasis on outcomes that matter to patients. Questions are selected for their relevance to clinical practice by section advisors and contributors, in collaboration with primary care clinicians and patient groups. Each new issue of *Clinical Evidence* will include new questions as well as updates of existing questions. Readers can suggest new clinical questions using the feedback slips to be found at the back of the book and on the *Clinical Evidence* website www.clinicalevidence.org, or by writing directly to *Clinical Evidence*.

SEARCHING AND APPRAISING THE LITERATURE
For each question, the literature is searched using the Cochrane Library, Medline, Embase and, occasionally, other electronic databases, looking first for good systematic reviews of RCTs; then for good RCTs published since the search date of the review. Where we find no good recent systematic reviews, we search for individual RCTs. The date of the search is recorded in the methods section for each topic. Of the studies that are identified in the search, we select and summarise only a small proportion. The selection is done by critically appraising the abstracts of the studies identified in the search, a task performed independently by two information scientists using validated criteria similar to those of Sackett, et al[5] and Jadad.[6,7] Where the search identifies more than one or two good reviews or trials, we select those we judge to be the most robust or relevant, using the full text of the article. Where we identify few or no good reviews or trials, we include other studies but highlight their limitations. Contributors, who are chosen for their expertise in the field and their skills in epidemiology, are asked to review our selection of studies, and to justify any additions or exclusions they wish to make.

Our search strategy and critical appraisal criteria are available on our web site www.clinicalevidence.org.

SUMMARISING THE EVIDENCE, PEER REVIEW, AND EDITING
The contributors summarise the evidence relating to each question. Each topic is then peer reviewed by the section advisors, and by at least three external expert clinicians. The revised text is then extensively edited by editors with clinical and epidemiological training, and data are checked against the original study reports.

Feedback

Despite the extensive peer review and quality checks described above, we expect that the text will contain some errors and inconsistencies. Please let us know of any you find, either by using the response form at the back of the book or at www.evidence.org/response.htm, or by contacting *Clinical Evidence* directly (by post, via our web site, or by e-mail to CEfeedback@bmjgroup.com.

REFERENCES

1. Enkin M, Keirse M, Renfrew M, et al. *A guide to effective care in pregnancy and childbirth*. Oxford: Oxford University Press, 1998.
2. Zhang J, Yu KF. What is the relative risk?: A method of correcting the odds ratio in cohort studies of common outcomes. *JAMA* 1998;280:1690–1691.
3. Demets DL. Methods for combining randomized clinical trials: strengths and limitations. *Stat Med* 1987;6:341–348.
4. Smith R. Beyond conflict of interest. *BMJ* 1998;317:219–292.
5. Sackett DL, Haynes RB, Guyatt GH, Tugwell P. *Clinical Epidemiology: A basic science for clinical medicine*. 2nd ed. Boston: Little Brown, 1991.
6. Jadad A. Assessing the quality of RCTs: Why, what, how and by whom? In: Jadad A. *Randomised Controlled Trials*. London: BMJ Books, 1998:45–60.
7. Jadad AR, Moore RA, Carroll D, Jenkinson C, et al. Assessing the quality of reports of randomized clinical trials: is blinding necessary? *Control Clin Trials* 1996;17:1–12.

Absolute risk (AR) This is the probability that an individual will experience the specified outcome during a specified period. It lies in the range 0 to 1. In contrast to common usage, the word 'risk' may refer to adverse events (such as myocardial infarction), or desirable events (such as cure).

Absolute risk reduction (ARR) The absolute difference in risk between the experimental and control groups in a trial. It is used when the risk in the control group exceeds the risk in the experimental group, and is calculated by subtracting the AR in the experimental group from the AR in the control group. This figure does not give any idea of the proportional reduction between the two groups; for this, relative risk reduction (RRR) is needed — see below.

Absolute risk increase (ARI) The absolute difference in risk between the experimental and control groups in a trial. It is used when the risk in the experimental group exceeds the risk in the control group, and is calculated by subtracting the AR in the control group from the AR in the experimental group. This figure does not give any idea of the proportional increase between the two groups; for this, relative risk increase (RRI) is needed (see below).

Bias Systematic deviation of study results from the true results, due to the way(s) in which the study is conducted.

Case control study A study design that examines a group of people who have experienced an event (usually an adverse event) and a group of people who have not experienced the same event, and looks at how exposure to suspect (usually noxious) agents differed between the two groups. This type of study design is most useful for trying to ascertain the cause of rare events, such as rare cancers.

Clinically significant A finding that is clinically important. Here, 'significant' takes its everyday meaning of 'important' (compare

with statistically significant, see below). Where the word 'significant' or 'significance' is used without qualification in the text, it is being used in its statistical sense.

Cohort study A non-experimental study design that follows a group of people (a cohort), and then looks at how events differ among people within the group. A study that examines two cohorts, one that has been exposed to a suspect agent or treatment, and one that has not been exposed, is useful for trying to ascertain whether exposure is likely to cause specified events (often adverse).

Prospective cohort studies (which track participants forward in time) are more reliable than retrospective cohort studies (which look back in time to ascertain whether or not participants were exposed to the agent in question).

Completer analysis Analysis of data from only those participants who remained at the end of the study. Compare with intention to treat analysis, which uses data from all participants who enrolled (see below).

Confidence interval (CI) The 95% confidence interval (or 95% confidence limits) would include 95% of results from studies of the same size and design. This is close but not identical to saying that the true size of the effect (never exactly known) has a 95% chance of falling within the confidence interval. If the 95% CI for a relative risk or an odds ratio crosses 1, the effect size is likely to lie in a range where risk is either increased or decreased.

Controls in a randomised controlled trial refer to the participants in its comparison group. They are allocated either to placebo, to no treatment, or to the standard treatment.

Cross sectional study A study design that involves surveying a population about an exposure, or condition, or both, at one point in time. It can be used for assessing prevalence of a condition in the population.

Effect size Many methods are used to quantify the size of an effect. For dichotomous outcomes, relative risk and odds ratio are examples. Typically, the term effect size is used for continuous variables (such as pain scores or height), where the standardised mean difference or weighted mean difference (see below) are commonly used.

Event The occurrence of a dichotomous outcome that is being sought in the study (such as myocardial infarction, death, or a four-point improvement in pain score).

Experimental study A study in which the investigator studies the effect of intentionally altering one or more factors under controlled conditions.

False negative A person with the target condition (defined by the gold standard) who has a negative test result.

False positive A person with the target condition (defined by the gold standard) who has a positive test result.

Hazard ratio (HR) This is broadly equivalent to relative risk, but is used when the risk is not constant with respect to time. If however, the assumption is made that the risks remain in proportion between population groups in a study, then although the absolute risks (hazards) may alter as time passes, the hazard ratio between groups remains constant. The term is typically used in the context of survival over time and is then broadly equivalent to the relative risk of death. If the hazard ratio is 0.5 then the relative risk of dying in one group is half the risk of dying in the other group.

Heterogeneity In the context of meta-analysis, heterogeneity means dissimilarity between studies. It can be due to use of different statistical methods (statistical heterogeneity), or evaluation of different types of patients, treatments or outcomes (clinical heterogeneity). Heterogeneity may render pooling of data in meta-analysis unreliable or inappropriate.

Homogeneity Similarity (see heterogeneity).

Incidence The number of new cases of a condition occurring in a population over a specified period of time.

Intention to treat analysis Analysis of data from all participants who were enrolled into the study as if they had remained in the group into which they were randomised, regardless of whether they actually remained until the end or withdrew from the trial. Compare with completer analysis (see above).

Likelihood ratio The ratio of the probability that an individual with the target condition has a specified test result to the probability that an individual without the target condition has the same specified test result.

Meta-analysis A statistical technique that summarises the results of several studies in a single weighted estimate, in which more weight is given to results from larger studies.

Morbidity Rate of illness but not death.

Mortality Rate of death.

Negative likelihood ratio (LR−) The ratio of the probability that an individual with the target condition has a negative test result to the probability that an individual without the target condition has a negative test result. This is the same as the ratio of number of the false negatives to the number of true negatives, and the same as the ratio (1-sensitivity/specificity).

Negative predictive value (NPV) The chance of not having a disease given a negative test result (not to be confused with specificity, which is the other way round, see below)

Number needed to treat (NNT) One measure of treatment effectiveness. It is the number of people you would need to treat with a specific intervention for a given period of time to prevent one additional adverse outcome or achieve one additional beneficial outcome. NNT can be calculated as 1/ARR (see appendix 2).

Number needed to harm (NNH) One measure of treatment harm. It is the number of people you would need to treat with a specific intervention for a given period of time to cause one additional adverse outcome. NNH can be calculated as 1/ARI.

Odds The odds of an event happening is defined as the probability that an event will occur, expressed as a proportion of the probability that the event will not occur.

Odds ratio (OR) One measure of treatment effectiveness. It is the odds of an event happening in the experimental group, expressed as a proportion of the odds of an event happening in the control group. The closer the OR is to one, the smaller the difference in effect between the experimental intervention and the control intervention. If the OR is greater (or less) than one, then the effects of the treatment are more (or less) than those of the control treatment. Note that the effects being measured may be adverse (e.g. death or disability) or desirable (e.g. survival). When events are rare, the OR is analogous to the relative risk (RR), but as event rates increase, the OR and RR diverge.

Odds reduction The complement of odds ratio (1-OR), similar to the relative risk reduction (RRR) when events are rare.

P value The probability that an observed difference occurred by chance, if it is assumed that there is in fact no underlying difference between the means of the observations. If this probability is less than 1 in 20 (which is when the P value is less than 0.05), then the result is conventionally regarded as being "statistically significant".

Placebo A biologically inert treatment given to the control participants in trials.

Positive likelihood ratio (LR+) The ratio of the probability that an individual with the target condition has a positive test result to the probability that an individual without the target condition has a positive test result. This is the same as the ratio of number of the false negatives to the number of true negatives, and the same as the ratio (1-sensitivity/specificity).

Positive predictive value (PPV) The chance of having a disease given a positive test result (not to be confused with sensitivity, which is the other way round, see below).

Power A study has adequate power if it can reliably detect a clinically important difference (for instance, between two treatments) if one actually exists. The power of a study is increased when it includes more events or when its measurement of outcomes is more precise.

Prevalence The proportion of people with a finding or disease in a given population at a given time.

Publication bias occurs when studies with positive results being more likely to be published than studies with negative results, so making it appear from surveys of the published literature that treatments are more effective than is truly the case.

Randomised controlled trial (RCT) A trial in which participants are randomly assigned to two groups: one (the experimental group) receiving the intervention that is being tested, and the other (the comparison or control group) receiving an alternative treatment or placebo. This design allows assessment of the relative effects of interventions.

Regression analysis Given data on a dependent variable and one or more independent variables, regression analysis involves finding the "best" mathematical model to describe or predict the dependent variable as a function of the independent variable(s). There are several regression models that suit different needs. Common forms are linear, logistic, and proportional hazards.

Relative risk (RR) The number of times more likely (RR greater than 1) or less likely (RR less than 1) an event is likely to happen in one group compared with another. It is analogous to the odds ratio (OR) when events are rare, and is the ratio of the absolute risk for each group.

Relative risk increase (RRI) The proportional increase in risk between experimental and control participants in a trial.

Relative risk reduction (RRR) The proportional reduction in risk between experimental and control participants in a trial. It is the complement of the relative risk (1-RR).

Sensitivity The chance of having a positive test result given that you have a disease (not to be confused with positive predictive value (PPV), which is the other way around, see above).

Significant By convention taken to mean statistically significant at the 5% level (see statistically significant).

Specificity The chance of having a negative test result given that you do not have a disease (not to be confused with negative predictive value (NPV), which is the other way around, see above).

Standardised mean difference (SMD) A measure of effect size used when outcomes are continuous (such as height, weight, or symptom scores) rather than dichotomous (such as death or myocardial infarction). The mean differences in outcome between the groups being studied are standardised to account for differences in scoring methods (such as pain scores). The measure is a ratio, and therefore has no units.

Statistically significant means that the findings of a study are unlikely to be due to

chance. Significance at the commonly cited 5% level (P < 0.05) means that the observed result would occur by chance in only 1 in 20 similar studies. Where the word "significant" or "significance" is used without qualification in the text, it is being used in this statistical sense.

Systematic review A review in which all the trials on a topic have been systematically identified, appraised, and summarised according to predetermined criteria. It can, but need not, involve meta-analysis as a statistical method of adding together and numerically summarising the results of the trials that meet minimum quality criteria.

True negative A person without the target condition (defined by the gold standard) who has a negative test result.

True positive A person with the target condition (defined by the gold standard) who also has a positive test result.

Validity The soundness or rigour of a study. A study is valid if the way it is designed and carried out means that the results are unbiased and give you an accurate estimate of the effect that is being measured.

Weighted mean difference (WMD) A measure of effect size used when outcomes are continuous (such as symptom scores or height) rather than dichotomous (such as death or myocardial infarction). The mean differences in outcome between the groups being studied are weighted to account for different sample sizes and differing precision between studies. The WMD is an absolute figure, and so takes the units of the original outcome measure.

Last updated Issue 3

Shamir Mehta and Salim Yusuf

INTERVENTIONS

Key Messages

- Good evidence from systematic reviews of RCTs supports the following interventions in people presenting with symptoms of acute myocardial infarction:
  - Aspirin (at least 160 mg chewed and swallowed immediately and continued
    daily for at least a few years and perhaps lifelong).
  - Thrombolytic treatment (streptokinase ± intravenous/subcutaneous hep-
    arin or tissue plasminogen activator [tPA] + intravenous heparin) in people
    with ST elevation on their presenting electrocardiogram (ECG).
  - β blocker (started intravenously within hours of infarction and continued
    orally for several years) in people without contraindications.
  - ACE inhibitor (started within 24 hours of infarction and continued daily) for
    about a month in people at low risk of death, and for several months in
    people with heart failure at any time during hospital admission or with a left
    ventricular ejection fraction less than 40%.
  - Nitrates (shown to be safe for symptomatic relief in this setting, but to have
    at most a modest effect on mortality).
- Systematic reviews of RCTs have found no evidence of mortality benefit from
  calcium channel blockers during or after acute myocardial infarction; there is
  potential for increased mortality in people with heart failure.
- One systematic review of RCTs has found that, in high risk people who present
  early (< 4 hours after onset of symptoms) and have ST elevation, primary
  percutaneous transluminal coronary angioplasty (PTCA) is more effective than
  thrombolytic treatment, provided it can be performed quickly (< 90 minutes
  after hospital arrival) by an experienced operator and staff in a high volume
  centre.

DEFINITION	Acute myocardial infarction (AMI) is the sudden occlusion of a coronary artery leading to myocardial death.
INCIDENCE/ PREVALENCE	AMI is one of the most common causes of mortality in both developed and developing nations. In 1990, ischaemic heart disease was the leading cause of death worldwide, accounting for about 6.3 million deaths. The age standardised incidence varies among and within countries.[1] Each year, about 900 000 people in the USA experience an AMI, and about 225 000 of them die. About half of these people die within 1 hour of symptoms and before reaching a hospital emergency room.[2] Event rates increase with age for both sexes and are higher in men than women, and in poorer than richer people at all ages. The incidence of death from AMI has fallen in many Western countries over the past 20 years.
AETIOLOGY/ RISK FACTORS	The immediate mechanism of AMI is rupture of an atheromatous plaque causing thrombosis and occlusion of coronary arteries and myocardial death. Factors that may convert a stable plaque into an unstable plaque (the "active plaque") have yet to be fully elucidated; however, shear stresses, inflammation, and autoimmunity have been proposed. The changing rates of coronary heart disease in different populations are only partly explained by changes in the standard risk factors for ischaemic heart disease (particularly fall in blood pressure and smoking).
PROGNOSIS	AMI may lead to a host of mechanical and electrical complications, including death, ventricular dysfunction, congestive heart failure, cardiogenic shock, fatal and non-fatal arrhythmia, valvular dysfunction, or myocardial rupture.
AIMS	To relieve pain; to restore blood supply to heart muscle; to reduce incidence of complications (such as congestive heart failure, myocardial rupture, valvular dysfunction, fatal and non-fatal arrhythmia); to prevent recurrent ischaemia and infarction; and to decrease mortality.
OUTCOMES	**Efficacy outcomes:** Rates of major cardiovascular events, including death, recurrent AMI, refractory ischaemia, and stroke. **Safety outcomes:** Rates of major bleeding and intracranial haemorrhage.
METHODS	We searched Medline, Embase, and Cochrane electronic databases in July 1998 to identify relevant systematic reviews. Individual high quality trials published after the last acceptable systematic review were also selected. *Clinical Evidence* update search and appraisal December 1999.

> **QUESTION** Which treatments improve outcomes in acute myocardial infarction?

> **OPTION** ASPIRIN AND OTHER ANTIPLATELET TREATMENTS

One systematic review of RCTs has found that, in people with AMI, aspirin reduces mortality (one life saved per 40 people treated during the acute phase), reinfarction (one fewer non-fatal reinfarction per 100 people treated), and stroke (one fewer non-fatal stroke per 300 people treated). The evidence suggests an optimal dose of aspirin of 160–325 mg acutely, followed by long term treatment with at least 75 mg/day indefinitely.

Benefits: **Aspirin versus placebo:** We found one systematic review (search date 1990), which identified nine RCTs in 18 773 people treated with antiplatelet agents or placebo soon after the onset of AMI and for a period of at least 1 month afterwards.[3] The absolute and relative benefits found in the systematic review are shown in figure 1, p 14. The largest of the trials involved 17 187 people with suspected AMI randomised to receive either placebo or aspirin (162.6 mg) chewed and swallowed on the day of AMI and continued daily for 1 month.[4] In subsequent long term follow up, the mortality benefit was maintained for up to 4 years.[5] In the systematic review, the most widely tested aspirin regimens were 75–325 mg/day.[3] Doses throughout this range seemed similarly effective, with no evidence that "higher" doses were more effective (500–1500 mg/day: odds reduction compared with placebo 21%, 95% CI 14% to 27%) than "medium" doses (160–325 mg/day: odds reduction 28%, 95% CI 22% to 33%) or "lower" doses (75–160 mg/day: odds reduction 26%, 95% CI 5% to 42%). There was insufficient evidence for efficacy of doses below 75 mg/day. One study found that administering a loading dose of 160–325 mg/day achieved a prompt antiplatelet effect.[6]

Harms: In the largest trial, there was no significant increase in rates of cerebral haemorrhage or bleeds requiring transfusion (0.4% on aspirin and placebo).[4] There was a small absolute excess of "minor" bleeding (ARI 0.6%, 95% CI not available, P < 0.01).

Comment: None.

OPTION   **THROMBOLYTIC TREATMENT**

Systematic reviews of RCTs have found that prompt thrombolytic treatment (within 6 hours and perhaps up to 12 hours and longer after the onset of symptoms) reduces mortality in people with AMI and ST elevation or bundle branch block on their presenting ECG. Fifty six people would need treatment in the acute phase to prevent one additional death. Strokes, intracranial haemorrhage, and major bleeds are more common in people given thrombolysis; with one additional stroke for every 250 people treated and one additional major bleed for every 143 people treated. The reviews have found that intracranial haemorrhage is more common in people of advanced age and low body weight, those with hypertension on admission, and those given tPA rather than another thrombolytic agent.

Benefits: **Thrombolytic treatment versus placebo:** We found one systematic review (published in 1994), which identified nine RCTs, each including at least 1000 people with suspected AMI who received either thrombolytic treatment or placebo (total n = 58 600).[7] Baseline ECGs showed ST segment elevation in 68% of people, and ST segment depression, T wave abnormalities, or no abnormality in the rest. Mortality was reduced by thrombolytic treatment (AR 9.6% with thrombolysis, 11.5% with placebo; ARR 1.9%; RRR 18%, 95% CI 13% to 23%; NNT in the acute phase 56, 95% CI 43 to 77). Greatest benefit was found in the large group of people presenting with ST elevation (RRR 21%, 95% CI not available) or bundle branch block (RRR 25%). **Timing of treatment:** The earlier thrombolytic treatment was given, the greater the absolute benefit (see figure 2, p 15). For each hour of delay the absolute risk reduction for death decreased by 0.16% (ARR for death if given within 6 hours of symptoms 3%; ARR for death if given 7–12 hours after onset of symptoms 2%).[8] Too few people in the systematic review received treatment more than 12 hours after the onset of symptoms to determine whether the benefits of thrombolytic treatment given after 12 hours would outweigh the risks. Extrapolation of the data (see figure 2, p 15) suggests that, at least for people with ST elevation, there may be some net benefit of treatment between 12 and 18 hours after symptom onset (ARR for death 1%). **Type of infarct:** Reduced rates of death were seen in people with all types of infarct, but the benefit was several times greater in those with anterior infarction (ARR 3.7%) compared with those with inferior infarction (ARR 0.8%) or infarctions in other zones (ARR 2.7%). **Different thrombolytic agents:** One systematic review[8] (published in 1997) identified three large RCTs comparing streptokinase versus tPA (see table 1, p 13).[9–11] The first trial was unblinded and in people with ST elevation and symptoms of AMI for less than 6 hours. Participants were first randomised to intravenous tPA 100 mg over 3 hours or streptokinase 1.5 MU over 1 hour, and then further randomised to subcutaneous heparin 12 500 U twice daily beginning 12 hours later, or no heparin. It found heparin added no significant benefit (AR of death in hospital 8.5% v 8.9% on no heparin; RRR 0.05, 95% CI −0.04 to +0.14).[9] In the second trial, people with suspected AMI presenting within 24 hours of symptoms were randomised to receive either streptokinase 1.5 MU over 1 hour, tPA 0.6 MU/kg every 4 hours, or anisoylated plasminogen streptokinase activator complex (APSAC) 30 U/3 minutes, and then further randomised to subcutaneous heparin 12 500 U starting at 7 hours and continued for 7 days, or no heparin. All received aspirin on admission. At 35 days, mortality was similar among the three regimens (streptokinase 10.6%, APSAC 10.5%, tPA 10.3%), and the addition of heparin made no significant difference (AR of death 10.3% v 10.6% on no heparin).[10] The third trial was unblinded and in people with ST segment elevation presenting within 6 hours of symptom onset. Participants were randomised to one of four regimens: streptokinase 1.5 MU over 1 hour plus subcutaneous heparin 12 500 U twice daily starting 4 hours after thrombolytic treatment; streptokinase 1.5 MU over 1 hour plus intravenous heparin 5000 U bolus followed by 1000 U/hour; accelerated tPA 15 mg bolus then 0.75 mg/kg over 30 minutes followed by 0.50 mg/kg over 60 minutes, plus intravenous heparin 5000 U bolus then 1000 U/hour; or tPA 1.0 mg/kg over 60 minutes, 10% given as a bolus, plus streptokinase 1.0 MU over 60 minutes.[11] Meta-analysis of the three trials, weighted by sample size, found no significant difference in the combined outcome of any stroke or death unrelated to stroke (ARs 9.4% for streptokinase only regimens v 9.2% for tPA based regimens, including the combined tPA and streptokinase arm in the third trial; ARR for tPA v streptokinase 0.2%, 95% CI −0.2% to +0.5%; RRR 2.1%).[8]

Harms: **Stroke/intracerebral haemorrhage:** The risk of stroke was increased by thrombolytic treatment given in the acute phase (ARI compared with placebo 0.4%, 95% CI 0.2% to 0.5%; NNH 250).[7]

In the third trial comparing different thrombolytic treatments, the overall incidence of intracerebral haemorrhage was 0.7% and of stroke 1.4%, of which 31% were severely disabling and 50% were intracerebral haemorrhages. The risk of haemorrhagic stroke was higher with tPA (AR 0.72%) than with streptokinase and subcutaneous heparin (AR 0.49%) or with streptokinase and intravenous heparin (AR 0.54%, P = 0.03 for tPA compared with combined streptokinase arms).[11] **Predictive factors for stroke/intracranial haemorrhage:** Multivariate analysis of data from a large database of people who experienced intracerebral haemorrhage after thrombolytic treatment identified four independent predictors of increased risk of intracerebral haemorrhage: age ≥ 65 years (OR 2.2, 95% CI 1.4 to 3.5), weight < 70 kg (OR 2.1, 95% CI 1.3 to 3.2), hypertension on admission (OR 2.0, 95% CI 1.2 to 3.2), and use of tPA rather than another thrombolytic agent (OR 1.6, 95% CI 1.0 to 2.5). Absolute risk of intracranial haemorrhage was 0.26% on streptokinase in the absence of risk factors, and 0.96%, 1.32%, and 2.17% in people with one, two, or three risk factors.[12] Analysis of 592 strokes in 41 021 people from the trials found seven factors to be predictors of intracerebral haemorrhage: advanced age, lower weight, history of cerebrovascular disease, history of hypertension, higher systolic or diastolic pressure on presentation, and use of tPA rather than streptokinase.[13,14] **Major bleeding:** The risk of major bleeding was increased by thrombolytic treatment given in the acute phase (ARI compared with placebo 0.7%; 95% CI 0.6% to 0.9%; NNH 143).[7] Bleeding was most common in people undergoing procedures (coronary artery bypass grafting or PTCA). Spontaneous bleeds were observed most often in the gastrointestinal tract.[11]

Comment: The evidence suggests that it is far more important to administer prompt thrombolytic treatment than to debate which thrombolytic agent should be used. A strategy of rapid use of any thrombolytic in a broad population is likely to lead to the greatest impact on mortality. When the results of RCTs are taken together, tPA based regimens do not seem to confer a significant advantage in the combined outcome of any stroke and death (unrelated to stroke) over streptokinase. The legitimacy of combining the results of the three trials can be questioned, as the selection criteria and protocols differed in important aspects (see systematic review[8] for arguments to justify combining the results of these trials despite their apparent differences).

OPTION	β BLOCKERS

Systematic reviews of RCTs have found that oral β blockers given within hours of infarction reduce both mortality and reinfarction in people with AMI. Adding β blockers to thrombolytic treatment confers additional benefit.

Benefits: **Given within hours of infarction:** We found three systematic reviews (search date 1997, published in 1985 and 1987), which identified 27 RCTs of early use of β blockers.[15–17] The older reviews found that, within 1 week of treatment, β blockers significantly reduced the risk of death compared with placebo (RRR 13%, 95% CI 2% to 25%).[16,17] The greatest benefit was found with early

Cardiovascular disorders

treatment (RRR for death with treatment within the first 2 days was about 25%). Incidence of other major vascular events was also reduced (RRR for the combined outcome of death, non-fatal cardiac arrest, or non-fatal reinfarction 16%, 1110 events v 1298 events, 95% CI not available, P < 0.001). The largest of these trials compared intravenous atenolol 5–10 mg given immediately followed by 100 mg orally given daily for 7 days versus standard treatment (no β blocker) in 16 027 people with AMI.[18] After 7 days, atenolol reduced vascular mortality compared with control (AR 3.89% on atenolol v 4.57% in the controls; ARR 0.7%; RRR 15%, 95% CI 12% to 27%; NNT 147). The trial found more benefit in people with ECG evidence of AMI at entry (in people with ECG suggesting anterior infarction, inferior infarction, both, or bundle branch block, AR of death 5.33% on atenolol, 6.49% for controls; ARR 1.16%; NNT 86, 95% CI not available). People older than 65 years and those with large infarcts had the most benefit.[19] **In people receiving thrombolytic treatment:** We found one trial that compared early versus delayed metoprolol in 1434 people with AMI receiving tPA.[19] Early treatment began on day one (intravenous then oral) and delayed treatment on day six (oral). At 6 days, participants receiving early treatment had significantly lower rates of reinfarction (AR 2.7% early v 5.1% delayed, 95% CI not available, P = 0.02) and recurrent chest pain (AR 18.8% v 24.1%, P < 0.02). There were no early (6 days) or late (1 year) differences observed in mortality or left ventricular ejection fraction between the two groups. **Long term use:** See beta blockers under secondary prevention of ischaemic cardiac events, p 83.

Harms: People with asthma or severe congestive cardiac failure were excluded from most trials. Many of the early trials tended to enrol people at low risk of death soon after AMI. In people given immediate rather than delayed β blockers following tPA, there was a non-significantly increased frequency of heart failure during the initial admission to hospital (15.3% v 12.2%, P = 0.10).[19] The presence of first degree heart block and bundle branch block was associated with an increased frequency of adverse events.

Comment: β Blockers may reduce rates of cardiac rupture and ventricular fibrillation. This may explain why people older than 65 years and those with large infarcts benefited most, as they also have higher rates of these complications. The trials were mostly conducted in the prethrombolytic era. The trial comparing early versus delayed β blockade following thrombolysis was too small to rule out an effect on mortality of β blockers when added to thrombolysis.[19] The findings from the most recent review are compatible with the older reviews.[15] It will be appraised for the next issue of Clinical Evidence.

OPTION   ANGIOTENSIN CONVERTING ENZYME (ACE) INHIBITORS

One systematic review of four large RCTs has found that ACE inhibitors used within 24 hours of onset of symptoms reduce mortality in people with AMI. The question of whether ACE inhibitors should be offered to everyone presenting with AMI or only to people with signs of heart failure remains unresolved.

Benefits: **In all people after an AMI:** We found one systematic review (published in 1998, 4 large RCTs, each including > 1000 participants), comparing ACE inhibitors versus placebo given to all people irrespective of clinical heart failure or left ventricular dysfunction, within 36 hours of the onset of symptoms of AMI. Data from 98 496 people were pooled.[20] After 30 days, ACE inhibitors reduced all cause mortality compared with placebo (AR 7.1% in the ACE inhibitor group v 7.6% in the control group; RRR 7%, 95% CI 2% to 11%; NNT 200 to save one life by 30 days). Most of this benefit was in the first 7 days after AMI. The absolute benefit was particularly large in some high risk groups: people in Killip class 2–3 (clinically moderate to severe heart failure at first presentation; RRR 9.1%; NNT 71, 99% CI 36 to 10 000), people with heart rates > 100 beats/minute at entry (RRR 14.5%; NNT 44, 99% CI 25 to 185), and people with an anterior AMI (RRR 12.8%; NNT 94, 99% CI 56 to 303). ACE inhibitors also reduced the incidence of non-fatal cardiac failure (AR 14.6% v 15.2%, 95% CI not available; P = 0.01). **In selected people after an AMI:** A selective strategy was tested in three trials.[21–23] Treatment was restricted to people with clinical heart failure, objective evidence of left ventricular dysfunction, or both, and was started a few days after AMI (n = about 6000). These trials found consistently that long term treatment with ACE inhibitors in this selected population was associated with a significant reduction in mortality and reinfarction (RRRs from one trial[20]: for cardiovascular death 21%, 95% CI 5% to 35%; for development of severe heart failure 37%, 95% CI 20% to 50%; for congestive heart failure requiring admission to hospital 22%, 95% CI 4% to 37%; and for recurrent AMI 25%, 95% CI 5% to 40%).

Harms: The systematic review found an excess of persistent hypotension (AR 17.6% v 9.3%, 95% CI for difference not available; P < 0.01) and renal dysfunction (AR 1.3% v 0.6%; P < 0.01) in people given ACE inhibitors.[20] The relative and absolute risks of these adverse effects were uniformly distributed across both the high and lower cardiovascular risk groups.

Comment: The largest benefits of ACE inhibitors in AMI are seen when treatment is started within 24 hours. The evidence does not answer the question of which people with an AMI should be offered ACE inhibitors, and for how long after AMI it remains beneficial to start treatment with an ACE inhibitor.

OPTION NITRATES

RCTs performed before and during the thrombolytic era have found that intravenous nitrates are safe in the acute management of symptoms in people with AMI, but may reduce mortality only slightly.

Benefits: **Without thrombolysis:** We found one systematic review (published 1988, 10 RCTs comparing intravenous nitroglycerine or nitroprusside v placebo, 2000 people with AMI).[24] The trials were all conducted in the prethrombolytic era. Nitrates reduced the relative risk of death by 35% (95% CI 16% to 55%). The observed benefit of nitrates seemed to be mostly during the acute hospitalisation period, with modest or little long term survival benefit. **With aspirin/ thrombolysis:** During the thrombolytic era, two large RCTs compared nitrates given acutely versus placebo in 58 050 and 17 817 people with AMI (90% received aspirin and about 70% received thrombolytic treatment).[25,26] In one trial, people received oral controlled release mononitrate 30–60 mg/day.[25] In the other, people received intravenous nitroglycerine for 24 hours followed by transdermal nitroglycerine 10 mg daily.[25] Neither trial found a significant improvement in survival, either in the total sample or in subgroups of people at different risk of death. Nitrates were a useful adjunctive treatment to help control symptoms in people with AMI.

Harms: The systematic review and the large trials found no significant harm associated with routine use of nitrates in people with AMI.[24–26]

Comment: The two large trials had features that may have caused them to not find a benefit even if one exists: a large proportion of people took nitrates outside the study, there was a high rate of concurrent use of other hypotensive agents; people were relatively low risk; and nitrates were not titrated to blood pressure and heart rate.[25,26]

OPTION CALCIUM CHANNEL BLOCKERS

RCTs have found that calcium channel blockers given to people within the first few days of an AMI do not reduce deaths, and may increase deaths in people with reduced left ventricular function.

Benefits: **Dihydropyridine calcium channel blockers:** We found no systematic review. We found two large RCTs comparing short acting nifedipine versus placebo in people treated within the first few days of AMI.[27,28] Neither found evidence of benefit and both found trends towards increased mortality on nifedipine. One trial was terminated prematurely because of lack of efficacy. It found a 33% increase in mortality on nifedipine that did not reach significance.[28] There are insufficient data on sustained release nifedipine, amlodipine, or felodipine in this setting. **Verapamil:** We found no systematic review. We found one RCT comparing placebo versus verapamil started intravenously on admission for AMI then continued orally for 6 months in 1436 people.[29] At 6 months, there was no significant difference in mortality (AR 12.8% verapamil v 13.9% placebo) and at 12 months no significant difference in reinfarction (AR 7% v 8.3%) or mortality (AR 15.2% v 16.4%).

Harms: Two systematic reviews of trials of any kind of calcium channel blockers in people with AMI found a non-significant increase in mortality of about 4% and 6%.[30,31] One trial in 2466 people with AMI compared diltiazem 60 mg orally four times daily started 3–15 days after AMI versus placebo.[32] Overall there was no effect on total mortality or reinfarction between the two groups, but subgroup analysis found a 41% increase in death or reinfarction in people with congestive heart failure (RRI 1.41, 95% CI 1.01 to 1.96).

Comment: None.

OPTION PRIMARY PERCUTANEOUS TRANSLUMINAL CORONARY ANGIOPLASTY (PTCA) VERSUS THROMBOLYSIS

One systematic review of RCTs has found that, in the short term, primary PTCA is at least as effective as (and possibly superior to) thrombolysis in

the treatment of AMI, in terms of reducing mortality, reinfarction, and haemorrhagic stroke. However, the trials were conducted mainly in high volume, specialist centres. The effectiveness of PTCA compared with thrombolysis in less specialist centres remains to be defined.

Benefits: We found one systematic review (published in 1997, 10 RCTs of primary PTCA v thrombolysis in people with AMI, n = 2606).[33] None of the trials had sufficient power to detect mortality reductions individually. **Death and reinfarction:** The review found reduced mortality with primary PTCA versus thrombolysis at 30 days after intervention (ARs 4.4% for primary PTCA, 6.5% for thrombolysis; ARR 2.1%; OR 0.66, 95% CI 0.46 to 0.94; NNT 48).[33] The effect was similar regardless of which thrombolysis regimen was used. There was also a significant reduction in the combined end point of death and reinfarction with PTCA (OR 0.58, 95% CI 0.44 to 0.76). The largest single trial compared primary PTCA versus accelerated tPA in 1138 people with AMI (with ST elevation on the ECG) who presented within 12 hours of symptom onset.[34] At 30 days, there was no significant difference in mortality between the two groups (AR 5.7% v 7.0%), but primary PTCA significantly reduced the primary end point of death, non-fatal AMI, or non-fatal disabling stroke (AR 9.6% v 13.7% on tPA; OR 0.67, 95% CI 0.47 to 0.97). This effect was substantially attenuated by 6 months.

Harms: **Stroke:** The review found that PTCA was associated with a signifi-cant reduction in the risk of all types of stroke (AR 0.7% v 2.0%) and haemorrhagic stroke (AR 0.1% v 1.1%).[32] In the largest trial, the collective rate of haemorrhagic stroke in people given thrombolysis was 1.1%, substantially higher than that observed in trials compar-ing thrombolysis with placebo.[34] This may have been because the trials summarised above were in older people and used tPA. However, the lower rates of haemorrhagic stroke with primary PTCA were consistent across almost all trials, and this may be the major advantage of PTCA over thrombolysis.

Comment: Although collectively the trials found an overall short term reduction in deaths with PTCA compared with thrombolysis, there were several pitfalls common to individual trials, most of which may have inflated the benefit of PTCA.[35] Trials comparing PTCA with thrombolysis could not be easily blinded, and ascertainment of end points that required some judgement, such as reinfarction or stroke, may have been influenced by the investigators' knowledge of the treatment allocation (only one trial had a blinded adjudication events commit-tee). Also, people allocated to PTCA were discharged 1–2 days earlier than those allocated to thrombolysis, which favoured PTCA by reducing the time for detection of in hospital events. In addition, the trials conducted before the largest trial[34] should be viewed as hypothesis generating, in that the composite outcome (death, reinfarction, and stroke) was not prospectively defined, and atten-tion was only placed on these end points after there seemed to be some benefit on post hoc analysis. The results are also based on short term outcomes only and do not provide information on collective long term benefit. For example, in the largest trial, the composite end point was significant at 30 days, but with a wide degree of uncertainty, and this was substantially attenuated to a non-significant difference by 6 months.[34] The lower mortality and reinfarction rates reported with primary PTCA are promising but not conclusive, and the real benefits may well be smaller. Only in a minority of centres that perform a high volume of PTCA and in the hands of experienced interventionalists may primary PTCA be clearly superior to thrombolytic treatment. Elsewhere, primary PTCA may be of greatest benefit in people with contraindications to thrombolysis, in people in cardiogenic shock, or in people where the mortality reduction with thrombolysis is modest and the risk of intracranial haemorrhage is increased, for example, elderly people.[36] The value of PTCA over thrombolysis in people presenting to hospital more than 12 hours after onset of chest pain remains to be tested.

REFERENCES

1. Murray C, Lopez A. Mortality by cause for eight regions of the world: global burden of disease study. *Lancet* 1997;349:1269–1276.
2. National Heart, Lung, and Blood Institute. *Morbidity and mortality: chartbook on cardiovascular, lung, and blood diseases.* Bethesda, Maryland: US Department of Health and Human Services, Public Health Service, National Institutes of Health; May 1992.
3. Antiplatelet Trialists' Collaboration. Collaborative overview of randomised trials of antiplatelet therapy I: prevention of death, myocardial infarction, and stroke by prolonged antiplatelet therapy in various categories of people. *BMJ* 1994;308:81–106. Search date, trials available at March 1990; primary sources Medline, Current Contents.
4. Second International Study of Infarct Survival (ISIS-2) Collaborative Group. Randomized trial of intravenous streptokinase, oral aspirin, both or neither among 17–187 cases of suspected acute myocardial infarction. *Lancet* 1988;ii:349–360.
5. Baigent BM, Collins R. ISIS-2: four year mortality of 17187 patients after fibrinolytic and antiplatelet therapy in suspected acute myocardial infarction study [abstract]. *Circulation* 1993;(suppl I):I-291.
6. Patrignani P, Filabozzi P, Patrono C. Selective cumulative inhibition of platelet thromboxane production by low-dose aspirin in healthy subjects. *J Clin Invest* 1982;69:1366–1372.
7. Fibrinolytic Therapy Trialists' (FTT) Collaborative Group. Indications for fibrinolytic therapy in suspected acute myocardial infarction: collaborative overview of early mortality and major morbidity results of all randomized trials of more than 1000 patients. *Lancet* 1994;343:311–322. Search date and primary sources not stated.
8. Collins R, Peto R, Baigent BM, Sleight DM. Aspirin, heparin and fibrinolytic therapy in suspected acute myocardial infarction. *N Engl J Med* 1997;336:847–860. Search date and primary sources not stated.
9. Gruppo Italiano per lo studio della streptochinasi nell'infarto miocardico (GISSI). GISSI-2: a factorial randomised trial of alteplase versus streptokinase and heparin versus no heparin among 12–490 patients with acute myocardial infarction. *Lancet* 1990;336:65–71.
10. Third International Study of Infarct Survival (ISIS-3) Collaborative Group. ISIS-3: a randomised comparison of streptokinase vs tissue plasminogen activator vs anistreplase and of aspirin plus heparin vs aspirin alone among 41–299 cases of suspected acute myocardial infarction. *Lancet* 1992;339:753–770.
11. The GUSTO Investigators. An international randomized trial comparing four thrombolytic strategies for acute myocardial infarction. *N Engl J Med* 1993;329:673–682.
12. Simoons MI, Maggioni AP, Knatterud G, et al. Individual risk assessment for intracranial hemorrhage during thrombolytic therapy. *Lancet* 1993;342:523–528.
13. Gore JM, Granger CB, Simoons MI, et al. Stroke after thrombolysis: mortality and functional outcomes in the GUSTO-1 trial. *Circulation* 1995; 92:2811–2818.
14. Berkowitz SD, Granger CB, Pieper KS, et al. Incidence and predictors of bleeding after contemporary thrombolytic therapy for myocardial infarction. *Circulation* 1997;95:2508–2516.
15. Freemantle N, Cleland J, Young P, Mason J, Harrison J. Beta Blockade after myocardial infarction: systematic review and meta regression analysis. *BMJ* 1999;318:1730–1737.
16. Yusuf S, Peto R, Lewis S, et al. Beta-blockade during and after myocardial infarction: an overview of the randomized trials. *Prog Cardiovasc Dis* 1985;27:355–371. Search date not stated; primary sources computer-aided search of the literature; manual search of reference lists and enquiries to colleagues about relevant papers.
17. Sleight P for the ISIS Study Group. Beta blockade early in acute myocardial infarction. *Am J Cardiol* 1987;60:6A–12A.
18. First International Study of Infarct Survival (ISIS-1). Randomised trial of intravenous atenolol among 16–027 cases of suspected acute myocardial infarction. *Lancet* 1986;ii:57–66.
19. Roberts R, Rogers WJ, Mueller HS, et al. Immediate versus deferred beta-blockade following thrombolytic therapy in patients with acute myocardial infarction: results of the thrombolysis in myocardial infarction (TIMI) II-B study. *Circulation* 1991;83:422–437.
20. ACE inhibitor Myocardial Infarction Collaborative Group. Indications for ACE inhibitors in the early treatment of acute myocardial infarction: systematic overview of individual data from 100 000 patients in randomised trials. *Circulation* 1998;97:2202–2212. Search date not stated; primary source collaboration group of principal investigators of all randomized trials who collated individual patient data.
21. Pfeffer MA, Braunwald E, Moye LA, et al. Effect of captopril on mortality and morbidity in patients with left ventricular dysfunction after myocardial infarction. *N Engl J Med* 1992; 327:669–677.
22. The Acute Infarction Ramipril Efficacy (AIRE) Study Investigators. Effect of ramipril on mortality and morbidity of survivors of acute myocardial infarction with clinical evidence of heart failure. *Lancet* 1993;342:821–828.
23. The Trandolapril Cardiac Evaluation (TRACE) Study

Group. A clinical trial of the angiotensin-converting-enzyme inhibitor trandolapril in patients with left ventricular dysfunction after myocardial infarction. *N Engl J Med* 1995;333:1670–1676.

24. Yusuf S, Collins R, MacMahon S, Peto R. Effect of intravenous nitrates on mortality in acute myocardial infarction: an overview of the randomised trials. *Lancet* 1988;1:1088–1092. Search date not stated; primary sources literature, colleagues, investigators, and pharmaceutical companies.

25. Fourth International Study of Infarct Survival (ISIS-4) Collaborative Group. ISIS-4: a randomised factorial trial assessing early oral captopril, oral mononitrate, and intravenous magnesium sulphate in 58,050 patients with suspected acute myocardial infarction. *Lancet* 1995;345:669–685.

26. Gruppo Italiano per lo studio della streptochinasi nell'infarto miocardico (GISSI). GISSI-3: effects of lisinopril and transdermal glyceryl trinitrate singly and together on 6-week mortality and ventricular function after acute myocardial infarction. *Lancet* 1994;343:1115–1122.

27. Wilcox RG, Hampton JR, Banks DC, et al. Early nifedipine in acute myocardial infarction: the TRENT study. *BMJ* 1986;293:1204–1208.

28. Goldbourt U, Behar S, Reicher-Reiss H, et al. Early administration of nifedipine in suspected acute myocardial infarction: the secondary prevention reinfarction Israel nifedipine trial 2 study. *Arch Intern Med* 1993;153:345–353.

29. The Danish Study Group on Verapamil in Myocardial Infarction. Verapamil in acute myocardial infarction. *Eur Heart J* 1984;5:516–529.

30. Yusuf S, Furberg CD. Effects of calcium channel blockers on survival after myocardial infarction. *Cardiovasc Drugs Ther* 1987;1:343–344. Search dates and primary sources not stated.

31. Teo KK, Yusuf S, Furberg CD. Effects of prophylactic antiarrhythmic drug therapy in acute myocardial infarction: an overview of results from randomized controlled trials. *JAMA* 1993;270:1589–1595. Search date not stated; primary sources Medline, and correspondence with investigators and pharmaceutical companies.

32. The Multicenter Diltiazem Post Infarction Trial Research Group. The effect of diltiazem on mortality and reinfarction after myocardial infarction. *N Engl J Med* 1988;319:385–392.

33. Weaver WD, Simes RJ, Betriu A, et al. Comparison of primary coronary angioplasty and intravenous thrombolytic therapy for acute myocardial infarction: a quantitative review. *JAMA* 1997;278:2093–2098. Search date March 1996; primary sources Medline and scientific session abstracts of stated journals.

34. The GUSTO IIb Angioplasty Substudy Investigators. A clinical trial comparing primary coronary angioplasty with tissue plasminogen activator for acute myocardial infarction. *N Engl J Med* 1997;336:1621–1628.

35. Yusuf S, Pogue J. Primary angioplasty compared to thrombolytic therapy for acute myocardial infarction [editorial]. *JAMA* 1997;278:2110–2111.

36. Van de Werf F, Topol EJ, Lee KL, et al. Variations in patient management and outcomes for acute myocardial infarction in the United States and other countries: results from the GUSTO trial. *JAMA* 1995;273:1586–1591.

Shamir Mehta
Interventional Cardiologist and
Clinical Scholar

Salim Yusuf
Professor of Medicine

Director, Division of Cardiology
McMaster University
Hamilton, Ontario
Canada

Competing interests: SM has received a fee for speaking at symposia. SY has received funds for research and speaking from a variety of pharmaceutical companies related and unrelated to any product discussed here.

TABLE 1 Direct randomised comparisons of the standard streptokinase regimen with various tPA based fibrinolytic regimens in patients with suspected AMI in the GISSI-2, ISIS-3, and GUSTO-1 trials (see text, p 4).[9–11]

Trial and treatment	Number of participants randomised	Any stroke Absolute number (%)	Any death Absolute number (%)	Death not related to stroke[†] Absolute number (%)	Stroke or death Absolute number (%)
GISSI-2[‡]					
Streptokinase	10 396	98 (0.9)	958 (9.2)	916 (8.8)	1014 (9.8)
t-PA	10 372	136 (1.3)	993 (9.6)	931 (9.0)	1067 (10.3)
Effect/1000 people treated with t-PA instead of streptokinase		3.7 ± 1.5 more	3.6 ± 4.0 more	1.7 ± 4.0 more	5.3 ± 4.2 more
ISIS-3[§]					
Streptokinase	13 780	141 (1.0)	1455 (10.6)	1389 (10.1)	1530 (11.1)
t-PA	13 746	188 (1.4)	1418 (10.3)	1325 (9.6)	1513 (11.0)
Effect/1000 people treated with t-PA instead of streptokinase		3.5 ± 1.3 more	2.4 ± 3.7 fewer	4.4 ± 3.6 fewer	1.0 ± 3.8 fewer
GUSTO-1[¶]					
Streptokinase (subcutaneous heparin)	9841	117 (1.2)	712 (7.3)	666 (6.8)	783 (8.0)
Streptokinase (intravenous heparin)	10 410	144 (1.4)	763 (7.4)	709 (6.8)	853 (8.2)
t-PA alone	10 396	161 (1.6)	653 (6.3)	585 (5.6)	746 (7.2)
t-PA plus streptokinase	10 374	170 (1.6)	723 (7.0)	647 (6.2)	817 (7.9)
Effect/1000 people treated with t-PA-based regimens instead of streptinokinase		3.0 ± 1.2 more	6.6 ± 2.5 fewer	8.6 ± 2.4 fewer	5.5 ± 2.6 fewer
$\chi^2/2$ heterogeneity of effects between 3 trials		0.7	5.6	7.0	5.4
P value		0.3	0.06	0.03	0.07

TABLE 1 Continued

Weighted average of all 3 trials*
Effect/1000 patient treated with t-PA-based regimens instead of streptokinase

3.3 ± 0.8 more	2.9 ± 1.9 fewer	4.9 ± 1.8 fewer	1.6 ± 1.9 fewer
P value			
< 0.001	> 0.1	0.01	0.4

Values are numbers (%). This table should not be used to make direct non-randomised comparisons between the absolute event rates in different trials, because the patient populations may have differed substantially in age and other characteristics. Deaths recorded throughout the first 35 days are included for GISSI-2 and ISIS-3 and throughout the first 30 days for GUSTO-1. Numbers randomised and numbers with follow up are from the ISIS-3 report[10] and GUSTO-1[11] (supplemented with revised GUSTO-1 data from the National Auxiliary Publications Service), and numbers with events and the percentages (based on participants with follow up) are from the ISIS-3 report[10] and Van de Werf, et al.[36] Plus-minus values are ± SD. In all three trials, streptokinase was given in an intravenous infusions of 1.5 million units over a period of 1 hour.

†Death not related to stroke was defined as death without recorded stroke.

‡In the GISSI-2 trial, the t-PA regimen involved an initial bolus of 10 mg, followed by 50 mg in the first hour and 20 mg in each of the second and third hours.

§In the ISIS-3 trial, the t-PA regimen involved 40 000 clot-lysis units per kilogram of body weight as an initial bolus, followed by 360 000 units per kilogram in the first hour and 67 000 units per kilogram in each of the next 3 hours.

¶In the GUSTO-1 trial, the t-PA alone regimen involved an initial bolus of 15 mg, followed by 0.75 mg per kilogram (up to 50 mg) in the first 30 minutes and 0.5 mg per kilogram (up to 35 mg) in the next hour; in the GUSTO-1 trial the other t-PA based regimen involved 0.1 mg of t-PA per kilogram (up to 9 mg) as an initial bolus and 0.9 mg per kilogram (up to 81 mg) in the remainder of the first hour, plus 1 million units of streptokinase in the first hour.

*The weights are proportional to the sample sizes of the trials, so this average gives most weight to the GUSTO-1 trial and least to the GISSI-2 trials.[9] Reproduced from Collins R, Peto R, Baigent BM, Sleight DM. Aspirin, heparin and fibrinolytic therapy in suspected AMI. *N Engl J Med* 1997;336:847–860, with permission of the publisher.

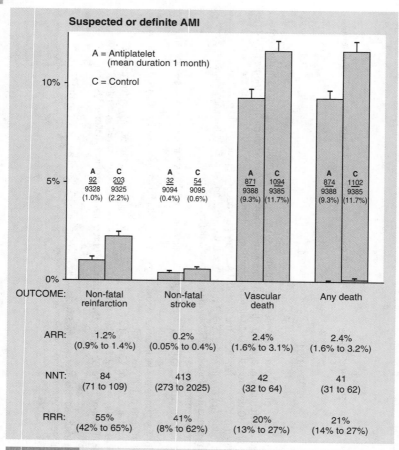

Suspected or definite AMI

A = Antiplatelet (mean duration 1 month)

C = Control

OUTCOME:	Non-fatal reinfarction	Non-fatal stroke	Vascular death	Any death
	A 92 / 9328 (1.0%) — C 203 / 9325 (2.2%)	A 32 / 9094 (0.4%) — C 54 / 9095 (0.6%)	A 871 / 9388 (9.3%) — C 1094 / 9385 (11.7%)	A 874 / 9388 (9.3%) — C 1102 / 9385 (11.7%)
ARR:	1.2% (0.9% to 1.4%)	0.2% (0.05% to 0.4%)	2.4% (1.6% to 3.1%)	2.4% (1.6% to 3.2%)
NNT:	84 (71 to 109)	413 (273 to 2025)	42 (32 to 64)	41 (31 to 62)
RRR:	55% (42% to 65%)	41% (8% to 62%)	20% (13% to 27%)	21% (14% to 27%)

FIGURE 1 Absolute effects of antiplatelet treatment on various outcomes in people with a prior suspected or definite acute myocardial infarction.[3] The columns show the absolute risks over 1 month for each category; the error bars are the upper 95% confidence interval. In "any death" column non-vascular deaths are represented by lower horizontal lines. The table displays for each outcome the absolute risk reduction (ARR), the number of people needing treatment for 1 month to avoid one additional event (NNT), and the relative risk reduction (RRR), with their 95% CIs (see text, p 3). Published with permission.[3]

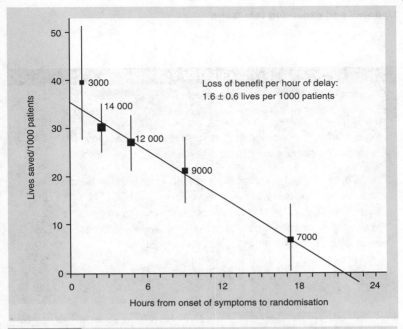

FIGURE 2 **Absolute number of lives saved at 1 month per 1000 people receiving thrombolytic treatment plotted against the time from the onset of symptoms to randomisation among 45 000 people with ST segment elevation or bundle branch block.[7] Numbers along the curve are the number of people treated at different times (see text, p 4). Published with permission.[8]**

Changing behaviour

Updated and expanded this issue

Margaret Thorogood, Melvyn Hillsdon and Carolyn Summerbell

INTERVENTIONS

*In terms of producing the intended behavioural change.
See glossary, p 31

Key Messages

Smoking

- Systematic reviews of RCTs found that simple, one off advice from a physician during a routine consultation was associated with 2% of smokers quitting smoking and not relapsing for 1 year when compared with no advice; additional encouragement or support might increase (by a further 3%) the effectiveness of the advice. RCTs found that individual advice from a psychologist compared with no advice achieved a similar quit rate (3%). One systematic review of RCTs found that trained counsellors, who were neither doctors nor nurses, increased quit rates by 4% compared with minimal intervention. One systematic review found that smoking cessation advice from trained nurses compared with usual care or control increased the rate of quitting, but by less than 1%. One systematic review found that brief advice delivered in primary care increased the quit rate by 3% compared to control, and by indirect comparison that intensive advice might approximately double the quit rate.

- One systematic review of RCTs and one subsequent RCT found that nicotine replacement was an effective additional component of cessation strategies in smokers who smoked at least 10 cigarettes daily. We found no clear evidence that any method of delivery of nicotine is more effective than others. We found limited evidence from three RCTs with follow up of 2–6 years that the additional benefit of nicotine replacement therapy on quit rates reduces with time.

- One systematic review of RCTs found no evidence that acupuncture increased rates of smoking cessation at 12 months.

- One systematic review of antidepressants used as part of a smoking cessation programme found that buproprion increased quit rates. The same systematic review found that moclobemide and anxiolytics did not significantly increase quit rates.

- One systematic review of RCTs found very limited evidence that exercise might increase smoking cessation.

- Two systematic reviews found that in pregnant women antismoking interventions without nicotine replacement were as effective as nicotine replacement in healthy non-pregnant women.

- One systematic review and one RCT found that antismoking interventions had a greater impact in people at higher risk of smoking related disease.

- One systematic review has found that training health professionals to give antismoking advice increases the effectiveness of antismoking interventions.

Physical activity and diet

- We found weak evidence from systematic reviews and subsequent RCTs that counselling sedentary people increased their physical activity compared with no intervention. One RCT found that exercise advice delivered in the home by physiotherapists increased physical activity in women over 80 years and reduced their risk of falling.

  - Systematic reviews found that advice on cholesterol lowering diet (that is, advice to lower fat intake or increase the ratio of polyunsaturated to saturated fatty acid) led to a small reduction in blood cholesterol concentrations in the long term (6 months or more).

  - Systematic reviews and one RCT found that salt restriction significantly reduced blood pressure in people with hypertension. The same reviews and RCT found limited evidence that salt restriction was effective in preventing hypertension. The RCT found limited evidence that advice on restricting salt intake was less effective than advice on weight reduction in preventing hypertension.

- Systematic reviews found a combination of advice on diet and exercise supported by behaviour therapy was probably more effective than either diet or exercise advice alone in the treatment of obesity, and might lead to sustained weight loss.

DEFINITION	Cigarette smoking, diet, and level of physical activity are important in the aetiology of many chronic diseases. Individual change in behaviour has the potential to decrease the burden of chronic disease, particularly cardiovascular disease.
INCIDENCE/ PREVALENCE	In the developed world, the decline in smoking has slowed and the prevalence of regular smoking is increasing in young people. A sedentary lifestyle is becoming increasingly common and the prevalence of obesity is increasing rapidly.
AIMS	To encourage individuals to reduce or abandon unhealthy behaviours and to take up healthy behaviours; to support the maintenance of these changes in the long term.
OUTCOMES	Ideally the outcomes considered would be clinical, and would relate to the underlying conditions (longevity, quality of life, rate of stroke, or myocardial infarction). However, most studies report proxy outcomes, such as the proportion of people changing behaviour (for example, stopping smoking) in a specified period.
METHODS	*Clinical Evidence* update search and appraisal May 2000. Recent appropriate systematic reviews were identified as well as subsequent RCTs. Systematic reviews and RCTs included are those with at least 6 months of follow up.

QUESTION Which interventions reduce cigarette smoking?

OPTION COUNSELLING

Systematic reviews of RCTs have found that simple, one off advice from a physician during a routine consultation is associated with 2% of smokers quitting smoking and not relapsing for 1 year. Additional encouragement or support may increase (by a further 3%) the effectiveness of the advice. Individual advice from a psychologist achieves a similar quit rate (3%), and advice from trained nurse counsellors, or from trained counsellors who are neither doctors nor nurses, increases quit rates compared with minimal intervention.

Benefits: We found four systematic reviews.[1–4] One (search date not given, 17 RCTs, 14 438 smokers) evaluated simple advice from physicians. The advice was typically of less than 5 minutes duration. It found that 1.9% of smokers (95% CI 0.1% to 2.8%) stopped smoking as a direct result of the advice and did not relapse for at least 1 year.[1] Rates of cessation in the control groups ranged from 1.1% to 14.1% and in the intervention groups from 1.5% to 14.5%. The results were similar when the analysis was confined to the six trials in which cessation was confirmed by biochemical markers. Ten trials tested the effect of additional support, such as additional visits and encouragement or demonstrations of exhaled carbon monoxide in the person's breath. There was a high degree of heterogeneity (with rates of cessation ranging from −0.5% to +29%) but the overall estimate of smokers quitting for 1 year was 5% (95% CI 1% to 8%). Five trials of individual sessions with a psychologist found that the number of smokers quitting at 1 year as a result of advice was 2.8% (95% CI 1.3% to 4.2%). The second systematic review (search date 1998) of interventions provided by counsellors trained in smoking cessation (other than doctors and nurses) used a broad definition of counselling including all contacts with a smoker that lasted at least 10 minutes. Eleven trials were included, of which six had follow up for at least 1 year, while the rest had a minimum follow up of 6 months. The review found that counselling increased the rate of quitting (263/1381 [14%] quit with counselling v 194/1899 [10%] with control, OR of quitting 1.55, 95% CI 1.27 to 1.90).[2] The third review (search date 1999) considered the effectiveness of smoking interventions delivered by a nurse. Nineteen trials were identified, with four having a follow up period of less than 1 year. It found that advice from a nurse increased the rate of quitting (621/4689 [13.2%] quit with advice v 402/3223 [12.5%] with control, OR 1.43, 95% CI 1.24 to 1.6).[3] The final systematic review (search date 1995) identified 23 trials of smoking advice in general practice.[4] In 20 of the trials, a general practitioner gave advice, although nurses or counsellors were also involved in four of these trials. In three trials, the advice was given solely by a nurse or health visitor. Smoking cessation was measured for between 6 months and 2 years. There was significant heterogeneity because of the inclusion of two trials (both involving only general practitioners) with notably larger effects. When these two trials were excluded, the review found that advice increased the odds of smoking cessation (935/9361 [9.7%] quit with advice v 513/7952 [6.8%] with control, OR 1.32, 95% CI 1.18 to 1.48). The review found that (by indirect comparisons) intensive advice was more effective than brief advice (616/7651 [8%] quit with brief advice v 391/6486 [6%] with control, OR for quitting after brief advice 1.27, 95% CI 1.11 to 1.45; with intensive advice 319/2070 [15.4%] quit v 122/1106 [11.0%], OR after intensive advice 1.46, 95% CI 1.18 to 1.80). Fifty smokers would need to be given brief advice (or 25 smokers given intensive advice) for one additional person to quit for at least 6 months.[4]

Harms: We found no evidence of harm.

Comment: The effects of advice may be considered disappointingly small, but a year on year reduction of 2% in the number of smokers would represent a significant public health gain (see smoking cessation under primary prevention, p 51).

OPTION   NICOTINE REPLACEMENT

One systematic review and one subsequent RCT have found that nicotine replacement is an effective component of cessation strategies in smokers who smoke at least 10 cigarettes a day. Fifteen such smokers would have to be treated with nicotine replacement to produce one extra non-smoker at 12 months, but this overestimates effectiveness, since

relapse will continue after 12 months. Higher dose (4 mg) gum is more effective than lower dose (2 mg) gum in very dependent smokers. We found no clear evidence that any one method of delivery of nicotine is more effective, or evidence of further benefit after 8 weeks' treatment with patches. Long term relapse may occur in people who quit, but the review found that the rate of relapse was not greater in those who quit with the aid of nicotine replacement. Abstinence after 1 week is a strong predictor of 12 month abstinence.

Benefits: **Abstinence at 12 months:** We found one systematic review and one subsequent RCT.[5,6] The systematic review (search date 1999) identified 49 trials of nicotine gum, 32 trials of nicotine transdermal patches, four of nicotine intranasal spray, four of inhaled nicotine, and two of sublingual tablet.[5] All forms of nicotine replacement were more effective than placebo. When the abstinence rates for all trials were pooled according to the longest duration of follow up available, the odds of abstinence were increased by 72% (95% CI 60% to 84%) with nicotine replacement compared with placebo. Seventeen per cent of smokers allocated to nicotine replacement successfully quit, compared with 10% in the control group. The review found no significant difference in benefit between different forms of nicotine replacement (OR for abstinence 1.63 for nicotine gum to 2.27 for nicotine nasal spray). In trials that directly compared 4 mg with 2 mg nicotine gum, the higher dose improved abstinence in highly dependent smokers (pooled OR of abstinence 2.27, 95% CI 1.69 to 4.22). The review found no evidence of a difference in effectiveness for 16 hour patches versus 24 hour patches, and no difference in effect in trials where the dose was tapered compared with those where the patches were withdrawn abruptly. Use of the patch for 8 weeks was as effective as longer use, and there was very weak evidence in favour of nicotine replacement in relapsed smokers. One trial in 3585 people found that abstinence at 1 week was a strong predictor of 12 month abstinence (25% of those abstinent at 1 week were abstinent at 12 months v 2.7% of those not abstinent at 1 week).[6] One meta-analysis of relapse rates in nicotine replacement trials found that nicotine replacement increased abstinence at 12 months, but that the addition of nicotine replacement did not significantly affect relapse rates between 6 weeks and 12 months.[7] **Longer term abstinence:** Three recent trials[8–10] have found that nicotine replacement does not affect long term abstinence. In one RCT, which compared nicotine spray versus placebo, 47 people abstinent at 1 year were followed for up to a further 2 years and 5 months, after which there was still a significant, although smaller, difference in abstinence (in longer term 15.4% abstinent with nicotine spray v 9.3% with placebo, NNT for one extra person to abstain 7 at 1 year v 11 at 3.5 years).[8] The second trial compared 5 months of nicotine patches plus nicotine spray versus the same patches plus a placebo spray. It found no significant difference between treatments after 6 years (16.2% abstinent with nicotine spray v 8.5% with placebo spray, P = 0.08).[9] The third trial compared patches delivering different nicotine doses versus placebo patches. The trial followed everyone that quit at 6 weeks for a further 4 to 5 years, and found no significant difference in relapse between the groups. Overall, 73% of people who quit at 6 weeks relapsed.[10]

Harms: Nicotine gum has been associated with hiccups, gastrointestinal disturbances, jaw pain, and orodental problems. Nicotine transdermal patches have been associated with skin sensitivity and irritation. Nicotine inhalers and nasal spray have been associated with local irritation at the site of administration. Nicotine sublingual tablets have been reported to cause hiccups, burning, and smarting sensations in the mouth, sore throat, coughing, dry lips, and mouth ulcers.[11]

Comment: Nicotine replacement may not represent an "easy cure" for nicotine addiction, but it does improve the cessation rate. The evidence suggests that the majority of smokers attempting cessation fail at any one attempt, or relapse over the next 5 years. Multiple attempts may be needed.

| OPTION | ACUPUNCTURE | New |

One systematic review of RCTs has found no evidence that acupuncture increases rates of smoking cessation at 12 months.

Benefits: We found one systematic review (search date 1999, 18 RCTs, 3772 people) comparing acupuncture with sham acupuncture, other treatment or no treatment. Only five trials (2535 people) reported abstinence after at least 12 months.[12] The review found that acupuncture versus control treatment produced no significant reduction in smoking cessation at 12 months (OR 1.02, 95% CI 0.72 to 1.43).

Harms: None were documented.

Comment: None.

| OPTION | PHYSICAL EXERCISE | New |

One systematic review of RCTs found limited evidence that exercise might increase smoking cessation.

Benefits: We found one systematic review (search date 1999, 8 RCTs)[13] of exercise compared with control interventions. Four small RCTs in the review reported point prevalence of non-smoking at 12 months and found no significant benefit from exercise, but these studies were insufficiently powered to exclude a clinically important effect. One RCT in 281 women found that three exercise sessions per week for 12 weeks plus a cognitive behaviour programme (see glossary, p 31) improved continuous abstinence from smoking at 12 months compared with the behaviour programme alone (16/134 [12%] with exercise v 8/147 [5%] with control; ARR 6.5%, 95% CI −19% to +0.0%; RR 2.2, 95% CI 0.98 to 4.5).[14]

Harms: None were documented.

Comment: None.

OPTION ANTIDEPRESSANT AND ANXIOLYTIC TREATMENT New

One systematic review has found that quit rates are significantly increased by buproprion, but not by moclobemide or anxiolytics.

Benefits: We found one systematic review (search date 1999, 3230 people in eight RCTs of antidepressants and 945 people in six RCTs of anxiolytics).[15] Only five of the RCTs of antidepressants (1985 people) reported abstinence after at least 12 months. The review found that buproprion 300 mg daily (an antidepressant) increased cessation at 12 months compared with control treatment (four RCTs; AR quitting 21% with buproprion v 8% with control; OR 2.73, 95% CI 1.90 to 3.94; NNT 8). Another RCT in the review found that combined buproprion plus a nicotine patch was more efficacious than a patch alone (OR 2.65, 95% CI 1.58 to 4.45), but not more effective than buproprion alone. One RCT of moclobemide (an antidepressant) found no significant difference in abstinence at 12 months. Four RCTs of anxiolytics (626 people) found no significant increase in abstinence at 12 months with anxiolytics versus control treatment.

Harms: Headache, insomnia, and dry mouth were reported in people using buproprion.[15] The largest RCT found that discontinuation rates caused by adverse events were 3.8% with placebo, 6.6% for nicotine replacement therapy, 11.9% for buproprion, and 11.4% for buproprion plus nicotine replacement therapy.[16] Anxiolytics may cause dependence and withdrawal problems, tolerance, paradoxical effects, and impair driving ability.

Comment: None.

QUESTION Are smoking cessation interventions more effective in people at high risk of smoking related disease?

OPTION IN PREGNANT WOMEN

Two systematic reviews of RCTs have found that the effect of antismoking interventions in pregnant women increased abstinence rates and decreased the risk of giving birth to low birthweight babies. The increase in abstinence with non-nicotine replacement interventions was similar to the increase found in trials of nicotine replacement in men and non-pregnant women.

Benefits: We found two systematic reviews.[1,17] One (search date 1999) identified 34 trials of smoking cessation interventions in pregnancy. It found that smoking cessation programmes improved abstinence (OR of abstinence in late pregnancy with antismoking programmes v no programmes 0.53, 95% 0.47 to 0.60).[17] The findings were similar if the analysis was restricted to trials in which abstinence was confirmed by means other than self reporting. The review also found that antismoking programmes reduced the risk of low birth weight babies, but found no evidence of an effect on the rates of very low birthweight babies or perinatal mortality, although the power to detect such effects was low (OR for low birthweight babies 0.80, 95% CI 0.69 to 0.99). The review calculated that of 100 smokers attending a first antenatal visit, 10 stopped spontaneously and a further 6–7 stopped as the result of a smoking cessation programme. Five included trials examined the effects of interventions to prevent relapse in 800 women who had quit smoking. Collectively, these found no evidence that these interventions reduced relapse rate.[17] One earlier systematic review (search date not given) identified 10 trials of antismoking interventions in 4815 pregnant women.[1] It included one trial of physician advice, one trial of advice by a health educator, one trial of group sessions, and seven trials of behaviour therapy based on self help manuals. Cessation rates among trials ranged from 1.9–16.7% in the control groups and from 7.1–36.1% in the intervention groups. The review found that antismoking interventions increased the rate of quitting (ARI with intervention v no intervention 7.6%, 95% CI 4.3% to 10.8%).[1]

Harms: None documented.

Comment: Some women quit smoking before their first antenatal visit, and the majority of these will remain abstinent. In women who are still smoking at their first antenatal visit, advice to stop smoking improves abstinence rates, but most women continue to smoke. Two trials of nicotine replacement are currently under way.[17]

OPTION IN PEOPLE AT HIGH RISK OF DISEASE

One systematic review of RCTs has found that antismoking advice improves smoking cessation in men at high risk of cardiovascular events. One trial also found a greater effect in men and women with early chronic obstructive lung disease.

Benefits: We found no trials in which the same intervention was used in high and low risk people. We found one systematic review (search date not given, four trials, 13 208 healthy men at high risk of heart disease)[1] and one subsequent RCT.[18] The systematic review found that antismoking advice improved smoking cessation rates compared with control interventions (ARI of smoking cessation 21%, 95% CI 10% to 31%; NNT 5, 95% CI 4 to 10).[1] One early trial, which was included in the review, used non-random allocation in 223 men after myocardial infarction. The intervention group was given intensive advice by the therapeutic team while in the coronary care unit. The trial found that the self reported cessation rate at 1 year or more was higher in the intervention group than the control group (63% quit in the intervention group v 28% in the control group; ARI of quitting 36%, 95% CI 23% to 48%).[19] The subsequent RCT compared postal advice on smoking cessation versus no intervention in men aged 30–45 years with either a history of asbestos exposure, or forced expiratory volume in 1 second (FEV_1) in the lowest quartile for their age. Postal advice increased the self reported sustained cessation rate at 1 year compared with no intervention (5.6% with postal advice v 3.5%; P < 0.05; NNT 48).[18]

Harms: None were documented.

Comment: There was heterogeneity in the four trials included in the review, partly because of a less intense intervention in one trial and the recording of a change from cigarettes to other forms of tobacco as success in another. One of the included trials was weakened by use of self reported smoking cessation as an outcome and non-random allocation to the intervention.[19]

| QUESTION | Does training of professionals increase the effectiveness of smoking cessation interventions? |

One systematic review has found that antismoking interventions are more effective if the health professionals delivering the interventions have received training. One trial has shown training pharmacy staff has a small effect on over the counter sales of nicotine replacement therapy. One extra ex-smoker can be expected for about 50 people advised by a trained clinician compared with an untrained clinician.

Benefits: We found one systematic review and one subsequent RCT.[20,21] The systematic review (search date 1998) identified eight trials of training medical practitioners and one trial of training dental practitioners to give antismoking advice. All the trials took place in the USA. The training was provided on a group basis, and variously included lectures, videotapes, role plays, and discussion. The importance of setting quit dates and offering follow up was emphasised in most of the training programmes. The review found that training health professionals improved quit rates. Three trials used prompts and reminders to practitioners to deploy smoking cessation techniques and found higher quit rates.[20] One RCT in Scotland used sequential allocation of pharmacy personnel to a 2 hour training workshop in giving support to smokers in quitting, or to no training. Customers wanting to quit smoking in the pharmacies with trained staff were found to be significantly more likely to buy a nicotine replacement product (97.8% v 92.5%, P = 0.0085).[21]

Harms: None were documented.

Comment: The systematic review should be interpreted with caution because there were variations in the way the anlysis allowed for the unit of randomisation. A revised cochrane review is available in The Cochrane Library, Issue 3, 2000. It will be included in the next issue of *Clinical Evidence*.

| QUESTION | Which interventions increase physical activity in sedentary people? |

| OPTION | COUNSELLING |

We found weak evidence from systematic reviews and subsequent RCTs that sedentary people can be encouraged to increase their physical activity. Interventions that encourage moderate rather than vigorous exercise, and do not require attendance at a special facility, may be more successful. Increases in walking in previously sedentary women can be sustained over at least 10 years. Brief advice from a physician is probably not effective in increasing physical activity.

Benefits: We found two systematic reviews and six subsequent RCTs.[22–29] One review (search date 1996) identified 11 RCTs of single factor physical activity promotion in 1699 people, all based in the USA.[22] Seven trials evaluated advice to undertake exercise from home (mainly walking, but including jogging and swimming), and six evaluated advice to undertake facility based exercise (including jogging and walking on sports tracks, endurance exercise, games, swimming, and exercise to music classes). An increase in activity in the intervention groups was seen in trials in which home based moderate exercise was encouraged and regular brief follow up of participants was provided. In most of the trials, participants were self selected volunteers, so the effects of the interventions may have been exaggerated. Another systematic review compared "lifestyle" physical activity interventions with either standard exercise treatment or a control group.[23] Lifestyle interventions were defined as those concerned with the daily accumulation of moderate or vigorous exercise as part of everyday life. The review found two RCTs, one of which found more self reported physical activity in the lifestyle group than a standard exercise group; the other (n = 235) found no difference in physical activity between the groups. Three of the additional trials[24–26] involved primary care delivered interventions, all of which failed to show any significant changes in self reported physical activity at follow up compared with controls. One quasi-randomised trial tested the effect of brief physician advice plus a mailed leaflet on physical activity in 776 people in a primary care setting. After 12 months, the trial found no difference in self reported activity between intervention and control groups.[27] One recent trial of encouraging walking in 125 women found no difference in walking levels at 30 months' follow up between subjects receiving an 8 week behavioural intervention and those receiving a 5 minute telephone call and written information about the benefits of exercise, although both groups increased walking.[28] One further trial aimed at changing levels of physical activity compared a primary care physician's offer of an appointment with an exercise development officer versus a postal leaflet control group. At 8 months' follow up the number of sedentary people in the intervention group was significantly lower than the control group.[29] One trial of encouraging women to increase walking found significantly increased walking in the intervention group. Ten year follow up of 86% of the original 229 women in the trial found that women who had been encouraged to walk reported significantly more walking (median estimated calorie expenditure from self reported amount of walking 1344 kcal/week in women given encouragement *v* 924 kcal/week in women not encouraged to walk, P = 0.01).[30]

Harms: None of the reviews, or the trials, reported any incidences of harm from taking up exercise.

Comment: Self reporting of effects by people in a trial, especially where blinding to interventions is not possible (as is the case with advice or encouragement), is a potential source of bias. Several trials are in progress, including one in the UK, in which people in primary care have been randomised to two different methods of encouraging an increase in walking, or to a no intervention arm. One ongoing multisite trial in the USA has randomised 874 people to one of three experimental counselling interventions.[31]

QUESTION What are effects of exercise advice in high risk people?

OPTION IN WOMEN AGED OVER 80 YEARS

One RCT found exercise advice increased physical activity in women aged over 80 years and decreased the risk of falling.

Benefits: We found no systematic review. One RCT in 233 women aged over 80, conducted in New Zealand, compared four visits from a physiotherapist who advised a course of 30 minutes of home based exercises three times a week that was appropriate for the individual, versus a similar number of social visits.[32] After 1 year, women who had received physiotherapist visits were significantly more active than women in the control group, and 42% were still completing the recommended exercise programme at least three times a week. The mean annual rate of falls in the intervention group was 0.87 compared with 1.34 in the control group, a difference of 0.47 falls per year (95% CI 0.04 to 0.90).

Harms: No additional harms in the intervention group were reported.

Comment: None.

QUESTION What are the effects on blood cholesterol of advice aimed at lowering blood cholesterol?

OPTION COUNSELLING

Systematic reviews have found that advice on eating a cholesterol lowering diet (that is, advice to reduce fat intake or increase the polyunsaturated to saturated fatty acid ratio in the diet) leads to a small reduction in blood cholesterol concentrations in the long term (6 months or more). We found evidence of a dose response, in that dietary advice recommending more stringent reduction in fat and cholesterol intake lowered blood cholesterol more than less stringent advice. We found no evidence to support the effectiveness of such advice in primary care.

Benefits: **Effects on blood cholesterol:** We found three systematic reviews[11,33,34] and one subsequent RCT that reported biochemical rather than clinical end points.[35] None of these systematic reviews included evidence after 1996. One review (search date 1993) identified five trials of cholesterol lowering dietary advice (principally advice from nutritionists or specially trained counsellors) with follow up for 9–18 months.[33] It found a reduction in blood cholesterol concentration in the intervention group of 0.22 mmol/l (95% CI 0.05 to 0.39 mmol/l) compared with the control group. However, there was significant heterogeneity (P < 0.02), with two outlying studies — one showing no effect and one showing a larger effect. This review excluded trials in people at high risk of heart disease. Another systematic review (search date 1996) identified 13 trials of more than 6 months' duration and included people at high risk of heart disease.[11] It found that dietary advice reduced blood cholesterol (mean reduction in blood cholesterol concentration with advice 4.5%, 95% CI 3.9% to 5.1%; given a mean baseline cholesterol of 6.3 mmol/l, mean absolute reduction about

To continue receiving Clinical Evidence......

We hope that you enjoy receiving this **complimentary** issue of *Clinical Evidence.* The UnitedHealth Foundation is pleased to be able to provide you with this Issue and has made a commitment to provide copies of the next Issue.

In order to receive the next issue, please provide us with the information requested below, or if you would prefer you may e-mail us at uhfce@uhc.com or call us at 1-877-485-8074.

Sincerely,
William W. McGuire, M.D.
UnitedHealth Foundation

Name _____

Address _____

City _____

Specialty _____

e-mail address: _____

UNITEDHEALTH
MN008-T500
PO BOX 1459
MINNEAPOLIS MN 55440-1459

MN008-T500
UNITEDHEALTH FOUNDATION
PO BOX 1459
MINNEAPOLIS MN 55440-1459

$ 0.20
PLACE
POSTCARD
POSTAGE
HERE

0.3 mmol/l). The third systematic review (search date 1995, one trial,[36] 76 people) found no significant difference between brief versus intensive advice from a general practitioner and dietician on blood cholesterol at 1 year.[34] The subsequent RCT compared advice on healthy eating versus no intervention in 95 men and 91 women at high risk of CHD. At 1 year, it found no significant differences between groups in total and low density lipoprotein (LDL) cholesterol concentrations for either sex, even though the reported percentage of energy from fat consumed by both women and men in the advice group decreased significantly compared with that reported by the women and men in the control group.[35] These results may reflect bias caused by self-reporting of dietary intake. **Effects on clinical outcomes:** We found two systematic reviews that reported on morbidity and mortality.[11,37] The first compared 13 separate and single dietary interventions.[11] It found no significant effect of dietary interventions on total mortality (OR 0.93, 95% CI 0.84 to 1.03) or coronary heart disease (CHD) mortality (OR 0.93, 95% CI 0.82 to 1.06), but found a reduction in non-fatal myocardial infarction (OR 0.77, 95% CI 0.67 to 0.90). The second systematic review (27 studies including 40 intervention arms, 30 901 person years) found dietary advice to reduce or modify dietary fat versus no dietary advice had no significant effect on total mortality (HR 0.98, 95% CI 0.86 to 1.12) or cardiovascular disease (CVD) mortality (HR 0.98, 95% CI 0.77 to 1.07), but significantly reduced CVD events (HR 0.84, 95% CI 0.72 to 0.99).[37] RCTs in which people were followed for more than 2 years showed significant reductions in the rate of CVD events. The relative protection from CVD events was similar in both high and low risk groups, but was significant only in high risk groups.

Harms: We found no evidence about harms.

Comment: The finding of a 0.2–0.3 mmol/l reduction in blood cholesterol in the two systematic reviews accords with the findings of a meta-analysis of the plasma lipid response to changes in dietary fat and cholesterol.[38] The analysis included data from 244 published studies (trial duration 1 day to 6 years) and concluded that adherence to dietary recommendations (30% energy from fat, < 10% saturated fat, and < 300 mg cholesterol per day) compared with average US dietary intake would reduce blood cholesterol by about 5%.

QUESTION   **Does dietary advice to reduce sodium intake lead to a sustained fall in blood pressure?**

Systematic reviews and RCTs have found that salt restriction reduces blood pressure in people with normal blood pressure, and in people with hypertension. The effect was more pronounced in older people. We found no evidence of effects on morbidity and mortality.

Benefits: We found three systematic reviews about the long term effects of advice to restrict salt.[33,39,40] The first systematic review (search date 1993, five trials with follow up for 9–18 months) compared dietary advice (mainly from nutritionists or specially trained counsellors) with control treatment. It found that the advice slightly reduced systolic blood pressure (change in blood pressure: −1.9 mm Hg systolic, 95% CI −3.0 to −0.8 mm Hg), but not diastolic blood pressure (−1.2 mm Hg, 95% CI −2.6 to +0.2 mm Hg).[33] The second review (eight RCTs in adults over 44 years with and without hypertension) found no clearly significant systolic blood pressure changes after at least 6 months' follow up with advice on salt restriction versus no dietary advice either in people with hypertension (−2.9 mm Hg, 95% CI −5.8 to 0.0 mm Hg) or in people without hypertension (−1.3 mm Hg, 95% CI −2.7 to +0.1 mm Hg). Small but significant changes in mean diastolic blood pressure were found in people with hypertension (2.1 mm Hg, 95% CI −4.0 to −0.1 mm Hg) but not in people without hypertension (−0.8 mm Hg, 95% CI −1.8 to +0.2 mm Hg).[39] The definitions of hypertension varied between the trials. The third review found that in people aged over 44 years defined as having hypertension, a reduction in sodium intake of 100 mmol per day resulted in a decrease of 6.3 mm Hg in systolic blood pressure and 2.2 mm Hg in diastolic pressure.[40] For younger people with hypertension, the systolic fall was 2.4 mm Hg and the diastolic fall was negligible.[41] Three RCTs of salt restriction followed people without hypertension for over 12 months. The largest (181 people) found that advice on restricting salt was less effective in preventing hypertension than advice on weight reduction.

Harms: None reported.

Comment: None.

QUESTION	What are the effects of lifestyle interventions to achieve sustained weight loss?

Systematic reviews and subsequent RCTs have found that a combination of advice on diet and exercise, supported by behaviour therapy, is probably more effective in achieving weight loss than either diet or exercise advice alone. A low energy, low fat diet is the most effective lifestyle intervention for weight loss. RCTs have found no significant differences in weight loss between interventions to promote physical activity. Weight regain is likely, but weight loss of 2–6 kg may be sustained over at least 2 years.

Benefits: We found three systematic reviews,[42–44] and eight additional RCTs.[45–52] One systematic review (search date 1996) identified 99 studies, including some that tested either dietary or physical activity interventions with or without a behaviour intervention component. The combination of diet and exercise in conjunction with behavioural therapy produced greater weight loss than diet alone. This finding, however, was based on the results of one RCT in which a mean weight loss of 3.8 kg at 1 year was observed in a group receiving diet guidelines and behaviour intervention compared with a significantly different mean loss of 7.9 kg in a group receiving the same intervention plus a programme of walking.[42] The second systematic review of the detection, prevention, and treatment of obesity (published in 1999, 11 RCTs and additional prospective cohort studies) included eight RCTs that compared dietary prescriptions with exercise, counselling, or behavioural therapy for the treatment of obesity, and three RCTs that compared dietary counselling alone with no intervention. In both comparisons, initial weight loss was followed by gradual weight regain once treatment had stopped (mean difference in weight change at least 2 years after baseline: 2–6 kg for dietary prescription trials, and 2–4 kg for dietary counselling trials).[43] The third systematic review of RCTs and observational studies found similar results; it found that a combination of diet and exercise, supported by behaviour therapy, was more effective than any one or two of these individual interventions.[44] One additional RCT compared advice on an energy restricted diet to advice on a fat restricted diet.[49] Weight loss was greater on an energy restricted diet than on the fat restricted diet at 6 months (−11.2 kg v −6.1 kg, P < 0.001) and at 18 months (−7.5 kg v −1.8 kg, P < 0.001). Five RCTs focused on physical activity.[45–47,51,52] The heterogeneity of interventions makes pooling of data inappropriate, but no major differences were found between the various behaviour therapies and exercise regimes. One RCT[48] found behavioural choice treatment (see glossary, p 31) versus standard behaviour therapy (see glossary, p 31) resulted in greater weight loss at 12 months (−10.1 kg v −4.3 kg, P < 0.01). One RCT (166 people) compared standard behaviour therapy plus support from friends with standard behaviour therapy without support. It found no additional weight loss at 16 months with social support from friends (−4.7 kg v −3.0 kg, P < 0.3).[50]

Harms: The systematic reviews and RCTs provided no evidence about harms resulting from diet or exercise for weight loss.

Comment: None.

QUESTION What are the effects of lifestyle interventions to maintain weight loss? New

One systematic review and additional RCTs have found that most types of maintenance strategy result in smaller weight gains or greater weight losses compared with no contact. Strategies that involve personal contact with a therapist, family support, multiple interventions, or are weight focused appear most effective.

Benefits: We found one systematic review[42] and five additional RCTs.[53–57] The systematic review included 21 studies of different types and combinations of interventions. It found that increased contact with a therapist in the long term produced smaller weight gain or greater weight loss. The review found that additional self help peer groups, self management techniques, or involvement of the family or spouse may increase weight loss. The largest weight loss was seen in programmes using multiple strategies. Two small RCTs (102 people[53] and 100 people in two trials[57]) assessed simple strategies without face to face contact with a therapist. Frequent phone contacts, optional food provision, continued self monitoring, urge control, or relapse prevention did not reduce the rate of weight regain. One small RCT (117 people) found that phone contacts plus house visits did reduce the rate of weight regain compared with no intervention (3.65 kg v 6.42 kg, P = 0.048).[54] One small RCT (67 people) found that people on a weight focused programme maintained weight loss better than those on an exercise focused programme (0.8 kg v 4.4 kg, P < 0.01).[55] One five year RCT in 489 menopausal women compared behavioural intervention in two phases aimed at lifestyle changes in diet and physical activity with lifestyle assessment. People in the intervention group were encouraged to lose weight during the first 6 months (phase I), and thereafter maintain this weight loss for a further 12 months (phase II) The intervention resulted in weight loss compared to control during the first 6 months (−8.9 lb v −0.8 lb, P < 0.05), most of which was sustained over phase II (−6.7 lb v +0.6 lb, P < 0.05).[56]

Harms: We found no direct evidence that interventions designed to maintain weight loss are harmful.

Comment: Weight regain is common. The resource implication of providing long term maintenance of any weight loss may be a barrier to the routine implementation of maintenance programmes.

QUESTION **What are the effects of lifestyle advice to prevent weight gain?** *New*

One small RCT found that low intensity education increased weight loss. An extension of this RCT found no significant effect on weight gain from a mailed newsletter with or without a linked financial incentive.

Benefits: We found three systematic reviews,[42,43,58] which included the same two RCTs.[59,60] The second RCT was an extension of the first. The first RCT (219 people) compared low intensity education with a financial incentive to maintain weight versus an untreated control group. It found significantly greater average weight loss in the intervention group than in the control group (−2.1 lb v −0.3 lb, P = 0.03).[59] The second RCT (228 men and 998 women) compared a monthly newsletter versus the newsletter plus a lottery incentive versus no contact. There was no difference in weight gain after 3 years between the groups (1.6 kg v 1.5 kg v 1.8 kg).[60]

Harms: None reported.

Comment: None

QUESTION **What are the effects of training professionals in promoting reduction of body weight** *New*

One systematic review of poor quality RCTs has found little evidence on the sustained effect of interventions to improve health professionals' management of obesity. One subsequent small RCT found limited evidence that training for primary care doctors in nutrition counselling plus a support programme reduced body weight of the people in their care over 1 year.

Benefits: We found one systematic review[61] (search date 1998, 12 studies of five had follow up over 1 year) and one subsequent RCT.[62] The studies in the review were heterogeneous and poor quality. The subsequent RCT (45 people) compared nutrition counselling training plus a support programme for primary care doctors versus usual care.[62] The nutrition supported intervention compared with usual care increased weight loss at 1 year (additional weight loss 2.3 kg, P < 0.001).

Harms: None reported.

Comment: The doctors were randomly allocated to treatment but the analysis of results was based on the patients in the care of those doctors. No allowance was made for cluster bias. This increases the chance that the additional weight loss could have occurred by chance.

GLOSSARY

Cognitive behaviour programme Traditional cognitive behavioural topics (e.g. self-monitoring, stimulus control, coping with cravings and high risk situations, stress management, and relaxation techniques) along with topics of particular importance to women (e.g. healthy eating, weight management, mood management, and managing work and family).

Behavioural choice treatment A cognitive behavioural intervention based on a decision making model of women's food choice. This relates situation specific eating behaviour to outcomes and goals using decision theory. The outcomes and goals governing food choice extend beyond food related factors to include self esteem and social acceptance.

Standard behaviour therapy A behavioural weight management programme that incorporates moderate calorie restriction to promote weight loss.

Substantive changes since last issue

Smoking cessation In people at high risk of disease. One new trial comparing postal advice on smoking cessation versus no intervention found that postal advice increased the self reported cessation rate.[18]

Effects of dietary advice to reduce or modify fat intake and lower blood cholesterol: counselling One new systematic review found a significant reduction in cardiovascular events, but no reduction in overall or cardiovascular mortality.[37] One new RCT found no significant benefit of intervention programmes in primary care.[36]

Diet and blood pressure Two new systematic reviews[39,40] and one RCT[41] found that salt restriction reduces blood pressure in people with hypertension. The same reviews and RCT found limited evidence that salt restriction was effective in preventing hypertension. The RCT found that advice on restricting salt intake was less effective than advice on weight reduction in preventing hypertension.[41]

Interventions to change lifestyle and sustain weight loss Five new RCTs of various types and combinations of interventions.[48–52] Overall, more personal contact in the long term reduced weight gain or increased weight loss.

REFERENCES

1. Law M, Tang JL. An analysis of the effectiveness of interventions intended to help people stop smoking. *Arch Intern Med* 1995;155:1933–1941. Search date not specified but before 1995; primary sources Medline and Index Medicus; dates not given, but selected trials range from 1967 to 1993.

2. Lancaster T, Stead LF. Individual behavioural counselling for smoking cessation. In: The Cochrane Library, Issue 1, 2000. Oxford: Update Software. Search date October 1998; primary sources Cochrane Tobacco Addiction Group Trials Register to October 1998.

3. Rice VH, Stead LF. Nursing interventions for smoking cessation. In: The Cochrane Library, Issue 1, 2000. Oxford: Update Software. Search date May 1999; primary sources Cochrane Tobacco Addiction Group Trials Register to May 1999, and Cinahl 1983 to May 1999.

4. Ashenden R, Silagy C, Weller D. A systematic review of the effectiveness of promoting lifestyle change in general practice. *Family Practice* 1997; 14:160–176. Search date May 1995; primary sources Medline, Psychlit, Sociofile, Cinahl,

Embase, and Drug; all searched from the year of their inception up to May 1995.

5. Silagy C, Mant D, Fowler G, Lancaster T. Nicotine replacement therapy for smoking cessation. In: The Cochrane Library, Issue 1, 2000. Oxford: Update Software.

6. Tonneson P, Paoletti P, Gustavsson G, et al. Higher dose nicotine patches increase one year smoking cessation rates: results from the European CEASE trial. *Eur Respir J* 1999;13:238–246.

7. Stapleton J. Cigarette smoking prevalence, cessation and relapse. *Stat Methods Med Res* 1998;7:187–203. Search date and primary sources not given.

8. Stapleton JA, Sutherland G, Russell MA. How much does relapse after one year erode effectiveness of smoking cessation treatments? Long term follow up of a randomised trial of nicotine nasal spray. *BMJ* 1998;316:830–831.

9. Blondal T, Gudmundsson J, Olafsdottir I, et al. Nicotine nasal spray with nicotine patch for smoking cessation: randomised trial with six years follow up. *BMJ* 1999;318:285–289.

10. Daughton DM, Fortmann SP, Glover ED, et al. The

smoking cessation efficacy of varying doses of nicotine patch delivery systems 4 to 5 years post-quit day. *Prev Med* 1999;28:113–118.

11. Ebrahim S, Davey Smith G. *Health promotion in older people for the prevention of coronary heart disease and stroke*. Health promotion effectiveness reviews series, No 1. London: Health Education Authority, 1996.

12. White AR, Rampes H, Ernst E. Acupuncture for smoking cessation. In: The Cochrane Library, Issue 2, 2000. Oxford: Update Software. Search date 1999; primary sources Cochrane Tobacco Addiction Group Register, Medline, PsychLit, Dissertation Abstracts, Health Planning and Administration, SocialSciSearch, Smoking and Health, Embase, Biological Abstracts and Drug.

13. Ussher MH, Taylor AH, West R, McEwen A. Does exercise aid smoking cessation? *Addiction* 2000; 95:199–208.

14. Marcus BH, Albrecht AE, King TK, et al. The efficacy of exercise as an aid for smoking cessation in women. *Arch Intern Med* 1999;159: 1229–1234.

15. Hughes JR, Stead LF, Lancaster T. Anxiolytics and antidepressants for smoking cessation. In: The Cochrane Library, Issue 2, 2000. Oxford: Update Software. Search date 1999; primary sources specialised register of the Cochrane Tobacco Addiction Group.

16. Jorenby DE, Leischow SJ, Nides MA, et al. A controlled trial of sustained-release bupropion. A nicotine patch, or both for smoking cessation. *N Engl J Med* 1999;340:685–691.

17. Lumley J, Oliver S, Waters E. Interventions for promoting smoking cessation during pregnancy. In: Cochrane Library, Issue 1, 2000. Oxford: Update Software. Search date October 1998; primary sources Cochrane Tobacco Addiction Group Trials Register to October 1998.

18. Humerfelt S, Eide GE, Kvale G, et al. Effectiveness of postal smoking cessation advice: a randomized controlled trial in young men with reduced FEV_1 and asbestos exposure. *Eur Respir J* 1998;11: 284–290.

19. Burt A, Thornley P, Illingworth D, et al. Stopping smoking after myocardial infarction. *Lancet* 1974; 1:304–306.

20. Lancaster T, Silagy C, Fowler G, Spiers I. Training health professionals in smoking cessation. In: The Cochrane Library, Issue 3, 1998. Oxford: Update Software; primary sources specialised register of the Cochrane Tobacco Addiction Group 1966–1998.

21. Sinclair HK, Bond CM, Lennox AS, et al. Training pharmacists and pharmacy assistants in the stage of change model of smoking cessation: a randomised controlled trial in Scotland. *Tobacco Control* 1998;7:253–261.

22. Hillsdon M, Thorogood M. A systematic review of physical activity promotion strategies. *Br J Sports Med* 1996;30:84–89. Search date 1996; primary sources Medline, Excerpta Medica, Sport, SCISearch 1966 to 1996; hand search of reference lists.

23. Dunn AL, Anderson RE, Jakicic JM. Lifestyle physical activity interventions. History, short- and long-term effects and recommendations. *Am J Prev Med* 1998;15:398–412. Search date not given; primary sources Medline, Current Contents, Biological Abstracts, The Johns Hopkins Medical Institutions Catalog, Sport Discus, and Grateful Med.

24. Goldstein MG, Pinto BM, Marcus BH, et al. Physician-based physical activity counseling for middle-aged and older adults: a randomised trial. *Ann Behaviour Med* 1999;1:40–47.

25. Harland J, White M, Drinkwater C, et al. The Newcastle exercise project: a randomised controlled trial of methods to promote physical activity in primary care. *BMJ* 1999;319:828–832.

26. Taylor, A, Doust, J, Webborn, N. Randomised controlled trial to examine the effects of a GP exercise referral programme in Hailsham, East Sussex, on modifiable coronary heart disease risk factors. *J Epidemiol Community Health* 1998;52: 595–601.

27. Bull F, Jamorozik K. Advice on exercise from a family physician can help sedentary patients to become active. *Am J Prev Med* 1998;15:85–94.

28. Chen A, Sallis J, Castro C, et al. A home-based behavioral intervention to promote walking in sedentary ethnic minority women: project WALK. *Womens Health* 1998;4:19–39.

29. Stevens W, Hillsdon M, Thorogood M, McArdle D. Cost-effectiveness of a primary care based physical activity intervention in 45–74 year old men and women; a randomised controlled trial. *Br J Sports Med* 1998;32:236–41.

30. Pereira MA, Kriska AN, Day RD, et al. A randomized walking trial in postmenopausal women. *Arch Intern Med* 1998;158:1695–1701.

31. King A, Sallis JF, Dunn AL, et al. Overview of the activity counselling trial (ACT) intervention for promoting physical activity in primary health care settings. *Med Sci Sports Exerc* 1998;30:1086–1096.

32. Campbell AJ, Robertson MC, Gardner MM, et al. Randomised controlled trial of a general practice programme of home based exercise to prevent falls in elderly women. *BMJ* 1997;315:1065–1069.

33. Brunner E, White I, Thorogood M, et al. Can dietary interventions change diet and cardiovascular risk factors? A meta-analysis of randomised controlled trials. *Am J Public Health* 1997;87:1415–1422. Search date July 1993; primary sources computer and manual searches of databases and journals. No further details given.

34. Tang JL, Armitage JM, Lancaster T, et al. Systematic review of dietary intervention trials to lower blood total cholesterol in free living subjects. *BMJ* 1998;316:1213–1220. Search date 1996; primary sources Medline, Human Nutrition, Embase, and Allied and Alternative Health 1966 to 1995; hand search of Am J Clin Nutr, and reference list checks.

35. Stefanick ML, Mackey S, Sheehan M, et al. Effects of diet and exercise in men and postmenopausal women with low levels of HDL cholesterol and high levels of LDL cholesterol. *N Engl J Med* 1998;339:12–20.

36. Tomson Y, Johannesson M, Aberg H. The costs and effects of two different lipid intervention programmes in primary health care. *J Intern Med* 1995;237:13–17.

37. Hooper L, Summerbell C, Higgins J, et al. Dietary advice, modification or supplementation aimed at lipid lowering for prevention of cardiovascular disease in patients with and without ischaemic heart disease. The Cochrane Library, Issue 2, 2000. Oxford: Update Software. Search date 1999, primary sources Cochrane Library, Medline, Embase, CAB Abstracts, CVRCT registry, related Cochrane groups' trial registers, trials known to experts in the field and biographies.

38. Howell WH, McNamara DJ, Tosca MA, et al. Plasma lipid and lipoprotein responses to dietary fat and cholesterol: a meta-analysis. *Am J Clin Nutr* 1997;65:1747–1764. Search date 1994; primary source Medline 1966 to February 1994, hand search of selected review publications and bibliographies.

39. Ebrahim S, Davey Smith G. Lowering blood

pressure: a systematic review of sustained effects of non-pharmacological interventions. *J Public Health* 1998;2:441–448.

40. Fodor JG, Whitmore B, Leenen F, Larochelle P. Recommendations on dietary salt. *Can Med Assoc J* 1999;160(suppl 9):S29–34.

41. He J, Whelton PK, Appel LJ, et al. Long-term effects of weight loss and dietary sodium reduction on incidence of hypertension. *Hypertension* 2000;35:544–549.

42. Wing R, Epstein LH, Paternostro-Bayles M, et al. Exercise in a behavioural weight control program for obese patients with type 2 (non insulin dependent) diabetes. *Diabetologica* 1988;31: 902–909.

43. Douketis JD, Feightner JW, Attia J, Feldman WF. Periodic health examination, 1999 update. Detection, prevention and treatment of obesity. Canadian Task Force on Preventive Health Care. *Can Med Assoc J* 1999;160:513–525. Search date April 1999; primary sources Medline (1996 to April 1998); Current Contents (1966 to 1999); and hand search of references.

44. The National Heart, Lung, and Blood Institute. Clinical guidelines on the identification, evaluation, and treatment of overweight and obesity in adults. Bethesda Maryland: National Institutes of Health, 1998; website http://www.nhlbi.nih.gov/nhlbi/ guidelns/ob_home.htm

45. Wing RR, Polley BA, Venditti E, et al. Lifestyle intervention in overweight individuals with a family history of diabetes. *Diabetes Care* 1998;21:350– 359.

46. Anderson RE, Wadden TA, Barlett SJ, et al. Effects of lifestyle activity v structured aerobic exercise in obese women. *JAMA* 1999;281:335–340.

47. Jakicic JM, Winters C, Lang W, Wing RR. Effects of intermittent exercise and use of home exercise equipment on adherence, weight loss, and fitness in overweight women. *JAMA* 1999;282:1554– 1560.

48. Sbrocco T, Nedegaard RC, Stone JM, Lewis EL. Behavioural choice treatment promotes continuing weight loss. *J Consult Clin Psychol* 1999;67:260– 266.

49. Harvey-Berino J. Calorie restriction is more effective for obesity treatment than dietary fat restriction. *Ann Behav Med* 1999;21:35–39.

50. Wing RR, Jeffery RW. Benefits of recruiting participants with friends and increasing social support for weight loss and maintenance. *J Consult Clin Psychol* 1999;67:132–138.

51. Jeffery RW, Wing RR, Thorson C, Burton LR. Use of personal trainers and financial incentives to increase exercise in a behavioural weight loss program. *J Consult Clin Psychol* 1998;66:777– 783.

52. Craighead LW, Blum MD. Supervised exercise in behavioural treatment for moderate obesity. *Behav Ther* 1989;20:49–59.

53. Bonato DP, Boland FJ. A comparison of specific strategies for long-term maintenance following a behavioural treatment program for obese women. *Int J Eat Disord* 1986;5:949–958.

54. Hillebrand TH, Wirth A. Evaluation of an outpatient care program for obese patients after an inpatient treatment. *Prav Rehab* 1996;8(2):83–87.

55. Leermakers EA, Perri MG, Shigaki CL, Fuller PR. Effects of exercise-focused versus weight-focused maintenance programs on the management of obesity. *Addict Behav* 1999;24:219–227.

56. Simkin-Silverman LR, Wing RR, Boraz, MA, Meilan EN, Kuller LH. Maintenance of cardiovascular risk factor changes among middle-aged women in a lifestyle intervention trial. *Women's Health: Research on Gender, Behaviour, and Policy* 1998; 4:255–271.

57. Wing RR, Jeffery RW, Hellerstedt WL, Burton LR. Effect of frequent phone contacts and optional food provision on maintenance of weight loss. *Ann Behav Med* 1996;18:172–176.

58. Hardeman W, Griffin S, Johnston M, et al. Interventions to prevent weight gain: a systematic review of psychological models and behaviour change methods. *Int J Obesity* 2000;4:131–143.

59. Forster JL, Jeffery RW, Schmid TL, Kramer FM. Preventing weight gain in adults: a pound of prevention. *Health Psychol* 1988;7:515–525.

60. Jeffery RW, French SA. Preventing weight gain in adults: the pound of prevention study. *Am J Public Health* 1999;89:747–751.

61. Harvey EL, Glenny A, Kirk SFL, Summerbell CD. Improving health professionals' management and the organisation of care for overweight and obese people. In: The Cochrane Library, Issue 1, 2000. Oxford: Update Software. Search date January 1998; primary sources specialised registers of the Cochrane Effective Practice and Organisation of Care Group May 1997; The Cochrane Depression, Anxiety and Neurosis Group August 1997; The Cochrane Diabetes Group August 1997; The Cochrane Controlled Trials Register September 1997; MEDLINE 1966 to January 1998; EMBASE 1988 to December 1997; Cinahl 1982 to November 1997; PsychLit 1974 to December 1997; Sigle 1980 to November 1997; Sociofile 1974 to October 1997; Dissertation Abstracts 1861 to January 1998; Conference Papers Index 1973 to January 1998; Resource Database in Continuing Medical Education and hand searched seven key journals and contacted experts in the field.

62. Ockene IS, Hebert JR, Ockene JK, et al. Effect of physician-delivered nutrition counseling training and an office-support program on saturated fat intake, weight, and serum lipid measurements in a hyperlipidemic population: Worcester area trial for counseling in hyperlipidemia (WATCH). *Arch Intern Med* 1999;159:725–731.

Margaret Thorogood
Reader in Public Health and
Preventative Medicine

Melvyn Hillsdon
Lecturer in Health Promotion

London School of Hygiene and Tropical
Medicine, University of London
London
UK

Carolyn Summerbell
Reader in Human Nutrition
School of Health
University of Teesside
Middlesbrough
UK

Competing interests: None declared.

Cardiovascular disorders

Updated this issue

Robert McKelvie

INTERVENTIONS

Beneficial
ACE inhibitors 38
Digoxin (improves morbidity in
  people already receiving diuretics
  and ACE inhibitors). 41
β Blockers 42
Spironolactone in severe heart
  failure. 44

Likely to be beneficial
Multidisciplinary interventions. . .36
Exercise 37
Angiotensin II receptor blockers .40
Amiodarone 45
Implantable cardiac
  defibrillators 45

Unlikely to be beneficial
Calcium channel blockers 44

Likely to be ineffective or harmful
Positive inotropes (non-digitalis) .41
Non-amiodarone antiarrhythmic
  drugs 45

To be covered in future issues of
  Clinical Evidence
Aspirin
Anticoagulants
Vasodilators
Coronary revascularisation
Atheroma risk factor modification
Management of diastolic
  dysfunction

See glossary, p 48

Key Messages

Non-drug treatments

- We found conflicting evidence for multidisciplinary care. One systematic review of RCTs has found that multidisciplinary approaches to nutrition, patient counselling, and education reduce hospital admissions, may improve quality of life, and enhance patient knowledge. However, the review excluded one large RCT that found that multidisciplinary follow up increased readmission rates.

- RCTs found that prescribed exercise training improved functional capacity and quality of life, and reduced the rate of adverse cardiac events.

Drug and invasive treatments

- One systematic review and recent RCTs have found that angiotensin converting enzyme (ACE) inhibitors reduce mortality, admission to hospital for heart failure, and ischaemic events in people with heart failure. Relative benefits are similar in different groups of people, but absolute benefits are greater in people with severe heart failure.

- RCTs found no evidence of a difference between angiotensin II receptor blockers and ACE inhibitors in their effects on functional capacity and symptoms, but trials were too small to rule out clinically important differences. One

RCT found that angiotensin II receptor blockers were at least as good as ACE inhibitors for reducing clinical events (death or admission to hospital).

- RCTs have found that positive inotropic drugs improve symptoms but do not reduce mortality. Many of the non-digoxin positive inotropic drugs may increase mortality. Only digoxin has been found to improve morbidity in people already receiving diuretics and ACE inhibitors.

- Systematic reviews have found strong evidence that adding a β blocker to ACE inhibitors decreases the rate of death and admission to hospital. The reviews found less robust evidence that β blockers improve exercise capacity and reduce all cause mortality.

- We found no evidence supporting the use of calcium channel blockers in heart failure.

- One RCT found that, in people with severe heart failure, adding an aldosterone receptor antagonist to ACE inhibitor treatment reduced mortality compared with ACE inhibitors alone.

- Systematic reviews found weak evidence suggesting that amiodarone may reduce mortality in people with heart failure.

- Evidence extrapolated from one systematic review in people treated after a myocardial infarction suggests that non-amiodarone antiarrhythmic drugs may increase mortality in people with heart failure.

- RCTs have found good evidence that, in people with asymptomatic left ventricular systolic dysfunction (LVSD), ACE inhibitors delay the onset of symptomatic heart failure and reduce cardiovascular events.

DEFINITION Heart failure occurs when abnormality of cardiac function causes failure of the heart to pump blood at a rate sufficient for metabolic requirements, or maintains cardiac output only with a raised filling pressure. It is characterised clinically by breathlessness, effort intolerance, fluid retention, and poor survival. It can be caused by systolic or diastolic dysfunction and is associated with neurohormonal changes.[1] Left ventricular systolic dysfunction (LVSD) is defined as left ventricular ejection fraction (LVEF) below 0.40. It can be symptomatic or asymptomatic. Defining and diagnosing diastolic heart failure can be difficult. Recently proposed criteria include evidence of: (1) heart failure, (2) normal or mildly abnormal left ventricular systolic function, (3) abnormal left ventricular relaxation, filling, diastolic distensibility, or diastolic stiffness.[2] The clinical usefulness of these criteria is limited by ability to standardise the third criterion. A diagnostic scheme based on the degree of diagnostic certainty has been proposed.[3] A person meeting all three criteria would have definite diastolic heart failure while people meeting only the first and second conditions would have possible diastolic heart failure.

INCIDENCE/ The incidence and prevalence of heart failure increase with age.
PREVALENCE Under 65 years of age the incidence is 1/1000 men per year and 0.4/1000 women per year. Over 65 years, incidence is 11/1000 men per year and 5/1000 women per year. Under 65 years the prevalence of heart failure is 1/1000 men and 1/1000 women; over 65 years the prevalence is 40/1000 men and 30/1000 women.[4] The prevalence of asymptomatic LVSD is 3% in the general population.[5–7] The mean age of people with asymptomatic LVSD is lower than that for symptomatic individuals. Both heart failure and asymptomatic LVSD are more common in men.[5–7]

AETIOLOGY/ RISK FACTORS	Coronary artery disease is the most common cause of heart failure.[4] Other common causes include hypertension and idiopathic dilated congestive cardiomyopathy. After adjustment for hypertension, the presence of left ventricular hypertrophy remains a risk factor for the development of heart failure. Other risk factors include cigarette smoking, hyperlipidaemia, and diabetes mellitus.[5]
PROGNOSIS	The prognosis of heart failure is poor, with 5 year mortality ranging from 26 to 75%.[4] Up to 16% of people are readmitted with heart failure within 6 months of first admission. In the USA it is the leading cause of hospital admission among people over 65 years old.[4] In people with heart failure, a new myocardial infarction increases the risk of death (RR 7.8, 95% CI 6.9 to 8.8); 34% of all deaths in people with heart failure are preceded by a major ischaemic event.[8] Sudden death, mainly caused by ventricular arrhythmias, is responsible for 25–50% of all deaths, and is the most common cause of death in people with heart failure.[9] The presence of asymptomatic LVSD increases an individual's risk of having a cardiovascular event. One large prevention trial found that, for a 5% reduction in ejection fraction, the risk ratio for mortality was 1.20 (95% CI 1.13 to 1.29), for hospital admission for heart failure was 1.28 (95% CI 1.18 to 1.38), and for development of heart failure was 1.20 (95% CI 1.13 to 1.26).[5]
AIMS	To relieve symptoms; to improve quality of life; to reduce morbidity and mortality, with minimum adverse effects.
OUTCOMES	Functional capacity (assessed by the New York Heart Association [NYHA] functional classification or more objectively by using standardised exercise testing or the 6 minute walk test);[10] quality of life (assessed with questionnaires);[11] mortality; adverse effects of treatment. Proxy measures of clinical outcome (e.g. LVEF, hospital readmission rates) are used here only when clinical outcomes are unavailable.
METHODS	*Clinical Evidence* update search and appraisal May 2000 using the medical subject headings of heart failure (congestive), epidemiology, prevalence, incidence, prognosis, and treatment, to identify RCTs and systematic reviews that met *Clinical Evidence* quality criteria.

QUESTION What are the effects of non-drug treatments?

OPTION MULTIDISCIPLINARY INTERVENTIONS

We found conflicting evidence. One systematic review of RCTs has found that multidisciplinary approaches to nutrition, patient counselling, and education reduce hospital admissions, may improve quality of life, and enhance patient knowledge. However, the review excluded a large RCT, which found that multidisciplinary follow up increased readmission rates.

Benefits: We found one systematic review (published in 1999), which identified seven RCTs in 1164 people with heart failure treated for 1–6 months with either a multidisciplinary programme or conventional care alone.[12] The multidisciplinary programme included non-drug treatments such as nutrition advice, counselling, patient education, and exercise training. Six of the RCTs (666 people) were chosen for analysis in the systematic review. The RCTs found that multidisciplinary programmes reduced hospital use, and improved quality of life, functional capacity, patient satisfaction, and compliance with diet and medication compared with conventional care. The four RCTs (543 people) that reported hospital readmissions over 1–6 months found significant reductions with the intervention (AR 89/286 [31%] for intervention, 116/257 [45%] for control; ARR 14%, 95% CI 6% to 21%; RRR 31%, 95% CI 13% to 47%; NNT 7, 95% CI 5 to 17). The seventh RCT was excluded from analysis in the systematic review, but it is not clear how this study differs from those included, apart from its findings. The seventh study included 504 men with heart failure who received conventional follow up or an intensive follow up with their primary care physician and a nurse. This RCT found an increased hospital readmission rate over 6 months in the intervention group compared with controls (AR of readmission 130/249 [52%] for intervention, 106/255 [42%] for control; ARI 11%, 95% CI 2% to 19%; RRI 26%, 95% CI 5% to 46%). Combination of the results of this study with the others found that the intervention had no definite effect compared with control (ARs 219/535 [41%] for intervention, 222/512 [43%] for control; ARR 2.4%, 95% CI –3.6% to +8.2%; RRR 5.6%, 95% CI –8% to +19%).

Harms: We found no reports of harm associated with multidisciplinary management.[12]

Comment: Studies were small, involved highly selected patient populations, and were usually performed in academic centres so results may not generalise to smaller community centres. The systematic review excluded, without *a priori* exclusion criteria, a seventh RCT that found different effects. Interventions varied among studies, and relative merits of each strategy are unknown. Studies generally lasted less than 6 months, and it is not known how well people adhere to treatment over the longer term. Larger studies are needed to define the effects on mortality and morbidity of longer term multidisciplinary interventions.

OPTION   EXERCISE

RCTs have found that prescribed exercise training improves functional capacity and quality of life. One recent RCT has also found that exercise significantly reduces adverse cardiac events.

Benefits: We found one non systematic review, one systematic review and one overview of RCTs from a collaborative group of exercise training in people with heart failure.[13–15] They identified a few small RCTs, which reported only proxy outcomes (maximum exercise time (see glossary, p 48), oxygen uptake, various biochemical measures, and unvalidated symptom scores) in a small number of people over a few weeks. No significant adverse effects were found. One recent RCT published since the reviews included 99 people with heart failure (88 men, 11 women). Fifty people were allocated to 12 months of exercise training and 49 to a control group with no exercise.[16] After 12 months, compared with control, exercise improved quality of life (P < 0.001), fatal or non-fatal cardiac events, mortality, and hospital readmission for heart failure (cardiac events: AR 17/50 [34%] for training, 37/49 [76%] for control; ARR 42%, 95% CI 20% to 58%; RRR 55%, 95% CI 27% to 77%; NNT 2, 95% CI 2 to 5; mortality: AR 9/50 [18%] for training, 20/49 [41%] for control; RRR 56%, 95% CI 13% to 80%; NNT 4, 95% CI 3 to 19; readmission: AR 5/50 [10%] for training, 14/49 [29%] for control; ARR 19%, 95% CI 3% to 25%; RRR 65%, 95% CI 12% to 88%; NNT 5, 95% CI 4 to 30).[16]

Harms: The two systematic reviews and the collaborative overview reported no important adverse effects associated with prescribed exercise training.[13–15]

Comment: The studies were small, involved highly selected patient populations, and were performed in well resourced academic centres. The results may not generalise to smaller community centres. The specific form of exercise training varied among studies and the relative merits of each strategy are unknown. The studies generally lasted less than 1 year and long term effects are unknown. Larger studies over a longer period are needed.

QUESTION What are the effects of drug treatments in heart failure?

OPTION ANGIOTENSIN CONVERTING ENZYME (ACE) INHIBITORS

One systematic review and recent RCTs have found that, in symptomatic patients with a low ejection fraction, ACE inhibitors significantly reduce mortality, hospital admissions for heart failure, and ischaemic events. Benefits are found in different types of people with heart failure.

Benefits: We found one systematic review of ACE inhibitors versus placebo in heart failure (published 1995, 32 RCTs, outcome measures included total mortality assessed by intention to treat, 7105 people).[17] Trial duration varied from 3 to 42 months. Entry criteria were usually equivalent to a NYHA functional class (see glossary, p 48) II or worse. The review found that ACE inhibitors reduced mortality compared with placebo (OR 0.77, 95% CI 0.67 to 0.88; pooled data AR for death 611/3870 [16%] for ACE inhibitor group, 709/3235 [22%] for placebo group; ARR 6%, 95% CI 4% to 8%; NNT 16, 95% CI 13 to 22). Relative reductions in mortality were similar in different subgroups (stratified by age, sex, cause of heart failure, and NYHA class). Relative reduction was greater for progressive heart failure (OR 0.69, 95% CI 0.58 to 0.83) rather than sudden or presumed arrhythmic death (OR 0.91, 95% CI 0.73 to 1.12) or fatal myocardial infarction (OR 0.82, 95% CI 0.60 to 1.11). ACE inhibitors also reduced the composite outcome of total death or hospital admission for heart failure (OR 0.65, 95% CI 0.57 to 0.74; for pooled data, ARs 854/3810 [22%] for ACE inhibitor group, 1036/3178 [33%] for placebo group; ARR 10%, 95% CI 8% to 12%; NNT 10, 95% CI 8 to 12). Relative reduction of mortality or hospital admission was greater at follow up at 90 days or less (reported by 30 trials, OR 0.53, 95% CI 0.44 to 0.63) than at follow up of more than 90 days (reported by 10 trials, OR 0.76, 95% CI

0.66 to 0.88). One subsequent non-systematic review identified two further RCTs.[9] The first trial randomised people after myocardial infarction with clinically apparent heart failure (but no measurement of systolic function) to ACE inhibitor or placebo. It found that ACE inhibitors reduced mortality (170/1014 [17%] deaths with ACE inhibitor, 222/992 [22%] with placebo; ARR 6%, 95% CI 2% to 9%; RRR 25%, 95% CI 10% to 41%; NNT 18, 95% CI 12 to 44).[9] The second trial, comparing an ACE inhibitor (trandolapril) versus placebo for 24–50 months in 1749 people with clinical heart failure after myocardial infarction, found that trandolapril reduced mortality (AR 304/876 [35%] on ACE inhibitor, 369/873 [42%] on placebo; ARR 8%, 95% CI 3% to 12%; RRR 22%, 95% CI 9% to 33%; NNT 13, 95% CI 8 to 33) and decreased the proportion of people who developed worse heart failure (14% v 20%; RRR 29%, 95% CI 10% to 42%; NNT 19, 95% CI 12 to 51). Individual trials that studied high risk groups found that ACE inhibitors significantly reduced some ischaemic event rates. One RCT in people with left ventricular dysfunction found that, compared with placebo, ACE inhibitors reduced myocardial infarction (combined fatal or non-fatal myocardial infarction: AR 9.9% v 12.3%; RRR 23%, 95% CI 2% to 39%), hospital admission for angina (AR 15% v 19%; RRR 27%, 95% CI 12% to 40%), and the combined end point of cardiac death, non-fatal myocardial infarction, or hospital admission for angina (AR 43% v 51%; RRR 23%, 95% CI 14% to 32%).[8] Effects on hospital readmissions were observed shortly after starting ACE inhibitor treatment, although effects on ischaemic events were not apparent for at least 6 months and peaked at 36 months. **Dosage:** We found one recent large RCT that compared low dose lisinopril (2.5 mg or 5.0 mg daily) versus high dose lisinopril (32.5 mg or 35 mg daily) in 3164 people with NYHA class II-IV heart failure.[18] It found no significant difference in overall mortality but found that high dose lisinopril reduced the combined outcome of death or hospital admission for any reason, and reduced admissions for heart failure (overall mortality: 717/1596 [44.9%] with low dose v 666/1568 [42.5%] with high dose, hazard ratio 0.92, 95% CI 0.80 to 1.03; risk of death or hospital admission for any reason, 1338 events with low dose [AR 83.8%] v 1250 events with high dose [AR 79.7%], hazard ratio 0.88, 95% CI 0.82 to 0.96; hospital admissions for heart failure: 1576 admissions with low dose v 1199 admissions with high dose, ARR 24%, no 95% CI given, P = 0.002). **Comparison of different ACE inhibitors:** The systematic review found similar benefits with different ACE inhibitors.[17]

Harms: We found no systematic review. The main adverse effects documented in large trials were cough, hypotension, hyperkalaemia, and renal dysfunction. Compared with placebo, ACE inhibitors increased the incidence of cough (37% v 31%; ARI 7%, 95% CI 3% to 11%; RRI 23%, 95% CI 11% to 35%; NNH 14, 95% CI 9 to 31), dizziness or fainting (57% v 50%; ARI 7%, 95% CI 3% to 11%; RRI 14%, 95% CI 6% to 21%; NNH 14, 95% CI 9 to 32), increased creatinine concentrations above 177 µmol/l (10.7% v 7.7%; ARI 3%, 95% CI 0.6% to 6%; RRI 38%, 95% CI 9% to 67%; NNH 34, 95% CI 17 to 158), and increased potassium concentrations above 5.5 mmol/l (ARs 6.4% v 2.5%; ARI 4%, 95% CI 2% to 7%; RRI 156%, 95% CI 92% to 220%; NNH 26, 95% CI 15 to 55).[19] Angioedema was not found to be more common with ACE inhibitors than placebo (3.8% taking enalapril v 4.1% taking placebo; ARI 0.3%, 95% CI −1.4% to +1.5%).[19] The trial comparing low and high doses of lisinopril found that most adverse effects were more common with high dose (no P value reported; dizziness: 12% with low dose v 19% with high dose; hypotension: 7% with low dose v 11% with high dose; worsening renal function: 7% with low dose v 10% with high dose; significant change in serum potassium concentration 7% with low dose v 7% with high dose), although there was no difference in withdrawal rates between groups (17% discontinued with high dose v 18% with low dose). The trial found that cough was less commonly experienced with high dose compared with low dose lisinopril (cough: 13% with low dose v 11% with high dose).

Comment: The relative beneficial effects of ACE inhibitors were similar in different subgroups of people with heart failure. Most RCTs evaluated left ventricular function by assessing LVEF, but some studies defined heart failure clinically, without measurement of left ventricular function in people at high risk of developing heart failure (soon after myocardial infarction).

| OPTION | ANGIOTENSIN II RECEPTOR BLOCKERS |

One RCT found that angiotensin II receptor antagonists improved symptoms compared with placebo. RCTs have found no evidence that angiotensin II receptor blockers alter functional capacity or symptoms compared with ACE inhibitors, but the trials were too small to rule out clinically important differences. We found moderate evidence from one RCT that angiotensin II receptor blockers are as effective as ACE inhibitors in reducing all cause mortality.

Benefits: We found no systematic review. **Versus placebo:** We found one meta-analysis of a non-systematic review [20] and one additional RCT.[21] The review included three RCTs (890 people) all of 12 weeks duration comparing losartan with placebo in people with heart failure NYHA class II and III. It found a significant reduction in mortality with losartan (AR 11/616 [1.8%] losartan v 13/274 [4.7%] placebo; OR 0.34, 95% CI 0.14 to 0.80). The additional RCT (844 people) compared 12 weeks of candesartan cilexetil (4 mg daily, n = 208 v 8 mg daily, n = 212 v 16 mg daily, n = 213) versus placebo (n = 211) on exercise capacity and symptoms in people with heart failure NYHA class II and III.[21] It found that candesartan cilexetil 16 mg daily improved exercise time in a standardised symptom limited bicycle ergonometry exercise compared with placebo (47.2 v 30.8 seconds, P = 0.046). All doses of candesartan cilexetil significantly improved the Dyspnoea Fatigue Index score (see glossary, p 48) compared with placebo (P < 0.001). **Versus ACE inhibitors:** We found one systematic review (3 RCTs, 1004 people).[20] Two of the RCTs compared losartan with enalapril (116 people with NYHA class II and III, 8 weeks' duration; 166 people with NYHA class III and IV, 12 weeks' duration). The third RCT compared losartan with captopril (722 people with NYHA Grade II and III, 48 weeks' duration). When the results of these trials were combined, there was no significant reduction in mortality when losartan was compared with ACE inhibitors (AR 25/538 [4.6%] with losartan v 34/466 [7.3%] with ACE inhibitors; OR 0.60, 95% CI 0.34 to 1.04).

Harms: We found no systematic review. The RCT comparing different doses of candesartan cilexetil with placebo found no evidence of a difference among groups for serious adverse events (placebo 4.7%; 4 mg 1.4%; 8 mg 5.7%; 16 mg 5.6%) or withdrawal because of adverse events (placebo 4.3%; 4 mg 1.9%; 8 mg 4.7%; 16 mg: 5.6%).[21]

Comment: None of the trials of an angiotensin II receptor blocker compared with an ACE inhibitor was designed with mortality as the primary end point. A further trial is in progress comparing losartan with captopril. In people who are truly intolerant of an ACE inhibitor the evidence supports the use of an angiotensin II receptor blocker with the expectation, at the very least, of symptomatic improvement of the heart failure. Pilot studies have examined the efficacy, tolerability, and safety of combining angiotensin II receptor blockers and ACE inhibitors in people with symptomatic heart failure.[22,23] Larger studies are in progress.

OPTION **POSITIVE INOTROPIC AGENTS**

We found no evidence that positive inotropic drugs other than digoxin reduce mortality and morbidity in people with heart failure, and most RCTs found that they increased mortality. One well designed RCT found that digoxin decreased the rate of hospital admissions for worsening heart failure in people already receiving diuretics and ACE inhibitors, although it found no evidence of an effect on mortality.

Benefits: **Digoxin:** We found one systematic review, which included 13 RCTs of digoxin versus placebo over 3–24 weeks in 1138 people with heart failure and sinus rhythm,[24] and one recent large RCT.[25] The systematic review found that six of the 13 RCTs enrolled people without assessment of ventricular function and may have included some people with mild or no heart failure. Other limitations of the older trials included crossover designs and small sample sizes. The systematic review found symptomatic improvement in people who were in sinus rhythm, with heart failure, but did not find a definite effect on mortality (clinical worsening of heart failure in 52/628 [8.3%] with digoxin v 131/631 [20.8%] with placebo; ARR 12.5%, 95% CI 9.5% to 14.7%; RRR 60%, 95% CI 46% to 71%; mortality 16/628 [2.5%] with digoxin v 15/631 [2.4%] with placebo; ARR −0.2%, 95% CI −2.6% to +1.1%; RRR −7%, 95% CI −113% to +47%). The subsequent large RCT randomised 6800 people (88% men, mean age 64 years, NYHA class I-III, 94% already taking ACE inhibitors, 82% taking diuretics) to blinded additional treatment with either digoxin or placebo for a mean of 37 months.[25] Digoxin did not reduce all cause mortality compared with placebo (AR 1181/3397 [34.8%] with digoxin v 1194/3403 [35.1%] with placebo; ARR 0.3%, 95% CI −2.0% to +2.6%; RRR 0.9%, 95% CI −6% to +7%). The number of people admitted to hospital for worsening heart failure was substantially reduced in the digoxin group as was the combined outcome of death or hospital admission caused by worsening heart failure (admission for heart failure: AR 910/3397 [27%] for digoxin, 1180/3403 [35%] for placebo; ARR 8%, 95% CI 6% to 10%; RRR 23%, 95% CI 17% to 28%; NNT over 37 months to avoid one hospital admission for heart failure 13 people, 95% CI 10 to 17; admission or death due to heart failure: AR 1041/3397 [31%] for digoxin, 1291/3403 [38%] for placebo; ARR 7.3%, 95% CI 5.1% to 9.4%; RRR 19%, 95% CI 13% to 25%; NNT 14, 95% CI 11 to 20). **Other inotropic agents:** Non-digitalis inotropic agents have been evaluated in RCTs including up to 3600 people. Some of these studies found improved functional capacity and quality of life but not consistently across all studies. We found no evidence that positive inotropic agents decrease mortality; most RCTs found increased risk of death (see harms below).

Harms: We found no systematic review. **Digoxin:** The RCT in 6800 people found that more participants had suspected digoxin toxicity in the digoxin group versus placebo (11.9% v 7.9%; ARI 4%, 95% CI 2.4% to 5.8%; RRI 50%, 95% CI 30% to 73%; NNH 25, 95% CI 17 to 42).[25] The trial found no evidence that digoxin increased the risk of ventricular fibrillation or tachycardia compared with placebo (AR 37/3397 [1.1%] with digoxin, 27/3403 [0.8%] with placebo; ARI 0.3%, 95% CI −0.1% to +1.0%; RRI 37%, 95% CI −16% to +124%). Rates of supraventricular arrhythmia and second or third degree atrioventricular block were higher with digoxin than placebo (supraventricular arrhythmia: AR 2.5% with digoxin, 1.2% with placebo; ARI 1.3%, 95% CI 0.5% to 2.4%; RRI 108%, 95% CI 44% to 199%, NNH 77, 95% CI 42 to 190; second or third degree atrioventricular block: AR 1.2% v 0.4%; ARI 0.8%, 95% CI 0.2% to 1.8%; RRI 193%, 95% CI 61% to 434%; NNH 126, 95% CI 56 to 402). **Other inotropic agents:** RCTs have found that non-digitalis positive inotropic agents increase mortality compared with placebo.[9] One RCT assessed mortality over 6 months in 1088 people with heart failure treated with milrinone or placebo and found an increase in all cause mortality for people taking milrinone (ARs 168/561 [30%] for milrinone, 127/527 [24%] for placebo; ARI 6%, 95% CI 0.5% to 12%; RRI 24%, 95% CI 2% to 49%; NNH 17, 95% CI 8 to 193).[26] Another RCT of 3833 people with heart failure found an increase in mortality for those taking 60 mg vesnarinone per day versus placebo for 9 months (ARs 292/1275 [23%] for 60 mg vesnarinone, 242/1280 [19%] for placebo; ARI 4%, 95% CI 1% to 8%; RRI 21%, 95% CI 4% to 40%; NNH 25, 95% CI 13 to 126).[9]

Comment: None.

OPTION   β BLOCKERS

We found strong evidence from systematic reviews of RCTs that adding β blockers to standard treatment with ACE inhibitors in people with moderate heart failure reduces the rate of death or hospital admission. The reviews found less robust evidence that β blockers improve exercise capacity.

Benefits: We found six systematic reviews and two recent large RCTs [27,28] of the effects of β blockers in heart failure. One systematic review (published in 1998, 18 RCTs of β blockers versus placebo, 1.5–44 months, 3023 people with heart failure) obtained details of outcomes directly from trial investigators.[29] The participants had idiopathic dilated cardiomyopathy (n = 1718) or ischaemic heart disease (n = 1513). Trials in people after AMI were excluded. Most participants had NYHA class II or III symptoms. The systematic review found strong evidence that β blockers reduced the combined outcome of death or admission to hospital (AR 239/1486 [16%] on β blockers, 293/1155 [25%] on placebo; ARR 9%, 95% CI 7% to 12%; RRR 37%, 95% CI 26% to 46%; NNT 11, 95% CI 9 to 15). The result was robust to the addition of neutral results from further trials. The review also found that addition of β blockers reduced total mortality compared with placebo (AR 130/1718 [8%] for β blockers, 156/1305 [12%] for placebo; ARR 4%, 95% CI 2% to 6%; RRR 37%, 95% CI 21% to 50%; NNT 23, 95% CI 17 to 40) and improved NYHA class. These results were less robust (the conclusion could be altered by addition or removal of only one moderate sized study). The two recent RCTs found stronger evidence of reduced mortality from the additional use of β blockers compared with placebo in heart failure. The first randomised 2647 people with heart failure (NYHA class III-IV) to additional bisoprolol or placebo.[27] The trial was stopped early because the bisoprolol group showed significant reduction in all cause mortality and sudden deaths (all cause mortality: AR after 1.3 years 156/1327 [11.8%] for bisoprolol, 228/1320 [17.3%] for placebo; ARR 5.5%, 95% CI 3.0% to 7.6%; RRR 32%, 95% CI 18% to 44%; NNT 18, 95% CI 13 to 33; sudden death: AR 48/1327 [3.6%] for bisoprolol, 83/1320 [6.3%] for placebo; ARR 2.7%, 95% CI 1.2% to 3.7%; RRR 42%, 95% CI 19% to 60%; NNT 37, 95% CI 27 to 86). The other trial randomised 3991 people with heart failure (NYHA class II-IV) to additional controlled release metoprolol or placebo.[28] It was stopped early because the metoprolol group showed significant reduction in all cause mortality, sudden death, and death due to worsening heart failure (all cause mortality: AR after 1 year 145/1990 [7.3%] for metoprolol, 217/2001 [10.8%] for placebo; ARR 3.6%, 95% CI 1.9% to 4.9%; RRR 33%, 95% CI 18% to 45%; NNT 28, 95% CI 20 to 52; sudden death: AR 79/1990 [4.0%] for metoprolol, 132/2001 [6.6%] for placebo; ARR 2.6%, 95% CI 1.4% to 3.6%; RRR 40%, 95% CI 21% to 54%; NNT 38, 95% CI 28 to 72; deaths from worsening heart failure: ARs 30/1990 [1.5%] for metoprolol, 58/2001 [2.9%] for placebo; ARR 1.4%, 95% CI 0.6% to 1.9%; RRR 48%, 95% CI 20% to 67%; NNT 72, 95% CI 52 to 177).

Harms: Fears that β blockers may cause excessive problems with worsening heart failure, bradyarrhythmias, or hypotension have not been confirmed. In one trial the overall drug discontinuation rate for adverse reactions was 7.8% in the placebo group and 5.7% in the carvedilol group.[29] The findings from the trial of metoprolol were similar, with the study drug discontinued in 13.9% of the controlled release metoprolol group and in 15.3% of the placebo group (RR 0.91, 95% CI 0.78 to 1.06).[27]

Comment: Good evidence was found for the use of β blockers in people with moderate symptoms (NYHA class II-III) receiving standard treatment including ACE inhibitors. The value of β blockers needs clarification in NYHA class IV, in heart failure with preserved ejection fraction, in asymptomatic LVSD, and in heart failure after AMI.

OPTION CALCIUM CHANNEL BLOCKERS

We found no evidence that calcium channel blockers are of benefit in people with heart failure.

Benefits: **After myocardial infarction:** See calcium channel blockers under acute myocardial infarction, p 1. **Other heart failure:** We found one non-systematic review of three RCTs in 1790 people with heart failure.[9] One RCT compared amlodipine versus placebo over 14 months in 1153 people with heart failure (NYHA class III-IV, LVEF < 0.30) already treated with diuretics, digoxin, and ACE inhibitors.[30] No significant difference in the primary combined end point of all cause mortality and hospital admission for cardiovascular events was found (AR 222/571 [39%] for amlodipine, 246/582 [42%] for placebo; ARR 3.4%, 95% CI −2.3% to +8.8%; RRR 8%, 95% CI −6% to +21%). Subgroup analysis of people with primary cardiomyopathy found a reduction in combined mortality and hospital admission, and all cause mortality alone (admission or death: AR 58/209 [28%] for amlodipine, 78/212 [37%] for placebo; ARR 9.0%, 95% CI 0.1% to 37%; RRR 25%, 95% CI 0.2% to 45%; NNT 11, 95% CI 6 to 1107; all cause mortality AR 45/209 [22%] for amlodipine, 74/212 [35%] for placebo; ARR 13%, 95% CI 5% to 20%; RRR 38%, 95% CI 15% to 57%; NNT 7, 95% CI 5 to 19). There was no significant difference in the subgroup with heart failure caused by coronary artery disease. One recent RCT compared diltiazem versus placebo in 186 people with idiopathic dilated cardiomyopathy (NYHA class I-III).[9] It found no evidence of a difference in survival between the two groups in those who did not have a heart transplant, although people on diltiazem had improved cardiac function, exercise capacity, and subjective quality of life. A third RCT compared felodipine versus placebo in 451 people with mild heart failure (NYHA class II-III).[9] No significant adverse or beneficial effect was found.

Harms: Calcium channel blockers have been found to exacerbate symptoms of heart failure or increase mortality in people with pulmonary congestion after myocardial infarct or ejection fraction less than 0.40 (see calcium channel blockers under acute myocardial infarction, p 1).[9]

Comment: Many of the RCTs were underpowered and had wide confidence intervals. An RCT is in progress to test the hypothesis that amlodipine decreases mortality in people with primary dilated cardiomyopathy.

OPTION ALDOSTERONE RECEPTOR ANTAGONISTS

One recent large RCT of people with severe heart failure (on usual treatment including ACE inhibitor) has found that adding an aldosterone receptor antagonist (spironolactone) further decreases mortality.

Benefits: We found no systematic review. We found one RCT of spironolactone (25 mg daily) versus placebo in 1663 people with heart failure (NYHA class III-IV, LVEF < 0.35, all taking ACE inhibitors and loop diuretics and most taking digoxin).[31] The trial was stopped early because of a significant reduction in the primary end point of all cause mortality for spironolactone versus placebo after 2 years (mortality AR 284/822 [35%] for spironolactone, 386/841 [46%] for placebo; ARR 11%, 95% CI 7% to 16%; RRR 25%, 95% CI 15% to 34%; NNT 9, 95% CI 6 to 15).

Harms: The trial found no evidence that spironolactone in combination with an ACE inhibitor may result in an increased incidence of clinically significant hyperkalaemia. Gynaecomastia or breast pain was reported in 10% of men given spironolactone and 1% of men given placebo.[31]

Comment: The RCT was large and well designed. As only NYHA functional class III-IV patients were randomised into the study, these data cannot necessarily be generalised to people with milder heart failure.

| OPTION | ANTIARRHYTHMIC TREATMENT |

Systematic reviews have found weak evidence that amiodarone reduces total mortality in people with heart failure. One systematic review of RCTs has found good evidence that the implantable cardiac defibrillator (ICD) reduces mortality in people with heart failure who have experienced a cardiac arrest. The review found conflicting evidence for prophylactic implantation of ICDs in people at risk of arrhythmia. Other antiarrhythmic agents may increase mortality in people with heart failure.

Benefits: **Amiodarone:** We found two systematic reviews of the effects of amiodarone versus placebo in heart failure.[32,33] The most recent identified 10 RCTs in 4766 people with a wide range of conditions including symptomatic and asymptomatic heart failure, ventricular arrhythmia, recent myocardial infarction, and recent cardiac arrest.[32] Eight of these studies reported the number of deaths. The review found that treatment with amiodarone over 3–24 months reduced the risk of death from any cause compared with placebo or conventional treatment (AR 436/2262 [19%] for amiodarone, 507/2263 [22%] for control; ARR 3%, 95% CI 0.8% to 5.3%; RRR 14%, 95% CI 4% to 24%; NNT 32, 95% CI 19 to 126). This review did not perform any subgroup analyses to reveal the effect of amiodarone on people with heart failure. The earlier systematic review found eight RCTs of prophylactic amiodarone versus placebo or usual care in 5101 people after myocardial infarction and five RCTs in 1452 people with heart failure.[33] Mean follow up was 16 months. Analysis of data from all 13 RCTs found a lower total mortality with amiodarone than control (10.9% v 12.3% dead per year). The effect was significant with some methods of calculation (fixed effects model: OR 0.87, 95% CI 0.78 to 0.99) but not with others (random effects model: OR 0.85, 95% CI 0.71 to 1.02). The effect of amiodarone was significantly greater in RCTs that compared amiodarone versus usual care than in placebo controlled RCTs. Deaths classified as arrhythmic death or sudden death were significantly reduced by amiodarone compared with placebo (OR 0.71, 95% CI 0.59 to 0.85). Subgroup analysis found a significant effect of amiodarone in the five heart failure RCTs (19.9% deaths per year v 24.3% in the placebo group; OR 0.83, 95% CI 0.70 to 0.99). **Implantable cardiac defibrillators:** We found three RCTs examining the effects of ICDs in people with left ventricular dysfunction. The first trial randomised 1016 people to an ICD or antiarrhythmic drug treatment (mainly amiodarone).[34] People included in this study had been resuscitated from ventricular fibrillation or been cardioverted from sustained ventricular tachycardia; they also had either syncope or other serious cardiac symptoms, along with a LVEF of ≤0.40. ICDs improved survival at 1, 2, and 3 years compared with antiarrhythmic treatment (ICD v antiarrhythmic; 1 year survival: 89.3% v 82.3%; 2 year survival 81.6% v 73.7%; 3 year survival 75.4% v 64.1%). The second trial included 196 people with NYHA class I-III heart failure and previous myocardial infarction, a LVEF ≤0.35, a documented episode of asymptomatic unsustained ventricular tachycardia and inducible non-suppressible ventricular tachyarrhythmia on electrophysiologic study.[35] Ninety five people received an implantable defibrillator and 101 received conventional medical treatment. The trial found that ICDs reduced mortality compared with conventional treatment over a mean follow up of 27 months (15 deaths in ICD group [11 from cardiac cause] and 39 deaths in the conventional therapy group [27 from cardiac cause], HR for overall mortality 0.46, 95% CI 0.26 to 0.82). The third trial included 1055 people aged less than 80 years who were scheduled for coronary artery bypass surgery, had a left ventricular ejection less than 0.36, and had electrocardiographic abnormalities. They were randomised to ICD (900 people) at the time of bypass surgery or to no ICD (454 people).[36] The trial found no significant difference in all cause mortality between the two groups over a mean follow up of 32 months (101 deaths [71 from cardiac causes] in ICD group v 95 deaths [72 from cardiac causes] in control group, HR 1.07, 95% CI 0.81 to 1.42). **Other antiarrhythmics:** Apart from β blockers, other antiarrhythmic drugs seem to increase mortality in people at high risk (see antiarrhythmics under secondary prevention of ischaemic cardiac events, p 83).

Harms: **Amiodarone:** Amiodarone was not found to increase the non-arrhythmic death rate (OR 1.02, 95% CI 0.87 to 1.19).[33] In placebo controlled RCTs, after 2 years 41% of people in the amiodarone group and 27% in the placebo group had permanently discontinued study medication.[33] In 10 RCTs of amiodarone versus placebo, amiodarone increased the odds of reporting adverse drug reactions compared with placebo (OR 2.22, 95% CI 1.83 to 2.68). Nausea was the most common adverse effect. Hypothyroidism was the most common serious adverse effect (7.0% of amiodarone treated group versus 1.1% of controls). Hyperthyroidism (1.4% v 0.5%), peripheral neuropathy (0.5% v 0.2%), lung infiltrates (1.6% v 0.5%), bradycardia (2.4% v 0.8%), and liver dysfunction (1.0% v 0.4%) were all more common in the amiodarone group.[33] **Implantable cardiac defibrillators:** RCTs found that the main adverse effects of ICDs were infection (about 5%), pneumothorax (about 2%), bleeding requiring further operation (about 1%), serious haematomas (about 3%), cardiac perforation (about 0.2%), problems with defibrillator lead (about 7%), and malfunction of defibrillator generator (about 3%).[34-36] **Other antiarrhythmics:** These agents (particularly class I antiarrhythmics) may increase mortality (see antiarrhythmics under secondary prevention of ischaemic cardiac events, p 83).

Comment: **Amiodarone:** RCTs of amiodarone against usual treatment found larger effects than placebo controlled trials.[33] These findings suggest bias; unblinded follow up may be associated with reduced usual care or improved adherence with amiodarone. Further studies are required to assess the effects of amiodarone treatment on mortality and morbidity in people with heart failure. **Implantable cardiac defibrillators:** The RCTs were all in people with previous ventricular arrhythmias. It is uncertain whether asymptomatic ventricular arrhythmia is in itself a predictor of sudden death in people with moderate or severe heart failure.[37] The role of ICDs in other groups of people with heart failure awaits evaluation. Several RCTs of prophylactic ICD treatment are ongoing in people with heart failure and in survivors of acute myocardial infarction.[38]

QUESTION	What are the effects of ACE inhibitors in people at high risk of heart failure?

RCTs have found good evidence that ACE inhibitors can delay development of symptomatic heart failure and reduce the frequency of cardiovascular events in people with asymptomatic LVSD, and in people with other cardiovascular risk factors for heart failure.

Benefits: **In people with asymptomatic LVSD:** We found no systematic review but found two RCTs.[39,40] One large RCT examined ACE inhibitors versus placebo over 40 months in people with asymptomatic LVSD (LVEF < 0.35).[39] It found no evidence that ACE inhibitors significantly decreased total mortality and cardiovascular mortality compared with placebo (all cause mortality: AR 313/2111 [14.8%] for ACE inhibitor v 334/2117 [15.8%] for placebo; ARR 0.9%, 95% CI −1.3% to +2.9%; RRR 6%, 95% CI −8% to +19%; cardiovascular mortality: AR 265/2111 [12.6%] for ACE inhibitor v 298/2117 [14.1%] for placebo; ARR 1.5%, 95% CI −0.6% to +3.3%; RRR 11%, 95% CI −4% to +24%). During the study, more people assigned to the placebo than to the enalapril group received digoxin, diuretics, or ACE inhibitor that were not part of the study protocol, which may have contributed to the lack of significant difference in mortality between the two groups. Compared with placebo, ACE inhibitors reduced symptomatic heart failure, reduced hospital admission for heart failure, and reduced fatal or non-fatal myocardial infarction (symptomatic heart failure: AR 438/2111 [21%] for ACE inhibitor v 640/2117 [30%] for placebo; ARR 9.5%, 95% CI 7% to 12%; RRR 31%, 95% CI 23% to 39%; NNT 11, 95% CI 9 to 14; admission for heart failure: AR 306/2111 [15%] for ACE inhibitor v 454/2117 [21%] for placebo; ARR 7%, 95% CI 5% to 9%; RRR 32%, 95% CI 23% to 41%; NNT 14, 95% CI 11 to 21; fatal or non-fatal myocardial infarction: AR 7.6% for ACE inhibitor, 9.6% for placebo; ARR 2%, 95% CI 0.4% to 3.4%; RRR 21%, 95% CI 4% to 35%).[8,39] A second trial in asymptomatic people after myocardial infarction with documented LVSD found that ACE inhibitors (captopril) reduced mortality and reduced risk of ischaemic events compared with placebo.[40] **In people with other risk factors:** We found one large RCT that compared ramipril 10 mg daily versus placebo in 9297 high risk people (people with vascular disease or diabetes plus one other cardiovascular risk factor) who were not known to have LVSD or heart failure, for a mean of 5 years.[41] It found that ramipril reduced the risk of heart failure (AR for heart failure 9.0% with ramipril v 11.5% with placebo; RR 0.77, 95% CI 0.67 to 0.87; P < 0.001). Ramipril also reduced the combined risk of myocardial infarction or stroke or cardiovascular death, reduced the risk of these outcomes separately, and reduced all cause mortality (see ACE inhibitors in people at high risk, p 83). During the trial, 496 people underwent echocardiography; 2.6% of these people were found to have ejection fraction less than 0.40. Retrospective review of records found that left ventricular function had been documented in 5193 people; 8.1% had a reduced ejection fraction.

Harms: We found no systematic review. The first RCT over 40 months found that a high proportion of people in both groups reported adverse effects (76% in the enalapril group versus 72% in the placebo group).[39] Dizziness or fainting (46% v 33%) and cough (34% v 27%) were reported more often in the enalapril group (no P value reported). The incidence of angioedema was the same (1.4%) in both groups. Study medication was permanently discontinued by 8% of the participants in the enalapril group versus 5% in the placebo group (no P value reported).

Comment: Asymptomatic LVSD is prognostically important, but we found no prospective studies that have assessed the usefulness of screening to detect its presence.

GLOSSARY

Dyspnoea Fatigue Index Measures impact of breathlessness on ability to carry out activities of daily living, with a scale from 0 to 12.

Exercise time This is the total time in seconds that a person is able to pedal in a standardised symptom limited bicycle ergonometry exercise test.

NYHA class Classification of severity by symptoms. Class I: No limitation of physical activity; ordinary physical activity does not cause undue fatigue or dyspnoea. Class II: Slight limitation of physical activity; comfortable at rest, but ordinary physical activity results in fatigue or dyspnoea. Class III: Limitation of physical activity; comfortable at rest, but less than ordinary activity causes fatigue or dyspnoea. Class IV: Unable to carry on any physical activity without symptoms; symptoms are present even at rest; if any physical activity is undertaken, symptoms are increased.

Substantive changes since last issue

Angiotensin II receptor blockers One new systematic review;[20] no change in conclusions.

REFERENCES

1. Poole-Wilson PA. History, definition, and classification of heart failure. In: Poole-Wilson PA, Colucci WS, Massie BM, Chatterjee K, Coats AJS, eds. *Heart failure. Scientific principles and clinical practice*. London: Churchill Livingston, 1997:269–277.

2. Working Group Report. How to diagnose diastolic hear failure: European Study Group on Diastolic Heart Failure. *Eur Heart J* 1998;19:990–1003.

3. Vason RS, Levy D. Defining diastolic heart failure: a call for standardized diagnostic criteria. *Circulation* 2000;101:2118–2121.

4. Cowie MR, Mosterd A, Wood DA, et al. The epidemiology of heart failure. *Eur Heart J* 1997; 18:208–225.

5. McKelvie RS, Benedict CR, Yusuf S. Prevention of

congestive heart failure and management of asymptomatic left ventricular dysfunction. *BMJ* 1999;318:1400–1402.

6. Bröckel U, Hense HW, Museholl M, et al. Prevalence of left ventricular dysfunction in the general population [abstract]. *J Am Coll Cardiol* 1996;27(suppl A):25.

7. Mosterd A, deBruijne MC, Hoes A, et al. Usefulness of echocardiography in detecting left ventricular dysfunction in population-based studies (the Rotterdam study). *Am J Cardiol* 1997;79; 103–104.

8. Yusuf S, Pepine CJ, Garces C, et al. Effect of enalapril on myocardial infarction and unstable angina in patients with low ejection fractions. *Lancet* 1992;340:1173–1178.

9. Gheorghiade M, Benatar D, Konstam MA, et al. Pharmacotherapy for systolic dysfunction: a review of randomized clinical trials. *Am J Cardiol* 1997; 80(suppl 8B):14–27H.

10. Bittner V, Weiner DH, Yusuf S, et al, for the SOLVD Investigators. Prediction of mortality and morbidity with a 6-minute walk test in patients with left ventricular dysfunction. *JAMA* 1993;270:1702–1707.

11. Rogers WJ, Johnstone DE, Yusuf S, et al, for the SOLVD Investigators. Quality of life among 5 025 patients with left ventricular dysfunction randomized between placebo and enalapril. The studies of left ventricular dysfunction. *J Am Coll Cardiol* 1994;23:393–400.

12. Rich MW. Heart failure disease management: a critical review. *J Card Fail* 1999;5:64–75. Search dates 1983 to 1998; primary sources Medline; references in published articles.

13. Miller TD, Balady GJ, Fletcher GF. Exercise and its role in the prevention and rehabilitation of cardiovascular disease. *Ann Behav Med* 1997;19: 220–229.

14. Dracup K, Baker DW, Dunbar SB, et al. Management of heart failure. II. Counseling, education and lifestyle modifications. *JAMA* 1994; 272:1442–1446. Search date 1993; primary sources Medline; Embase.

15. European Heart Failure Training Group. Experience from controlled trials of physical training in chronic heart failure. Protocol and patient factors in effectiveness in the improvement in exercise tolerance. *Eur Heart J* 1998;19:466–475.

16. Belardinelli R, Georgiou D, Cianci G, et al Randomized, controlled trial of long-term moderate exercise training in chronic heart failure. Effects on functional capacity, quality of life, and clinical outcomes. *Circulation* 1999;99:1173–1182.

17. Garg R, Yusuf S, for the Collaborative Group on ACE Inhibitor Trials. Overview of randomized trials of angiotensin-converting enzyme inhibitors on mortality and morbidity in patients with heart failure. *JAMA* 1995;273:1450–1456. Search date 1994; primary sources Medline; correspondence with investigators and pharmaceutical firms.

18. Packer M, Poole-Wilson PA, Armstrong PW, et al, on behalf of the ATLAS Study Group. Comparative effects of low and high doses of the angiotensin-converting enzyme inhibitor, lisinopril, on morbidity and mortality in chronic heart failure. *Circulation* 1999;100:2312–2318.

19. SOLVD Investigators. Effect of enalapril on survival in patients with reduced left ventricular ejection fractions and congestive heart failure. *N Engl J Med* 1991;325:293–302.

20. Sharma D, Buyse M, Pitt B, et al. and the Losartan Heart Failure Mortality Meta-analysis Study Group. Meta-analysis of observed mortality data from all-controlled, double-blind, multiple-dose studies of losartan in heart failure. *Am J Cardiol* 2000;85:187–192.

21. Riegger GAJ, Bouzo H, Petr P, et al, for the Symptom, Tolerability, Response to Exercise Trial of Candesartan Cilexetil in Heart Failure (STRETCH) Investigators. Improvement in exercise tolerance and symptoms of congestive heart failure during treatment with candesartan cilexetil. *Circulation* 1999;100:2224–2230.

22. McKelvie R, Yusuf S, Pericak D, et al., for the RESOLVD Investigators. Comparison of candesartan, enalapril, and their combination in congestive heart failure: randomized evaluation of strategies for left ventricular dysfunction (RESOLVD pilot study). *Circulation* 1999;100:1056–1064.

23. Hamroff G, Katz SD, Mancini D, et al. Addition of angiotensin II receptor blockade to maximal angiotensin-converting enzyme inhibition improves exercise capacity in patients with severe congestive heart failure. *Circulation* 1999;99: 990–992.

24. Kraus F, Rudolph C, Rudolph W. Wirksamkeit von Digitalis bei Patienten mit chronischer Herzinsuffizienz und Sinusrhythmus. *Herz* 1993; 18:95–117. Search date 1992; primary source Medline.

25. Digitalis Investigation Group. The effect of digoxin on mortality and morbidity in patients with heart failure. *N Engl J Med* 1997;336:525–533.

26. Packer M, Carver JR, Rodeheffer RJ, et al, for the PROMISE Study Research Group. Effect of oral milrinone on mortality in severe chronic heart failure. *N Engl J Med* 1991;325:1468–1475.

27. CIBIS-II Investigators and Committees. The cardiac insufficiency bisoprolol study II (CIBIS-II): a randomised trial. *Lancet* 1999;353:9–13.

28. MERIT-HF Study Group. Effect of metoprolol CR/XL in chronic heart failure: metoprolol CR/XL randomised intervention trial in congestive heart failure. *Lancet* 1999;353:2001–2007.

29. Lechat P, Packer M, Chalon S, et al. Clinical effects of β-adrenergic blockade in chronic heart failure. A meta-analysis of double-blind, placebo-controlled, randomized trials. *Circulation* 1998;98: 1184–1191. Search date not stated; primary sources Medline; reference lists; colleagues; pharmaceutical industry.

30. Packer M, O'Connor CM, Ghali JK, et al, for the Prospective Randomized Amlodipine Survival Evaluation Study Group. Effect of amlodipine on morbidity and mortality in severe chronic heart failure. *N Engl J Med* 1996;335:1107–1114.

31. Pitt B, Zannad F, Remme WJ, et al, for the Randomized Aldactone Evaluation Study Investigators. The effects of spironolactone on morbidity and mortality in patients with severe heart failure. *N Engl J Med* 1999;341:709–717.

32. Piepoli M, Villani GQ, Ponikowski P,et al. Overview and meta-analysis of randomised trials of amiodarone in chronic heart failure. *Int J Cardiol* 1998;66:1–10. Search date 1997; primary sources unspecified computerised literature database.

33. Amiodarone Trials Meta-Analysis Investigators. Effect of prophylactic amiodarone on mortality after acute myocardial infarction and in congestive heart failure: meta-analysis of individual data from 6500 patients in randomised trials. *Lancet* 1997; 350:1417–1424.

34. The Antiarrhythmic versus Implantable Defibrillators (AVID) Investigators. A comparison of antiarrhythmic-drug therapy with implantable defibrillators I patients resuscitated from near-fatal ventricular arrhythmias. *N Engl J Med* 1997;337: 1576–1583.

35. Moss AJ, Hall WJ, Cannom DS, et al. Improved survival with an implanted defibrillator in patients with coronary disease at high risk for ventricular arrhythmia. *N Engl J Med* 1996;335:1933–1940.

36. Bigger JT for The Coronary Artery Bypass Graft (CABG) Patch Trial Investigators. Prophylactic use of implanted cardiac defibrillators in patients at high risk for ventricular arrhythmias after coronary-artery bypass graft surgery. *N Engl J Med* 1997; 337:1569–1575.

37. Teerlink JR, Jalaluddin M, Anderson S, et al. Ambulatory ventricular arrhythmias in patients with heart failure do not specifically predict an increased risk of sudden death. *Circulation* 2000; 101:40–46.

38. Connolly SJ. Prophylactic antiarrhythmic therapy for the prevention of sudden death in high-risk patients: drugs and devices. *Eur Heart J* 1999(suppl C):31–35.

39. SOLVD Investigators. Effect of enalapril on mortality and the development of heart failure in asymptomatic patients with reduced left ventricular ejection fractions. *N Engl J Med* 1992; 327:685–691.

40. Rutherford JD, Pfeffer MA, Moyé LA, et al. Effects of captopril on ischaemic events after myocardial infarction. *Circulation* 1994;90:1731–1738.

41. The Heart Outcome Prevention Evaluation Study Investigators. Effects of an angiotensin-converting-enzyme inhibitor, ramipril, on cardiovascular events in high-risk patients. *N Engl J Med* 2000; 342:145–153.

Robert McKelvie
Associate Professor of Medicine
McMaster University
Hamilton, Ontario
Canada

Competing interests: None declared.

INTERVENTIONS

Key Messages

Exercise

- Observational studies have found that moderate to high physical activity reduces coronary heart disease (CHD) and stroke. They also found that sudden death after strenuous exercise was rare, more common in sedentary people, and did not outweigh the benefits.

Diet

- Observational studies have found that consumption of fruit and vegetables is associated with reduced ischaemic vascular disease.
- RCTs have found no evidence that β carotene supplements are effective and have found that they may be harmful.
- We found insufficient evidence to support antioxidant supplements in healthy people.

Smoking

- Observational studies have found a strong association between smoking and overall mortality and ischaemic vascular disease.
- Several large cohort studies have found that the increased risk associated with smoking falls after stopping smoking.

SPECIFIC INTERVENTIONS

In people with raised blood pressure

- We found prospective evidence that lifestyle interventions reduce blood pressure but insufficient evidence that these interventions reduce mortality or morbidity.
- Systematic reviews have found good evidence that drug treatment reduces blood pressure.
- Trials of drug treatment have found a greater reduction in blood pressure compared with trials of lifestyle changes, although we found no head to head comparisons.
- Systematic reviews have found that the main determinant of benefit of treatment for hypertension is the pretreatment absolute cardiovascular disease risk.
- The evidence of beneficial effects on mortality and morbidity is strongest for diuretics and then β blockers.
- We found no direct evidence on effects of lowering blood pressure beyond 140/80 mm Hg.
- Systematic reviews have found that, in people over age 60 years with systolic blood pressures greater than 160 mm Hg, lowering systolic blood pressure decreased total mortality and fatal and non-fatal cardiovascular events.

Antithrombotic drugs

- We found insufficient evidence to identify which asymptomatic individuals would benefit overall and which would be harmed by regular treatment with aspirin.
- One RCT found that the benefits and harms of oral anticoagulation among individuals without symptoms of cardiovascular disease were finely balanced and that net effects were uncertain.

To lower cholesterol

- Systematic reviews have found that reducing cholesterol concentration in asymptomatic people lowers the rate of cardiovascular events but have found no evidence that cholesterol rduction by any method reduces overall death rate in people at low baseline risk of cardiovascular events.

■ Systematic reviews and RCTs have found that combined use of cholesterol lowering diet and lipid lowering drugs reduces cholesterol concentration more than lifestyle interventions alone.

DEFINITION	Primary prevention in this context is the long term management of people at increased risk but with no evidence of cardiovascular disease. Clinically overt ischaemic vascular disease includes acute myocardial infarction (AMI), angina, stroke, and peripheral vascular disease. Many adults have no symptoms or obvious signs of vascular disease, even though they have atheroma and are at increased risk of ischaemic vascular events because of one or more risk factors (see aetiology below).
INCIDENCE/ PREVALENCE	In the USA, around 42% of all deaths are from vascular disease. AMI and its sequelae remain the most common single cause of death.
AETIOLOGY/ RISK FACTORS	Identified major risk factors for ischaemic vascular disease include increasing age, male sex, raised low density lipoprotein cholesterol, reduced high density lipoprotein cholesterol, raised blood pressure, smoking, diabetes, family history of cardiovascular disease, obesity, and sedentary lifestyle. For many of these risk factors, observational studies show a continuous gradient of increasing risk of cardiovascular disease with increasing levels of the risk factor, with no obvious threshold level. Although by definition event rates are higher in high risk people, of all ischaemic vascular events that occur in the population, most occur in people with intermediate levels of absolute risk because there are many more of them than there are people at high risk; see appendix 1.[1]
PROGNOSIS	About half of people who suffer an AMI die within 28 days, and two thirds of AMIs occur before the person reaches hospital.[2] The benefits of intervention in unselected people with no evidence of cardiovascular disease (primary prevention) are small because in such people the baseline risk is small. However, absolute risk of ischaemic vascular events varies dramatically, even among people with similar levels of blood pressure or cholesterol. Estimates of absolute risk can be based on simple risk equations or tables (see appendix 1).[3,4]
AIMS	To reduce mortality and morbidity from cardiovascular disease, with minimum adverse effects.
OUTCOMES	Incidence of fatal and non-fatal cardiovascular events (including coronary, cerebrovascular, renal, and eye disease, and heart failure). Surrogate outcomes include changes in levels of individual risk factors, such as blood pressure.
METHODS	*Clinical Evidence* update search and appraisal May 2000.

Primary prevention

| QUESTION | Does physical activity reduce the risk of vascular events in asymptomatic people? |

Charles Foster, Michael Murphy

Updated this issue

We found strong observational evidence that moderate to high levels of physical activity reduce the risk of non-fatal and fatal CHD and stroke. People who are physically active (those who undertake moderate levels of activity daily or almost daily) typically experience 30–50% reductions in relative risk of CHD compared with people who are sedentary, after adjustment for other risk factors. The absolute risk of sudden death after strenuous activity is small (although greatest in people who are habitually sedentary) and does not outweigh observed benefits.

Benefits: **Effects of physical activity on CHD:** We found no RCTs. Three systematic reviews published between 1989 and 1992 evaluated observational studies and found increased risk of CHD in sedentary compared with active people.[5–7] Since 1992, 17 large, well conducted prospective, non-randomised studies, with follow up periods ranging from 18 months to 29 years, have specifically examined the association between physical activity and risk of non-fatal or fatal CHD.[8–24] The studies found that risk declined with increasing levels of physical activity (for examples of activity levels see table 1, p 78) (AR for CHD death in people with sedentary lives (rare or no physical activity) 70 per 10 000 person years v 40 per 10 000 person years in people with the highest level of activity (> 3500 kcal per week), absolute benefit of high levels of physical activity 30 lives saved per 10 000 person years). **Effects of physical fitness on CHD:** We found no RCTs. One systematic review (published in 1992) identified seven large, well designed prospective, non-randomised studies of the effects of physical fitness on CHD.[25] All used reproducible measures of physical fitness. Five studies adjusted for other CHD risk factors. These found an increased risk of death from CHD in people with low levels of physical fitness compared with those with high levels (RR of death lowest quartile v highest quartile ranged from 1.2 to 4.0). Most studies reported only baseline measures of physical fitness, thus not accounting for changes in fitness. One recent large follow up study found lower risk among people who increased their fitness level (RR for CVD death compared with those whose level of fitness did not change 0.48, 95% CI 0.31 to 0.74).[26] **Effects of physical activity on stroke:** We found no RCTs and no systematic review of observational studies. We found 12 observational studies (published between 1990 and 1999), based on 3680 strokes among North American, Japanese, and European populations.[27–40] Most of these found that moderate activity was associated with reduced risk of stroke compared with inactivity (RR of stroke, moderate activity v inactivity about 0.5). One cohort study from Japan found that "heavy" physical activity reduced the risk of stroke compared with "moderate" activity (RR of stroke, "heavy" v "moderate" activity about 0.3; P < 0.05).[38] In most studies, the benefits were greater in older people and in men. Most studies were conducted in white men in late middle age, which potentially limits their applicability to other groups of people. The results usually persisted after adjustment for other known risk factors for stroke (blood pressure, blood lipids, body mass index, and smoking) and after exclusion of people with pre-existing diseases that might limit physical activity and increase risk of stroke. The more recent studies found maximum reduction in the risk of stroke with moderate as opposed to high levels of physical exercise levels.

Harms: No direct evidence of harm was reported in the studies described. We found two studies in people who had experienced non-fatal myocardial infarction, conducted in the USA and Germany. Each involved more than 1000 events and found that 4–7% of these events occurred within 1 hour of strenuous physical activity.[41–43] Strenuous activity was estimated to have raised the relative risk of AMI between two and sixfold in the hour after activity, with risks returning to baseline after that. However, the absolute risk remained low, variously estimated at six deaths per 100 000 middle aged men per year[44] or 0.3 to 2.7 events per 10 000 person hours of exercise.[45] Both studies found that the relative risk of AMI after strenuous activity was much higher in people who were habitually sedentary (RR 107, 95% CI 67 to 171) compared with the relative risk in those who engaged in heavy physical exertion on five or more occasions per week (RR 2.4, 95% CI 1.5 to 3.7).[41] Injury is likely to be the most common adverse event, but we found too few population data to quantify its risk.

Comment: Findings from these observational studies should be interpreted with caution. The studies varied in definitions of levels of activity and fitness. The level of activity or fitness experienced by each participant was not experimentally assigned by an investigator (as in an RCT) but resulted from self selection. Active (or fit) participants are likely to differ from inactive (or unfit) participants in other ways that also influence their risk of cardiovascular disease. Confounding of this type can be partially controlled by adjustment for other known risk factors (such as age, smoking status, and body mass index), but it is likely that some residual confounding will remain, which could overestimate the effect of exercise. The studies have found that the absolute risk of sudden death during or immediately after physical activity is small and does not outweigh the observed benefits.

QUESTION What intensity and frequency of physical activity improves fitness?

Charles Foster, Michael Murphy

Updated this issue

Small RCTs have found that at least moderate intensity exercise (equivalent to brisk walking) is necessary to improve fitness. We found insufficient evidence on the effects of short bouts of exercise several times a day compared with longer daily bouts.

Benefits: **Intensity:** We found no systematic review. Numerous small RCTs of varying quality have been conducted in different subpopulations. In general, these found that over a period of 6–12 months, low intensity activity programmes produced no measurable changes in maximum oxygen consumption (Vo_2max), whereas moderate intensity activity programmes (equivalent to brisk walking) typically produced improvements of 20% in oxygen consumption in sedentary people. Table 1 gives the intensity of effort required for a range of physical activities, p 78. Two recent RCTs compared structured aerobic exercise (such as step classes and aerobics classes) with lifestyle activity programmes (such as regular walking and using stairs instead of elevators) among obese women[46] and sedentary men and women.[47] Both studies reported similar, significant changes in measures of cardiovascular fitness and blood pressure with each intervention, and these changes were sustained for at least 2 years after intervention. One prospective follow up study of women previously involved in a randomised trial of physical activity found that women who start a programme of regular walking maintain higher levels of physical activity 10 years after the intervention.[48] **Frequency:** We found no systematic review. One RCT in 36 men compared 8 weeks of a single daily session of 30 minutes of exercise versus three daily sessions of 10 minutes each.[49] It found no significant difference in fitness benefit between groups.

Harms:	None reported.
Comment:	None.

QUESTION What are the effects of dietary interventions on the risk of heart attack and stroke in asymptomatic people?

Andy Ness

Updated this issue

OPTION EATING MORE FRUIT AND VEGETABLES

Cohort studies have found that eating more fruit and vegetables reduces the risk of heart attack and stroke. The size and nature of any real protective effect is uncertain.

Benefits: **Ischaemic heart disease:** We found no RCTs. We found three systematic reviews of observational studies.[50-52] With addition of recently published studies[53-60] to those reported in the first review,[50] a protective association was observed for ischaemic heart disease in 14 of 24 cohort studies. In the second review, the authors calculated a summary measure of the protective association of 15% between those above the 90th centile and those below the 10th centile for fruit and vegetable consumption.[51] In the third review the authors estimated that increased intake of fruit and vegetables of around 150 g per day was associated with a reduced risk of CHD of between 20–40%.[52] The validity of these estimates has been questioned. One large, high quality cohort study found that eating more vegetables was associated with decreased coronary mortality (≥ 117 g vegetables per day $v < 61$ g vegetables per day RRR 34%, 95% CI 4% to 54%; for fruit, the association was more modest and not significant (≥ 159 g fruit per day $v < 75$ g fruit per day RRR 23, 95% CI −12% to +46%).[61] **Stroke:** We found no RCTs but we found two systematic reviews examining the evidence from observational studies for stroke.[50,52] With addition of recently published studies[53,58,62–66] to those reported in the first review,[50] a protective association was observed in 10 of 15 cohort studies for stroke. In the second review the authors estimated that increased intake of fruit and vegetables of around 150 g per day was associated with a reduced risk of stroke of 0–25%.[52] The basis for this estimate is not clear. One large, high quality cohort study in US health professionals found that increased fruit and vegetable intake was associated with a decreased risk of ischaemic stroke (RRR per daily serving of fruit and vegetables 6%, 95% CI 1% to 10%; RRR in the fifth of the population eating the most fruit and vegetables v the fifth eating the least 31%, 95% CI 8% to 48%).[67]

Harms: None were identified.

Comment: Lack of trial evidence and deficiencies in the data available from observational studies mean that the size and nature of any real protective effect is uncertain.[68,69] The observed associations could be the result of confounding as people who eat more fruit and vegetables often come from higher socioeconomic groups and adopt other healthy lifestyles.[70]

OPTION ANTIOXIDANTS

Updated this issue

We found no evidence of benefit from β carotene supplements, and RCTs suggest that they may be harmful. Other antioxidant supplements may be beneficial, but we found insufficient trial evidence to support their use.

Benefits: **β Carotene:** We found one systematic review of prospective studies and RCTs (search date not given, published 1997), which did not pool data because of heterogeneity among studies.[71] Most prospective cohort studies of β carotene found a modest protective association with increased intake,[71–74] although several large trials of β carotene supplementation found no evidence of benefit.[74,75] **Vitamin C:** We found two systematic reviews,[71,76] which mostly included the same studies, and five subsequent prospective studies.[57,63,68,77,78] Three of 14 cohort studies found a significant protective association between vitamin C and CHD, and two of nine studies found a protective association between vitamin C and stroke. We found no large trials of vitamin C supplementation alone. Two large trials of multivitamin supplements have been carried out in Linxian, China.[71,79–81] One trial (that was included in the reviews) was carried out in 29 584 participants drawn from the general population who were randomised by using a factorial design to one of four arms: arm A–retinol (10 000 IU) and zinc (22.5 mg); arm B–riboflavin (5.2 mg) and niacin (40 mg); arm C–ascorbic acid (120 mg) and molybdenum (30 µg); arm D–carotene (15 mg), selenium (50 µg), and vitamin E (30 mg). After 6 years the trial found that the treatment assigned to people in arm D reduced all cause mortality and death due to stroke (RRR for death from any cause arm D v other arms 9%, 95% CI 1% to 16%). It found no reduction in stroke or all cause mortality among the other arms.[71] The other trial (subsequent to the reviews) included 3318 people with oesophageal dysplasia who were randomised to placebo or a multivitamin supplement that contained 14 vitamins and 12 minerals, including vitamin C (180 mg), vitamin E (60 IU [1 IU = 0.67 mg], β carotene (15 mg), and selenium (50 µg). After 6 years it found that the supplement did not significantly reduce stroke or death from all causes (RRR for all cause mortality 7%, 95% CI −16% to +25%; RRR for stroke 33%, 95% CI −7% to +63%).[79,80] **Vitamin E:** We found one systematic review and additional prospective studies.[71] Eight large cohort studies (5 of which were included in the review) have examined the association between vitamin E intake and ischaemic heart disease. Six found a significant protective association,[71,77,82] whereas two found no significant association.[57,83] In three studies the protective association was with dietary vitamin E.[71,82] In the others it was either wholly or mainly with vitamin E supplements.[71,83] In the review, the largest RCT of vitamin E alone versus placebo (in 29 133 Finnish smokers) found that vitamin E did not significantly reduce mortality compared with placebo (RRR for death 2%, 95% CI −9% to +5%) after 5–8 years. (See above for the results of the Linxian trials.[71,79–81]) Two cohort studies found no association between vitamin E intake and stroke.[78,84] **Antioxidant minerals:** We found little epidemiological evidence about the cardioprotective effect of copper, zinc, or manganese on the heart.[85] Cohort studies reported an increased risk of ischaemic heart disease in people with low blood selenium concentrations.[86] Most of these were carried out in Finland, a country with low intakes of antioxidants.[87] (See also the results of the Linxian trials, p 57).[71,79–81] **Flavonoids:** We found no systematic review. We found five cohort studies,[65,87–90] three of which reported a reduced risk of ischaemic heart disease with increased flavonoid intake.[65,87,88] One of three observational studies reported a reduced risk of stroke with increased flavonoid intake.[65,66,84]

Harms: Several large trials found that β carotene supplements may increase cardiovascular mortality (pooled data from four RCTs, RRI for cardiovascular death 12%, 95% CI 4% to 22%).[74] Explanations for these results include use of the wrong isomer, the wrong dose, or a detrimental effect on other carotenoid levels.[91,92]

Comment: Trials of antioxidants such as β carotene and vitamin E have not produced any evidence of benefit. Routine use of antioxidant supplements is not justified by the currently available evidence. More trials of antioxidant supplementation are under way.[93] **Vitamin E:** Cohort studies have found no association between rates of ischaemic heart disease and vitamin E levels,[73] but blood concentrations of vitamin E are a poor marker of intake,[94] and storage of blood samples may have led to errors in measurement of vitamin E concentrations.[73] The large trial in Finnish smokers was designed to examine the effects of vitamin E and other supplements on cancer incidence. Cardiovascular end points were not primary outcomes.[95]

QUESTION   By how much does smoking cessation, or avoidance of starting smoking, reduce risk?

Julian J Nicholas, Thomas Kottke

Last updated Issue 3

Observational studies have found that cigarette smoking is strongly related to overall mortality. We found evidence from both observational and randomised studies that cigarette smoking increases the risk of CHD and stroke. The evidence is strongest for stroke.

Benefits: Several large cohort studies examining the effects of smoking have been extensively reviewed by the US surgeon general[96] and the UK Royal College of Physicians.[97] The reviews concluded that cigarette smoking was causally related to disease and that smoking cessation substantially reduced the risk of cancer, respiratory disease, CHD, and stroke. **Death from all causes:** The longest prospective cohort study, in 34 439 male British doctors whose smoking habits were periodically assessed over 40 years (1951–1991), found a strong association between smoking and increased mortality. It found that smokers were about three times more likely to die in middle age (45–64 years) and twice as likely to die in older age (65–84 years) compared with lifelong non-smokers (95% CIs not given).[98] The prospective nurses' health study followed 117 001 middle aged female nurses for 12 years. It found that the total mortality in current smokers was nearly twice that in lifelong non-smokers (RR of death 1.87, 95% CI 1.65 to 2.13).[99] **CHD:** One review (published in 1990) identified 10 cohort studies, involving 20 million person years of observation.[96] All studies found a higher incidence of CHD among smokers (pooled RR of death from CHD compared with non-smokers 1.7, 95% CI not available).[96] People smoking more than 20 cigarettes per day were more likely to have a coronary event (RR 2.5, 95% CI not given).[97] Middle aged smokers were more likely to experience a first non-fatal AMI compared with people who had never smoked (RR in men 2.9, 95% CI 2.4 to 3.4; RR in women 3.6, 95% CI 3.0 to 4.4).[100,101] One RCT of advice encouraging smoking cessation in 1445 men aged 40–59 years found that more men given advice to stop smoking gave up cigarettes (mean absolute reduction in men continuing to smoke after advice v control 53%). The trial found no evidence that men given advice to stop had a significantly lower mortality from CHD (RRR 18%, 95% CI −18% to +43%).[102] The wide confidence intervals mean that there could have been anything from a 43% decrease to an 18% increase in rates of CHD death in men given advice to quit, regardless of whether they actually gave up smoking. **Stroke:** One systematic review (published in 1989) found 32 studies (17 cohort studies with concurrent or historical controls, 14 case control studies, and one hypertension intervention trial). It found good evidence that smoking was associated with an increased risk of stroke (RR of stroke in cigarette smokers v non-smokers 1.5, 95% CI 1.4 to 1.6).[103] Smoking was associated with an increased risk of cerebral infarction (RR 1.92, 95% CI 1.71 to 2.16) and subarachnoid haemorrhage (RR 2.93, 95% CI 2.48 to 3.46), but no increased risk of intracerebral haemorrhage (RR 0.74, 95% CI 0.56 to 0.98). The relative risk of stroke in smokers versus non-smokers was highest in those aged under 55 years (RR 2.9, 95% CI 2.40 to 3.59) and lowest in those aged over 74 years (RR 1.11, 95% CI 0.96 to 1.28).

Harms: We found no evidence that stopping smoking increases mortality in any subgroup of smokers.

Comment: We found no evidence of publication or other overt bias that may explain the observed association between smoking and stroke.

Cardiovascular disorders

There was a dose-response curve between the number of cigarettes smoked and the relative risk for stroke, consistent with a causal relation. The absolute risk reduction from stopping smoking will be highest for those with the highest absolute risk of vascular events.

QUESTION	How quickly do risks diminish when smokers stop smoking?

Julian J Nicholas, Thomas Kottke

Last updated Issue 3

Observational studies have found that the risk of death and cardiovascular events falls when people stop smoking. The risk can take many years to approach that of non-smokers, particularly in those with a history of heavy smoking.

Benefits: **Death from all causes:** In people who stopped smoking, observational studies found that death rates fell gradually to lie between those of lifelong smokers and people who had never smoked. Estimates for the time required for former smokers to bring their risk of death in line with people who had never smoked varied among studies but may be longer than 15 years.[104] Actuarial projections from one study among British doctors predicted that life expectancy would improve even among people who stopped smoking in later life (65 years and over).[98] **CHD:** Observational studies found that, in both male and female ex-smokers, the risk of coronary events rapidly declined to a level comparable with that of people who had never smoked after 2–3 years and was independent of the number of cigarettes smoked before quitting.[96] **Stroke:** The US surgeon general's review of observational studies found that the risk of stroke decreased in ex-smokers compared with smokers (RR of stroke, smokers v ex-smokers 1.2, 95% CI not available) but remained raised for 5–10 years after cessation compared with those who had never smoked (RR of stroke ex-smokers v never smokers 1.5, 95% CI not available).[96] One recent study in 7735 middle aged British men found that 5 years after smoking cessation the risk of stroke in previously light smokers (< 20 cigarettes per day) was identical to that of lifelong non-smokers, but the risk in previously heavy smokers (> 21 cigarettes per day) was still raised compared with lifelong non-smokers (RR of stroke, previously heavy smokers v never smokers 2.2, 95% CI 1.1 to 4.3).[105] One observational study in 117 001 middle aged female nurses also found a fall in risk on stopping smoking and found no difference between previously light and previously heavy smokers (RR in all former smokers 2–4 years after stopping smoking 1.17, 95% CI 0.49 to 2.23).[99]

Harms: We found no evidence that stopping smoking increases mortality in any subgroup of smokers.

Comment: For a review of the evidence on methods of changing smoking behaviour, see secondary prevention of ischaemic cardiac events, p 83.

Cindy Mulrow, Rod Jackson

Updated this issue

OPTION   PHYSICAL ACTIVITY

**One systematic review of RCTs has found that aerobic exercise reduces
blood pressure (see table 2, p 79).**

Benefits: We found no RCTs examining the effects of exercise on morbidity,
mortality, or quality of life. One systematic review (published in
1996) identified 29 RCTs examining effects of blood pressure. The
trials compared at least 4 weeks of regular aerobic exercise versus
no exercise in 1533 sedentary adults with normal blood pressure
aged 18–79 years.[106] Exercise regimens included walking, jogging,
cycling, or both, often lasting 45–60 minutes per session, for 3 days
a week (mean exercise intensity about 60–70% of Vo_2max). Compared with non-exercising control groups, groups randomised to
aerobic exercise reduced their systolic blood pressure by
4.7 mm Hg (95% CI 4.4 to 5.0 mm Hg) and diastolic blood pressure
by 3.1 mm Hg (95% CI 3.0 to 3.3 mm Hg). Greater reductions were
seen in people with higher initial blood pressures. Trials with
interventions lasting longer than 6 months' duration in adults aged
45 years or over with hypertension found smaller mean reductions
in blood pressure but with wide confidence intervals (systolic
reduction 0.8 mm Hg, 95% CI 5.9 mm Hg reduction to 4.2 mm Hg
increase).[107]

Harms: Musculoskeletal injuries may occur, but their frequency was not
documented.

Comment: Many adults find aerobic exercise programmes difficult to sustain.
The clinical significance of the observed reductions in blood pressure is uncertain. The type and amount of exercise most likely to
result in benefits are unclear, with some recent studies showing
some benefits with simple increases in lifestyle activity. One cohort
study in 173 men with hypertension found that "regular heavy
activity several times weekly" compared with no or limited spare
time physical activity reduced all cause and cardiovascular mortality
(all cause mortality RR 0.43, 95% CI 0.22 to 0.82; cardiovascular
mortality RR 0.33, 95% CI 0.11 to 0.94).[108]

OPTION   LOW FAT, HIGH FRUIT AND VEGETABLE DIET

**One RCT found that a low fat, high fruit and vegetable diet modestly
reduced blood pressure (see table 2, p 79).**

Benefits: We found no systematic review and no RCTs examining the effects
of low fat, high fruit and vegetable diet on morbidity or mortality in
people with primary hypertension. For evidence from cohort studies
in asymptomatic people in general see, p 56. One RCT in 459
adults with systolic blood pressures of < 160 mm Hg and diastolic
blood pressures of 80–90 mm Hg compared effects of three diets

on blood pressure (control diet low in both magnesium and potassium v fruit and vegetable diet high in both potassium and magnesium v combination of the fruit and vegetable diet with a low fat diet high in both calcium and protein).[109] After 8 weeks the fruit and vegetable diet reduced systolic and diastolic blood pressure compared with the control diet (mean change in systolic blood pressure $-2.8\,mm\,Hg$, 97.5% CI -4.7 to $-0.9\,mm\,Hg$; mean change in diastolic blood pressure $-1.1\,mm\,Hg$, 97.5% CI $-2.4\,mm\,Hg$ to $+0.3\,mm\,Hg$). The combination diet also reduced systolic and diastolic blood pressure compared with the control diet (mean change in systolic blood pressure $-5.5\,mm\,Hg$, 97.5% CI $-7.4\,mm\,Hg$ to $-3.7\,mm\,Hg$; mean change in diastolic blood pressure $-3.0\,mm\,Hg$, 97.5% CI -4.3 to $-1.6\,mm\,Hg$).

Harms: We found no direct evidence that a low fat, high fruit and vegetable diet is harmful.

Comment: The trial was of short duration and participants were supplied with food during the intervention period.[109] Other studies have found that long term maintenance of particular diets is difficult for many people, although low fat, high fruit and vegetable diets may have multiple benefits (see changing behaviour, p 16).

OPTION   REDUCED ALCOHOL CONSUMPTION

One systematic review of RCTs has found inconclusive evidence regarding effects of alcohol reduction on blood pressure.

Benefits: We found no RCTs examining the effects of reducing alcohol consumption on morbidity or mortality. Over 60 population studies have reported associations between alcohol consumption and blood pressure; the relation was found to be generally linear, although several studies reported a threshold effect at around two to three standard drinks a day.[110] Any adverse effect of up to two drinks per day on blood pressure was found to be either small or non-existent. One systematic review of seven trials in 751 people with hypertension (mainly men) found that data were inconclusive on the benefits of reducing alcohol among moderate to heavy drinkers (25–50 drinks weekly).[111]

Harms: We found no direct evidence that reducing alcohol intake to as few as two drinks a day was harmful.

Comment: Most data were from observational studies. RCTs were small and lacked reliable information about adherence. Substantial reductions in alcohol use in both control and intervention groups were observed, with limited ability to detect differences between groups.

OPTION   SALT RESTRICTION

One systematic review of RCTs has found that salt restriction may lead to modest reductions in blood pressure, with more benefit in people older than 45 years than in younger people (see table 2, p 79).

Benefits: We found no RCT examining the effects of salt restriction on morbidity or mortality. We found one systematic review (published in 1998), which identified 58 trials examining effects of blood pressure in 2161 people with hypertension aged 23–73 years (mean age 49 years).[112] We also found one subsequent RCT lasting 30 months in 875 men and women with hypertension 60–80 years (mean age 66 years).[113] Interventions were low salt diets, with or without weight reduction. People in the control groups took their usual diet. Changes in salt intake varied among trials in the systematic review; a mean reduction in sodium intake of 118 mmol (6.7 g) per day for 28 days led to reductions of 3.9 mm Hg (95% CI 3.0 to 4.8 mm Hg) in systolic blood pressure and 1.9 mm Hg (95% CI 1.3 to 2.5 mm Hg) in diastolic blood pressure.[112] The subsequent trial in elderly people found that a mean decrease in salt intake of about 40 mmol (2.35 g) per day reduced systolic blood pressure by 2.6 mm Hg (95% CI 0.4 to 4.8 mm Hg) and diastolic blood pressure by 1.1 mm Hg (95% CI 0.3 mm Hg rise in diastolic to 2.5 mm Hg fall). An earlier systematic review (published in 1996) identified 28 RCTs in 1131 people with hypertension. It found that lesser reductions of 60 mmol per day led to smaller reductions in systolic/diastolic blood pressure of 2.2 mm Hg/0.5 mm Hg and found greater effects in trials, in which mean age was > 45 years (6.3/2.2 mm Hg).[114]

Harms: We found no direct evidence that low salt diets may increase morbidity or mortality. Epidemiological data conflict, with one observational study suggesting that very low salt intakes may be associated with increased incidence of myocardial infarction in middle aged men.[115]

Comment: Small trials tended to report larger reductions in systolic and diastolic blood pressure than larger trials. This is consistent with publication bias or less rigorous methodology in small trials.[114]

OPTION SMOKING CESSATION

Epidemiological data clearly identify that smoking is a significant risk factor for cardiovascular disease (see option, p 58). We found no direct evidence that stopping smoking decreases blood pressure in people with hypertension.

Benefits: We found no direct evidence that stopping smoking reduces blood pressure in people with hypertension, although we found good evidence that in general, smoking cessation reduces risk of cardiovascular disease (see option, p 58).

Harms: We found insufficient evidence in this context.

Comment: None.

OPTION WEIGHT LOSS

One systematic review of RCTs has found that modest weight reductions of 3–9% of body weight are achievable in motivated middle aged and older adults, and may lead to modest reductions in blood pressure in obese people with hypertension. Many adults find it difficult to maintain weight loss (see table 2, p 79).

Benefits: We found no RCTs examining the effects of weight loss on morbidity and mortality. One systematic review (published in 1998) identified

18 RCTs examining effects on blood pressure in 2611 middle aged people (mean age 50 years, mean weight 85 kg, mean blood pressures 152/98 mm Hg, 55% men).[116] Caloric intakes ranged from 450 to 1500 kcal per day; most diets led to weight reductions of 3–9% of body weight. Combined data from the six trials that did not vary antihypertensive regimens during the intervention period found that reducing weight reduced systolic and diastolic blood pressures (mean reduction in systolic pressure, weight loss v no weight loss 3 mm Hg, 95% CI 0.7 to 6.8 mm Hg; mean reduction in diastolic blood pressure 2.9 mm Hg diastolic, 95% CI 0.1 to 5.7 mm Hg). Trials that allowed adjustment of antihypertensive regimens found that lower doses and fewer antihypertensive drugs were needed in the weight reduction groups compared with control groups.

Harms: We found no direct evidence that intentional gradual weight loss of less than 10% of body weight is harmful in obese adults with hypertension.

Comment: None.

OPTION **POTASSIUM SUPPLEMENTATION**

One systematic review of RCTs has found that a daily potassium supplementation of about 60 mmol (2000 mg, which is roughly the amount contained in 5 bananas) is feasible for many adults and reduces blood pressure a little (see table 3, p 79).

Benefits: We found no RCTs examining the effects of potassium supplementation on morbidity or mortality. One systematic review (published in 1997) of 21 RCTs compared effects on blood pressure of potassium supplements (60–100 mmol potassium chloride daily) versus placebo or no supplement in 1560 adults (aged 19–79 years) with hypertension.[117] It found that, compared with the control interventions, potassium supplements reduced systolic and diastolic blood pressures (mean decrease in systolic blood pressure with potassium supplements 4.4 mm Hg systolic, 95% CI 2.2 to 6.6 mm Hg; mean decrease in diastolic blood pressure 2.5 mm Hg diastolic, 95% CI 0.1 to 4.9 mm Hg).

Harms: We found no direct evidence of harm in people without kidney failure and in people not taking drugs that increase serum potassium concentration. Gastrointestinal adverse effects such as belching, flatulence, diarrhoea, or abdominal discomfort occurred in 2–10% of people.[117]

Comment: None.

OPTION **FISH OIL SUPPLEMENTATION**

One systematic review of RCTs has found that fish oil supplementation in large doses of 3 g per day modestly lowers blood pressure (see table 3, p 79).

Benefits: We found no RCTs examining the effects of fish oil supplementation on morbidity or mortality. One systematic review (published in 1993) found seven RCTs (mostly of short duration), which compared effects on blood pressure of fish oil (usually 3 g daily as capsules) versus no supplements or "placebo" in 339 people (mainly middle aged white men, mean age 50 years) with hypertension.[118] The contents of placebo capsules varied among trials. Some used oil mixtures containing omega-3 polyunsaturated fatty acids, some without. The review found that fish oil supplements reduced blood pressure compared with control interventions (mean decrease in blood pressure in treatment group v control group 4.5 mm Hg systolic, 95% CI 1.2 to 7.8 mm Hg, and 2.5 mm Hg diastolic, 95% CI 0.6 to 4.4 mm Hg).

Harms: Belching, bad breath, fishy taste, and abdominal pain occurred in about a third of people taking high doses of fish oil.[118]

Comment: The trials were of short duration and used high doses of fish oil. Such high intake may be difficult to maintain. We found no evidence of beneficial effect on blood pressure at lower intakes.

OPTION CALCIUM SUPPLEMENTATION

We found insufficient evidence on the effects of calcium supplementation specifically in people with hypertension. One systematic review of RCTs in people both with and without hypertension found that calcium supplementation may reduce systolic blood pressure by small amounts (see table 3, p 79).

Benefits: We found no RCTs examining the effects of calcium supplementation on morbidity or mortality. One systematic review (published in 1999) found 42 RCTs examining effects of calcium supplementation (500–2000 mg daily) versus placebo or no supplements on blood pressure in 4560 middle aged adults with hypertension and normal blood pressure.[119] It found that calcium supplements reduced blood pressure by a small amount (mean systolic blood pressure reduction, supplement v control 1.4 mm Hg, 95% CI 0.7 to 2.2 mm Hg; mean diastolic reduction 0.8 mm Hg, 95% CI 0.2 to 1.4 mm Hg).

Harms: Adverse gastrointestinal effects, such as abdominal pain, were generally mild and varied among particular preparations.

Comment: Data relating specifically to people with hypertension are limited by few studies with small sample sizes and short durations.

OPTION MAGNESIUM SUPPLEMENTATION

We found limited and conflicting evidence on the effect of magnesium supplementation on blood pressure in people with hypertension and normal magnesium concentrations.

Benefits: We found no RCTs examining the effects of magnesium supplementation on morbidity or mortality. A few small, short term RCTs found mixed results on effects on blood pressure reduction (see table 3, p 79).

Harms: Inadequate data.

Comment: None.

Cardiovascular disorders

QUESTION What are the effects of drug treatment in primary hypertension?

Cindy Mulrow, Rod Jackson

Updated this issue

OPTION ANTIHYPERTENSIVE DRUGS VERSUS PLACEBO

Many systematic reviews of RCTs have found that drug treatment decreases the risk of fatal and non-fatal stroke, cardiac events, and total mortality in specific populations of people. The biggest benefit is seen in people with highest baseline risk of cardiovascular disease.

Benefits: We found many systematic reviews. One (published in 1996) summarised 17 RCTs of at least 1 year's duration with morbidity and mortality outcomes in 37 000 people.[120] Reductions in systolic/diastolic blood pressure varied but averaged around 12–16/5–10 mm Hg. There was evidence of benefit in total death rate, cardiovascular death rate, stroke, major coronary events, and congestive cardiac failure, but the absolute results depended on age and the severity of the hypertension (see below). The biggest benefit was seen in those with the highest baseline risk. The trials mainly compared placebo versus diuretics (usually thiazides with the addition of amiloride or triamterene) and versus β blockers (usually atenolol or metoprolol) in a stepped care approach. One systematic review (search date 1999, 8 RCTs, n = 15 693) found that, in people over 60 years old with systolic hypertension, treatment of systolic pressures greater than 160 mm Hg decreased total mortality and fatal and non-fatal cardiovascular events. Absolute benefits were greater in men than women, in people aged over 70, and in those with prior cardiovascular events or wider pulse pressure. The relative hazard rates associated with a 10 mm Hg higher initial systolic blood pressure were 1.26 (P = 0.0001) for total mortality, 1.22 (P = 0.02) for stroke, but only 1.07 (P = 0.37) for coronary events. Active treatment reduced total mortality (RR 0.87, 95% CI 0.78 to 0.98, P = 0.02).[121] We found only one published, large, well designed, placebo controlled RCT of a long acting dihydropyridine calcium channel blocker in people with hypertension, in which a total of 4695 people (aged at least 60 years with isolated systolic hypertension but no severe cardiovascular or other disease) were randomised to treatment for about 2 years with either placebo or nitrendipine.[122] The baseline risk of fatal or non-fatal cardiovascular events was 3.4% per year. It found that nitrendipine reduced the risk of cardiovascular events compared with placebo (RR 31%, 95% CI 14% to 45%; NNT to avoid cardiovascular event per year 94, no 95% CI given). A randomised double blind trial involving 9297 high risk people with evidence of vascular disease or diabetes and one other cardiovascular risk factor, but without heart failure, found that ramipril (an angiotensin converting enzyme [ACE] inhibitor) versus placebo reduced overall mortality (10.4% v 12.2%; RR 0.84, 95% CI 0.75 to 0.95), myocardial infarction (9.9% v 12.3%; RR 0.80, 95% CI 0.70 to 0.90), and stroke (3.4% v 4.9%; RR 0.68, 95% CI 0.56 to 0.84). About half of the participants had hypertension; mean baseline blood pressure was 139/79 mm Hg and ramipril over 5 years decreased blood pressure on average 3/2 mm Hg compared with placebo.[123] **Target diastolic blood pressure:** We found one trial in 18 790 people with a mean age of 62 years and diastolic blood pressures between 100–115 mm Hg, which aimed to evaluate the effects on cardiovascular risk of target diastolic blood pressures of 90, 85, and 80 mm Hg.[124] However, mean achieved diastolic blood pressures were 85, 83, and 81 mm Hg, which limited power to detect differences among groups. There were no significant differences in major cardiovascular events among the three groups.

Harms:	**Mortality and major morbidity:** One systematic review of RCTs comparing diuretics and β blockers versus placebo found no increase in non-cardiovascular mortality in treated people.[120] One systematic review of nine case control and three cohort studies found that long term diuretic use may be associated with an increased risk of renal cell carcinoma (OR in case control studies 1.55, 95% CI 1.4 to 1.7).[125] Absolute risks cannot be calculated from these studies, but renal cell carcinoma is rare, so the absolute risk increase of any real effect would be correspondingly small. Renal cell carcinoma can cause hypertension; this fact may have confounded the results of these studies. **Quality of life and tolerability:** One systematic review and several recent trials found that quality of life was not adversely affected and may be improved in those who remain on treatment.[126,127]

Comment:	Trials included people who were healthier than the general population, with lower rates of cardiovascular risk factors, cardiovascular disease, and comorbidity. People with higher cardiovascular risk can expect greater short term absolute risk reduction than seen in the trials, whereas people with major competing risks such as terminal cancer or end stage Alzheimer's disease can expect smaller risk reduction. In the systematic review,[120] five of the trials were in middle aged adults with mild to moderate hypertension. Seven of the trials were in people older than 60 years. On average, every 1000 person years of treatment in older adults prevented five strokes (95% CI 2 to 8), three coronary events (95% CI 1 to 4), and four cardiovascular deaths (95% CI 1 to 8). Drug treatment in middle aged adults prevented one stroke (95% CI 0 to 2) for every 1000 person years of treatment and did not significantly affect coronary events or mortality.

OPTION COMPARING ANTIHYPERTENSIVE DRUG TREATMENTS

Updated this issue

Two systematic reviews have found that initial treatment with diuretics or β blockers reduces mortality and morbidity with minimal adverse effects. RCTs found no significant morbidity or mortality advantages of ACE inhibitors or calcium channel blockers over diuretics and β blockers. RCTs have found that an ACE inhibitor reduces rates of death, myocardial infarction, and stroke in high risk persons. One RCT found that a thiazide diuretic is superior to an α blocker in reducing cardiovascular events, particularly congestive heart failure.

Benefits: **β blockers versus diuretics:** One systematic review (published in 1997) identified RCTs comparing effects of high and low dose diuretics and β blockers in over 48 000 people.[128] A second systematic review (published in 1998) was limited to 10 RCTs in 16 164 elderly people.[129] These reviews did not summarise direct comparisons of diuretics versus β blockers but compared results of trials that used diuretics as first line agents versus results of trials that used β blockers as first line agents. The reviews found no significant difference between diuretics and β blockers for lowering blood pressure. They found that diuretics reduced coronary events, but found no evidence that β blockers reduced coronary events. **β blockers versus ACE inhibitors:** One single blind trial (10 985 people aged 25–66 years) found that an ACE inhibitor (captopril) was no more effective than conventional treatment (diuretics or β blockers) in reducing cardiovascular morbidity or mortality. Captopril increased the risk of stroke compared with β blockers (125 people would need to be treated with ACE inhibitor rather than β blocker for one extra stroke to occur, 95% CI 69 to 651 people). However, the methods of the trial may limit the validity of results (see comment below).[130] **Comparison of β blockers, diuretics, ACE inhibitors, and calcium channel antagonists:** One unblinded RCT compared diuretics and/or β blockers versus calcium channel antagonists (felodipine or isradipine) versus ACE inhibitors (enalapril or lisinopril) in 6600 people aged 70–84 years. It found no significant difference in blood pressure control or cardiovascular morbidity or mortality.[131] **Comparison of α blockers and diuretics:** A randomised, double blind trial in high risk people with hypertension (n = 24 335) found no differences in coronary heart disease outcomes between doxazosin, an α blocker, compared with chlorthalidone. However, doxazosin compared with chlorthalidone increased the total number of cardiovascular events (4 year rate 25% v 22%; RR 1.25, 95% CI 1.17 to 1.33) and, in particular, increased congestive heart failure (4 year rate 8% v 4%; RR 2.04 95% CI 1.79 to 2.32).[132] **Drug treatment in people with diabetes:** See cardiovascular disease in diabetes, p 295.

Harms: **Quality of life and tolerability:** In the three long term, double blind comparisons of low dose diuretics, β blockers, ACE inhibitors, and calcium channel blockers, tolerability and overall quality of life indicators tended to be more favourable for diuretics and β blockers than for newer drugs.[133–135] One systematic review (published in 1999) of RCTs comparing thiazides versus β blockers found that thiazides were associated with fewer withdrawals because of adverse effects (RR 0.69, 95% CI 0.63 to 0.76).[136] Adverse effects are agent specific. The recent unblinded RCT comparing diuretics, β blockers, calcium channel antagonists, and ACE inhibitors found that after 5 years of follow up, 26% of people receiving felodipine or isradipine reported ankle oedema, 30% receiving enalapril or lisonopril reported cough, and 9% receiving diuretics and/or β blockers reported cold hands and feet.[131] **Major harm controversies:** Case control, cohort, and randomised studies suggest that short and intermediate acting dihydropyridine calcium channel blockers, such as nifedipine and isradipine, may increase cardiovascular morbidity and mortality.[137]

Comment: Results of the large ACE inhibitor trial reported above warrant cautious interpretation because a flaw in the randomisation process resulted in unbalanced groups.[130]

Jeffrey L Probstfield, Michael Pignone

Updated this issue

We found no direct evidence that cholesterol reduction lowers overall mortality in people with no existing cardiovascular symptoms. RCTs have found that benefit is related to an individual's baseline risk of cardiovascular events and to the degree of cholesterol lowering rather than to the individual's absolute cholesterol concentration (see figure 1, p 83). Systematic reviews have found that, in people with a high baseline risk, cholesterol reduction improves outcomes (see secondary prevention of ischaemic cardiac events; cholesterol reduction, p 83).

Benefits: We found many reviews of the effects of cholesterol lowering on cardiovascular event rates, CHD mortality, and total mortality. Most concluded that cholesterol reduction lowered cardiovascular events but that there was little evidence that cholesterol reduction lowers overall mortality when used in people with no existing cardiovascular symptoms (primary prevention).[138,139,140] **Statins:** We found two systematic reviews that considered the effect of HMG-CoA reductase inhibitors (statins) versus placebo on clinical outcomes in people given long term (≥ 6 months) treatment. The first found five major trials and another 18 smaller RCTs.[140] The second (search date 1998) included five large RCTs, of mean duration 5.4 years, in a total of 30 817 people. [141] Both systematic reviews pooled analyses of two large primary prevention trials (13 200 people). These trials were powered to detect differences in composite end points. They found that, after at least 4 years of treatment, statins compared with placebo did not significantly reduce all cause mortality (OR 0.87, 95% CI 0.17 to 1.06) or CHD mortality (OR 0.73, 95% CI 0.51 to 1.05), but did reduce major coronary events (OR 0.66, 95% CI 0.57 to 0.76) and cardiovascular mortality (OR 0.68, 95% CI 0.50 to 0.93). In the large statin trials included in the review, the absolute risk reduction for CHD events, CHD mortality, and total mortality varied with the baseline risk in the placebo group of each trial (see figure 1, p 83).[142–146] The effect of statins seemed to be fully explained by their lipid lowering ability.[147] **Other treatments:** We found no systematic review specifically in people with low baseline risk. We found one systematic review (search date 1996), which did not differentiate primary and secondary prevention and included RCTs of any cholesterol lowering intervention, irrespective of duration, as long as mortality data were reported. It found 59 RCTs in a total of 173 160 people receiving drug treatments (statins, n–3 fatty acids, fibrates, resins, hormones, or niacin) alone, dietary intervention alone, or surgery (ileal bypass) alone.[148] Overall, baseline risk was similar in people allocated to all interventions. Among non-surgical treatments, the review found that only statins reduced CHD mortality (RR v control: 0.69, 95% CI

0.59 to 0.80 for statins; 0.44, 95% CI 0.18 to 1.07 for n–3 fatty acids; 0.98, 95% CI 0.78 to 1.24 for fibrates; 0.71, 95% CI 0.51 to 0.99 for resins; 1.04, 95% CI 0.93 to 1.17 for hormones; 0.95, 95% CI 0.83 to 1.10 for niacin; 0.91, 95% CI 0.82 to 1.01 for diet), and that only statins and n–3 fatty acids reduced all cause mortality (RR v control: 0.79, 95% CI 0.71 to 0.89 for statins; 0.68, 95% CI 0.53 to 0.88 for n–3 fatty acids; 1.06, 95% CI 0.78 to 1.46 for fibrates; 0.85, 95% CI 0.66 to 1.08 for resins; 1.09, 95% CI 1.00 to 1.20 for hormones; 0.96, 95% CI 0.86 to 1.08 for niacin; 0.97, 95% CI 0.81 to 1.15 for diet). **Low fat diet:** See changing behaviour, p 16.

Harms: Specific harms of statins are discussed in secondary prevention of ischaemic cardiac events, p 83.

Comment: The CHD event rate in the placebo group of the two large primary prevention trials using statins was 0.6%[142] and 1.5 %[146] per year. If the 17% relative reduction in total mortality observed in the higher risk West of Scotland trial is real, then about 110 high risk people without known CHD would need to be treated for 5 years to save one life. We found no RCTs evaluating the effect of statins in asymptomatic people aged over 75 years. Several large studies are under way.[149]

QUESTION What is the role of antithrombotic treatment in asymptomatic people?

Cathie Sudlow

Updated this issue

OPTION ANTIPLATELET TREATMENT

We found the role of antiplatelet treatment in individuals without symptoms of cardiovascular disease to be uncertain. We found insufficient evidence from RCTs to identify which individuals would benefit overall and which would be harmed by regular treatment with aspirin (see tables 4 and 5, pp 80, 81).

Benefits: We found two systematic reviews.[124,150–152] **In low risk people:** One systematic review of RCTs of antiplatelet treatment (published in 1994) included nearly 30 000 individuals with no clinically apparent arterial disease. Most participants were involved in two large trials of aspirin versus control among male doctors in the UK (aspirin dose 500 mg daily) and the USA (aspirin dose 325 mg every other day).[150,153,154] **In people with identifiable risk factors for cardiovascular events:** Since the review, two further RCTs of aspirin versus control among asymptomatic individuals with identifiable risk factors for vascular events have been published.[124,152] One was a 2 x 2 factorial RCT of aspirin 75 mg daily versus placebo and of low intensity oral anticoagulation with warfarin (target international normalised ratio [INR] 1.5) versus placebo, among around 5000 men aged 45–69 years. People were recruited from the general population, were in the top 20–25% of a distribution of CHD risk score, and were followed for around 6 years.[152] The other RCT also used a factorial design, with comparisons of aspirin 75 mg daily versus placebo and of three different intensities of blood pressure reduction among about 19 000 individuals with hypertension, most whom had no history of vascular disease.[124] Data on vascular events (non-fatal myocardial infarction, non-fatal stroke, or vascular death) from the primary prevention trials are summarised in table 4, p 81. Antiplatelet treatment produced a 13% (95% CI 5% to 20%) proportional reduction in the odds of a vascular event, corresponding to the avoidance of only about one vascular event per 1000 individuals treated per year. There was a clear reduction in myocardial infarction: among the three trials in the 1994 overview, the odds of a non-fatal myocardial infarction were reduced by 29% (95% CI 14% to 41%); in one RCT the rate of all (fatal or non-fatal) ischaemic heart disease was reduced by 20% (95% CI 1% to 35%); and in the other RCT, the rate of all myocardial infarction was reduced by 36% (95% CI 15% to 51%). Although antiplatelet treatment seemed to reduce the risk of ischaemic stroke, it also seemed to increase the risk of haemorrhagic stroke. In the 1994 overview, the odds of a non-fatal stroke were increased by 21% (95% CI 0% to 38%); in one RCT, there was a non-significant reduction in the rate of all stroke of 3% (95% CI −45% to +35%), and in the other, there was a non-significant reduction in the rate of all stroke of 2% (95% CI −24% to +22%). The second systematic review (search date 1998, 5 RCTs) of aspirin versus placebo in the primary prevention of stroke and other major vascular events included over 52 000 people. It found aspirin reduced the risk of myocardial infarction (RR 0.74, 95% CI 0.68 to 0.82) but had no significant effect on stroke (RR 1.08, 95% CI 0.95 to 1.24.[151]

Harms: Serious, potentially life threatening bleeding is the most important adverse effect of antiplatelet treatment. Intracranial bleeds are uncommon, but they are often fatal and usually cause substantial disability in survivors. Major extracranial bleeds occur mainly in the gastrointestinal tract may require hospital admission or blood transfusion but do not generally result in permanent disability and are rarely fatal. Table 5 shows the approximate excess annual rates for intracranial and major extracranial bleeds (see table 5, p 81).

Comment: Individuals in primary prevention trials were at much lower risk of vascular events (average 1% per year in the control group) than the high risk people with clinical manifestations of cardiovascular disease that were included in the first overview (average 9% per year in the control group).[150] The absolute benefit of aspirin was therefore small and, as it was of similar magnitude to the risks of bleeding, the net effects were statistically uncertain. The size and direction of the effects of aspirin in particular individuals may well depend on specific factors, such as age, blood pressure, smoking status, or history of diabetes mellitus. At present there is insufficient information to identify which individuals would benefit overall and which would be harmed by regular treatment with aspirin. Further information will soon become available from an RCT comparing aspirin 100 mg daily versus placebo among 40 000 apparently healthy postmenopausal women,[155] and subsequently from a detailed overview of individual participant data from all available trials.

| OPTION | ANTICOAGULANT TREATMENT |

We found evidence from one RCT that the benefits and risks of low intensity oral anticoagulation among individuals without evidence of cardiovascular disease are finely balanced, and the net effects are uncertain.

Benefits:
We found no systematic review. We found one RCT assessing anticoagulation (with a low target INR of 1.5) among individuals without evidence of cardiovascular disease.[152] It found that the proportional effects of warfarin were similar among people allocated aspirin or placebo, and overall warfarin non-significantly reduced the odds of a vascular event over about 6.5 years compared with placebo (253 events in 2762 people allocated to warfarin, AR 9.2% v 288 events in 2737 people allocated to placebo, AR 10.5%; mean ARR warfarin v placebo about 2 events per 1000 individuals per year; reduction in odds of vascular event warfarin v placebo 14%, 95% CI −2% to +28%). Compared with placebo, warfarin reduced the rate of all ischaemic heart disease by 21% (95% CI 4% to 35%), but had no significant effect on the rate of the stroke (increase in AR 15%, 95% CI −22% to +68%) or other causes of vascular death.

Harms:
Allocation to warfarin was associated with a non-significant excess of about 0.4 intracranial bleeds per 1000 individuals per year (14/2762 [0.5%] warfarin v 7/2737 [0.3%] placebo) and a non-significant excess of extracranial bleeds of about 0.5 per 1000 individuals per year (21/2545 [0.8%] warfarin v 12/2540 [0.5%] placebo).

Comment:
As is the case for aspirin, the benefits and risks of low intensity oral anticoagulation among people without evidence of cardiovascular disease are finely balanced. The number of individuals randomised to date is only around 10% of the number included in primary prevention trials of aspirin (see above), and so the reliable identification of those who may benefit from such treatment will require further large scale randomised evidence.

Substantive changes since last issue

Eating more fruit and vegetables: Ischaemic heart disease Three new cohort studies;[58–60] conclusions unchanged.

Eating more fruit and vegetables: Stroke Two new cohort studies;[58,66] conclusions unchanged.

Antioxidants: Stroke One new cohort study;[66] conclusions unchanged.

Antihypertensive drugs versus placebo One new systematic review summarising randomised trials in people over 60 years with systolic hypertension found treatment of systolic pressures greater than 160 mm Hg decreased total mortality.[121] One new RCT found ramipril (an ACE inhibitor) reduced deaths, myocardial infarction, and stroke in high risk participants with evidence of vascular disease or diabetes and one other cardiovascular risk factor, but without heart failure.[123]

Comparing antihypertensive drug treatments One large double blind RCT found no differences in coronary heart disease outcomes between doxazosin (an α blocker) and chlorthalidone. However, compared with chlorthalidone, doxazosin increased the total number of cardiovascular events and congestive heart failure.[132]

Lowering cholesterol in asymptomatic people: Statins in people under 75 years One additional systematic review; conclusions unchanged.[140]

REFERENCES

1. Heller RF, Chinn S, Pedoe HD, Rose G. How well can we predict coronary heart disease? Findings of the United Kingdom heart disease prevention project. *BMJ* 1984;288:1409–1411.
2. Tunstall-Pedoe H, Morrison C, Woodward M, Fitzpatrick B, Watt G. Sex differences in myocardial infarction and coronary deaths in the Scottish MONICA population of Glasgow 1985 to 1991: presentation, diagnosis, treatment, and 28-day case fatality of 3991 events in men and 1551 events in women. *Circulation* 1996;93: 1981–1992.
3. Anderson KV, Odell PM, Wilson PWF, Kannel WB. Cardiovascular disease risk profiles. *Am Heart J* 1991;121:293–298.
4. National Health Committee. Guidelines for the management of mildly raised blood pressure in New Zealand. Wellington Ministry of Health, 1993 http://www.nzgg.org.nz/library/gl_complete/ bloodpressure/table1.cfm
5. Powell KE, Thompson PD, Caspersen CJ, Kendrick JS. Physical activity and the incidence of coronary heart disease. *Ann Rev Public Health* 1987;8: 253–287. Search date 1995; primary sources computerised searches of personal files, *J Chronic Dis* 1983–1985 and *Am J Epidemiol* 1984–1985.
6. Berlin JA, Colditz GA. A meta-analysis of physical activity in the prevention of coronary heart disease. *Am J Epidemiol* 1990;132:612–628. Search date not stated; primary sources review articles and Medline.
7. Eaton CB. Relation of physical activity and cardiovascular fitness to coronary heart disease. Part I: A meta-analysis of the independent relation of physical activity and coronary heart disease. *J Am Board Fam Pract* 1992;5:31–42. Search date not stated; primary source Medline.
8. Fraser GE, Strahan TM, Sabate J, Beeson WL, Kissinger D. Effects of traditional coronary risk factors on rates of incident coronary events in a low-risk population: the Adventist health study. *Circulation* 1992;86:406–413.
9. Lindsted KD, Tonstad S, Kuzma JW. Self-report of physical activity and patterns of mortality in Seventh-Day Adventist men. *J Clin Epidemiol* 1991;44:355–364.
10. Folsom AR, Arnett DK, Hutchinson RG, Liao F, Clegg LX, Cooper LS. Physical activity and incidence of coronary heart disease in middle-aged women and men. *Med Sci Sports Exerc* 1997;29:901–909.
11. Jensen G, Nyboe J, Appleyard M, Schnohr P. Risk factors for acute myocardial infarction in Copenhagen, II: Smoking, alcohol intake, physical activity, obesity, oral contraception, diabetes, lipids, and blood pressure. *Eur Heart J* 1991;12: 298–308.
12. Simonsick EM, Lafferty ME, Phillips CL, et al. Risk due to inactivity in physically capable older adults. *Am J Public Health* 1993;83:1443–1450.
13. Haapanen N, Miilunpalo S, Vuori I, Oja P, Pasanen M. Association of leisure time physical activity with the risk of coronary heart disease, hypertension and diabetes in middle-aged men and women. *Int J Epidemiol* 1997;26:739–747.
14. Sherman SE, D'Agostino RB, Cobb JL, Kannel WB. Does exercise reduce mortality rates in the elderly? Experience from the Framingham heart study. *Am Heart J* 1994;128:965–672.
15. Rodriguez BL, Curb JD, Burchfiel CM, et al. Physical activity and 23-year incidence of coronary heart disease morbidity and mortality among middle-aged men: the Honolulu heart program. *Circulation* 1994;89:2540–2544.
16. Eaton CB, Medalie JH, Flocke SA, Zyzanski SJ, Yaari S, Goldbourt U. Self-reported physical activity predicts long-term coronary heart disease and all-cause mortalities: 21-year follow-up of the Israeli ischemic heart disease study. *Arch Fam Med* 1995;4:323–329.
17. Stender M, Hense HW, Doring A, Keil U. Physical activity at work and cardiovascular disease risk: results from the MONICA Augsburg study. *Int J Epidemiol* 1993;22:644–650.
18. Leon AS, Myers MJ, Connett J. Leisure time physical activity and the 16-year risks of mortality from coronary heart disease and all-causes in the multiple risk factor intervention trial (MRFIT). *Int J Sports Med* 1997;18(suppl 3):208–315.
19. Rosolova H, Simon J, Sefrna F. Impact of cardiovascular risk factors on morbidity and mortality in Czech middle-aged men: Pilsen longitudinal study. *Cardiology* 1994;85:61–68.
20. Luoto R, Prattala R, Uutela A, Puska P. Impact of unhealthy behaviors on cardiovascular mortality in Finland, 1978–1993. *Prev Med* 1998;27:93–100.
21. Woo J, Ho SC, Yuen YK, Yu LM, Lau J. Cardiovascular risk factors and 18-month mortality and morbidity in an elderly Chinese population aged 70 years and over. *Gerontology* 1998;44: 51–55.
22. Gartside PS, Wang P, Glueck CJ. Prospective assessment of coronary heart disease risk factors: The NHANES I epidemiologic follow-up study (NHEFS) 16-year follow-up. *J Am Coll Nutr* 1998; 17:263–269.
23. Dorn JP, Cerny FJ, Epstein LH, Naughton J, et al. Work and leisure time physical activity and mortality in men and women from a general population sample. *Ann Epidemiol* 1999;9:366–373.
24. Hakim AA, Curb JD, Petrovitch H, et al. Effects of walking on coronary heart disease in elderly men: the Honolulu heart program. *Circulation* 1999; 100:9–13.
25. Eaton CB. Relation of physical activity and cardiovascular fitness to coronary heart disease, part II: cardiovascular fitness and the safety and efficacy of physical activity prescription. *J Am Board Fam Pract* 1992;5:157–165. Search date not stated; primary sources Medline and hand searches.
26. Blair SN, Kohl HW 3rd, Barlow CE, Paffenbarger RS Jr, Gibbons LW, Macera CA. Changes in physical fitness and all-cause mortality: a prospective study of healthy and unhealthy men. *JAMA* 1995;273:1093–1098.
27. Sacco RL, Gan R, Boden-Albala B, et al. Leisure-time physical activity and ischemic stroke risk: the Northern Manhattan stroke study. *Stroke* 1998; 29:380–387.
28. Shinton R. Lifelong exposures and the potential for stroke prevention: the contribution of cigarette smoking, exercise, and body fat. *J Epidemiol Community Health* 1997;51:138–143.
29. Gillum RF, Mussolino ME, Ingram DD. Physical activity and stroke incidence in women and men. The NHANES I epidemiologic follow-up study. *Am J Epidemiol* 1996;143:860–869.
30. Kiely DK, Wolf PA, Cupples LA, Beiser AS, Kannel WB. Physical activity and stroke risk: the Framingham study [correction appears in *Am J Epidemiol* 1995;141:178]. *Am J Epidemiol* 1994; 140:608–620.
31. Abbott RD, Rodriguez BL, Burchfiel CM, Curb JD. Physical activity in older middle-aged men and reduced risk of stroke: the Honolulu heart program. *Am J Epidemiol* 1994;139:881–893.
32. Haheim LL, Holme I, Hjermann I, Leren P. Risk

factors of stroke incidence and mortality: a 12-year follow-up of the Oslo study. *Stroke* 1993; 24:1484–1489.

33. Wannamethee G, Shaper AG. Physical activity and stroke in British middle aged men. *BMJ* 1992; 304:597–601.

34. Menotti A, Keys A, Blackburn H, et al. Twenty-year stroke mortality and prediction in twelve cohorts of the seven countries study. *Int J Epidemiol* 1990; 19:309–315.

35. Lindenstrom E, Boysen G, Nyboe J. Risk factors for stroke in Copenhagen, Denmark. II. Lifestyle factors. *Neuroepidemiology* 1993;12:43–50.

36. Lindenstrom E, Boysen G, Nyboe J. Lifestyle factors and risk of cerebrovascular disease in women: the Copenhagen City heart study. *Stroke* 1993;24:1468–1472.

37. Folsom AR, Prineas RJ, Kaye SA, Munger RG. Incidence of hypertension and stroke in relation to body fat distribution and other risk factors in older women. *Stroke* 1990;21:701–706.

38. Nakayama T, Date C, Yokoyama T, Yoshiike N, Yamaguchi M, Tanaka H. A 15.5-year follow-up study of stroke in a Japanese provincial city: the Shibata study. *Stroke* 1997;28:45–52.

39. Lee IM, Hennekens CH, Berger K, Buring JE, Manson JE. Exercise and risk of stroke in male physicians. *Stroke* 1999;30:1–6.

40. Evenson KR, Rosamond WD, Cai J, et al. Physical activity and ischemic stroke risk: the atherosclerosis in communities study. *Stroke* 1999;30:1333–1339.

41. Mittleman MA, Maclure M, Tofler GH, Sherwood JB, Goldberg RJ, Muller JE. Triggering of acute myocardial infarction by heavy physical exertion. Protection against triggering by regular exertion: determinants of myocardial infarction onset study investigators. *N Engl J Med* 1993;329:1677–1683.

42. Willich SN, Lewis M, Lowel H, Arntz HR, Schubert F, Schroder R. Physical exertion as a trigger of acute myocardial infarction: triggers and mechanisms of myocardial infarction study group. *N Engl J Med* 1993;329:1684–1690.

43. Pate RR, Pratt M, Blair SN, et al. Physical activity and public health. A recommendation from the Centers for Disease Control and Prevention and the American College of Sports Medicine. *JAMA* 1995;273:402–407.

44. Thompson PD. The cardiovascular complications of vigorous physical activity. *Arch Intern Med* 1996;156:2297–2302.

45. Oberman A. Exercise and the primary prevention of cardiovascular disease. *Am J Cardiol* 1985;55:10–20.

46. Andersen RE, Wadden TA, Bartlett SJ, Zemel B, Verde TJ, Franckowiak SC. Effects of lifestyle activity vs structured aerobic exercise in obese women: a randomized trial. *JAMA* 1999;281:335–340.

47. Dunn AL, Marcus BH, Kampert JB, Garcia ME, Kohl HW, Blair SN. Comparison of lifestyle and structured interventions to increase physical activity and cardiorespiratory fitness: a randomized trial. *JAMA* 1999;281:327–434.

48. Pereira MA, Kriska AM, Day RD, Cauley JA, LaPorte RE, Kuller LH. A randomized walking trial in postmenopausal women: effects on physical activity and health 10 years later. *Arch Intern Med* 1998;158:1695–1701.

49. DeBusk RF, Stenestrand U, Sheehan M, Haskell WL. Training effects of long versus short bouts of exercise in healthy subjects. *Am J Cardiol* 1990; 65:1010–1013.

50. Ness AR, Powles JW. Fruit and vegetables and cardiovascular disease: a review. *Int J Epidemiol* 1997;26:1–13. Search date 1995; primary

sources Medline, Embase, and hand searches of personal bibliographies, books, reviews, and citations in located reports.

51. Law MR, Morris JK. By how much does fruit and vegetable consumption reduce the risk of ischaemic heart disease? *Eur J Clin Nutr* 1998; 52:549–556. Search date not stated; primary sources Medline, Science Citation Index, and hand searches of review articles.

52. Klerk M, Jansen MCJF, van't Veer P, Kok FJ. *Fruits and vegetables in chronic disease prevention.* Wageningen: Grafisch Bedrijf Ponsen and Looijen, 1998. Search date 1998; primary sources Medline, Current Contents, and Toxline.

53. Key TJA, Thorogood M, Appleby PN, Burr ML. Dietary habits and mortality in 11 000 vegetarians and health conscious people: results of a 17 year follow up. *BMJ* 1996;313:775–779.

54. Pietinen P, Rimm EB, Korhonen P, et al. Intake of dietary fibre and risk of coronary heart disease in a cohort of Finnish men. *Circulation* 1996;94: 2720–2727.

55. Mann JI, Appleby PN, Key TJA, Thorogood M. Dietary determinants of ischaemic heart disease in health conscious individuals. *Heart* 1997;78:450–455.

56. Geleijnse M. Consumptie van groente en fruit en het risico op myocardinfarct 1997. Basisrapportage. Rotterdam: Erasmus Universiteit (cited in appendix XIII of review by Klerk).

57. Todd S, Woodward M, Tunstall-Pedoe H, Bolton-Smith C. Dietary antioxidant vitamins and fiber in the etiology of cardiovascular disease and all-cause mortality: results from the Scottish heart health study. *Am J Epidemiol* 1999;150:1073–1080.

58. Bazzano L, Ogden LG, Vupputuri S, Loria C, Myers L, Whelton PK. Fruit and vegetable intake reduces cardiovascular mortality: results from the NHANES I epidemiologic follow-up study (NHEFS). 40th Annual Conference Cardiovascular Epidemiology and Prevention [abstract] *Circulation* 2000;8–8.

59. Lui S, Manson JE, Cole SR, Willett WC, Buring JE. Fruit and vegetable intake and risk of cardiovascular disease. 40th Annual Conference Cardiovascular Epidemiology and Prevention [abstract] *Circulation* 2000;30–31.

60. Lui S, Lee I-M, Ajani U, Lui SR, Buring JE, Manson JE. Vegetable consumption and risk of coronary heart disease in men: results from the physicians health study. 40th Annual Conference Cardiovascular Epidemiology and Prevention [abstract] *Circulation* 2000;30–31.

61. Knekt P, Reunanen A, Jarvinen R, Heliovaara M, Aromaa A. Antioxidant vitamin intake and coronary mortality in a longitudinal population study. *Am J Epidemiol* 1994;139:1180–1189.

62. Keli SO, Hertog MGL, Feskens EJM, Kromhout D. Dietary flavonoids, antioxidant vitamins, and incidence of stroke. *Arch Intern Med* 1996;156: 637–642.

63. Daviglus ML, Orencia AJ, Dyer AR, et al. Dietary vitamin C, beta-carotene and 30-year risk of stroke: results from the Western Electric study. *Neuroepidemiology* 1997;16:69–77.

64. Ascherio A, Rimm EB, Hernan MA, et al. Prospective study of potassium intake and risk of stroke among US men. *Can J Cardiol* 1997;13: 44B.

65. Yochum L, Kushi LH, Meyer K, Folsom AR. Dietary flavonoid intake and risk of cardiovascular disease in postmenopausal women. *Am J Epidemiol* 1999; 149:943–949.

66. Knekt P, Isotupa S, Rissanen H, et al. Quercetin intake and the incidence of cerebrovascular disease. *Eur J Clin Nutr* 2000;54:415–417.

67. Joshipura KJ, Ascherio A, Manson JE, et al. Fruit

and vegetable intake in relation to risk of ischemic stroke. *JAMA* 1999;282:1233–1239.

68. Ness AR, Powles JW. Does eating fruit and vegetables protect against heart attack and stroke? *Chem Indus* 1996;792–794.

69. Ness AR, Powles JW. Dietary habits and mortality in vegetarians and health conscious people: several uncertainties exist. *BMJ* 1997;314:148.

70. Serdula MK, Byers T, Mokhad AH, Simoes E, Mendleim JM, Coates RJ. The association between fruit and vegetable intake and chronic disease risk factors. *Epidemiology* 1996;7:161–165.

71. Lonn EM, Yusuf S. Is there a role for antioxidant vitamins in the prevention of cardiovascular disease? An update on epidemiological and clinical trials data. *Can J Cardiol* 1997;13:957–965. Search date not stated; primary sources Medline, science citation index, handsearching.

72. Jha P, Flather M, Lonn E, Farkouh M, Yusuf S. The antioxidant vitamins and cardiovascular disease: a critical review of epidemiological and clinical trial data. *Ann Intern Med* 1995;123:860–872.

73. Roxrode KM, Manson JE. Antioxidants and coronary heart disease: observational studies. *J Cardiovasc Risk* 1996;3:363–367.

74. Egger M, Schneider M, Davey Smith G. Spurious precision? Meta-analysis of observational studies. *BMJ* 1998;316:140–144.

75. Gaziano JM. Randomized trials of dietary antioxidants in cardiovascular disease prevention and treatment. *J Cardiovasc Risk* 1996;3:368–371.

76. Ness AR, Powles JW, Khaw KT. Vitamin C and cardiovascular disease—a systematic review. *J Cardiovasc Risk* 1997;3:513–521. Search date 1996; primary sources Medline, Embase, and hand searches of personal bibliographies, books, reviews and citations in located reports.

77. Klipstein-Grobusch K, Geleijnse JM, den Breeijen JH, et al. Dietary antioxidants and risk of myocardial infarction in the elderly: the Rotterdam study. *Am J Clin Nutr* 1999;69:261–266.

78. Ascherio A, Rimm EB, Hernan MA, et al. Relation of consumption of vitamin E, vitamin C, and carotenoids to risk for stroke among men in the United States. *Ann Intern Med* 1999;130:963–970.

79. Li J, Taylor PR, Li B, et al. Nutrition intervention trials in Linxian, China: multiple vitamin/mineral supplementation, cancer incidence, and disease-specific mortality among adults with esophageal dysplasia. *J Natl Cancer Inst* 1993;85:1492–1498.

80. Mark SD, Wang W, Fraumeni JF, et al. Lowered risks of hypertension and cerebrovascular disease after vitamin/mineral supplementation. *Am J Epidemiol* 1996;143:658–664.

81. Mark SD, Wang W, Fraumeni JFJ, et al. Do nutritional supplements lower the risk of stroke or hypertension? *Epidemiology* 1998;9:9–15.

82. Losonczy KG, Harris TB, Havlik RJ. Vitamin E and vitamin C supplement use and risk of all-cause and coronary mortality in older persons: the established populations for epidemiologic studies of the elderly. *Am J Clin Nutr* 1996;64:190–196.

83. Sahyoun NR, Jacques PF, Russell RM. Carotenoids, vitamin C and E, and mortality in an elderly population. *Am J Epidemiol* 1996;144:501–511.

84. Keli SO, Hertog MGL, Feskens EJM, Kromhout D. Dietary flavonoids, antioxidant vitamins, and incidence of stroke. *Arch Intern Med* 1996;156:637–642.

85. Houtman JP. Trace elements and cardiovascular disease. *J Cardiovasc Risk* 1996;3:18–25.

86. Nève J. Selenium as a risk factor for cardiovascular disease. *J Cardiovasc Risk* 1996;3:42–47.

87. Hertog MGL, Feskens EJM, Holliman PCH, Katan MB, Kromhout D. Dietary antioxidant flavonoids and risk of coronary heart disease: the Zutphen elderly study. *Lancet* 1993;342:1007–1011.

88. Knekt P, Jarvinen R, Reunanen A, Maatela J. Flavonoid intake and coronary mortality in Finland: a cohort study. *BMJ* 1996;312:478–481.

89. Rimm EB, Katan MB, Ascherio A, Stampfer MJ, Willett WC. Relation between intake of flavonoids and risk for coronary heart disease in male health professionals. *Ann Intern Med* 1996;125:384–389.

90. Hertog MGL, Sweetnam PM, Fehily AM. Antioxidant flavonols and ischemic heart disease in a Welsh population of men: the Caerphilly study. *Am J Clin Nutr* 1997;65:1489–1494.

91. Doering WV. Antioxidant vitamins, cancer, and cardiovascular disease. *N Engl J Med* 1996;335:1065.

92. Pietrzik K. Antioxidant vitamins, cancer, and cardiovascular disease. *N Engl J Med* 1996;335:1065–1066.

93. Hennekens CH, Gaziano JM, Manson JE, Buring JE. Antioxidant vitamin cardiovascular disease hypothesis is still promising, but still unproven: the need for randomised trials. *Am J Clin Nutr* 1995;62(suppl):1377–1380.

94. Bates CJ, Thurnham DI, Bingham SA, Margetts BM, Nelson M. Biochemical markers of nutrient intake. In: Margetts BM, Nelson M, eds. *Design concepts in nutritional epidemiology*. Oxford: Oxford Medical Publications, 1991.

95. The Alpha-Tocopherol Beta Carotene Cancer Prevention Study Group. The effect of vitamin E and beta carotene on the incidence of lung cancer and other causes in male smokers. *N Engl J Med* 1994;330:1029–1035.

96. US Department of Health and Human Services. *The health benefits of smoking cessation: a report of the Surgeon General*. Rockville, Maryland: US Department of Health and Human Services, Public Health Service, Centers for Disease Control: 1990. DHHS Publication (CDC) 90–8416.

97. Royal College of Physicians. *Smoking and health now*. London: Pitman Medical and Scientific Publishing, 1971.

98. Doll R, Peto R, Wheatley K, Gray R, Sutherland I. Mortality in relation to smoking: 40 years' observations on male British doctors. *BMJ* 1994;309:901–911.

99. Kawachi I, Colditz GA, Stampfer MJ, et al. Smoking cessation in relation to total mortality rates in women: a prospective cohort study. *Ann Intern Med* 1993;119:992–1000.

100. Rosenberg L, Kaufman DW, Helmrich SP, Shapiro S. The risk of myocardial infarction after quitting smoking in men under 55 years of age. *N Engl J Med* 1985;313:1511–1514.

101. Rosenberg L, Palmer JR, Shapiro S. Decline in the risk of myocardial infarction among women who stop smoking. *N Engl J Med* 1990;322:213–217.

102. Rose G, Hamilton PJ, Colwell L, Shipley MJ. A randomised controlled trial of anti-smoking advice: 10-year results. *J Epidemiol Community Health* 1982;36:102–108.

103. Shinton R, Beevers G. Meta-analysis of relation between cigarette smoking and stroke. *BMJ* 1989;298:789–794. Search date 1988; primary source index references from three studies on cigarette smoking and stroke on medicine 1965–1988.

104. Rogot E, Murray JL. Smoking and causes of death among US veterans: 16 years of

observation. *Public Health Rep* 1980;95:213–222.

105. Wannamethee SG, Shaper AG, Ebrahim S. History of parental death from stroke or heart trouble and the risk of stroke in middle-aged men. *Stroke* 1996;27:1492–1498.

106. Halbert JA, Silagy CA, Finucane P, Withers RT, Hamdorf PA. The effectiveness of exercise training in lowering blood pressure: a meta-analysis of randomised controlled trials of 4 weeks or longer. *J Hum Hypertens* 1997;11:641–649. Search date 1996; primary sources Medline, Embase, Science Citation Index.

107. Ebrahim S, Davey Smith G. Lowering blood pressure: a systematic review of sustained non-pharmacological interventions. *J Public Health Med* 1998;20:441–448. Search date 1995; primary source Medline.

108. Engstom G, Hedblad B, Janzon L. Hypertensive men who exercise regularly have lower rate of cardiovascular mortality. *J Hypertens* 1999;17:737–742.

109. Appel LJ, Moore TJ, Obarzanek E, et al. A clinical trial of the effects of dietary patterns on blood pressure. *N Engl J Med* 1997;336:1117–1124.

110. Beilin LJ, Puddey IB, Burke V. Alcohol and hypertension: kill or cure? *J Hum Hypertens* 1996;10(suppl 2):1–5.

111. Campbell NRC, Ashley MJ, Carruthers SG, et al. Recommendations on alcohol consumption. *Can Med Assoc J* 1999;(suppl 9):13–20. Search date 1996; primary source Medline.

112. Graudal NA, Galloe AM, Garred P. Effects of sodium restriction on blood pressure, renin, aldosterone, catecholamines, cholesterols, and triglyceride. *JAMA* 1998;279:1383–1391. Search date 1997; primary source Medline.

113. Whelton PK, Appel LJ, Espelland MA, et al. Sodium reduction and weight loss in the treatment of hypertension in older persons: a randomized controlled trial of non pharmacologic interventions in the elderly (TONE). *JAMA* 1998;279:839–846.

114. Midgley JP, Matthew AG, Greenwood CMT, Logan AG. Effect of reduced dietary sodium on blood pressure. *JAMA* 1996;275:1590–1597. Search date 1994; primary sources Medline, Current Contents.

115. Alderman MH, Madhavan S, Cohen H, Sealey JE, Laragh JH. Low urinary sodium associated with greater risk of myocardial infarction among treated hypertensive men. *Hypertension* 1995; 25:1144–1152.

116. Brand MB, Mulrow CD, Chiquette E, et al. Weight-reducing diets for control of hypertension in adults. In: The Cochrane Library, Issue 4. Oxford: Update Software, 1998. Search date 1997; primary source Cochrane Library, Medline.

117. Whelton PK, He J, Cutler JA, et al. Effects of oral potassium on blood pressure: meta-analysis of randomized controlled clinical trials. *JAMA* 1997; 277:1624–1632. Search date 1995; primary source Medline.

118. Morris MC, Sacks F, Rosner B. Does fish oil lower blood pressure? A meta-analysis of controlled clinical trials. *Circulation* 1993;88:523–533. Search date not given; primary source Index Medicus.

119. Griffith LE, Guyatt GH, Cook RJ, et al. The influence of dietary and nondietary calcium supplementation on blood pressure. *Am J Hypertens* 1999;12:84–92. Search date 1994; primary sources Medline, Embase.

120. Gueyffier F, Froment A, Gouton M. New meta-analysis of treatment trials of hypertension: improving the estimate of therapeutic benefit. *J Hum Hypertens* 1996;10:1–8. Search date 1997; primary source Medline.

121. Staessen JA, Gasowski J, Wang JG, et al. Risks of untreated and treated isolated systolic hypertension in the elderly: meta-analysis of outcome trials. *Lancet* 2000;355:865–872. Search date 1999; primary sources other systematic reviews and reports from collaborative trialists.

122. Staessen JA, Fagard R, Thijs L, et al. Randomised double-blind comparison of placebo and active treatment for older patients with isolated systolic hypertension. *Lancet* 1997;350: 757–764.

123. The Heart Outcomes Prevention Evaluation Study Investigators. Effects of an angiotensin-converting-enzyme inhibitor, ramipril, on cardiovascular events in high-risk patients. *N Engl J Med* 2000;342:145–53.

124. Hansson L, Zanchetti AZ, Carruthers SG, et al. Effects of intensive blood pressure lowering and low-dose aspirin in patients with hypertension: principal results of the hypertension optimal treatment (HOT) trial. *Lancet* 1998;351:1755–1762.

125. Grossman E, Messerli FH, Goldbourt U. Does diuretic therapy increase the risk of renal cell carcinoma? *Am J Cardiol* 1999;83:1090–1093. Search dates 1966 to 1998; primary sources Medline.

126. Beto JA, Bansal VK. Quality of life in treatment of hypertension: a meta-analysis of clinical trials. *Am J Hypertens* 1992;5:125–133. Search date 1990; primary sources Medline, ERIC.

127. Croog SH, Levine S, Testa MA. The effects of antihypertensive therapy on quality of life. *N Engl J Med* 1986;314:1657–1664.

128. Psaty BM, Smith NS, Siscovick DS, et al. Health outcomes associated with antihypertensive therapies used as first line agents: a systematic review and meta-analysis. *JAMA* 1997;277:739–745. Search date 1995; primary source Medline.

129. Messerli FH, Grossman E, Goldbourt. Are beta blockers efficacious as first-line therapy for hypertension in the elderly? A systematic review. *JAMA* 1998;279:1903–1907. Search date 1998; primary source Medline.

130. Hansson L, Lindholm LH, Niskanen L et al. Effect of angiotensin-converting-enzyme inhibition compared with conventional therapy on cardiovascular morbidity and mortality in hypertension: the captopril prevention project (CAPP) randomised trial. *Lancet* 1999;353:611–616.

131. Hansson L, Lindholm L, Ekbom T, et al. Randomised trial of old and new antihypertensive drugs in elderly patients: cardiovascular mortality and morbidity the Swedish trial in old patients with hypertension-2 study. *Lancet* 1999;354: 1751–1756.

132. The ALLHAT Officers and Coordinators for the ALLHAT Collaborative Research Group. Major cardiovascular events in hypertensive patients randomized to doxazosin vs chlorthalidone: the antihypertensive and lipid-lowering treatment to prevent heart attack trial (ALLHAT). *JAMA* 2000; 283:1967–1975.

133. Neaton JD, Grimm RH, Prineas RJ, et al. Treatment of mild hypertension study: final results. *JAMA* 1993;270:713–724.

134. Materson BJ, Reda DJ, Cushman WC, et al. Single drug therapy for hypertension in men. *N Engl J Med* 1993;328:914–921.

135. Philipp T, Anlauf M, Distler A, Holzgreve H, Michaelis J, Wellek S. Randomised, double blind, multicentre comparison of hydrochlorothiazide, atenolol, nitrendipine, and enalapril in

antihypertensive treatment: results of the HANE study. *BMJ* 1997;315:154–159.

136. Wright JM, Lee CH, Chambers CK. Systematic review of antihypertensive therapies: does the evidence assist in choosing a first line drug? *Can Med Assoc J* 1999;161:25–32. Search date 1998; primary sources Medline 1996 to 1997, Cochrane Library to 1998.

137. Cutler JA. Calcium channel blockers for hypertension—uncertainty continues. *N Engl J Med* 1998;338:679–680.

138. Katerndahl DA, Lawler WR. Variability in meta-analytic results concerning the value of cholesterol reduction in coronary heart disease: a meta-meta-analysis. *Am J Epidemiol* 1999; 149:429–441. Search date 1995; primary sources Medline and meta-analysis bibliographies.

139. Froom J, Froom P, Benjamin M, Benjamin BJ. Measurement and management of hyperlipidemia for the primary prevention of coronary heart disease. *J Am Board Fam Pract* 1998;11:12–22.

140. Ebrahim S, Davey Smith G, McCabe CCC, et al. What role for statins? A review and economic model. *Health Technology Assessment* 1999;3: 19;1–91. Search dates 1997; primary sources Medline, Cochrane Controlled Trials Register, and personal contact with investigators working in the field of cholesterol lowering.

141. LaRosa JC, He J, Vupputuri S. Effect of statins on risk of coronary disease: a meta-analysis of randomized controlled trials. *JAMA* 1999;282: 2340–2346. Search date 1998; primary sources Medline, bibliographies and authors' reference files.

142. Downs JR, Clearfield M, Weis S, et al. Primary prevention of acute coronary events with lovastatin in men and women with average cholesterol levels: results of the AFCAPS/TexCAPS. *JAMA* 1998;279:1615–1622.

143. Scandinavian Simvastatin Survival Study Group. Randomized trial of cholesterol lowering in 4444 patients with coronary heart disease: the Scandinavian simvastatin survival study (4S). *Lancet* 1995;344:1383–1389.

144. Long-term Intervention with Pravastatin in Ischemic Disease (LIPID) Study Program. Prevention of cardiovascular events and death with pravastatin in patients with coronary heart disease and a broad range of initial cholesterol levels. *N Engl J Med* 1998;339:1349–1357.

145. Sacks FM, Pfeffer MA, Moye LA, et al for the Cholesterol and Recurrent Events Trial Investigators. Effect of pravastatin on coronary events after myocardial infarction in patients with average cholesterol levels. *N Engl J Med* 1996; 335:1001–1009.

146. Shepherd J, Cobbe SM, Ford I, et al for the West

of Scotland Coronary Prevention Study Group. Prevention of coronary heart disease with pravastatin in men with hypercholesterolemia. *N Engl J Med* 1995;333:1301–1307.

147. Gould AL, Rossouw JE, Santanello NC, Heyse JF, Furberg CD. Cholesterol reduction yields clinical benefit: impact of statin trials. *Circulation* 1998; 97:94–52.

148. Bucher HC, Griffith LE, Guyatt G. Systematic review on the risk and benefit of different cholesterol-lowering interventions. *Arterioscler Thromb Vasc Biol* 1999:19;187–195. Search date October 1996; primary sources Medline, Embase, and hand searches of bibliographies.

149. Carlsson CM, Carnes M, McBride PE, Stein JH. Managing dyslipidaemia in older adults. *J Am Geriatr Society* 1999;47:1458–1465.

150. Antiplatelet Trialists' Collaboration. Collaborative overview of randomised trials of antiplatelet therapy—I: prevention of death, myocardial infarction, and stroke by prolonged antiplatelet therapy in various categories of patients. *BMJ* 1994;308:81–106. Search date 1990; primary sources Medline, Current Contents, hand searches of reference lists of trials and review articles, journal abstracts and meeting proceedings, trial register of the International Committee on Thrombosis and Haemostasis, and personal contacts with colleagues and antiplatelet manufacturers.

151. Hart RG, Halperin JL, McBride R, Benavente O, Man-Son-Hing M, Kronmal RA. Aspirin for the primary prevention of stroke and other major vascular events. Meta-analysis and hypotheses. *Arch Neurol* 2000;57:326–332. Search date 1998; primary sources unspecified computerised medical databases 1980 to 1998, Cochrane Collaboration registry 1998, and hand searched references of Antiplatelet Trialists' Collaboration publications.

152. Medical Research Council's General Practice Research Framework. Thrombosis prevention trial: randomised trial of low-intensity anticoagulation with warfarin and low dose aspirin in the primary prevention of ischaemic heart disease in men at increased risk. *Lancet* 1998;351:233–241.

153. Peto R, Gray R, Collins R, et al. Randomised trial of prophylactic daily aspirin in British male doctors. *BMJ* 1988;296:313–316.

154. Steering Committee of the Physicians' Health Study Research Group. Final report on the aspirin component of the ongoing physicians' health study. *N Engl J Med* 1989;321:129–135.

155. Buring JE, Hennekens CH for the Women's Health Study Group. Women's health study: summary of the study design. *J Myocardial Ischemia* 1992;4:27–29

Michael Murphy
Director, ICRF General Practice Research Group

Charles Foster
British Heart Foundation Scientist

Cathie Sudlow
Specialist Registrar in Neurology
Department of Neurology, Derriford Hospital
Plymouth
UK

Rod Jackson
Associate Professor of Epidemiology
University of Auckland
Auckland
New Zealand

Julian Nicholas
Resident Physician
Mayo Clinic
Rochester
USA

Cindy Mulrow
Professor of Medicine
University of Texas Health Science Center
San Antonio
USA

Andy Ness
Senior Lecturer in Epidemiology
University of Bristol
Bristol
UK

Michael Pignone
Associate Professor of Medicine
Division of General Internal Medicine,
University of North Carolina
Chapel Hill
USA

Competing interests: CF, CS, MM none declared. CM has participated in multicentre research trials evaluating antihypertensive agents that were funded by industry.

TABLE 1 Examples of common physical activities by intensity of effort required in multiples of the resting rate of oxygen consumption during physical activity. Based on table from Pate et al (see text, p 56).[43]

Activity type	Light activity (< 3.0 METs)	Moderate activity (3.0–6.0 METs)	Vigorous activity (> 6.0 METs)
Walking	Slowly (1–2 mph)	Briskly (3–4 mph)	Briskly uphill or with a load
Swimming	Treading slowly	Moderate effort	Fast treading or swimming
Cycling	–	For pleasure or transport (≤ 10 mph)	Fast or racing (> 10 mph)
Golf	Power cart	Pulling cart or carrying clubs	–
Boating	Power boat	Canoeing leisurely	Canoeing rapidly (> 4 mph)
Home care	Carpet sweeping	General cleaning	Moving furniture
Mowing lawn	Riding mower	Power mower	Hand mower
Home repair	Carpentry	Painting	–

mph, miles per hour; METs, work metabolic rate/resting metabolic rate; 1 MET represents the rate of oxygen consumption of a seated adult at rest.

TABLE 2 Effectiveness of lifestyle interventions for lowering blood pressure in people with primary hypertension: results of RCTs (see text, pp 61, 62, 63).

Intervention	Mean decrease in syst/diast BP (mmHg)	Number of RCTs (people)	Participants	Duration (weeks)	Mean change in targeted factor
Exercise	5/3	29 (1533)	80% male, age 28–72	> 4	50 mins aerobic 3 x a week
Low fat high fruit and vegetable diet	5.5/3*	1 (459)	50% male, mean age 44	8	
Weight loss	3/3	18 (2611)	55% male, mean age 50	2–52	3–9% of body weight
Salt restriction	4/2	58 (2161)	Mean age 49	1–52	118 mmol/day
	2/0.5	28 (1131)	Mean age 47	4	60 mmol/day

* Data presented for 459 people with systolic BP below 160 mmHg and diastolic BP 80 to 95 mmHg; for the subgroup of 133 people with systolic BP ≥140 mmHg or diastolic BP ≥90 mmHg, the mean decrease of BP was 11.4/5.5; syst/diast BP, systolic/diastolic blood pressure.

TABLE 3 Effectiveness of dietary supplementation for lowering blood pressure in people with primary hypertension: results of RCTs (see text, pp 64, 65).

Intervention	Decrease in syst/diast BP (mmHg)	Number of RCTs (people)	Participants	Duration	Change in targeted factor
Potassium supplement	4.4/2.5	21 (1560)	Age 19–79	1–24 weeks	60–100 mmol/day
Fish oil supplement	4.5/2.5	7 (339)	Mean age 50	Mean 8 weeks	3 g/day or more
Calcium supplement	2/0	12 (383)	Not clear	8 weeks median	800–1500 mg/day

TABLE 4 Effects of antiplatelet treatment (mainly aspirin) on vascular events (non-fatal myocardial infarction, non-fatal stroke, or vascular death) in RCTs among individuals without evidence of cardiovascular disease (see text, pp 70, 71).

Trials*	Antiplatelet (events/patients) (%)	Controls (events/patients) (%)	Odds ratio (CI†)	Approx average duration of treatment (years)	Approx control group risk (per year)	Approx vascular events avoided per 1000 patients treated per year (95% CI)
APT[150] (3 trials)	652/14 608 (4.5%)	708/14 604 (4.8%)	0.90 (0.77 to 1.05)	5.2‡	0.9%	0.7
TPT[152]	211/2545 (8.3%)	250/2540 (9.8%)	0.83 (0.64 to 1.07)	6.4	1.5%	2.4
HOT[124]	315/9399 (3.4%)	368/9391 (3.9%)	0.85 (0.70 to 1.04)	3.8	1.0%	1.5
All trials	**1178/26553 (4.4%)**	**1326/26535 (5.0%)**	**0.87 (0.80 to 0.95)**	**5.0‡**	**1.0%**	**1.1 (0.4 to 1.8)**

*Published data from TPT and HOT; data provided by trialists for trials in the APT overview.
†99% CI for 1994 APT overview, TPT and HOT; 95% CI for "all trials".
‡Weighted by study size. The proportional effects of aspirin were similar in the absence or presence of warfarin, so the data presented are not stratified by warfarin allocation. Heterogeneity of ORs between five trials: χ^2 (4 df) = 4.5; NS.

TABLE 5 Effects of aspirin on intracranial bleeds and major extracranial bleeds in RCTs among individuals without evidence of cardiovascular disease (see text, pp 70, 71).

	Antiplatelet (events/patient) (%)	Controls (events/patients) (%)	Approx average duration of treatment (years)	Approx excess bleeds per 1000 patients treated per year (95% CI)
Intracranial bleeds				
APT[150] (2 trials)	44/14466 (0.3%)	24/14454 (0.2%)	5.2	
TPT[152]	12/2545 (0.5%)	6/2540 (0.2%)	6.4	
HOT[124]	14/9399 (0.1%)	165/9391 (0.2%)	3.8	
All trials	**70/26410 (0.3%)**	**45/26385 (0.2%)**	**5.0**	**0.2 (0.02 to 0.4)**
Major extracranial bleeds				
APT[150] (2 trials)	69/14466 (0.5%)	49/14454 (0.3%)	5.2	
TPT[152]	20/2545 (0.8%)	13/2540 (0.5%)	6.4	
HOT[124]	122/9399 (1.3%)	63/9391 (0.7%)	3.8	
All trials	**211/26410 (0.8%)**	**125/26385 (0.5%)**	**5.0**	**0.7 (0.4 to 0.9)**

Primary prevention

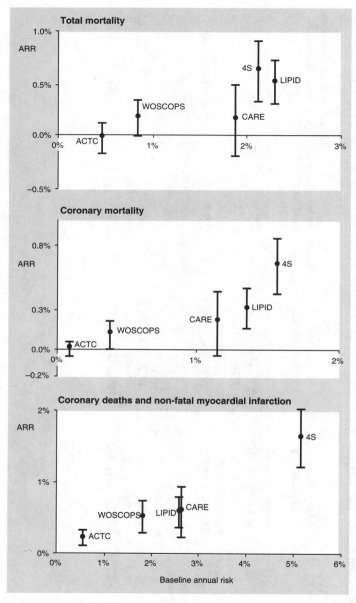

Effects of cholesterol lowering: relation between the ARR (for annual rates of total mortality, coronary heart disease mortality and coronary deaths and non-fatal myocardial infarction in patients treated with statins) and the baseline risk of those events in the placebo group for each of the five large statin trials (ACTC = AFCAPS/TexCAPS[142], 4S[143], LIPID[144], CARE[145], WOSCOPS[146]) (see text, p 69).

Updated this issue

Clinical Evidence writers on secondary prevention of ischaemic cardiac events

Key Messages

Antithrombotic treatment

- One collaborative overview has found that antiplatelet treatment reduces the risk of serious vascular events. Evidence from this overview and subsequent RCTs suggests that aspirin 75 mg daily is as effective as higher doses. We found no clear evidence that any other antiplatelet regimen is definitely superior to medium dose aspirin (that is, 75–325 mg daily) in the prevention of vascular events. One systematic review found that clopidogrel is a safe and effective alternative to aspirin.

■ One systematic review has found that anticoagulants produce a similar reduction in the risk of serious vascular events to that produced by aspirin. However, aspirin is associated with a lower risk of haemorrhage compared with oral anticoagulants. The systematic review found no clear evidence that the addition of oral anticoagulants to aspirin produced additional benefit.

Other drug treatments

■ Systematic reviews have found that:
  • β Blockers reduce the risk of all causes of mortality, coronary mortality, recurrent non-fatal myocardial infarction (MI), and sudden death in people after MI.
  • In people who have had an MI with or without left ventricular dysfunction, ACE inhibitors reduce rates of death, hospitalisation for congestive heart failure, and recurrent non-fatal MI.
  • Using class I antiarrhythmic agents after MI increases the risk of cardiovascular mortality and sudden death.
  • Amiodarone reduces the risk of sudden death and marginally reduces overall mortality in people at high risk of death after MI. We found limited evidence that D-sotalol may be harmful rather than beneficial in this setting.
  • Calcium channel blockers do not reduce mortality in people after MI or with chronic coronary heart disease. Diltiazem and verapamil may reduce rates of reinfarction and refractory angina in people after MI who do not have heart failure.

■ Data from the only large well designed RCT of hormone replacement therapy (HRT) published to date provide no evidence that it reduces major cardiovascular events in postmenopausal women with established coronary artery disease, despite strong evidence from RCTs that HRT improves some cardiovascular risk factors.

Cholesterol reduction

■ One systematic review has found that lowering cholesterol with statins substantially reduces the risk of cardiovascular mortality and morbidity with no evidence of an increase in non-cardiovascular mortality.

Blood pressure reduction

■ We found no direct evidence of the effects of lowering blood pressure in people with established coronary heart disease. Observational studies and extrapolation from trials of blood pressure reduction in people with no history of ischaemic cardiac events support the lowering of blood pressure in those with concomitant risk factors that put them at higher risk. The evidence for benefit is strongest for β blockers.

Non-drug treatments

■ The role of vitamin E, β carotene, and vitamin C remains unclear.

■ RCTs have found that advising people with coronary artery disease to eat more fish (particularly fatty fish) or more fruit and vegetables, bread, pasta, potatoes, olive oil, and rapeseed margarine (that is, a more Mediterranean diet) may result in a substantial survival benefit. We found no strong evidence from RCTs for a beneficial effect of low fat or high fibre diets on major non-fatal coronary heart disease events or coronary heart disease mortality.

- Systematic reviews have found that cardiac rehabilitation improves coronary risk factors and reduces the risk of major cardiac events in people after MI. The role of exercise alone in reducing the risk of adverse cardiovascular outcomes is not clear.

- We found no RCTs of the effects of smoking cessation on cardiovascular events in people with coronary heart disease. Epidemiological studies have found that people with coronary heart disease who stop smoking rapidly reduce their risk of recurrent coronary events or death. The use of nicotine patches seems safe in people with coronary heart disease.

- One systematic review of mainly poor quality RCTs has found that psychological and stress management may decrease rates of MI or cardiac death in people with coronary heart disease.

Surgical treatments

- RCTs performed up to the mid 1980s found that, compared with medical treatment, coronary artery bypass grafting carried a greater risk of death in the first year but reduced the risk of death from coronary artery disease at 5 and 10 years. Greatest benefit occurred in people with more severe disease (multivessel disease, left ventricular dysfunction, or MI). We found no evidence of increased protection against subsequent MI. One more recent RCT, using modern techniques and with optimal background medical treatment, found even greater superiority of surgical revascularisation over non-invasive treatment.

- RCTs found that, in comparison with percutaneous transluminal coronary angioplasty (PTA), intracoronary stents afforded superior acute and long term clinical and angiographic results.

DEFINITION	Secondary prevention in this context is the long term management of people with a prior acute myocardial infarction (MI), and of people at high risk of ischaemic cardiac events for other reasons such as a history of angina or coronary surgical procedures.
INCIDENCE/ PREVALENCE	Coronary artery disease is the leading cause of death in developed countries and is becoming a major cause of mortality and morbidity in developing countries. There are pronounced international, regional, and temporal differences in death rates. In the USA, the prevalence of overt coronary artery disease approaches 4%.[1]
AETIOLOGY/ RISK FACTORS	Most ischaemic cardiac events are associated with atheromatous plaques that can cause acute obstruction of coronary vessels. Atheroma is more likely in elderly people, in those with established coronary artery disease, and in those with risk factors (such as smoking, hypertension, high cholesterol, diabetes mellitus).
PROGNOSIS	Almost half of those who suffer an acute MI die before they reach hospital. Of those hospitalised, 7–15% die in hospital and another 7–15% die during the following year. Observational studies suggest a decline in 1 year mortality in the last decade of life.[2] People who survive the acute stage of MI fall into three prognostic groups, based on their baseline risk (see table 1, p 112):[3–5] high (20% of all survivors), moderate (55%), and low (25%) risk. Long term prognosis depends on the degree of left ventricular dysfunction, the presence of residual ischaemia, and the extent of any electrical instability. Further risk stratification procedures include evaluation of left ventricular function (by echocardiography or nuclear ventriculography) and of myocardial ischaemia (by non-invasive stress

testing).[5-9] Those with low left ventricular ejection fraction, ischaemia, or poor functional status may be evaluated further by cardiac catheterisation.[10]

AIMS	To improve long term survival and quality of life; to prevent (recurrent) MI, unstable angina, left ventricular dysfunction, heart failure, and sudden cardiac death; and to restore and maintain normal activities.
OUTCOMES	Mortality (total, cardiovascular, coronary, sudden death, non-cardiovascular), morbidity (MI, severe angina, and stroke), or quality of life.
METHODS	*Clinical Evidence* update search and appraisal May 2000.

QUESTION What are the effects of antithrombotic treatment?

Cathie Sudlow

Updated this issue

OPTION ANTIPLATELET TREATMENT

One collaborative overview has found that prolonged antiplatelet treatment reduces the risk of serious vascular events in people at high risk of ischaemic cardiac events. Along with subsequent RCTs, it found that, for prolonged use, aspirin 75 mg daily is as effective as higher doses. We found no clear evidence that any other antiplatelet regimen is superior to medium dose aspirin (that is, 75–325 mg daily) to prevent vascular events, although one RCT has found that clopidogrel appears to be a safe and effective alternative.

Benefits: **Antiplatelet treatment versus control:** One collaborative overview, published in 1994, found that a month or more of antiplatelet treatment significantly reduced the odds of a vascular event (non-fatal MI, non-fatal stroke, or vascular death) by about one quarter compared with control, among about 70 000 people at high risk of occlusive arterial disease (odds reduction 27%, 95% CI 24% to 30%).[11] Most of these people were at high risk of ischaemic cardiac events, and some people (including those with a history of MI, those with stable angina, and those who had undergone coronary revascularisation procedures) were at particularly high risk. Among the 20 000 people with a prior MI, antiplatelet treatment prevented 18 non-fatal recurrent MIs, six non-fatal strokes, and 13 vascular deaths per 1000 people treated for about 2 years. The review also found that antiplatelet treatment reduced all cause mortality (see figure 1, p 113). **Different daily doses of aspirin:** Around two thirds of the RCTs in the overview involved an aspirin regimen, and medium dose aspirin (75–325 mg daily) was the most widely tested of these. Indirect comparisons found that daily doses of < 160 mg (mostly 75–150 mg), 160–325 mg, and 500–1500 mg prevented similar proportions of vascular events among high risk people, while direct comparisons also showed that daily aspirin doses of 75–325 mg or 500–1500 mg were similarly effective.[11] One additional recent RCT directly compared lower doses of aspirin (81 mg or 325 mg daily) with higher doses (650 mg or 1300 mg) in almost

3000 people at high risk of cardiovascular events. It found no significant difference between lower and higher doses for rate of stroke, MI or death (5.4% with lower dose v 7.0% with higher; P = 0.07).[12] The review found only limited evidence for the effectiveness of daily doses of aspirin of less than 160 mg. One subsequent RCT compared aspirin 75 mg daily with placebo in 2000 people with unstable angina.[13] It found that a daily dose of aspirin 75 mg reduced the composite outcome of MI or sudden death compared with placebo (RRR 34%, 95% CI 24% to 49%). **Alternative antiplatelet regimens to aspirin:** The 1994 review found no evidence that any antiplatelet regimen was more effective than medium dose aspirin alone in the prevention of vascular events.[11] One systematic review of randomised trials (search date March 1999) comparing either ticlopidine or clopidogrel with aspirin found four trials among 22 656 people at high risk of vascular disease (including 6000 presenting with recent MI).[14] Most of these people were included in large trial of clopidogrel (75 mg daily) versus aspirin (325 mg daily).[15] Compared with aspirin, the thienopyridines reduced the odds of a vascular event by 9% (OR 0.91; 95% CI 0.84 to 0.98; 2P = 0.01), but there was substantial uncertainty about the size of any additional benefit (11 events prevented per 1000 people treated for about 2 years, (95% CI 2 to 19 events).[14]

Harms: Bleeding is the most important adverse effect of antiplatelet treatment. The 1994 overview found that the excess risk of intracranial bleeding with antiplatelet treatment was small (at most one or two bleeds per 1000 people per year) in trials of long term treatment.[11] Antiplatelet treatment produced a small but significant excess of non-fatal major extracranial bleeds (three bleeds per 1000 people), but there was no clear excess of fatal extracranial bleeds.[11] In one RCT directly comparing two different doses of aspirin, 1200 mg daily was associated with more gastrointestinal bleeding than 325 mg daily,[16] although we found no good evidence for a variation in gastrointestinal bleeding risk in the range 75–325 mg daily. The systematic review of randomised trials of the thienopyridine derivatives versus aspirin found that the thienopyridines produced significantly less gastrointestinal haemorrhage and upper gastrointestinal upset than aspirin. However, they increased the odds of skin rash and of diarrhoea: ticlopidine by about twofold and clopidogrel by about one third. Ticlopidine (but not clopidogrel) increased the odds of neutropenia.[14] Observational studies have also found that ticlopidine is associated with thrombocytopenia and thrombotic purpura.[17,18] We found no clear evidence of an excess of haematological adverse side effects with clopidogrel.[19,20]

Comment: Among people at high risk of cardiac events, the large absolute reductions in serious vascular events far outweighed any absolute risks.

OPTION	ORAL ANTICOAGULANTS IN THE ABSENCE OF ANTIPLATELET TREATMENT

One systematic review has found that high or moderate intensity oral anticoagulants given alone reduce the risk of serious vascular events in

people with coronary artery disease, but were associated with substantial risks of bleeding. Oral anticoagulants require regular monitoring for intensity of anticoagulant effect.

Benefits: One systematic overview of the effects of oral anticoagulation in people with coronary artery disease found 16 trials of high intensity anticoagulation (INR > 2.8) versus control in 10 056 people, and four trials of moderate intensity anticoagulation (INR 2–3) versus control in 1365 people. Antiplatelet therapy was not routinely given in any of these 20 trials. The review found that high intensity anticoagulation reduced the odds of the combined outcome of death, MI or stroke compared with control (odds reduction 43%, 95% CI 37% to 49%, about 98 events avoided per 1000 people treated). Compared with control, moderate intensity anticoagulation reduced these odds by a somewhat smaller, non-significant amount.[21] In direct comparisons of high or moderate intensity oral anticoagulation with aspirin, the effects on death, MI or stroke were similar (OR 1.04; 95% CI 0.80 to 1.34).[21]

Harms: Compared with control, high intensity anticoagulation increased the odds of major (mainly extracranial) bleeding about sixfold (OR 6.0, 95% CI 4.4 to 8.2, absolute increase of 39 events per 1000 people treated), and moderate intensity anticoagulation also increased the odds of major bleeding about eightfold (OR 7.7, 95% CI 3.3 to 17.6).[21] Compared with aspirin, high or moderate intensity oral anticoagulation increased the odds of major bleeding more than twofold (OR 2.4, 95% CI 1.6 to 3.6).[21]

Comment: Oral anticoagulants provide substantial protection against vascular events in the absence of antiplatelet therapy, but the risks of serious bleeding are higher than for antiplatelet treatment, and regular monitoring is required. Medium dose aspirin provides similar protection, but is safer and easier to use; see antiplatelet treatment, p 86.

OPTION   ORAL ANTICOAGULANTS IN ADDITION TO ANTIPLATELET TREATMENT

One systematic review found no evidence that the addition of low intensity oral anticoagulation (target INR < 1.5) to aspirin produces additional benefit. The effects of adding a more intensive anticoagulant regimen (target INR 2–3) are uncertain.

Benefits: One systematic overview found six RCTs that examined the effects of adding an oral anticoagulant regimen to aspirin in 8915 people with coronary artery disease. Three of these trials assessed the addition of a low intensity (target INR < 1.5) regimen to aspirin in a total of 8435 people, and found no significant reduction in the odds of death, MI or stroke (OR 0.91; 95% CI 0.79 to 1.06).[21] Trials assessing the addition of a moderate intensity (INR 2–3) oral anticoagulant regimen to aspirin were too small (total n = 480) to produce reliable estimates of efficacy and safety.[21]

Harms: Too few major bleeds have been recorded in RCTs to quantify reliably the effects of adding oral anticoagulants to aspirin. The review found a non-significant excess of major bleeds produced by the addition of low intensity oral anticoagulation to aspirin (OR 1.29; 95% CI 0.96 to 1.75), as well as by the addition of more intense anticoagulation (OR 1.88; 95% CI 0.59 to 6.00).[21]

Comment: The issue of whether adding a moderately intense oral anticoagulant regimen to aspirin provides additional net benefit to people at high risk of ischaemic cardiac events is being assessed in several ongoing RCTs (CHAMP, WARIS-2, ASPECT-2).

QUESTION **What are the effects of other drug treatments?**

Eva Lonn

Updated this issue

OPTION β BLOCKERS

We found strong evidence from systematic reviews of RCTs that β blockers reduce the risk of all cause mortality, coronary mortality, recurrent non-fatal MI, and sudden death in people after MI. Most benefit was seen in those at highest risk of death after an MI (> 50 years old; previous MI, angina pectoris, hypertension, or treatment with digitalis; transient mechanical or electrical failure; higher heart rate at study entry). About a quarter of people suffered adverse effects.

Benefits: **Survival and reinfarction:** One systematic review, published in 1993, identified 26 RCTs in over 24 000 people in whom β blockers were started orally within days or weeks of an acute MI (late intervention trials) and continued for between 6 weeks to 3 years. Most trials followed participants for 1 year. The review found improved survival in people given β blockers (RRR 23%, 95% CI 14% to 30%).[22] One prior systematic review, published in 1985, identified 24 RCTs of long term use of β blockers after MI. It found that, compared with placebo, β blockers reduced total mortality (RRR about 20%, NNT 48), sudden death (RRR about 30%, NNT 63), and non-fatal reinfarction (RRR about 25%, NNT 56).[23] **Anginal symptoms:** We found no good RCTs evaluating the antianginal effects of β blockers in people after MI. One trial found atenolol more effective than placebo in people with chronic stable effort angina or silent ischaemia.[24] **Different types of β blockers:** The earlier review found no differences between β blockers with and without cardioselectivity or membrane stabilising properties, but it raised concerns about the lack of efficacy of β blockers with intrinsic sympathomimetic activity in long term management after MI.[23] One RCT in 607 people at high risk after MI found that acebutolol, a β blocker with moderate partial agonist activity, decreased 1 year mortality compared with placebo (AR of death: 11% with placebo, 6% with acebutolol; RRR 48%, 95% CI 9% to 71%).[25] **Effects in different subgroups:** One systematic review (search date 1983) evaluated 1 year mortality in clinically relevant subgroups.[26] It identified nine RCTs comparing placebo with β blockers started > 24 hours after onset of symptoms of acute MI and continued for 9–24 months. Pooled analysis of individual person data (n = 13 679) found that the beneficial effects of β blockers on mortality seemed comparable in men and women. The highest absolute benefit from β blockers was seen in subgroups with the highest baseline risks (that is, those with the highest mortality on placebo): those over 50 years of age; those with a history of previous MI, angina pectoris, hypertension, or treatment with digitalis; those with transient signs or symptoms of mechanical or electrical failure in the early phases of MI; and those with a higher heart rate at study entry. Low risk subgroups had smaller absolute benefit, which was inconsistent across trials.

Harms: Adverse effects include shortness of breath, bronchospasm, bradycardia, hypotension, heart block, cold hands and feet, diarrhoea, fatigue, reduced sexual activity, depression, nightmares, faintness, insomnia, blacking out, and hallucinations. Rates vary in different studies. One RCT reported an absolute risk increase for any adverse effect on propranolol compared with placebo of 24% (95% CI not available). Serious adverse effects were uncommon and only a small proportion of people withdrew as a result.[27]

Comment: Continued benefit has been reported from the use of β blockers up to 6 years after MI (ARR for mortality 5.9%, 95% CI not available, P = 0.003; RRR 18%). However, the study was not blinded after 33 months.

OPTION   ANGIOTENSIN CONVERTING ENZYME (ACE) INHIBITORS

In people who have had an MI and have left ventricular dysfunction, there is strong evidence from a systematic review of RCTs that ACE inhibitors reduce rates of death, hospitalisation for congestive heart failure, and recurrent non-fatal MI. The effects of ACE inhibitors in people who have had an MI but do not have left ventricular dysfunction have not yet been adequately evaluated.

Benefits: **In people with low left ventricular ejection fraction:** One systematic review,[28] published in 1997, identified three RCTs comparing placebo with ACE inhibitors (captopril, ramipril, or trandolapril) started 3–16 days after acute MI and continued for 15–42 months. It analysed individual data from 5966 people with a recent MI and with clinical manifestations of congestive heart failure or moderate left ventricular dysfunction (left ventricular ejection fraction ≥35–40%). ACE inhibitors significantly reduced rates of death (RRR 26%, 95% CI 17% to 34%; NNT 17 people treated for about 2 years to prevent one death), hospitalisation for congestive heart failure (RRR 27%, 95% CI 15% to 37%; NNT 28), and recurrent non-fatal MI (RRR 20%, 95% CI 6% to 31%; NNT 43). **In people without impaired ventricular function or evidence of congestive heart failure:** We found no systematic review. We found one large RCT in 9297 people at high risk of cardiovascular events, which found that the ACE inhibitor ramipril (10 mg/day) reduced the composite primary outcome of cardiovascular death, stroke or MI compared with placebo over an average of 4.7 years (RRR for composite outcome, ramipril v placebo 22%, NNT 26; RRR for cardiovascular death 26%, NNT 50; RRR for MI 20%, NNT 42; RRR for stroke 32%, NNT 67; RRR for death from all causes 16%, NNT 56). In addition, the trial found that ramipril reduced the need for revascularisation procedures and reduced heart failure related outcomes (need for revascularisation: RRR 15%, no CI provided; heart failure related outcomes: RRR 23%, no CI provided). The trial found benefit of ACE inhibitor over placebo in all subgroups examined, including women and men, people over and under 65 years of age, those with and without a history of coronary artery disease, with and without a history of hypertension, with and without a history of diabetes, with and without a history of peripheral vascular disease, with and without a history of cerebrovascular disease, and those with and without microalbuminuria at study entry.[29] **In people with diabetes:** We found one RCT (see cardiovascular disease in diabetes under antihypertensive treatment, p 295).[30]

Harms: The major adverse effects reported in these trials were cough (ARI versus placebo of 5–10%), dizziness, hypotension (5–10%), renal failure ($< 3\%$), hyperkalaemia ($< 3\%$), angina, syncope, diarrhoea (2%) and, for captopril, alteration in taste (2% of captopril users).[28]

Comment: There are several other ongoing large RCTs evaluating the use of ACE inhibitors in people without clinical manifestations of heart failure and with no or with mild impairment in left ventricular systolic function. These include one trial of trandolapril in 8000 people with coronary artery disease, and one trial of perindopril in 10 500 people with stable coronary artery disease.[31]

OPTION   CLASS I ANTIARRHYTHMIC AGENTS (QUINIDINE, PROCAINAMIDE, DISOPYRIMIDE, ENCAINIDE, FLECAINIDE, MORIZICINE)

One systematic review of RCTs has found that the use of class I antiarrhythmic agents after MI increases the risk of cardiovascular mortality and sudden death.

Benefits: None (see harms below).

Harms: One systematic review, published in 1993, identified 51 RCTs comparing placebo with class I antiarrhythmic drugs, given both acutely and later in the management of MI, in 23 229 people.[22] The review found that the antiarrhythmic agents increased mortality (AR of death 5.6% v 5.0% with placebo, OR 1.14, 95% CI 1.01 to 1.28). One RCT compared encainide or flecainide with placebo in 1498 people with MI and with asymptomatic or mildly symptomatic ventricular arrhythmia. After 10 months of follow up, it found that these agents increased the risk of death or cardiac arrest (RR 2.38, 95% CI 1.59 to 3.57), equivalent to one additional death or cardiac arrest for every 17 people treated for about 10 months with encainide or flecainide rather than placebo.[32]

Comment: The evidence implies that these drugs should not be used in people after MI or with significant coronary artery disease.

OPTION   CLASS III ANTIARRHYTHMIC AGENTS (AMIODARONE, D-SOTALOL)

Two systematic reviews of RCTs have found that amiodarone reduces the risk of sudden death and marginally reduces overall mortality in people at high risk of death after MI. Limited evidence on the effects of D-sotalol suggests that it may be harmful rather than beneficial in this setting.

Benefits: One systematic review, published in 1997, analysed individual person data from 13 RCTs of amiodarone in high risk people. A total of 6553 people were involved; 78% with a recent MI from eight trials, and 22% with congestive heart failure from five trials.[33] Most trials were placebo controlled with a mean follow up of about 1.5 years. Participants were selected with a recent MI and a high risk of death from cardiac arrhythmia (based on low left ventricular ejection fraction, frequent ventricular premature depolarisations or non-sustained ventricular tachycardia, but no history of sustained symptomatic ventricular tachycardia or ventricular fibrillation). Participants with congestive heart failure were symptomatic but stable and did not have a recent MI, although in most cases the heart failure was ischaemic in origin. All trials used a loading dose of amiodarone (400 mg/day for 28 days or 800 mg/day for 14 days) followed by a maintenance dose (200–400 mg/day). Amiodarone significantly reduced total mortality (ARs 10.9% per year on amiodarone, 12.3% per year with placebo; RRR 13%, 95% CI 1% to 22%; NNT 71 people treated per year to avoid one additional death) and rates of sudden cardiac death (RRR 29%, 95% CI 15% to 41%; NNT 59). Amiodarone had similar effects in the post MI and congestive heart failure studies. Comparable findings emerged from another systematic review, published in 1997, which reviewed amiodarone trials in 5864 people with MI, congestive heart failure, left ventricular dysfunction, or cardiac arrest.[34]

Harms: Adverse events leading to discontinuation of amiodarone, and expressed per 100 person years, were hypothyroidism (7.0 v 1.1 on placebo; OR 7.3), hyperthyroidism (1.4 v 0.5; OR 2.5), peripheral neuropathy (0.5 v 0.2; OR 2.8), lung infiltrates (1.6 v 0.5; OR 3.1), bradycardia (2.4 v 0.8; OR 2.6), and liver dysfunction (1.0 v 0.4; OR 2.7).[33]

Comment: The reviews' conclusions are probably specific to amiodarone.[33,34] One RCT found increased mortality with the class III antiarrhythmic agent D-sotalol compared with placebo in 3121 people with MI and left ventricular dysfunction (ARs for death 5% v 3.1%; RR 1.65, 95% CI 1.15 to 2.36). The trial was terminated prematurely after less than 1 year of follow up.[35] The two largest RCTs of amiodarone after MI found a favourable interaction between β blockers and amiodarone with additional reduction in cardiac mortality.[36,37]

OPTION   CALCIUM CHANNEL BLOCKERS

One systematic review of RCTs found no benefit from calcium channel blockers in people after MI or with chronic coronary heart disease. Diltiazem and verapamil may reduce rates of reinfarction and refractory angina in people after MI who do not have heart failure.

Benefits: One systematic review (search date 1993) identified 24 RCTs of calcium channel blockers (including dihydropyridines, diltiazem, and verapamil) administered early or late during the course of acute MI or unstable angina and continued in the intermediate or long term.[22] Two of the trials used angiographic regression of coronary stenosis as an outcome in people with stable coronary heart disease treated with calcium channel blockers. The review found no significant difference in the absolute risk of death compared with placebo (AR 9.7% v 9.3%; ARI on calcium channel blockers compared with placebo 0.4%, 95% CI −0.4% to +1.2%; OR 1.04, 95% CI 0.95 to 1.14). **Diltiazem and verapamil:** The review found no significant effect compared with placebo (OR 0.95, 95% CI 0.82 to 1.09).[22] Three trials comparing diltiazem or verapamil with placebo reported benefit on active treatment (decreased rates of recurrent infarction and refractory angina) but only for those people without signs or symptoms of heart failure. For those with clinical manifestations of heart failure, the trends were towards harm.[38–40] **Dihydropyridines:** The review found no significant effect compared with placebo (OR 1.16, 95% CI 0.99 to 1.35). Several individual RCTs of dihydropyridines found increased mortality, particularly when these agents were started early in the course of acute MI and in the absence of β blockers.

Harms: Adverse effects reported of verapamil and diltiazem include atrioventricular block, atrial bradycardia, new onset heart failure, hypotension, dizziness, oedema, rash, constipation, and pruritus.

Comment: Newer generation dihydropyridines, such as amlodipine and felodipine, have not been well studied in people after MI but have been found to be safe in people with heart failure, including heart failure of ischaemic origin.

OPTION   **HORMONE REPLACEMENT THERAPY**

We found no clear evidence from RCTs that HRT reduces major cardiovascular events in postmenopausal women with established coronary artery disease, despite strong evidence from RCTs that HRT improves some cardiovascular risk factors.

Benefits: **Combined oestrogen and progestins:** We found no systematic review. One large RCT has evaluated the effects of oestrogens plus progestins on clinical outcomes in 2763 postmenopausal women with coronary heart disease.[41] It compared placebo with conjugated equine oestrogen 0.625 mg/day plus medroxyprogesterone acetate 2.5 mg/day for an average of 4.1 years, and found no differences in rates of non-fatal MI or deaths caused by coronary heart disease (event occurred in 172 women with HRT and 176 women with placebo; RRR compared with placebo 1%, 95% CI −2.2% to +2.0%). It also found no difference in the other secondary cardiovascular outcomes (coronary revascularisation, unstable angina, congestive heart failure, resuscitated cardiac arrest, stroke or transient ischaemic attack, and peripheral arterial disease) or in all cause mortality. **Oestrogen alone:** We found no good RCTs of oestrogen alone (without progestins) in the secondary prevention of coronary heart disease in postmenopausal women. One RCT found that high dose oestrogen (5 mg conjugated equine oestrogens/day) was associated with increased risk of MI and thromboembolic events in men with pre-existing coronary heart disease.[42]

Harms: Pooled estimates from observational studies found an increased risk of endometrial cancer (RR > 8) and of breast cancer (RR 1.25 to 1.46) when oestrogen was used for over 8 years. In most observational studies the addition of progestins prevented endometrial cancer but not breast cancer. The risk of venous thromboembolism, including pulmonary embolism and deep vein thrombosis, was three to four times higher with HRT than without. However, because the incidence of venous thromboembolism is low in postmenopausal women, the absolute increase in risk was only about one to two additional cases of venous thromboembolism in 5000 users per year.[43] In the RCT described above,[41] more women in the HRT than in the placebo group experienced venous thromboembolism (34/172 v 12/176; OR 2.89, 95% CI 1.50 to 5.58) and gall bladder disease (84/172 v 62/176; OR 1.38, 95% CI 0.84 to 1.38).

Comment: Many observational studies have found reduced rates of clinical events caused by coronary heart disease in postmenopausal women using HRT, especially in women with pre-existing coronary heart disease. Hormone users experienced 35–80% fewer recurrent events than non-users.[44,45] Meanwhile, several RCTs have found that HRT improves cardiovascular risk factors.[46] It is not known whether studies longer than 4 years would show a benefit.

QUESTION What are the effects of cholesterol reduction?

Mike Pignone

Updated this issue

Systematic reviews and large subsequent RCTs have found that lowering cholesterol in people at high risk of ischaemic coronary events substantially reduces the risk of cardiovascular mortality and morbidity. One systematic review of primary and secondary prevention trials has found that statins constitute the single most effective type of treatment for reducing cholesterol and reducing cardiovascular risk. The absolute benefits increased as baseline risk increased, but did not seem to be influenced by the individual's absolute cholesterol concentration. We found no direct evidence for effects in people over 75, or for effects of combined treatments to reduce cholesterol and other cardiovascular risk factors.

Benefits: **Statins:** We found one systematic review (search date 1998) that considered the effect of HMG-CoA reductase inhibitors (statins) compared with placebo on clinical outcomes in people given long term (≥ 4 years) treatment.[47] It found five large RCTs, of mean duration 5.4 years, in a total of 30 817 people. Combining the three secondary prevention trials, the review found that statins reduced CHD mortality, cardiovascular mortality, and all cause mortality compared with control (CHD mortality: OR 0.71, 95% CI 0.63 to 0.80; cardiovascular mortality: OR 0.73, 95% CI 0.66 to 0.82; all cause mortality: 0.77, 95% CI 0.70 to 0.85). Combining primary and secondary prevention, it found that statins compared with control reduced total cholesterol, LDL, and triglycerides, and increased HDL cholesterol (mean reduction 20% total cholesterol, 28% LDL, 13% triglycerides; mean increase 5% HDL), and reduced major coronary events (RRR 31%, 95% CI 26% to 35%, ARR 3.6%, 95% CI 2.9% to 4.3%, NNT 28, 95% CI 23 to 34) and all cause mortality (RRR 21%, 95% CI 14% to 28%, ARR 16%, 95% CI 11% to 22%, NNT 61, 95% CI 45 to 95). Absolute risk reduction increased as baseline risk increased in primary prevention (see figure 1 in primary prevention, p 51). Differences between the baseline cholesterol concentration seemed to play no role in determining the results of the trials, in the ranges studied to date. **Effects of statins in different groups of people:** Combining data from primary and secondary prevention trials, the review found that, compared with placebo, statins reduced coronary events by a similar proportional amount in men (reduction in OR 31%, 95% CI 26% to 35%; ARR 3.7%, 95% CI 2.9% to 4.4%) and in women (reduction in OR 29%, 95% CI 31% to 42%; ARR 3.3%, 95% CI 1.3% to 5.2%), and in people under 65 (reduction in OR 31%, 95% CI 24% to 36%; ARR 3.2% 95% CI 2.4% to 4.0%), and in people over the age of 65 (reduction in OR 32%, 95% CI 23% to 39%; ARR 4.4%, 95% CI 3.0% to 5.8%). The reduction of CHD events in women involved more non-fatal and fewer fatal events than in men. One large trial found an insignificant increase in the relative risk of overall mortality with statins compared with placebo for the subgroup of women, but the confidence interval was wide (RR 1.16, 95% CI 0.68 to 1.99).[48] Other trials have not yet reported overall mortality results for women. **Intensity of statin treatment:** We found one RCT that compared aggressive reduction of cholesterol with lovastatin and, if necessary, cholestyramine (aiming for target LDL 1.6–2.2 mmol/l [60–85 mg/dl]) with more moderate reduction (target LDL 3.4–3.7 mmol/l [130–140mg/dl]) with the same drugs, in 1351 people with a history of saphenous vein coronary artery bypass graft. The trial found that aggressive treatment reduced the risk of needing repeat revascularisation at 4 years (6.5% with aggressive treatment v 9.2% with moderate treatment, P = 0.03).[47] **Other treatments:** We found one systematic review (search date 1996), which did not differentiate primary and secondary prevention, and included RCTs of any cholesterol lowering intervention, irrespective of duration, as long as mortality data was reported. It found 59 RCTs in a total of 173 160 people receiving drug treatments (statins, n–3 fatty acids, fibrates, resins, hormones, or niacin) alone, dietary intervention alone, or surgery (ileal bypass) alone.[49] Overall, baseline risk was similar among all intervention groups. Among non-surgical treatments, the review found that only statins reduced CHD mortality, and that only statins and n–3 fatty acids reduced all cause mortality (RR of CHD mortality, treatment v control 0.69, 95% CI 0.59 to 0.80 for statins; 0.44, 95% CI 0.18 to 1.07 for n–3 fatty acids; 0.98, 95% CI 0.78 to 1.24 for fibrates; 0.71, 95% CI 0.51 to 0.99 for resins; 1.04, 95% CI 0.93 to 1.17 for hormones; 0.95, 95% CI 0.83 to 1.10 for niacin; 0.91, 95% CI 0.82 to 1.01 for diet. RR of all cause mortality, treatment v control 0.79, 95% CI 0.71 to 0.89 for statins; 0.68, 95% CI 0.53 to 0.88 for n–3 fatty acids; 1.06, 95% CI 0.78 to 1.46 for fibrates; 0.85, 95% CI 0.66 to 1.08 for resins; 1.09, 95% CI 1.00 to 1.20 for hormones; 0.96, 95% CI 0.86 to 1.08 for niacin; 0.97, 95% CI 0.81 to 1.15 for diet). One subsequent RCT compared gemfibrozil with placebo in 2531 men with coronary heart disease and a low level of HDL-C (< 1 mmol/l).[50] After a median of 5.1 years the composite outcome of non-fatal MI or death from coronary heart disease was lower with gemfibrozil than placebo (ARs 219/1264 [17.3%] for gemfibrozil v 275/1267 [21.7%] for placebo; ARR 4.4%, 95% CI 1.4% to 7%; RRR 20%, 95% CI 6% to 32%; NNT 23, 95% CI 14 to 73). **Cholesterol lowering versus angioplasty:** We found no systematic review. One RCT found that aggressive lipid lowering treatment was as effective as PTA for reducing ischaemic events, although anginal symptoms were reduced more by PTA (see PTA versus medical treatment, p 104).

Harms: Total non-cardiovascular events, total and tissue specific cancers, and accident and violent deaths have been reported in statin trials. However, the systematic review of long term statin trials found no significant difference between statins and placebo in terms of non-cardiovascular mortality, cancer incidence, asymptomatic elevation of creatine kinase (> 10 times upper reference limit), or elevation of transaminases (> 3 times upper reference limit) during a mean of 5.4 years of treatment (OR of event, statin v placebo 0.93, 95% CI 0.81 to 1.07 for non-cardiovascular mortality; 0.99, 95% CI 0.90 to 1.08 for cancer; 1.25, 95% CI 0.83 to 1.89 for creatine kinase rise; 1.13, 95% CI 0.95 to 1.33 for transaminase rise).[47] We found no evidence of additional harm associated with cholesterol lowering in elderly people, or in people following acute MI.

Comment: The evidence indicates that, in a wide range of clinical contexts, the RRR depends on the size of the fall in cholesterol and is not otherwise dependent on the method by which cholesterol is lowered. The absolute benefit over several years of lowering cholesterol will therefore be greatest in people with the highest baseline risk of an ischaemic cardiac event. Even if the RRR attenuates at older age, the ARR for ischaemic cardiac events may be higher in elderly people than in younger individuals. However, long term benefit for cholesterol lowering has not yet been directly shown in those > 75 years old. Additional information may be provided by the Heart Protection Study (20 000 participants, completion 2000, simvastatin),[51] the Women's Health Initiative (48 000 participants, completion 2007, diet, up to age 79 years),[52] and the Antihypertensive and Lipid Lowering Treatment to Prevent Heart Disease Trial (10 000 participants, completion 2002, pravastatin, no upper age limit).[53] It is not known whether cholesterol reduction will provide benefit for those with initial cholesterol concentrations lower than those selected in the published trials. We found no evidence to indicate whether starting statin treatment immediately after acute infarction provides additional benefits. We found no large direct comparisons of cholesterol modifying drugs; it remains unclear whether any one drug has advantages over others in subgroups of high risk people with particular lipid abnormalities. Since the main aim of treatment is to reduce absolute risk (rather than to reduce the cholesterol to any particular concentration), treatments aimed at lowering cholesterol need evaluating for effectiveness in comparison and in combination with other possible risk factor interventions in each individual.

Eva Lonn

Updated this issue

We found no direct evidence of the effects of blood pressure lowering in people with established coronary heart disease. Observational studies, and extrapolation of primary prevention trials of blood pressure reduction, support the lowering of blood pressure in those at high risk of ischaemic coronary events. The evidence for benefit is strongest for β blockers, although not specifically in people with raised blood pressure. The target blood pressure in these people is not clear.

Benefits: We found no systematic review and no RCTs designed specifically to examine blood pressure reduction in those with established coronary heart disease. Prospective epidemiological studies have established that blood pressure continues to be a risk factor for cardiovascular events in people who have already experienced MI. Prospective follow up of 5362 men who reported prior MI during screening for one large RCT found no detectable association between systolic blood pressure and coronary heart disease mortality, and increased coronary heart disease mortality for those with lowest diastolic blood pressure in the first 2 years of follow up.[54] After 15 years there were highly significant linear associations between both systolic and diastolic blood pressure and increased risk of coronary heart disease mortality (stronger relation for systolic blood pressure), with apparent benefit for men with blood pressure maintained at levels lower than the arbitrarily defined "normal" levels. Experimental evidence of benefit from lowering of blood pressure in those with coronary heart disease requires extrapolation from primary prevention trials, since trials of antihypertensive treatment in elderly people[55–57] are likely to have included people with preclinical coronary heart disease. Mortality benefit has been established for β blockers after MI (see option, p 89), for verapamil and diltiazem after MI in those without heart failure (see calcium channel blockers, p 92), and for ACE inhibitors after MI, especially in those with heart failure (see ACE inhibitors, p 90).

Harms: Some observational studies have found increased mortality among those with low diastolic blood pressure.[58] Trials in elderly people of blood pressure lowering for hypertension or while treating heart failure[59] found no evidence of a J shaped relation between blood pressure and death.

Comment: Without specific studies comparing different antihypertensive treatments, the available evidence is strongest for a beneficial effect of β blockers when treating survivors of an MI who have raised blood pressure. We found no specific evidence about the target level of blood pressure.

QUESTION What are the effects of non-drug treatments?

Andy Ness, Eva Lonn

Updated this issue

OPTION DIETARY INTERVENTIONS

RCTs have found that advising people with coronary heart disease to eat more fish (particularly oily fish), more fruit and vegetables, bread, pasta, potatoes, olive oil, and rapeseed margarine (that is, a more Mediterranean diet) may result in a substantial survival benefit. We found no strong evidence from RCTs for a beneficial effect of low fat or high fibre diets on major non-fatal coronary heart disease events or coronary heart disease mortality.

Benefits: **Low fat diets:** One systematic review, published in 1998, found no evidence that allocation to a low fat diet reduced mortality from coronary heart disease in people after MI (RR 0.94, 95% CI 0.84 to 1.06).[60] One large RCT randomised 2033 middle aged men with a recent MI to three dietary arms: fat advice (to eat less fat); fibre advice (to eat more cereal fibre); and fish advice (to eat at least two portions of fatty fish a week).[61] Advice to reduce fat was complicated and, though fat intake reduced only slightly in the fat advice group, fruit and vegetable intake increased by around 40 g per day.[62] There was, however, no clear reduction in mortality (unadjusted RR at 2 years for death from any cause 0.97, 95% CI 0.75 to 1.27). **High fibre diets:** In the trial, people advised to eat more fibre doubled their intake, but survival was non-significantly worse (unadjusted RR at 2 years for death from any cause 1.23, 95% CI 0.95 to 1.60). **High fish diets:** In the trial, those advised to eat more fish ate three times as much fish, although about 14% could not tolerate the fish and were given fish oil capsules. Those given fish advice were significantly less likely to die within 2 years (RRR 29%, 95% CI 7% to 46%; NNT 30). In a second trial, 11 324 people who had survived a recent MI were randomised to receive 1 g daily of n-3 PUFA (fish oil) or no fish oil. Those given fish oil were less likely to die within 3.5 years (RRR 0.14, 95% CI 0.03 to 0.24).[63] **Mediterranean diet:** One RCT compared advice to eat a Mediterranean diet (more bread, more vegetables, more fruit, more fish, and less meat), and to replace butter and cream with rapeseed margarine with usual dietary advice in 605 middle aged people with a recent MI.[64] There were several dietary differences between the groups. Fruit intake, for example, was around 50 g/day higher in the intervention group than the control group. After 27 months the trial was stopped prematurely because of better outcomes in the intervention group. There were 20 deaths in the control group and eight in the intervention group (adjusted RRR of death 70%, 95% CI 18% to 89%; NNT 25 over 2 years).

Harms: No major adverse effects have been reported.

Comment: Diets low in saturated fat and cholesterol can lead to 10–15% reductions in cholesterol concentrations in highly controlled settings, such as in metabolic wards.[65] In people in the community, the effects are more modest: 3–5% reductions in cholesterol concentrations in general population studies and 9% reductions in people after MI.[60,66-68] Several RCTs of intensive dietary intervention in conjunction with multifactorial risk reduction treatment found decreased progression of anatomic extent of coronary heart disease on angiography.[69] A trial of advice to eat more fruit and vegetables in men with angina is under way (Burr M, personal communication). **Effect on cardiovascular risk factors:** Other studies have investigated the effects of dietary interventions on cardiovascular risk factors rather than the effect on cardiovascular morbidity and mortality. One systematic review (search date 1992) suggested that garlic may reduce cholesterol by about 10%.[70] Some trials in this review had methodological flaws. More recent reports published in 1998 found no effects of garlic powder or garlic oil on cholesterol concentrations.[71,72] One systematic review (search date 1991) reported modest reductions in cholesterol levels of 2–5% from oats and psyllium enriched cereals (high fibre diets), although we found no evidence that high fibre diets reduce mortality in people with CHD.[69] One systematic review of soy protein also reported modest reductions in cholesterol concentrations.[73]

OPTION	ANTIOXIDANT VITAMINS (VITAMIN E, β CAROTENE, VITAMIN C)

The role of vitamin E, β carotene, and vitamin C in the long term management of people at high risk for ischaemic cardiac events remains unclear.

Benefits:

We found no systematic review of RCTs. **Vitamin E and β carotene:** Four large RCTs have looked at vitamin E in people with coronary artery disease.[63,75-77] The first recruited 2002 people with angiographically proven ischaemic heart disease.[74] The dose of vitamin E was high (400 IU or 800 IU) and the duration of follow up short (a median of 510 days). The trial found that vitamin E reduced non-fatal coronary events (RRR 77%, 95% CI 53% to 89%), but also found a non-significant increase in coronary death (RRI 18%, −0.4% to +127%) and all cause mortality. The second trial, in 29 133 male Finnish smokers, compared β carotene and vitamin E supplements with placebo. The dose of vitamin E (50 mg/day) was smaller than that used in the first trial. In the subgroup analysis of data from the 1862 men with prior MI, the trial found that vitamin E reduced non-fatal MI (RRR 38%, 95% CI 4% to 59%) but non-significantly increased coronary death (RRI 33%, 95% CI −14% to +105%).[76] There were significantly more deaths from coronary heart disease on β carotene than placebo. In the third trial,[63] 11 324 people were randomised in a factorial design to receive either vitamin E (300 mg) daily or no vitamin E (as well as being randomised to receive fish oil). After 3.5 years there was a small and non-significant reduction in the risk of cardiovascular death and deaths from all causes in those who received vitamin E compared with those who did not (RRR all cause mortality 0.92%, 95% CI 0.82% to 1.04%). There was no significant change in the rate of non-fatal coronary events in those who received vitamin E (RRI 40%, 95% CI −12% to +22%).[61] The fourth and most recent trial enrolled 9 541 people at high cardiovascular risk, of which 80% had prior clinical manifestations of coronary artery disease (the remainder had other athersoclerotic vascular disease manifestations or diabetes with at least one additional cardiovascular risk factor). The trial compared natural source Vitamin E (D-alpha tocopherol acetate) 400 IU/day with placebo and followed participants for an average of 4.7 years.[77] It found no significant differences in any cardiovascular outcomes between vitamin E and placebo (AR of major fatal or non-fatal cardiovascular event 16.2% with vitamin E v 15.5% with placebo, P = NS; AR for cardiovascular death 7.2% with vitamin E v 6.9% with placebo, P = NS; AR for non-fatal MI 11.2% v 11.0% with placebo, P = NS; AR for stroke 4.4% with vitamin E v 3.8% with placebo, P = NS; AR for death from any cause 11.2% with vitamin E v 11.2% with placebo, P = NS). Pooled analysis from all four of these major RCTs found no evidence that vitamin E altered cardiovascular events and all cause mortality compared with placebo when given for 1.3 to 4.5 years. **Vitamin C:** We found three small RCTs comparing vitamin C with placebo. The first RCT randomised 538 people admitted to an acute geriatric unit to vitamin C (200 mg daily) or placebo for 6 months.[79] The second RCT randomised 297 elderly people with low vitamin C levels to vitamin C (150 mg daily for 12 weeks then 50 mg daily) or placebo for 2 years.[80] The third RCT randomised 199 elderly people to vitamin C (200 mg daily) or placebo for 6 months.[81] The three trials were small and brief, and their combined results provide no evidence of any substantial early benefit of vitamin C supplementation (RRI for mortality for vitamin v placebo 8%, 95% CI −7% to +26%).

Harms: Two of the three trials of vitamin E reported non-significant increases in the risk of coronary death (see benefits above).[75,76] Four large RCTs of β carotene supplementation in primary prevention found no cardiovascular benefits, and two of the trials raised concerns about increased mortality (RRI for cardiovascular death, β carotene v placebo 12%, 95% CI 4% to 22%) and cancer rates.[82]

Comment: One systematic review of epidemiological studies, published in 1997, found consistent associations between increased dietary or supplemental intake of vitamin E, or both, and lower cardiovascular risk and less consistent associations for β carotene and vitamin C.[82] Most observational studies of antioxidants have excluded people with pre-existing disease.[83,84]

OPTION   CARDIAC REHABILITATION INCLUDING EXERCISE

Systematic reviews of RCTs have found that cardiac rehabilitation improves coronary risk factors and reduces the risk of major cardiac events in people after MI. The role of exercise alone in reducing the risk of adverse cardiovascular outcomes is not clear.

Benefits: **Cardiac rehabilitation:** Three systematic reviews identified RCTs of cardiac rehabilitation including exercise in people after MI. Rehabilitation included medical evaluation, prescribed exercise, cardiac risk factor modification, education, and counselling. The reviews found 20–25% reductions in cardiovascular deaths in the treatment groups.[85–87] One review identified 22 RCTs in 4554 people with a recent MI. After a mean follow up of 3 years, there were significant reductions in total mortality (RRR 20%, no CI given), cardiovascular mortality (RRR 22%, no CI given), and fatal reinfarction (RRR 25%, no CI given), but no significant difference in rates of non-fatal reinfarction.[86] **Exercise alone:** One more recent qualitative systematic review, published in 1995, found that rehabilitation with exercise alone had little effect on rates of non-fatal MI or overall mortality but a small beneficial effect on angina.[80]

Harms: No study documented an increased risk of reinfarction or other adverse cardiovascular outcomes for exercise rehabilitation compared with control. Rates of adverse cardiovascular outcomes (syncope, arrhythmia, MI, or sudden death) were low (2–3/100 000 person hours) in supervised rehabilitation programmes, and rates of fatal cardiac events during or immediately after exercise training were reported in two older surveys as ranging from 1/11 6 400 to 1/78 4 000 person hours.[78]

Comment: The three reviews included RCTs performed before the widespread use of thrombolytic agents and β blockers after MI. Most participants were men under 70 years of age. Other interventions aimed at risk factor modification were often provided in the intervention groups (including nutritional education, counselling in behavioural modification, and, in some trials, lipid lowering medications). We found no strong evidence that exercise training and cardiac rehabilitation programmes increased the proportion of people returning to work after MI.

OPTION   SMOKING CESSATION

We found no RCTs of the effects of smoking cessation on cardiovascular events in people with coronary heart disease. Moderate evidence from epidemiological studies indicates that people with coronary heart disease who stop smoking rapidly reduce their risk of recurrent coronary events or death. The use of nicotine patches seems safe in people with coronary heart disease.

Benefits: We found no RCTs evaluating the effects of smoking cessation on coronary mortality and morbidity. Many observational studies found that people with coronary heart disease who stop smoking rapidly reduce their risk of cardiac death and MI (RRR about 50% for recurrent coronary events or premature death compared with continuing smokers)[88] (see smoking cessation under primary prevention, p 51). The studies found that about half of the benefits occur in the first year of stopping smoking, followed by a more gradual decrease in risk, reaching the risk of never smokers after several years of abstinence.[88] Among people with peripheral arterial disease and stroke, smoking cessation has been shown in observational studies to be associated with improved exercise tolerance, decreased risk of amputation, improved survival, and reduced risk of recurrent stroke.

Harms: Two recent RCTs found no evidence that nicotine replacement using transdermal patches in people with stable coronary heart disease increased cardiovascular events.[89,90]

Comment: One RCT compared the impact of firm and detailed advice to stop smoking in 125 survivors of acute MI versus conventional advice in

85 people.[91] Allocation to the intervention or control group was determined by day of admission. At follow up over 1 year after admission, 62% of the intervention group and 28% of the control group were non-smokers. Mortality and morbidity were not reported.

OPTION   PSYCHOLOGICAL AND STRESS MANAGEMENT INTERVENTIONS

One systematic review of mainly poor quality RCTs has found that psychological and stress management may decrease rates of MI or cardiac death in people with coronary heart disease.

Benefits:
One systematic review, published in 1996, found 23 RCTs in a total of 3180 people with coronary artery disease; 2024 people received one of a diverse range of psychosocial treatments and 1156 people received usual treatment.[92] Mortality data were available in only 12 studies. Compared with control interventions, psychosocial interventions were associated with a 41% reduction in mortality (OR 1.70, 95% CI 1.09 to 2.64) and a 46% reduction in non-fatal events in the first 2 years of follow up after MI (OR 1.84, 95% CI 1.12 to 2.99).[92]

Harms:
No specific harms were reported.

Comment:
These results should be interpreted with caution because of the methodological limitations of the individual RCTs and the use of a diverse range of interventions (relaxation, stress management, counselling). The RCTs were generally small, with short follow up, and used non-uniform outcome measures. Methods of concealment allocation were not assessed. The authors of the review acknowledged the strong possibility of publication bias but made no attempt to quantify it. The results were inconsistent across trials.[93] Several observational studies have found that depression and social isolation (lack of social and emotional support) are independent predictors of mortality and non-fatal coronary heart disease events in people after MI.[94]

QUESTION   What are the effects of surgical treatments?

Charanjit Rihal

Updated this issue

OPTION   CORONARY ARTERY BYPASS GRAFTING (CABG) VERSUS MEDICAL TREATMENT

RCTs performed up to the mid 1980s found that, in comparison with medical treatment, CABG carried a greater risk of death in the first year but reduced the risk of death from coronary artery disease at 5 and 10 years. Greatest benefit occurred in people with more severe disease (multivessel disease, left ventricular dysfunction, or MI). There was no evidence of increased protection against subsequent MI. Data from a more recent RCT, using modern techniques and with optimal background medical treatment, suggest even greater superiority of revascularisation.

Benefits: One systematic review, published in 1994, analysed individual data from 2649 people with coronary heart disease in seven RCTs comparing CABG with medical treatment. Participants, most of whom were middle aged men with multivessel disease but good left ventricular function, were enrolled from 1972 to 1984 (97% were male, 82% 41–60 years old, 80% with ejection fraction > 50%, 60% with prior MI, and 83% with two or three vessel disease).[95] Participants who were assigned to CABG also received medical treatment, and 40% of participants assigned to initial medical treatment underwent CABG in the following 10 years. One subsequent RCT compared medical treatment with revascularisation (CABG or PTA) in 558 people with asymptomatic but definite ischaemia (positive exercise test or ambulatory electrocardiogram).[96] **Mortality and MI:** The systematic review found that participants assigned to an initial strategy of CABG had reduced mortality at 5 years (RRR compared with participants assigned to an initial strategy of medical treatment 39%, 95% CI 23% to 52%), 7 years (RRR 32%, 95% CI 17% to 44%), and 10 years (RRR 17%, 95% CI 2% to 30%).[95] In the subsequent RCT, mortality at 2 years was significantly lower after routine revascularisation (AR of death 1.1% v 6.6% and 4.4% in the two medical groups, P < 0.02).[96] No overall impact of CABG on subsequent infarction was found either in individual trials or in the systematic review, possibly because those assigned to surgery had increased rates of infarction in the perioperative period (see harms below). In the RCT, revascularisation reduced rates of death or MI compared with medical treatment (AR of MI or death 4.7% with revascularisation v 8.8% and 12.1% with medical treatment, P < 0.04).[96] **Other non-fatal end points:** Most trials did not prospectively collect data on readmission rates, recurrent angina, or quality of life. **Effects in different people:** The systematic review found that the relative benefits were similar in participants with different baseline risk (OR for death 0.61 if left ventricular function normal and 0.59 if abnormal). The absolute benefit of CABG was greatest in people with an abnormal ejection fraction, because the baseline risk of death was twice as high in this group (ejection fraction > 50%, ARR of death over 5 years 5%; ejection fraction < 50%, ARR 10%). Both absolute and relative mortality benefits were higher in people with a greater number of diseased coronary arteries, especially those with three vessel disease (OR of death 0.58, P < 0.001), and those with left main coronary artery disease (OR 0.32, P = 0.004) or any involvement of the left anterior descending coronary artery (OR 0.58), even if only one or two vessels were involved.[95]

Harms: **Perioperative complications:** In the systematic review, of the 1240 participants who underwent CABG, 40 (3.2%) died and 7.1% had documented non-fatal MI within 30 days of the procedure. At 1 year, the estimated incidence of death or MI was 11.6% with CABG and 8% with medical treatment (RRI 45%, 95% CI 18% to 103%).[95] Since the diagnosis of MI after CABG is difficult, its true incidence may be higher. In the recent RCT, after 2 years of follow up, rates of death or MI were significantly lower in those assigned to routine revascularisation (AR for death 1.1% v 6.6% and 4.4% for the two medical groups, P < 0.02; AR for death or MI 4.7% v 12.1% and 8.8% in the two medical groups, P < 0.04).[96]

Comment: The results of the systematic review may not be generalisable to current practice. Participants were 65 years or younger, but over half of CABG procedures are now performed on people over 65. Almost all participants were male. High risk people such as those with severe angina and left main coronary artery stenosis were under represented. Internal thoracic artery grafts were used in less than 5% of participants. Lipid lowering agents (particularly HMG-CoA reductase inhibitors) and aspirin were used infrequently (aspirin used in 3% of participants at enrolment). Only about half of participants were taking β blockers. The systematic review may underestimate the real benefits of CABG in comparison with medical treatment alone since medical and surgical treatment for coronary artery disease were not mutually exclusive; by 5 years 25% of people receiving medical treatment had undergone CABG surgery and by 10 years 41% had undergone CABG surgery. The underestimate of effect would be greatest among people at high risk. People with previous CABG have not been studied in RCTs, although they now represent a growing proportion of those undergoing CABG.

OPTION **CORONARY PERCUTANEOUS TRANSLUMINAL ANGIOPLASTY (PTA) VERSUS MEDICAL TREATMENT FOR STABLE CORONARY ARTERY DISEASE**

RCTs have found that in people with stable coronary artery disease, in comparison with medical treatment, coronary PTA is more effective for alleviating angina pectoris, myocardial ischaemia, and improving exercise tolerance. However, it is associated with increased risk of MI during and soon after the procedure, emergency CABG, and repeat procedures for restenosis. The RCTs found no evidence that PTA reduces the overall risk of MI or death in people with unstable angina.

Benefits: We found no systematic review. We found three good RCTs comparing angioplasty with medical treatment.[97-100] **Mortality, MI, and unstable angina:** The first RCT included 212 people followed for a mean of 5 years. It found no significant difference in rates of death (AR 9.5% for PTA v 10.3% for medical groups, P = NS) or non-fatal MI (7.6% v 6.5%, P = NS).[100] However, more people initially assigned to medical treatment underwent PTA or CABG during follow up (35.5% v 13.3%, P < 0.0001) or presented with unstable angina (25.2% v 6.7%, P = 0.001). The second RCT found a significant increase in rates of death or MI with PTA (AR by 3 years with PTA 6.3% v 3.3% on medical treatment; ARI 3%, 95% CI 0.4% to 5.7%). The higher rate of death or MI with PTA was attributable to one death and seven procedure related MIs.[100] The third RCT assigned 341 people with stable, mild coronary artery disease and mild angina to PTA plus standard medical therapy or to aggressive lipid lowering therapy with atorvastatin.[99] LDL cholesterol levels fell in both groups, but more so in people given atorvastatin (mean LDL cholesterol reduced to 2.0 mmol/l with atorvastatin v 3.0 mmol/l with PTA). Over a mean follow up period of 18 months the PTA group experienced more cardiac events (defined as cardiac death or arrest, CABG, PTA, stroke, or worsening angina) than the atorvastatin group, but the difference fell just short of being significant (ARs 37/177 [21%] for PTA versus 22/164 [13%] for the atorvastatin group; ARR 8%, 95% CI −0.7% to +13%; RRR 36%, 95% CI −3% to

+62%). **Angina pectoris:** In the first RCT, although PTA was technically successful in only 80% of people, it led to a higher proportion of participants free of angina at 6 months (64% v 46%, P < 0.01), fewer monthly anginal episodes in those who were still symptomatic, lower use of medication, and greater improvement in duration of treadmill exercise, even though concomitant antianginal medications were discontinued before the test (improvement 2.1 v 0.5 minutes, P < 0.0001).[98] In the second RCT, angina pectoris and treadmill exercise time improved significantly in both groups at 3 months, but more so with PTA (ARR of moderate to severe angina [grade 2 or worse] for PTA v medical treatment over 3 months 16.5%; NNT 6). At 3 years, the ARR for angina had fallen to 7.6% because people with severe symptoms in both groups underwent PTA for symptom control.[99] The third RCT found that PTA signifi- cantly improved angina compared with atorvastatin (improvement in angina over 18 months 95/177 [54%] for PTA v 67/164 [41%] for atorvastatin; ARI 13%, 95% CI 2% to 23%; RRI 24%, 95% CI 4% to 42%; NNT 8, 95% CI 4 to 46).[97] **Effects in different people:** Antianginal benefit from PTA was limited to people with moderate to severe (grade 2 or worse) angina (20% lower incidence of angina and 1 minute longer treadmill exercise times compared with medi- cal treatment); people with mild symptoms at enrolment derived no significant improvement in symptoms.[99]

Harms: Procedural death and MI, as well as repeat procedures for resteno- sis, are the main hazards of PTA. In the first RCT, two (1.9%) emergency CABG operations and five (4.8%) MIs occurred at the time of the procedure. By 6 months, the PTA group had higher rates of CABG surgery (7% v 0%) and non-protocol PTA (15.2% v 10.3%).[98,101] In the second RCT, the higher rate of death or MI with PTA was attributable to one death and seven procedure related MIs.[99]

Comment: PTA has become one of the most commonly performed invasive procedures. We found good evidence that it treats the symptoms of angina pectoris, but we found no evidence that it reduces the overall incidence of death or MI in people with stable angina. This is likely to be because of the risk of complications during and soon after the procedure, and the fact that most PTAs are performed for single vessel disease.

| OPTION | CORONARY PTA VERSUS CABG FOR MULTIVESSEL DISEASE |

One systematic review of RCTs has found no evidence of a difference in efficacy between PTA and CABG in low to medium risk people, in terms of rates of death and MI, and quality of life. However, these trials were too small to exclude a 20–30% difference in mortality. PTA is associated with a greater need for repeat procedures. The largest of these trials found that people with diabetes (specifically, those treated with oral hypoglycaemic drugs or insulin) who also have multivessel coronary disease have better long term survival following CABG than PTA.

Benefits: One systematic review, published in 1995, identified eight RCTs in 3371 people with multivessel disease.[102] We found one subse- quent RCT that included 1829 people.[103] **Angina pectoris:** In all trials at 1 year, the prevalence of moderate to severe angina pectoris (grade 2 or worse) was significantly higher after PTA than after CABG (RR 1.6, 95% CI 1.3 to 1.9). After 3 years this difference had decreased as rates of repeat revascularisation increased in the people allocated to PTA (RR 1.2, 95% CI 1.0 to 1.5). **Mortality:** When results from all nine trials were pooled, there was no significant difference in all cause mortality between groups (AR 7.3% after PTA v 6.8%; OR 1.09, 95% CI 0.88 to 1.35).[103] The largest of these trials found that in participants being treated for diabetes CABG reduced mortality more than PTA both after 5 years (AR of death with CABG 19.4% v 34.5% with PTA; P = 0.003)[103] and after 7 years (AR of death with CABG 23.6% v 44.3% with PTA; P = 0.0011). Such a difference was not observed among non-diabetics or any other subgroup.[104] **Death or MI:** In all trials, the combined end point of death or MI was not significantly different between groups (AR 13.8% v 13.4%, OR 1.05, 95% CI 0.89 to 1.23).[105] The largest of these trials, in people with diabetes treated with insulin or oral hypoglycaemic agents, found that after a mean follow up of 7.7 years freedom from death or MI was similar following CABG or PTA, 75.3% CABG v 73.5% PTA, p = 0.46.[104] **Repeat procedures:** In all trials, the need for repeat procedures was significantly higher in people with PTA (AR 44% v 6.0% in people allocated to CABG, OR 7.9, 95% CI 6.9 to 9.0).[99] **Quality of life:** Subsequent analysis of the trial data has found significant improvements in quality of life measures and return to employment after both PTA and CABG but no difference between groups over 3–5 years of follow up.[106,107]

Harms: See harms of PTA versus medical treatment, p 105. CABG is more invasive than PTA, but PTA is associated with a greater need for repeat procedures.

Comment: Although no major differences in death or MI were observed in the nine RCTs, these trials enrolled people at relatively low risk of cardiac events. It is therefore premature to conclude that PTA and CABG are equivalent for all people with multivessel disease. Fewer than 20% of participants had left ventricular dysfunction, almost 70% had one or two vessel disease, and observed mortality was only 2.6% for the first year, and 1.1% per year thereafter. Participants enrolled in the largest trial more closely approximated to moderate risk people, but this was caused primarily by the higher proportion of participants with diabetes mellitus.[103] Even in that trial nearly 60% of participants had two vessel coronary artery disease. Finally, even though nine trials have been performed, the total enrolment of 5200 falls short of what would be needed to show mortality differences of 20–30% among people at low and moderate risk. Large mortality differences between the two procedures (40–50%) are unlikely.

OPTION CORONARY PTA VERSUS INTRACORONARY STENTS

RCTs have found that, in comparison with coronary PTA, intracoronary stents afford superior acute and long term clinical and angiographic results.

Benefits: We found no systematic review. **For disease of native coronary arteries:** We found three RCTs comparing elective stenting with

PTA.[98–109] At 12 months, intracoronary stents significantly reduced the risk of recurrent angina (13% v 30%, P = 0.04) but not of death, MI, or need for CABG.[104] At 6 months, all three trials found a lower prevalence of angiographic restenosis (31% v 42%, P = 0.046; 22% v 32%, P = 0.02; and 17% v 40%, P = 0.02), and a lower rate of repeat PTA (13.5% v 23.3%, RR 0.58, 95% CI 0.40 to 0.85).[109] **For saphenous vein graft lesions in people with prior CABG:** We found one RCT comparing elective stents with standard balloon angioplasty in 220 people.[110] Acute angiographic results were better with stents than balloon angioplasty. At 6 months there was no significant difference in rates of restenosis (37% v 46%, P = 0.24), but the overall incidence of death, MI, CABG, or repeat PTA was lower in the stent group (27% v 42%, P = 0.03). **For treatment of chronic total occlusions:** Chronic occlusions of the coronary arteries are particularly prone to restenosis and reocclusion following PTA. We found three RCTs comparing PTA alone with PTA followed by insertion of stents.[111–113] One trial involved 119 people with chronic total occlusion and found that stenting reduced angina and angiographic restenosis compared with PTA alone (57% of the stent group were angina free at 6 month follow up versus 24% of the PTA only group, 95% CI not available, P < 0.001; restenosis [> 50% stenosis on follow up angiography] occurred in 74% of PTA and 32% of people with a stent, P < 0.001). Repeat procedures were undertaken less often among people with a stent than among people receiving PTA (22% v 42%, P = 0.025).[111] In the second trial involving 110 participants, those treated with stents experienced less ischaemia (14% v 46%, P = 0.002), had less restenosis (32% v 68%, P < 0.001), and underwent fewer repeat procedures (5.3% v 22%, P = 0.038) by 9 months.[112] The third RCT in 110 participants found that, at angiographic follow up after 4 months, those with stents experienced less restenosis (26% v 62%, P = 0.01), less reocclusion (2% v 1%, P = 0.05), and fewer repeat PTAs (24% v 55%, P = 0.05). No deaths or CABG surgeries occurred in either group. The incidence of MI was low in both groups (0% stent v 2% PTA, P = NS).[113] **For treatment of restenosis after initial PTA:** We found one RCT of coronary stenting compared with balloon angioplasty for treatment of restenosis in 383 people. During 6 months of follow up, the stent group experienced fewer recurrent restenoses (18% v 32%, P = 0.03) and repeat procedures (10% v 27%, P = 0.001). Survival free of MI or repeat revascularisation was 84% in the stent group and 72% in the PTA group (P = 0.04).[114]

Harms: Initially, aggressive combination antithrombotic and anticoagulant regimens were used because of a high incidence of stent thrombosis and MI. These regimens led to a high incidence of arterial access site bleeding.[108] More recently, improved stent deployment techniques and use of aspirin and ticlopidine have reduced both stent thrombosis and arterial access site bleeding.[110,115] Currently, the risk of stent thrombosis is less than 1%.[109,115,116] Haemorrhage (particularly femoral artery bleeding) was more frequent after stenting than PTA alone,[111] but occurred in less than 3% following stenting when antiplatelet drugs were used without long term anticoagulants.

Comment: It remains to be determined if stenting influences the relative benefits and harms of percutaneous procedures compared with CABG.

Substantive changes since last issue

Antiplatelet treatment One systematic review found that thienopyridines (ticlopidine or clopidogrel) reduced the odds of a vascular event compared with aspirin but there was substantial uncertainty about the size of any additional benefit.[14] The review found that clopidogrel was safer than ticlopidine.

Effects of cholesterol reduction: Effects of statins in different groups of people One large trial found from sub-group analysis no significant effect on all cause mortality of statins in women but the trial had low power and the confidence interval was wide.[50]

Surgical treatments: Coronary PTA versus CABG for multivessel disease One large RCT found improved survival in people with diabetes 7 years after CABG v PTA.[104]

REFERENCES

1. Greaves EJ, Gillum BS. 1994 Summary: national hospital discharge survey. Advance data from Vital and Health Statistics, no. 278. Hyattsville, Maryland: National Center for Health Statistics, 1996.

2. Rouleau JL, Talajic M, Sussex B, et al. Myocardial infarction patients in the 1990s – their risk factors, stratification and survival in Canada: the Canadian assessment of myocardial infarction (CAMI) study. *J Am Coll Cardiol* 1996;27:1119–1127.

3. Shaw LJ, Peterson ED, Kesler K, Hasselblad V, Califf RM. A meta-analysis of predischarge risk stratification after acute myocardial infarction with stress electrocardiographic, myocardial perfusion, and ventricular function imaging. *Am J Cardiol* 1996;78:1327–1337. Search date 1995; primary sources Medline 1980 to 1995, and hand search of bibliographies of review articles published 1985 to 1995.

4. Kudenchuk PJ, Maynard C, Martin JS, et al. Comparison, presentation, treatment and outcome of acute myocardial infarction in men versus women (the myocardial infarction triage and intervention registry). *Am J Cardiol* 1996;78:9–14.

5. The Task Force on the Management of Acute Myocardial Infarction of the European Society of Cardiology. Acute myocardial infarction: pre-hospital and in-hospital management. *Eur Heart J* 1996;17:43–63.

6. Peterson ED, Shaw LJ, Califf RM. Clinical guideline: part II. Risk stratification after myocardial infarction. *Ann Intern Med* 1997;126:561–582.

7. The Multicenter Postinfarction Research Group. Risk stratification and survival after myocardial infarction. *N Engl J Med* 1983;309:331–336.

8. American College of Cardiology/American Heart Association Task Force on Practice Guidelines (Committee on Exercise Testing). ACC/AHA guidelines for exercise testing. *J Am Coll Cardiol* 1997;30:260–315.

9. Fallen E, Cairns J, Dafoe W, et al. Management of the postmyocardial infarction patient: a consensus report – revision of the 1991 CCS guidelines. *Can J Cardiol* 1995;11:477–486.

10. Madsen JK, Grande P, Saunamaki, et al. Danish multicenter randomized study of invasive versus conservative treatment in patients with inducible ischemia after thrombolysis in acute myocardial infarction (DANAMI). *Circulation* 1997;96:748–755.

11. Antiplatelet Trialists' Collaboration. Collaborative overview of randomised trials of antiplatelet therapy – I: prevention of death, myocardial infarction, and stroke by prolonged antiplatelet therapy in various categories of patients. *BMJ* 1994;308:81–106. Search date; trials available at March 1990; primary source Medline; Current Contents; hand search of journals, reference lists and conference proceedings; authors of trials and drug manufacturers.

12. Taylor DW, Barnett HJM, Haynes RB, et al, for the ASA and Carotid Endarterectomy (ACE) Trial Collaborators. Low-dose and high-dose acetylsalicylic acid for patients undergoing carotid endarterectomy: a randomised controlled trial. *Lancet* 1999;353:2179–2184.

13. Juul-Möller S, Edvardsson N, Jahnmatz B, Rosen A, Soreneson S, Omblus R, for the Swedish Angina Pectoris Aspirin Trial (SAPAT) Group. Double-blind trial of aspirin in primary prevention of myocardial infarction in patients with stable chronic angina pectoris. *Lancet* 1992;340:1421–1425.

14. Hankey GJ, Sudlow CLM, Dunbabin DW. Thienopyridine derivatives (ticlopidine, clopidogrel) versus aspirin for preventing stroke and other serious vascular events in high vascular risk patients. In: The Cochrane Library, Issue 1, 2000. Oxford: Update software. Search date March/July 1999; primary sources Medline July 1999; Embase July 1999; Cochrane Stroke Group Register March 1999; Antithrombotics Trialists' database March 1999; authors of trials; and drug manufacturers.

15. CAPRIE Steering Committee. A randomised, blinded, trial of clopidogrel versus aspirin in patients at risk of ischaemic events. *Lancet* 1996; 348:1329–1339.

16. Farrell B, Godwin J, Richards S, Warlow C. The United Kingdom transient ischaemic attack (UK-TIA) aspirin trial: final results. *J Neurol Neurosurg Psychiatry* 1991;54:1044–1054.

17. Moloney BA. An analysis of the side effects of ticlopidine. In: Hass WK, Easton JD, eds. *Ticlopidine, Platelets and Vascular Disease.* New York: Springer, 1993:117–139.

18. Bennett CL, Davidson CJ, Raisch DW, Weinberg PD, Bennett RH, Feldman MD. Thrombotic thrombocytopenic purpura assoicated with ticlopidine in the setting of coronary artery stents and stroke prevention. *Arch Int Med* 1999; 159: 2524–2528.

19. Bennett CL, Connors JM, Carwile JM, Moake JL, Bell WR, Tarantolo SR, McCarthy LJ, Sarode R, Hatfield AJ, Feldman MD, Davidson CJ, Tsai HM. Thrombotic thrombocytopenic purpura associated with clopidogrel. *N Engl J Med* 2000; 342: 1773–1777.

20. Hankey GJ. Clopidogrel and thrombotic

thrombocytopenic purpura. *Lancet* 2000; 356: 269–270.

21. Anand SS, Yusuf S. Oral anticoagulant therapy in patients with coronary artery disease: a meta-analysis. *JAMA* 1999;282:2058–2067.

22. Teo KK, Yusuf S, Furberg CD. Effects of prophylactic antiarrhythmic drug therapy in acute myocardial infarction. *JAMA* 1993;270:1589–1595. Search date 1993; primary sources Medline 1960 to 1993; hand search of reference lists; details of unpublished trials sought from pharmaceutical industry/other investigators.

23. Yusuf S, Peto R, Lewis J, Collins R, Sleight P. Beta blockade during and after myocardial infarction: An overview of the randomized trials. *Prog Cardiovasc Dis* 1985;27:335–371. No details of search date or primary sources given.

24. Pepine CJ, Cohn PF, Deedwania PC, et al for the ASIST Study Group. Effects of treatment on outcome in mildly symptomatic patients with ischemia during daily life: the atenolol silent ischemia study (ASIST). *Circulation* 1994;90:762–768.

25. Boissel J-P, Leizerovicz A, Picolet H, et al, for the APSI Investigators. Secondary prevention after high-risk acute myocardial infarction with low-dose acebutolol. *Am J Cardiol* 1990;66:251–260.

26. The Beta-Blocker Pooling Project Research Group. The beta-blocker pooling project (BBPP): subgroup findings from randomized trials in post infarction patients. *Eur Heart J* 1988;9:8–16. Search date placebo controlled trials published by December 1983; details of primary sources not given.

27. Beta-blocker Heart Attack Trial Research Group. A randomized trial of propranolol in patients with acute myocardial infarction: I. Mortality results. *JAMA* 1982;247:1707–1714.

28. Flather M, Kober L, Pfeffer MA, et al. Meta-analysis of individual patient data from trials of long-term ACE-inhibitor treatment after acute myocardial infarction (SAVE, AIRE, and TRACE studies). *Circulation* 1997;96(suppl 1):I–706. No details of search date or primary sources given.

29. The Heart Outcomes Prevention Evaluation (HOPE) Investigators. Effects of an angiotensin-converting enzyme inhibitor, ramipril, on cardiovascular events in high-risk patients. *N Engl J Med* 2000; 342;145–153.

30. Heart Outcomes Prevention Evaluation (HOPE) Investigators. Effects of ramipril on cardiovascular and microvascular outcomes on people with diabetes mellitus: results of the hope study and MICRO-HOPE substudy. *Lancet* 2000;355:253–259.

31. Yusuf S, Lonn E. Anti-ischaemic effects of ACE inhibitors: review of current clinical evidence and ongoing clinical trials. *Eur Heart J* 1998;19(suppl J):J36–44.

32. Echt DS, Liebson PR, Mitchell LB, et al. Mortality and morbidity in patients receiving encainide, flecainide, or placebo. *N Engl J Med* 1991;324: 781–788.

33. Amiodarone Trials Meta-Analysis Investigators. Effect of prophylactic amiodarone on mortality after acute myocardial infarction and in congestive heart failure: meta-analysis of individual data from 6500 patients in randomised trials. *Lancet* 1997; 350:1417–1424. No details of search date or primary sources given.

34. Sim I, McDonald KM, Lavori PW, Norbutas CM, Hlatky MA. Quantitative overview of randomized trials of amiodarone to prevent sudden cardiac death. *Circulation* 1997;96:2823–2829. Search date 1997; primary sources Medline and Biosis 1985 to March 1997.

35. Waldo AL, Camm AJ, de Ruyter H, et al for the SWORD Investigators. Effect of d-sotalol on mortality in patients with left ventricular dysfunction after recent and remote myocardial infarction. *Lancet* 1996;348:7–12.

36. Cairns JA, Connolly SJ, Roberts R, Gent M, for the Canadian Amiodarone Myocardial Infarction Arrhythmia Trial Investigators. Randomized trial of outcome after myocardial infarction in patients with frequent or repetitive ventricular premature depolarisations: CAMIAT. *Lancet* 1997;349:675–682.

37. Julian DG, Camm AJ, Janse MJ, et al for the European Myocardial Infarct Amiodarone Trial Investigators. Randomised trial of effect of amiodarone on mortality in patients with left-ventricular dysfunction after recent myocardial infarction: EMIAT. *Lancet* 1997;349:667–674.

38. Gibson R, Boden WE, Theroux P et al. Diltiazem and reinfarction in patients with non-Q-wave myocardial infarction. *N Engl J Med* 1986;315: 423–429.

39. The Multicenter Diltiazem Postinfarction Trial Research Group. The effect of diltiazem on mortality and reinfarction after myocardial infarction. *N Engl J Med* 1988;319:385–392.

40. The Danish Study Group on Verapamil in Myocardial Infarction. Effect of verapamil on mortality and major events after acute myocardial infarction: the Danish verapamil infarction trial II (DAVIT II). *Am J Cardiol* 1990;66:779–785.

41. Hulley S, Grady D, Bush T, et al. Randomized trial of estrogen plus progestin for secondary prevention of coronary heart disease in postmenopausal women. *JAMA* 1998;280:605–613.

42. Coronary Drug Research Project Research Group. The coronary drug project: initial findings leading to modifications of its research protocol. *JAMA* 1970;214:1303–1313.

43. Daly E, Vessey MP, Hawkins MM, Carson JL, Gough P, Marsh S. Risk of venous thromboembolism in users of hormone replacement therapy. *Lancet* 1996;348:977–980.

44. Newton KM, LaCroix AZ, McKnight B, et al. Estrogen replacement therapy and prognosis after first myocardial infarction. *Am J Epidemiol* 1997; 145:269–277.

45. Sullivan JM, El-Zeky F, Vander Zwaag R, et al. Effect on survival of estrogen replacement therapy after coronary artery bypass grafting. *Am J Cardiol* 1997;79:847–850.

46. The Writing Group for the PEPI Trial. Effects of estrogen or estrogen/progestin regimens on heart disease risk factors in postmenopausal women. *JAMA* 1995;273:199–208.

47. Miettinen TA, Pyorala K, Olsson AG, Musliner TA, Cook TJ et al. Cholesterol-lowering therapy in women and elderly patients with myocardial infarction or angina pectoris: findings from the Scandinavian Simvastatin Survival Study (4S). *Circulation* 1997;96:4211–4218.

48. LaRosa JC, He J, Vupputuri S. Effect of statins on risk of coronary disease: A meta-analysis of randomized controlled trials. *JAMA* 1999;282: 2340–2346. Search date 1998; primary sources Medline, bibliographies and authors' reference files.

49. Bucher HC, Griffith LE, Guyatt G. Systematic review on the risk and benefit of different cholesterol-lowering interventions. *Arterioscler Thromb Vasc Biol* 1999;19:187–195. Search date October 1996; primary sources Medline, Embase, bibliographic searches.

50. Rubins HB, Robins SJ, Collins D, et al. Gemfibrozil for the secondary prevention of coronary heart disease in men with low levels of high-density lipoprotein cholesterol. *N Engl J Med* 1999;341: 410–418.

51. The Cholesterol Treatment Trialists' (CTT) Collaboration. Protocol for a prospective collaborative overview of all current and planned randomized trials of cholesterol treatment regimens. *Am J Cardiol* 1995;75:1130–1134.

52. The Women's Health Initiative Study Group. Design of the women's health initiative clinical trial and observational study. *Control Clin Trials* 1998; 19:61–109.

53. Davis BR, Cutler JA Gordon DJ, et al for the ALLHAT Research Group. Rationale and design for the antihypertensive and lipid lowering treatment to prevent heart attack trial (ALLHAT). *Am J Hypertens* 1996;9:342–360.

54. Flack JM, Neaton J, Grimm R, et al. Blood pressure and mortality among men with prior myocardial infarction. *Circulation* 1995;92;2437–2445.

55. Dahlof B, Lindholm LH, Hansson L, et al. Morbidity and mortality in the Swedish trial in old patients with hypertension (STOP-hypertension). *Lancet* 1991;338:1281–1285.

56. Medical Research Council Working Party. MRC trial on treatment of hypertension in older adults: principal results. *BMJ* 1992;304:405–412.

57. Systolic Hypertension in Elderly Patients (SHEP) Cooperative Research Group. Prevention of stroke by antihypertensive treatment in older persons with isolated systolic hypertension. *JAMA* 1991; 265:3255–3264.

58. D'Agostini RB, Belanger AJ, Kannel WB, et al. Relationship of low diastolic blood pressure to coronary heart disease death in presence of myocardial infarction: the Framingham study. *BMJ* 1991;303:385–389.

59. Pfeffer MA, Braunwald E, Moye LA, et al on behalf of the SAVE investigators. Effect of captopril on mortality and morbidity in patients with left ventricular dysfunction after myocardial infarction: results of the survival and ventricular enlargement trial. *N Engl J Med* 1992;327:669–677.

60. NHS Centre for Reviews and Dissemination, University of York. Cholesterol and coronary heart disease: screening and treatment. *Eff Health Care* 1998;4:Number 1. Search date and primary sources not given.

61. Burr ML, Fehily AM, Gilbert JF, et al. Effects of changes in fat, fish, and fibre intakes on death and myocardial reinfarction: diet and reinfarction trial (DART). *Lancet* 1989;2:757–761.

62. Fehily AM, Vaughan-Williams E, Shiels K, et al. The effect of dietary advice on nutrient intakes: evidence from the diet and reinfarction trial (DART). *J Hum Nutr Dietetics* 1989;2:225–235.

63. GISSI-Prevenzione Investigators. Dietary supplementation with n-3 polyunsaturated fatty acids and vitamin E after myocardial infarction: results of the GISSI-Prevenzione. *Lancet* 1999; 354:447–455.

64. de Lorgeril M, Renaud S, Mamelle N, et al. Mediterranean alpha-linolenic acid-rich diet in secondary prevention of coronary heart disease. *Lancet* 1994;343:1454–1459.

65. Clarke R, Frost C, Collins R, et al. Dietary lipids and blood cholesterol: quantitative meta-analysis of metabolic ward studies. *BMJ* 1997;314:112–117. Search date 1995; primary sources Medline 1960 to 1995, hand search of reference lists and nutrition journals.

66. Tang JL, Armitage JM, Lancaster T, et al. Systematic review of dietary intervention trials to lower blood total cholesterol in free-living subjects. *BMJ* 1998;316:1213–1220. Search date 1997; primary sources Medline, Human Nutrition, Embase, and Allied and Alternative Medicine 1966 to 1997, hand searching the *Am J Clin Nutr*; and references of review articles.

67. Brunner E, White I, Thorogood M, et al. Can dietary interventions change diet and cardiovascular risk factors? A meta-analysis of randomized controlled trials. *Am J Public Health* 1997;87:1415–1422. Search date 1993; primary sources Medline 1966 to July 1993, and manual search of selected journals.

68. Ebrahim S, Davey SG. *Health promotion in older people for the prevention of coronary heart disease and stroke.* London: Health Education Authority, 1996.

69. Waters D. Lessons from coronary atherosclerosis "regression" trials. *Cardiol Clin* 1996;14:31–50.

70. Silagy C, Neil A. Garlic as a lipid lowering agent: a meta-analysis. *J R Coll Physicians Lond* 1994;28:39–45. Search date July 1992; primary sources Medline 1966 to July 1992; Alternative Medicine database; authors of published studies; manufacturers; and hand searched references.

71. Isaacson JL, Moser M, Stein EA, et al. Garlic powder and plasma lipids and lipoproteins. *Arch Intern Med* 1998;158:1189–119.

72. Berthold HK, Sudhop T, von Bergmann K. Effect of a garlic oil preparation on serum lipoproteins and cholesterol metabolism. *JAMA* 1998;279:1900–1902.

73. Ripsin CM, Keenan JM, Jacobs DR Jr, et al. Oat products and lipid lowering: a meta-analysis. *JAMA* 1992;267:3317–3325. Search date 1991; primary sources Medline 1966 to 1991; unpublished trials solicited form all known investigators of lipid-oats association.

74. Anderson J, Johnstone B, Cooke-Newell M. Meta-analysis of the effects of soy protein intake on serum lipids. *N Engl J Med* 1995;333:276–282. No details of search date or primary sources given.

75. Stephens NG, Parsons A, Schofield PM, et al. Randomised controlled trial of vitamin E in patients with coronary disease: Cambridge heart antioxidant study (CHAOS). *Lancet* 1996;347:781–786.

76. Rapola JM, Virtamo J, Ripatti S, et al. Randomised trial of α-tocopherol and β-carotene supplements on incidence of major coronary events in men with previous myocardial infarction. *Lancet* 1997;349:1715–1720.

77. The Heart Outcomes Prevention Evaluation Study Investigators. Vitamin E supplementation and cardiovascular events in high-risk patients. The Heart Outcomes Prevention Evaluation Study Investigators. *N Engl J Med* 2000;342:154–160.

78. Wenger NK, Froelicher NS, Smith LK, et al. *Cardiac rehabilitation and secondary prevention.* Rockville, Maryland: Agency for Health Care Policy and Research and National Heart, Lung and Blood Institute, 1995. Search date and primary source not given.

79. Wilson TS, Datta SB, Murrell JS, Andrews CT. Relation of vitamin C levels to mortality in a geriatric hospital: a study of the effect of vitamin C administration. *Age Aging* 1973;2:163–170.

80. Burr ML, Hurley RJ, Sweetnam PM. Vitamin C supplementation of old people with low blood levels. *Gerontol Clin* 1975;17:236–243.

81. Hunt C, Chakkravorty NK, Annan G. The clinical and biochemical effects of vitamin C supplementation in short-stay hospitalized geriatric patients. *Int J Vitam Nutr Res* 1984;54:65–74.

82. Lonn EM, Yusuf S. Is there a role for antioxidant vitamins in the prevention of cardiovascular diseases? An update on epidemiological and clinical trials data. *Can J Cardiol* 1997;13:957–965. Search date 1996; primary sources Medline 1965 to 1996; and one reference from 1997.

83. Jha P, Flather M, Lonn E, Farkouh M, Yusuf S. The antioxidant vitamins and cardiovascular disease: a

critical review of epidemiologic and clinical trial data. *Ann Intern Med* 1995;123:860–872.

84. Ness AR, Powles JW, Khaw KT. Vitamin C and cardiovascular disease: a systematic review. *J Cardiovasc Risk* 1997;3:513–521. Search date not given; primary sources Medline, experts, and hand searched references.

85. Oldridge NB, Guyatt GH, Fisher MS, Rimm AA. Cardiac rehabilitation after myocardial infarction: combined experience of randomized clinical trials. *JAMA* 1988;260:945–950. Search date not specified; primary sources Medline.

86. O'Connor GT, Buring JE, Yusuf S, et al. An overview of randomized trials of rehabilitation with exercise after myocardial infarction. *Circulation* 1989;80: 234–244. No details of search date or primary sources given.

87. Berlin JA, Colditz GA. A meta-analysis of physical activity in the prevention of coronary heart disease. *Am J Epidemiol* 1990;132:612–628. No details of search date or primary sources given.

88. US Department of Health and Human Services. *The health benefits of smoking cessation: a report of the surgeon general*. Bethesda, Maryland: US DHSS, 1990.

89. Working Group for the Study of Transdermal Nicotine in Patients with Coronary Artery Disease. Nicotine replacement therapy for patients with coronary artery disease. *Arch Intern Med* 1994; 154:989–995.

90. Joseph AM, Norman SM, Ferry LH, et al. The safety of transdermal nicotine as an aid to smoking cessation in patients with cardiac disease. *N Engl J Med* 1996;335:1792–1798.

91. Burt A, Thornley P, Illingworth D, White P, Shaw TRD, Turner R. Stopping smoking after myocardial infarction. *Lancet* 1974;1:304–306.

92. Linden W, Stossel C, Maurice J. Psychosocial interventions in patients with coronary artery disease: a meta-analysis. *Arch Intern Med* 1996; 156:745–752. No details of search date or primary sources given.

93. US Department of Health and Human Services. Cardiac rehabilitation. AHCPR Publication No 96–0672, 1995;121–128.

94. Hemingway H, Marmot M. Psychosocial factors in the primary and secondary prevention of coronary heart disease: a systematic review. In Yusuf S, Cairns JA, Camm AJ, Fallen EL, Gersh BJ, eds. *Evidence based cardiology*. London: BMJ Books, 1998. Search date 1996; primary sources Medline 1966 to 1996; manual searching of bibliographies of retrieved articles and review articles.

95. Yusuf S, Zucker D, Peduzzi P, et al. Effect of coronary artery bypass graft surgery on survival: overview of 10-year results from randomized trials by the coronary artery bypass graft surgery trialists collaboration. *Lancet* 1994;344:563–570. No search date or primary sources given.

96. Davies RF, Goldberg AD, Forman S, et al. Asymptomatic cardiac ischemia pilot (ACIP) study two-year follow-up: outcomes of patients randomized to initial strategies of medical therapy versus revascularization. *Circulation* 1997;95: 2037–2043.

97. Fischman DL, Leon MB, Bain DS, et al. A randomized comparison of coronary-stent placement and balloon angioplasty in the treatment of coronary artery disease. *N Engl J Med* 1994;331:496–501.

98. Parisi AF, Folland ED, Hartigan P. A comparison of angioplasty with medical therapy in the treatment of single-vessel coronary artery disease. *N Engl J Med* 1992;326:10–16.

99. RITA-2 Trial Participants. Coronary angioplasty versus medical therapy for angina: the second randomized intervention treatment of angina (RITA-2) trial. *Lancet* 1997;350:461–468.

100. Pitt B, Waters D, Brown WV et al. Aggressive lipid-lowering therapy compared with angioplasty in stable coronary artery disease. *N Engl J Med* 1999;341:70–76.

101. Morris KG, Folland ED, Hartigan PM, Parisi AF. Unstable angina in late follow-up of the ACME trial. *Circulation* 1995;92(suppl I):I–725.

102. Pocock SJ, Henderson RA, Rickards AF, et al. Meta-analysis of randomized trials comparing coronary angioplasty with bypass surgery. *Lancet* 1995;346:1184–1189. No details of search date or primary sources given.

103. Bypass Angioplasty Revascularization Investigation (BARI) Investigators. Comparison of coronary bypass surgery with angioplasty in patients with multivessel disease: *N Engl J Med* 1996;335:7–225.

104. The BARI Investigators. Seven-Year Outcome in the Bypass Angioplasty Revascularization Investigation (BARI) By Treatment and Diabetic Status. *J Am Coll Cardiol* 2000;35:1122–1129.

105. Rihal CS, Gersh BJ, Yusuf S. Chronic coronary artery disease: coronary artery bypass surgery vs percutaneous transluminal coronary angioplasty vs medical therapy. In: Yusuf S, Cairns JA, Camm JA, Fallen EL, Gersh BJ, eds. *Evidence based cardiology*. London: BMJ Books, 1998.

106. Hlatky MA, Rogers WJ, Johnstone I, et al. Medical care costs and quality of life after randomization to coronary angioplasty or coronary bypass surgery. *N Engl J Med* 1997; 336:92–99.

107. Wihrborg P. Quality of life after coronary angioplasty or bypass surgery. *Eur Heart J* 1999; 20:653–658.

108. Serruys PW, de Jaeger P, Kiemeneij F, A comparison of balloon-expandable-stent implantation with balloon angioplasty in patients with coronary artery disease. *N Engl J Med* 1994;33:489–495.

109. Versaci F, Gaspardone A, Tomai F, Crea F, Chiariello L, Gioffre PA. A comparison of coronary-artery stenting with angioplasty for isolated stenosis of the proximal left anterior descending coronary artery. *N Engl J Med* 1997; 336:817–822.

110. Savage MP, Douglas JS, Fischman DL, et al. Stent placement compared with balloon angioplasty for obstructed coronary bypass grafts. *N Engl J Med* 1997;337:740–747.

111. Sirnes P, Golf S, Yngvar M, et al. Stenting in chronic coronary occlusion (SICCO): a randomized controlled trial of adding stent implantation after successful angioplasty. *J Am Coll Cardiol* 1996;28:1444–1451.

112. Rubartelli P, Niccoli L, Verna E, et al. Stent implantation versus balloon angioplasty in chronic coronary occlusions: results from the GISSOC trial. *J Am Coll Cardiol* 1998;32:90–96.

113. Sievert H, Rohde S, Utech A, et al. Stent or angioplasty after recanalization of chronic coronary occlusions? (the SARECCO trial). *Am J Cardiol* 1999;84:386–390.

114. Erbel R, Haude M, Hopp HW, et al. Coronary artery stenting compared with balloon angioplasty for restenosis after initial balloon angioplasty. *N Engl J Med* 1998;23:1682–1688.

115. Schomig A, Neumann EF, Kastrati A, et al. A randomized comparison of antiplatelet and anticoagulation therapy after the placement of intracoronary stents. *N Engl J Med* 1996;334: 1084–1089.

116. Leon MB, Baim DS, Gordon P, et al. Clinical and angiographic results from the stent anticoagulation regimen study (STARS). *Circulation* 1996;94:I–685.

Cardiovascular disorders

Cathie Sudlow
Specialist Registrar in Neurology
Department of Neurology
Derriford Hospital
Plymouth
UK

Eva Lonn
Associate Professor of Medicine
Hamilton General Hospital
Hamilton
Canada

Michael Pignone
Division of General Internal Medicine
University of North Carolina
Chapel Hill, NC
USA

Andrew Ness
Senior Lecturer in Epidemiology
University of Bristol
Bristol
UK

Charanjit Rihal
Consultant Cardiologist
Mayo Clinic and Mayo Foundation
Rochester
USA

Competing interests: CS, AN, CR none declared. JLP
has been reimbursed and received honoraria from the
Merck Company. EL has received honoraria for
delivering lectures from different companies, including
Hoechst Marion Roussel, the Merck Company, and
Parke-Davies; research grants have been part awarded
by Hoechst Marion Roussel and the Medical Research
Council of Canada.

TABLE 1	Prognostic groups for people who survive the acute stage of MI (see text, p 85).	

Baseline risk	One year mortality	Clinical markers[3–5]
High	10–50%	Older age; history or previous MI; reduced exercise tolerance (New York Heart Association functional classes II–IV) before admission; clinical signs of heart failure in the first 2 days (Killip classes IIb, III, and IV) or persistent heart failure on days 3–5 after infarction; early increased heart rate; persistent or early appearance of angina at rest or with minimal exertion; and multiple or complex ventricular arrhythmias during monitoring in hospital.
Moderate	10%	–
Low	2–5%	Younger age (< 55 years), no previous MI, an event free course during the first 5 days after MI.[3]

Prior MI (not acute MI)

A = Antiplatelet (mean 2 years)
C = Control

Adjusted % of patients (+1SD)

OUTCOME:	Non-fatal reinfarction	Non-fatal stroke	Vascular death	Any death
	A 460/9877 (4.7%)	A 82/8375 (1.0%)	A 797/9877 (8.1%)	A 910/9877 (9.2%)
	C 645/9914 (6.5%)	C 129/8372 (1.5%)	C 933/9914 (9.4%)	C 1029/9914 (10.4%)
Benefit per 1000:	18 (12 to 25)	6 (2 to 9)	13 (5 to 22)	12 (2 to 21)
% odds reduction:	31% (21 to 39%)	39% (20 to 54%)	15% (5 to 33%)	12% (2 to 20%)

FIGURE 1 The absolute effects of antiplatelet treatment on various outcomes in people with prior MI: results of a systematic review.[11] The columns show the absolute risks over 2 years for each outcome. The error bars represent standard deviations. In the "any death" column, non-vascular deaths are represented by lower horizontal lines (see text, p 86).

Cardiovascular disorders

Updated and expanded this issue

Gord Gubitz and Peter Sandercock

INTERVENTIONS

Key Messages

Systematic reviews of RCTs have found that:

■ Stroke rehabilitation units reduce death and severe disability.

■ Thrombolysis reduces the risk of dependency, but increases the risk of death (both from intracranial haemorrhage and from any cause).

■ Early use of aspirin after a known ischaemic stroke reduces the chance of death and dependency and improves the chance of complete recovery.

■ We found no evidence that immediate systemic anticoagulation improves outcome after ischaemic stroke.

■ Blood pressure reduction soon after acute ischaemic stroke has not been adequately tested in large scale RCTs, and may be harmful.

■ RCTs have found no evidence that calcium channel antagonists, lubeluzole, GABA agonists, glycine antagonists or N-methyl-D-glutamine (NMDA) antagonists improve clinical outcomes in people with acute ischaemic stroke.

■ We found no evidence of benefit from surgical evacuation of cerebral or cerebellar haematomas.

DEFINITION	Stroke is characterised by rapidly developing clinical symptoms and signs of focal, and at times global, loss of cerebral function lasting more than 24 hours or leading to death, with no apparent cause other than that of vascular origin.[1] Ischaemic stroke is defined as stroke caused by vascular insufficiency (such as cerebrovascular thromboembolism) rather than haemorrhage.
INCIDENCE/ PREVALENCE	Stroke is the third most common cause of death in most developed countries.[2] It is a worldwide problem; about 4.5 million people die from stroke each year. Stroke can occur at any age, but half of all strokes occur in people over 70 years old.[3]
AETIOLOGY/ RISK FACTORS	About 80% of all acute strokes are caused by cerebral infarction, usually resulting from thrombotic or embolic occlusion of a cerebral artery.[4] The remainder are caused either by intracerebral or subarachnoid haemorrhage.
PROGNOSIS	About 10% of all people with acute ischaemic strokes will die within 30 days of stroke onset.[5] Of those who survive the acute event, about 50% will experience some level of disability after 6 months.[6]
AIMS	To achieve rapid restoration and maintenance of blood supply to the ischaemic area in the brain; to minimise brain damage and hence impairment, disability, and secondary complications.
OUTCOMES	Risk of death or dependency (generally assessed as the proportion of people dead or requiring physical assistance for transfers, mobility, dressing, feeding, or toileting 3–6 months after stroke onset[6]); quality of life.
METHODS	*Clinical Evidence* update search and appraisal May 2000.

QUESTION   What are the effects of specialised care in people with stroke?

One systematic review of RCTs has found that people with stroke who are managed in specialist stroke rehabilitation units are more likely to be alive and living at home a year after the stroke than those managed in general medical wards, and that stroke unit care reduces time spent in hospital. Observational studies found that these results were reproducible in routine clinical settings.

Benefits: We found one systematic review (search date 1998) that identified 20 RCTs in 3864 people with stroke comparing specialised stroke rehabilitation units versus conventional care [7]. In most trials, the specialised stroke rehabilitation unit consisted of a designated area or ward, although some trials used a mobile "stroke team". Participants in these trials were usually transferred to stroke care within the first or second week following stroke onset. People cared for in a stroke rehabilitation unit had lower rates of death or dependency after a median follow up of 1 year (RRR 10%, 95% CI 5% to 15%; NNT 16, 95% CI 10 to 43) (see figure 1, p 125). The length of stay was calculated differently for many of the trials, so the consequent heterogeneity between results limits generalisability. Overall, length of stay in the stroke unit group was reduced by about 2–11 days. Since the review, two of the included trials have published follow-up data. One RCT (n = 220) found that care in a combined acute and rehabilitation unit compared with care in general wards increased the proportion of people able to live at home 10 years after their stroke (ARR 11%, 95% CI 1.9% to 20%; NNT 9, 95% CI 5 to 52).[8] The second RCT (n = 220) compared treatment in a 15 bed multidisciplinary stroke rehabilitation unit versus treatment in general medical wards.[9] Five years after the stroke, the risk of death or disability for people treated in the stroke unit was reduced (RR 0.91, 95% CI 0.83 to 0.99).

Harms: No detrimental effects attributable to stroke units were reported.

Comment: Although the proportional reduction in death or dependency seems larger with thrombolysis, stroke unit care is applicable to most stroke patients, whereas thrombolysis is applicable only to a small proportion. The systematic review did not provide data on which aspects of the multidisciplinary approach led to improved outcome, although one limited retrospective analysis of one of the RCTs found that several factors, including early mobilisation, increased use of oxygen, intravenous saline solutions, and antipyretics may have been responsible.[10] Most of the trials excluded the most mild and severe strokes. Following publication of the systematic review,[7] prospective observational data have been collected in one large series of over 14 000 people in 80 Swedish hospitals.[11] In this series, people admitted to stroke units had reduced dependence at 3 months (RRR 6%, 95% CI 1% to 11%). Although biases are inherent in such observational data, the findings suggest that the results of the meta-analysis may be reproducible in routine clinical settings.

QUESTION What are the effects of medical treatment in acute ischaemic stroke?

OPTION THROMBOLYSIS

We found little evidence on the balance between benefits and harms from thrombolysis in acute ischaemic stroke. One systematic review found that thrombolysis given soon after acute ischaemic stroke reduced overall risk of death and dependency in the long term, but that this benefit was achieved at the cost of an increased short term risk of fatal intracranial haemorrhage. It remains unclear which people are most likely to benefit or be harmed.

Benefits: We found one systematic review (search date in 1999) comparing thrombolytic treatment versus placebo given soon after the onset of stroke.[12] It identified 17 RCTs in a total of 5216 highly selected people. All trials included a computed tomography (CT) or magnetic resonance scan before randomisation to exclude intracranial haemorrhage or other non-stroke disorders. The systematic review included information on three different thrombolytic agents: streptokinase, urokinase, and recombinant tissue plasminogen activator (rt-PA), but direct comparison of different thrombolytic drugs was not possible. Two trials used intra-arterial administration and the rest used the intravenous route. Thrombolysis reduced the risk of being dead or dependent at the end of the studies (ARR 4.2%, 95% CI 1.2% to 7.2%; RRR 7%, 95% CI 3% to 12%; NNT 24, 95% CI 14 to 83) (see figures 1 and 2, p 125). In the subset of trials assessing intravenous rt-PA, the findings were similar (ARR 5.7%, 95% CI 2.0% to 9.4%; RRR 10%, 95% CI 4% to 16%; NNT 18, 95% CI 11 to 50).

Harms: **Fatal intracranial haemorrhage:** In the systematic review, thrombolysis increased fatal intracranial haemorrhage compared with placebo (ARI 4.4%, 95% CI 3.4% to 5.4%; RRI 396%, 95% CI 220% to 668%; NNH 23, 95% CI 19 to 29).[12] In the subset of trials assessing intravenous rt-PA, the findings were similar (ARI 2.9%, 95% CI 1.7% to 4.1%; RRI 259%, 95% CI 102% to 536%; NNH 34, 95% CI 24 to 59). **Death:** In the systematic review, thrombolytic treatment increased the risk of death by the end of the follow up period compared with placebo (ARI 3.3%, 95% CI 1.2% to 5.4%; RRI 23%, 95% CI 10% to 38%; NNH 30, 95% CI 19 to 83).[12] This excess of deaths was offset by fewer people being alive but dependent 6 months after stroke onset. The net effect was a reduction in the number of people who were dead or dependent.

Comment: There was no significant heterogeneity of treatment effect overall, but heterogeneity of results was noted for the outcomes of death, and death or dependency at final follow up among the eight trials evaluating intravenous rt-PA.[12] Explanations may include the concomitant use of antithrombotic agents (aspirin or heparin) within the first 24 hours of thrombolysis, stroke severity, the presence of early ischaemic changes on CT scan, and the time from stroke onset to randomisation. A subgroup analysis of the small amount of available data suggested that thrombolysis may be more beneficial if given within 3 hours of symptom onset, but the duration of the "therapeutic time window" could not be determined reliably. Most of the trial data related to outcome at 3 months; only one trial reported 1 year outcome data.[13] We found little evidence about which people are most and least likely to benefit from thrombolysis. One ongoing RCT is evaluating rt-PA (given within 6 hours of event) versus placebo in acute ischaemic stroke.[14]

OPTION ASPIRIN

One systematic review of RCTs has found that antiplatelet treatment with aspirin started within 48 hours of acute ischaemic stroke reduces the risk of death and dependence, as does the continued long term use of aspirin (see aspirin under stroke prevention, p 126). Most people included in the systematic review had a CT scan to exclude haemorrhage before treatment was started; in such people aspirin was beneficial. There is less evidence about the effect of aspirin in people who have not been scanned first.

Benefits: **Early use of aspirin:** We found one systematic review (search date in 1999).[15] This identified eight RCTs comparing antiplatelet treatment started within 14 days of the stroke versus placebo in 41 325 people with definite or presumed ischaemic stroke; 98% of the data in the systematic review came from two large RCTs testing aspirin 160–300 mg daily started within 48 hours of stroke onset.[16,17] Most people had an ischaemic stroke confirmed by CT scan before randomisation, but people who were conscious could be randomised before CT scan if the stroke was very likely to be ischaemic on clinical grounds. Treatment duration varied from 10–28 days. Aspirin started within the first 48 hours of acute ischaemic stroke reduced death or dependency at 6 months' follow up (RRR 3%, 95% CI 1% to 5%; NNT 77, 95% CI 43 to 333) (see figure 1, p 125). The number needed to treat for one extra person to make a complete recovery from their stroke was 91 (95% CI 50 to 500). **Long term treatment (3 years):** See aspirin under stroke prevention, p 126.

Harms: Aspirin caused an excess of about two intracranial and four extracranial haemorrhages per 1000 people treated, but these small risks were more than offset by the reductions in death and disability from other causes both in the short term[15] and in the long term.[18] Common adverse effects of aspirin (such as dyspepsia and constipation) were dose related.[19]

Comment: We found no clear evidence that any one dose of aspirin is more effective than any other in the treatment of acute ischaemic stroke. One recent metaregression analysis of the dose response effect of aspirin on stroke found a uniform effect of aspirin in a range of doses from 50–1500 mg/day.[20] People unable to swallow safely after a stroke may be given aspirin as a suppository.

OPTION   IMMEDIATE SYSTEMIC ANTICOAGULATION

One systematic review of RCTs has found that comparing immediate treatment with systemic anticoagulants (including unfractionated heparin, low molecular weight heparin, heparinoids, or specific thrombin inhibitors) with usual care but not including systemic anticoagulants offers no short or long term improvement in acute ischaemic stroke. The risk of deep venous thrombosis and pulmonary embolus is reduced, but this benefit is offset by a dose dependent risk of intracranial and extracranial haemorrhage.

Benefits: **Death or dependency:** We found one systematic review (search date in 1999).[21] It identified 21 RCTs in 23 427 people comparing unfractionated heparin, low molecular weight heparin, heparinoids, oral anticoagulants, or specific thrombin inhibitors versus usual care but not including systemic anticoagulants. Over 80% of the data came from one trial, which randomised people with any severity of stroke to treatment with either subcutaneous heparin or placebo, usually after exclusion of haemorrhagic stroke by CT scan.[17] The found no significant difference in the proportion of people dead or dependent in the treatment and control groups at the end of follow up (3–6 months after the stroke, ARR 0.4%, 95% CI –0.9% to +1.7%; RRR 0%, 95% CI –2% to +3%) (see figure 1, p 125). There was no clear short or long term benefit of anticoagulants in any prespecified subgroup, including those with stroke of presumed cardioembolic origin, or with each of the types of anticoagulant tested, although the numbers of people randomised to treatment with agents other than subcutaneous unfractionated heparin were small (so that random error may have obscured any real differences between anticoagulant regimens). **Deep venous thrombosis and pulmonary embolism:** The systematic review included 10 small heterogeneous RCTs that assessed the effects of anticoagulants in 916 people at high risk of deep venous thrombosis after their stroke.[21] Anticoagulation reduced the risk of deep vein thrombosis compared with control (ARR 29%, 95% CI 24% to 35%; RRR 64%, 95% CI 54% to 71%; NNT 3, 95% CI 2 to 4). The systematic review (total n > 22 000) found that anticoagulants reduced the development of symptomatic pulmonary embolism compared with control (ARR 0.3%, 95% CI 0.1% to 0.6%; RRR 38%, 95% CI 16% to 54%; NNT 333, 95% CI 167 to 1000).[21] No trial sought pulmonary emboli systematically by performing investigations in all people to rule out silent events. The frequency of reported pulmonary emboli was low and varied among RCTs, so there may have been under-ascertainment.

Harms:
The systematic review found that anticoagulation slightly increased symptomatic intracranial haemorrhages within 14 days of starting treatment compared with control (ARI 0.93%, 95% CI 0.68% to 1.18%; RRI 163%, 95% CI 95% to 255%; NNH 108, 95% CI 85 to 147).[21] The large trial of subcutaneous heparin found that this effect was dose dependent (symptomatic intracranial haemorrhage by using medium dose compared with low dose heparin for 14 days, RRI 143%, 95% CI 82% to 204%; NNH 97, 95% CI 68 to 169).[17] The review also found a dose dependent increase in major extracranial haemorrhages after 14 days of treatment with anticoagulants (ARI 0.91%, 95% CI 0.67% to 1.15%; RRI 231%, 95% CI 136% to 365%; NNH 109, 95% CI 87 to 149).[21]

Comment:
We are aware of a recently completed trial of the low molecular weight heparin tinzaparin; full publication of results is awaited.[22] Alternative treatments to prevent deep venous thrombosis and pulmonary embolism after acute ischaemic stroke include aspirin and compression stockings. The evidence relating to these will be reviewed in a future issue of Clinical Evidence.

OPTION BLOOD PRESSURE REDUCTION

One systematic review of RCTs has found no evidence that blood pressure reduction is of benefit in people with acute ischaemic stroke, but suggests that treatment may be harmful.

Benefits:
We found one systematic review (search date 1997), which identified three RCTs comparing blood pressure lowering treatment versus placebo in 113 people with acute stroke.[23] Several different antihypertensive agents were used. The trials collected insufficient clinical data to allow an analysis of the relation between changes in blood pressure and clinical outcome.

Harms:
Two placebo controlled RCTs have suggested that people treated with antihypertensive agents may have a worse clinical outcome and increased mortality. The first compared the calcium channel antagonist nimodipine in 295 people with acute ischaemic stroke. The trial was stopped prematurely because of an excess of unfavourable neurological outcomes in the nimodipine treated group. Exploratory analyses confirmed that this negative correlation was related to reductions in mean arterial blood pressure (P = 0.02) and diastolic blood pressure (P = 0.0005).[24] The second evaluated β blockers (atenolol or propranolol) in 302 people

with acute ischaemic stroke. There was a non-significant increase in death for patients taking β blockers, and no difference in the proportion of patients achieving a good outcome.[25] One systematic review (search date 1994) evaluated nine placebo controlled RCTs of nimodipine in 3719 people with acute stroke; no net benefit was found.[26] A second review (published in 1998) of 24 trials of calcium antagonists in 6894 people found a non-significant increase in the risk of death (RRR 8%, 95% CI 1% reduction to 18% increase).[27] Although treatment with calcium antagonists in these trials was intended for neuroprotection, blood pressure was lower in the treatment group in several trials.

Comment: Population based data suggest a direct and continuous association between blood pressure and the risk of recurrent stroke.[28] However, acute blood pressure lowering in acute ischaemic stroke may lead to increased cerebral ischaemia. The systematic review[24] identified several ongoing RCTs, and a collaboration to collect further information has been formed.[29] In addition, we identified two additional ongoing RCTs not included in the systematic review.[30,31]

OPTION NEUROPROTECTIVE AGENTS

Systematic reviews have found no evidence that calcium channel blockers, GABA agonists, glycine antagonists, or NMDA antagonists improve clinical outcomes in people with acute ischaemic stroke. RCTs have found no evidence that lubeluzole, which inhibits presynaptic glutamate release, improves clinical outcomes in people with acute ischaemic stroke.

Benefits: We found no systematic reviews evaluating the general effectiveness of neuroprotective agents in acute ischaemic stroke. **Calcium channel antagonists:** We found one systematic review (search date 1999), which included 28 trials in a total of 7521 people with acute ischaemic stroke.[32] It found that calcium channel antagonists did not significantly reduce the risk of poor outcome (including death) at the end of the follow up period compared with placebo (ARI of poor outcome 4.9%, 95% CI −2.5% to +7.3%; RRI 4%, 95% CI −2% to +9%). **GABA agonists:** We found one systematic review (search date 1999) evaluating the GABA analogue piracetam, which included three trials in a total of 1002 people with acute ischaemic stroke.[33] It found no significant difference between treatment and control groups for the number of people dead or dependent at the end of follow up (ARI 0.2%, 95% CI −6.0% to +6.4%; RRI 0%, 95% CI −11% to +9%). We found one RCT, which compared the GABA agonist clomethiazole versus placebo in 1360 people with acute stroke.[34] It found no significant effect on achievement of functional independence (ARR 1.5%, 95% CI −4.0% to +6.6%; RRR 3.0%, 95% CI −7% to +13%). **Lubeluzole:** We found two RCTs assessing lubeluzole, an inhibitor of presynaptic glutamate release.[35,36] Intention to treat analysis of the first trial (n = 721) found that lubeluzole did not significantly reduce mortality at 12 weeks (AR 20.7 % with lubeluzole v 25.2% with placebo; ARR 4.5%, P = NS; RRR 18%, 95% CI −7% to +37%). The second trial (n = 725; 365 people randomised to lubeluzole, 360 to placebo) also found no significant difference in mortality at 12 weeks between lubeluzole and placebo (intention to treat analysis: ARR 0.6%, 95% CI −4.8% to +7.4%; RRR 3%, 95% CI −22% to +29%). A third trial has been completed, and full publication is awaited.[37] **Glycine antagonists:** We found abstracts of two RCTs evaluating the glycine antagonist GV150526 against placebo.[38,39] The first randomised 1804 people and found no significant difference in death or functional outcome.[38] The second randomised 1605 people and also found no significant difference in functional outcome at the end of follow up.[39] **NMDA antagonists:** Two recent RCTs evaluating the NMDA antagonist (see glossary, p 122) CGS19775 found no significant difference in the proportion of people with a Barthel Index Score over 60, but data were limited as the trials were terminated because of adverse outcomes after only 31% of the total planned patient enrolment.[40]

Harms:
In the systematic review of calcium antagonists, indirect and limited comparisons of intravenous versus oral administration of calcium antagonist found no significant difference in adverse events (ARI of adverse events, intravenous v oral 2.3%, 95% CI −0.9% to +3.7%; RRI 17%, 95% CI −3% to +41%).[32] In the systematic review of piracetam, there was a non-significant increase in death with piracetam versus placebo, which was no longer apparent after correction for imbalance in stroke severity.[33] Lubeluzole has also been noted to have adverse outcomes, especially at higher doses. One phase II trial of lubeluzole in 232 people was terminated prematurely because of an excess of deaths in the arm randomised to a higher dosage of drug.[41] This problem has not been noted with the lower drug dosages used in the published phase III studies.[35,36] The trials of CGS19775 were terminated after enrolling 567 people because of greater early mortality in the CGS19775 groups.[40]

Comment:
A systematic review is being developed to assess all of the lubeluzole data.[42] Another systematic review[43] is being developed for tirilazad, a steroid derivative that has shown no evidence of clinical benefit in one major trial that was terminated prematurely on the advice of the independent monitoring committee.[44] The effects of the cell membrane precursor citicholine have been evaluated in a number of small trials, and a systematic review is in progress.[45] Systematic reviews are also being developed for antioxidants,[46] and for excitatory amino acid modulators.[46] Several RCTs are ongoing, including one trial of intravenous magnesium sulphate[47] and another assessing the role of diazepam (a GABA agonist).[48]

QUESTION   **What are the effects of surgical treatment for intracerebral haematomas?**

OPTION   EVACUATION

We found that the balance between benefits and harms has not been clearly established for the evacuation of supratentorial haematomas. We found no evidence from RCTs on the role of evacuation or ventricular shunting in people with infratentorial haematoma whose conscious level is declining.

Benefits:
For supratentorial haematomas: We found one systematic review of RCTs (search date 1998),[49] as well as one systematic

review (search date 1997) that also assessed information from case series.[50] Both systematic reviews assessed the same four RCTs comparing surgery (craniotomy in 3 trials and endoscopy in 1) versus best medical treatment in 354 people with primary supratentorial intracerebral haemorrhage. Neither review found any significant short or long term differences in death or disability for surgically treated people (ARI 3.3%, 95% CI −5.9% to +12.5%; RRI 5%, 95% CI −7% to +19%). **For infratentorial haematomas:** We found no evidence from systematic reviews or RCTs on the role of surgical evacuation or ventricular shunting.[51]

Harms: The systematic reviews[49,50] found that for the 254 people randomised to craniotomy rather than best medical treatment, there was increased death and disability (ARI 12%, 95% CI 1.8% to 22%; RRI 17%, 95% CI 2% to 34%; NNH 8, 95% CI 5 to 56). For the 100 people randomised to endoscopy rather than best medical practice there was no significant effect on death and disability (RRR 24%, 95% CI −2% to +44%).

Comment: Current practice is based on the consensus opinion that people with infratentorial (cerebellar) haematomas whose conscious level is declining probably benefit from evacuation of the haematoma. The systematic reviews identified several ongoing RCTs assessing the evacuation of supratentorial haematomas.

GLOSSARY

NMDA antagonist Glutamate can bind to N-methyl-D-aspartate (NMDA) receptors on cell surfaces. One hypothesis proposed that glutamate released during a stroke can cause further harm to neurones by stimulating the NMDA receptors. NMDA antagonists block these receptors.

Substantive changes since last issue

Stroke rehabilitation units Two RCTs with 5 and 10 year follow up data; no change in conclusions.[8,9]

Neuroprotective agents: glycine antagonists Two RCTs reported in abstract form show no net benefit versus placebo.[38,39]

Neuroprotective agents: NMDA antagonists Two RCTs terminated early owing to greater early mortality in patients receiving the NMDA antagonist.[40]

REFERENCES

1. Hatano S. Experience from a multicentre stroke register: a preliminary report. *Bull World Health Organ* 1976;54:541–553.
2. Bonita R. Epidemiology of stroke. *Lancet* 1992; 339:342–344.
3. Bamford J, Sandercock P, Dennis M, Warlow C, Jones L, McPherson K. A prospective study of acute cerebrovascular disease in the community: the Oxfordshire community stroke project, 1981–1986. 1. Methodology, demography and incident cases of first ever stroke. *J Neurol Neurosurg Psychiatry* 1988;51:1373–1380.
4. Bamford J, Dennis M, Sandercock P, Burn J, Warlow C. A prospective study of acute cerebrovascular disease in the community: the Oxfordshire community stroke project, 1981–1986. 2. Incidence, case fatality rates and overall outcome at one year of cerebral infarction, primary intracerebral and subarachnoid haemorrhage. *J Neurol Neurosurg Psychiatry* 1990;53:16–22.
5. Bamford J, Dennis M, Sandercock P, Burn J,

Warlow C. The frequency, causes and timing of death within 30 days of a first stroke: the Oxfordshire community stroke project. *J Neurol Neurosurg Psychiatry* 1990;53:824–829.
6. Wade DT. Functional abilities after stroke: measurement, natural history and prognosis. *J Neurol Neurosurg Psychiatry* 1987;50:177–182.
7. Stroke Unit Trialists' Collaboration. Organised inpatient (stroke unit) care for stroke. In: The Cochrane Library, Issue 4, 1999. Oxford: Update Software. Search date June 1998; primary sources Cochrane Collaboration Stroke Group; reference lists of relevant articles; contact with colleagues; preliminary findings publicised at stroke conferences in the UK, Scandinavia, Germany, Netherlands, Switzerland, Spain, Canada and South America.
8. Indredavik B, Bakke RPT, Slordahl SA, Rokseth R, Haheim LL. Stroke unit treatment. 10-year follow-up. *Stroke* 1999;30:1524–1527.
9. Lincoln NB, Husbands S, Trescoli C, Drummond AER, Gladman JRF, Berman P. Five year follow up

of a randomised controlled trial of a stroke rehabilitation unit. *BMJ* 2000;320:549.

10. Indredavik B, Bakke RPT, Slordahl SA, Rokseth R, Haheim LL. Treatment in a combined acute and rehabilitation stroke unit. Which aspects are most important. *Stroke* 1999;30:917–923.

11. Stegmayr B, Asplund K, Hulter-Asberg K, et al. Stroke units in their natural habitat: can results of randomized trials be reproduced in routine clinical practice? For the risk-stroke collaboration. *Stroke* 1999;30:709–714.

12. Wardlaw JM, del Zoppo G, Yamaguchi T. Thrombolysis for acute ischaemic stroke. In: The Cochrane Library, Issue 4, 1999. Oxford: Update Software. Search date March 1999; primary sources Cochrane Collaboration Stroke Group; Medline; Embase; the Ottawa Stroke Trials Registry; references quoted in thrombolysis papers; direct contact with principal investigators of trials attendance at international conferences on acute stroke; abstracts of other neurological and cerebrovascular symposia as published in journals; and colleagues and pharmaceutical companies.

13. Kwiatkowski T, Libman R, Frankel M, et al. Effects of tissue plasminogen activator for acute ischemic stroke at one year. National Institute of Neurological Disorders and stroke recombinant tissue plasminogen activator stroke study group. *N Engl J Med* 1999;340:1781–1787.

14. The Third International Stroke Trial (IST-3). Protocol URL: http://www.dcn.ed.ac.uk/csrg.

15. Gubitz G, Sandercock P, Counsell C. Antiplatelet therapy for acute ischaemic stroke. In: The Cochrane Library, Issue 4, 1999. Oxford: Update Software. Search date March 1999; primary sources Cochrane Collaboration Stroke Group; Register of the Antiplatelet Trialists Collaboration June 1998; MedStrategy 1995; pharmaceutical companies marketing antiplatelet agents.

16. CAST. Randomised placebo-controlled trial of early aspirin use in 20 000 patients with acute ischaemic stroke. CAST (Chinese acute stroke trial) collaborative group. *Lancet* 1997;349:1641–1649.

17. International Stroke Trial Collaborative Group. The international stroke trial (IST): a randomised trial of aspirin, heparin, both or neither among 19 435 patients with acute ischaemic stroke. *Lancet* 1997;349:1569–1581.

18. Antiplatelet Trialists' Collaboration. Collaborative overview of randomised trials of antiplatelet therapy I: prevention of death, myocardial infarction and stroke by prolonged antiplatelet therapy in various categories of patients. *BMJ* 1994;308:81–106. Search date 1990; primary sources Medline and Current Contents.

19. Slattery J, Warlow CP, Shorrock CJ, Langman MJS. Risks of gastrointestinal bleeding during secondary prevention of vascular events with aspirin – analysis of gastrointestinal bleeding during the UK-TIA trial. *Gut* 1995;37:509–511.

20. Johnson ES, Lanes SF, Wentworth CE, Satterfield MH, Abebe BL, Dicker LW. A metaregression analysis of the dose-response effect of aspirin on stroke. *Arch Intern Med* 1999;159:1248–1253.

21. Gubitz G, Sandercock P, Counsell C, Signorini D. Anticoagulants for acute ischaemic stroke. In: The Cochrane Library, Issue 4, 1999. Oxford: Update Software. Search date March 1999; primary sources Cochrane Collaboration Stroke Group; MedStrategy 1995; Antithrombotic therapy trialists' collaboration trials register August 1998; and manufacturers of anticoagulants.

22. Bath P for the TAIST Investigators. Tinzaparin in Acute Ischaemic Stroke Trial (TAIST). *Cerebrovasc Dis* 2000;10(suppl 2):81.

23. Blood Pressure in Acute Stroke Collaboration (BASC). Interventions for deliberately altering blood pressure in acute stroke. In: The Cochrane Library, Issue 4, 1999. Oxford: Update Software. Search date May 1997; primary sources Cochrane Stroke Group trials register to 1997; Ottawa Stroke Trials Registry to 1994; Medline 1965 to May 1997; Embase 1981 to May 1997; ISI; handsearch of existing review articles; and researchers in the field and pharmaceutical companies contacted.

24. Wahlgren NG, MacMahon DG, DeKeyser J, Ingredavik B, Ryman, T. Intravenous nimodipine west European stroke trial (INWEST) of nimodipine in the treatment of acute ischaemic stroke. *Cerebrovasc Dis* 1994;4:204–210.

25. Barer DH, Cruickshank JM, Ebrahim SB, Mitchell JRA. Low dose beta blockade in acute stroke (BEST trial): an evaluation. *BMJ* 1988;296:737–741.

26. Mohr JP, Orgogozo JM, Harrison MJG, et al. Meta-analysis of oral nimodipine trials in acute ischaemic stroke. *Cerebrovasc Dis* 1994;4:197–203. Search date 1994; primary source Bayer database.

27. Horn J, Orgogozo JM, Limburg M. Review on calcium antagonists in ischaemic stroke; mortality data. *Cerebrovasc Dis* 1998;8(suppl 4):27.

28. Rodgers A, MacMahon S, Gamble G. Blood pressure and risk of stroke patients with cerebrovascular disease. *BMJ* 1996;313:147.

29. Bath F, Bath P. What is the correct management of blood pressure in acute stroke? The blood pressure in acute stroke collaboration. *Cerebrovasc Dis* 1997;7:205–213.

30. Schrader J, Rothemeyer M, Luders S, Kollmann K. Hypertension and stroke – rationale behind the ACCESS trial. *Basic Res Cardiol* 1998;93(suppl 2):69–78.

31. Bath P, Bath F for the ENOS Investigators. Efficacy of Nitric Oxide in Stroke (ENOS) Trial – A prospective large randomised controlled trial in acute stroke (abstract). *Cerebrovasc Dis* 2000; 10(suppl 2);8.

32. Horn J, Limburg M. Calcium antagonists for acute ischemic stroke. In: The Cochrane Library, Issue 1, 2000. Oxford: Update Software. Search date March 1999; primary source Cochrane Stroke Review Group Trials Register to March 1999.

33. Ricci S, Celani MG, Cantisani AT, Righetti E. Piracetam for acute ischaemic stroke. In: The Cochrane Library, Issue 1, 2000. Oxford: Update Software. Search date January 1999; primary sources Cochrane Stroke Review Group trials register to January 1999; Medline 1965 to January 1999; Embase 1980 to January 1999; BIDIS ISI 1981 to January 1999; handsearch of 15 journals and manufacturers contacted.

34. Wahlgren NG, Ranasinha KW, Rosolacci T, et al. Clomethiazole acute stroke study (CLASS): results of a randomised, controlled trial of clomethiazole versus placebo in 1360 acute stroke patients. *Stroke* 1999;30:21–28.

35. Grotta J, for the US and Canadian Lubeluzole Stroke Study Group. Lubeluzole treatment for acute ischaemic stroke. *Stroke* 1997;28:2338–2346.

36. Diener HC. Multinational randomised controlled trail of lubeluzole in acute ischaemic stroke. *Cerebrovasc Dis* 1998;8:172–181.

37. Wessel TC. Determinants of outcome in the lubeluzole clinical trial (abstract). In: Proceedings of the Seventh Annual Conference on ischemic stroke. Advances in novel therapeutic development. Washington DC. November 19–20, 1998. IBC USA Conferences Inc, Southborough, MA.

38. Lees K, Asplund K, Carolei A, et al for the GAIN International Investigators. GV150526 in the acute treatment of acute stroke: Gain International. *Cerebrovasc Dis* 2000;10(suppl 2):106.

39. Sacco R for the GAIN Americas Collaborative Group. GV150526 in the treatment of acute stroke: Results of the GAIN Americas Trial. *Cerebrovasc Dis* 2000;10(suppl 2):106.

40. Davis S, Lees K, Albers G, et al for the ASSIST Investigators. Selfotel in acute ischemic stroke. Possible neurotoxic effects of an NMDA antagonist. *Stroke* 2000;31:347–354.

41. Wahlgren NG, MacMahon DG, De Keyser J, Indredavik B, Ryman T for the INWEST Study Group. Intravenous nimodipine west European stroke trial (INWEST) of nimodipine in the treatment of acute ischaemic stroke. *Cerebrovasc Dis* 1994;4:204–210.

42. Gandolfo C, Conti M. Lubeluzole for acute ischemic stroke (Cochrane Protocol). In: The Cochrane Library, Issue 1, 2000. Oxford: Update Software (in press).

43. Bath P for the Tirilazad International Steering Committee. Tirilazad for acute ischaemic stroke (Cochrane Protocol). In: The Cochrane Library, Issue 2, 2000. Oxford: Update Software (in press).

44. The RANTTAS Investigators. A randomized trial of tirilazad mesylate in patients with acute stroke (RANTTAS). *Stroke* 1996;27:1453–1458.

45. Saver JL, Wilterdink J. Choline precursors for acute and subacute ischemic and hemorrhagic stroke

(Cochrane Protocol). In: The Cochrane Library, Issue 1, 2000. Oxford: Update Software (in press).

46. Cochrane Stroke Review Group. Department of Clinical Neurosciences, Western General Hospital, Crewe Road, Edinburgh, UK EH4 2XU. URL: http://www.dcn.ed.ac.uk/csrg.

47. Muir KW, Lees KR. IMAGES. Intravenous magnesium efficacy in stroke trial (abstract). *Cerebrovasc Dis* 1996;6:75P383.

48. Lodder, J, van Raak L, Kessels F, Hilton A. Early GABA-ergic Activation Study in Stroke (EGASIS). *Cerebrovasc Dis* 2000;10(suppl 2):80.

49. Prasad K , Shrivastava A. Surgery for primary supratentorial intracerebral haemorrhage. In: The Cochrane Library, Issue 4, 1999. Oxford: Update Software. Search date August 1998; primary sources Cochrane Collaboration Stroke Group; reference lists of all identified trials, and handsearching of specialist journals and monographs.

50. Hankey G, Hon C. Surgery for primary intracerebral hemorrhage: is it safe and effective? A systematic review of case series and randomised trials. *Stroke* 1997;28:2126–2132. Search date January 1996 to June 1997; primary sources Medline; references and reports cited in identified articles, and all published epidemiological studies and reviews were also examined.

51. Treatment of primary intracerebral haemorrhage. In: Warlow CP, Dennis MS, van Gijn J, et al, eds. *Stroke: a practical guide to management*. Oxford: Blackwell Science,1996:435.

Gord Gubitz
Assistant Professor
Division of Neurology
Dalhousie University
Halifax
Canada

Peter Sandercock
Professor of Neurology
Neurosciences Trials Unit
University of Edinburgh
Edinburgh
UK

Competing interests: GG, none declared. PS has received honoraria for lectures, funds for research, funds for members of his staff, and fees for single consultancies from Glaxo Wellcome, Boehringer Ingelheim, and Sanofi/BMS. PS has also received a grant from Glaxo Wellcome to undertake a clinical trial.

FIGURE 1 The proportional effects of different interventions on "death or dependency" at the end of scheduled follow up: results of systematic reviews.[7,12,16,17] The data refer only to benefits and not to harms (see text, p 115).

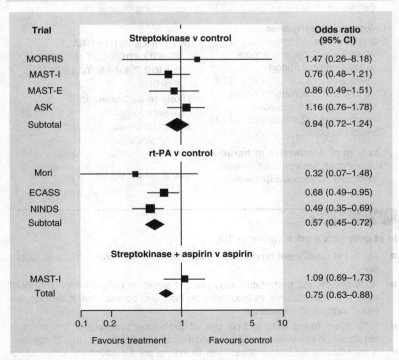

FIGURE 2 Effect of thrombolysis on death and dependency at end of trial follow up: results of a systematic review of RCTs (see text , p 116).[12]

Cardiovascular disorders

Updated this issue

Clinical Evidence writers on secondary prevention of stroke

INTERVENTIONS

Key Messages

In people with a prior stroke or TIA

- We found insufficient randomised evidence for routine blood pressure reduction.

- RCTs have found that statins may prevent stroke in people with a history of coronary heart disease. In those with no history of coronary heart disease, we found inconclusive evidence.

- RCTs have found that routine use of prolonged antiplatelet treatment is beneficial unless there is a clear contraindication, and that aspirin 75 mg daily is as effective as higher doses. We found no good evidence that any other antiplatelet regimen is superior to medium dose aspirin (75–325 mg daily) in the prevention of vascular events.

- RCTs have found that clopidogrel or the combination of aspirin and dipyridamole are safe and effective alternatives to medium dose aspirin.

© *Clinical Evidence* 2000;4:126–143.

- One systematic review found that ticlopidine or clopidogrel reduced the odds of a vascular event compared with aspirin but there was substantial uncertainty about the size of any additional benefit.
- We found no evidence of benefit from anticoagulation in people in sinus rhythm, but an increased risk of serious bleeding.
- One systematic review has found that carotid endarterectomy reduces the risk of major stroke in people with moderate and severe carotid stenosis provided the risks of imaging and surgery are small.
- We found that the role of percutaneous transluminal angioplasty (PTA) has not been adequately evaluated.

In people with atrial fibrillation and a prior stroke or TIA

- Systematic reviews and RCTs have found that anticoagulants reduce the risk of stroke, provided there is a low risk of bleeding and careful monitoring. Aspirin reduces the risk of stroke, but less effectively than anticoagulants. These findings support the use of aspirin in people with atrial fibrillation and contraindications to anticoagulants.

In people with atrial fibrillation but no other major risk factors for stroke

- Systematic reviews and RCTs have found that anticoagulants are of net benefit, provided there is a low risk of bleeding and careful monitoring. Aspirin is a reasonable alternative in people with contraindications to anticoagulants.

DEFINITION	Prevention in this context is the long term management of people with a prior stroke or transient ischaemic attack (TIA), and of people at high risk of stroke for other reasons such as atrial fibrillation. **Stroke:** See definition under stroke management, p 114. **TIA:** Similar to a mild ischaemic stroke except that symptoms last for less than 24 hours.[1]
INCIDENCE/ PREVALENCE	See incidence/prevalence under stroke management, p 114.
AETIOLOGY/ RISK FACTORS	See aetiology under stroke management, p 114. Risk factors for stroke include prior stroke or TIA, increasing age, hypertension, diabetes, cigarette smoking, and emboli associated with atrial fibrillation, artificial heart valves or myocardial infarction. The relation with cholesterol is less clear; an overview of prospective studies among healthy middle aged individuals found no association between total cholesterol and overall stroke risk.[2] However, one review of prospective observational studies in eastern Asian people found that cholesterol was positively associated with ischaemic stroke but negatively associated with haemorrhagic stroke.[3]
PROGNOSIS	People with a history of stroke or TIA are at high risk of all vascular events, such as myocardial infarction, but are at particular risk of subsequent stroke (about 10% in the first year and about 5% per year thereafter; see figure 1, p 143 and figure 1 in secondary prevention of ischaemic cardiac events, p 83.[4,5] People with intermittent atrial fibrillation treated with aspirin should be considered at similar risk of stroke, compared to people with sustained atrial fibrillation treated with aspirin (rate of ischaemic stoke per year, intermittent v sustained, 3.2% v 3.3%).[6]
AIMS	To prevent death or disabling stroke, as well as other serious non-fatal outcomes, especially myocardial infarction, with minimal adverse effects from treatment.

OUTCOMES	Rates of death, dependency, myocardial infarction, and stroke.
METHODS	*Clinical Evidence* update search and appraisal May 2000. Recent appropriate systematic reviews were identified as well as more recent RCTs.

QUESTION **What are the effects of interventions in people with prior stroke or TIA?**

OPTION BLOOD PRESSURE REDUCTION

Cathie Sudlow

We found insufficient evidence for routine blood pressure reduction among people with a prior stroke or TIA, but a large, ongoing RCT will provide further information.

Benefits: We found two overviews[7,8] and three subsequent RCTs.[9–11] One overview of RCTs of antihypertensive treatment (generally comprising a diuretic, a β blocker, or both), in around 48 000 people with hypertension, most of whom had no history of vascular disease, found that a reduction of about 10–12/5–6 mmHg in systolic/diastolic blood pressure over 2–3 years reduced the odds of stroke by 38% (95% CI 31% to 45%).[7] The results of a subsequent RCT of the calcium channel antagonist nitrendipine versus placebo in 4695 elderly people with systolic hypertension were similar: a reduction of about 10/5 mmHg over 2 years reduced the risk of stroke by 42% (95% CI 17% to 60%).[9] In the overview, the proportional effects of treatment on stroke were similar among people with differing degrees of hypertension, among middle aged and elderly people, and among people with or without a prior stroke or TIA.[8] Two of the trials (including around 500 people) specifically aimed to assess the effects of blood pressure reduction among people with hypertension with a prior stroke or TIA. These two trials were included in an overview of four RCTs of antihypertensive treatment versus placebo in around 3000 people with a history of a cerebrovascular event (with or without hypertension). Similar, but statistically uncertain, results were obtained: an average diastolic blood pressure reduction of 3 mmHg for about 3 years was associated with a non-significant reduction in the odds of stroke of 19% (95% CI −1% to +39%).[8] In a preliminary report (yet to be confirmed) from a further trial in China, in which 5665 people with a prior stroke or TIA were randomised to receive either the diuretic indapamide or placebo, reducing diastolic blood pressure by about 2 mm Hg over 2 years was associated with a reduction in stroke incidence (RRR 29%, 95% CI 12% to 42%).[10] We found one large RCT in 9297 people at high risk of vascular disease, of whom about 1000 had a history of stroke or TIA and about half had hypertension. It found that, compared with placebo, about 5 years of ramipril (an angiotensin converting enzyme [ACE] inhibitor) reduced diastolic blood pressure by an average of 2 mmHg, reduced risk of stroke by 31% (95% CI 16% to 44%), and reduced the risk of combined outcome of stroke, myocardial infarction, or cardiovascular death by 22% (95% CI 14% to 30%). The results for the primary outcome were similar among those with or without a prior stroke or TIA, and among those with or without hypertension.[11]

Harms:
In people with a history of stroke, reports of an apparently J-shaped relationship between blood pressure and subsequent stroke have led to concerns that blood pressure reduction may actually increase the risk of recurrent stroke, perhaps because of reduced cerebral perfusion.[12] However, preliminary analyses of data from over 15 000 people with a history of cerebrovascular or coronary events included in trials in the systematic review found a positive relation between usual diastolic blood pressure and the subsequent risk of stroke; for every 5 mmHg decrease in usual diastolic blood pressure there was about a 15% proportional reduction in stroke risk. These analyses found no evidence of any threshold below which a lower diastolic blood pressure was not associated with a lower stroke risk.[12,13] The RCTs found no evidence that reducing diastolic blood pressure was hazardous, at least down to about 80 mmHg.[7]

Comment:
There is persisting uncertainty about the net effects of blood pressure reduction among people with a previous cerebrovascular event. Further information will be provided by a large RCT that is currently assessing the balance of benefits and risks of treatment with the ACE inhibitor perindopril among 6000 people with a history of stroke or TIA.[8]

OPTION   CHOLESTEROL REDUCTION

Cathie Sudlow

We found insufficient evidence about the effects of routinely reducing cholesterol in people with a prior stroke or TIA. Evidence from large RCTs suggests benefit from reducing cholesterol with a statin in people with prior stroke or TIA who also have a definite history of coronary heart disease (see table 1, p 142).

Benefits:
We found three overviews[14–16] and one subsequent RCT.[17] Systematic reviews of early trials found no evidence that reducing mean total cholesterol by around 11% with a fibrate, resin, or dietary regimen significantly altered stroke, but found that reducing mean total cholesterol by about 21% with a statin reduced the relative odds of stroke by 24%, (and reduced the relative odds of coronary heart disease by a third) (see table 1, p 142).[14,15,18] We found two small, early RCTs that directly assessed effects of reducing cholesterol in people with a prior stroke or TIA. The drug used (clofibrate in both cases) produced only a small fall in the mean cholesterol, and the results were inconclusive.[19,20] Large RCTs have assessed the effects of reducing cholesterol on coronary heart disease risk, in many thousands of people, both in those with a history of coronary heart disease and in healthy people. These trials did not specifically aim to include people with a prior stroke or TIA, but many reported on stroke as an outcome.[14,15,18] One recent, large RCT assessed the effects of treatment designed to raise HDL cholesterol and lower triglycerides. It compared gemfibrozil versus placebo, given over about 5 years, in 2531 men with coronary heart disease and low HDL cholesterol. It found that gemfibrozil increased HDL cholesterol (by about 6%), reduced triglycerides, did not change LDL choles-

Cardiovascular disorders

terol, and reduced total cholesterol (by about 4%). Compared with placebo, gemfibrozil produced a significant reduction in coronary heart disease (RRR 22%, 95% CI 7% to 35%), but a non-significant reduction in stroke (RRR 25%, 95% CI –6% to +47%).[17]

Harms: The trials found uncertain effects of statins on fatal stroke (95% CI ranging from an increase of about a half to a one third reduction), (see table 1, p 142)[14] possibly because lowering cholesterol may slightly increase the risk of haemorrhagic stroke, which is more likely to be fatal.[3] Only two large scale statin trials reported haemorrhagic stroke separately, but there were too few events (n = 10) to draw any conclusions.[21,22]

Comment: A planned prospective overview of individual participant data from all RCTs of cholesterol reduction will provide a reliable summary of the overall effects of reducing cholesterol concentrations among different groups of people, including those with a prior stroke or TIA.[23]

OPTION ANTIPLATELET TREATMENT

Cathie Sudlow

RCTs have found that prolonged antiplatelet treatment is beneficial for people with a prior (presumed ischaemic) stroke or TIA, unless there is a clear contraindication. We found no clear evidence that any other antiplatelet regimen is superior to medium dose aspirin (75–325 mg daily) in the prevention of vascular events. Aspirin 75 mg daily is as effective as higher doses in the long term prevention of vascular events, but it remains unclear whether doses lower than 75 mg daily are sufficient. RCTs have found that clopidogrel or the combination of aspirin and dipyridamole are safe and effective alternatives to medium dose aspirin.

Benefits: **Antiplatelet treatment versus control:** One systematic review (published in 1994), which included 70 000 people at high risk of occlusive arterial disease found that, compared with no antiplatelet treatment, a month or more of antiplatelet treatment reduced the odds of a vascular event (non-fatal myocardial infarction, non-fatal stroke, or vascular death) by about a quarter (odds reduction 27%, 95% CI 24% to 30%, P < 0.0001).[5] The review included about 10 000 people with a prior (presumed ischaemic) stroke or TIA, among whom about 20 non-fatal strokes, nine non-fatal myocardial infarctions, and 11 vascular deaths were prevented per 1000 people treated with antiplatelet treatment for about 3 years. There was also a clear reduction in all cause mortality (see figure 1, p 143)[5] **Different daily doses of aspirin:** Around two thirds of the RCTs in the 1994 review involved an aspirin regimen, and medium dose aspirin (75–325 mg daily) was the most widely tested. Direct comparisons among 2425 high risk people found the effects on vascular events of daily doses of 75–325 mg or 500–1500 mg to be similar.[5] One subsequent RCT in 2849 people undergoing carotid endarterectomy also found no significant difference in the rate of stroke, myocardial infarction, or death between lower doses (81 mg or 325 mg daily) and higher doses (650 mg or 1300 mg daily, AR 5.4% with lower doses v 7.0% with higher doses; P = 0.07).[24] Indirect comparisons in the 1994 review found that daily doses of < 160 mg (mostly 75–150 mg), 160–325 mg, and 500–1500 mg had similar effects in preventing vascular events.[5] The inclusion of data from two subsequent large RCTs among high risk people (one of them including almost 1400 people with a prior ischaemic stroke or TIA[25]) assessing a daily dose of exactly 75 mg versus control,[25,26] showed that this aspirin dose significantly reduced vascular events (odds reduction 29%, 95% CI 17% to 39%).[5] We found more limited evidence for effects of doses under 75 mg daily. One RCT, which included about 6000 people with prior stroke or TIA, found that, compared with placebo, aspirin 50 mg daily reduced the combined outcome of stroke or death by 13% (95% CI 1% to 25%).[27] A second RCT directly compared aspirin 30 mg daily versus 283 mg daily, and found no evidence of a difference in effect in about 3000 people with recent TIA or minor ischaemic stroke, although the trial could not rule out a clinically important difference.[28] **Dipyridamole and aspirin:** The 1994 review found no clear evidence that any regimen was more effective than medium dose aspirin alone in the prevention of vascular events. It found that adding dipyridamole to aspirin did not seem to produce a reduction in vascular events compared with aspirin alone, but the possibility of a small additional benefit was not excluded.[5] One more recent RCT found that, although adding dipyridamole to aspirin 50 mg daily significantly reduced stroke (RRR about 23%), the combination did not significantly reduce the combined risk of stroke or death (RRR 13%, P = NS).[27] A detailed review of all trials that have assessed the addition of dipyridamole to aspirin is in preparation.[29] **Thienopyridines (clopidogrel and ticlopidine):** One systematic review of RCTs (4 RCTs, 22 656 people at high risk of vascular disease, including 9840 with a TIA or ischaemic stroke) compared either ticlopidine or clopidogrel with aspirin.[30] Most people were included in a large trial of clopidogrel (75 mg daily) versus aspirin (325 mg daily).[31] Compared with aspirin, the thienopyridines reduced the odds of a vascular event by 9% (OR 0.91; 95% CI 0.84 to 0.98), but there was substantial uncertainty about the size of any additional benefit (11 events prevented per 1000 people treated for about 2 years, 95% CI 2 to 19 events).[30]

Harms: Potentially life threatening bleeding is the most important adverse effect of antiplatelet treatment. **Intracranial haemorrhages:** These are uncommon, but often fatal, and usually cause significant disability in survivors. The 1994 overview found that any excess risk of intracranial bleeding with antiplatelet treatment was small, at most one or two per 1000 people per year in trials of long term treatment.[5] **Extracranial haemorrhages:** Unlike intracranial events, extracranial bleeds are much less likely to cause permanent disability or death. The 1994 review found that antiplatelet treatment was significantly associated with a small excess of three per 1000 non-fatal major extracranial bleeds, but no clear excess of fatal extracranial bleeds.[5] **Different doses of aspirin:** In a direct randomised comparison, aspirin 1200 mg daily was associated with more gastrointestinal bleeding than 325 mg daily.[32] We found no definite evidence for any clinically relevant variation in gastrointestinal bleeding risk in the range 75–325 mg daily. However, it seems reasonable to choose the lowest conveniently available dose in this range. **Neutropenia with thienopyridines:** The systematic review found that the thienopyridines produced significantly less gastrointestinal haemorrhage and upper gastrointestinal upset than aspirin. However, they increased the odds of skin rash and of diarrhoea (ticlopidine by about twofold and clopidogrel by about one third). Ticlopidine (but not clopidogrel) increased the odds of neutropenia.[30]

Comment: In people with a prior stroke or TIA, the large absolute reductions in serious vascular events produced by antiplatelet treatment far outweighed any absolute hazards.

OPTION	LONG TERM ORAL ANTICOAGULATION FOR PEOPLE IN NORMAL SINUS RHYTHM

Gord Gubitz, Peter Sandercock

One systematic review of RCTs did not find that long term oral anticoagulation reduced the risk of stroke recurrence after presumed ischaemic stroke in people in normal sinus rhythm. Risk of fatal intracranial and extracranial haemorrhage was increased.

Benefits: We found one systematic review, updated in 1997, which evaluated nine small trials (mean duration 1.8 years) comparing oral anticoagulants (warfarin, dicoumarol, phenindione) versus placebo.[33] The review included 1214 people in normal sinus rhythm with previous non-embolic presumed ischaemic stroke or TIA, and found no clear benefit of anticoagulation on death or dependency (ARR 4%, 95% CI −6% to +14%; RRR 5%, 95% CI −9% to +18 %), or on mortality or recurrent stroke.

Harms: By the end of the trials, the systematic review found a significantly increased risk of fatal intracranial haemorrhage (ARI 2%, 95% CI 0.4% to 3.6%; RRI 151%, 95% CI 12% to 460%; NNH 49 people treated with anticoagulants over 1.8 years for one additional non-fatal extracranial haemorrhage, 95% CI 27 to 240).[30] The risk of fatal and non-fatal extracranial haemorrhage was also increased by anticoagulants compared with placebo (ARI 5.1%, 95% CI 3.0% to 7.2%; RRI 486%, 95% CI 139% to 1332%; NNH 20, 95% CI 14 to 33). **Warfarin versus aspirin:** One RCT compared aspirin versus oral anticoagulant (target international normalised ratio [INR] 3.0 to 4.5) in 1316 people for around 14 months after TIA or non-disabling stroke.[34] The trial was stopped early because of an excess number of poor outcomes (almost exclusively related to cerebral haemorrhage) in the anticoagulant group compared with control (AR 12.4% anticoagulant v 5.4% control; ARI 7%, 95% CI 4% to 10%; NNH 14, 95% CI 10 to 25).

Comment: The trials in the systematic review all had major methods problems, including poor monitoring of anticoagulation.[33] All were completed before introducing routine computed tomography (CT) scanning, which means that people with primary haemorrhagic strokes could have been included. The systematic review could not therefore provide a reliable and precise overall estimate of the balance of risk and benefit regarding death or dependency. Most people in the trial comparing warfarin and aspirin did have a CT scan, but an adverse outcome was still seen with anticoagulants. Two further RCTs are in progress: one compares a lower intensity of adjusted dose warfarin (to maintain an INR of 1.4–2.8) with aspirin 325 mg four times daily within 30 days after stroke and treated for at least 2 years,[35] while the other assesses warfarin (to maintain an INR of 2.0 to 3.0) versus aspirin (any dose between 30–325 mg) versus aspirin plus dipyridamole (400 mg daily).[36]

| OPTION | CAROTID ENDARTERECTOMY FOR PEOPLE WITH RECENT CAROTID TERRITORY ISCHAEMIA |

Gord Gubitz, Peter Sandercock

One systematic review has found that carotid endarterectomy reduces the risk of major stroke and death in people with a recent carotid territory TIA or non-disabling ischaemic stroke who have moderate or severe symptomatic stenosis of the ipsilateral carotid artery. People with milder degrees of stenosis do not benefit from endarterectomy. Evidence from another systematic review suggests a possible benefit in people with asymptomatic but severe stenosis, but the results of a new large scale trial are awaited.

Benefits:
People with symptomatic stenosis: We found one recently published systematic review,[37] which included data from three RCTs comparing carotid surgery versus control treatment in 6143 people with a recent neurological event in the territory of a stenosed ipsilateral carotid artery. Ninety six per cent of these data came from two large RCTs.[38,39] Participants were randomised within 4 and 6 months of the onset of vascular symptoms. The trials used different methods to measure degree of stenosis. The trials included 1247 people with severe stenosis (70–99%,[39] 80–99%[38]), 1259 people with moderate stenosis (50–69%,[39] 70–79%[38]), and 3397 people with mild stenosis (< 50%,[39] < 70%[38]). The degree of benefit from surgery was related to the degree of stenosis. For people with severe stenosis, there was a significant decrease in the subsequent risk of major stroke or death (ARR 6.7%, 95% CI 3.2% to 10.0%; RRR 48%, 95% CI 27% to 63%; NNT 15, 95% CI 10 to 31). People with moderate stenosis also benefited (ARR 4.7%, 95% CI 0.8% to 8.7%; RRR 27%, 95% CI 5% to 44%; NNT 21, 95% CI 11 to 125). People with mild stenosis did not benefit from surgery but had an increased risk of stroke (RRI 20%, 95% CI 0% to 44%). In the trial with longer follow up, the annual risk of stroke after 3 years was not significantly different between people who had had surgery and those who had not.[38] In the other trial people with severe stenosis had a durable benefit from endartectomy at 8 years follow up.[40]
People with asymptomatic stenosis: We found one systematic review, published in 1998, including five trials with 2440 people evaluating carotid endarterectomy for asymptomatic carotid stenosis (no carotid territory TIA or minor stroke within past few months).[41] Carotid endarterectomy versus medical treatment reduced the risk of ipsilateral stroke or death (AR 7.4% over 3 years in the medical group v 4.7% in the surgical group; ARR 2.7%; 95% CI 0.8% to 4.6%; NNT 37 95% CI 22 to 125). Although the risk of perioperative stroke or death from carotid surgery for people with asymptomatic stenosis seems to be lower (2.7%) than in people with symptomatic stenosis, the risk of stroke or death without

surgery in asymptomatic people is relatively low and so, for most people, the balance of risk and benefit from surgery remains unclear.[41]

Harms: **People with symptomatic stenosis:** The systematic review of endarterectomy for symptomatic stenosis found that carotid surgery was associated with a definite risk of recurrent stroke or death.[37] In the systematic review, the relative risk of disabling stroke or death within 30 days of randomisation was 2.5 (95% CI 1.6 to 3.8). A second systematic review of 36 studies, published in 1997, identified several risk factors for operative stroke and death from carotid endarterectomy, including female sex, occlusion of the contralateral internal carotid artery, stenosis of the ipsilateral external carotid artery, and systolic blood pressure > 180 mmHg.[42] Endarterectomy is also associated with other troublesome postoperative complications, including wound infection (3%), wound haematoma (5%), and lower cranial nerve injury (5–7%). **People with asymptomatic stenosis:** Given the low prevalence of severe carotid stenosis in the general population, there is concern that screening asymptomatic people may result in more strokes than it prevents.[43]

Comment: **People with symptomatic stenosis:** The two RCTs contributing most of the data to the systematic review[38,39] used different techniques to measure the degree of carotid stenosis, but conversion charts are available and were used in the systematic review.[37] The trials, as well as observational studies,[4] found that risk of recurrent stroke was highest around the time of the symptomatic event. **People with asymptomatic stenosis:** A large scale trial is ongoing, and aims to confirm or refute the findings of the systematic review described above.[44]

OPTION   CAROTID PERCUTANEOUS TRANSLUMINAL ANGIOPLASTY

Gord Gubitz, Peter Sandercock

We found that carotid PTA has not been adequately assessed in people with a recent carotid territory TIA or non-disabling ischaemic stroke who have severe stenosis of the ipsilateral carotid artery.

Benefits: We found no systematic review or placebo controlled RCTs. **Carotid PTA:** One RCT compared "best medical treatment" plus carotid PTA versus best medical treatment plus carotid endarterectomy in 504 people with a recent carotid territory TIA or non-disabling ischaemic stroke with stenosis of the ipsilateral carotid artery.[45] Too few people were randomised between angioplasty and best medical care to provide reliable estimates of efficacy. Preliminary data have been published in abstract form, suggesting that rates of stroke or death at 30 days were similar in endarterectomy and PTA groups. Three year outcome data have also been published in abstract form,[46] finding that although there was a significant increase in restenosis in people undergoing PTA (21% v 5% of people undergoing endarterectomy, P < 0.0001), there was no difference between the two groups in rates of disabling stroke or death, or ipsilateral stroke. **Vertebral artery PTA:** The RCT randomised only 16 people between vertebral PTA and best medical treatment. This did not provide enough data for reliable estimates of efficacy.[45]

Harms: We found insufficient randomised data upon which to comment. Analysis of the safety data of the RCT has not yet been published.[45]

Comment: An ongoing RCT is comparing carotid revascularisation endarterectomy versus stenting.[47]

QUESTION **What are the effects of anticoagulant and antiplatelet treatment in people with atrial fibrillation?**

Gord Gubitz, Peter Sandercock, Gregory Lip

Systematic reviews have found that people with atrial fibrillation at high risk of stroke (see glossary, p 138) and with no contraindications benefit from anticoagulation. Antiplatelet agents are less effective than warfarin, and are associated with a lower bleeding risk, but are a reasonable alternative if warfarin is contraindicated or if risk of ischaemic stroke is low. The best time to begin anticoagulation after an ischaemic stroke is unclear.

Benefits: Three risk strata have been identified based on evidence derived from one systematic review of five RCTs,[48] and one subsequent RCT.[49] **In people with atrial fibrillation at high risk of stroke, adjusted dose warfarin:** We found three systematic reviews examining the effect of warfarin in different groups of people with atrial fibrillation at high risk of stroke.[48,50,51] The first (updated in 1995) identified two RCTs comparing warfarin with placebo in 1053 people with chronic non-rheumatic atrial fibrillation and a history of prior stroke or TIA.[50] A total of 98% of the people came from one double blind RCT,[52] which began treatment within 3 months of a minor stroke or TIA, and randomised 669 people to anticoagulant (target INR 2.5 to 4.0) or aspirin or placebo. Follow up was more than 2 years. It found that anticoagulants reduced the risk of recurrent stroke (ARR 13.7%, 95% CI 7.3% to 20.1%; RRR 61%, 95% CI 37% to 75%; NNT 7 over 1 year, 95% CI 5 to 14). The second (published in 1994) included five RCTs comparing warfarin with placebo in 2461 elderly people with atrial fibrillation and a variety of stroke risks.[48] Follow up was for a mean of 1.5 years. The review found that anticoagulation reduced the risk of stroke (ARR 4.4%, 95% CI 2.8% to 6.0%; RRR 68%, 95% CI 50% to 79%; NNT 23 over 1 year, 95% CI 17 to 36). The third (search date 1999, 16 RCTs, n = 9874) included six trials (n = 2900) of adjusted dose warfarin compared with no anticoagulation in high risk people.[51] It found that adjusted dose warfarin reduced stroke (ARR 2.7% per year for primary prevention, 8.4% per year for secondary prevention; RRR 62%, 95% CI 48% to 72%). The same review found adjusted dose warfarin reduced overall relative risk for all stroke by 36% (95% CI 14% to 52%) compared with aspirin, but the effect varied widely among the five included randomised trials, none of which were blinded (2837 people). See comment. **Minidose warfarin:** We found no systematic review or RCTs of low dose warfarin regimens in people with atrial fibrillation and a recent transient ischaemic attack or acute stroke. We found one trial which compared the use of low, fixed dose warfarin (target INR 1.2–1.5) plus aspirin (325 mg per day) with standard adjusted dose warfarin treatment (target INR 2.0–3.0) in 1044 people with atrial fibrillation at high risk of stroke.[49] Adjusted dose warfarin was associated with a significantly lower rate of both ischaemic stroke or systemic embolism (ARR 6.0%, 95% CI 3.4% to 8.6%; NNT 17, 95% CI 12 to 29) and of disabling or fatal stroke (ARR 3.9%, 95% CI 1.6% to 6.1%; NNT 26, 95% CI 16 to 63). We found three additional RCTs,[53–55] which aimed to evaluate adjusted dose warfarin versus low dose warfarin and aspirin, but were stopped prematurely when the results of the earlier trial[49] were published. Analyses of the optimal anticoagulation intensity for stroke prevention in atrial fibrillation found that stroke risk was substantially increased at INR levels below 2.[56,57] **Antiplatelet treatment:** We found one systematic review and a subsequent RCT comparing warfarin versus antiplatelet regimens in people with atrial fibrillation and a prior TIA or stroke. The systematic review (updated in 1995)[58] included data from one trial comparing warfarin (target INR 2.5 to 4.0) with aspirin (300 mg) in elderly people with atrial fibrillation and a prior history of stroke or TIA.[52] Both agents reduced the risk of recurrent stroke, although warfarin was more effective (ARs 22.6% for aspirin, 8.9% for warfarin; ARR 14%, 95% CI 7% to 20%; RRR 61%, 95% CI 36% to 76%; NNT 7, 95% CI 5 to 14). The subsequent RCT compared warfarin (INR 2.0–3.5) with indobufen (a reversible inhibitor of cylcooxygenase) in 916 people within 15 days of stroke onset.[59] It did not find any significant difference in the rate of recurrent stroke between the two groups (AR 5% for indobufen, 4.0% for warfarin; ARR 1.0%, 95% CI −1.7% to +3.7%). Pooling the data from the two trials shows benefits with either agent, although the absolute risk of recurrent stroke with warfarin (5.6%) is less than with antiplatelet agents (10.8%). The absolute risk reduction with warfarin compared with antiplatelet agents was 5.2% (95% CI 2.3% to 8.1%), corresponding to a number needed to treat with warfarin to avoid a stroke of 19 (95% CI 12 to 43). We found no systematic review dealing exclusively with people in atrial fibrillation with additional risk factors but no history of stroke or TIA. We found one systematic review,[60] published in 1997, involving 2574 people in three RCTs comparing aspirin versus control. This included one RCT of people with prior stroke or TIA. Aspirin reduced the risk of stroke, although the confidence interval included the possibility of no benefit (RRR 21%, 95% CI 0% to 38%). **In people with atrial fibrillation at moderate risk of stroke:** See glossary, p 138. We found no RCT that considered this group specifically. **In people with atrial fibrillation at low risk of stroke, anticoagulants:** See glossary, p 139. We found one systematic review[48] comparing warfarin with placebo in people with atrial fibrillation and a variety of stroke risks. It found that the annual stroke rate for people with atrial fibrillation younger than 65 years of age without a history of hypertension, previous stroke or TIA, or diabetes was the same (1% per year) for those treated with warfarin or placebo. **Antiplatelet agents:** We found two systematic reviews. The first[61] (2 RCTs, 1680 people) compared aspirin to placebo in people with atrial fibrillation but without previous stroke or TIA. People with either intermittent (paroxysmal) or sustained (constant) ECG confirmed non-valvular atrial fibrillation were included. The mean age was 68 years in the first trial and 74 years in the second trial. Overall, 30% were over 75 years. Aspirin did not produce significantly lower rates of ischaemic stroke (OR 0.71, 95% CI 0.46 to 1.10), all stroke (OR 0.70, 95% CI 0.45 to 1.08), all disabling or fatal stroke (OR 0.88, 95% CI 0.48 to 1.58), and the composite end point of stoke, myocardial infarction (MI) or vascular death (OR 0.76, 95% CI 0.54 to 1.05). For primary prevention among people with an average stroke rate of 4.5% per year, about 10 strokes would be prevented annually for every 1000 people given aspirin. The second systematic review includes the two trials analysed in the first review plus four additional trials, three of which were considered but excluded by the first review. The average rate of stroke among people assigned to placebo was 5.2% for primary prevention and 12.9% for secondary prevention. Meta-analysis found aspirin reduced the risk of stroke (RRR 22%, 95% CI 2 to 28%; ARR for primary prevention 1.5% per year [NNT 67]; ARR for secondary prevention 2.5% per year [NNT 40], CIs not provided).[51] A full evaluation of these systematic reviews will be included in *Clinical Evidence* Issue 5 (see comment below).

Harms: The major risk associated with anticoagulants and antiplatelet agents was haemorrhage. In the systematic review evaluating elderly people with variable risk factors for stroke, the absolute risk of major bleeding was 1% for placebo, 1% for aspirin, and 1.3% for warfarin.[48] The absolute risk of intracranial haemorrhage increased from 0.1% per year with control to 0.3% per year with warfarin.[51] The absolute risks were three times higher in people who had bled previously. Both bleeding and haemorrhagic stroke were more common in people aged over 75. The risk of death after a major bleed ranged from 13–33% and risk of subsequent morbidity in those who survived a major bleed was 15%. The risk of bleeding was associated with an INR > 3, fluctuating INRs, and uncontrolled hypertension. In the systematic review evaluating people with prior stroke or TIA, major extracranial bleeding was more frequent with anticoagulation than with placebo (ARI 4.9%, 95% CI 1.6% to 8.2%; RRI 518%, 95% CI 41% to 2607%; NNH 20, 95% CI 12 to 63).[50] The studies were too small to define the rate of intracranial haemorrhage (none occurred in the two RCTs). In the systematic review comparing anticoagulants and antiplatelet agents,[58] major extracranial bleeding was more frequent with anticoagulation (ARI 4.9%, 95% CI 1.6% to 8.2%; RRI 564%, 95% CI 52% to 2811%; NNH 20, 95% CI 12 to 63). The studies were too small to define the rate of intracranial haemorrhage (in the one RCT, none of the people on anticoagulant and one person on aspirin had an intracranial bleed). The two systematic reviews comparing aspirin with placebo found no increase in major haemorrhage with aspirin but the number of haemorrhagic events was small.[51,61]

Comment: As well as the trade offs between benefits and harms, each person's treatment preferences should be considered when deciding how to treat.[62–67] We found net benefit of anticoagulation for people in atrial fibrillation who have had a TIA or stroke, or who are over 75 years of age and at a high risk of stroke. We found less clear cut evidence for those aged 65–75 at high risk, and for those with moderate risk (that is, over age 65 not in a high risk group; those under age 65 with clinical risk factors), or for those at low risk (under age 65 with no other risk factors). The benefits of warfarin in the

RCTs may not translate into effectiveness in clinical practice.[68,69] In the RCTs, most strokes in people randomised to warfarin occurred while they were not in fact taking warfarin, or were significantly underanticoagulated at the time of the event. People in the RCTs were highly selected (< 10%, range 3–40% of eligible people were randomised); many were excluded after assessments for the absence of contraindications and physicians' refusal to enter them into the study. Many of the studies were not double blinded and some had decreased inter-rater agreement for "soft" neurological end points. The frequent monitoring of warfarin treatment under trial conditions and motivation of people/investigators was probably more than that seen in usual clinical practice. The best time to start anticoagulation after an ischaemic stroke is unclear. Three recent systematic reviews have been published that update, summarise and further clarify the role of antithrombotic agents in people with atrial fibrillation.[51–53] The first systematic review[61] included 2313 people from five RCTs comparing oral anticoagulants versus usual care but without anticoagulation in people with non-valvular chronic atrial fibrillation and no history of TIA or stroke. In four trials the mean age was 67–68 years, and in the fifth it was 74 years. Overall the mean age was 69 years with 20% of people over 75 years. A total of 45% of people had hypertension, 15% had diabetes and 15% had a prior history of myocardial infarction. About half (1154 people) were randomised to receive adjusted dose oral anticoagulation with estimated mean INRs between 2.0 and 2.6 during a follow up period which averaged 1.5 years per participant. Oral anticoagulation was associated with large, highly significant reductions in ischaemic stroke (OR 0.34, 95% CI 0.23 to 0.52), all stroke (OR 0.39, 95% CI 0.26 to 0.59), all disabling or fatal stroke (OR 0.47, 95% CI 0.28 to 0.80), and the combined endpoint of all stroke, MI or vascular death (OR 0.56, 95% CI 0.42 to 0.76). However, the ARR was modest with about 25 strokes, MIs or vascular deaths prevented per year for every 1000 people given oral anticoagulants. The second systematic review [61] compared aspirin to placebo (two RCTs, 1680 people with atrial fibrillation but without previous stroke or TIA. The third systematic review[51] considered trials of adjusted dose warfarin versus placebo, antiplatelet therapy versus placebo, adjusted dose warfarin compared with aspirin, adjusted dose warfarin versus other antithrombotic regimens and other randomised comparisons. Initial assessment of these meta-analyses indicates no substantial change in the evidence. There is increased evidence about the need to identify the baseline risk of individuals and to use antithrombotic therapy judiciously. A full evaluation of these systematic reviews will be included in *Clinical Evidence* Issue 5.[61]

GLOSSARY

People at high risk of stroke People of any age with a previous TIA or stroke or a history of rheumatic vascular disease, coronary artery disease, congestive heart failure, and/or impaired left ventricular function or echocardiography; and people aged 75 and over with hypertension, diabetes, or both.

People at moderate risk of stroke People over age 65 who are not in the high risk group; and people under age 65 with clinical risk factors, including diabetes, hypertension, peripheral arterial disease, and ischaemic heart disease.

People at low risk of stroke All other people under age 65 with no history of stroke, TIA, embolism, hypertension, diabetes, or other clinical risk factors.

Substantive changes since last issue

Cholesterol reduction One new overview of RCTs; no change in conclusion.[16]

Antiplatelet treatment One new systematic review found either ticlopidine or clopidogrel reduced the odds of a vascular event compared with aspirin but there was substantial uncertainty about the size of any additional benefit.[30]

In people with atrial fibrillation at high risk of stroke, adjusted dose warfarin One new systematic review comparing adjusted dose warfarin with no anticoagulation in high risk patients. It found that adjusted dose warfarin reduced stroke. No change in conclusions. The same review found adjusted dose warfarin reduced overall relative risk for all stroke compared with aspirin, but the effect varied widely among the five included randomised trials, none of which were blinded.[51]

In people with atrial fibrillation at low risk of stroke, antiplatelet agents Two new systematic reviews, trials included and findings varied.[51,61]

REFERENCES

1. Hankey GJ, Warlow CP. *Transient ischaemic attacks of the brain and eye.* London: WB Saunders, 1994.
2. Prospective Studies Collaboration. Cholesterol, diastolic blood pressure, and stroke: 13,000 strokes in 450,000 people in 45 prospective cohorts. *Lancet* 1995;346:1647–1653.
3. Eastern Stroke and Coronary Heart Disease Collaborative Research Group. Blood pressure, cholesterol, and stroke in eastern Asia. *Lancet* 1998;352:1801–1807.
4. Warlow CP, Dennis MS, van Gijn J, et al. Predicting recurrent stroke and other serious vascular events. In: *Stroke. A practical guide to management.* Oxford. Blackwell Science, 1996:545–552.
5. Antiplatelet Trialists' Collaboration. Collaborative overview of randomised trials of antiplatelet therapy – I: prevention of death, myocardial infarction, and stroke by prolonged antiplatelet therapy in various categories of patients. *BMJ* 1994;308:81–106.
6. Hart RG, Pearce LA, Rothbart RM, McAnulty JH, Asinger RW, Halperin JL. Stroke with intermittent atrial fibrillation: incidence and predictors during aspirin therapy. Stroke Prevention in Atrial Fibrillation Investigators. *J Am Coll Cardiol* 2000; 35:183–187.
7. Collins R, MacMahon S. Blood pressure, antihypertensive drug treatment and the risks of stroke and of coronary heart disease. *Br Med Bull* 1994;50:272–298.
8. PROGRESS Management Committee. Blood pressure lowering for the secondary prevention of stroke: rationale and design of PROGRESS. *J Hypertension* 1996;14(suppl 2):S41–46.
9. Staessen JA, Fagard R, Thijs L, et al for the Systolic Hypertension in Europe (Syst–Eur) Trial Investigators. Randomised double-blind comparison of placebo and active treatment for older patients with isolated systolic hypertension. *Lancet* 1997;350:757–764.
10. PATS Collaborating Group. Post-stroke antihypertensive treatment study: a preliminary result. *Chinese Med J* 1995;108:710–717.
11. The Heart Outcomes Prevention Evaluation Study Investigators. Effects of an angiotensin-converting-enzyme inhibitor, ramipril, on death from cardiovascular causes, myocardial infarction, and stroke in high-risk patients. *N Engl J Med* 2000; 342:145–153.
12. Rodgers A, MacMahon S, Gamble G, Slattery J, Sandercock P, Warlow C for the United Kingdom Transient Ischaemic Attack Collaborative Group. Blood pressure and risk of stroke in patients with cerebrovascular disease. *BMJ* 1996;313:147.
13. Neal B, Clark T, MacMahon S, Rodgers A, Baigent C, Collins R on behalf of the Antithrombotic Trialists' Collaboration. Blood pressure and the risk of recurrent vascular disease. *Am J Hypertension* 1998;11:25A–26A.
14. Hebert PR, Gaziano M, Hennekens CH. An overview of trials of cholesterol lowering and risk of stroke. *Arch Intern Med* 1995;155:50–55. Search dates and primary sources not specified.
15. Hebert PR, Gaziano JM, Chan KS, Hennekens CH. Cholesterol lowering with statin drugs, risk of stroke, and total mortality: an overview of randomized trials. *JAMA* 1997;278:313–321. Search date 1995; primary sources not specified but searched 1985 to 1995; Cholesterol and Current Events (CARE) data added in October 1996.
16. Di Mascio R, Marchioli R, Tognoni G. Cholesterol reduction and stroke occurrence: an overview of randomized clinical trials. *Cerebrovasc Dis* 2000; 10:85–92.
17. Rubins HB, Robins SJ, Collins D, et al. Gemfibrozil for the secondary prevention of coronary heart disease in men with low levels of high-density lipoprotein cholesterol. *N Engl J Med* 1999;341: 410–418.
18. The long-term intervention with pravastatin in ischaemic disease (LIPID) study group. Prevention of cardiovascular events and death with pravastatin in patients with coronary heart disease and a broad range of initial cholesterol levels. *N Engl J Med* 1998;339:1349–1357.
19. Acheson J, Hutchinson EC. Controlled trial of clofibrate in cerebral vascular disease. *Atherosclerosis* 1972;15:177–183.
20. Anonymous. The treatment of cerebrovascular disease with clofibrate. Final report of the Veterans' Administration Cooperative Study of Atherosclerosis, neurology section. *Stroke* 1973; 4:684–693.
21. Plehn JF, Davis BR, Sacks FM, et al for the CARE Investigators. Reduction of stroke incidence after myocardial infarction with pravastatin: the cholesterol and recurrent events (CARE) study. *Circulation* 1999;99:216–223.
22. Scandinavian Simvastatin Survival Study Group. Randomised trial of cholesterol lowering in 4444 patients with coronary heart disease: the Scandinavian simvastatin survival study (4S).

Cardiovascular disorders

Lancet 1994;344:1383–1389.

23. Cholesterol Treatment Trialists' Collaboration. Protocol for a prospective collaborative overview of all current and planned randomized trials of cholesterol treatment regimens. Am J Cardiol 1995;75:1130–1134.

24. Taylor DW, Barnett HJM, Haynes RB, et al, for the ASA and Carotid Endarterectomy (ACE) Trial Collaborators. Low-dose and high-dose acetylsalicylic acid for patients undergoing carotid endarterectomy: a randomised controlled trial. Lancet 1999;353:2179–2184.

25. SALT Collaborative Group. Swedish aspirin low-dose trial (SALT) of 75 mg aspirin as secondary prophylaxis after cerebrovascular ischaemic events. Lancet 1991;338:1345–1349.

26. Juul-Möller S, Edvardsson N, Jahnmatz B, Rosen A, Soreneson S, Omblus R, for the Swedish Angina Pectoris Aspirin Trial (SAPAT) Group. Double-blind trial of aspirin in primary prevention of myocardial infarction in patients with stable chronic angina pectoris. Lancet 1992;340:1421–1425.

27. Diener HC, Cunha L, Forbes C, Sivenius J, Smets P, Lowenthal A. European secondary prevention study 2: dipyridamole and acetylsalicylic acid in the secondary prevention of stroke. J Neurol Sci 1996;143:1–13.

28. The Dutch TIA Study Group. A comparison of two doses of aspirin (30 mg vs 283 mg a day) in patients after a transient ischaemic attack or minor ischaemic stroke. N Engl J Med 1991;325:1261–1266.

29. Sudlow C, Baigent C, on behalf of the Antithrombotic Trialists' Collaboration. Different antiplatelet regimens in the prevention of vascular events among patients at high risk of stroke: new evidence from the antithrombotic trialists' collaboration. Seventh European Stroke Conference, Edinburgh, May, 1998. Cerebrovasc Dis 1998;8(suppl 4):68.

30. Hankey GJ, Sudlow CLM, Dunbabin DW. Thienopyridine derivatives (ticlopidine, clopidogrel) versus aspirin for preventing stroke and other serious vascular events in high vascular risk patients. In: The Cochrane Library, Issue 1, 2000. Oxford: Update software. Search date March 1999; primary sources Cochrane Stroke Group Trials Register; Antithrombotic Trialists' database and contacted Sanofi pharmacological company.

31. CAPRIE Steering Committee. A randomised, blinded, trial of clopidogrel versus aspirin in patients at risk of ischaemic events. Lancet 1996;348:1329–1339.

32. Farrell B, Godwin J, Richards S, Warlow C. The United Kingdom transient ischaemic attack (UK-TIA) aspirin trial: final results. J Neurol Neurosurg Psychiatry 1991;54:1044–1054.

33. Liu M, Counsell C, Sandercock P. Anticoagulants for preventing recurrence following ischaemic stroke or transient ischaemic attack. In: The Cochrane Library, Issue 4, 1999. Oxford: Update software. Search date not stated; primary source Cochrane Stroke Group Trials Register, and contact with companies marketing anticoagulant agents.

34. The Stroke Prevention in Reversible Ischaemia Trial (SPIRIT) Study Group. A randomised trial of anticoagulant versus aspirin after cerebral ischemia of presumed arterial origin. Ann Neurol 1997;42:857–865.

35. Mohr J for the WARSS Group. Design considerations for the warfarin-antiplatelet recurrent stroke study. Cerebrovasc Dis 1995;5:156–157.

36. De Schryvfer E for the ESPRIT Study Group. ESPRIT: mild anticoagulation, acetylsalicylic acid plus dipyridamole or acetylsalicylic acid alone after cerebral ischaemia of arterial origin [abstract]. Cerebrovasc Dis 1998;8(suppl 4):83.

37. Cina C, Clase C, Haynes R. Carotid endarterectomy for symptomatic stenosis. In: The Cochrane Library, Issue 4, 1999. Oxford: Update software. Search date March 1999; primary sources Cochrane Stroke Group Specialised Register of Trials; Medline 1996 to October 1998; Embase 1990 to May 1997; Healthstar and Serline 1996 to May 1997; Cochrane Controlled Trials Register to 1998; DARE to 1998; Best Evidence 1991 to 1996.

38. European Carotid Surgery Trialists' Collaborative Group. Randomised trial of endarterectomy for recently symptomatic carotid stenosis: final results of the MRC European carotid surgery trial. Lancet 1998;351:1379–1387.

39. North American Symptomatic Carotid Endarterectomy Trial Collaborators. Beneficial effect of carotid endarterectomy in symptomatic patients with high-grade carotid stenosis. N Engl J Med 1991;325:445–453.

40. Barnett HJ, Taylor DW, Eliasziw M, et al. Benefit of carotid endartectomy in patients with symptomatic moderate or severe stenosis. North American symptomatic carotid endartectomy trial collaborators. N Engl J Med 1998;339:1415–1425.

41. Benavente O, Moher D, Pham B. Carotid endarterectomy for asymptomatic carotid stenosis: a meta-analysis. BMJ 1998;317:1477–1480. Search dates 1966 to 1998, primary sources Medline, CCTR Ottawa Stroke Trials Register, Current Contents, and hand searching.

42. Rothwell P, Slattery J, Warlow C. Clinical and angiographic predictors of stroke and death from carotid endarterectomy: systematic review. BMJ 1997;315:1571–1577.

43. Whitty C, Sudlow C, Warlow C. Investigating individual subjects and screening populations for asymptomatic carotid stenosis can be harmful. J Neurol Neurosurg Psychiatry 1998;64:619–623.

44. Halliday A, Thomas D, Manssfield A. The asymptomatic carotid surgery trial (ACST). Rationale and design. Eur J Vascular Surg 1994;8:703–710.

45. Brown MM, for the CAVATAS Investigators. Results of the carotid and vertebral artery transluminal angioplasty study (CAVATAS) [abstract]. Cerebrovasc Dis 1998;8(suppl 4):21.

46. Brown M, Pereira A, McCabe D. Carotid and vertebral transluminal angioplasty study (CAVATAS): 3 year outcome data [abstract]. Cerebrovasc Dis 1999;9(suppl 1):66.

47. Al-Mubarek N, Roubin G, Hobson R, Ferguson R, Brott T, Moore W. Credentialing of Stent Operators for the Carotid Revascularization Endarterectomy vs Stenting Trial (CREST) [abstract]. Stroke 2000;31:292.

48. Atrial Fibrillation Investigators. Risk factors for stroke and efficacy of antithrombotic therapy in atrial fibrillation. Arch Intern Med 1994;154:1449–1457.

49. Stroke Prevention in Atrial Fibrillation Investigators. Adjusted-dose warfarin versus low-intensity, fixed-dose warfarin plus aspirin for high-risk patients with atrial fibrillation: stroke prevention in atrial fibrillation III randomised clinical trial. Lancet 1996;348:633–638.

50. Koudstaal P. Anticoagulants for preventing stroke in patients with nonrheumatic atrial fibrillation and a history of stroke or transient ischemic attack. In: The Cochrane Library, Issue 4, 1999. Oxford: Update software. Search date not stated; primary source Cochrane Stroke Group Trials Register, and contact with trialists.

51. Hart R, Benavente O, McBride R, Pearce L. Antithrombotic therapy to prevent stroke in patients with atrial fibrillation: a meta-analysis. *Ann Intern Med* 1999;131:492–501. Search date 1999; primary sources Medline, Cochrane Database and Antithrombotic Trialists Collaboration.

52. European Atrial Fibrillation Trial Study Group. Secondary prevention in non-rheumatic atrial fibrillation after transient ischaemic attack or minor stroke. *Lancet* 1993;342:1255.

53. Pengo V, Zasso Z, Barbero F, et al. Effectiveness of fixed minidose warfarin in the prevention of thromboembolism and vascular death in nonrheumatic atrial fibrillation. *Am J Cardiol* 1998; 82:433–437.

54. Gullov A, Koefoed B, Petersen P, et al. Fixed minidose warfarin and aspirin alone and in combination vs adjusted-dose warfarin for stroke prevention in atrial fibrillation. Second Copenhagen Atrial Fibrillation, Aspirin, and Anticoagulation Study. *Arch Intern Med* 1998; 158:1513–1521.

55. Vermeer F, Langenberg M, Hellemons B, Lodder J, Schouten H van Ree J, Knottnerus J. Primary prevention of arterial thrombo-embolism in non-rheumatic atrial fibrillation: Results of the PATAF study. *Eur Heart J* 1998;19(suppl):154.

56. The European Atrial Fibrillation Trial Study Group. Optimal oral anticoagulant therapy in patients with nonrheumatic atrial fibrillation and recent cerebral ischemia. *N Engl J Med* 1995;333:5–10.

57. Hylek, EM, Skates, SJ, Sheehan, MA, Singer, DE. An analysis of the lowest effective intensity of prophylactic anticoagulation for patients with nonrheumatic atrial fibrillation. *N Engl J Med* 1996;335:540–546.

58. Koudstaal P. Anticoagulants versus antiplatelet therapy for preventing stroke in patients with nonrheumatic atrial fibrillation and a history of stroke or transient ischemic attacks. In: The Cochrane Library, Issue 4, 1999. Oxford: Update Software. Search date not stated; primary source Cochrane Stroke Group Trials Register, and contact with trialists.

59. Morocutti, C, Amabile G, Fattapposta F, et al for the SIFA Investigators. Indobufen versus warfarin in the secondary prevention of major vascular events in nonrheumatic atrial fibrillation. *Stroke* 1997;28:1015–1021.

60. Atrial Fibrillation Investigators. The efficacy of aspirin in patients with atrial fibrillation: analysis of pooled data from 3 randomized trials. *Arch Intern Med* 1997;157:1237–1240.

61. Benavente O, Hart R, Koudstaal, P, Laupacis A, McBride R. Antiplatelet therapy for preventing stroke in patients with non-valvular atrial fibrillation and no previous history of stroke or transient ischemic attacks. In: The Cochrane Library, Issue 1,2000. Oxford: Update software. Search date June 1999; primary sources Medline, Cochrane Register of Trials, and reference lists of relevant articles.

62. Lip G. Thromboprophylaxis for atrial fibrillation. *Lancet* 1999;353:4–6.

63. Ezekowitz M, Levine J. Preventing stroke in patients with atrial fibrillation. *JAMA* 1999;281: 1830–1835.

64. Hart R, Sherman D, Easton D, Cairns J. Prevention of stroke in patients with nonvalvular atrial fibrillation. *Neurology* 1998;51:674–681.

65. Feinberg W. Anticoagulation for prevention of stroke. *Neurology* 1998;51(suppl 3):S20–S22.

66. Albers G. Choice of antithrombotic therapy for stroke prevention in atrial fibrillation. Warfarin, aspirin, or both? *Arch Intern Med* 1998;158: 1487–1491.

67. Nademanee K, Kosar E. Long-term antithrombotic treatment for atrial fibrillation. *Am J Cardiol* 1998; 82:37N–42N.

68. Gubitz G, Hadorn DC, Bassett K, Kazanjian A. Anticoagulation in chronic non-valvular atrial fibrillation: a critical appraisal and meta-analysis. *Can J Cardiol* 1997;13:811–815.

69. Blakely J. Anticoagulation in chronic nonvalvular atrial fibrillation: appraisal of two meta-analyses. *Can J Cardiol* 1998;14:945–948.

Cathie Sudlow
Specialist Registrar in Neurology
Department of Neurology
Derriford Hospital
Plymouth
UK

Gord Gubitz
Assistant Professor
Division of Neurology
Delahouise University
Halifax
Canada

Peter Sandercock
Professor in Neurology
Neurosciences Trials Unit
University of Edinburgh
Edinburgh
UK

Gregory Lip
Consultant Cardiologist and
Reader in Medicine
City Hospital
Birmingham
UK

Competing interests: CS, GG none declared. PS has received honoraria for lectures, funds for research, funds for members of his staff, and fees for single consultancies from Glaxo Wellcome, Boehringer Ingelheim, Sanofi/BMS. GL is UK principal investigator for the ERAFT Trial (Knoll) and has been reimbursed by various pharmaceutical companies for attending several conferences, running educational programmes and research projects.

TABLE 1 Effects of cholesterol lowering on risk of stroke: results of two systematic review of RCTs of non-statin interventions and statins in the primary and secondary prevention of coronary heart disease* (see text, p 129).

Overview	Number of		Mean reduction in cholesterol (%)	Summary OR (95% CI) for active treatment v control	
	Participants	Strokes		Fatal or non-fatal stroke	Fatal stroke
Non-statin interventions					
1995 overview (11 trials)[14]	36 000	435	11%	0.99 (0.82 to 1.21)	1.10 (0.79 to 1.54)
Statin interventions					
1997 overview (14 trials)[15] + LIPID trial[18]	38 000	827	21%	0.76 (0.66 to 0.87)	0.99 (0.67 to 1.45)
Subtotal, primary prevention trials	8 000	108	20%	0.80 (0.54 to 1.16)	–
Subtotal, secondary prevention trials	30 000	719	22%	0.75 (0.65 to 0.87)	–

* The findings of other published overviews are consistent with the results shown here.

PRIOR STROKE or TIA

A = Antiplatelet therapy (mean 3 years)

C = Control

	A	C	A	C	A	C	A	C
	109	163	479	600	497	562	675	780
	5654	5681	5837	5870	5837	5870	5837	5870
	(1.9%)	(2.9%)	(8.2%)	(10.2%)	(8.5%)	(9.6%)	(11.6%)	(13.3%)

OUTCOME:	Non-fatal myocardial infarction	Non-fatal stroke recurrence	Vascular death	Any death
Benefit per 1000:	9 (4 to 15)	20 (9 to 31)	11 (1 to 21)	17 (5 to 29)
%odds reduction:	36% (17 to 52%)	23% (11 to 33%)	14% (1 to 25%)	16% (5 to 25%)

FIGURE 1 Absolute effects of antiplatelet treatment on various outcomes in patients with a prior stroke or TIA: results of a systematic review.[5] The columns show the absolute risks over 3 years for each outcome; the error bars represent standard deviations. In the "any death" column, non-vascular deaths are represented by lower horizontal lines (see text, pp 127, 130). Adapted with permission.[5]

Cardiovascular disorders

Updated this issue

David Fitzmaurice, FD Hobbs and Richard McManus

INTERVENTIONS

Beneficial

To be covered in future issues of
Clinical Evidence
Thrombolysis for pulmonary
embolism
Compression stockings for DVT
Oral antithrombotic agents (such as
glycoprotein IIb/IIIa antagonists)
Inferior vena cava filters
Thromboembolism in pregnancy

Key Messages

Proximal DVT

- One RCT found that combined intravenous unfractionated heparin and oral anticoagulant reduced recurrent thromboembolic events in people with proximal DVT compared with oral anticoagulants alone.

- One systematic review found good evidence that longer duration of anticoagulation was associated with significantly fewer recurrent DVTs, and limited evidence that longer duration of anticoagulation was associated with a significant increase in the incidence of major haemorrhage.

- Systematic reviews have found that low molecular weight heparin is at least as effective as unfractionated heparin in reducing the incidence of recurrent thromboembolic disease.

- Systematic reviews have found that low molecular weight heparin is at least as safe as unfractionated heparin for the treatment of DVT.

Isolated calf vein thrombosis

- One RCT has found that warfarin plus unfractionated herparin reduces the risk of recurrence in isolated calf vein thrombosis compared with unfractionated heparin alone.

- We found insufficient evidence on optimal duration or intensity of anticoagulation.

Pulmonary embolism

■ One RCT has found that combined treatment with oral anticoagulant plus intravenous unfractionated heparin reduces mortality compared with unfractionated herparin alone. One RCT found no evidence of a difference in the benefits and harms of low molecular weight heparin and unfractionated heparin in people with pulmonary embolism.

Duration of warfarin treatment

■ Evidence for intensity and duration of treatment has been extrapolated from studies in people with proximal DVT and any venous thromboembolism. One systematic review found good evidence of a significant reduction in recurrent venous thromboembolism with longer duration of anticoagulation, and limited evidence of increased risk of major haemorrhage with longer periods of anticoagulation. The absolute risk of recurrent venous thromboembolism decreases with time whereas the relative risk reduction with therapy remains constant. Harms of therapy, including major haemorrhage, continue during prolonged treatment. People with thromboembolism have different risk profiles and it is likely that the optimal duration of anticoagulation will vary between people.

Intensity of warfarin treatment

■ One RCT in people with a first episode of idiopathic venous thromboembolism treated for 3 months with warfarin found no significant difference in recurrence between treatment targeted at an INR of 2.0–3.0 or 3.0–4.5. Treatment targeted at the higher INR was associated with a greater risk of bleeding.

DEFINITION | **Venous thromboembolism** is any thromboembolic event occurring within the venous system, including DVT and pulmonary embolism. **Deep vein thrombosis (DVT) is a radiologically** confirmed partial or total thrombotic occlusion of the deep venous system of the legs sufficient to produce symptoms of pain or swelling. **Proximal DVT** affects the veins above the knee (popliteal, superficial femoral, common femoral, and iliac veins). **Isolated calf vein thrombosis** is confined to the deep veins of the calf and does not affect the veins above the knee. **Pulmonary embolism** is radiologically confirmed partial or total thromboembolic occlusion of pulmonary arteries, sufficient to cause symptoms of breathlessness, chest pain, or both. **Post-thrombotic syndrome** is oedema, ulceration, and impaired viability of the subcutaneous tissues of the leg occurring after DVT. **Recurrence** refers to symptomatic deterioration due to a further (radiologically confirmed) thrombosis, after a previously confirmed thromboembolic event, where there had been an initial partial or total symptomatic improvement. **Extension** refers to a radiologically confirmed new, constant, symptomatic intraluminal filling defect extending from an existing thrombosis.

INCIDENCE/ PREVALENCE | We found no reliable data on the incidence/prevalence of DVT or pulmonary embolism in the UK. Scandinavian data suggest an annual incidence of 1.6–1.8 per 1000 people in the general population.[1,2] One postmortem study extrapolated that 600 000 people develop pulmonary embolism each year in the USA, of whom 60 000 die as a result.[3]

AETIOLOGY/ RISK FACTORS | Risk factors for DVT include immobility, surgery (particularly orthopaedic), malignancy, smoking, pregnancy, older age, and inherited and acquired prothrombotic clotting disorders.[4] The evidence for these factors is mainly observational and this includes an association with the oral contraceptive pill but the ARI of death due to venous thromboembolism when taking any combined oral contraception is small – 1 to 3 per million women per year[5] The principal causal factor for the development of pulmonary embolism is the presence of DVT.[4]

PROGNOSIS
Symptomatic calf vein thrombosis in people not having surgery has an annual recurrence rate of over 25%.[6,7] There is a 40–50% risk of proximal extension, with the attendant risk of pulmonary embolisation assumed to be the same as for proximal vein thrombosis in these people.[8] The complications of proximal DVT are fatal or non-fatal pulmonary embolism, recurrent venous thrombosis, and the post-thrombotic syndrome. Historically, one observational study found a 20% mortality from pulmonary emboli in people in hospital with untreated DVT.[9] One non-systematic review of observational studies found that, in people after surgery who have a asymptomatic calf vein DVT, the rate of fatal pulmonary embolism was 13–15%.[10] The incidence of other complications without treatment is not known. Continuing risk is related to the presence of thrombotic risk factors.[11] People given unfractionated heparin usually require hospitalisation and require regular blood tests for dose adjustment, whereas low molecular weight heparin can be administered in primary or ambulatory care and blood tests are not required routinely because the dose is fixed.

AIMS
To prevent thrombus extension; to prevent the post-thrombotic syndrome and pulmonary embolisation; and to reduce recurrence and mortality, with minimal adverse effects of treatment.

OUTCOMES
Rates of symptomatic recurrence, post-thrombotic syndrome, symptomatic pulmonary embolism, and death. Proxy outcomes include radiological evidence of clot extension or pulmonary embolism.

METHODS
Clinical Evidence update search and appraisal May 2000. Several papers identified from personal sources from 1999 and 2000 were also included. Observational studies were used for estimating incidence, prevalence, and adverse event rates. RCTs were included only if cases and outcomes were objectively defined, and if the trial provided dose ranges (with adjusted dosing schedules for oral anticoagulation and unfractionated heparin) and independent, blinded outcome assessment.

QUESTION   What are the effects of treatments for proximal DVT?

OPTION   ANTICOAGULATION

We found no RCTs comparing warfarin with placebo. One RCT found that combined warfarin and intravenous unfractionated heparin for initial treatment reduced recurrence compared with warfarin alone. One systematic review found that longer duration of anticoagulation was associated with significantly fewer recurrences. Systematic reviews have found that low molecular weight heparin is at least as effective as unfractionated heparin in reducing the incidence of recurrent

thromboembolic disease. We found evidence from systematic reviews that low molecular weight heparin is at least as safe as unfractionated heparin for the treatment of DVT.

Benefits: **Warfarin versus placebo:** We found no RCTs. **Warfarin plus heparin:** One RCT in 120 people with proximal DVT found that combined intravenous unfractionated heparin (UFH) plus warfarin reduced recurrence compared with warfarin alone at interim analysis at 6 months, and as a result the trial was stopped (rate of recurrence 12/60 [20%] with warfarin alone v 4/60 [6.7%] with combined treatment, P = 0.058; NNT 8, 95% CI 4 to 71).[12] One person in the combined treatment group committed suicide at 6 months. There were two cancer related deaths, confirmed by post mortem examination, in the group treated with warfarin alone, one in week 11 and the other in week 12. **Duration of anticoagulation:** We found one systematic review of four RCTs (search date 2000, n = 1500).[13] Two RCTs included people with a first episode of venous thromboembolism, one RCT was in people with a second episode of venous thromboembolism, and the fourth RCT was in people with acute proximal deep vein thrombosis. The periods of treatment compared were different in all four RCTs; 4 weeks versus 3 months, 6 weeks versus 6 months, 3 months versus 27 months and 6 months versus 4 years. In all RCTs vitamin K antagonist dosages were adjusted to achieve an INR between 2.0 and 3.0. The individual RCTs all showed significant protection from prolonged treatment. Combining these, 91/742 (12%) of people in the short arm had thromboembolic complications compared with 7/758 (0.9%) in the long arm (OR 0.15, 95% CI 0.10 to 0.23). None of the individual RCTs found a significant reduction in mortality for the entire period following randomisation. Analysis of the pooled data found a non-significant reduction in mortality favouring prolonged treatment (OR 0.70, 95% CI 0.45 to 1.09). **Intensity of anticoagulation:** We found one RCT comparing warfarin with INR targets of 2.0 to 3.0 with 3.0 to 4.5 for 12 weeks following an initial course of intravenous heparin in people with a first episode of idiopathic venous thromboembolism. It found similar recurrence rates at 10 months for both INR target ranges (recurrence rate 1/47 [2.1%] with lower target range v 1/49 [2%] with higher range, P = NS). However, there were significantly more haemorrhagic events in the higher target group (2/47 [4.3%] v 11/49 [22.4%], P = 0.015).[14] **Abrupt versus gradual discontinuation of warfarin:** We found one RCT in 41 people with DVT that compared abrupt withdrawal of warfarin with an additional month of warfarin at a fixed low dose of 1.25 mg/day. It found no evidence of a difference in recurrence rates between the two groups (recurrence occurred in three people who stopped warfarin abruptly compared with one person who reduced warfarin gradually, P = NS).[15] **Low molecular weight heparin versus unfractionated heparin:** We found two systematic reviews confined to symptomatic proximal DVT.[16,17] One (search date 1993, 16 RCTs, n = 2045) found that low molecular weight heparin (LMWH) reduced thrombus extension compared with unfractionated heparin (ARs not given; OR for thrombus extension 0.45, 95% CI 0.25 to 0.81).[16] The other review (search date 1994, 10 RCTs, n = 1424) found that, compared with unfractionated heparin, low molecular weight heparin reduced symptomatic thromboembolic complications (ARs not given; RR 0.47, 95% CI 0.27 to 0.82) and mortality RR 0.53, 95% CI 0.31 to 0.90).[17] We also found three systematic reviews comparing low molecular weight heparin with unfractionated heparin in people with radiologically confirmed symptomatic venous thromboembolism, and one subsequent RCT. [18–21] The first (search date 1999, 14 RCTs, n = 4754) included five studies (blinded and unblinded, n = 1636) which examined proximal thrombosis.[21] Analysis of these trials showed statistically significant reductions in thrombotic complications (LMWH v UFH; ARs 39/814 [4.8%] v 64/822 [7.8%]; OR 0.60, 95% CI 0.40 to 0.89). Overall mortality was also reduced (LMWH v UFH; ARs 44/814 [5.4%] v 68/822 [8.3%]; OR 0.64, 95% CI 0.43 to 0.93). Eight of the 14 RCTs in the systematic review included people with symptomatic deep venous thrombosis of the leg without symptoms of pulmonary embolism, and these accounted for approximately 75% of all participants. Analysis of the seven RCTs that concealed treatment allocation found no significant difference between treatments for rates of recurrent venous thromboembolism during treatment (ARs 34/1569 [2.2%] v 43/1595 [2.7%]; OR 0.80, 95% CI 0.51 to 1.26), or at the end of follow up (ARs 75/1671 [4.5%] v 92/1693 [5.4%], OR 0.82, 95% CI 0.60 to 1.12), or overall mortality (ARs 123/1671 [7.4%] v 150/1694 [8.9%]; OR 0.82, 95% CI 0.64 to 1.05) or major haemorrhage. Wider analysis that included unblinded trials, and so is likely to be more biased, found that low molecular weight heparin reduced overall mortality and major haemorrhage compared with unfractionated heparin (see harms below). The second and third systematic reviews included many of the same trials as the first. Results were similar with no differences between UFH and LMWH for recurrent venous thromboembolism or pulmonary embolism, and an unexplained, significant difference in favour of LMWH for total mortality when data was pooled.[19,20] We also found one open RCT not included in the systematic reviews which compared 294 people with acute proximal DVT who received intravenous standard heparin in the hospital (n = 98) or low molecular weight heparin subcutaneously twice daily administered primarily at home (outpatients) or alternatively in hospital (n = 97), or subcutaneous calcium heparin (n = 99) administered at home. No significant differences were found between groups. DVT was observed in 6.1% of people in the LMWH group, in 6.2% in the standard heparin group, and in 7.1% in the subcutaneous calcium heparin group.[21] See stroke management; systemic anticoagulation, p 114.

Harms: **Warfarin:** Two non-systematic reviews of RCTs and cohort studies found annual bleeding rates of 0–4.8% (fatal bleeding) and 2.4–8.1% (major bleeds).[22,23] Rates depended on how bleeding was defined and the intensity of anticoagulation. Major bleeding was associated with underlying predisposing causes such as trauma, surgery and occult carcinoma. In the systematic review of four RCTs comparing length of anticoagulation, none of the individual studies found a significant increase in bleeding complications during prolonged treatment for venous thromboembolism compared with shorter treatment.[13] The periods of treatment were different in all four RCTs and the populations studied had different types of venous thromboembolism (see benefits above). However, pooling these studies, 9/758 (2.5%) of patients on prolonged treatment had a major haemorrhage compared with 4/742 (0.5%) in the short arm (OR 3.75; 95% CI 1.63 to 8.62). We found one systematic review of four RCTs. One RCT found that higher levels of bleeding were also associated with higher target INRs.[24] One retrospective observational cohort study in 6814 people treated with warfarin found a 32% increase in all bleeding and a 46% increase in major bleeds for every 10 years of age above 40 years.[25] One study in 2745 people being treated with warfarin (inception cohort, 2011 person years) reported lower annual rates for fatal, major, and minor bleeds (0.25%, 1.1%, and 6.2%).[26] It found that, compared with INR less than 4.5, an INR greater than 4.5 increased the risk of bleeding (RR for all bleeds 7.9, 95% CI 5.4 to 11.5) **Heparin:** One systematic review found an incidence of heparin induced thrombocytopenia of 1.18% in 3306 patients treated for at least 5 days with no difference between low molecular weight or unfractionated heparin (LMWH v UFH, RR 0.85, 95% CI 0.45 to 1.62).[19] One systematic review of low molecular weight heparin compared with unfractionated heparin in venous thromboembolism found in blinded RCTs a non-significant difference between LMWH and UFH for major haemorrhage (ARs 27/1791 [1.5%] v 39/1827 [2.1%]; OR 0.71, 95% CI 0.43 to 1.15).[18] Pooling of blinded and unblinded studies in this systematic review found that low molecular weight heparin and unfractionated heparin both carried a 1–2% risk of major haemorrhage when given for up to 10 days.[18] In the analysis of the five studies (blinded and unblinded, n = 1636), which examined proximal thrombosis, a significant reduction in major haemorrhage was found (LMWH v UFH; 8/814 [1.0%] v 19/822 [2.3%]; OR 0.44, 95% CI 0.21 to 0.95). The second and third systematic reviews, covering many of the same trials, found similar significant reductions in major haemorrhage.[19,20] One of the systematic reviews in people with DVT found that, compared with low molecular weight heparin, unfractionated heparin was associated with higher rates of clinically important bleeding (ARs not given; RR unfractionated v low molecular weight heparin 2.48, 95% CI 1.27 to 6.67) and death (see benefits above).[11]

Comment: **Studies evaluating harm:** These varied in regard to diagnostic criteria, definitions of adverse events, and intensity of anticoagulation, making interpretation difficult. **Duration of warfarin therapy:** The absolute risk of recurrent venous thromboembolism decreases with time whereas the relative risk reduction with therapy remains constant. Harms of therapy, including major haemorrhage, continue during prolonged treatment. Individual people have different risk profiles and it is likely that the optimal duration of anticoagulation will vary between people. **Differences between low molecular weight heparins:** We found no trials comparing different low molecular weight heparins.

Thromboembolism

| QUESTION | What are the effects of treatment for isolated calf vein thrombosis? |

| OPTION | ANTICOAGULATION |

One RCT found that, in isolated calf vein thrombosis, warfarin plus unfractionated intravenous heparin (INR 2.5–4.2) reduced rates of proximal extension compared with heparin alone. We found insufficient evidence on optimal duration or intensity of anticoagulation.

Benefits:
Anticoagulation: We found no systematic review and no good placebo controlled RCTs. We found one RCT that compared unfractionated intravenous heparin for at least 5 days with or without 3 months of warfarin. It found that heparin plus warfarin reduced proximal extension of clot at 1 year compared with heparin alone (proximal extension occurred in 1/23 people with heparin plus warfarin v 9/28 people with heparin alone; ARR 28%, 95% CI 8.6 to 47.0, P < 0.02).[6] **Duration and intensity of anticoagulation:** We found insufficient evidence in people with isolated calf vein thrombosis.

Harms:
See harms of anticoagulation, under treatments for proximal DVT, p 148.

Comment:
Many reported cases of isolated calf vein thrombosis are asymptomatic but detected radiologically for research purposes. We found very limited evidence on the clinical significance of asymptomatic calf vein thrombosis. Similarly, studies into the incidence of pulmonary embolism associated with isolated calf vein thrombosis detected asymptomatic embolism by ventilation–perfusion scanning, and it is not clear what the clinical significance of these findings are.

| QUESTION | What are the effects of treatments for pulmonary embolism? |

| OPTION | ANTICOAGULATION |

One small RCT found that heparin plus warfarin significantly reduced mortality in people with pulmonary embolism, compared with no anticoagulant treatment. Two RCTs found that low molecular weight heparin was at least as effective as unfractionated heparin in people with pulmonary embolism.

Benefits:
Anticoagulation: We found no systematic review. We found one RCT in 35 people with pulmonary embolism comparing heparin plus warfarin with no anticoagulation. It found that anticoagulation reduced mortality (0/16 deaths [0%] with anticoagulation v 5/19 deaths [26%] with no anticoagulation; NNT 4, 95% CI 2 to 16).[27] We found no RCTs investigating heparin versus placebo, warfarin versus placebo, or heparin and warfarin versus heparin alone or warfarin alone. **Duration and intensity of anticoagulation:** We found no direct evidence in people with pulmonary embolism alone. Evidence for intensity and duration of treatment has been extrapolated from studies in people with proximal DVT and any venous

thromboembolism. These trials found that while bleeding rates are increased by higher INR target ranges (INR 3.0–4.5), recurrence rates are not significantly different compared with a lower range (INR 2.0–3.0) and that longer courses of anticoagulation reduced recurrence compared with shorter courses (see benefits of antico-agulation under treatments for isolated calf vein thrombosis, p 150). **Low molecular weight heparin versus unfractionated heparin:** We found no systematic review. We found two RCTs. The first compared subcutaneous LMWH with intravenous heparin in 612 people with symptomatic pulmonary embolism who did not receive thrombolysis or embolectomy. The trial found no significant difference between treatments for rates of death (AR 14/308 [4.5%] with heparin v 12/304 [3.9%] with tinzaparin; P = NS), or recurrent thromboembolism (6/308 [1.9%] with heparin v 5/304 [1.6%] with tinzaparin, P = NS).[28] The second RCT compared fixed dose subcutaneous given once daily with dose adjusted intravenous heparin in people with proximal DVT. Of 200 patients at study entry without signs or symptoms of pulmonary embolism but with high probability lung scan findings, none of the 97 who received low molecular weight heparin had new episodes of venous thromboem-bolism compared with 7 (6.8%) of 103 patients who received intravenous heparin (P = 0.01).[24]

Harms: The first RCT found no difference between UFH and LMWH for major haemorrhage (UFH 5/308 [1.6%] v LMWH 3/304 [1.0%]; P = NS).[28] The second trial found that major bleeding associated with initial therapy occurred in one patient who was given low molecular weight heparin and in two patients given intravenous heparin (P = NS).[24] However, the incidence of major haemorrhage is low and the number of participants in these trials was too small to detect a significant difference. See also harms of treatments for proximal DVT.

Comment: None.

Substantive changes since last issue

Proximal DVT: Duration of anticoagulation One new systematic review; conclu-sions unchanged.[13]
Low molecular weight heparin versus unfractionated heparin One updated systematic review[21], two new systematic reviews in people with venous throm-boembolism (mainly proximal DVT).[19,20] One new additional RCT in people with proximal DVT; conclusions unchanged.[14]
Pulmonary embolism: Low molecular weight heparin versus unfractionated heparin One additional RCT; conclusions unchanged.[24]

Footnote
Congenital deficiency of protein C, protein S, antithrombin III, Factor V Leiden mutation, and acquired conditions such as antiphospholipid antibody syndrome and systematic lupus erythematosus are associated with an increased risk of venous thromboembolism.

REFERENCES

1. Nordstrom M, Linblad B, Bergqvist D, Kjellstrom. A prospective study of the incidence of deep-vein thrombosis within a defined urban population. *Arch Intern Med* 1992;326:155–160.

2. Hansson PO, Werlin L, Tibblin G, Eriksson H. Deep

vein thrombosis and pulmonary embolism in the general population. *Arch Intern Med* 1997;157: 1665–1670.

3. Rubinstein I, Murray D, Hoffstein V. Fatal pulmonary emboli in hospitalised patients: an

autopsy study. *Arch Intern Med* 1988;148:1425–1426.

4. Hirsh J, Hoak J. Management of deep vein thrombosis and pulmonary embolism. *Circulation* 1996;93:2212–2245.

5. Farley TMM, Meirik O, Chang CL, Marmot MG, Poulter NR. Effects of different progestogens in low oestrogen oral contraceptives on venous thromboembolic disease. *Lancet* 1995;346:1582–1588.

6. Lagerstedt C, Olsson C, Fagher B, Oqvist B, Albrechtsson U. Need for long term anticoagulant treatment in symptomatic calf vein thrombosis. *Lancet* 1985;334:515–518.

7. Lohr J, Kerr T, Lutter K, Cranley R, Spirtoff K, Cranley J. Lower extremity calf thrombosis: to treat or not to treat? *J Vasc Surg* 1991;14:618–623.

8. Kakkar VV, Howe CT, Flanc C, Clarke MB. Natural history of postoperative deep vein thrombosis. *Lancet* 1969;2:230–232.

9. Zilliacus H. On the specific treatment of thrombosis and pulmonary embolism with anticoagulants, with a particular reference to the post thrombotic sequelae. *Acta Med Scand* 1946;170:1–221.

10. Giannoukas AD, Labropoulos N, Burke P, Katsamouris A, Nicolaides AN. Calf deep vein thrombosis: a review of the literature. *Eur J Vasc Endovasc Surg* 1995;10:398–404.

11. Lensing AWA, Prandoni P, Prins MH, Buller HR. Deep-vein thrombosis. *Lancet* 1999;353:479–485.

12. Brandjes DPM, Heijboer H, Buller HR, Rijk M, Jagt H, ten Cate JW. Acenocoumarol and heparin compared with acenocoumarol alone in the initial treatment of proximal-vein thrombosis. *N Engl J Med* 1992;327:1485–1489.

13. Hutten BA, Prins MH. Duration of treatment with vitamin K antagonists in symptomatic venous thromboembolism. Cochrane Library. Issue 3, 2000. Oxford: Update software. Search date January 2000; primary sources Medline 1966 to January 2000; Embase 1980 to January 2000; hand-searching relevant journals and personal contacts.

14. Hull R, Hirsh J, Jay RM, et al. Different intensities of oral anticoagulant therapy in the treatment of proximal vein thrombosis. *N Engl J Med* 1982;307:1676–1681.

15. Ascani A, Iorio A, Agnelli G. Withdrawal of warfarin after deep vein thrombosis: effects of a low fixed dose on rebound thrombin generation. *Blood Coagul Fibrinolysis* 1999;10:291–295.

16. Leisorovicz A, Simonneau G, Decousous H, Boissel JP. Comparison of efficacy and safety of low molecular weight heparins and unfractionated heparin in initial treatment of deep venous thrombosis: a meta-analysis. *BMJ* 1994;309:299–304. Search date December 1993; primary sources Medline and hand searched references.

17. Lensing AWA, Prins MH, Davidson BL, Hirsh J. Treatment of deep venous thrombosis with low-molecular weight heparins. *Arch Intern Med* 1995;

155:601–607. Search date 1994; primary sources Medline 1984 to 1994; manual search and hand searched references.

18. Van den Belt AGM, Prins MH, Lensing AWA, et al. Fixed dose subcutaneous low molecular weight heparins versus adjusted dose unfractionated heparin for venous thromboembolism. Cochrane Library. Issue 4, 1999. Oxford: Update software. Search date July 1999; primary sources Medline 1966 to July 1999, Embase 1980 to July 1999, and LILACS (dates not given); contacted researchers and pharmaceutical companies; and hand searched references.

19. Dolovich LR, Ginsberg JS, Douketis JD, Holbrook AM, Cheah G. A meta-analysis comparing low-molecular-weight heparins with unfractionated heparin in the treatment of venous thromboembolism. *Arch Int Med* 2000;160:181–188. Search date 1996; primary sources Medline 1986 to 1996; HEALTH 1975 to 1996; and Cochrane Library 1997, Issue 1; and hand searched references.

20. Bijsterveld NR, Hettiarachchi R, Peters R, Prins MH, Levi M, Buller HR. Low-molecular weight heparins in venous and arterial thrombotic disease. *Thrombosis & Haemostasis* 1999; 82(Suppl 1):139–147. Search date 1999; primary sources Medline 1996 to 1999; Embase 1996 to 1999; principial study investigators; and hand searched references.

21. Belcaro G, Nicolaides AN, Cesarone MR, Laurora G, De Sanctis MT et al. Comparison of low-molecular-weight heparin, administered primarily at home, with unfractionated heparin, administered in hospital, and subcutaneous heparin, administered at home for deep-vein thrombosis. *Angiology* 1999;50:781–787.

22. Landefeld CS, Beyth RJ. Anticoagulant related bleeding: clinical epidemiology, prediction, and prevention. *Am J Med* 1993;95:315–328.

23. Levine MN, Hirsh J, Landefeld CS, Raskob G. Haemorrhagic complications of anticoagulant treatment. *Chest* 1992;102(suppl):352–363.

24. Hull RD, Raskob GE, Brant RF, Pineo GF, Elliott G et al. Low-molecular-weight heparin vs heparin in the treatment of patients with pulmonary embolism. American-Canadian Thrombosis Study Group. *Arch Int Med* 2000;160:229–236.

25. van der Meer FJM, Rosendaal FR, Vandenbroucke, Briet E. Bleeding complications in oral anticoagulant therapy. *Arch Intern Med* 1993;153:1557–1562.

26. Palareti G, Leali N, Coccheri S, et al. Bleeding complications of oral anticoagulant treatment: an inception-cohort, prospective collaborative study (ISCOAT). *Lancet* 1996;348:423–428.

27. Barrit DW, Jordan SC. Anticoagulant drugs in the treatment of pulmonary embolism: a controlled trial. *Lancet* 1960;i:1309–1312.

28. Simonneau G, Sors H, Charbonnier B, et al. A comparison of low-molecular weight heparin with unfractionated heparin for acute pulmonary embolism. *N Engl J Med* 1997;337:663–669.

David Fitzmaurice
Senior Lecturer

FD Hobbs
Professor

Richard McManus
Clinical Research Fellow

Department of Primary Care and General Practice, The Medical School, University of Birmingham Birmingham UK

Competing interests: DF and RM none declared. FDH has been reimbursed for speaking at symposia.

Cardiovascular disorders

Updated this issue

Madhu Natarajan

INTERVENTIONS

Beneficial
Aspirin 155
Low molecular weight heparins
    added to aspirin. 158

Likely to be beneficial
Glycoprotein IIb/IIIa inhibitors . .156
Unfractionated heparin added to
    aspirin 157

Trade off between benefits and harms
Ticlopidine 155
Hirudin. 158

Unknown effectiveness
Nitrates 159
β Blockers 159
Routine early invasive treatment for
    all people with unstable
    angina 160

Unlikely to be beneficial
Calcium channel blockers 159

To be covered in future issues of *Clinical Evidence*
Clopidogrel

Key Messages

- One systematic review of RCTs has found that aspirin reduces the risk of death or myocardial infarction (MI) in people with unstable angina.

- One RCT found that ticlopidine was significantly more effective than conventional treatment (without aspirin) in unstable angina, but was associated with a significant risk of neutropenia.

- RCTs have found that glycoprotein IIb/IIIa inhibitors may improve outcome in people who undergo early percutaneous interventions when added to aspirin plus heparin, or heparin alone.

- Two systematic reviews have found that the effect of adding unfractionated heparin to aspirin is marginal. We found strong evidence from two systematic reviews that adding low molecular weight heparins (LMWH) to aspirin significantly reduces the short term rates of death and MI in people with unstable angina. One systematic review found no significant difference in benefits between LMWH and unfractionated heparin. One systematic review comparing short term treatment with LMWH versus unfractionated heparin found no significant difference in the frequency of major bleeding, and found that long term LMWH is associated with a significant increase in the risk of major bleeding compared with placebo.

- RCTs have found that hirudin versus unfractionated heparin in people also taking aspirin reduces short term but not medium term rates of death or MI.

- One systematic review of RCTs has found no evidence that calcium channel blockers prevent death or MI in people with unstable angina.

Unstable angina

- We found that the effects of nitrates or β blockers in people with unstable angina have not yet been adequately evaluated.

- Three RCTs have found little evidence that routine early invasive treatment reduces mortality compared with initial medical treatment plus later, more selective intervention.

DEFINITION Unstable angina is distinguished from stable angina, acute MI, and non-cardiac pain, by the pattern (characteristic pain present at rest or on lower levels of activity) or severity (recently increasing intensity, frequency, or duration) of symptoms, and the absence of persistent ST elevation on a resting electrocardiogram (ECG). Unstable angina includes a variety of different clinical patterns: angina at rest of up to 1 week's duration; angina increasing in severity to moderate or severe pain; non-Q wave MI; and post-MI angina continuing for more than 24 hours.

INCIDENCE/ PREVALENCE In industrialised countries the annual incidence of unstable angina is about six per 10 000 people in the general population.

AETIOLOGY/ RISK FACTORS Risk factors are the same as for other manifestations of ischaemic heart disease: older age, previous atheromatous cardiovascular disease, diabetes mellitus, smoking cigarettes, hypertension, hypercholesterolaemia, male sex, and a family history of ischaemic heart disease. Unstable angina can also occur in association with other disorders of the circulation, including heart valve disease, arrhythmia, and cardiomyopathy.

PROGNOSIS In people taking aspirin, the incidence of serious adverse outcomes (such as death, acute MI, or refractory angina requiring emergency revascularisation) is 5–10% within the first 7 days and about 15% at 30 days. Between 5% and 14% of people with unstable angina die in the year after diagnosis, with around half of these deaths occurring within 4 weeks of diagnosis. No single factor identifies people at higher risk of an adverse event. Risk factors include severity of presentation (e.g. duration of pain, rapidity of progression, evidence of heart failure), medical history (e.g. previous unstable angina, acute MI, left ventricular dysfunction), other clinical parameters (e.g. age, diabetes), ECG changes (e.g. severity of ST segment depression, deep T wave inversion, transient ST elevation), biochemical parameters (e.g. troponin concentration), and change in clinical status (e.g. recurrent chest pain, silent ischaemia, haemodynamic instability).

AIMS To relieve pain and ischaemia; to prevent death and MI; to identify people at high risk requiring revascularisation; to facilitate early hospital discharge in people at low and medium risk; to modify risk factors; to prevent death, MI, and recurrent ischaemia after discharge from hospital, with minimum adverse effects.

OUTCOMES Rate of death or MI (often measured at 2, 7, and 30 days, and 6 months after randomisation); adverse effects of treatment. Some RCTs include rates of refractory ischaemia or readmission for unstable angina.

METHODS *Clinical Evidence* update search and appraisal May 2000.

OPTION   ASPIRIN

One systematic review of RCTs has found that aspirin alone reduces the risk of death and MI in people with unstable angina. The evidence suggests no added cardiovascular benefit, and possible added harm, from doses of aspirin over 325 mg daily.

Benefits: One systematic review (published in 1994) compared antiplatelet treatment versus placebo in 100 000 people in 145 RCTs.[1] Seven of these trials included a total of 4000 people with unstable angina. The review found at 6 months that antiplatelet treatment (mostly medium dose aspirin, 75–325 mg daily) reduced the combined outcome of vascular death, MI, or stroke (AR 14% on placebo v 9% on antiplatelet treatment; RRR 35%, 95% CI 21% to 49%). This means that 20 people would need to be treated with aspirin rather than placebo to prevent one additional event in 6 months (NNT 20, 95% CI 15 to 34). Individual trials within the systematic review showed consistent benefit from daily aspirin in terms of reduced deaths and MI.

Harms: People taking doses of aspirin ranging from 75 to 1200 mg daily had no significant adverse events, including gastrointestinal intolerance or bleeding.[1] However, the sum of the evidence suggests no added cardiovascular benefit, and greater incidence of gastrointestinal effects, for aspirin doses greater than 325 mg daily. Some people are allergic to aspirin.

Comment: The systematic review covered a wide range of people with different morbidities and levels of risk. Its results should be generalisable to routine practice.[1] People with unstable angina who are allergic or who do not respond to aspirin will need alternative antiplatelet treatment.

OPTION   TICLOPIDINE

One RCT found that ticlopidine was more effective than conventional treatment (without aspirin) in people with unstable angina, but it was associated with a significant risk of neutropenia. Ticlopidine may therefore be an alternative in people who are intolerant of, or allergic to, aspirin.

Benefits: We found no systematic review of ticlopidine in unstable angina. One RCT (published in 1990) compared ticlopidine versus conventional treatment without aspirin in 652 people (72% male) with unstable angina treated within 48 hours of admission.[2] At 6 months, there were significantly fewer vascular deaths or non-fatal MI in people taking ticlopidine (RRR compared with control 46%, 95% CI 12% to 81%; NNT for 6 months 16, 95% CI 9 to 62). We found no trial of ticlopidine versus aspirin in the treatment of unstable angina.

Harms: Reversible neutropenia was reported in 1–2% of people taking ticlopidine. Other adverse effects include diarrhoea and rash.

Comment: Ticlopidine is an alternative for people with unstable angina who are intolerant of, or allergic to, aspirin. A large study is currently comparing clopidogrel plus aspirin versus aspirin alone in this group of people.

OPTION GLYCOPROTEIN IIB/IIIA PLATELET RECEPTOR INHIBITORS

RCTs have found that adding parenteral glycoprotein IIb/IIIa inhibitors to unfractionated heparin alone or unfractionated heparin plus aspirin reduces deaths and MI. However, this was in the context of high rates of early percutaneous interventions.

Benefits: We found no systematic review, but we found three RCTs which examined adding intravenous glycoprotein IIb/IIIa inhibitors to standard treatment,[3–5] and three RCTs which compared a glycoprotein IIb/IIIa inhibitor versus heparin.[3,5,6] The primary end points varied, but all trials included data on death rates and MI at 30 days (see table 1, p 164). **Added to heparin or aspirin or both:** We found one RCT with three treatment arms comparing tirofiban, heparin, or both, as an infusion for a mean of 72 hours in 1915 people with unstable angina or non-Q wave MI.[3] The arm in which people were receiving tirofiban alone was stopped early because of excess mortality at 7 days (AR of death at 7 days, 4.6% with tirofiban alone v 1.1% with heparin alone). The trial found that compared with heparin alone, tirofiban plus heparin reduced rates of death, MI, or refractory ischaemia (at 7 days, AR 12.9% with tirofiban + heparin v 17.9% with heparin, RR 0.68, 95% CI 0.53 to 0.88, P = 0.004; at 30 days, AR 18.5% with tirofiban + heparin v 22.3% with heparin, P = 0.03; at 6 months, AR 27.7% with tirofiban + heparin v 32.1% with heparin, P = 0.02). Early angiography and intervention were encouraged in this trial. We found another RCT, which compared eptifibatide plus heparin plus aspirin versus heparin plus aspirin in 9461 people with unstable angina. The trial found modest benefit when eptifibatide was added to aspirin and unfractionated heparin (deaths and non-fatal MI at 30 days, eptifibatide 11.6% v placebo 16.7%, P = 0.01). No benefit was seen in people with low rates of intervention with percutaneous transluminal coronary angioplasty (PTCA).[4] A smaller RCT (2282 people), which included five treatment arms, compared high dose lamifiban with and without heparin versus low dose lamifiban with and without heparin versus heparin plus placebo. The trial found that rates of ischaemic events were similar with high dose lamifiban plus heparin versus heparin plus placebo, but that the combination of low dose lamifiban and heparin reduced ischaemic events (AR of ischaemic event at 6 months, 12.6% with low dose lamifiban + heparin v 17.9% with heparin + placebo, P = 0.025). **Versus heparin:** One RCT compared intravenous tirofiban versus heparin for 48 hours in 3232 people who were already receiving aspirin.[6] The primary composite end point of death, MI, or refractory ischaemia at 48 hours was significantly lower on tirofiban (AR 3.8% v 5.6%; RRR 33%, 95% CI 8% to 52%), but at 30 days there was no significant difference in the end point of death or MI (see table 1, p 164). The RCT that included five treatment arms (high and low dose lamifiban ± heparin versus heparin + placebo) was able to compare low and high dose lamifiban alone versus heparin. The trial found no significant difference in combined outcome of death or non-fatal MI at 30 days between heparin alone, low dose lamifiban alone, or high dose lamifiban alone (AR of death or MI, 11.7% with heparin v 10.6% with low dose lamifiban v 12.0% with high dose lamifiban, P = 0.668).[5] However, at 6 months there were significantly fewer deaths or MI in people on low dose lamifiban alone, compared with high dose lamifiban alone or heparin alone (AR of death or MI, 13.7% with low dose lamifiban v 16.4% with high dose lamifiban v 17.9% with heparin). One further RCT, which included three arms (tirofiban v heparin v both) found that tirofiban alone increased mortality at 7 days compared with other treatments.[3] This arm of the trial was therefore stopped early (see top of benefits section above).[3]

Harms: No difference was reported in rates of major bleeding between tirofiban and heparin (AR 0.4% in both groups).[6] When high dose lamifiban was added to heparin, there were more intermediate or major bleeds than with heparin alone (AR 12.1% v 5.5%, P = 0.002), although bleeding rates were similar with low dose lamifiban plus heparin compared with heparin plus placebo.[5] Reversible thrombocytopenia occurred more frequently with tirofiban than with heparin (AR 1.1% v 0.4%, P = 0.04).[6]

Comment: The smaller trial of adding a glycoprotein IIb/IIIa inhibitor to standard treatment[5] suggests that a "dose ceiling" may exist beyond which escalation of dose results in higher bleeding complications with no increase in efficacy.

QUESTION **What are the effects of antithrombin treatments?**

OPTION UNFRACTIONATED HEPARIN

Updated this issue

Two systematic reviews of six small RCTs have found benefit from adding unfractionated heparin to aspirin in people with unstable angina, but this may have occurred by chance.

Benefits: **Added to aspirin:** We found two systematic reviews that met our quality criteria. Both included the same six RCTs in 1353 people with unstable angina who were treated with either heparin and aspirin or aspirin alone for 2–7 days.[7,8] The first review (published in 1996) found that the risk of death or MI during treatment with heparin plus aspirin was less than that for aspirin alone (AR 55/698 [8%] 68/655 [10%]); but the differences could have arisen by chance (OR 0.67, 95% CI 0.44 to 1.02).[7] The second review (published in 2000) used a different statistical method for meta-analysis and found a result that just reached statistical significance (OR 0.67, 95% CI 0.45 to 0.99).[8] The first systematic review also found no significant difference between the two groups (from 4 RCTs with data available) in the rate of death or MI at 12 weeks (AR 12% on heparin + aspirin v 14% on aspirin alone; RR 0.82, 95% CI 0.56 to 1.20).[7] **Versus LMWH:** See benefits of LMWH, p 158.

Harms: Major bleeding occurred in 0.4% of people on aspirin and 1.5% of those on aspirin plus heparin (RR 1.89, 95% CI 0.66 to 5.38).[7]

Unstable angina

Comment: In this situation it is not clear which statistical method is preferred.

OPTION	LOW MOLECULAR WEIGHT HEPARINS

Updated this issue

One systematic review found that aspirin plus LMWH is more effective than aspirin alone in the first 30 days after an episode of unstable angina. One systematic review found no significant difference in benefits between LMWH and unfractionated heparin. One systematic review comparing short term treatment with LMWH versus unfractionated heparin found no significant difference in the frequency of major bleeding, and found that long term LMWH is associated with a significant increase in the risk of major bleeding compared with placebo.

Benefits: **Adding LMWH to aspirin:** We found one systematic review[8] (search date not stated, 2 RCTs, 1639 people), which compared LMWH for up to 7 days versus placebo or untreated control. The review found a reduction in death or MI with LMWH (OR 0.34, 95% CI 0.20 to 0.58). The same systematic review found five RCTs (12 099 people) comparing long term LMWH versus placebo. The review found no benefit of long term LMWH given for up to 90 days (OR for death or MI, LMWH v placebo 0.98, 95% CI 0.81 to 1.17). **Versus unfractionated heparin:** We found one systematic review[8] of five RCTs (12 171 people), which compared an equal duration (maximum 8 days) of LMWH versus unfractionated heparin. The review found no significant difference between treatments (OR for death or MI, LMWH v unfractionated heparin 0.88, 95% CI 0.69 to 1.12).

Harms: One systematic review comparing LMWH versus unfractionated heparin found no significant difference in the frequency of major bleeds between treatments (OR 1.00, 95% CI 0.64 to 1.57)[8] (see harms of unfractionated heparin, p 157). Long term LMWH versus placebo is associated with a significant increase in the risk of major bleeding (OR 2.26, 95% CI 1.63 to 3.14), equivalent to an excess of 12 bleeds for every 1000 people treated.[8]

Comment: LMWH may be more attractive than unfractionated heparin for routine short term use because coagulation monitoring is not required and it can be self-administered after discharge.

OPTION	HIRUDIN

RCTs have found that in people with unstable angina taking aspirin, rates of death and MI are significantly lower during infusion of hirudin than during infusion of unfractionated heparin. However, no added benefit is found once the infusion stops. Longer durations of hirudin infusion (> 72 hours) are currently being evaluated. Compared with heparin, hirudin causes significantly more major bleeds requiring transfusion but no more life threatening bleeds or haemorrhagic strokes.

Benefits: We found no systematic review. **Versus unfractionated heparin:** Three large RCTs in more than 19 000 people with unstable angina taking aspirin compared R-hirudin versus unfractionated heparin given for 2–3 days.[9–11] A pooled analysis of these trials found reduced risk of cardiovascular death or MI at the end of the 72-hour treatment period (AR 233/9615 [2.4%] for hirudin, 315/9446 [3.3%] for heparin; ARR 0.9%, 95% CI 0.5% to 1.3%; RRR 27%, 95% CI 14% to 39%), with some loss of this early benefit at 7 days (RRR 17%, 95% CI 6% to 27%) and 35 days (RRR 9%, 95% CI 0% to 17%).

Harms: In the largest RCT, hirudin versus unfractionated heparin was associated with a significant increase in the need for transfusion (AR 10.2% v 8.4%, P = 0.01), and a trend for increased extracranial haemorrhage (AR 10.2% v 8.6%, P = 0.06) and intracranial haemorrhage (AR 0.2% v 0.02%, P = 0.06).[9] In the second largest RCT, hirudin was associated with an excess of major bleeding (AR 1.2% v 0.7%; RR 1.71, 95% CI 1.13 to 2.58) but no increase in life threatening bleeds or strokes at day 7.[11] The smallest RCT reported no haemorrhagic strokes and no difference in the rate of major bleeds (about 1% in all groups).[10] Hirudin was associated with a higher rate of minor bleeding (AR 16.2% low dose hirudin [LDHir] v 21.3% medium dose hirudin [MDHir] v 10.5% heparin; RR LDHir v heparin 1.54, 95% CI 1.03 to 2.31; RR MDHir v heparin 2.03, 95% CI 1.39 to 2.96).[10]

Comment: Whether longer duration of treatment has greater benefits is the target of future trials (S Yusuf, personal communication). Two of the trials gave doses of hirudin in proportion to the body weight, but gave heparin as a fixed dose.[9,10]

QUESTION What are the effects of anti-ischaemic treatments?

OPTION NITRATES, β BLOCKERS, AND CALCIUM CHANNEL BLOCKERS

The effects of nitrates, β blockers, and calcium channel blockers on rates of death or MI have not yet been adequately evaluated in people with unstable angina. Short acting dihydropyridine calcium channel blockers may increase mortality.

Benefits: **Nitrates:** We found no systematic reviews or RCTs of nitrates versus placebo in unstable angina. We found one RCT in 162 people with unstable angina of intravenous glyceryl trinitrate versus placebo for 48 hours. Those receiving glyceryl trinitrate had fewer episodes of chest pain, less severe episodes (pain lasting ≥ 20 minutes), and less need for additional sublingual glyceryl trinitrate.[12] We found one RCT comparing intravenous glyceryl trinitrate, heparin, and glyceryl trinitrate plus heparin versus placebo in 200 people with unstable angina within 6 months of PTCA. The trial found that recurrent angina occurred significantly less frequently in people treated with glyceryl trinitrate alone and glyceryl trinitrate plus heparin compared with placebo, but there was no benefit from heparin alone or additional benefit from combination treatment (P < 0.003 for glyceryl trinitrate alone and for glyceryl trinitrate plus heparin v placebo).[13] **β Blockers:** We found no systematic review of β blockers versus placebo in unstable angina. We found two RCTs. The first trial randomised 338 people with rest angina not receiving β blocker treatment to nifedipine, metoprolol, both, or neither in a double blind, placebo controlled fashion.[14] The main outcome was recurrent angina or MI within 48 hours. Metoprolol was significantly more effective than nifedipine. The second trial randomly assigned 81 people with unstable angina on "optimal doses" of nitrates and nifedipine to placebo or at least 160 mg/day of propranolol.[15] The incidence of cardiac death, MI, and requirement for coronary artery bypass grafting or percutaneous coronary interventions at 30 days did not differ between the two groups (propranolol 16/42 v placebo 18/39, P = NS). People taking propranolol had a lower cumulative probability of experiencing recurrent rest angina over the first 4 days of the trial. The mean number of clinical episodes of angina, duration of angina, glyceryl trinitrate requirement, and ischaemic ST changes by continuous ECG monitoring was also lower. **Calcium channel blockers:** We found one systematic review (published in 1989). It found that that calcium channel blockers reduced symptoms and ischaemia but had no effect on rates of MI or death.[16]

Harms: Hypotension is a potential adverse effect of nitrates. However, both older and more recent large RCTs in people with other ischaemic conditions showed that nitrates were safe and well tolerated when used judiciously in clinically appropriate doses. Potential adverse effects of β blockers include bradycardia, exacerbation of reactive airways disease, and hypoglycaemia in diabetics. Observational studies have reported increased mortality with short acting dihydropyridine calcium channel blockers (such as nifedipine) in people with coronary heart disease.[17,18]

Comment: We found no good evidence that anti-ischaemic drugs (nitrates, β blockers, calcium channel blockers) prevent death or MI. By consensus, until further data are available intravenous nitrates remain a first line treatment together with heparin and aspirin in unstable angina.

QUESTION   What are the effects of invasive treatments?

OPTION   EARLY ROUTINE CARDIAC CATHETERISATION AND REVASCULARISATION

RCTs have found that early invasive treatment reduces symptoms and promotes early discharge compared with early conservative treatment in people with unstable angina. However, they found that early invasive treatment did not reduce rates of death and MI. We found insufficient evidence to ascertain whether certain people (e.g. those who are refractory to medical treatment) are more likely than others to benefit from early invasive treatment.

Benefits: We found no systematic review. Three RCTs have compared early routine angiography/revascularisation versus medical treatment alone.[19-22] The largest, most recent trial (2457 people with unstable angina) compared early invasive treatment (within the first 7 days) versus non-invasive treatment plus planned coronary angiography, followed by placebo controlled long term dalteparin for 3 months, using a factorial randomisation protocol.[22] All people were initially treated with open-label dalteparin or standard heparin for up to 72 hours after admission. In people randomised to invasive treatment, 96% underwent cardiac catheterisation, and 71%

underwent revascularisation within the first 10 days. The trial found that compared with early non-invasive treatment, early invasive treatment reduced the risk of the primary end point of combined death and MI at 6 months (113/1207 [9.4%] v 148/1226 [12.1%]; RR 0.78, 95% CI 0.62 to 0.98), but did not significantly reduce mortality at six months (23/1207 [1.9%] with early invasive treatment v 36/1226 [2.9%] with non-invasive treatment; RR 0.65, 95% CI 0.39 to 1.09). The trial also found that invasive treatment significantly reduced angina and readmission rates (presence of angina at 6 months, 256/1174 [22%] with invasive treatment v 455/1177 [39%] with non-invasive treatment; RR 0.56, 95% CI 0.50 to 0.64, P < 0.001; readmission during 6 month period, 357/1167 [31%] with invasive treatment v 594/1204 [49%] with non-invasive treatment, RR 0.62, 95% CI 0.60 to 0.69, P < 0.001). The second trial used a factorial design to compare tissue plasminogen activator versus placebo, and early invasive treatment (cardiac catheterisation at 18–48 hours) versus early conservative treatment, in 1473 people with unstable angina presenting within 24 hours of ischaemic chest discomfort.[19,20] All people received aspirin and unfractionated heparin. Within 6 weeks, 64% of people randomised to conservative treatment underwent cardiac catheterisation, 26% underwent percutaneous transluminal coronary angioplasty, and 24% underwent coronary artery bypass grafting. At 6 weeks, there was no significant difference in the composite end point (death, MI, or a symptom limited exercise stress test) (invasive 18.1% v conservative 16.2%, P = 0.78). However, invasive treatment significantly reduced readmission (7.8% v 14.1%, P < 0.001), total duration of all readmissions (total 365 days v 930 days, P < 0.001), and need for antianginal medications (P < 0.02). At 1 year, there was no significant difference in rates of death or MI (invasive 10.8% v conservative 12.2%, P = 0.42), but the lower numbers of repeat hospital admissions and hospital days with invasive treatment persisted. The third and smallest trial compared invasive versus conservative treatment in 920 people.[21] Over 23 months of follow up (range 12–44 months) there was no significant difference in the combined primary end point of death or MI (RR 0.87, 95% CI 0.68 to 1.10).

Harms: The largest, most recent RCT found that early invasive treatment increased major bleeding compared with early non-invasive treatment, but found no significant difference between treatments for ischaemic or haemorrhagic stroke (major bleeds, AR 1.6% with invasive treatment v 0.7% with non-invasive treatment, P value not given).[22] The second RCT reported no differences in complication rates (death, MI, emergency coronary artery bypass grafting, abrupt vessel closure, haemorrhage, serious hypotension) between invasive and conservative treatment (14% v 13%, P = 0.38).[19,20] In the smallest RCT, people who underwent early invasive treatment were significantly more at risk of death or MI at hospital discharge (36 v 15 people, P = 0.004), 30 days after randomisation (48 v 26 people, P = 0.012), and at 1 year (111 v 85 people, P = 0.05).[21]

Comment: All trials have reported only short term and medium term follow up, so we cannot exclude a long term difference in effect between early invasive and early non-invasive strategies. It is not clear yet whether there are subgroups of people that benefit particularly from either invasive or conservative treatment. Advances in catheterisation and revascularisation technology and periprocedural management may reduce the early risks of invasive treatment in the future.

Substantive changes since last issue

Unfractionated heparin One new systematic review; no change in conclusions.[8]
Low molecular weight heparin One new systematic review. Long term treatment with LMWH confers no benefit and is associated with a significant increase in the risk of major bleeding compared with placebo.[8]
Nitrates New RCT; no change in conclusions.[13]

REFERENCES

1. Antiplatelet Trialists' Collaboration. Collaborative overview of randomised trials of antiplatelet therapy. I: Prevention of death, myocardial infarction, and stroke by prolonged antiplatelet therapy in various categories of patients. *BMJ* 1994;308:81–106. Trials available in March 1990 were included; primary sources Medline, Current Contents.
2. Balsano F, Rizzon P, Violi F, et al and the Studio della Ticlopidina nell'Angina Instabile Group. Antiplatelet treatment with ticlopidine in unstable angina: a controlled multicentre clinical trial. *Circulation* 1990;82:17–26.
3. PRISM-PLUS Study Investigators. Inhibition of the platelet glycoprotein IIb/IIIa receptor with tirofiban in unstable angina and non-Q-wave myocardial infarction. *N Engl J Med* 1998;338:1488–1497.
4. Pursuit Trial Investigators. Inhibition of platelet glycoprotein IIb/IIIa with eptifibatide in patients with acute coronary syndromes. *N Engl J Med* 1998;339:436–443.
5. PARAGON Investigators. International, randomized, controlled trial of lamifiban (a platelet glycoprotein IIb/IIIa inhibitor), heparin, or both in unstable angina. *Circulation* 1998;97:2386–2395.
6. PRISM Study Investigators. A comparison of aspirin plus tirofiban with aspirin plus heparin for unstable angina. *N Engl J Med* 1998;338:1498–1505.
7. Oler A, Whooley MA, Oler J, Grady D. Adding heparin to aspirin reduces the incidence of myocardial infarction and death in patients with unstable angina: a meta-analysis. *JAMA* 1996; 276:811–815. Search date 1995; primary sources Medline 1966 to September 1995, hand search of reference lists, consultation with experts.
8. Eikelboom JW, Anand SS, Malmberg K, et al. Unfractionated heparin and low molecular weight heparin in acute coronary syndrome without ST elevation: a meta-analysis. *Lancet* 2000;355: 1936–1942. Search date not stated. Primary sources Medline and Embase, reference lists of published papers were scanned, experts canvassed for unpublished trials, personal data.
9. GUSTO IIb Investigators. A comparison of recombinant hirudin with heparin for the treatment of acute coronary syndromes. *N Engl J Med* 1996; 335:775–782.
10. OASIS Investigators. Comparison of the effects of two doses of recombinant hirudin compared with heparin in patients with acute myocardial ischemia without ST elevation: a pilot study. *Circulation* 1997;96:769–777.
11. OASIS-2 Investigators. Effects of recombinant hirudin (lepirudin) compared with heparin on death, myocardial infarction, refractory angina, and revascularisation procedures in patients with acute myocardial ischaemia without ST elevation: a randomised trial. *Lancet* 1999;353:429–38.
12. Karlberg KE, Saldeen T, Wallin R, et al. Intravenous nitroglycerine reduces ischaemia in unstable angina pectoris: a double-blind placebo-controlled study. *J Intern Med* 1998;243:25–31.
13. Douchet S, Malekinapour M, Theroux P, et al. Randomized trial comparing intravenous nitroglycerin and heparin for treatment of unstable angina secondary or restenosis after coronary artery angioplasty. *Circulation* 2000;101:955–961.
14. HINT Research Group. Early treatment of unstable angina in the coronary care unit: a randomized, double blind, placebo controlled comparison of recurrent ischaemia in patients treated with nifedipine or metoprolol or both. *Br Heart J* 1986; 56:400–413.
15. Gottlieb SO, Weisfeldt ML, Ouyang P, et al. Effect of the addition of propranolol to therapy with nifedipine for unstable angina pectoris: a randomized, double-blind, placebo-controlled trial. *Circulation* 1986;73:331–337.
16. Held PH, Yusuf S, Furberg CD. Calcium channel blockers in acute myocardial infarction and unstable angina: an overview. *BMJ* 1989;299: 1187–1192. Search date not stated; primary sources not specified in detail.
17. Furberg CD, Psaty BM, Meyer JV. Nifedipine: dose-related increase in mortality in patients with coronary heart disease. *Circulation* 1995;92: 1326–1331. Search date and primary sources not specified.
18. WHO-ISH Study. Ad hoc subcommittee of the liaison committee of the World Health Organisation and the International Society of Hypertension: effects of calcium antagonists on the risks of coronary heart disease, cancer and bleeding. *J Hypertens* 1997:15:105–115.
19. The TIMI IIIB Investigators. Effects of tissue plasminogen activator and a comparison of early invasive and conservative strategies in unstable angina and non-Q-wave myocardial infarction. results of the TIMI IIIB trial. *Circulation* 1994;89: 1545–1556.
20. Anderson V, Cannon CP, Stone PH, et al for the TIMI IIIB Investigators. One-year results of the thrombolysis in myocardial infarction (TIMI) IIIB clinical trial: a randomized comparison of tissue-type plasminogen activator versus placebo and early invasive versus early conservative strategies in unstable angina and non-Q wave myocardial

infarction. *J Am Coll Cardiol* 1995;26:1643–1650.

21. Boden WE, O'Rourke RA, Crawford MH, et al for the VANQWISH Trial Investigators. Outcomes in patients with acute non-Q-wave myocardial infarction randomly assigned to an invasive as compared with a conservative management strategy. *N Engl J Med* 1998;338:1785–1792.

22. Yusuf S, Zucker D, Peduzzi P, et al. Effect of coronary artery bypass graft surgery on survival: overview of 10-year results from randomized trials by the coronary artery bypass graft surgery trialists collaboration. *Lancet* 1994;344:563–570.

Madhu Natarajan
Division of Cardiology
McMaster University
Hamilton
Canada

Competing interests: None declared.

TABLE 1 Effects of glycoprotein IIb/IIIa inhibitors in unstable angina and non-Q wave myocardial infarction: results of main RCTs (see text, p 156).

Trial	Total participants	Comparison	Odds reduction for death or MI at 30 days* (95% CI)	NNT to avoid one additional death or MI at 30 days
PRISM-PLUS[3]	1570	Tirofiban + heparin v heparin alone	30% (4% to 49%)	31
PURSUIT[4]	10948	Eptifibatide + heparin v heparin alone	11% (1.3% to 20%)	67
PARAGON[5]	2282	Lamifiban + heparin v heparin alone	4% (−32% to +30%)	N/A
PRISM[6]	3232	Aspirin + tirofiban v aspirin + heparin	20% (−5% to +39%)	N/A

* = 1-OR, equivalent to RRR; NA, not applicable; MI, myocardial infarction.

Updated this issue

Paddy O'Neill

QUESTIONS

INTERVENTIONS

TREATMENT

Likely to be beneficial
Non-steroidal anti-inflammatory
drugs (NSAIDs) 166

**Trade off between benefits and
harms**
Antibiotics 167

Unlikely to be beneficial
Antibiotics in children under 2
years old with uncomplicated
acute otitis media (AOM) . . .167

Unknown effectiveness
Paracetamol. 166

PREVENTION

**Trade off between benefits and
harms**
Long term antibiotic
prophylaxis 169
Xylitol syrup or gum 171

**To be covered in future issues of
*Clinical Evidence***
Myringotomy
Surgery

Covered elsewhere in this issue
Otitis media with effusion, p 279

Key Messages

Treatment

- We found limited evidence from one RCT that non-steroidal anti-inflammatory drugs (NSAIDs) may be more effective than placebo in relieving pain. The trial found no significant difference between paracetamol and placebo. The dosing regimen for paracetamol may not have been optimal and the trial may not have been adequately powered to rule out a difference.

- We found conflicting evidence from two systematic reviews on the effects of antibiotics in uncomplicated acute otitis media (AOM). Rates of adverse effects are almost doubled in children taking antibiotics compared with placebo. We found no clear evidence favouring a particular antibiotic.

- One systematic review and one subsequent RCT have found no evidence that antibiotics improve outcome in children aged less than 2 years with uncomplicated AOM.

- One systematic review found greater immediate benefit but no difference in long term outcome with 10 day courses of antibiotics compared with shorter (5 day) courses.

Prevention

- One systematic review found that long term antibiotic prophylaxis has a modest effect in preventing recurrence of AOM. One subsequent RCT found no significant difference between antibiotic prophylaxis and placebo.

- We found insufficient evidence on which antibiotic to use, for how long, and how many episodes of AOM justify treatment.

- We found limited evidence from one RCT that xylitol syrup or gum was effective in preventing AOM, but had significant adverse effects.

© *Clinical Evidence* 2000;4:165–172.

Acute otitis media

DEFINITION	Otitis media is inflammation in the middle ear. Subcategories include acute otitis media (AOM), otitis media with effusion (also known as "glue ear", p 279), recurrent AOM, and chronic suppurative otitis media. AOM presents with systemic and local signs and has a rapid onset. The persistence of an effusion beyond 3 months without signs of infection defines otitis media with effusion, whereas chronic suppurative otitis media is characterised by continuing inflammation in the middle ear causing otorrhoea and a perforated tympanic membrane.
INCIDENCE/ PREVALENCE	AOM is common, with a high morbidity and low mortality. In the UK about 30% of children under 3 years old visit their general practitioner with AOM each year, and 97% receive antimicrobial treatment.[1] By 3 months of age, 10% of children have had an episode of AOM. It is the most common reason for outpatient antimicrobial treatment in the USA.[2]
AETIOLOGY/ RISK FACTORS	The most common bacterial causes for AOM are *Streptococcus pneumoniae (S pneumoniae)*, *Haemophilus influenzae*, and *Moraxella catarrhalis*. The incidence of penicillin resistant *S pneumoniae* has risen, but rates differ between countries. The most important risk factors are young age and attendance at day care centres such as nursery schools. Others include white race, male sex, and a history of enlarged adenoids, tonsillitis, or asthma. Other aetiological factors include multiple previous episodes, bottle feeding, a history of ear infections in parents or siblings, and use of a soother or pacifier. The evidence for an effect of environmental tobacco smoke is controversial.[1]
PROGNOSIS	In about 80% of children the condition resolves in about 3 days without antibiotic treatment. Complications are rare but include hearing loss, mastoiditis, meningitis, and recurrent attacks.[1]
AIMS	To reduce the severity and duration of pain and other symptoms, to prevent complications, and to minimise adverse effects of treatment.
OUTCOMES	Pain control (in infants this can be assessed by proxy measures such as parental observation of distress/crying and analgesic use); incidence of complications such as deafness (usually divided into short and long term hearing loss), recurrent attacks of AOM, mastoiditis, and meningitis; resolution of otoscopic appearances; incidence of adverse effects of treatment.
METHODS	*Clinical Evidence* update search and appraisal May 2000.

QUESTION   What are the effects of treatments?

OPTION   ANALGESIA

One RCT found that non-steroidal anti-inflammatory drugs (NSAIDs) were more effective than placebo in relieving pain. The trial found no significant difference between paracetamol and placebo. The dosing

**regimen for paracetamol may not have been optimal and the trial may
have been too small to rule out a difference.**

Benefits: We found no systematic review. We found one double blind multi-
             centre RCT comparing three times daily treatment with ibuprofen,
             paracetamol, or placebo for 48 hours in 219 children aged 1–6
             years with otoscopically diagnosed AOM.[3] All children received
             antibiotic treatment with ceflacor. The proportions of children still
             experiencing pain by the second day were 7% on NSAIDs, 10% on
             paracetamol, and 25% on placebo. Compared with placebo, ibu-
             profen was significantly more effective (P < 0.01) but paracetamol
             was not (P value not quoted). There was no significant difference
             between placebo and active treatments for other outcomes
             (appearance of the tympanic membrane, rectal temperature, and
             parental assessment).

Harms: All treatments were well and equally tolerated.

Comment: The trial may have been too small to detect a significant difference
             between paracetamol and placebo. The lack of significant differ-
             ence may also be explained by the use of a three times daily
             regimen, since paracetamol is usually given four times daily. The
             evidence from this trial may be further limited because the assess-
             ment of the child's pain relief was based on parental observation,
             using a scale of 0 or 1.

OPTION   ANTIBIOTICS

**We found conflicting evidence from systematic reviews. The more recent
review found that antibiotics reduce the proportion of children still in pain
at 2–7 days and reduce the risk of developing contralateral AOM. The
review found that antibiotics have no effect on pain within 24 hours, and
no effect on incidence of AOM or deafness at 1 month. Rates of adverse
effects were almost doubled in children on antibiotics compared with
placebo. We found no clear evidence favouring a particular antibiotic. One
systematic review and one subsequent RCT have found no evidence that
antibiotics improve outcomes in children aged under 2 years with
uncomplicated AOM.**

Benefits: **Versus placebo or no treatment:** We found two systematic
             reviews.[4,5] The first (search date June 1992) identified four RCTs
             comparing antibiotics versus placebo or no treatment in 535
             children aged 4 months to 18 years with AOM.[5] Co-intervention with
             analgesics and other symptomatic relief was allowed in most trials.
             Rate of treatment success (absence of all presenting symptoms
             and signs at around 7–14 days after treatment started) was
             significantly greater on active treatment (AR 13.7% v 81%; ARR
             67.3%, no CI quoted). The second systematic review (search date
             March 1999) identified nine RCTs comparing early use of antibiotics
             versus placebo in children aged 7 months to 15 years with AOM.[4]
             Most trials did not state the time interval between onset of symp-
             toms and starting treatment: the two that did stated 1–24 hours
             and about 30 hours. Four studies reported pain outcomes 24 hours
             after presentation (n = 717). All four found that antibiotic treatment
             was no more effective than placebo (RR 1.02 95% CI 0.85 to
             1.22). Nine trials found that, 2–7 days after presentation, fewer

children were still in pain after treatment with antibiotics compared with placebo (106/1043 children in pain after antibiotics v 145/1005 after placebo, ARR 4.8%, 95% CI 2.1% to 7.5%; RR 0.67, 95% CI 0.53 to 0.85), and fewer children experienced contralateral AOM (35/329 with antibiotic v 56/337 with placebo, ARR 5.9%, 95% CI 1.0% to 10.8%; RR 0.65, 95% CI 0.45 to 0.94). The trial found no significant difference in the rate of subsequent attacks of AOM (187/864 with antibiotics v 175/804 with placebo; RR 1.00, 95% CI 0.83 to 1.19), abnormal tympanometry at 1 month (85/234 with antibiotic v 91/238 with placebo; RR 0.94, 95% CI 0.74 to 1.19) or abnormal tympanometry at 3 months (38/182 with antibiotic v 49/188 with placebo; RR 0.80, 95% CI 0.55 to 1.16). Only 1/1962 children developed mastoiditis (in a penicillin treated group).[4] **Choice of antibiotic regimen:** The first systematic review (search date June 1992) identified 33 RCTs of antibiotics in 5400 children aged 4 months to 18 years with AOM.[5] Compared with placebo or no treatment, the rate of treatment success (absence of all presenting signs and symptoms of AOM at around 7–14 days after treatment was started) was significantly higher with penicillin (ARI 15.7%, 95% CI 4.7% to 26.7%), ampicillin/amoxicillin (ARI 13%, 95% CI 6.8% to 19%), and for any antibiotic (ARI 13.7%, 95% CI 8.2% to 19.2%). The review found no significant differences between antimicrobial agents in rate of treatment success at 7–14 days or of middle ear effusion at 30 days. **Antibiotics in children aged under 2 years:** We found one systematic review and one subsequent RCT. The review (search date 1997) found four RCTs in 741 children with AOM under the age of 2 years, which compared antibiotics versus placebo alone or versus placebo with myringotomy.[6] The outcome measured was symptomatic clinical improvement. The review found no significant difference between the two groups (OR 1.31, 95% CI 0.83 to 2.08). The subsequent RCT compared amoxicillin (40 mg/kg per day in three doses) versus placebo in 240 children aged 6 months to 2 years. The trial found that amoxicillin reduced persistence of symptoms after 4 days (69/117 [59%] children had persistent symptoms with amoxicillin v 89/123 [72%] with placebo; ARR 13%, 95% CI 1% to 25%, P = 0.03) and slightly reduced duration of fever (mean duration with amoxicillin 2 days v 3 days with placebo, mean reduction 1 day, no CI given, P = 0.004). However, the trial found that amoxicillin did not alter duration of pain, otoscopic appearances at 4 days or clinically judged treatment failure rate after 11 days (mean duration of pain or crying: 8 days with amoxicillin v 9 days with placebo, P = 0.43; otoscopic appearance: 88/114 [77%] not improved with amoxicillin v 99/120 [83%] with placebo; ARR 6%, 95% CI , -4% to +16%, P = 0.30; treatment failure defined as persistent symptoms or eardrum signs: 72/112 [64%] with amoxicillin v 84/120 [70%] with placebo; ARR 6%, 95% CI -6% to +18, P = 0.35).[7]

Harms: The first review gave no information on adverse events.[5] In the second review, antibiotics were associated with a near doubling of the risk of vomiting, diarrhoea, or rashes (RR 1.55, 95% CI 1.11 to 2.16).[4] The recent RCT in children under 2 years found no significant difference in rates of diarrhoea developing after either 4 or 10 days of antibiotics or placebo (day 4: 20/117 [17%] children developed diarrhoea with amoxicillin v 12/123 [10%] with placebo,

ARI 7%, 95% CI −2% to +16%; day 10: 14/117 [12%] with amoxicillin v 10/123 [8%] with placebo, ARI 4%, 95% CI −4% to +12%). Three children withdrew from the placebo group because of skin rashes and two from the antibiotic group because of diarrhoea.[7]

Comment: The first review[5] excluded two placebo controlled trials that were included in the second,[4] on the basis that they included myringotomy as part of treatment. This may have biased results in favour of antibiotic treatment and may explain the higher absolute risk reduction quoted in the first review. We found inadequate evidence for the effectiveness of antibiotics in areas where the incidence of complicating mastoiditis is high. Children with AOM aged under 2 years are at greater risk of a poorer outcome than older children.

OPTION   SHORT VERSUS LONGER COURSES OF ANTIBIOTICS

One systematic review found greater immediate benefit but no difference in long term outcome with 10 day courses of antibiotics compared with shorter (5 day) courses.

Benefits: We found one systematic review[8] and one subsequent RCT.[9] The systematic review (search date 1997) identified 32 RCTs of antibiotic treatment in children aged 4 weeks to 18 years with AOM.[9] Treatment failure, relapse, or reinfection at an early evaluation (8–19 days) were significantly more likely with shorter courses of antibiotics (5 days) than with longer courses (8–10 days) (OR compared with longer courses 1.52, 95% CI 1.17 to 1.98). However, by 20–30 days there were no significant differences between treatment groups (OR 1.22, 95% CI 0.98 to 1.54). The more recent prospective double blind RCT included 385 younger children (mean age 13.3 months, range 4–30 months) with newly diagnosed AOM.[9] They were given either amoxycillin/clavulanate in three divided doses for 10 days or for 5 days, followed by 5 days of placebo. Clinical success or failure was assessed at 12–14 days, then again at 28–42 days after starting treatment. Intention to treat analysis found that the 10 day regimen increased clinical success on days 12–14 compared with the 5 day regimen (ARI 11.5%, 95% CI 2.8% to 19.2%). However, by days 28–42 there was no significant difference in clinical success between the two groups (P = 0.34).

Harms: One RCT of amoxicillin plus clavulanate in 868 children aged between 2 months and 12 years reported diarrhoea in 26.7% of children on three times daily treatment for 10 days, compared with 9.6% in children on twice daily treatment for 10 days (P < 0.0001), and 8.7% in children on twice daily treatment for 5 days (P < 0.0001).[10] No P value was quoted for the comparison between 10 and 5 day twice daily treatments. The trial made no mention of other adverse effects.

Comment: The 5 day treatment group did not receive a placebo from days 6–10, which may have biased the results.[10]

Acute otitis media

| QUESTION | What are the effects of preventive interventions? |

| OPTION | LONG TERM ANTIBIOTIC TREATMENT |

One systematic review found that long term antibiotic prophylaxis has a modest effect in preventing recurrences of AOM. However, one subsequent RCT found no significant difference between antibiotic prophylaxis and placebo. We found insufficient evidence on which antibiotic to use, for how long, and how many episodes of AOM justify treatment.

Benefits: **Versus placebo:** We found one systematic review and one subsequent RCT. The systematic review (search date April 1993) identified 33 RCTs comparing antibiotics versus placebo to prevent recurrent AOM and otitis media with effusion.[11] Nine of the trials (n = 945) looked at recurrent AOM only. It was not clear from the review which of the studies referred only to children; four either included the word "children" in the title or appeared in paediatric journals. Most studies defined recurrent AOM as at least three episodes of AOM in 6 months. The most commonly used antibiotics were amoxicillin, cotrimoxazole, and sulfamethoxazole, given for 3 months to 2 years. All nine studies showed a lower rate of recurrence with antibiotic treatment, although in seven the difference was not significant. Overall, the review found that antibiotics slightly reduced recurrence of AOM (AR of recurrence per patient per month 0.08 with antibiotics v 0.19 with placebo; ARR 11%, 95% CI 3% to 19%; NNT per month to prevent one acute episode 9, 95% CI 5 to 33). The later RCT included 194 children aged 3 months to 6 years with three documented episodes of AOM within the preceding 6 months, who were randomised to amoxycillin 20 mg/kg per day either once or twice daily, or placebo.[12] The children were followed up monthly if asymptomatic, or within 3–5 days if they had symptoms of upper respiratory tract infection, for up to 90 days. The trial found that antibiotics were no more effective than placebo in preventing recurrent AOM (RR of remaining AOM free, diagnosed by otoscopy and tympanometry 1.00, 95% CI 0.66 to 1.52 using completer analysis, 36 lost to follow up). Including those lost to follow up yielded similar results, whether these children's outcomes were assumed in favour of placebo or in favour of antibiotics. **Choice and duration of antibiotic:** The systematic review found no significant difference in rate of recurrence between antibiotics. Greater treatment effect was seen with treatment lasting less than 6 months, but the confidence intervals overlapped (ARR for recurrence with courses < 6 months 21%, 95% CI 7% to 49%; ARR with courses > 6 months 4%, 95% CI 1% to 9%).[11]

Harms: The studies gave no information on harms.

Comment: None.

We found limited evidence that xylitol syrup or gum reduces the incidence of AOM. Adverse effects included abdominal discomfort.

Benefits: We found no systematic review, but found one RCT in 857 children (54% boys) that compared xylitol sugar given five times daily for 3 months in the form of syrup, chewing gum or lozenges, versus placebo.[13] Children deemed too young to chew gum (mean age 2.2 years) were allocated to xylitol syrup (10 g xylitol per day, n = 159) or a control syrup (0.5 g of xylitol per day, n = 165). Children deemed old enough to chew gum (mean age 4.6 years) were given xylitol chewing gum (8.4 g xylitol per day, n = 179), control chewing gum (0.5 g of xylitol per day, n = 178) or xylitol lozenges (10 g xylitol per day, n = 176). Each time the child showed any signs of acute respiratory infection, AOM was excluded using tympanometry and otoscopy. Follow up was for 3 months. The trial found that children who received xylitol syrup were less likely than those receiving control syrup to have one or more episodes of AOM (RRR 30%, 95% CI 4.6% to 55%). Chewing xylitol gum reduced the incidence of AOM compared with control gum (RRR 40%, 95% CI 10% to 71%) but xylitol lozenges were not significantly more effective than control gum (RRR 20%, 95% CI 13% to 51%).

Harms: Abdominal discomfort was reported as a reason for dropping out, and the overall drop out rate in the xylitol group was twice as high as for those receiving placebo (13% *v* 7%; RR 1.8, 95% CI 1.2 to 2.8). We found no evidence about long term effects of xylitol.

Comment: The children in this study received xylitol or the control intervention five times daily, a regimen that might be difficult to maintain long term. We found no evidence about optimum duration of treatment.

REFERENCES

1. Froom J, Culpepper L, Jacobs M, et al. Antimicrobials for acute otitis media? A review from the

2. Del Mar C, Glasziou P, Hayem M. Are antibiotics indicated as initial treatment for children with acute otitis media? A meta-analysis. *BMJ* 1997; 314:1526–1529. Search date 1966 to August 1994; primary sources Medline, Current Contents.

3. Bertin L, Pons G, d'Athis P, et al. A randomized double blind multicentre controlled trial of ibuprofen versus acetaminophen and placebo for symptoms of acute otitis media in children. *Fundam Clin* International Primary Care Network. *BMJ* 1997;315:98–102.*Pharmacol* 1996;10: 387–392.

4. Glasziou PP, Hayem M, Del Mar CB. Antibiotic use for acute otitis media in children. In: The Cochrane Library, Issue 4, 1999. Oxford: Update Software. Search date 1958 to January 1999, updated March 1999; primary sources Cochrane Controlled Trials Register, Medline, Index Medicus, Current Contents, and reference lists of articles

5. Rosenfeld RM, Vertrees JE, Carr J, et al. Clinical efficacy of antimicrobial drugs for acute otitis media: meta-analysis of 5400 children from thirty-three randomised trials. *J Pediatr* 1994;124:355–367. Search date 1966 to June 1992; primary sources Medline, Current Contents.

6. Damoiseaux RA, van Balen FAM, Hoes AW, de Melker RA. Antibiotic treatment of acute otitis

media in children under two years of age: evidence based? *Huisarts en Wetenschap* 1999; 354–357. Search date January 1997; primary sources Medline 1966 to January 1997, Embase 1974 to January 1997 and hand searched references.

7. Damoiseaux RA, van Balen FA, Hoes AW, Verheij TJ, de Melker RA. Primary care based randomised, double blind trial of amoxicillin versus placebo for acute otitis media in children aged under 2 years. *BMJ* 2000;320:350–354.

8. Kozyrskj AL, Hildes Ripstein E, Longstaffe SEA, et al. Treatment of acute otitis media with a shortened course of antibiotics: a meta-analysis. *JAMA* 1998;279:1736–1742. Primary sources Medline 1966 to 1997, Embase 1974 to 1997, Current Contents, Science Citation Index.

9. Cohen R, Levy C, Boucherat M, Langue J, de la Rocque F. A multicenter randomized, double blind trial of 5 versus 10 days of antibiotic therapy for acute otitis media in young children. *J Pediatr* 1998;133:634–639.

10. Hoberman A, Paradise JL, Burch DJ, et al. Equivalent efficiency and reduced occurrence of diarrhoea from a new formulation of amoxycillin/ clavulanate potassium (Augmentin) for treatment of acute otitis media in children. *Pediatr Infect Dis J* 1997;16:463–470.

11. Williams RL, Chalmers TC, Stange KC, Chalmers FT, Bowin SJ. Use of antibiotics in preventing

recurrent acute otitis media and in treating otitis media with effusion: a meta-analytic attempt to resolve the brouhaha. *JAMA* 1993;270:1344–1351. [Published erratum appears in *JAMA* 1994; 27:430.] Search date 1966 to April 1993; primary sources Medline, Current Contents.

12. Roark R, Berman S. Continuous twice daily or once daily amoxycillin prophylaxis compared with placebo for children with recurrent acute otitis media. *Pediatr Infect Dis J* 1997;16:376–378.

13. Uhari M, Kontiokari T, Niemela MA. Novel use of xylitol sugar in preventing acute otitis media. *Pediatrics* 1998;102:879–884.

Paddy O'Neill
General Practitioner
Norton Medical Centre
Stockton on Tees
UK

Competing interests: None declared.

QUESTIONS

INTERVENTIONS

TREATING ACUTE SEVERE CHILDHOOD ASTHMA
Beneficial
Oxygen 175
Ipratropium bromide added to
β_2 agonists 175
Spacer devices for delivery of
β_2 agonists (as effective as
nebulisers) 176
Systemic corticosteroids 176

Likely to be beneficial
Intravenous theophylline 177

SINGLE AGENT PROPHYLAXIS IN CHILDREN WITH ASTHMA
Beneficial
Inhaled corticosteroids 177
Oral theophylline 177
Inhaled sodium cromoglycate . . .178
Inhaled long acting β_2
agonists 178

TREATING ACUTE WHEEZE IN INFANCY
Unknown effectiveness
β_2 agonists 179
Inhaled anticholinergic drugs . .180
Oral corticosteroids 181

PROPHYLAXIS IN WHEEZING INFANTS
Unknown effectiveness
Inhaled corticosteroids 177
Oral theophylline 177
Inhaled sodium cromoglycate . .178

To be covered in future issues of
Clinical Evidence
Effects of treatments in chronic
asthma inadequately controlled
by regular low dose inhaled
steroids
Oral leukotriene receptor
antagonists

Key Messages

Treating acute severe childhood asthma

- Strong consensus suports the use of oxygen for acute, severe asthma. We found one prospective cohort study suggesting that it is effective.

- One systematic review of RCTs has found that adding ipratropium bromide to β_2 agonists in acute severe asthma leads to marginal improvement.

- One systematic review of RCTs has found no difference between nebuliser and metered dose inhaler plus spacer for delivering β_2 agonists in acute severe asthma, in children old enough to use a spacer.

- Systematic reviews of RCTs have found that systemic corticosteroids in acute asthma reduce the likelihood of hospital admission and length of hospital stay.

- We found conflicting evidence from one systematic review and one large RCT on the effects of intravenous theophylline in acute severe asthma.

Prophylaxis in childhood asthma

- One systematic review of RCTs has found that prophylactic inhaled corticosteroids improve symptoms compared with placebo.
- RCTs have found that prophylactic inhaled steroids are more effective than oral theophylline, sodium cromoglycate, and inhaled long acting β_2 agonists.
- One systematic review of long term follow up studies has found no evidence of growth retardation in asthmatic children treated with inhaled steroids, although short term studies found reduced growth velocity in some children.

Treatment and prophylaxis in infants with wheeze

- We found evidence on the effects of treatment and prophylaxis in wheezy infants to be weak and conflicting, perhaps because of the difficulty in distinguishing asthmatic from non-asthmatic wheezing in infancy (see bronchiolitis, p 183).

DEFINITION	**Childhood asthma** is characterised by chronic or recurrent cough and wheeze. The diagnosis is confirmed by demonstrating reversible airway obstruction in children old enough to perform peak flow measurements or spirometry. Diagnosing asthma in children requires exclusion of other causes of recurrent respiratory symptoms. **Wheezing in infancy** may be caused by acute viral infection (see bronchiolitis, p 183), episodic viral associated wheeze, or asthma, and these are not easy to distinguish clinically.
INCIDENCE/ PREVALENCE	Survey data suggest that the prevalence of wheeze, shortness of breath, and diagnosed asthma are rising in children, over and above a recognised tendency for asthma to be diagnosed more readily. One questionnaire study from Aberdeen, Scotland, surveyed 2510 children aged 8–13 years in 1964 and 3403 children in 1989. Over the 25 years, prevalence of wheeze rose from 10.4% to 19.8%; episodes of shortness of breath from 5.4% to 10.0%; and diagnosis of asthma from 4.1% to 10.2%.[1] One prospective cohort study (826 neonates followed up at 3 and 6 years of age) found that 34% of the overall sample had had at least one wheezing illness before age 3, 14% wheezed before age 3 and were still wheezing at age 6, and 15% reported a wheezing illness in the past year at age 6 but had not wheezed before age 3.[2]
AETIOLOGY/ RISK FACTORS	Asthma is more common in children with a personal or family history of atopy. Precipitating factors are known to include infection, house dust mites, allergens from pet animals, exposure to tobacco smoke, and anxiety.
PROGNOSIS	One retrospective cohort study of wheezing in the first year of life found that 14% of children with one attack and 23% of children with four or more attacks (recalled at age 5) had experienced at least one wheezing illness in the past year at age 10.[3]
AIMS	To reduce or abolish cough and wheeze; to attain best possible lung function; to reduce the risk of severe attacks; to minimise sleep disturbance and absence from school; to minimise adverse effects of treatment; and to allow normal growth.
OUTCOMES	Wheeze; cough; nights disturbed by asthma; days lost from school or normal activities; hospital admission; duration of stay in hospital; lung function tests (peak expiratory flow rate [PEFR]) and forced

expiratory volume in one second (FEV_1); blood oxygen saturation in acute attacks; airway hyper-responsiveness, measured using methacholine challenge tests.

METHODS   *Clinical Evidence* update search and appraisal May 2000.

QUESTION   **How effective are treatments for acute severe asthma in children?**

OPTION   OXYGEN

One prospective cohort study and clinical experience support the need for oxygen in acute severe asthma.

Benefits: We found no systematic review or RCTs. One double blind, prospective cohort study (280 children) found that decreased oxygen saturation upon entry to an emergency department was correlated with increased rates of hospital admission or subsequent readmission and administration of more intravenous aminophylline and steroids. Odds ratios for admission/readmission were 35 (95% CI 11 to 150) with arterial oxygen saturation 91% or less compared with 96% or more; and 4.2 (95% CI 2.2 to 8.8) with arterial oxygen saturation of 92–95% compared with 96% or more.[4]

Harms: We found no evidence of harm.

Comment: An RCT of oxygen in acute asthma would be considered unethical. Although the cohort study does not directly address whether oxygen should be given therapeutically, it does suggest, along with clinical experience, that oxygen should continue to be given promptly to children with acute severe asthma.[4]

OPTION   IPRATROPIUM BROMIDE ADDED TO β_2 AGONISTS

We found good evidence from one systematic review and one subsequent RCT that combination treatment with an anticholinergic agent plus a β_2 agonist improves lung function and may reduce admission rates compared with a β_2 agonist alone, or placebo.

Benefits: We found one systematic review (search date 1997, 10 RCTs, participants aged 18 months to 17 years) comparing combined inhaled anticholinergics plus β_2 agonists versus β_2 agonists alone.[5] Two RCTs found that, compared with β_2 agonists alone, combination treatment improved FEV_1 in children with milder asthma at 1 hour (WMD 16%, 99% CI 2% to 30%) and 2 hours (WMD 17.5%, 99% CI 0.4% to 35%), but found no evidence of a reduction in admission rate. With multiple dose protocols for severe exacerbations (5 RCTs), combination treatment was found to reduce the rate of hospital admission (OR 0.6, 99% CI 0.3 to 1.1, NNT 11) and improve FEV_1 by 9.8% of predicted (99% CI 5% to 14% of predicted). One subsequent placebo controlled RCT (90 children aged 6–18) found a greater rate of improvement in lung function with combination treatment (between 30 and 120 minutes: mean increase in PEFR 22.7% *v* 15.4%; mean increase in FEV_1 19.5% *v* 14.3%, P = 0.0001 for all results) but no reduction in rates of admission.[6]

Asthma in children

Harms: No difference in the rate of adverse effects was noted in either study.

Comment: None.

OPTION   **SPACER WITH METERED DOSE INHALER VERSUS NEBULISER**

One systematic review of RCTs found no difference between a metered dose inhaler plus spacer and nebulisation for delivering β_2 agonists in children with acute asthma who are old enough to use a spacer.

Benefits: We found one systematic review (search date 1998), which identified 12 RCTs comparing nebuliser with metered dose inhaler with spacer for the administration of β_2 agonists to children with acute asthma.[7] Six RCTs studied children aged over 2 years, excluding life threatening cases, and three studied children under 5 years. The review found no significant difference in hospital admission rates (OR 0.71, 95% CI 0.23 to 2.23), but one large RCT (152 children, aged 2 years and older) found that time spent in the emergency department was lower in children treated with spacers (WMD −32 minutes, 95% CI −24–50 minutes).[8] The rate of increase in pulse rate was higher with nebulisers (WMD 10% from baseline, 95% CI 5.9% to 14.1% from baseline). Two RCTs reported blood gas results showing less deterioration with spacer than with nebuliser. No outcomes were worse with spacer.

Harms: There were no reports of serious adverse effects with either mode of delivery.[7]

Comment: These findings suggest that, in children old enough to use a spacer, metered dose inhalers plus spacers could be substituted for nebulisation in the treatment of acute asthma in emergency departments and hospital wards.

OPTION   **SYSTEMIC CORTICOSTEROIDS**

Two systematic reviews of RCTs have found that systemic corticosteroids reduce the likelihood of hospital admission and improve lung function.

Benefits: We found two systematic reviews. One review (search date February 1991) identified two placebo controlled RCTs in children, both evaluating the need for hospital stay after acute asthma.[9] The first RCT (30 children) found reduced admission rates with methylprednisolone (OR 0.42, 95% CI 0.0 to 1.0). The second RCT found reduced length of hospital stay for children on prednisolone (median length of stay 24 hours v 39 hours; P = 0.0011). The second review (updated in 1997) identified two different RCTs (61 children). It found that pulmonary function test scores improved with steroids (WMD 14.3, 95% CI 5.4 to 23.3).[10]

Harms: We found few adverse effects reported for short courses of systemic corticosteroids. Several case reports and case series have associated systemic corticosteroid treatment with severe varicella infection. One case control study (167 cases, 134 controls) in otherwise immunocompetent children with complicated and uncomplicated varicella infection did not find significant risk attributable to corticosteroid exposure (OR 1.6, 95% CI 0.2 to 16.9).[11]

Comment: None.

| OPTION | INTRAVENOUS THEOPHYLLINE |

We found conflicting evidence of benefit from one systematic review of small RCTs and one subsequent large RCT. Treatment was frequently discontinued because of adverse effects.

Benefits: We found one systematic review (search date 1994, 6 small RCTs, 164 children aged 1.5–18 years), which found no significant benefit from treatment with intravenous theophylline in addition to other routine treatment (mean difference in FEV_1 +39%; $P = 0.25$).[12] One more recent RCT (163 children aged 1–19 with acute severe asthma, 43% admitted to intensive care) found greater improvement in FEV_1 at 6 hours (mean difference in FEV_1 10.4%, 95% CI 4% to 17%), less additional oxygen needed in the first 30 hours (median 18 v 6 hours; $P = 0.015$), and reduced likelihood of intubation in children receiving intravenous aminophylline compared with placebo (AR 0% v 6%; $P = 0.027$).[13]

Harms: Theophylline has well known serious adverse effects (cardiac arrhythmia, convulsion) if therapeutic blood concentrations are exceeded. In the recent RCT, 32% of children receiving aminophylline had their infusion discontinued because of adverse effects, mainly nausea and vomiting.[13]

Comment: The trials in the review were too small to exclude a clinically important effect.

| QUESTION | What are the effects of single agent prophylaxis in childhood asthma? |

Prophylactic inhaled steroids, oral theophylline, and inhaled sodium cromoglycate have all been found to improve symptoms and lung function in children with asthma when compared with placebo (see comment below). RCTs have found that inhaled steroids are more effective than theophylline, sodium cromoglycate, or inhaled long acting β_2 agonists for improving symptoms and lung function in children with asthma. Two systematic reviews of studies with long term follow up have found no evidence of growth retardation in asthmatic children treated with inhaled steroids. Some shorter term studies detected reduced growth velocity.

Benefits: **Inhaled corticosteroids versus placebo:** We found one systematic review of 24 RCTs (search date 1996, 1087 children, 10/24 trials in pre-school children, duration 4–88 weeks) comparing regular inhaled steroids versus placebo.[14] Overall, it found that steroids improved symptom score, reduced β_2 agonist and oral steroid use, and improved peak flow rate (overall weighted relative improvement in symptom score 50%, 95% CI 49% to 51%; reduction in β_2 agonist use 37%, 95% CI 36% to 38%; reduction in oral steroid use 68%, 95% CI 66% to 70%; weighted mean overall improvement in PEFR 11% predicted, 95% CI 9.5% to 12.5% predicted). **Inhaled corticosteroids versus theophylline:** We found no systematic review. One double blind, placebo controlled RCT (195 children aged 6–16 years, followed up for 12 months) compared oral theophylline versus inhaled beclomethasone (360 µg daily).[15] It found that beclomethasone gave similar symptom control with less use of bronchodilators and oral steroids. **Inhaled corticosteroids versus sodium cromoglycate:** We found no systematic review. Several small comparative RCTs have found sodium cromoglycate to be less effective than inhaled steroids in improving symptoms and lung function. **Inhaled corticosteroids versus inhaled long acting β_2 agonists:** We found no systematic review. We found two large RCTs comparing beclomethasone 200 µg twice daily versus salmeterol 50 µg twice daily given for 1 year. The first trial, in 67 children aged 6–16 years, found that beclomethasone was more effective than salmeterol in improving FEV_1, reducing rescue bronchodilator usage, and reducing airway hyper-responsiveness (FEV_1: mean change with salmeterol –4.5% of predicted, 95% CI –9.0% to +0.1%; mean change with beclomethasone, about 10% of predicted, 95% CI not given; mean difference beclomethasone v salmeterol, 14.2% of predicted, 95% CI 8.3% to 20.0% predicted; average rescue salbutamol usage: 0.44 uses per day with salmeterol, 0.07 with beclomethasone, P < 0.001).[16] In addition, the trial found that over the treatment period both treatments improved symptom scores and PEFR, but with no significant difference between treatments at 1 year (improvement in morning PEFR 49 l/minute with salmeterol, 61 l/minute with beclomethasone; 3% of children asymptomatic prior to trial with salmeterol v 6% with beclomethasone; 36% after trial with salmeterol v 55% with beclomethasone). There were two exacerbations in the beclomethasone group compared with 17 in the salmeterol group. The second trial randomised 241 children aged 6–14 to beclomethasone (81 children), salmeterol (80 children) or placebo (80 children).[17] It found that beclomethasone was more effective in reducing airway hyper-responsiveness than salmeterol (P = 0.003). Beclomethasone reduced rescue bronchodilator use and treatment withdrawals due to exacerbations (P < 0.001 and P = 0.03) compared with placebo, but salmeterol did not (P = 0.09 and P = 0.55). Both treatments improved spirometric indices compared with placebo, but the differences between beclomethasone and salmeterol were not significant.

Harms: **Inhaled steroids:** One systematic review (search date December 1996) found no significant adverse effects, including no documented effects on growth (monitored in 8 studies) or adrenal function (monitored in 12 studies).[14] Observational studies found little or no biochemical evidence of change in bone metabolism with inhaled steroids. Two cross sectional studies used a slit lamp to screen for lenticular changes in 198 children taking long term inhaled steroids.[15,18] The only case of posterior subcapsular cataract was in a child who had also received several prolonged courses of oral steroids. **Effects of inhaled steroids on growth:** Another systematic review (search date January 1993) identified 21 studies that reported height for age in asthmatic children treated with steroids. No evidence of growth impairment was found in the 12 studies involving beclomethasone (331 children).[19] A more recent review found three RCTs comparing the effects of beclomethasone and non-steroidal medication on linear growth in children with asthma (200 µg twice daily, duration up to maximum 54 weeks) suggesting a short term decrease in linear growth of -1.54 cm per year.[20] One RCT of inhaled beclomethasone (360 µg daily) compared with oral theophylline for 1 year.[21] There was a significant difference in rate of growth, more notable in boys, with the theophylline group have a greater rate of growth (mean rate of growth in pre-pubescent boys 4.3 cm/year v 6.2 cm/year). This effect was not sufficient to be noticed by the children or their parents, and no child was withdrawn from the study on this account. The two trials comparing beclomethasone with salmeterol found a similar slowing in linear growth with beclomethasone (growth over year of treatment 5.4 cm and 6.1 cm in the salmeterol groups, 4.0 cm and 4.7 cm in beclomethasone groups, P = 0.004, P = 0.007).[16,17] One controlled, prospective parallel group study compared 216 children treated with 400–600 µg budesonide daily with 62 children treated with theophylline or sodium cromoglycate, with 3–5 years' follow up.[22] No evidence of growth impairment with budesonide was found. **Theophylline:** One RCT found that continuous oral theophylline was associated with a higher frequency of headache, gastric irritation, and tremor than beclomethasone (360 µg daily).[21] One systematic review (12 studies, 340 children) of the behavioural and cognitive effects of theophylline found no evidence of significant adverse effects.[23] **Sodium cromoglycate:** Sodium cromoglycate may cause cough, throat irritation, and bronchoconstriction, but no long term adverse effects have been reported. **Inhaled long acting β_2 agonists:** These agents, in common with other β_2 agonists may occasionally cause tremor or tachycardia. Three large RCTs found no evidence of important adverse effects from salmeterol over 1 year.[16,17,24]

Comment: Evidence on the effects of oral leukotriene receptor antagonists in comparison with inhaled steroids, and on the relative effects of the options for stepping up treatment in children with symptoms of asthma inadequately controlled on regular low dose inhaled steroids, will be reviewed in a future issue of *Clinical Evidence*. **Theophylline and cromoglycate versus placebo:** Numerous RCTs have shown that these agents are effective compared with placebo for prophylaxis in childhood asthma.

QUESTION What are the effects of treatment for acute wheezing in infancy?

OPTION β_2 AGONISTS DELIVERED BY NEBULISER OR METERED DOSE INHALER/SPACER

We found conflicting evidence from RCTs. Transient hypoxia may be caused by nebulised bronchodilators, particularly with air driven nebulisers, and seems less likely when using metered dose inhalers/spacers (see bronchiolitis, p 183).

Benefits: We found no systematic review. We found many hospital based RCTs of nebulised β_2 agonists compared with normal saline in infants and young children with acute wheezing. Some, but not all, have found short term improvements in clinical respiratory distress scores with β_2 agonists.[25] We found no large RCTs with clinical outcomes. Small RCTs with physiological rather than clinical end points found that giving β_2 agonists by metered dose inhaler with spacer to wheezy infants was effective, with less likelihood than nebulisation to show transient adverse effects on lung function.[26,27] A large single blind RCT based in an inner city hospital emergency department in Santiago, Chile compared nebulised salbutamol 0.25 mg/kg three times in 1 hour with salbutamol by MDI/spacer two puffs five times in 1 hour in the treatment of moderate to severe wheezing in 123 children aged 1–24 months (mean age 8 months). Treatment was repeated for a second hour together with intramuscular betamethasone in children assessed as non-responders after the first hour. Withholding of β_2 agonist treatment from a control group was considered unethical. Success of treatment as measured by reduction in clinical severity score after 1 hour was 71% (nebuliser group) and 90% (spacer group) and at 2 hours 94% (nebuliser group) and 100% (spacer group). Only one child (in the nebuliser group) was hospitalised due to treatment failure.[28]

Harms: Some infants have transiently decreased oxygen saturation after nebulisation, especially with air driven nebulisers.[25] Nebulised β_2 agonists are known to cause tachycardia, tremor, and hypokalaemia, but serious adverse effects are rare.

Comment: None.

OPTION   **INHALED ANTICHOLINERGIC DRUGS**

We found limited and conflicting evidence from one systematic review of small RCTs on the effects of inhaled anticholinergic drugs for clinical outcomes.

Benefits: We found one systematic review (search date 1998, 321 children, 6 RCTs) of anticholinergic drugs for wheeze in children under 2 years.[29] One included RCT found that adding ipratropium bromide to β_2 agonists resulted in fewer children receiving further treatment 45 minutes after initial treatment in the emergency room (OR 0.22, 95% CI 0.08 to 0.61), but a second similar study found no additional benefit. A third included RCT (31 hospitalised children) comparing ipratropium bromide versus placebo found no difference in the duration of hospitalisation (WMD −0.4 days, 95% CI −1.4 to +0.61). Adding ipratropium bromide to β_2 agonist had no effect on duration of hospitalisation compared with β_2 agonist alone (WMD −0.4 days, 95% CI −1.41 to +0.61). In one home based, 2 month crossover trial, parents preferred regular nebulised ipratropium bromide to nebulised water, but there was no significant reduction in the frequency of reported symptoms during treatment.[29]

Harms: No evidence of harm specific to the use of anticholinergic agents was found in these studies.

Comment: The studies were too small to exclude a clinically important effect of ipratropium bromide.

OPTION **ORAL CORTICOSTEROIDS**

We found no evidence that oral steroids improve outcomes in acute wheezing in infancy.

Benefits: We found no systematic review. One outpatient study compared oral prednisolone with placebo (38 acutely wheezing children aged 3–17 months, including 30 children previously admitted with wheeze). It found no significant differences in outcome between the two groups in the 56 episodes studied.[30]

Harms: No important adverse effects were identified.

Comment: Acute infantile wheezing may be due to bronchiolitis. This is often difficult to separate from other acute wheezing, and is dealt with elsewhere (see bronchiolitis, p 183).

QUESTION **What are the effects of prophylaxis in wheezing infants?**

We found weak and conflicting evidence.

Benefits: We found no systematic review. We found inconsistent results of placebo controlled trials on inhaled steroids in recurrent or persistent infant wheezing. Some found improvements in symptom scores and reduced administration of additional treatments. Other studies did not find beneficial effect. We found a greater tendency for positive findings in studies of older children and in studies involving administration by metered dose inhaler and spacer rather than nebuliser. We found no RCTs of continuous oral theophylline in infants, and the small numbers of trials with inhaled sodium cromoglycate were mainly negative.

Harms: We found no good evidence on the long term safety of treatment with continuous inhaled steroids in infancy. Known effects of using nebuliser and face masks include oral candidiasis and thinning of facial skin.

Comment: Administering inhaled treatments to infants is difficult and dependent upon dosage and inhaler device. RCTs of treatment for infant wheezing used a variety of drugs, dosages, and devices, and were sometimes conducted on populations with differing proportions of children with asthma rather than other types of infant wheeze. These factors may explain the inconsistent results.

Substantive changes since last issue

Single agent prophylaxis Additional data available on effects of inhaled steroids on growth; no change in conclusions.[20]

β_2 agonist by nebuliser or spacer Additional RCT identified on β agonists; no change in conclusions.[28]

REFERENCES

1. Russell G, Ninan TK. Respiratory symptoms and atopy in Aberdeen school children: evidence from two surveys 25 years apart. *BMJ* 1992;304:873–875.
2. Martinez FD, Wright AL, Taussig L, et al. Asthma and wheezing in the first six years of life. *N Engl J Med* 1995;333:132–138.
3. Park ES, Golding J, Carswell F, et al. Pre-school

wheezing and prognosis at 10. *Arch Dis Child* 1986;61:642–646.
4. Geelhoed GC, Landau LI, Le Souef PN. Evaluation of SaO2 as a predictor of outcome in 280 children presenting with acute asthma. *Ann Emerg Med* 1994;23:1236–1241.
5. Plotnick LH, Ducharme FM. Efficacy and safety of combined inhaled anticholinergics and β_2 agonists

in the initial management of acute paediatric asthma. In: The Cochrane Library, Issue 1, 1999. Oxford: Update Software. Search dates 1997; primary sources Medline 1966 to 1997; Embase 1980 to 1997; Cinahl 1982 to 1997; handsearch of bibliographies of references; pharmaceutical companies contacted for details of unpublished trials and personal contact.

6. Qureshi F, Zaritsky A, Lakkis H. Efficacy of nebulised ipratropium in severely asthmatic children. *Ann Emerg Med* 1997;29:205–211.

7. Cates CJ. Comparison of holding chambers and nebulisers for β-agonists in acute asthma. In: The Cochrane Library, Issue 1, 1999. Oxford: Update Software. Search date February 1998; primary sources Medline; Cochrane Airways Review Group Register 1966 to February 1998.

8. Chou KJ, Cunningham SJ, Crain EF. Metered-dose inhalers with spacers vs nebulizers for pediatric asthma. *Arch Pediatr Adolesc Med* 1995;149: 201– 205.

9. Rowe BH, Kelleher JL, Oxman AD. Effectiveness of steroid therapy in acute exacerbations of asthma: a meta-analysis. *Am J Emerg Med* 1992;10:301– 310. Search date February 1991; primary sources Medline 1966 to February 1991; Science Citation Search 1980 to 1990; and content experts, review articles, textbooks.

10. Rowe BH, Spooner CH, Ducharme FM, Bretzlaff JA, Bota GW. The effectiveness of corticosteroids in the treatment of acute exacerbations of asthma: a meta-analysis of their effect on relapse following acute assessment. In: The Cochrane Library, Issue 1, 1999. Oxford: Update Software. Search dates May 1997; primary sources Cochrane Airways Group Register 1966 to May 1997.

11. Patel H, Macarthur C, Johnson D. Recent corticosteroids use and the risk of complicated varicella in otherwise immunocompetent children. *Arch Pediatr Adolesc Med* 1996;150:409–414.

12. Goodman DC, Littenberg B, O'Connor GT, et al. Theophylline in acute childhood asthma: a meta-analysis of its efficacy. *Pediatr Pulmonol* 1996;21: 211–218. Search date May 1994; primary sources Medline 1966 to May 1994.

13. Yung M, South M. Randomised controlled trial of aminophylline for severe acute asthma. *Arch Dis Child* 1998;79:405–410.

14. Calpin C, Macarthur C, Stephens D, et al. Effectiveness of prophylactic inhaled steroids in childhood asthma: a systematic review of the literature. *J Allergy Clin Immunol* 1997;100:452– 457. Search date December 1996; primary source Medline.

15. Simons FE, Persaud MP, Gillespie CA, et al. Absence of posterior subcapsular cataracts in young patients treated with inhaled corticosteroids. *Lancet* 1993;342:776–778.

16. Verberne A, Frost C, Roorda R, et al. One year treatment with salmeterol compared with beclomethasone in children with asthma. *Am J Respir Crit Care Med* 1997;156:688–695.

17. Simons FER and the Canadian Beclomethasone Diproprionate – Salmeterol Xinafoate Study Group. A comparison of beclomethasone, salmeterol and placebo in children with asthma. *N Engl J Med* 1997;337:1659–1665.

18. Abuektish F, Kirkpatrick JN, Russell G. Posterior subcapsular cataract and inhaled steroid therapy. *Thorax* 1995;50:674–676.

19. Allen DB, Mullen M, Mullen B. A meta-analysis of the effect of oral and inhaled steroids on growth. *J Allergy Clin Immunol* 1994;93:967–976. Search date January 1993; primary sources literature search of leading medical journals 1956 to 1993.

20. Sharek PJ, Bergman DA. Beclomethasone for asthma in children: effects on linear growth. In: The Cochrane Library, Issue 2000. Oxford: Update Software. Search date March 1999; primary sources Cochrane Airways Group Asthma Trials Register.

21. Tinkelman DG, Reed C, Nelson H, et al. Aerosol beclomethasone diprionate compared with theophylline as primary treatment of chronic, mild to moderately severe asthma in children. *Pediatrics* 1993;92:64–77.

22. Agertoft L, Pedersen S. Effects of long-term treatment with an inhaled corticosteroid on growth and pulmonary function in asthmatic children. *Respir Med* 1994;88:373–381.

23. Stein MA, Krasowski M, Leventhal BL, et al. Behavioural and cognitive effects of theophylline and caffeine. *Arch Pediatr Adolesc Med* 1996:50: 284–288. Search date not given; primary sources Medline, PsycLIT, Dissertation Abstracts, and hand searched references.

24. Lenney W, Pedersen S, Boner AL, Ebbutt A, Jenkins M, on behalf of an international study group. Efficacy and safety of salmeterol in childhood asthma. *Eur J Pediatr* 1995;154:983– 990.

25. Alario AJ, Lewander W, Dennehy P, et al. The efficacy of nebulised metaproterenol in wheezing infants and young children. *Am J Dis Child* 1992; 146:412–418.

26. Kraemer R, Frey U, Sommer CW, et al. Short term effect of albuterol, delivered via a new auxiliary device, in wheezy infants. *Am Rev Respir Dis* 1991;144:347–351.

27. Yuksel B, Greenough A. Comparison of the effects on lung function of different methods of bronchodilator administration. *Respir Med* 1994; 88:22.

28. Rubilar L, Castro-Rodrguez JA, Girardi G. Randomized controlled trial of salbutamol via metered-dose inhaler with spacer verus nebuliser for acute wheezing in children less than 2 years of age. *Pediatr Pulmonol* 2000;29:264–269.

29. Everard M, Kurian M. Anticholinergic drugs for wheeze in children under the age of two years. Cochrane Collaboration. In: The Cochrane Library, Issue 1, 1999. Oxford: Update Software. Search date 1998; primary sources Cochrane Airways Group Register 1966 to May 1998; hand search of respiratory care and paediatric journals.

30. Webb M, Henry R, Milner AD. Oral corticosteroids for wheezing attacks under 18 months. *Arch Dis Child* 1986;61:15–19.

Duncan Keeley
General Practitioner
Thame
Oxfordshire
UK

Competing interests: The author has received occasional consultancy fees or assistance with organisation of, or travel to, meetings from companies including Allen and Hanburys, Astra, MSD, Zeneca, 3M, and Boots.

Updated this issue

Nancy Tang and Elaine Wang

INTERVENTIONS

TREATMENT
Unknown effectiveness

Unlikely to be beneficial

PREVENTION
Beneficial

Unknown effectiveness

To be covered in future issues of
  Clinical Evidence
Oxygen
Surfactant, in the context of
  bronchopulmonary dysplasia

See glossary, p 190

Key Messages

Treatment

- Two small, good quality systematic reviews of RCTs have found that inhaled bronchodilators improve overall clinical scores in children in the short term, although they found no evidence that bronchodilators reduce admission rates or improve oxygen saturation.

- One systematic review and seven RCTs found limited and conflicting evidence on the effects of corticosteroids in children with bronchiolitis.

- One RCT found no evidence that routine use of antibiotics improved clinical scores in children with bronchiolitis.

- One systematic review of small RCTs found no evidence that ribavirin reduces mortality or the risk of respiratory deterioration in children admitted to hospital with respiratory syncytial virus (RSV) bronchiolitis. One additional RCT found no evidence that ribavirin reduces duration of ventilation or hospital stay in children intubated for bronchiolitis.

- We found insufficient evidence to determine the effect of immunoglobulin treatment on clinical outcomes for children with bronchiolitis.

Preventing transmission in hospital

■ We found no evidence from RCTs that cohort segregation, handwashing, or the wearing of gowns, masks or eye-nose goggles by carers reduced transmission rates between children in hospital.

Prevention in high risk children

■ One systematic review of RCTs has found that, in children born prematurely, in children with bronchopulmonary dysplasia, and in children with a combination of risk factors, prophylactic respiratory syncytial virus immunoglobulin or monoclonal antibody reduces admission rates to hospital and intensive care.

DEFINITION	Bronchiolitis is a virally induced acute bronchiolar inflammation that is associated with signs and symptoms of airway obstruction. Diagnosis is based on clinical findings. Clinical manifestations include fever, rhinitis (inflammation of the nasal mucosa), tachypnoea, expiratory wheezing, cough, rales, use of accessory muscles, apnoea (absence of breathing), dyspnoea (difficulty in breathing), alar flaring (flaring of the nostrils), and retractions (in-drawing of the intercostal soft tissues on inspiration). Clinically, disease severity (see glossary, p 190) of bronchiolitis may be classified as mild, moderate, or severe.
INCIDENCE/ PREVALENCE	Bronchiolitis is the most common lower respiratory tract infection in infants, occurring in a seasonal pattern with highest incidence in the winter in temperate climates[1] and in the rainy season in warmer countries. Each year in North America, about 21% of infants have lower respiratory tract disease and 6–10 per 1000 infants require admission to hospital for bronchiolitis (1%–2% of children under 12 months of age[2]). The peak rate of admission occurs in infants aged between 2–6 months.[3]
AETIOLOGY/ RISK FACTORS	Respiratory syncytial virus (RSV) is responsible for bronchiolitis in 70% of cases. This figure reaches 80–100% in the winter months. However, in early spring, parainfluenza virus type 3 is often responsible.[1]
PROGNOSIS	**Morbidity and mortality:** Disease severity is directly related to the size of the infant, and proximity and frequency of contact with infective infants. Children at increased risk of morbidity and mortality are those with congenital heart disease, chronic lung disease, history of premature birth, hypoxia, and age less than 6 weeks.[4] Other factors associated with a prolonged or complicated hospital stay include a history of apnoea or respiratory arrest, pulmonary consolidation as shown on a chest radiograph, and (in North America) native American or Inuit race.[5] The risk of death within 2 weeks is high for children with congenital heart disease (3.4%) or chronic lung disease (3.5%) compared with other groups combined (0.1%).[4] Rates of admission to the intensive care unit (ICU) (range 31% to 36%) and need for mechanical ventilation (range 11% to 19%) is similar among all high risk groups.[4] The percentage of these children needing oxygen supplementation is also high (range 63% to 80%).[4] In contrast, mortality in children with bronchiolitis, but without these risk factors, is less than 1%, and rates of ICU admission and ventilation in such children are markedly lower (15% and 8%).[6] **Long term prognosis:** Information on long term prognosis varies depending on inception cohort. One small prospective

study of two matched cohorts (one with bronchiolitis, n = 25; one without, n = 25) found no evidence that bronchiolitis requiring outpatient treatment was associated with an increased risk of asthma in the long term.[7] Possible confounding factors include differences in illness severity, smoke exposure, and crowding.[8] We found one prospective study in 50 randomly selected infants admitted with bronchiolitis, followed up by questionnaire for 5 years, and a visit in the fifth year. It found a doubling of asthma incidence compared with the general population, although there was large (30%) loss to follow up, and no matched control group.[9]

AIMS	To decrease morbidity and mortality, shorten hospital stay, and prevent transmission of infection, with minimum adverse effects.
OUTCOMES	Death rate; rate of intubation or admission to ICU; clinical score (clinical score is a subjective, unvalidated measure that is based on judgements made by the clinician); rates of clinical and serological infection.
METHODS	*Clinical Evidence* update search and appraisal May 2000. Studies were appraised independently by the two authors and then reviewed again together to resolve differences by consensus. Titles were scanned and, if the article seemed relevant, the abstract was obtained and appraised to determine if the complete article was to be reviewed.

QUESTION What are the effects of treatment for children with bronchiolitis?

OPTION BRONCHODILATORS (INHALED SALBUTAMOL, INHALED EPINEPHRINE/ADRENALINE)

Two small, good quality systematic reviews of RCTs have found that inhaled bronchodilators achieve short term improvement in overall clinical scores in children treated in hospitals, emergency departments, and outpatient clinics, although they found no evidence that bronchodilators reduced admission rates or improved oxygen saturation.

Benefits: We found two systematic reviews. The first (updated in 1998) found eight RCTs in a total of 485 children treated in outpatient clinics or the emergency department and after admission to hospital.[10] The second review (search date 1995) found five RCTs in 251 children treated in outpatient clinics.[11] Four RCTs were common to both reviews. The first review found that, in the short term, bronchodilators improved clinical scores in children with mild and moderately severe bronchiolitis (RR for lack of improvement in clinical score, bronchodilator *v* placebo, 0.76, 95% CI 0.60 to 0.95).[10] Both reviews found no evidence that bronchodilators improved oxygen saturation by a clinically important amount (effect size for oxygen saturation 0.14, 95% CI −0.04 to +0.33;[10] mean difference in oxygen saturation 1.2%, 95% CI 0.8% to 1.6%[11]). Both reviews found no evidence that bronchodilators versus placebo reduced admission rates in children treated in outpatient clinics or the emergency department (RR 0.85, 95% CI 0.47 to 1.53;[10] 23 children treated with bronchodilator admitted *v* 21 with placebo, P = NS[11]).

Bronchiolitis

Harms: One systematic review reported tachycardia, increased blood pressure, decreased oxygen saturation, flushing, hyperactivity, prolonged cough, and tremor following use of bronchodilators. The review did not report frequency of adverse events.[10] The second review did not report on harms.[11]

Comment: None of the trials used respiratory failure as an outcome. Discrepancies in primary studies included differences in study populations, such as inclusion of sedated children, short duration of follow up, and validity of clinical scores. Results of individual trials were contradictory. Bronchodilators may improve the clinical appearance of a child through a general stimulatory effect rather than by improving respiratory function.[12]

OPTION   CORTICOSTEROIDS

One systematic review and seven RCTs found limited and conflicting evidence on the effects of corticosteroids in children with bronchiolitis.

Benefits: We found one systematic review[13] (6 RCTs, search date 1999; 347 children in hospital) and seven additional RCTs of corticosteroids versus placebo in children with bronchiolitis.[14–20] Three of the additional RCTs had been mentioned in the systematic review but excluded because of data inconsistency,[18] treatment outside hospital,[19] or failure to report the outcome markers sought by the systematic review.[20] The systematic review found no significant difference in the mean length of stay in all the RCTs that reported length of stay (5 RCTs; mean −0.43 days, 95% CI −1.05 to +0.18 days), in the four RCTs with clearly identified randomisation methods (mean −0.35 days, 95% CI −0.84 to +0.14 days) and after exclusion of RCTs that included children with previous wheezing (4 RCTs; mean −0.29 days, 95% CI −0.71 to +0.13 days).[13] Interpretation of the effect of corticosteroids versus placebo on clinical symptoms found by the systematic review is difficult (see comment below). The RCTs in the systematic review reported different clinical scales at varying times after starting treatment. The scales usually included measurements of oxygen saturation, wheezing, accessory muscle use, and respiratory rate. Results 72 hours after starting treatment were too heterogeneous for analysis. Only three RCTs (197 children) provided results for 24 hours after starting treatment. The systematic review pooled the standardised effect size for clinical scores from these three RCTs and found that corticosteroids versus placebo produced a significant improvement (1.60, 95% CI 1.28 to 1.92). Six of the seven additional RCTs comparing corticosteroids versus placebo reported a clinical score: all found no significant difference for corticosteroids (355 children) versus placebo.[14–17,19,20]

Harms: The acute adverse effects of oral steroids are well documented, and include hyperglycaemia and immunosuppression. The trials did not give information on these.

Comment: The evidence presented in the published systematic review[13] is difficult to interpret because some of the RCTs did not exclude children with a history of wheezing who may have asthma, a condition likely to respond to steroids. The clinical scales used in the

RCTs included oxygen saturation, but the clinical relevance of changes in this item are unclear. Even if the results are accepted at face value, the clinical significance of an effect size of 1.6 is unclear. Another systematic review is under way (E Wang, personal communication, 2000). We found inadequate evidence to evaluate the effects of systemic versus inhaled corticosteroids.

OPTION	ROUTINE ANTIBIOTICS

One unblinded RCT found no evidence that routine antibiotics are of clinical benefit in children admitted to hospital with bronchiolitis and uncomplicated RSV pneumonia, although the study was not powerful enough to rule out an effect.

Benefits: We found no systematic review. We found one unblinded RCT comparing the routine use of antibiotics versus no antibiotics (no placebo) in 138 children admitted to hospital with clinically apparent pneumonia, 45% of whom were diagnosed with RSV infection. It found no significant difference between treatment groups in the proportion infected with RSV. It found no evidence that antibiotics reduced duration of hospital stay or respiratory rate, or improved clinical symptoms, clinical signs or radiographic assessment scores for pulmonary disease.[21]

Harms: The trial did not report on harms, although potential risks include superinfection with resistant bacteria and drug reactions.

Comment: The trial was unblinded and used block randomisation (children randomised in groups of 20). This reduces confidence in the results. Two children initially treated without antibiotics were switched to antibiotics owing to complicating purulent infections.

OPTION	RIBAVIRIN

One systematic review of small RCTs found no evidence that ribavirin reduced mortality or the risk of respiratory deterioration in children admitted to hospital with RSV bronchiolitis. One additional RCT found no evidence that ribavirin reduced duration of ventilation or hospital stay in children intubated for bronchiolitis.

Benefits: We found one systematic review (search date 1995, update 1997, 8 small RCTs, 250 children) and one subsequent RCT. The review found that, in children and infants hospitalised with RSV bronchiolitis, ribavirin did not significantly reduce mortality or the risk of respiratory deterioration compared with placebo (rate of respiratory depression with ribavirin v placebo 4/56 [7.1%] v 11/60 [18.3%], RR 0.42, 95% CI 0.16 to 1.34; mortality with ribavirin v placebo 3/56 [5.4%] v 6/43 [13.9%], RR 0.42, 95% CI 0.13 to 1.44).[22] The high mortality in both groups may have been due to severe disease at baseline. The RCT published after the review compared ribavirin aerosol versus placebo in 41 children within 24 hours of intubation for severe bronchiolitis. It found no difference in duration of ventilation (102 hours, 95% CI 37 to 167 hours with ribavirin v 126 hours, 95% CI 47 to 205 hours with placebo, P = 0.29) or hospital stay (256 hours, 95% CI 131 to 381 hours with ribavirin v 295 hours, 95% CI 171 to 419 hours; P = 0.32).[23]

Bronchiolitis

Harms: We found no prospective data. The review and RCTs did not report on harms. We found case reports of headaches and contact lens dysfunction in carers. Ribavirin has been reported to be associated with acute bronchospasm in treated children. The standard aerosol is sticky, and clogging of ventilatory equipment has been reported.[24]

Comment: We found one small prospective study, which compared pulmonary function tests in 54 children who had previously been randomised to inpatient treatment with ribavirin or placebo. It found no evidence of long term differences in outcome, although the study was not powerful enough to rule out a difference.[25]

OPTION **IMMUNOGLOBULINS (POOLED IMMUNOGLOBULINS, RSV IG)**

We found no evidence from small, low powered RCTs that immunoglobulins improve clinical outcomes in children admitted to hospital with bronchiolitis.

Benefits: We found no systematic review. We found five RCTs (4 using albumin solution as control, 1 using saline, total n = 335).[26–30] Two trials used pooled immunoglobulin, two trials used RSV Ig, and one trial used a synthetic monoclonal antibody. Neither trial using RSV Ig found evidence that RSV Ig shortened hospital stay compared with albumin (in high risk children (see glossary, p 190), mean duration of hospital stay RSV Ig v albumin 8.41 days v 8.89 days, P = NS; in non-high risk children, mean stay RSV Ig v albumin 4.58 days v 5.52 days, P = NS).[26,27] The third RCT found no evidence in 35 children that monoclonal antibody reduced hospital stay, duration of ventilation, or duration of treatment with supplemental oxygen (hospital stay, placebo v antibody 11.5 days, 95% CI 10.0 to 13.0 days v 14.5 days, 95% CI 12.4 to 16.6 days, P = 0.25; duration of oxygen treatment, placebo v antibody 9.5 days, 95% CI 7.9 to 11.1 days v 12.3 days, 95% CI 10.0 to 14.6 days, P = 0.47; duration of ventilation, placebo v antibody 6.2 days, 95% CI 4.7 to 7.7 days v 8.8 days, 95% CI 6.5 to 11.1 days, P = 0.45).[30] Neither of the remaining trials found any evidence that pooled immunoglobulin improved outcome in children with bronchiolitis.

Harms: The RCTs found that RSV Ig was associated with elevation of liver enzymes and anoxic spells (no frequency data given).[26] One open label RCT of prophylactic RSV Ig in 249 children found that adverse effects occurred in about 3% of treated children.[31] This trial and a subsequent analysis of the data found that effects included increased respiratory rate, mild fluid overload during the first infusion, urticarial reaction at the infusion site, mild decreases in oxygen saturation, and fever (no frequency data given).[31,32]

Comment: Four trials used albumin as control rather than placebo. The effects of albumin itself in bronchiolitis are not known.

QUESTION **What are the effects of measures to prevent transmission in hospital?**

OPTION NURSING INTERVENTIONS (COHORT SEGREGATION, HANDWASHING, GOWNS, MASKS, GLOVES, AND GOGGLES)

We found no direct evidence from RCTs that cohort segregation (see glossary, p 190), handwashing, use of gowns, masks, gloves, or goggles reduce nosocomial transmission of RSV to other children. Handwashing is a well established technique for reducing cross infection in other contexts, so RCTs may not be ethically feasible.

Benefits: We found no systematic review and no good quality RCTs examining effects of cohort segregation, handwashing, gowns, masks, gloves, or goggles, used either singly or in combination, on nosocomial transmission of bronchiolitis in children.

Harms: **Cohort segregation:** Potential risks of cohort segregation include misdiagnosing RSV infection and putting non-infected patients at risk by subsequent placement into the wrong cohort. **Handwashing:** Dermatitis is a well recognised adverse effect of repeated handwashing. **Other interventions:** No harms reported.

Comment: **Single nursing interventions:** We found four observational studies comparing nosocomial infection rates in separate series of children before and after introduction of cohort segregation, handwashing, gowns and masks, and goggles. No study adjusted results for variations in baseline incidence. Three found a lower incidence of transmission after introduction of cohort segregation alone, handwashing alone, and eye-nose goggles alone.[33–35] The fourth found no significant difference in transmission after introducing gowns and masks.[36] **Combinations of nursing interventions:** We found one RCT in 58 medical personnel caring for children admitted with bronchiolitis, which found no significant difference in nosocomial infection rate in staff when they used gowns and masks, in addition to handwashing (5/28 [18%] of those using gowns, masks, and handwashing v 4/30 [13%] in the control group; RR 1.3, 95% CI 0.4 to 3.6).[37] The trial did not report on transmission rates in the children. One non-randomised prospective trial in 233 children at risk of severe nosocomial infection compared transmission rates in wards adopting different nursing policies. It found that a combination of cohort segregation, gowns, and gloves reduced nosocomial transmission rates, compared with all other policies (cohort segregation alone, gown and gloves alone, no special precautions) taken together. However, the control interventions did not remain constant throughout the trial, the results were based on an interim analysis, and the definition of "at risk" children was not clearly stated.[38]

Child health

Bronchiolitis

QUESTION What are the effects of prophylactic measures in high risk children?

OPTION IMMUNOGLOBULIN

One systematic review of RCTs has found that, in children born prematurely, or children with bronchopulmonary dysplasia, prophylactic RSV Ig or monoclonal antibody given monthly reduces hospital admission. and admission to intensive care.

Benefits: We found one systematic review (updated March 1999, 4 RCTs, 2598 children) comparing monthly RSV Ig or monoclonal antibody versus placebo or no prophylaxis. Three of the trials used intravenous RSV Ig, and one used intramuscular monoclonal antibody. Two of the trials using RSV Ig were unblinded, and both of these used no prophylaxis as the control intervention. The review found that Ig reduced admission to hospital and intensive care but did not reduce the incidence of mechanical ventilation (OR prophylaxis v placebo for hospital admission 0.48, 95% CI 0.37 to 0.64; for ICU admission 0.47, 95% CI 0.29 to 0.77; for ventilation 0.99, 95% CI 0.48 to 2.07).[31]

Harms: See harms of immunoglobulins, p 188.

Comment: Premature infants included in the trials were children under 6 months old, with gestational age at birth less than either 32 or 35 weeks. Children with bronchopulmonary dysplasia were under 2 years old and still undergoing treatment for this anomaly. Planned subgroup analysis in the review found that prophylaxis reduced hospital admission in children whose only risk factor was prematurity (OR 0.27, 95% CI 0.15 to 0.49), and in children with bronchopulmonary dysplasia alone (OR 0.54, 95% CI 0.37 to 0.80), but not in children with cardiac comorbidity alone (OR 0.64, 95% CI 0.37 to 1.10).

GLOSSARY

Cohort segregation Children infected with different viral strains are segregated from each other and treated separately, with the aim of preventing cross infection.
Disease severity Mild: not requiring hospitalisation. Moderate: requiring hospitalisation but not intubation. Severe: requiring intubation or artificial ventilation.
High risk children Premature infants with or without bronchopulmonary dysplasia, or infants and children with congenital heart disease.

Substantive changes since last issue

Corticosteroids New systematic review; no change in conclusions.[13]

REFERENCES

1. Phelan P, Olinsky A, Robertson C. *Respiratory illness in children*. 4th ed. London: Blackwell Scientific Publications, 1994.
2. Gruber W. Bronchiolitis. In: Long S, Pickering L, Prober C, eds. *Principles and practice of pediatric infectious diseases*. 1st ed. New York: Churchill Livingstone, 1997:1821.
3. Glezen WP, Taber LH, Frank AL, Kessel JA. Risk of primary infection and reinfection with respiratory syncytial virus. *Am J Dis Child* 1986;140:543–546.
4. Navas L, Wang E, de Carvalho V, Robinson J, PICNIC. Improved outcome of respiratory syncytial virus infections in a high-risk hospitalized population of Canadian children. *J Pediatr* 1992; 121:348–354.
5. Wang EEL, Law BJ, Stephens D, PICNIC. Pediatric Investigators Collaborative Network on Infections in Canada (PICNIC) study of morbidity and risk factors with RSV disease. *J Pediatr* 1995;126: 212–219.
6. Wang EEL, Law BJ, Boucher F, et al. Pediatric Investigators Collaborative Network on Infections in Canada (PICNIC) study of admission and management variation in patients hospitalized with respiratory syncytial viral lower respiratory

infection. *J Pediatr* 1996;129:390–395.

7. McConnochie KM, Mark JD, McBride JT, et al. Normal pulmonary function measurements and airway reactivity in childhood after mild bronchiolitis. *J Pediatr* 1985;107:54–58.

8. McConnochie KM, Roghmann KJ. Parental smoking, presence of older siblings and family history of asthma increase risk of bronchiolitis. *Am J Dis Child* 1986;140:806–812.

9. Sly PD, Hibbert ME. Childhood asthma following hospitalization with acute viral bronchiolitis in infancy. *Pediatr Pulmonol* 1989;7:153–158.

10. Kellner JD, Ohlsson A, Gadomski AM, Wang EEL. Bronchodilators for bronchiolitis. In: The Cochrane Library, Issue 1, 2000. Oxford: Update Software. Search date June 1998; primary sources Medline from 1966; Embase from 1974; Reference Update, reference lists of articles, and files of two of the authors.

11. Flores G, Horwitz RI. Efficacy of beta 2-agonists in bronchiolitis: A reappraisal and meta-analysis. *Pediatrics* 1997;100:233–239. Search date 1995; primary sources Medline 1966 to January 1995, and hand searched references and selected journals.

12. Gadomski AM, Lichenstein R, Horton L, King J, Keane V, Permutt T. Efficacy of albuterol in the management of bronchiolitis. *Pediatrics* 1994;93: 907–912.

13. Garrison MM, Christakis DA, Harvey E, Cummings P, Davis RL. Systemic corticosteroids in infant bronchiolitis: A meta-analysis. *Pediatrics* 2000; 105:849. Search date 1999; primary sources Medline, Embase, Cochrane Clinical Trials Registry.

14. Richter H, Seddon P. Early nebulized budesonide in the treatment of bronchiolitis and the prevention of postbronchiolitic wheezing. *J Pediatr* 1998;132: 849–853.

15. Bulow SM, Nir M, Levin E. Prednisolone treatment for respiratory syncytial virus infection: a randomized controlled trial of 147 infants. *Pediatrics* 1999;104:77.

16. Tal A, Bavilski C, Yohai D, Bearman JE, Gorodischer R, Moses SW. Dexamethasone and salbutamol in the treatment of acute wheezing in infants. *Pediatrics* 1983;71:13–18.

17. Cade A, Brownlee KG, Conway, SP. Randomised placebo-controlled trial of nebulised corticosteroids in acute respiratory syncytial viral bronchiolitis. *Arch Dis Child* 2000;82:126–130.

18. Connolly JH, Field CM, Glasgow JF, Slattery CM, MacLynn DM. A double blind trial of prednisolone in epidemic bronchiolitis due to respiratory syncytial virus. *Acta Paediatr Scand* 1969;58: 116–120.

19. Berger I, Argaman Z, Schwartz SB. Efficacy of corticosteroids in acute bronchiolitis: short-term and long- term follow-up. *Pediatr Pulmonol* 1998; 26:162–166.

20. Leer JA, Green JL, Heimlich EM, et al. Corticosteroid treatment in bronchiolitis. A controlled collaborative study in 297 infants and children. *Am J Dis Child* 1969;117:495–503.

21. Fris B, Andersen P, Brenoe E, et al. Antibiotic treatment of pneumonia and bronchiolitis: a prospective randomised study. *Arch Dis Child* 1984;59:1038–1045.

22. Randolph AG, Wang EEL. Ribavirin for respiratory syncytial virus lower respiratory tract infection. In: The Cochrane Library, Issue 1, 2000. Oxford: Update Software. Search date 1997; primary sources Medline from 1975; hand searched references and noted experts contacted.

23. Guerguerian AM, Gauthier M, Lebel MH, Farrell CA, Lacroix J. Ribavirin in ventilated respiratory syncytial virus bronchiolitis. *Am J Respir Crit Care Med* 1999;160:829–834.

24. Johnson EM. Developmental toxicity and safety evaluations of ribavirin. *Pediatr Infect Dis J* 1997; 9(suppl):85–87.

25. Long CE, Voter KZ, Barker WH, Hall CB. Long term follow-up of children hospitalized with respiratory syncytial virus lower respiratory tract infection and randomly treated with ribavirin or placebo. *Pediatr Infect Dis J* 1997;16:1023–1028.

26. Rodriguez WJ, Gruber WC, Welliver RC, et al. Respiratory syncytial virus immune globulin intravenous therapy for RSV lower respiratory tract infection in infants and young children at high risk for severe RSV infections. *Pediatrics* 1997;99: 454–461.

27. Rodriguez WJ, Gruber WC, Groothuis JR, et al. Respiratory syncytial virus immune globulin treatment of RSV lower respiratory tract infection in previously healthy children. *Pediatrics* 1997; 100:937–942.

28. Hemming VG, Rodriguez W, Kim HW, et al. Intravenous immunoglobulin treatment of respiratory syncytial virus infections in infants and young children. *Antimicrob Agents Chemother* 1987;31:1882–1886.

29. Rimensberger PC, Burek-Kozlowska A, Morell A, et al. Aerosolized immunoglobulin treatment of respiratory syncytial virus infection in infants. Pediatr Infect Dis J 1996;15:209–216.

30. Malley R, DeVincenzo J, Ramilo O, et al. Reduction of respiratory syncytial virus (RSV) in tracheal aspirates in intubated infants by use of humanized monoclonal antibody to RSV F protein. *J Infect Dis* 1998;178:1555–1561.

31. Wang EEL, Tang NK. Immunoglobulin for preventing respiratory syncytial virus infection. In: The Cochrane Library. Issue 4, 1999. Oxford: Update Software. Search date March 1999; primary sources Cochrane Acute Respiratory Infections Trials Register, Medline, abstracts from the Pediatric Academy Meetings and the Interscience Conference on Antimicrobial Agents and Chemotherapy from 1994 to 1997.

32. Groothuis JR, Levin MJ, Rodriguez W, et al. Use of intravenous gamma globulin to passively immunize high-risk children against respiratory syncytial virus: safety and pharmacokinetics. *Antimicrob Agents Chemother* 1991;35:1469–1473.

33. Krasinski K, LaCouture R, Holzman R, Waithe E, Bonk S, Hanna B. Screening for respiratory syncytial virus and assignment to a cohort at admission to reduce nosocomial transmission. *J Pediatr* 1990;116:894–898.

34. Isaacs D, Dickson H, O'Callaghan C, Sheaves R, Winter A, Moxon ER. Handwashing and cohorting in prevention of hospital acquired infections with respiratory syncytial virus. *Arch Dis Child* 1991;66: 227–231.

35. Gala CL, Hall CB, Schnabel KC, et al. The use of eye-nose goggles to control nosocomial respiratory syncytial virus infection. *JAMA* 1986;256:2706–2708.

36. Hall CB, Douglas RG. Nosocomial respiratory syncytial virus infections: should gowns and masks be used? *Am J Dis Child* 1981;135:512–515.

37. Murphy D, Todd JK, Chao RK, Orr I, McIntosh K. The use of gowns and masks to control respiratory illness in pediatric hospital personnel. *J Pediatr* 1981;99:746–750.

38. Madge P, Paton JY, McColl JH, Mackie PLK. Prospective controlled study of four infection-control procedures to prevent nosocomial infection with respiratory syncytial virus. *Lancet* 1992;340: 1079–1083.

Bronchiolitis

Nancy Tang

Elaine Wang
Associate Professor

Hospital for Sick Children
University of Toronto and Aventis Pasteur
Toronto
Canada

Competing interests: None declared.

Updated this issue

David Creery and Kate Ackeman

INTERVENTIONS

*Although we found no direct
  evidence to support their use,
  widespread consensus holds that
  these interventions should be
  universally applied to children
  who have arrested, based on
  indirect evidence and
  extrapolation from adult data.
  Placebo controlled trials would
  be considered unethical.

Key Messages

- Outcome following out-of-hospital cardiorespiratory arrest in children is poor, and it is unclear at what stage intervention becomes futile.

- Prospective and retrospective observational studies have consistently found that out-of-hospital arrest in children where the cause is uncertain (fatal and near miss sudden infant death syndrome [SIDS]) has a far worse prognosis than arrest from any other cause.

- It is widely accepted that cardiopulmonary resuscitation (CPR) and ventilation should be undertaken in children who have arrested. Placebo controlled trials would be considered unethical. We found no prospective evidence on the effects of training parents to perform CPR.

- One RCT has found no evidence that endotracheal intubation improves survival or neurological outcome compared with bag-mask ventilation in children who have arrested in the community.

- We found no prospective evidence on the effects of bicarbonate, calcium, different doses of adrenaline (epinephrine), or direct current cardiac shock to improve the outcome of non-submersion out-of-hospital cardiorespiratory arrest in children.

Cardiorespiratory arrest

DEFINITION Non-submersion out-of-hospital cardiorespiratory arrest in children is a state of pulselessness and apnoea occurring outside of a medical facility and not apparently caused by submersion in water. The term "SIDS" refers to the sudden unexpected death of a child, usually between the ages of 1 month and 1 year, for which a thorough post-mortem examination fails to define an adequate cause of death.[1] Near miss SIDS refers to survival of a child after an unexpected arrest of unknown cause.

INCIDENCE/ PREVALENCE We found 11 studies reporting the incidence of non-submersion out-of-hospital cardiorespiratory arrest in children (see table 1, p 200).[2–12] Three of these studies were prospective; the others were retrospective.[2–9] Nine studies reported the incidence in the general population (both adults and children),[2–8,10,11] and seven reported the incidence in a paediatric population.[2,3,6–10] Incidence of arrests in the general population ranged from 2.2 to 5.7 per 100 000 per year (mean 3.1, 95% CI 2.0 to 4.2).[7] Incidence in children ranged from 6.9 to 18.0 arrests per 100 000 children per year (mean 11.0, 95% CI 7.0 to 15.1).[10] One prospective study in 300 children found that about 50% of out-of-hospital cardiorespiratory arrests occurred in children under 12 months, and about two thirds occurred in children under 18 months.[10]

AETIOLOGY/ RISK FACTORS We found 26 studies reporting the causes of non-submersion pulseless arrests in a total of 1574 children. The commonest causes of arrest were SIDS (39.1%), trauma (17.6%), chronic disease (7.1%), and pneumonia (4.2%) (see table 2, p 200).[2–11,13–28]

PROGNOSIS We found no systematic review that investigated non-submersion arrests alone. We found one systematic review (search dates 1970 to 1997, primary sources Medline and bibliographic search) that reported outcomes following CPR for both in-hospital and out-of-hospital arrests of any cause, including submersion in children.[29] Studies were excluded if they did not report on survival. The review found evidence from prospective and retrospective observational studies that out-of-hospital arrest of any cause in children carries a poorer prognosis than arrest within hospital (132/1568 children [8.4%] survived to hospital discharge after out-of-hospital arrest v 129/544 children [24%] after in-hospital arrests). About half of the survivors were involved in studies that reported on neurological outcome. Of these, survival with "good neurological outcome" (i.e. normal or mild neurological deficit) was higher in children who arrested in hospital, compared with those who arrested elsewhere (60/77 surviving children [78%] v 28/68 [41%]).[29] We found 26 studies in a total of 1734 children that reported only on out-of-hospital arrest (22 studies were included in the review; the remainder were published subsequent to the review search date).[2–11,13–28] Five of these studies were prospective in design;[10,11,14,20,22] the rest were retrospective. The overall survival rate following out of hospital arrest was 5% (87 children). Nineteen of these studies (n = 1140) found that, of the 48 surviving children, 12 (25%) had no or mild neurological disability, and 36 (75%) had moderate or severe neurological disability. Survival rates are listed according to cause of arrest (see table 2, p 200).

AIMS	To improve survival and minimise neurological sequelae in children suffering out-of-hospital cardiorespiratory arrest.
OUTCOMES	Out-of-hospital death rate; rate of death in hospital without return of spontaneous circulation; return of spontaneous circulation with subsequent death in hospital; and return of spontaneous circulation with successful hospital discharge with mild, moderate, severe, or no neurological sequelae; adverse effects of treatment.
METHODS	*Clinical Evidence* update search and appraisal May 2000. In addition, we searched citation lists of retrieved articles and relevant review articles. Studies reporting data on out-of-hospital arrest in adults that listed "adolescent" as a MeSH heading were also reviewed. Both authors reviewed the retrieved studies independently, and differences were resolved by discussion. We selected studies reporting data related to out-of-hospital cardiorespiratory arrests in children. Studies were excluded if data relating to submersion could not be differentiated from non-submersion data (except where we found no data relating exclusively to non-submersion arrest; in such cases we have included studies that did not differentiate these types of arrest, and have made it clear that such evidence is limited by this fact). Likewise, as the pathogenesis of arrest in adults appears to be different from arrest in children, studies were excluded if data relating to adults could not be differentiated from data relating to children.

QUESTION   What are the effects of treatments?

OPTION   AIRWAY MANAGEMENT AND VENTILATION

It is widely accepted that good airway management and rapid ventilation should be undertaken in a child who has arrested, and it would not be considered ethical to test its role in a placebo controlled trial.

Benefits:	We found no studies comparing airway management and ventilation versus no intervention.
Harms:	We found insufficient information.
Comment:	It would not be considered ethical to test the role of airway management and ventilation in a placebo controlled trial.

OPTION   INTUBATION VERSUS BAG-MASK VENTILATION

One controlled trial found no evidence of a difference in survival or neurological outcome between bag-mask ventilation and endotracheal intubation in children requiring airway management in the community.

Benefits:	We found no systematic review. One high quality controlled trial compared bag-mask ventilation versus endotracheal intubation (administered by paramedic staff trained in these techniques) in 830 children requiring airway management in the community, including 98 children who had arrested following submersion.[30] Treatments were not randomised; each was allocated on alternate days. Analysis was by intention to treat (see comment below). The trial found no significant difference in rates of survival or good

neurological outcome (normal, mild deficit, or no change from baseline function) between the two treatment groups (123/404 [30%] survived following bag-mask ventilation v 110/416 [26%] following intubation, OR 0.82, 95% CI 0.61 to 1.11; good neurological outcome achieved in 92/404 [23%] of children after bag-mask ventilation v 85/416 [20%] after intubation, OR 0.87, 95% CI 0.62 to 1.22).

Harms: The trial found that the time at the scene of the arrest was longer when intubation was intended, and this was the only significant determinant of a longer total time from dispatch of paramedic team to arrival at hospital (mean time at scene 9 minutes with bag-mask v 11 minutes with intubation, P < 0.001; mean total time 20 minutes with bag-mask v 23 minutes with intubation, P < 0.001).[30] However, the trial found no significant difference between bag-mask ventilation and intubation for complications common to both treatments (complications in 727 children for whom data available, bag-mask v intubation: gastric distension 31% v 7%, P = 0.20; vomiting 14% v 14%, P = 0.82; aspiration 14% v 15%, P = 0.84; oral or airway trauma 1% v 2%, P = 0.24). A total of 186 children across both treatment groups were thought by paramedical staff to be successfully intubated. Of these, oesophageal intubation occurred in three children (2%); the tube became dislodged in 27 children (14%, unrecognised in 12 children, recognised in 15); right main bronchus intubation occurred in 33 children (18%); and an incorrect size of tube was used in 44 children (24%). Death occurred in all but one of the children with oesophageal intubation or unrecognised dislodging of the tube.[30]

Comment: **Population characteristics:** The baseline characteristics of children did not differ significantly between groups in age, sex, ethnicity, or cause of arrest. The trial did not report the frequency of pulseless arrest versus respiratory arrest. **Intention to treat:** Intubation and bag-mask ventilation are not mutually exclusive. The study protocol allowed bag-mask ventilation before intubation and after unsuccessful intubation. Of 420 children allocated to intubation, 115 received bag-mask ventilation before intubation, 128 received bag-mask ventilation after attempted intubation, four were lost to follow up, and the remainder received intubation that was believed to be successful. Of 410 children allocated to bag and mask ventilation, 10 children were intubated successfully (although in violation of study protocol), nine received bag-mask ventilation after attempted intubation, six were lost to follow up, and the remainder received bag-mask ventilation in accordance with study protocol.[30]

OPTION INTRAVENOUS ADRENALINE (EPINEPHRINE)

Intravenous adrenaline (epinephrine) at "standard dose" (0.01 mg/kg) is a widely accepted treatment for establishing return of spontaneous circulation. We found no prospective evidence comparing adrenaline versus placebo or comparing standard or single doses versus high or multiple doses of adrenaline in children who have arrested in the community.

Benefits: We found no systematic review, no RCTs, and no prospective observational studies.

Harms:	We found no prospective data in this context.

Comment: **Versus placebo:** Standard dose adrenaline is a widely accepted treatment for arrests in children. Placebo controlled trials would be considered unethical. **High versus low dose:** Two small retrospective studies (total n = 128) found no evidence of a difference in survival to hospital discharge between low or single dose epinephrine and high or multiple dose adrenaline, although the studies were too small to rule out an effect.[7,9]

OPTION   INTRAVENOUS BICARBONATE

We found insufficient evidence on the effects of intravenous bicarbonate in cardiorespiratory arrest in children.

Benefits:	We found no RCTs.
Harms:	We found insufficient evidence.

Comment: Bicarbonate is widely believed to be effective in arrest associated with hyperkalaemic ventricular tachycardia or fibrillation, but we found no prospective evidence supporting this.

OPTION   INTRAVENOUS CALCIUM

We found insufficient evidence on the effects of intravenous calcium in cardiorespiratory arrest in children.

Benefits:	We found no RCTs.
Harms:	We found insufficient evidence.

Comment: Calcium is widely believed to be effective in arrest associated with hyperkalaemic ventricular tachycardia or fibrillation, but we found no prospective evidence supporting this.

OPTION   BYSTANDER CPR

It is widely accepted that CPR and ventilation should be undertaken in children who have arrested. Placebo controlled trials would be considered unethical. We found no prospective evidence on the effects of training parents to perform CPR. One systematic review of observational studies found that children who were witnessed having an arrest and who received bystander CPR were more likely to survive to hospital discharge.

Benefits: We found no RCTs. We found one systematic review of prospective and retrospective studies. This concluded that survival was improved in children who were witnessed to arrest and received CPR from a bystander. Of 150 witnessed arrests outside hospital, 19% survived to hospital discharge (28/150). Of those children who received bystander CPR, 20/76 (26%) survived to discharge.[29] The review did not report survival rates in children whose arrests were not witnessed, but the overall survival rate for out-of-hospital cardiac arrest was 8.4%. **Training parents to perform CPR:** We found no systematic review and no RCTs examining the effects of training parents to perform CPR in children who have arrested outside hospital.

Harms: Potential harms include those resulting from unnecessary chest compression after respiratory arrest with intact circulation.

Comment: The apparent survival rates for witnessed arrests and arrests with bystander initiated CPR may be artificially high because of inappropriate evaluation of true arrest.

OPTION   **DIRECT CURRENT CARDIAC SHOCK**

It is widely accepted that children who arrest outside hospital and are found to have ventricular fibrillation or pulseless ventricular tachycardia should receive direct current cardiac shock treatment. Placebo controlled trials would be considered unethical. We found insufficient evidence on the effects of direct current cardiac shock in children who have arrested in the community, regardless of the heart rhythm.

Benefits: We found no systematic review and no RCTs.

Harms: Insufficient evidence.

Comment: **In children with ventricular fibrillation:** One retrospective study in 29 children with ventricular fibrillation who had arrested out of hospital from a variety of causes, including submersion, found that of 27 children who were defibrillated, 11 survived (5 with no sequelae, 6 with severe disability). The five children with good outcome all received defibrillation within 10 minutes of arrest (time to defibrillation not given for those who died). Data on the two children who were not defibrillated were not presented.[31] **In children with asystole:** One retrospective study in 90 children with asystole (including those who had arrested after submersion) found that 49 (54%) had received direct current cardiac shock treatment. None of the children survived to hospital discharge, regardless of whether or not direct current cardiac shock was administered.[32] We found one systematic review of observational studies that recorded electrocardiogram (ECG) rhythm in a total of 1420 children who had arrested outside hospital. Bradyasystole or pulseless electrical activity was found in 73% whereas ventricular fibrillation (VF) or pulseless ventricular tachycardia (VT) were found in 10%.[29] The review found that survival after VF/VT arrest was higher than after asystolic arrest in children. Survival to discharge reported in the systematic review was 5% (39/802) for children with initial rhythm asystole and 30% (29/97) with initial rhythm VF/VT.[29]

REFERENCES

1. Gausche M, Barkin RM, eds. Sudden infant death syndrome (SIDS). In: Pediatric Emergency Medicine. Toronto: Mosby; 1997:1115–1116.
2. Eisenberg M, Bergner L, Hallstrom A. Epidemiology of cardiac arrest and resuscitation in children. Ann Emerg Med 1983;12:672–674.
3. Applebaum D, Slater PE. Should the Mobile Intensive Care Unit respond to pediatric emergencies? Clin Pediatr Phila 1986;25:620–623.
4. Tsai A, Kallsen G. Epidemiology of pediatric prehospital care. Ann Emerg Med 1987;16:284–292.
5. Thompson JE, Bonner B, Lower GM. Pediatric cardiopulmonary arrests in rural populations. Pediatrics 1990;86:302–306.
6. Safranek DJ, Eisenberg MS, Larsen MP. The epidemiology of cardiac arrest in young adults. Ann Emerg Med 1992;21:1102–1106.
7. Dieckmann RA, Vardis R. High-dose epinephrine in pediatric out-of-hospital cardiopulmonary arrest. Pediatrics 1995;95:901–913.
8. Kuisma M, Suominen P, Korpela R. Paediatric out-of-hospital cardiac arrests: epidemiology and outcome. Resuscitation 1995;30:141–150.
9. Ronco R, King W, Donley DK, Tilden SJ. Outcome and cost at a children's hospital following resuscitation for out-of-hospital cardiopulmonary arrest. Arch Pediatr Adolesc Med 1995;149:210–214.
10. Sirbaugh PE, Pepe PE, Shook JE, et al. A prospective, population-based study of the demographics, epidemiology, management, and outcome of out-of-hospital pediatric

cardiopulmonary arrest. *Ann Emerg Med* 1999; 33:174–184.

11. Friesen RM, Duncan P, Tweed WA, Bristow G. Appraisal of pediatric cardiopulmonary resuscitation. *Can Med Assoc J* 1982;126:1055–1058.

12. Hu SC. Out-of-hospital cardiac arrest in an oriental metropolitan city. *Am J Emerg Med* 1994;12:491–494.

13. Barzilay Z, Somekh E, Sagy M, Boichis H. Pediatric cardiopulmonary resuscitation outcome. *J Med* 1988;19:229–241.

14. Bhende MS, Thompson AE. Evaluation of an end-tidal CO_2 detector during pediatric cardiopulmonary resuscitation. *Pediatrics* 1995; 95:395–399.

15. Brunette DD, Fischer R. Intravascular access in pediatric cardiac arrest. *Am J Emerg Med* 1988;6: 577–579.

16. Clinton JE, McGill J, Irwin G, Peterson G, Lilja GP, Ruiz E. Cardiac arrest under age 40: etiology and prognosis. *Ann Emerg Med* 1984;13:1011–1015.

17. Hazinski MF, Chahine AA, Holcomb GW III, Morris JA, Jr. Outcome of cardiovascular collapse in pediatric blunt trauma. *Ann Emerg Med* 1994;23: 1229–1235.

18. Losek JD, Hennes H, Glaeser P, Hendley G, Nelson DB. Prehospital care of the pulseless, nonbreathing pediatric patient. *Am J Emerg Med* 1987;5:370–374.

19. Ludwig S, Kettrick RG, Parker M. Pediatric cardiopulmonary resuscitation. A review of 130 cases. *Clin Pediatr Phila* 1984;23:71–75.

20. Nichols DG, Kettrick RG, Swedlow DB, Lee S, Passman R, Ludwig S. Factors influencing outcome of cardiopulmonary resuscitation in children. *Pediatr Emerg Care* 1986;2:1–5.

21. O'Rourke PP. Outcome of children who are apneic and pulseless in the emergency room. *Crit Care Med* 1986;14:466–468.

22. Rosenberg NM. Pediatric cardiopulmonary arrest in the emergency department. *Am J Emerg Med* 1984;2:497–499.

23. Schindler MB, Bohn D, Cox PN, et al. Outcome of out-of-hospital cardiac or respiratory arrest in children. *N Engl J Med* 1996;335:1473–1479.

24. Sheikh A, Brogan T. Outcome and cost of open- and closed-chest cardiopulmonary resuscitation in pediatric cardiac arrests. *Pediatrics* 1994;93: 392–398.

25. Suominen P, Rasanen J, Kivioja A. Efficacy of cardiopulmonary resuscitation in pulseless paediatric trauma patients. *Resuscitation* 1998; 36:9–13.

26. Suominen P, Korpela R, Kuisma M, Silfvast T, Olkkola KT. Paediatric cardiac arrest and resuscitation provided by physician-staffed emergency care units. *Acta Anesthesiol Scand* 1997;41:260–265.

27. Torphy DE, Minter MG, Thompson BM. Cardiorespiratory arrest and resuscitation of children. *Am J Dis Child* 1984;138:1099–1102.

28. Walsh R. Outcome of pre-hospital CPR in the pediatric trauma patient. *Crit Care Med* 1994;22: A162.

29. Young KD, Seidel JS. Pediatric cardiopulmonary resuscitation: a collective review. *Ann Emerg Med* 1999;33:195–205. Search date 1966–1997; primary sources Medline and bibliographic search.

30. Gausche M, Lewis RJ, Stratton SJ, et al. Effect of out-of-hospital pediatric endotracheal intubation on survival and neurological outcome. *JAMA* 2000;283:783–790.

31. Mogayzel C, Quan L, Graves JR, Tiedeman D, Fahrenbruch C, Herndon P. Out-of-hospital ventricular fibrillation in children and adolescents: causes and outcomes. *Ann Emerg Med* 1995;25: 484–491.

32. Losek JD, Hennes H, Glaeser PW, Smith DS, Hendley G. Prehospital countershock treatment of pediatric asystole. *Am J Emerg Med* 1989;7:571–575.

David Creery
Children's Hospital of Eastern Ontario
Ottawa
Canada

Kate Ackerman
The Children's Hospital
Boston
USA

Competing interests: None declared.

TABLE 1 Incidence of non-submersion pre-hospital cardiorespiratory arrest in children* (see text, p 194).

Reference	Location	Year	Incidence per 100 000 people in total population	Incidence per 100 000 children
11	Manitoba, Canada	1982	2.93	–
2	King County, USA	1983	2.38	9.94
3	Jerusalem, Israel	1986	2.52	6.87
4	Fresno, USA	1987	5.74	–
5	Midwestern USA	1990	4.74	–
6	King County, USA	1992	2.42	10.07
12	Taipei, Taiwan	1994	1.29	–
7	San Francisco, USA	1995	2.18	16.14
8	Helsinki, Finland	1995	1.43	9.14
9	Birmingham, USA	1995	–	6.88
10	Houston, USA	1999	4.91	18.02

* Incidence represents arrests per 100 000 population per year.

TABLE 2 Causes of non-submersion pre-hospital cardiorespiratory arrest in children* (see text, p 194).

Cause	Number of arrests (%)	Number of survivors (%)
SIDS	691 (39.1)	1 (0.1)
Trauma	311 (17.6)	10 (3.2)
Chronic disease	126 (7.1)	9 (7.1)
Pneumonia	75 (4.2)	6 (8.0)
Non-accidental injury	23 (1.3)	2 (8.7)
Aspiration	20 (1.1)	0 (0)
Overdose	19 (1.1)	3 (15.8)
Other	309 (17.6)	28 (9.1)
Total	**1574 (88.1)**	**87 (3.7)**

*Figures represent the numbers of arrests/survivors in children with each diagnosis. SIDS, sudden infant death syndrome.

Updated and expanded this issue

Gregory Rubin

INTERVENTIONS

**Trade off between benefits and
harms**

*Not widely licensed for use in
children. Clinical use in adults
recently restricted due to heart
rhythm abnormalities.

Key Messages

- We found no direct evidence that increased fibre intake is effective in childhood constipation.
- Two small RCTs found that cisapride increased stool frequency and reduced gut transit time in children with constipation. Cisapride is not widely licensed for use in children; clinical use in adults is restricted due to heart arrhythmias.
- We found no placebo controlled trials of osmotic or stimulant laxatives. Small RCTs, comparing osmotic versus stimulant laxatives found limited evidence that both were effective. One small RCT found benefit from the addition of toilet training or biofeedback.
- Limited evidence from RCTs suggests short term but no long term benefit from adding biofeedback training to conventional treatment.

Constipation in children

DEFINITION Constipation is characterised by infrequent bowel evacuations, hard, small faeces, or difficult or painful defecation. The frequency of bowel evacuation varies from person to person.[1] Encopresis is defined as involuntary bowel movements in inappropriate places at least once a month for 3 months or more, in children aged 4 years and older.[2]

INCIDENCE/ PREVALENCE Constipation with or without encopresis is common in children. It accounts for 3% of consultations to paediatric outpatient clinics and 25% of paediatric gastroenterology consultations in the USA.[3] Encopresis has been reported in 1.5% of children at school entry.

AETIOLOGY/ RISK FACTORS No cause is discovered in 90–95% of children with constipation. The peak incidence is at 2–4 years of age. Psychosocial factors are often suspected, although most children with constipation are developmentally normal.[3] Chronic constipation can lead to progressive faecal retention, distension of the rectum, and loss of sensory and motor function. Organic causes for constipation are uncommon, but include Hirschsprung's disease (1/5000 births; male : female 4 : 1; constipation invariably present from birth), cystic fibrosis, anorectal physiological abnormalities, anal fissures, constipating drugs, dehydrating metabolic conditions, and other forms of malabsorption.[3]

PROGNOSIS Childhood constipation can be difficult to treat, and often requires prolonged support, explanation, and medical treatment. In one long term follow up study of children presenting under the age of 5 years, 50% recovered within 1 year and 65–70% recovered within 2 years; the remainder required laxatives for daily bowel movements or continued to soil for years.[3] It is not known what proportion continue to have problems into adult life, although adults presenting with megarectum or megacolon often have a history of bowel problems from childhood.

AIMS To remove faecal impaction and to restore a bowel habit in which stools are soft and passed without discomfort.

OUTCOMES Number of defecations per week; number of episodes of soiling per month; gut transit time; use of laxatives.

METHODS *Clinical Evidence* search and appraisal May 2000 using the following key terms: constipation, diet therapy, diagnosis, therapy, psychology, stimulant laxatives, dietary fibre, lactulose. The search was limited to infants and children. No systematic reviews were identified. Trials were selected for inclusion if they focused on the management of constipation or encopresis, or both; if they were relevant to primary health care; and if they included children without an organic cause for constipation.

QUESTION What are the effects of dietary and medical treatments?

OPTION INCREASED DIETARY FIBRE

We found no direct evidence of benefit from increasing dietary fibre intake on colonic transit time or cure of constipation in children.

Benefits: We found no systematic review or good RCTs of the effect of increasing dietary fibre on constipation in children. We found one RCT of the effect of laxatives plus advice about dietary fibre on chronic constipation and colonic transit time in 73 children with the same mean fibre intake as healthy controls but increased colonic transit time.[4] The study found that although advice significantly increased fibre intake, it did not significantly reduce colonic transit time or increase the cure of constipation at 6 months.

Harms: Adults who increase dietary fibre intake have reported abdominal pain and distension.

Comment: None.

OPTION CISAPRIDE

Two RCTs have found improvement in stool frequency and symptoms of constipation with cisapride after 8–12 weeks of treatment in an outpatient setting. We found no evidence from primary care settings. Cisapride has been suspended from the market in several countries because of adverse cardiac effects.

Benefits: We found no systematic review but found two RCTs. One RCT (69 children aged 4–18 years with idiopathic constipation) compared cisapride (0.3 mg/kg/day as a syrup) with placebo following clearance of accumulated stool. The RCT found that cisapride significantly increased stool frequency and decreased gut transit time after 8 weeks (mean stool frequency per week 6.75 v 1.31).[5] The second RCT (40 children, aged 2–16 years), analysed by intention to treat, showed significant benefit for cisapride over placebo at 12 weeks, as measured by a composite of improved stool frequency, absence of faecal soiling, and no use of other laxatives (improvement in composite index AR 14/20 [70%] with cisapride v 7/20 with placebo; RR 2.0, CI 1.03 to 3.88; NNT 3, 95% CI 1 to 24).[6]

Harms: RCTs did not report harms; see comment below.

Comment: Cisapride is licensed for use in children in the Republic of Ireland. Its license has been suspended in the UK and Germany, and its marketing stopped in the USA, due to association with heart rhythm abnormalities in adults.

OPTION OSMOTIC LAXATIVES

We found limited evidence that osmotic laxatives may increase stool frequency, and in infants result in normal stools. One small RCT found short term benefit from the addition of toilet training or biofeedback.

Benefits: We found no systematic review and no placebo controlled trials of osmotic laxatives in children. We found two small RCTs comparing the effects of lactitol versus lactulose on stool frequency and consistency in 51 and 39 children with constipation.[7,8] Both preparations resulted in a significant increase in stool frequency at 4 weeks and normal consistency of stools at 2 weeks compared with baseline.[7,8] One RCT of 220 non-breastfed, constipated infants (aged 0–6 months) compared 2% versus 4% lactulose mixed with an artificial milk preparation.[9] At 14 days, over 90% of parents in both groups reported easy passage of normal or thin consistency stools (P < 0.05 compared with baseline). **With toilet training or biofeedback:** One RCT in 87 children with encopresis compared medical treatment (enemas and laxatives) with and without toilet training.[10] A third arm of the trial evaluated biofeedback. Children receiving toilet training used significantly fewer laxatives and required fewer treatment sessions than those in the other two groups. Toilet training and biofeedback produced similar reductions in rates of soiling, which were greater than those achieved by medical treatment alone (P < 0.04).

Harms: One study found that children treated with lactulose experienced significantly more abdominal pain and flatus than those treated with lactitol.[7]

Comment: The benefits shown in these studies are comparisons of outcomes before and after treatment and were not necessarily due to the treatments.[7,8] Toilet training consisted of reinforcement and scheduling to promote response to the urge to defecate, and instruction and modelling to promote appropriate straining.[10]

OPTION   STIMULANT LAXATIVES

We found no placebo controlled RCT of their effects in children.

Benefits: We found no systematic review or placebo controlled RCT. Studies were all comparative and used multiple interventions, small sample sizes, or both. One quasi-randomised study (see Comment below) compared senna versus mineral oil concentrate in 37 children aged 3–12 years with chronic constipation.[11] The study found that senna versus mineral oil after six months was less effective in reducing involuntary faecal soiling (involuntary faecal soiling AR 8/18 [44%] with senna v differences were found in the number of children with relapses of constipation symptoms during the treatment period (relapses of constipation AR 12/19 [63%] with senna v 16/18 [89%] with mineral oil; RR 0.71 95% CI 0.48 to 1.04).[11] **With toilet training or biofeedback:** See osmotic laxatives above.[10]

Harms: None identified.

Comment: The study used last hospital number digit to randomise patients.[11]

OPTION   BIOFEEDBACK TRAINING

RCTs found short term benefit from adding biofeedback training to conventional treatment in childhood constipation. Two RCTs found no significant benefit after one year.

Benefits: We found no systematic review. Four RCTs compared conventional treatment with or without biofeedback in 87,[10] 192,[12] 129,[13] and 41[14] children with constipation, encopresis, or both. The biofeedback compared 2–6 weeks of training [14]or seminars [12]. Two studies found short term benefit in defecation dynamics,[12,14] and rates of soiling,[10] but none found significant improvement in soiling, stool frequency, or laxative use at 1 year or more.

Harms: None identified.

Comment: None.

Substantive changes since last issue

Cisapride One new RCT[6] supports evidence for efficacy in children. Cisapride is not widely licensed for use in this group. The clinical use of cisapride in adults has been greatly restricted due to adverse cardiac effects.

REFERENCES

1. Nelson R, Wagget J, Lennard-Jones JE, Barnes PRH. Constipation and megacolon in children and adults. In: Misiewicz JJ, Pounder RE, Venables CW. *Diseases of the gut and pancreas*. 2nd ed. Oxford: Blackwell Science, 1994.
2. American Psychiatric Association. *Diagnostic and statistical manual of mental disorders*. 4th ed. Washington, DC: American Psychiatric Association, 1994.
3. Loening-Baucke V. Chronic constipation in children. *Gastroenterology* 1993;105:557–1563.
4. Mooren GCAH, Van der Plas RN, Bossuyt PMM, Taminiau JAJM, Buller HA. The connection between dietary fibre intake and chronic constipation in children. *Ned Tijdschr Geneeskd* 1996;140:2036–2039.
5. Halibi IM. Cisapride in the management of chronic pediatric constipation. *J Pediatr Gastroenterol Nutr* 1999;28:199–202.
6. Nurko MD, Garcia-Aranda JA, Worona LB, Zlochisty O. Cisapride for the treatment of constipation in children: a double blind study. *J Pediatr* 2000;136:35–40.
7. Pitzalis G, Mariani P, Chiarini-Testa MR, et al. Lactitol in chronic idiopathic constipation of childhood. *Pediatr Med Chir* 1995;17:223–226.
8. Martino AM, Pesce F, Rosati U. The effects of lactitol in the treatment of intestinal stasis in

childhood. *Minerva Pediatr* 1992;44:319–323.
9. Hejlp M, Kamper J, Ebbesen F, Hansted C. Infantile constipation and allomin-lactulose. Treatment of infantile constipation in infants fed with breast milk substitutes: a controlled trial of 2% and 4% allomin-lactulose. *Ugeskr Laeger* 1990;152:1819–1822.
10. Cox DJ, Sutphen J, Borowitz S, et al. Contribution of behaviour therapy and biofeedback to laxative therapy in the treatment of pediatric encopresis. *Ann Behav Med* 1998;20:70–76.
11. Sondheimer JM, Gervaise EP. Lubricant versus laxative in the treatment of chronic functional constipation of children: a comparative study. *J Pediatr Gastroenterol Nutr* 1982;1:223–226.
12. Van der Plas RN, Benninga MA, B ller HA, et al. Biofeedback training in treatment of childhood constipation: a randomised controlled study. *Lancet* 1996;348:776–780.
13. Loening-Baucke V. Biofeedback treatment for chronic constipation and encopresis in childhood: long term outcome. *Pediatrics* 1995;96:105–111.
14. Loening BV. Modulation of abnormal defecation dynamics by biofeedback treatment in chronically constipated children with encopresis. *J Pediatr* 1990;116:214–222.

Gregory Rubin
Senior Lecturer in Primary Care
University of Sunderland
Sunderland
UK

Competing interests: None declared.

Croup

Updated this issue

Martin Osmond and David Evans

INTERVENTIONS

Key Messages

- We found that treatment of croup in primary care has not yet been evaluated adequately in RCTs.
- RCTs in primary paediatric assessment units (PAUs) have found that systemic steroids, nebulised steroids, and nebulised adrenaline (epinephrine) all improve symptoms. Systemic and nebulised steroids have also been found to reduce hospital admissions.
- RCTs have found no evidence of a difference between systemic and nebulised steroids, but the trials were too limited to rule out a clinically important difference.
- In children admitted to hospital, RCTs have found that systemic steroids, nebulised steroids in PAUs, and nebulised adrenaline all improve symptoms. Systemic and nebulised steroids have also been found to reduce hospital stay and reattendance.
- We found no good evidence to compare the effectiveness of systemic and nebulised steroids in hospitals.
- We found no good evidence to compare the effectiveness of nebulised adrenaline and steroids in hospitals.
- None of the RCTs we reviewed described any deaths in over 1000 infants with childhood croup, related either to croup itself or to any associated treatment.

DEFINITION	Croup is an acute clinical syndrome characterised by a harsh, barking cough, inspiratory stridor, and hoarse voice, caused by laryngeal or tracheal obstruction. Mild fever and rhinorrhoea may also be present. The most important differential diagnoses are acute epiglottitis, inhalation of a foreign body, and bacterial tracheitis.
INCIDENCE/ PREVALENCE	Croup occurs in about 3% of children aged under 6 years per year,[1] and causes 2–3% of hospital admissions in young children in the UK.[2] One retrospective Belgian study of 5–8 year olds found that 15.5% of children had suffered from croup, and 5% had experienced recurrent croup (3 or more episodes).[3]
AETIOLOGY/ RISK FACTORS	Croup is believed to be mainly viral in origin, but atopy plays a part in some children. The most common virus isolated is parainfluenza types 1, 2, or 3. Others include influenza, adenovirus, respiratory syncytial virus, and rhinovirus.
PROGNOSIS	Fewer than 2% of children with croup are admitted to hospital in the UK.[1] Of those admitted, only 0.5–1.5% require intubation. Mortality is low: of 208 children who were given artificial airways over a 10 year period, two died.[4] Symptoms of upper airway obstruction can be extremely distressing to the child and the family.
AIMS	To reduce suffering and distress, need for hospital admission, duration of hospital stay, rates of intubation, and mortality, without undue adverse effects.
OUTCOMES	Severity of symptoms and signs of upper airway obstruction, rates of hospital admission, visits to a medical practitioner or reattendance to accident and emergency department, intubation rates, mortality, and adverse effects of treatment. A commonly used definition of a clinically significant improvement is ≥ 2 points of the validated Westley croup score (maximum score, or most severe, 17)[5] within a predefined timescale. The Westley score comprises the sum of five clinical parameters: conscious level, cyanosis, stridor, air entry, and chest wall retractions. Intubation and death are rare in children with croup, so trials recruiting large numbers of children would be needed to exclude a difference in rates between interventions.
METHODS	*Clinical Evidence* update search and appraisal June 2000, covering croup, laryngotracheitis, and laryngotracheobronchitis. Data were extracted from trials that used randomisation (not quasi-randomisation) and intention to treat analysis. Common exclusion criteria were previous upper airway abnormalities, previous prolonged intubation, severe croup (cyanosis with impaired consciousness), and recent treatment with steroids. The conclusions presented below should not be applied to children with these clinical features. Most children in the studies were cared for in institutions with excellent staffing and monitoring facilities. RCTs performed in hospital settings studied children with more severe croup than those based in assessment units.

Croup

QUESTION	What are the effects of treatment in primary care settings?

We found insufficient evidence about the treatment of croup in primary care.

Benefits: We found no systematic review or RCTs evaluating interventions in acute childhood croup in primary care settings.

Harms: Insufficient data.

Comment: It is surprising that there is no evidence relating to children with croup in the primary care setting as this is where the great majority children with croup cases are treated.

QUESTION	What are the effects of treatment in primary paediatric assessment units?

OPTION	SYSTEMIC STEROIDS VERSUS PLACEBO IN PAEDIATRIC ASSESSMENT UNITS

Three RCTs found that a single dose of oral or intramuscular steroids significantly improved symptoms within 5 hours, reduced the likelihood of admission to hospital by 75%, and reduced the need for further treatment after discharge by 70%.

Benefits: We found two systematic reviews that included relevant trials of systemic steroids versus placebo for children with croup in paediatric assessment units (PAUs).[6,7] They did not, however, analyse these three trials[8–10] separately from other included studies. The three RCTs included 230 children seen at primary PAUs in Australia, Canada, and the USA. One compared a single intramuscular dose of 0.6 mg/kg dexamethasone given shortly after arrival in the assessment unit, versus placebo.[8] The others compared 0.15 mg/kg oral dexamethasone[9] and 0.6 mg/kg intramuscular dexamethasone[10] versus placebo in children ready for discharge from the assessment unit. **Symptom improvement:** Intramuscular dexamethasone (0.6 mg/kg) significantly improved the croup score within 5 hours (96 children; change in croup score: dexamethasone -2.9, placebo -1.3).[8] **Admission to hospital:** Intramuscular dexamethasone given shortly after arrival in the assessment unit reduced admissions to hospital (RR of admission compared with placebo 0.25, 95% CI 0.13 to 0.49; NNT to prevent one additional admission 2, 95% CI 1 to 3).[8] **Reattendance:** For the week after discharge, all three RCTs reported lower rates of reattendance to any medical practitioner or institution in children given steroids (RR for reattendance compared with placebo 0.33, 95% CI 0.19 to 0.56; NNT to prevent one additional child reattending 12, 95% CI 6 to 60).[8–10]

Harms: None reported.

Comment: The children were observed for up to 5 hours in a PAU before discharge was decided. Some children were treated with nebulised adrenaline.[10]

NEBULISED STEROIDS VERSUS PLACEBO IN PAEDIATRIC ASSESSMENT UNITS

RCTs have found that, compared with placebo, nebulised steroids reduce the likelihood of a poor response within 2–5 hours by more than half, and halve the risk of hospital admission.

Benefits: We found three systematic reviews,[6,7,11] which included four RCTs comparing nebulised steroids versus placebo for children with croup in PAUs.[8,12–14] The reviews, however, combined the results with RCTs of hospital based treatment. **Symptom improvement:** The four relevant RCTs (250 children) evaluated treatment in assessment units. They compared a single dose of inhaled steroids versus placebo, given after humidified oxygen.[8,12–14] Combined data from the three trials that dichotomised outcomes into either good (improvement in croup score of 2 or more) or poor response showed a significantly reduced likelihood of a poor response within 2–5 hours after treatment (RR 0.44, 95% CI 0.29 to 0.67).[12–14] **Admission to hospital:** Rate of admission was halved (RR 0.55, 95% CI 0.38 to 0.81; NNT to prevent 1 additional admission 4, 95% CI 3 to 8).[8,12–14] **Reattendance:** The trials found no evidence of a significant difference in rates of further admission (RR 0.74, 95% CI 0.26 to 2.08)[8,12–14] or consultations with other health practitioners (RR 0.86, 95% CI 0.34 to 2.19) in the week after discharge from the assessment unit.[8,12–14]

Harms: Nebulised steroids seem to be well tolerated. In one of these four trials, two neutropenic children suffered bacterial tracheitis after treatment with nebulised dexamethasone.[14]

Comment: We found insufficient evidence to compare regimens of nebulised steroids. In the trials, children were observed for up to 5 hours in the assessment unit, and all received humidified air or oxygen; in one trial, both groups also received oral dexamethasone 0.6 mg/kg.[13] One pilot RCT (in 17 hospitalised children) compared inhaled steroid (fluticasone propionate 1000 μg, 2 doses) versus placebo delivered by a metered dose inhaler and spacing device, as a potential treatment that could be given at home. The trial found no evidence of benefit, but was too low powered to rule out an effect.[15] We found another systematic review that did not analyse separately data from trials of nebulised steroids versus placebo.[6]

SYSTEMIC VERSUS NEBULISED STEROIDS IN PAEDIATRIC ASSESSMENT UNITS

RCTs have found that systemic dexamethasone and nebulised budesonide are equally effective in reducing symptoms. In one trial, oral dexamethasone reduced the rate of admission compared with nebulised budesonide.

Benefits: We found one systematic review,[7] which included a single RCT,[16] and we found two additional RCTs.[8,17] The RCTs compared oral dexamethasone 0.6 mg/kg versus nebulised budesonide 2 mg,[16,17] and intramuscular dexamethasone 0.6 mg/kg versus nebulised budesonide 4 mg[8] for 280 children with acute croup attending an assessment unit. The trials found no significant difference between nebulised budesonide and systemic dexamethasone in rates of symptom resolution or reattendance after discharge, although fewer children on oral dexamethasone were admitted (RR oral v nebulised steroids 0.53, 95% CI 0.34 to 0.81).[8]

Harms: None reported.

Comment: None.

OPTION   **NEBULISED ADRENALINE (EPINEPHRINE) IN PAEDIATRIC ASSESSMENT UNITS**

One small RCT found that nebulised adrenaline given in the assessment unit to children suffering from croup significantly improved symptoms within 30 minutes compared with placebo. Symptoms returned to preintervention severity in a third of children within 2 hours.

Benefits: We found no systematic review. **Adrenaline versus placebo:** We found one RCT comparing nebulised racemic adrenaline (0.5 mg/kg diluted to 2 ml with 0.9% sodium chloride) versus saline placebo in 54 children with stridor at rest seen in an assessment unit.[18] This trial found a significant improvement in croup scores 30 minutes after treatment with epinephrine (mean scores 2.0 v 3.6 on placebo; P < 0.01).[18] The trial found no significant reduction in duration of stay in the assessment unit (mean stay [range]: 11.5 hours [5–21] v 13.3 hours [6–24]). **Adrenaline combined with steroids:** We found no RCTs. Two prospective cohort studies have examined outcome in 115 children treated with nebulised adrenaline and dexamethasone 0.6 mg/kg in an assessment unit. Of the 55–66% who responded satisfactorily, all were discharged after 3–4 hours' observation, and none reattended for further medical care within 24–48 hours.[19,20]

Harms: We found no evidence of a significant difference in the harms after treatment with adrenaline or placebo. Of the children who had improved by 30 minutes, a considerable proportion relapsed, although there was no significant difference in the rate of relapse (return of croup scores to the pretreatment value) between the two groups (35% with adrenaline v 25% with placebo; RR adrenaline v placebo 1.41, 95% CI 0.36 to 5.51). This raises the question of whether children given nebulised adrenaline and then discharged may come to harm when symptoms recur. No children discharged in the RCT reattended for further treatment.[18] Children were observed for a minimum of 5 hours (up to 24 hours). During this time, 40% of treated children and 48% of controls were given a further dose of adrenaline, whereas 52% of treated children and 58% of controls received oral betamethasone (6 mg) before final discharge. These differences were not significant.

Comment: None.

| QUESTION | What are the effects of treatment in hospital? |

| OPTION | INHALATION OF HUMIDIFIED AIR/OXYGEN IN HOSPITAL |

The effectiveness of inhaling humidified air/oxygen has not been evaluated adequately.

Benefits: We found no systematic review. We found one RCT in 16 children, which compared up to 12 hours' care in a humidified atmosphere (air with relative humidity 87–95%) versus normal care.[21] The trial found no significant difference in recovery rates (mean croup scores at 6 hours were 3.1 v 3.8).

Harms: None reported.

Comment: The study was not blinded, and selection, performance, and detection biases remain possible.

| OPTION | SYSTEMIC STEROIDS VERSUS PLACEBO IN HOSPITAL |

RCTs have found that giving systemic corticosteroids to children admitted with croup significantly improves symptoms by 12 hours, and reduces hospital stay. Limited evidence suggests that a single dose of oral dexamethasone 0.3 mg/kg is as effective as 0.6 mg/kg in children admitted with croup.

Benefits: We found two systematic reviews,[22,11] which combined data from 11 relevant RCTs (904 children), and we found one additional RCT not included in either review (41 children).[23] The most common regimen was intramuscular or oral dexamethasone 0.3–0.6 mg/kg as a single dose on admission or repeated over 24–48 hours. **Symptom improvement:** RCTs that evaluated symptomatic improvement at 12–24 hours found that significantly more children responded to steroids than to placebo (response defined as ≥2 points improvement of croup score; RR of response 1.23, 95% CI 1.13 to 1.33; NNT to achieve response in one additional child 7, 95% CI 5 to 10). **Hospital stay:** Four RCTs evaluated duration of hospital stay. Three found a significant reduction in hospital stay on dexamethasone compared with placebo (median stay 20 v 13 hours,[17] mean stay 91 v 49 hours[24] and 9 v 3 days[23]). The fourth trial found no significant difference.[25] **Intubation rates:** Seven RCTs in the systematic review and two subsequent RCTs gave data on intubation rates.[17,22,23] Children given systemic steroids were less at risk of intubation than infants taking placebo (RR 0.21, 95% CI 0.06 to 0.69). This combined estimate is dominated by one small study with a much higher than average rate of intubation (5/32 children).[23]

Harms: Systemic steroids seem to be well tolerated. We found three RCTs (130 children) reporting rates of secondary bacterial infection.[23,25,26] These reported nine cases of pneumonia, one of septicaemia, one of bacterial tracheitis, one of otitis media, and one of sinusitis. Six cases were in treated children and seven in controls (RR for infection compared with placebo 0.94, 95% CI 0.33 to 2.69).

Comment: A significant reduction in time to symptom resolution may not reduce hospital stay, which is influenced by hospital policies and referral patterns, availability of treatment in the community, parental access to transportation and communications, and the tendency to discharge patients at a certain time each day.[27]

OPTION   HIGH VERSUS LOW DOSE SYSTEMIC STEROID REGIMENS IN HOSPITALS

Limited evidence suggests that a single dose of oral dexamethasone 0.3 mg/kg is as effective as 0.6 mg/kg in children admitted with croup.

Benefits: We found one systematic review,[7] which included one RCT comparing different single doses of oral dexamethasone (0.6 v 0.3 mg/kg and 0.3 v 0.15 mg/kg) in 120 children admitted with croup.[24] There were no significant differences in rate of improvement in croup score, duration of hospital stay, or intubation rates. However, children given the lower dose of dexamethasone were more likely to be given nebulised adrenaline than those given the higher dose (RR 2.32, 95% CI 1.02 to 5.28). We found no studies comparing other systemic regimens.

Harms: None reported.

Comment: None.

OPTION   NEBULISED STEROIDS VERSUS PLACEBO IN HOSPITAL

RCTs have found that children admitted with croup improve more rapidly, leave hospital sooner, and are less likely to reattend if given nebulised corticosteroids compared with children given placebo. We found insufficient evidence on the effect of nebulised steroids on intubation rates.

Benefits: We found one systematic review,[11] which included four RCTs comparing nebulised steroids with placebo for children admitted to hospital with croup (n = 252).[17,28-30] This review, however, combined the results with RCTs conducted in PAUs. **Symptom improvement:** One trial evaluated budesonide 1 mg, two doses 30 minutes apart.[28] The risk of an inadequate response by 2 hours was significantly reduced (RR 0.40, 95% CI 0.19 to 0.83; NNT to prevent one additional inadequate response 2, 95% CI 1 to 8). **Hospital stay:** Another trial compared nebulised budesonide 2 mg initially, followed by 1 mg every 12 hours, versus placebo and found a significant reduction in hospital stay (mean stay 36 v 55 hours).[29] The third RCT compared budesonide 2 mg single dose versus placebo and reported a significant reduction in the number of children staying in hospital for more than 24 hours (RR 0.37, 95% CI 0.16 to 0.88; NNT 3, 95% CI 2 to 14).[17] **Intubation rates:** Using data from the three trials, there was no significant effect on intubation rates (RR of intubation 0.18, 95% CI 0.01 to 3.67).[17,28,29] **Relapse rate:** The fourth trial compared nebulised budesonide 2 mg versus placebo given every 12 hours while in hospital.[30] The trial found that budesonide accelerated clinical improvement (decrease in croup score by 2 points or more) compared with placebo (P = 0.013), and reduced the rate of further medical attendance in the 3 days after discharge (reattendance rate 1/34 with budesonide v 7/32 with placebo; P = 0.02).

Harms: Nebulised steroids seem to be well tolerated. Two RCTs have reported adverse effects. One trial reported one episode of nausea and one episode of distress caused by firm application of the face mask for 10 minutes.[29] The other trial reported emotional distress in six out of 42 children treated with budesonide nebulisers and nine out of 40 children treated with placebo.[30] In four children with severe croup (1 treated with budesonide and 3 with placebo), this led to interventional treatment outside of the protocol (nebulised adrenaline).

Comment: The optimal regimen of nebulised steroids has not yet been established.

OPTION SYSTEMIC VERSUS NEBULISED STEROIDS IN HOSPITAL

We found no RCTs undertaken outside of PAUs of oral versus nebulised steroids for croup.

Benefits: We found no systematic review and no RCTs investigating the effects of oral versus nebulised steroids in hospital.

Harms: We found no evidence.

Comment: None.

OPTION NEBULISED ADRENALINE (EPINEPHRINE) IN HOSPITAL

One small RCT found that nebulised adrenaline given in the assessment unit to children suffering from croup significantly improved symptoms within 30 minutes compared with placebo. Symptoms returned to preintervention severity in a third of children within 2 hours.

Benefits: We found no systematic review. **Versus placebo:** We found three RCTs comparing nebulised adrenaline versus placebo in 53 children admitted to hospital with croup. Two trials did not show improvement with adrenaline but were too small to exclude a clinically significant difference.[31,32] The other small RCT compared aerosolised racemic adrenaline versus 0.9% sodium chloride placebo, both delivered by intermittent positive pressure breathing.[5] Children given adrenaline experienced greater reductions in croup score. The reduction was greatest within 30 minutes of treatment and was not apparent at 2 hours (mean croup scores at 30 minutes 1.7 v 3.1). **Nebuliser versus intermittent positive pressure breathing:** We found one RCT in 14 children comparing nebulised adrenaline delivered by intermittent positive pressure breathing versus nebulised adrenaline alone.[33] The trial found no significant difference in resolution of symptoms (mean croup scores at 30 minutes 3.1 v 2.4). **L-adrenaline versus racemic adrenaline:** We found one RCT comparing racemic adrenaline versus L-adrenaline in 31 children.[34] The trial found no significant difference in croup scores (mean scores at 30 minutes, 3.8 v 4.8).

Harms: There was no significant difference in the risk of cardiovascular adverse effects with L-adrenaline or racemic adrenaline. Three children receiving racemic adrenaline were intubated (RR of intubation with racemic *v* L-adrenaline 6.59, 95% CI 0.37 to 118).[34] Children given nebulised adrenaline need medical observation because symptoms may return to pretreatment severity (see harms under nebulised adrenaline in paediatric assessment units, p 210).

Comment: Racemic adrenaline comprises equal amounts of D- and L-isomers and was historically chosen in favour of the more readily available L-form in the belief that it caused fewer adverse cardiovascular effects.

OPTION NEBULISED ADRENALINE VERSUS STEROIDS IN HOSPITAL

We found no good evidence to compare the effectiveness of nebulised adrenaline and steroids.

Benefits: We found one systematic review,[7] which identified one RCT comparing nebulised adrenaline 4 mg versus nebulised budesonide 2 mg in 66 children admitted to hospital with croup.[35] This trial found no significant difference in duration of hospital stay (mean difference in hospital stay adrenaline *v* budesonide −5.8 hours, 95% CI −22.8 to +11.2) or in croup scores (mean change −2.9 *v* −1.7; P = 0.08). We found no RCTs comparing nebulised adrenaline versus oral steroids.

Harms: None reported.

Comment: Nebulised adrenaline and steroids may have an additive effect through different modes of action, although whether this leads to improved outcomes is unknown.

GLOSSARY

Primary paediatric assessment unit An emergency room or accident and emergency department with the facilities to monitor closely the clinical condition of a child with acute onset of inspiratory stridor.

Substantive changes since last issue

Systemic steroids versus placebo in paediatric assessment units Two new systematic reviews[6,7] of previously identified RCTs found; conclusions unaltered.
Nebulised steroids versus placebo in paediatric assessment units Three new systematic reviews[6,7,11] of previously identified RCTs found; conclusions unaltered.
Systemic versus nebulised steroids in paediatric assessment units One new systematic review[7] including one new RCT found; conclusions unaltered.
Systemic steroids versus placebo in hospital One new systematic review found;[11] conclusions unaltered.
Different systemic steroids regimens in hospital One new systematic review[7] of previously identified RCT found; conclusions unaltered.
Nebulised steroids versus placebo in hospital One new systematic review[11] of previously identified RCTs found; conclusions unaltered.
Systemic versus nebulised steroids in hospital Recategorisation of previously identified RCT; no evidence found for this option.
Nebulised adrenaline versus steroids in hospital One new systematic review[7] of one previously identified RCT found; conclusions unaltered.

REFERENCES

1. Denny FW, Murphy TF, Clyde WA Jr, Collier AM, Henderson FW. Croup: an 11-year study in a pediatric practice. *Pediatrics* 1983;71:871–876.

2. Phelan PD, Landau LI, Olinsily A. *Respiratory illness in children*. 2nd ed. Oxford: Blackwell Science, 1982:32–33.

3. Van Bever HP, Wieringa MH, Weyler JJ, et al. Croup and recurrent croup: their association with asthma and allergy. *Eur J Pediatr* 1999;158:253–257.

4. McEniery J, Gillis J, Kilham H, Benjamin B. Review of intubation in severe laryngotracheobronchitis. *Pediatrics* 1991;87:847–853.

5. Westley CR, Cotton EK, Brooks JG. Nebulized racemic epinephrine by IPPB for the treatment of croup: a double-blind study. *Am J Dis Child* 1978; 132:484–487.

6. Ausejo M, Saenz A, Pham B, et al. The effectiveness of glucocorticoids in treating croup: meta-analysis. *BMJ* 1999;319:595–600. Search date 1997; primary sources Cochrane Controlled Trials Register, Embase 1974 to August 1997, Medline 1966 to August 1997; letters to authors.

7. Ausejo M, Saenz A, Pham B, et al. Glucocorticoids for Croup. In: The Cochrane Library, Issue 1, 2000. Oxford: Update software. Search date 1997; primary sources Cochrane Controlled Trials Register, Embase 1974 to August 1997, Medline 1966 to August 1997, letters to authors. Substantially amended June 1999. [Q to A: what was amended?]

8. Johnson DW, Jacobson S, Edney PC, et al. A comparison of nebulised budesonide, intramuscular dexamethasone, and placebo for moderately severe croup. *N Engl J Med* 1998; 339:498–503.

9. Geelhoed GC, Turner J, Macdonald WBG. Efficacy of a small single dose of oral dexamethasone for outpatient croup: a double blind placebo controlled clinical trial. *BMJ* 1996;313:140–142.

10. Cruz MN, Stewart G, Rosenberg N. Use of dexamethasone in the outpatient management of acute laryngotracheitis. *Pediatrics* 1995;96:220–223.

11. Griffin S, Ellis S, Fitzgerald-Barron A, Rose J, Egger M. Nebulised steroid in the treatment of croup: a systematic review of randomised controlled trials. *Br J Gen Pract* 2000;50:135–141. Search date not specified; primary sources Cinahl, Cochrane Controlled Trials Register, Embase, Medline; hand searching of article bibliographies, pharmaceutical industry database.

12. Klassen TP, Feldman ME, Watters LK, Sutcliffe T, Rowe PC. Nebulized budesonide for children with mild-to-moderate croup. *N Engl J Med* 1994;331: 285–289.

13. Klassen TP, Watters LK, Feldman ME, Sutcliffe T, Rowe PC. The efficacy of nebulized budesonide in dexamethasone-treated outpatients with croup. *Pediatrics* 1996;97:463–466.

14. Johnson DW, Schuh S, Koren G, Jaffe DM. Outpatient treatment of croup with nebulized dexamethasone. *Arch Pediatr Adolesc Med* 1996; 150:349–355.

15. Jan Roorda R, Walhof CM. Effects of inhaled fluticasone propionate administered with metered dose inhaler and spacer in mild to moderate croup: A negative preliminary report. *Pediatr Pulmonol* 1998;25:114–117.

16. Klassen TP, Craig WR, Moher D, et al. Nebulized budesonide and oral dexamethasone for the treatment of croup: a randomized controlled trial. *JAMA* 1998;279:1629–1632.

17. Geelhoed GC, Macdonald WB. Oral and inhaled steroids in croup: a randomized, placebo-controlled trial. *Pediatr Pulmonol* 1995;20:355–361.

18. Kristjansson S, Berg-Kelly K, Winso E. Inhalation of racemic adrenaline in the treatment of mild and moderately severe croup. Clinical symptom score and oxygen saturation measurements for evaluation of treatment effects. *Acta Paediatr* 1994;83:1156–1160.

19. Ledwith CA, Shea LM, Mauro RD. Safety and efficacy of nebulized racemic epinephrine in conjunction with oral dexamethasone and mist in the outpatient treatment of croup. *Ann Emerg Med* 1995;25:331–337.

20. Kunkel NC, Baker MD. Use of racemic epinephrine, dexamethasone, and mist in the outpatient management of croup. *Pediatr Emerg Care* 1996;12:156–159.

21. Bourchier D, Dawson KP, Fergusson DM. Humidification in viral croup: a controlled trial. *Aust Paediatr J* 1984;20:289–291.

22. Kairys SW, Olmstead EM, O'Connor GT. Steroid treatment of laryngotracheitis: a meta-analysis of the evidence from randomized trials. *Pediatrics* 1989; 83:683–693. Search date June 1999; primary sources Medline, Embase, and Cochrane Library.

23. Sumboonnanonda A, Suwanjutha S, Sirinavin S. Randomized controlled trial of dexamethasone in infectious croup. *J Med Assoc Thai* 1997;80:262–265.

24. Geelhoed GC, Macdonald WBG. Oral dexamethasone in the treatment of croup: 0.15 mg/kg versus 0.3 mg/kg versus 0.6 mg/kg. *Pediatr Pulmonol* 1995;20:362–368.

25. Super DM, Cartelli NA, Broosks LJ, Lembo RM, Kumar ML. A prospective randomized double-blind study to evaluate the effect of dexamethasone in acute laryngotracheitis. *J Pediatr* 1989;115:323–329.

26. Kuusela AL, Vesikari T. A randomized double-blind, placebo-controlled trial of dexamethasone and racemic epinephrine in the treatment of croup. *Acta Paediatr Scand* 1988;77:99–104.

27. Kemper KJ. Medically inappropriate hospital use in a pediatric population. *N Engl J Med* 1988;318: 1033–1037.

28. Husby S, Agertoft L, Mortensen S, Pedersen S. Treatment of croup with nebulised steroid (budesonide): a double blind, placebo controlled study. *Arch Dis Child* 1993;68:352–355.

29. Godden CW, Campbell MJ, Hussey M, Cogswell JJ. Double blind placebo controlled trial of nebulised budesonide for croup. *Arch Dis Child* 1997;76: 155–158.

30. Roberts GW, Master VV, Staugas RE, et al. Repeated dose inhaled budesonide versus placebo in the treatment of croup. *J Paediatr Child Health* 1999;35:170–174.

31. Gardner HG, Powell KR, Roden VJ, Cherry JD. The evaluation of racemic epinephrine in the treatment of infectious croup. *Pediatrics* 1973;52:52–55.

32. Taussig LM, Castro O, Beaudry PH, Fox WW, Bureau M. Treatment of laryngotracheobronchitis (croup). *Am J Dis Child* 1975;129:790–793.

33. Fogel JM, Berg IJ, Gerber MA, Sherter CB. Racemic epinephrine in the treatment of croup: nebulization alone versus nebulization with intermittent positive pressure breathing. *J Pediatr* 1982;101:1028–1031.

34. Waisman Y, Klein BL, Boenning DA, et al. Prospective randomized double-blind study comparing L-epinephrine and racemic epinephrine aerosols in the treatment of laryngotracheitis (croup). *Pediatrics* 1992;89:302–306.

35. Fitzgerald D, Mellis C, Johnson M, et al. Nebulized budesonide is as effective as nebulized adrenaline in moderately severe croup. *Pediatrics* 1996;97: 722–725.

Martin Osmond
Associate Professor of Pediatrics
University of Ottawa
Ottawa
Canada

David Evans
Lecturer in Paediatrics and Child Health
University of Leeds
Leeds
UK

Competing interests: None declared.

New topic

Yadlapalli Kumar and Rajini Sarvananthan

INTERVENTIONS

Key Messages

- Small RCTs suggest prone and left lateral positioning reduce reflux but both are known risk factors for sudden infant death syndrome (SIDS).
- A small RCT found no significant differences between thickened feeds and placebo for reducing reflux or acidity.
- One small RCT found that sodium alginate improved parent reported symptoms of gastro-oesophageal reflux disease (GORD).
- RCTs of cisapride versus placebo found no consistent clinical benefits for childhood GORD, but cisapride is not widely licensed for use in children and clinical use in adults is restricted due to heart arrhythmias.
- One small RCT found cimetidine versus placebo was effective for GORD complicated by oesophagitis.
- We found insufficient evidence to comment on the use of proton pump inhibitors for GORD.
- We found insufficient evidence on the effect of surgical fundoplication. Although the majority of children improve surgical fundoplications, surgery is associated with significant mortality and morbidity.

DEFINITION
Gastro-oesophageal reflux disease (GORD) is the passive transfer of gastric contents into the oesophagus due to transient or chronic relaxation of the lower oesophageal sphincter.[1] A survey of 69 children with GORD attending a tertiary referral centre (median age 16 months) found that presenting symptoms were recurrent vomiting (72%), epigastric and abdominal pain (36%), feeding difficulties (29%), failure to thrive (28%), and irritability (19%).[2] Over 90% of children with GORD have vomiting before 6 weeks of age.[1] Rare complications of the condition include oesophagitis with haematemesis and anaemia, respiratory problems such as cough, apnoea and recurrent wheeze, and failure to thrive.[1] A small comparative study (n = 40) suggested that, when compared to healthy children, infants with GORD display slower development of feeding skills and problems affecting behaviour, swallowing, food intake, and mother–child interaction.[3]

INCIDENCE/ PREVALENCE
Gastro-oesophageal regurgitation is considered a problem if it is frequent and persistent.[1] Eighteen per cent of the general infant population has regurgitation.[4] In a study comparing the prevalence of GORD in children with respiratory dysfunction (n = 62) to a control group (n = 387), the prevalence of excessive gastro-oesophageal refux, diagnosed by pH-metric criteria, was 42% and 8%, respectively.[5]

AETIOLOGY/ RISK FACTORS
Factors favouring GORD are immaturity of the lower oesophageal sphincter, chronic relaxation of the sphincter, increased abdominal pressure, gastric distension, hiatus hernia, and oesophageal dysmotility.[1] Premature infants and children with severe neurodevelopmental problems or congenital oesophageal anomalies are particularly at risk.

PROGNOSIS
Regurgitation is considered benign and most cases resolve spontaneously by 12–18 months of age.[6] When GORD is due to hiatus hernia, however, 30% of cases persist until 4 years of age.[7]

AIMS
To relieve symptoms, maintain normal growth, prevent complications such as oesophagitis, and minimise adverse effects of treatment.

OUTCOMES
Clinical condition (in terms of symptoms and growth), parental distress; incidence of complications (e.g. oesophagitis). Reflux Index, a measure of the percentage of time with a low oesophageal pH (frequently < 4), is an intermediate outcome often used in RCTs. Clinical interpretation of the resulting data is problematic.

METHODS
We searched Best Evidence, CINAHL, the Cochrane Library, Embase and Medline (March 2000) for systematic reviews and RCTs relevant to gastrooesophageal reflux in children. All citations were reviewed and relevant papers ordered and scrutinized by both authors.

QUESTION **What are the effects of treatment for symptomatic gastro-oesophageal reflux?**

OPTION **DIFFERENT POSTURES**

We found two small RCTs that did not measure clinical outcomes. Both found that prone positioning significantly improved pH, compared with

supine positioning. A third small RCT in preterm infants found that prone positioning decreased the number of episodes of reflux. Prone positioning is associated with SIDS.

Benefits: We found no systematic review. We found no RCTs investigating the effects of posture on clinical symptoms. Three small RCTs all reported effects of posture on oesophageal pH variables such as Reflux Index. One RCT (crossover, n = 24, age < 5 months) found that the severity of GORD, expressed as Reflux Index, was significantly less in the prone and left lateral positions compared to the supine and right lateral positions (P < 0.001).[8] In this RCT, head elevation did not affect Reflux Index significantly. A second RCT (crossover, n = 15, age < 6 months) also found significantly less reflux in the prone position (head elevated in a harness) compared to supine positioning in an infant seat where the head and trunk were elevated to 60° (P < 0.001). Again results were expressed in terms that are difficult to interpret clinically (Reflux Index).[9] The third RCT (crossover, n = 18, < 37 weeks gestation but > 7 days old) compared prone versus left and right lateral positions over 24 hours.[10] Again the findings favoured the prone and left lateral positions (P < 0.001). This trial found the number of episodes of reflux to be less with prone positioning (mean prone 15.4 [SE 2.8] v mean left lateral 24.6 [SE 3.5] v mean right 41.6 [SE 4.6], P < 0.001).

Harms: None reported.

Comment: Both prone and left lateral positions are known risk factors for SIDS. In a large, prospective cohort study prone sleeping position compared with supine position was associated with an increased risk of SIDS (OR 4.47, 95% CI 1.30 to 15.43).[11] The side sleeping position was found to increase the risk of SIDS compared with the supine position (at 2 months, adjusted OR 6.57, 95% CI 1.71 to 25.2).[12]

OPTION   FEED THICKENERS

One small RCT found no significant difference between carob flour thickened feeds and a placebo thickener. A second small RCT found no significant difference between different thickeners.

Benefits: We found no systematic review. **Versus placebo:** We found two RCTs. The first (double blind, n = 20, age 1–16 weeks) compared feeds thickened with carob flour (locus bean gum preparation) versus Saint John's bread, which is free of fibre and polysaccharides.[13] Regurgitation, as documented by parents after 1 week of treatment, decreased, but the difference was not significant (mean regurgitation score 2.2 v 3.3). It is unclear how to interpret regurgitation scores. This RCT also found no significant decrease in the Reflux Index after 1 week. The second RCT compared dry rice cereal with isocaloric unthickened feeds but did not seek to report benefits (see harms of feed thickeners, p 220).[14] **Different thickeners:** We found one RCT (n = 24, age 5–11 months) that compared feeds thickened with carob flour versus a traditional formula thickened with rice flour.[15] At the end of the 2 week treatment period, babies receiving the carob flour formula had a significant decrease in both symptomatic score (mean percentage reduction 70.4% v 48.7%, P < 0.01) and number of episodes of emesis (58.1% v 34.1%, P < 0.05), recorded by parents.

Harms: The second RCT (n = 24, age 0–6 months) of thickened versus unthickened feeds found that coughing occurred more frequently after feedings thickened with dry rice cereal than after isocaloric unthickened feedings (cough salvos per hour, thickened feeds mean 3.1 [SE 0.8] v unthickened feeds mean 2.0 [SE 0.4], P = 0.034).[15]

Comment: None.

OPTION   SODIUM ALGINATE

One small RCT found that parents of children taking sodium alginate reported fewer episodes of regurgitation than those of infants given placebo.

Benefits: We found no systematic review. We found one RCT (n = 20, mean age 28 months, treatment duration 8 days).[16] Sodium alginate reduced episodes of regurgitation to 25–33% of the former level while no clinical improvement was noted with placebo (lactose powder). Sodium alginate significantly reduced all pH variables compared to placebo.

Harms: None reported.

Comment: The high sodium load of sodium alginate may be inappropriate in preterm babies.[17]

OPTION   CISAPRIDE

Small RCTs of cisapride versus placebo did not find consistent, clinically meaningful, effects for childhood GORD. Cisapride has been suspended from the market in several countries because of adverse cardiac effects.

Benefits: We found no systematic review but found five RCTs.[18–22] One trial of cisapride versus placebo for uncomplicated GORD (n = 95, age < 36 months) found that in the 72% of infants who completed the 2 week trial, there were no significant differences in crying, vomiting or gagging, overall symptom intensity score, or parental global evaluations.[18] The second RCT (n = 49, age 6 weeks to 2 years) found treatment to be acceptable (92% completed the 6-week RCT) but clinically ineffectual (no significant differences for parental or physician's global assessments).[19] The third RCT (double blind, duration 4 weeks, n = 30, age 3 months to 5 years) found that cisapride improved measures of pH more than placebo.[20] The fourth RCT (double blind placebo controlled, duration 16 days, n = 42, age 2–4 months) found no significant improvements in either reflux index or the more clinically meaningful number of reflux episodes per hour (mean cisapride 1.94 [SE 0.33] v mean placebo 2.31 [SE 0.23]).[21] The number of severe episodes of reflux significantly decreased for infants taking cisapride (mean cisapride 0.3 [SE 0.05] v mean placebo 0.59 [SE 0.16]). An RCT in children with GORD (n = 23, age < 1 year old) compared cisapride 0.15 mg/kg three times a day versus placebo for 4 weeks.[22] A significant response in both the frequency and severity of regurgitation was found. The same paper reports another RCT (n = 45) comparing cisapride 0.1 mg/kg three times a day versus cisapride 0.2 mg/kg three times a day, and placebo, for 3–4 weeks. A significant difference was found in clinical response, which was due mainly to the superior efficacy of the 0.2 mg/kg dose of cisapride over placebo.

Harms: None reported.

Comment: Cisapride is licensed for use in children in the Republic of Ireland. In the UK and Germany its license has been suspended and in the USA its marketing stopped, due to association with heart rhythm abnormalities in adults. A recent case control study (n = 201, age 1–12 months) found cisapride significantly prolonged the QTc interval on electrocardiogram in a subgroup of infants younger than 3 months whilst in older infants the difference was not significant.[23] Gastrointestinal adverse effects (borborygmi, cramps, and diarrhoea) occur in 2% of infants.[23] Rash, pruritus, urticaria, bronchospasm, extrapyramidal effects, headache, dose-related increases in urinary frequency, hyperprolactinaemia, and reversible liver function abnormalities are extremely rare.[23] Most macrolide antibiotics elevate plasma cisapride levels, which may be clinically significant.[23]

OPTION H$_2$ ANTAGONISTS

One small RCT found that cimetidine is an effective treatment for GORD complicated by oesophagitis in children.

Benefits: We found no systematic review. We found one RCT (double blind, 12 weeks duration) comparing cimetidine 30–40 mg/kg per day versus placebo (n = 37, age range 1 month to 14 years) in children with GORD complicated by oesophagitis.[24] More children improved on cimetidine (ARR 51% 95% CI 21% to 81%, NNT 2 95% CI 1.2 to 4.8). Improvement was defined in terms of either clinical or endoscopic findings. A second RCT in children with GORD (crossover, n = 27) compared different doses of cimetidine but reported only physiological outcomes (gastric pH, gastric acid supression).[25] We found no RCTs of ranitidine in children.

Harms: None reported.

Comment: Cimetidine has been reported to cause bradycardia in a small subgroup of patients and may increase cisapride plasma levels.[23] Bronchospasm, acute dystonic reactions, sinus node dysfunction, bradycardia, and increases in parasympathetic tone reactions have been reported with ranitidine.[23]

OPTION PROTON PUMP INHIBITORS (OMEPRAZOLE)

We found insufficient evidence on the effects of proton pump inhibitors on GORD.

Benefits: We found no systematic review or RCT. A small case series did not report clinical outcomes.[26]

Harms: None reported.

Comment: Proton pump inhibitors have been reported to cause hepatitis and omeprazole chronically elevates serum gastrin.[26]

OPTION   SURGERY

We found insufficient evidence on the effects of surgery on GORD. Although most children improve after fundoplications surgery is associated with significant mortality and morbidity.

Benefits: We found no systematic review or RCT comparing surgery with medical interventions, or one surgical procedure with another. We found a cohort study (n = 22) of children who had undergone anterior gastric fundoplication.[27] Twenty children (91%) remained asymptomatic by 2 years.

Harms: A retrospective review (n = 106) of modified Nissen's fundoplication showed a failure rate of 7.5% and, when neurologically impaired children were included, a long-term mortality of 7.8%.[28] If only neurologically normal children were considered, the mortality was 1.6% in the immediate postoperative period and 3.2% on long term follow up (3 deaths out of 62; all with associated congenital abnormalities).

Comment: Complications of surgical treatment include dumping, retching, intestinal obstruction, 'gas bloat', and recurrence of GORD.[17]

REFERENCES

1. Herbst JJ. *Textbook of Gastroenterology and Nutrition in Infancy*. 2nd ed. New York: Ravens Press, 1989:803–813.
2. Lee WS, Beattie RM, Meadows N, et al. Gastro-oesophageal reflux: Clinical profiles and outcome. *J Paediatr Child Health* 1999;35:568–571.
3. Mathisen B, Worrall L, Masel J. et al. Feeding problems in infants with gastro-oesophageal reflux disease: a controlled study. *J Paediatr Child Health* 1999;35:163–169.
4. Boulton TJ, Rowley MP. Nutritional studies during early childhood. III. Incidental observations of temperment, habits, and experiences of ill-health. *Aust Paediar J* 1979;15:87–90.
5. Sacré L, Vandenplas Y. Gastroesophageal reflux associated with respiratory abnormalities during sleep. *J Pediatr Gastroenterol Nutr* 1989;9:28–33.
6. Vandenplas Y, Belli D, Benhamou P, et al. A critical appraisal of current management practices for infant regurgitation – recommendations of a working party. *Eur J Pediatr* 1997;156:343–357.
7. Carre IJ. Natural history of partial thoracic stomach ("hiatus hernia") in children. *Arch Dis Child* 1959;34:344–353.
8. Tobin JM, McCloud P, Cameron DJS. Posture and gasro-oesophageal reflux: a case for left lateral positioning. *Arch Dis Child* 1997;76:254–258.
9. Orenstein SR, Whitington PF. Positioning for prevention of infant gastroesophageal reflux. *J Pediatr* 1983;103:534–537.
10. Ewer AK, James ME, Tobin JM. Prone and left lateral positioning reduce gastro-oesophageal reflux in preterm infants. *Arch Dis Child Fetal Neonatal Ed* 1999;81:F201–205.
11. Dwyer T, Ponsonby AB, Newman NM, et al. Prospective cohort study of prone sleeping position and sudden infant death syndrome. *Lancet* 1991;337:1244–1247.
12. Mitchell EA, Tuohy PG, Brunt JM, et al. Risk factors for sudden infant death syndrome following

the prevention campaign in New Zealand. *Pediatrics* 1997;100:835–840.
13. Vandenplas Y, Hachimi-Idrissi S, Casteels A, et al. A clinical trial with an "anti-regurgitation" formula. *Eur J Pediatr* 1994;153:419–423.
14. Orenstein SR, Shalaby TM, Putnam PE. Thickening feedings as a cause of increased coughing when used as therapy for gastroesophageal reflux in infants. *J Pediatr* 1992;121:913–915.
15. Borrelli O, Salvia G, Campanozzi A, et al. Use of a new thickened formula for treatment of symptomatic gastroesophageal reflux in infants. *Ital J Gastroenterol Hepatol* 1997;29:237–242.
16. Buts JP, Barudi C, Otte JB. Double-blind controlled study on the efficacy of sodium alginate (Gaviscon) in reducing gastroesophageal reflux assessed by 24 hour continuous pH monitoring in infants and children. *Eur J Pediatr* 1987;146:156–158.
17. Davies AEM, Sandhu BK. Diagnosis and treatment of gastro-oesophageal reflux. *Arch Dis Child* 1995;73:82–86.
18. Cohen RC, O'Loughlin EV, Davidson GP, et al. Cisapride in the control of symptoms in infants with gastroesophageal reflux:A randomised, double-blind, placebo-controlled trial. *J Pediatr* 1999;134:287–292.
19. Scott RB, Ferreira C, Smith L, et al. Cisapride in pediatric gasroesophageal reflux. *J Pediatr Gastroenterol Nutr* 1997;25:499–506.
20. Castro HE, Ferrero GB, Cortina LS, et al. Efectividad del cisapride en el tratamiento del reflujo gastroesofágico (RGE) en ni os. Valoración de un estudio a doble ciego. *Anales Esp Pediatr* 1994;40:5–8.
21. Vandenplas Y, de Roy C, Sacre L. Cisapride decreases prolonged episodes of reflux in infants. *J Pediatr Gastroenterol Nutr* 1991;12:44–47.
22. Van Eygen M, Van Ravensteyn H. Effect of cisapride on excessive regugitation in infants. *Clin Ther* 1989;11:669–677.

23. Vandenplas Y, Belli DC, Benatar A, et al. The role of cisapride in the treatment of pediatric gastroesophageal reflux. *J Pediatr Gastroenterol Nutr* 1999;28:518–528.

24. Cucchiara S, Gobio-Casali L, Balli F, et al. Cimetidine treatment of reflux esophagitis in children: An Italian multicentre study. *J Pediatr Gastro Nutr* 1989;8:150–156.

25. Lambert J, Mobassaleh M, Grand RJ. Efficacy of cimetidine for gastric acid supression in pediatric patients. *J Pediatr* 1992;120:474–478.

26. Gunasekaran TS, Hassall EG. Efficacy and safety of omeprazole for severe gastroesophageal reflux in children. *J Pediatr* 1993;123:148–154.

27. Bliss D, Hirschl R, Oldham K, et al. Efficacy of anterior gastric fundoplication in the treatment of gastroesophageal reflux in infants and children. *J Paediatr Surg* 1994;29:1071–1075.

28. Spillane AJ, Currie B, Shi E. Fundoplication in children: Experience with 106 cases. *Aust NZ J Surg* 1996;66:753–756.

Yadlapalli Kumar
Specialist Registrar in Paediatrics
Royal Liverpool Children's Hospital
NHS Trust
Liverpool
UK

Rajini Sarvananthan
Specialist Registrar in Paediatrics
St Luke's Hospital
Bradford
UK
Competing interests: None declared.

Infantile colic

New topic

Sally Wade and Teresa Kilgour

Key Messages

- One systematic review has found that dicyclomine reduces infantile colic but is associated with adverse events.
- One systematic review of RCTs found no evidence that simethicone reduced infantile colic.
- We found limited evidence from one small RCT that soya milk may reduce duration of crying compared with standard formula milk. We found insufficient evidence that other methods of eliminating cow's milk protein from the diet of infants are effective in reducing infantile colic.
- We found insufficient evidence from small RCTs on the effects of low lactose milk.
- We found limited evidence from small RCTs that herbal tea or sucrose solution were effective.
- One systematic review identified four small RCTs on modification of parental responses to the infant. Limited evidence suggests that less stimulation may reduce infantile colic.

DEFINITION	Infantile colic is characterised by excessive crying in an otherwise healthy baby. The crying typically starts in the first few weeks of life and ends by 4–5 months of age. Excessive crying is defined as crying that lasts at least 3 hours a day, for 3 days a week, for at least 3 weeks.[1]
INCIDENCE/ PREVALENCE	Infantile colic leads one in six families to consult a health professional. One population based study (409 breast or formula fed infants) found an incidence of infantile colic of 3.3–17.1%, depending on the definition used, and whether symptoms were reported prospectively or retrospectively. Using this definition, the incidence was 9%.[2] One RCT (89 breast and formula fed infants) found that, at 2 weeks of age, the incidence of crying more than 3 hours a day was 43% (formula fed) and 16% (breast fed) infants. The incidence at 6 weeks was 12% (formula fed) and 31% (breast fed).[3]
AETIOLOGY/ RISK FACTORS	The cause of infantile colic is unclear and may be part of the normal distribution of crying. Other possible factors are painful gut contractions, lactose intolerance, gas, or parental misinterpretation of normal crying.[1] One large survey found that older primigravid women, mothers in non-manual occupations, or those who stayed in full time education, had the greatest risk of reporting infantile colic.[4]
PROGNOSIS	We found no review that considered the prognosis for babies with colic. One study found that 29% of infants aged 1–3 months cried for more than 3 hours a day, but by 4–6 months of age, the prevalence had fallen to 7–11%.[5]
AIMS	To reduce infant crying and distress, and anxiety for the family.
OUTCOMES	Duration of crying (measured using dichotomous, ordinal, or continuous scales). Parents' perception of severity (recorded in a diary).
METHODS	We searched Cinahl, the Cochrane Library, Embase, and Medline in October 1999. We identified one high quality systematic review (search date 1996, 27 RCTs).[1] We reviewed all subsequent RCTs. The review authors had searched the Cochrane Library, Embase, and Medline and checked references for missing publications. They identified publications using reduction in crying or colic as the main outcome. Trials were excluded for the following reasons: infants studied had normal crying patterns, infants were older than 6 months, interventions lasted less than 3 days, trials had no control groups or had low Jadad (see glossary, p 229) quality scores.[6] Results were added from trials with different outcomes, which limits the value of the conclusions. Effect sizes of comparable interventions were calculated using a random effects model.

QUESTION What are the effects of treatments for infantile colic?

OPTION ANTICHOLINERGIC DRUGS

One systematic review has found that anticholinergic drugs (dicyclomine or dicycloverine) reduces infantile colic but is associated with adverse effects.

Benefits: We found one systematic review (search date 1996, 5 RCTs, 177 infants).[1] It added a variety of outcomes and found that anticholinergic drugs (most frequently dicyclomine 5 mg, four times daily) were more effective than placebo (effect size SMD 0.46, 95% CI 0.33 to 0.60) (see comment below). The clinical meaning of these data is unclear.

Harms: Two of the five RCTs compared harms of dicyclomine versus placebo. The first (crossover design, 30 infants) reported drowsiness in four infants on dicyclomine and one infant on placebo.[7] The second RCT (crossover design, 25 infants) reported loose stools or constipation in three infants on dicyclomine and one infant on placebo.[8] Case reports of harms included breathing difficulties, seizures, syncope, asphyxia, muscular hypotonia, and coma.[9]

Comment: Dicyclomine was used in four, and dicycloverine in one, of the five studies in the systematic review. Only one trial stated measures to make the control syrup taste the same as the drug syrup.[7] The value of the review is limited by summation of results of RCTs with different outcome measures, and by inclusion of crossover trials. The crossover design is unlikely to provide valid evidence because infantile colic is an unstable condition, and the effects of dicyclomine may continue even after a washout period.[10]

OPTION   SIMETHICONE

One systematic review found no evidence that simethicone reduces infantile colic.

Benefits: We found one systematic review (search date 1996, 3 RCTs, 136 infants).[1] It added different measures of outcome and found no evidence that simethicone was more effective than placebo. One RCT was of unsatisfactory quality. The second RCT (double blind crossover, 83 infants) compared 0.3 ml of simethicone before feeds versus placebo.[11] It found no significant difference for colic when rated by carers (response with simethicone 28%, with placebo 37%, response with both 20%. Effect size on five point scale −0.10, 95% CI −0.27 to +0.08). The third RCT (double blind crossover trial, 27 infants) compared simethicone with placebo and found no improvement as rated by parental interview, 24 hour diary, or behavioural observation (effect size 0.06, 95% CI −0.17 to +0.28).[12]

Harms: None reported.

Comment: The value of the conclusions is limited by summation of different outcomes and by inclusion of crossover design RCTs.

OPTION   REPLACEMENT OF COW'S MILK WITH SOYA OR CASEIN HYDROLYSATE

One small RCT found that soya replacement of standard formula milk was associated with reduced crying time. Another small RCT found no effect of multiple changes in infant diet between cow's milk formula and casein hydrolysate formula (hypoallergenic milk — see glossary, p 229).

Benefits: We found one systematic review, which identified two relevant RCTs.[1] One small RCT (19 infants) compared soya milk formula with standard milk formula.[13] It found that soya milk formula reduced crying compared with standard milk formula (duration of crying 4.3–12.7 hours [soya milk], 17.3–20.1 [formula milk]; mean difference 10.3 hours, 95% CI 4.3 to 16.2). One further RCT (double blind crossover, 17 infants) studied the effect of each of three changes of infant diet for 4 days. Colicky, bottle fed infants received casein hydrolysate and cow's milk alternatively. By the third change, there was no notable difference in the incidence of colic between groups, but 47% of infants left the study before completion.[14]

Harms: None reported.

Comment: The systematic review[1] also included RCTs that changed the diet of both mothers and infants. The mothers in the two RCTs were blinded to the milk the baby received, but it is possible they detected differences in smell and texture.

OPTION   LOW LACTOSE MILK

We found insufficient evidence from RCTs on the effects of low lactose milk.

Benefits: We found one systematic review and one small RCT. The systematic review (search date 1996)[1] included one RCT (double blind cross-over, 10 bottle fed infants), which compared pooled breast milk versus lactase treated breast milk, versus formula milk, versus lactase treated formula milk.[15] Five infants did not complete the trial. It found no evidence that low lactose diets reduced the time, severity, or duration of colic, as recorded by parents. The additional small crossover RCT (13 infants) compared lactase treated milk versus milk with placebo drops added.[16] It found that the lactase treated diet reduced crying time by an average of 1.14 hours a day (95% CI 0.23 to 2.05).

Harms: None reported.

Comment: Such small trials[15,16] (total of 23 infants) could not allow confident conclusions to be drawn. We found no evidence, other than their response to diet, that babies in the trials had confirmed lactose intolerance. The systematic review identified one further trial,[1,17] which will be considered in a future issue of *Clinical Evidence*.

OPTION   SUCROSE SOLUTION

We found limited evidence from one small RCT that sucrose solution may benefit infantile colic.

Benefits: We found no systematic review. We found one small RCT (crossover at 3–4 and 6–8 days, 19 infants), which compared 2 ml of 12% sucrose solution versus placebo, given to babies when they continued to cry despite comforting. The parents, blinded to the intervention, scored the effect of the treatment on a scale of 1 to 5.[18] The RCT found that parent rated improvement was more likely with sucrose than with placebo (sucrose 12/19 improved, AR 0.63;

placebo 1/19 improved, AR 0.05; ARI for improvement sucrose *v* placebo 58%, 95% CI 10% to 89%; RR of improvement with sucrose *v* placebo 12.0, 95% CI 3.0 to 17.9; NNT 2, 95% CI 1 to 10).

Harms: None reported.

Comment: None.

OPTION **HERBAL TEA**

We found limited evidence from one RCT included in a systematic review that herbal tea was effective for infantile colic.

Benefits: We found one systematic review (search date 1996), which identified one good quality RCT.[1,19] This trial compared a herbal tea preparation, containing extracts of chamomile, vervain, licorice, fennel, and balm mint in a sucrose solution, (33 infants) versus a sucrose control (35 infants). Parents gave these preparations up to three times daily in response to episodes of colic. Coding was known only to the pharmacist, and the taste and smell of the tea and placebo were similar. Parents rated the response using a symptom diary. The trial found that at 7 days, herbal tea eliminated colic in more infants than in sucrose controls (numbers reported colic free 19/33 [herbal tea], AR 0.58; 9/35 [sucrose], AR 0.26; ARI 32%, 95% CI 7% to 53%, RR of eliminating colic 2.23, 95% CI 1.27 to 3.08; NNT 3, 95% CI 2 to 14;).[19] One additional RCT, evaluating herbal drops, was not considered suitable for inclusion.[20]

Harms: None reported.

Comment: None.

QUESTION **What are the effects of modifying parental responses**

OPTION **BEHAVIOURAL MODIFICATION**

One systematic review has found conflicting evidence from four small RCTs on the effects of behavioural modification (see glossary, p 229) by parents in response to their baby's crying.

Benefits: We found one systematic review (search date 1996, 4 small RCTs).[1] **Focused counselling versus non-specific reassurance:** One RCT (22 infants) assessed maternal anxiety and the hours of crying each day by questionnaire. It found no evidence that counselling mothers about specific management techniques (responding to crying with gentle soothing motion, avoiding over stimulation, using a pacifier, and prophylactic carrying) was any better than providing them with reassurance (see glossary, p 229) and support.[21] **Focused counselling versus car ride simulation:** The same RCT allocated 16 infants (mean age 6.8 weeks) to car ride simulation for up to 1 hour. There were no important differences between this group and the control group (11 infants) for crying times or maternal anxiety.[21] **Focused counselling versus elimination of cow's milk protein:** Another RCT (20 infants) found that counselling parents to respond to their baby's cries by feeding, holding, offering a pacifier, stimulating, or putting the baby down to sleep, decreased duration and extent of crying more quickly than substitution of soya or cow's milk with hydrolysed casein formula. Mean decrease in crying (hours/day) as recorded by parent diary was 2.13 hours with counselling versus 1.16 hours with dietary change.[22] **Increased carrying versus general advice:** The third RCT (66 infants) randomised mothers of babies with colic to carry their infant, even when not crying, for at least an additional 3 hours a day, or to a general advice group (to carry, check baby's nappy, feed, offer pacifier, place baby near mother, or use background stimulation such as music). The first group carried their babies for 4.5 hours a day, compared with 2.6 hours a day in the general advice group. There was no effect on crying time (mean difference 3 minutes less, 95% CI 37 minutes less to 32 minutes more).[23] **Reducing stimulation versus non-specific interview:** The fourth RCT (42 infants, median age 10 weeks) allocated infants to a low stimulation group (mothers were advised to reduce stimulation by not patting, lifting, winding, jiggling, or reducing auditory stimulation), or to a group that was given an empathetic interview. For infants under 12 weeks, reduced stimulation improved colic more than for the controls (advice group 14/15 improved, [93%] v control group 6/12 improved [50%] ARI for improvement 43%, 95% CI 8% to 49%; RR 1.87, 95% CI 1.16 to 1.99; NNT 2, 95% CI 2 to 13;).[24] Improvement was defined as a score of +2 on a scale recording hours of crying a day and maternal distress. It is unclear if this scale has been validated.

Harms: None reported.

Comment: None.

GLOSSARY

Behavioural modification Changing the way parents respond to their baby's crying.

Hypoallergenic diet In bottle fed infants, a hypoallergenic diet uses a casein hydrolysate formula. In breast fed infants, a hypoallergenic diet involves a maternal diet free of artificial colourings, preservatives and additives, and low in common allergens (e.g. milk, egg, wheat, and nuts).

Jadad Scale This measures factors that impact on trial quality. Poor description of the factors, rated by low figures, are associated with greater estimates of effect. The scale includes three items: was the study described as randomised? (0–2); was the study described as double-blind? (0–2); was there a description of withdrawals and drop outs? (0–1).[6]

Reassurance Informing the parent that infantile colic is a self limiting condition resolving by 3–4 months of age, and is not caused by disease or any fault in parental care.

REFERENCES

1. Lucassen PLB, Assendelf WJJ, Gubbels JW, et al. Effectiveness of treatments for infantile colic: a systematic review. *BMJ* 1998;316:1563–1569. Search date 1996; primary sources Cochrane Controlled Trials Register, Embase, Medline, and reference searching.

2. Canivet C, Hagander B, Jakobsson I. Infantile colic—less common than previously estimated? *Acta Paediatr* 1996;85:454–458.

3. Lucas A, St James-Roberts I. Crying, fussing and colic behaviour in breast- and bottle-fed infants. *Early Hum Dev* 1998;53:9–19.

4. Crowcroft NS, Strachan DP. The social origins of infantile colic: questionnaire study covering 76 747 infants. *BMJ* 1997;314:1325–1328.

5. St James Roberts I, Halil A. Infant crying patterns in the first year: normal community and clinical

findings. *J Child Psychol Psychiatry* 1991;32:951–968.

6. Jadad AR, Moore RA, Carroll D, et al. Assessing the quality of reports of randomized clinical trials: is blinding necessary? *Control Clin Trials* 1996;17:1–12.

7. Hwang CP, Danielsson B. Dicyclomine hydrochloride in infantile colic. *BMJ* 1985;291:1014.

8. Gruinseit F. Evaluation of the efficacy of dicyclomine hydrochloride ("Merbentyl") syrup in the treatment of infantile colic. *Curr Med Res Opin* 1977;5:258–261.

9. Williams J, Watkin-Jones R. Dicyclomine: worrying symptoms associated with its use in some small babies. *BMJ* 1984;288:901.

10. Fleiss JL. The crossover study. In: Fleiss JL, ed. *The design and analysis of clinical experiments*. New York: John Wiley and Sons, 1986:

11. Metcalf TJ, Irons TG, Sher LD, et al. Simethicone in the treatment of infantile colic: a randomized, placebo-controlled, multicenter trial. *Pediatrics* 1994;94:29–34.

12. Danielsson B, Hwang CP. Treatment of infantile colic with surface active substance (simethicone). *Acta Paediatr Scand* 1985;74:446–450.

13. Campbell JPM. Dietary treatment of infantile colic: a double-blind study. *J R Coll Gen Pract* 1989;39:11–14.

14. Forsythe BWC. Colic and the effect of changing formulas: a double blind, multiple-crossover study. *J Pediatr* 1989;115:521–526.

15. Stahlberg MR, Savilahti E. Infantile colic and feeding. *Arch Dis Child* 1986;61:1232–1233.

16. Kearney PJ, Malone AJ, Hayes T, et al. A trial of lactase in the management of infant colic. *J Hum Nutr Diet* 1998;11:281–285.

17. Miller JJ, McVeagh P, Fleet GH, et al. Effect of yeast lactase enzyme on "colic" in infants fed human milk. *J Pediatr* 1990;117:261–263.

18. Markestad T. Use of sucrose as a treatment for infant colic. *Arch Dis Child* 1997;77:356–357.

19. Weizman Z, Alkrinawi S, Goldfarb D, et al. Herbal teas for infantile colic. *J Pediatr* 1993;122:650–654.

20. Jain SL, Tripathi SN. Clinical assessment of elcarim drops on colic, regurgitation, griping pain and constipation in infants in the age group below six months. *Med Surg* 1987;27:13–15.

21. Parkin PC, Schwartz CJ, Manuel BA. Randomised controlled trial of three interventions in the management of persistent crying of infancy. *Pediatrics* 1993;92:197–201.

22. Taubman B. Parental counseling compared with elimination of cow's milk or soy milk protein for the treatment of infant colic syndrome: a randomised trial. *Pediatrics* 1988;81:756–761.

23. Barr RG, McMullen SJ, Spiess H, et al. Carrying as a colic "therapy": a randomized controlled trial. *Pediatrics* 1991;87:623–630.

24. McKenzie S. Troublesome crying in infants: effect of advice to reduce stimulation. *Arch Dis Child* 1991;66:1416–1420.

Sally Wade
Staff Grade Community Paediatrician
Archer Street Clinic
Darlington
UK

Teresa Kilgour
Staff Grade Community Paediatrician
City Hospitals Sunderland
Sunderland
UK
Competing interests: None declared.

Updated this issue

Sara Bosson and Natalie Lyth

Key Messages

- One systematic review has found that desmopressin and imipramine are effective for short term symptom relief. The review found that desmopressin was associated with fewer adverse effects.
- One good quality RCT found that indomethacin was more effective than placebo for increasing the number of dry nights.
- A double blind crossover study in people with detrusor instability found significantly more dry nights with carbamazepine than with placebo. We found no evidence about the effects of carbamazepine in children with monosymptomatic nocturnal enuresis.
- One systematic review has found enuresis alarms to be effective for long term treatment of nocturnal enuresis, with drugs (especially desmopressin) and behavioural treatments providing some additional benefit.

DEFINITION Nocturnal enuresis is the involuntary discharge of urine at night in the absence of congenital or acquired defects of the central nervous system or urinary tract in a child aged 5 years or older.[1] Disorders that have bed wetting as a symptom (termed "nocturnal incontinence") can be excluded by a thorough history, examination, and urinalysis. "Monosymptomatic" nocturnal enuresis is characterised by night time symptoms only and accounts for 85% of cases. Nocturnal enuresis is defined as primary if the child has never been dry for a period of more than six months, and secondary if such a period of dryness preceded the onset of wetting.

INCIDENCE/ PREVALENCE Between 15% and 20% of 5 year olds, 7% of 7 year olds, 5% of 10 year olds, 2–3% of 12–14 year olds, and 1–2% of people aged 15 years and over wet the bed twice a week on average.[2]

AETIOLOGY/ RISK FACTORS Nocturnal enuresis is associated with several factors, including small functional bladder capacity, nocturnal polyuria, and arousal dysfunction. Linkage studies have identified associated genetic loci on chromosomes 8q, 12q, 13q, and 22q11.[3–6]

PROGNOSIS   Nocturnal enuresis has widely differing outcomes, from spontaneous resolution to complete resistance to all current treatments. About 1% of adults remain enuretic. Without treatment, about 15% of children with enuresis become dry each year.[7]

AIMS   To stay dry on particular occasions (e.g. when visiting friends); to reduce the number of wet nights; to reduce the impact of the enuresis on the child's lifestyle; to initiate successful continence; to avoid relapse, with minimal adverse effects.

OUTCOMES   Rate of initial success (defined as 14 consecutive dry nights); average number of wet nights per week; number of relapses after initial success; average number of wet nights after treatment has ceased.

METHODS   *Clinical Evidence* update search and appraisal May 2000. One large, high quality systematic review of 62 RCTs was identified as the best evidence currently available.[8]

QUESTION   What are the effects of treatments for short term relief of symptoms?

OPTION   DESMOPRESSIN, INDOMETHACIN, IMIPRAMINE, AND CARBAMAZEPINE

One systematic review has found that desmopressin and imipramine are both effective for rapid symptom relief, and that desmopressin has fewer adverse effects. One good quality RCT found that indomethacin was more effective than placebo at increasing the number of dry nights. A double blind crossover study in people with detrusor instability found significantly more dry nights with carbamazepine than with placebo.

Benefits: **Desmopressin, indomethacin, imipramine:** We found one high quality systematic review, which included a meta-analysis of good quality RCTs.[8] It found that treatment for up to six weeks with either intranasal (10–40 μg at night) or oral (200–400 μg at night) desmopressin, or imipramine (10–75 mg at night) was significantly more effective than placebo for achieving initial success (RR with desmopressin 4.6, 95% CI 1.4 to 15.0; with imipramine 4.2, 95% CI 1.2 to 15.0) (see table 1, p 235). One good quality RCT (n = 85, desmopressin *v* indomethacin *v* placebo) in children aged over 6 years with primary nocturnal enuresis found that indomethacin (100 mg daily) given by suppository was more effective than placebo over 3 weeks (mean number of dry nights: 8.9 with indomethacin *v* 3.8 with placebo, P < 0.005).[9] **Carbamazepine:** A double blind crossover study in 26 people selected for detrusor instability on videocystourethrography found that carbamazepine (200 mg at night) resulted in more dry nights than placebo over 30 days (mean number of dry nights: 18.8 with carbamazepine *v* 3.9 with placebo; P < 0.001).[9]

Harms: **Desmopressin:** In the systematic review,[8] seven out of 17 trials considering adverse effects found the following effects in a small number of children: anorexia, headache, rash, sight disturbance, upset stomach, unpleasant taste in the mouth, epistaxis, nasal discomfort. Rarely, water intoxication has been reported. **Imipramine:** In the same review,[8] nine out of 11 trials reported adverse effects with imipramine: anorexia, anxiety reaction, burning sensation, constipation, depression, diarrhoea, dizziness, drowsiness, dry mouth, headache, irritability, lethargy, sleep disturbance, upset stomach, vomiting. Imipramine has been reported as fatal in overdose. **Indomethacin:** The RCT reported no adverse effects.[10] **Carbamazepine:** The study reported no adverse effects.[9]

Comment: The systematic review included only studies of interventions used to remedy either primary or secondary nocturnal enuresis (incontinence was excluded by medical examination or explicitly mentioned in the inclusion/exclusion criteria of included RCTs), and included a systematic measurement of baseline wetting and outcomes.[8] The RCT of indomethacin also included a systematic measurement of baselines and outcomes.[10] Although the studies of indomethacin and carbamazepine did not show any adverse effects, they have well established adverse effect profiles. The study population in the RCT of carbamazepine versus placebo had proven detrusor instability; the results may not generalise to all children with nocturnal enuresis.[9]

QUESTION   What are the effects of treatments for long term management?

OPTION   ENURESIS ALARMS, DRY BED TRAINING, DRUG TREATMENTS, ALARM CLOCK

One systematic review has found that enuresis alarms achieve most initial success, are associated with lower relapse rates, and have fewest adverse effects. One RCT found that a simple alarm clock was effective for initial success when used for 16 weeks.

Benefits: We found a systematic review of 62 RCTs of interventions in people with primary or secondary nocturnal enuresis.[8] Table 1 summarises results of studies in children that compared behavioural, pharmacological, and non-drug treatments versus placebo, enuresis alarm, or no treatment controls (see table 1, p 235). Also included are the results from one additional RCT that compared a standard home alarm clock (to wake the child just before the usual time of enuresis) versus waking the child after three hours of sleep.[11]

Harms: **Medication:** See harms of desmopressin, indomethacin, imipramine, and carbamazepine, pp 232 and 233. **Enuresis alarms:** Four trials reported adverse effects, most commonly alarm failure, as well as failure to wake the person, false alarms, fright, and disturbance to others. **Standard home alarm clock:** None reported.

Comment: Medication acts rapidly (see desmopressin, indomethacin, imipramine, and carbamazepine, above) and may be an alternative where alarms are unacceptable.

QUESTION   What is the best age to start treatment?

We found insufficient evidence indicating the youngest age at which treatment becomes effective.

Benefits: We found no systematic review or RCTs.

Harms: We found no evidence.

Comment: Anecdotal experience suggests that reassurance is often all that is needed below the age of 7 years. Behavioural treatments, such as alarms, require motivation and commitment on the part of the child and parent. Anecdotal experience suggests that children under the age of 7 years may not exhibit the commitment needed. Minimum ages for which drugs are licensed vary according to local policy.

Substantive changes since last issue

Carbamazepine New crossover trial of carbamazepine and placebo in children with proven detrusor instability found significantly more dry nights with carbamazepine.[9]

REFERENCES

1. Forsythe WI, Butler R. 50 years of enuretic alarms; a review of the literature. *Arch Dis Child* 1991;64: 879–885.
2. Blackwell C. *A guide to enuresis: a guide to treatment of enuresis for professionals.* Bristol: Eric, 1989.
3. Eiberg H. Total genome scan analysis in a single extended family for primary nocturnal enuresis: Evidence for a new locus (ENUR 3) for primary nocturnal enuresis on chromosome 22q11. *Eur Urol* 1998;33:34–36.
4. Eiberg, H. Nocturnal enuresis is linked to a specific gene. *Scand J Urol Nephrol* 1995; 173(suppl):15–17.
5. Arnell H, Hjalmas M, Jagervall G, et al. The genetics of primary nocturnal enuresis: Inheritance and suggestion of a second major gene on chromosome 12q. *J Med Genet* 1997;34:360–365.
6. Eiberg H, Berendt I, Mohr J. Assignment of dominant inherited nocturnal enuresis (ENUR 1) to chromosome 13q. *Nat Genet* 1995;10:354–356.
7. Forsythe WI, Redmond A. Enuresis and spontaneous cure rate of 1129 enuretics. *Arch Dis Child* 1974;49:259–263.
8. Lister-Sharp D, O'Meara S, Bradley M, Sheldon TA. University of York. NHS Centre for Reviews and Dissemination. August 1997. *A systematic review of the effectiveness of interventions for managing childhood nocturnal enuresis.* CRD Report 11. Search date 1996; primary sources Cochrane Library, Medline, Embase, Psychlit.
9. Al Waili, NS. Carbamazepine to treat primary nocturnal enuresis: double-blind study. *Eur J Med Res* 2000;5:40–44.
10. Sener F, Hasanoglu E, Soylemezoglu O. Desmopressin versus indomethacin treatment in primary nocturnal enuresis and the role of prostaglandins. *Urology* 1998:52:878–881.
11. EL-Anany FG, Maghraby HA, Shaker SED, Abdel-Moneim AM. Primary nocturnal enuresis: a new approach to conditioning treatment. *Urology* 1999;53:405–409.

Sara Bosson
Staff Grade Community Paediatrician
Mancunian Community Health NHS Trust
Manchester
UK

Natalie Lyth
Staff Grade Community Paediatrician
Northallerton Health Service Trust
Northallerton
UK

Competing interests: SB, none declared. NL has been reimbursed for attending a symposium by Ferring Pharmaceuticals, the manufacturer of desmotabs.

TABLE 1 Effective treatments for enuresis: advantages and disadvantages (see text, p 233).[8]

	Initial success (14 consecutive dry nights)	Long term success	Evidence	Advantages	Disadvantages
Desmopressin	Four times more likely than with placebo (RR 4.6, 95% CI 1.4 to 15.0)	No better than placebo	Meta-analysis of three RCTs	Effective within days, safe, few adverse effects with appropriate pretreatment advice	Case reports of water intoxication
Imipramine (for 6 weeks)	Four times more likely than with placebo (RR 4.2, 95% CI 1.2 to 15.0)	No better than placebo (RR 1.1)	Meta-analysis of four RCTs	Effective within days	Risk of lethal overdose, frequent significant adverse effects
Alarm	Thirteen times more likely than with no treatment (RR 13.3, 95% CI 5.6 to 31.5)	31–61% still dry at 3 months. Nine times less likely relapse than with desmopressin	Meta-analysis of four RCTs	Safe	Takes longer to become dry, needs good cooperation from child and family
Alarm and medication	75% compared with 46% with alarm alone	Not studied	One RCT, n = 71 (not included in systematic review)	More rapid effect than alarm alone	Same adverse effects as medication
Dry bed training without alarm	No better than no treatment (RR 2.5, 95% CI 0.55 to 11.4)	No better than no treatment (RR 0.4, 95% CI 0.14 to 1.13)	One good quality RCT, n = 45	Safe	Requires high degree of motivation
Dry bed training with alarm	Ten times more likely than with no treatment (RR 10, 95% CI 2.69 to 37.24)	No better than alarm alone (RR 1.0, 95% CI 0.7 to 1.5)	One RCT, n = 45	Safe	Requires an even greater input from the family than either treatment alone
Standard home alarm clock	77.1% compared with 61.8% of children woken after 3 hours' sleep (RR 1.3, P = 0.03)	No better at 3 months than waking children after 3 hours' sleep (66% dry compared with 56% of control, P = 0.19)	One RCT, n = 125	Safe, does not require bed wetting to initiate alarm	None reported

Recurrent idiopathic epistaxis (nosebleeds)

New topic

Martin Burton and Robert Walton

QUESTIONS
Effects of treatments in children with recurrent idiopathic epistaxis . .237

INTERVENTIONS	
Trade off between benefits and harms Antiseptic creams . . . . .237 Silver nitrate cautery 238	Combination of chlorhexidine/neomycin cream and silver nitrate cautery . . .238

Key Messages

- One small RCT found that chlorhexidine/neomycin cream and silver nitrate cautery were of similar effectiveness. Some children found the smell and taste of the antiseptic cream unpleasant. All children found cautery painful despite the use of local anaesthesia.

- One small RCT found no advantage to adding once only silver nitrate cautery to standard treatment with a chlorhexidine/neomycin cream.

DEFINITION
Recurrent idiopathic epistaxis is recurrent, self limiting nasal bleeding in children for which no specific cause has been identified. There is no consensus on how frequent or severe recurrences need to be. A cross sectional study of a sample of 1218 children aged 11–14 years found that 8.6% had frequent episodes of epistaxis.[1] It is likely that most nosebleeds in children are not brought to the attention of health professionals, and that only the most severe are considered for treatment.

AETIOLOGY/ RISK FACTORS
In children, most epistaxis occurs from the anterior part of the septum in the region of Little's area.[2] Common local factors are inflammation of the nasal mucosa, excessive nasal dryness and trauma, including nose-picking.[2] Epistaxis caused by other specific local (e.g. tumours) or systemic factors (e.g. clotting disorders) is not considered here.

PROGNOSIS
Clinical experience suggests that recurrent epistaxis is less common in adolescents over 14 and that many children "grow out" of this problem.

AIMS
To reduce the number and severity of nosebleeds.

OUTCOMES
Number and severity of nosebleeds.

METHODS
Clinical Evidence search and appraisal February 2000. One author reviewed all RCTs and excluded those not relating to recurrent idiopathic epistaxis in children.

| QUESTION | What are the effects of treatments in children with recurrent idiopathic epistaxis? |

| OPTION | ANTISEPTIC CREAMS |

We found no placebo controlled trials. One small RCT found that chlorhexidine/neomycin cream and silver nitrate cautery were of similar effectiveness. Some children found the smell and taste of antiseptic cream unpleasant. All children found cautery painful despite the use of local anaesthesia.

Benefits:
We found no systematic review. **Versus placebo:** We found no RCTs. **Versus cautery:** We found one RCT, although the method of randomisation was not explicit. It involved 48 children, age 3–14 years, who had at least one nosebleed in the previous 4 weeks and a "history of repeated epistaxis".[3] They were randomised to antiseptic cream (chlorhexidine hydrochloride 0.1%, neomycin sulphate 3250 units/g) applied to both nostrils twice daily for 4 weeks (n = 24), or one episode of cautery (n = 24). Cautery was undertaken in secondary care using sliver nitrate applied on a stick to prominent vessels or bleeding points. After 8 weeks, this small study found no significant difference between treatments. About half of the children in both groups had complete resolution (no bleeding in past 4 weeks, RR 0.92, 95% CI 0.54 to 1.59). Rates of other outcomes were also similar between groups at 8 weeks: partial success (50% reduction in number of bleeds in past 4 weeks, 4/24 v 3/24), failure (less than 50% reduction in number of bleeds in past 4 weeks, 7/24 v 6/24) and lost at 8 weeks (1/24 v 2/24). **Plus cautery:** See silver nitrate cautery, p 238.

Child health

Harms: No adverse reactions were observed with antiseptic cream, but some children found the smell and taste unpleasant. No percentages were reported. Chlorhexidine/neomycin cream may cause occasional skin reactions. Some commercial antiseptic creams contain arachis (peanut) oil. All children undergoing cautery experienced pain even with the use of 5% cocaine as local anaesthetic.[3]

Comment: Both trials involving silver nitrate cautery were undertaken in the context of secondary care.[3,4] Silver nitrate cautery is also used in primary care. It is unknown if complication rates differ.

OPTION   SILVER NITRATE CAUTERY

We found no placebo controlled trials of cautery. Small short term trials in secondary care found no significant differences between silver nitrate cautery and an antiseptic preparation. One small RCT found no advantage to adding once only silver nitrate cautery to standard treatment with a chlorhexidine/neomycin cream. All children found cautery painful.

Benefits: We found no systematic review. **Versus placebo:** We found no RCTs. **Versus antiseptic cream:** See antiseptic creams, p 237. **Plus antiseptic cream:** One RCT (40 adults, 24 children) compared once only silver nitrate cautery plus chlorhexidine hydrochloride 0.1% neomycin sulphate 3250 units/g cream twice daily for 2 weeks with antiseptic cream alone. The study included too few children to allow conclusions to be drawn.[4]

Harms: The RCT reported no harms.[4] Recognised complications of cautery include septal perforation, although the incidence following unilateral cautery in children is not known. Simultaneous bilateral cautery in children is not recommended because of an expected increased risk of perforation.

Comment: See comment under antiseptic creams above.

REFERENCES

1. Rodeghiero F, Castaman G, Dini E. Epidemiological investigation of the prevalence of von Willebrand's disease. *Blood* 1987;69:454–459.
2. Watkinson JC, Epistaxis. In: Kerr AG, Mackay IS, Bull TR eds. *Scott-Brown's Otolaryngology*, Volume 4 Rhinology. Oxford: Butterworth-Heinemann, 1997;18:1–19
3. Ruddy J, Proops DW, Pearman K, Ruddy H. Management of epistaxis in children. *Int J Paediatr Otorhinolaryngol* 1991;21:139–142.
4. Murthy P, Nilssen ELK, Rao S, McClymont LG. A randomised clinical trial of antiseptic nasal carrier cream and silver nitrate cautery in the treatment of recurrent anterior epistaxis. *Clin Otolaryngol* 1999;228–231.

Martin Burton
Consultant Otolaryngologist
The Radcliffe Infirmary
Oxford
UK

Robert Walton
Honorary Senior Clinical Lecturer
Department of Public Health and
Primary Care, University of Oxford
Institute of Health Sciences
Oxford
UK

Competing interests: None declared.

Updated this issue

James Larcombe

Child health

QUESTIONS

INTERVENTIONS

Key Messages

- Antibiotic treatment is accepted clinical practice in children with acute urinary tract infection (UTI) and placebo controlled trials are considered unethical.

- We found little evidence on the effects of delaying treatment while results of microscopy or culture are awaited. Five retrospective studies found that medium to long term delays (4 days to 7 years) in treatment may be associated with an increased risk of renal scarring, but we found inconclusive evidence that shorter delays cause harm.

- One systematic review of RCTs has found that antibiotic treatment for 7 days or longer is more effective than shorter courses.

- One RCT found no evidence of a difference between oral and intravenous antibiotics for acute treatment in children under the age of 2 years with an uncomplicated first UTI.

- We found no evidence of benefit from routine diagnostic imaging of all children with a first UTI. We found indirect evidence suggesting that people at increased risk of future morbidity may benefit from investigation.

- Two small RCTs found that prophylactic antibiotics prevented recurrent UTI in children, particularly during the period of prophylaxis. We found inadequate evaluation of the long term benefits of prophylaxis, even in children with vesicoureteric reflux. We found insufficient evidence to comment on the optimum duration of prophylaxis.

- One systematic review and a later multicentre RCT found no evidence of differences between surgery for vesicoureteric reflux and medical management in the prevention of recurrence or complications from UTI.

DEFINITION UTI is defined by the presence of a pure growth of more than 10^5 colony forming units of bacteria per ml. Lower counts of bacteria may be clinically important, especially in boys and in specimens obtained by urinary catheter. Any growth of typical urinary pathogens is considered clinically important if obtained by suprapubic aspiration. In practice, three age ranges are usually considered on the basis of differential risk and different approaches to management: children under 1 year; young children (1 to 4, 5, or 7 years, depending on the information source); and older children (up to 12–16 years). Recurrent UTI is defined as a further infection by a new organism. Relapsing UTI is defined as a further infection with the same organism.

INCIDENCE/ PREVALENCE Boys are more susceptible before the age of 3 months; thereafter the incidence is substantially higher in girls. Estimates of the true incidence of UTI depend on rates of diagnosis and investigation. At least 8% of girls and 2% of boys will have a UTI in childhood.[1]

AETIOLOGY/ RISK FACTORS The normal urinary tract is sterile. Contamination by bowel flora may result in urinary infection if a virulent organism is involved or if the child is immunosuppressed. In neonates, infection may originate from other sources. *Escherichia coli* accounts for about three quarters of all pathogens. *Proteus* is more common in boys (about 30% of infections). Obstructive anomalies are found in 0–4% and vesicoureteric reflux in 8–40% of children being investigated for their first UTI.[2] Although vesicoureteric reflux is a major risk factor for adverse outcome, other as yet unidentified triggers may also need to be present.

PROGNOSIS After first infection, about half of girls have a further infection in the first year and three quarters within 2 years.[3] We found no figures for boys, but a review suggests that recurrences are common under 1 year of age but rare subsequently.[4] Renal scarring occurs in 5–15% of children within 1–2 years of their first UTI, although 32–70% of these scars are noted at the time of initial assessment.[2] The incidence of renal scarring rises with each episode of infection in childhood.[5] An RCT of medical versus surgical management of severe vesicoureteric reflux found that younger children (under 2 years) were at greater risk of renal scarring than older children, measured by dimercaptosuccinic acid (DMSA) scintigraphy, regardless of treatment allocation (AR for deterioration in DMSA scan over 5 years 21/86 younger children v 27/201 older children; RR 1.82, 95% CI 1.09 to 3.03).[6] Renal scarring is associated with future complications: poor renal growth; recurrent adult pyelonephritis; impaired glomerular function; early hypertension; and end stage renal failure.[7–10] A combination of recurrent urinary infection, severe vesicoureteric reflux, and the presence of renal scarring at first presentation is associated with the worst prognosis.

AIMS	To relieve acute symptoms; to eliminate infection; and to prevent recurrence, renal damage, and long term complications.
OUTCOMES	Short term: clinical symptoms and signs (dysuria, frequency, fever); urine culture; incidence of new renal scars. Long term: incidence of recurrent infection; prevalence of renal scarring; renal size and growth; renal function; prevalence of hypertension and renal failure.
METHODS	*Clinical Evidence update* search and appraisal May 2000. We gave priority to studies on the basis of their methods, relevance, and applicability.

What are the effects of treatment of acute urinary tract infection in children?

We found little evidence on the effects of giving early empirical treatment versus awaiting the results of microscopy or culture. Five retrospective studies found that delayed treatment may be associated with increased rates of renal scarring, but we found inconclusive evidence on the effects of shorter delays. Placebo controlled trials of antibiotics for symptomatic acute UTI in children would be considered unethical. One systematic review found that antibiotic treatment for 7 days or longer was more effective than short courses.

Benefits:
Immediate empirical versus delayed treatment: We found no RCTs comparing immediate empirical treatment versus treatment delayed while microscopy or culture results are awaited. Five retrospective observational studies found increased rates of scarring in children in whom diagnosis was delayed between 4 days (in acute UTI) to 7 years (when a child presented with chronic non-specific symptoms).[2] We found one RCT that compared oral versus intravenous antibiotic treatment for UTI in children under 2 years (see below). It found no evidence that children treated 24 hours after the onset of fever were at greater risk of renal scarring than children presenting within 24 hours (9/99 children presenting before 24 hours developed scarring v 19/159 children presenting later; RR 1.3, 95% CI 0.6 to 2.7; P = 0.29). However, this incidental analysis was done retrospectively.[11] **Long versus short courses:** We found one systematic review of 14 RCTs (search date not stated) comparing short course (single dose to 4 days) versus treatment of conventional duration (7–10 days).[12] It found two trials that were adequately powered to find an effect; both found that short courses were less effective than conventional treatment (data from the higher quality RCT: AR of failure to cure 37% with short course v 8% with long course; ARI short v long course 29%; RR 4.6, no 95% CI given; P < 0.01). The remaining 12 trials found no significant difference between long versus short courses but were too small to rule out a clinically important difference (see comment below). We found no RCTs comparing 5 day courses of antibiotics with other regimens. **Oral versus intravenous antibiotics:** We found one RCT in 309 children aged up to 2 years presenting with fever greater than 38.2 °C and their first UTI, confirmed from catheter specimen.[11] The trial compared oral cefixime for 14 days versus intravenous cefotaxime for 3 days plus 11 days of oral cefixime and found no significant difference between treatments for

mean duration of fever (24.7 hours with oral treatment v 23.9 hours with intravenous; P = 0.76), reinfection rate (132/153 children [86.3%] with oral treatment v 134/153 children [87.6%] with intravenous treatment; P = 0.28), incidence of renal scarring (intention to treat analysis: 15/153 [9.8%] with oral treatment [21 children not scanned] v 11/153 [7.2%] with intravenous treatment [13 children not scanned]; P = 0.21) and mean extent of scarring (7.9% of renal parenchyma with oral treatment v 8.6% with intravenous treatment).

Harms: **Long versus short courses:** The studies did not report comparative harms for long versus short courses of antibiotics nor for immediate versus delayed treatment. **Oral versus intravenous antibiotics:** We found weak evidence from a post-hoc subgroup analysis in children with grade III to IV (see glossary, p 245) reflux that renal scarring at 6 months may be more common with oral versus intravenous treatment (new renal scarring within 6 months: 8/24 children after oral antibiotics v 1/22 after intravenous antibiotics; ARI 29%, 95% CI 8% to 49%; NNH 3, 95% CI 2 to 13).[11]

Comment: We found no good evidence for predicting which children are at high risk of complications after an acute UTI. The RCT comparing oral versus intravenous antibiotics found retrospectively that new renal scarring after a first UTI was more common in children with vesicoureteric reflux than in children without (logistic regression model: AR of scarring 16/107 [15.0%] children with reflux v 10/165 [6.1%] children without; RR 2.47, 95% CI 1.17 to 5.24).[11] **Long versus short courses:** The systematic review comparing long versus short courses of antibiotics rigorously evaluated the methods of the included studies. It found that few studies accounted for confounding factors such as age, sex, and previous UTI. Those that considered these did so by selecting one subgroup only and not by stratifying children according to these factors which limits the generaliseability of the results. The 12 trials that found no evidence of a difference between long and short courses were too low powered to exclude a clinically important effect. **Oral versus intravenous antibiotics:** The trial comparing oral versus intravenous antibiotics excluded three of 309 children because investigators considered that the severity of symptoms in these children warranted intravenous treatment.[11]

QUESTION   **Which children benefit from diagnostic imaging?**

We found no evidence of benefit from routine diagnostic imaging of all children with a first UTI. We found indirect evidence suggesting that subgroups at increased risk of future morbidity may benefit from investigation.

Benefits: We found no RCTs. One systematic review of 63 descriptive studies (search date 1994) found no direct evidence that routine diagnostic imaging in children with UTI was effective.[2] The quality of studies was generally poor, and none included clinically important long term outcome measures.

Harms: The studies reported no evidence on harms. Potential harms include those relating to radiation, invasive procedures, and allergic reactions to contrast media.

Comment: Subgroups of children at high risk of future morbidity, including those with vesicoureteric reflux, may benefit from early investigation.[2] However, it may be difficult to identify such children clinically.[13] One prospective study found that the highest rates of renal scarring after pyelonephritis occurred between 1 and 5 years of age.[14] A further study found that presentation with pyelonephritic symptoms in older children is associated with higher rates of renal abnormalities.[15]

QUESTION What are the effects of preventive interventions?

OPTION PROPHYLACTIC ANTIBIOTICS

We found limited evidence from two small RCTs that prophylactic antibiotics reduce UTI recurrence in children, particularly during the period of prophylaxis. We found inadequate evaluation of the long term benefits of prophylaxis, even in children with vesicoureteric reflux. We found insufficient evidence to comment on the optimum duration of prophylaxis.

Benefits: **Versus no prophylaxis:** We found no systematic review. One RCT in 45 children (40 girls, 5 boys) with radiologically normal urinary tracts, no vesicoureteric reflux, and first or subsequent acute UTI compared 10 months' treatment with prophylactic antibiotics versus no treatment.[3] During the prophylaxis period, recurrent UTIs were reported in none of the children in the intervention group compared with 11 in the control group (AR 0% v 50%; ARR 50%, 95% CI not available). Twelve months after stopping prophylactic antibiotics, fewer children from the intervention group had experienced a UTI compared with those in the control group (AR 32% v 64%; ARR 27%, 95% CI −1.8% to +47%). One further double blind, crossover trial in 18 girls (one of whom had vesicoureteric reflux) aged 3–13 years found two episodes of infection in 1 year in girls taking antibiotics compared with 35 in the control groups (P < 0.01).[16] **Duration of prophylaxis:** We found no RCTs evaluating the optimum length of prophylaxis even in children with vesicoureteric reflux (although two studies of prolonged acute treatment were identified).[17]

Harms: Potential harms include those of using long term antibiotics. In one study, although gut flora were affected by treatment, E coli cultured from rectal swabs from 70% of children remained sensitive to the prophylactic antibiotic (co-trimoxazole).[18]

Comment: It may not be possible clinically to identify children who are at high risk of recurrent UTIs and long term damage.[19] Routine prophylaxis until the results of investigations are known may therefore be warranted.

OPTION SURGICAL CORRECTION FOR ANOMALIES OBSTRUCTING MICTURITION

We found no good studies evaluating surgical correction.

Benefits: We found no systematic review or RCTs.

Child health

Harms: Potential harms include the usual risks of surgery.

Comment: One small prospective study (271 children) suggested that children with minor anomalies do not develop renal scarring and may therefore not benefit from surgery.[20] Eight of 20 children with moderate degrees of vesicoureteric reflux had renal scars compared with none of the six children with minor anomalies. In the presence of major anomalies, the prevention of UTIs is not the prime motive of surgical intervention.

OPTION SURGICAL CORRECTION FOR VESICOURETERIC REFLUX

One systematic review and a later multicentre RCT found that, although surgery abolished reflux, there was no evidence of a difference between surgery and medical management in the prevention of recurrence or complications from UTIs. We found no evidence on the long term effects of surgical versus medical treatment for clinical outcomes.

Benefits: We found one systematic review of studies published before 1989, which included four RCTs comparing surgical correction in a total of 830 children with moderate/severe (grade III to V) vesicoureteric reflux versus medical management (continuous prophylactic antibiotics).[21] It found that surgery abolished reflux, but there were no significant differences in rates of subsequent UTIs, renal function, incidence of new renal scars, hypertension, or end stage renal failure among groups over a period of 6 months to 5 years. One later RCT in 132 children found that surgery reduced the incidence of pyelonephritis, although it found no significant difference in overall clinical outcome (pyelonephritis in 5/64 treated surgically versus 15/68 treated medically; ARR 14%, 95% CI 2% to 19%; RRR 65%, 95% CI 10% to 87%).[22] **Long term outcome:** We found no systematic review or RCTs.

Harms: The review gave no information on surgical complications, and none of the individual studies were designed to compare rates of adverse effects.[21] In one arm of the later RCT, seven of nine children who had postoperative obstruction developed evidence of renal scarring on DMSA scintigraphy. This may have negated an otherwise beneficial effect of surgery over medical management.[6]

Comment: Best results were obtained by centres handling the greatest number of cases.[23] Surgery is usually considered only in children with more severe vesicoureteric reflux (grade III to V), who are less likely to experience spontaneous resolution.[4,24] **Long term outcome:** We found one prospective cohort study in 226 children aged 5 days to 12 years who presented with UTI and were found to have grade III to IV vesicoureteric reflux.[7] It found that surgery was associated with a higher rate of resolution of reflux compared with medical treatment (AR of resolution from age 8 to 14 on micturating cystourethrography 29/33 managed surgically v 134/193 managed medically; ARR 19%, 95% CI 6% to 31%) but did not compare clinical outcomes.

GLOSSARY

Severity of vesicoureteric reflux:

Grade I Reflux into ureter only.

Grade II Reflux into ureter, pelvis, and calyces.

Grade III Mild/moderate dilatation or tortuosity of ureter, and mild/moderate dilatation of pelvis, but little or no forniceal blunting.

Grade IV As grade III, but with complete obliteration of forniceal angles, yet maintenance of papillary impressions in calyces.

Grade V Gross dilatation of ureters, pelvis, and calyces, and papillary impressions in calyces obliterated.

REFERENCES

1. Stark H. Urinary tract infections in girls: the cost-effectiveness of currently recommended investigative routines. *Pediatr Nephrol* 1997;11: 174–177.

2. Dick PT, Feldman W. Routine diagnostic imaging for childhood urinary tract infections: a systematic overview. *J Pediatr* 1996;128:15–22. Search date 1994; primary sources Medline 1966 to October 1994; hand searching of article bibliographies; and Current Contents.

3. Smellie JM, Katz G, Gruneberg RN. Controlled trial of prophylactic treatment in childhood urinary tract infection. *Lancet* 1978;ii:175–178.

4. Jodal U, Hansson S, Hjalmas K. Medical or surgical management for children with vesico-ureteric reflux? *Acta Paediatr Suppl* 1999;431: 53–61.

5. Jodal U. The natural history of bacteriuria in childhood. *Infect Dis Clin North Am* 1987;1:713–729.

6. Piepsz A, Tamminen-Mobius T, Reiners C, et al. Five-year study of medical and surgical treatment in children with severe vesico-ureteric reflux dimercaptosuccinic acid findings. International Reflux Study Group in Europe. *Eur J Pediatr* 1998; 157:753–758.

7. Smellie JM, Prescod NP, Shaw PJ, Risdon RA, Bryant TN. Childhood reflux and urinary infection: a follow-up of 10–41 years in 226 adults. *Pediatr Nephrol* 1998;12:727–736.

8. Berg UB. Long-term follow-up of renal morphology and function in children with recurrent pyelonephritis. *J Urol* 1992;148:1715–1720.

9. Martinell J, Claeson I, Lidin-Janson G, Jodal U. Urinary infection, reflux and renal scarring in females continuously followed for 13–38 years. *Pediatr Nephrol* 1995;104:379–136.

10. Jacobson S, Eklof O, Erikkson CG, Lins LE, Tidgren B. Development of hypertension and uraemia after pyelonephritis in childhood: 27 year follow up. *BMJ* 1989;299:703–706.

11. Hoberman A, Wald ER, Hickey RW, et al. Oral versus initial intravenous therapy for urinary tract infections in young febrile children. *Pediatrics* 1999;104:79–86.

12. Moffatt M, Embree J, Grimm P, Law B. Short-course antibiotic therapy for urinary tract infections in children: a methodological review of the literature. *Am J Dis Child* 1988;142:57–61.

No search date or primary sources given.

13. Smellie JM, Normand ICS, Katz G. Children with urinary infection: a comparison of those with and those without vesicoureteric reflux. *Kidney Int* 1981;20:717–722.

14. Benador D, Benador N, Slozman D, Mermillod B, Girardin E. Are younger patients at higher risk of renal sequelae after pyelonephritis? *Lancet* 1997; 349:17–19.

15. Rosenberg AR, Rossleigh MA, Brydon MP, Bass SJ, Leighton DM, Farnsworth RH. Evaluation of acute urinary tract infection in children by dimercaptosuccinic acid scintography: a prospective study. *J Urol* 1992;148:1746–1749.

16. Lohr JA, Nunley DH, Howards SS, Ford RF. Prevention of recurrent urinary tract infections in girls. *Pediatrics* 1977;59:562–565.

17. Garin EH, Campos A, Homsy Y. Primary vesico-ureteral reflux: a review of current concepts. *Pediatr Nephrol* 1998;12:249–256.

18. Smellie JM, Gruneberg RN, Leakey A, Atkin WS. Long term low dose co-trimoxazole in prophylaxis of childhood urinary tract infection: clinical aspects/bacteriological aspects. *BMJ* 1976;ii: 203–208.

19. Greenfield SP, Ng M, Gran J. Experience with vesicoureteric reflux in children: clinical characteristics. *J Urol* 1997;158:574–577.

20. Pylkannen J, Vilska J, Koskimies O. The value of childhood urinary tract infection in predicting renal injury. *Acta Paediatr Scand* 1981;70:879–883.

21. Shanon A, Feldman W. Methodological limitations in the literature on vesicoureteric reflux: a critical review. *J Pediatr* 1990;117:171–178. Search date 1988. Primary source: *Medline* 1972 to November 1988.

22. Weiss R, Duckett J, Spitzer A. Results of a randomized clinical trial of medical versus surgical management of infants and children with grades III and IV primary vesico-ureteral reflux (United States): the international reflux study in children. *J Urol* 1992;148:1667–1673.

23. Smellie JM. Commentary: management of children with severe vesicoureteral reflux. *J Urol* 1992;148:1676–1678.

24. Sciagra R, Materassi M, Rossi V, et al. Alternative approaches to the prognostic stratification of mild to moderate primary vesicoureteral reflux in children. *J Urol (Paris)* 1996;155:2052–2056.

James Larcombe
General Practitioner
Sedgefield
UK

Competing interests: None declared.

Digestive system disorders

Updated this issue

John Scholefield

INTERVENTIONS

Beneficial
Adjuvant chemotherapy in Dukes' type C colorectal cancer 247

Likely to be beneficial
Adjuvant chemotherapy in Dukes' type B colorectal cancer 247
Colonoscopy to detect metachronous cancers and polyps 249
3–5 yearly follow up 249
Total mesorectal excision 250

Trade off between benefits and harms
Preoperative radiotherapy 248

Unknown effectiveness
Preoperative versus postoperative radiotherapy 248

Unlikely to be beneficial
Annual or biannual follow up (no better than less frequent) . . .249

To be covered in future issues of *Clinical Evidence*
Surgery
Colonoscopic polypectomy
Chemotherapy via portal vein infusion
Immunotherapy
Specialist versus generalist surgical care
Liver resection for metastases

Key Messages

- RCTs have found that adjuvant chemotherapy improves 5 year survival by at least 5% in people with Dukes' type B and C tumours. The evidence of benefit in people with Dukes' type B tumours is less clear. We found no good data on harmful effects.

- We found limited evidence suggesting that annual or biannual follow up is no better than 3–5 yearly follow up in terms of detection of recurrence or survival. The harms of follow up are poorly understood.

- RCTs have found that, compared with surgery alone, preoperative radiotherapy significantly reduces the risk of local recurrence and can improve survival in some people with rectal cancer. About a third of people develop associated impairment of bowel function. One RCT found no significant survival benefit from short course preoperative radiotherapy compared with a longer course of postoperative radiotherapy.

- We found no RCTs that evaluated mesorectal excision for rectal cancer. Non-randomised studies suggest that it may reduce the rate of recurrence.

DEFINITION	Colorectal cancer is a malignant neoplasm arising from the lining (mucosa) of the large intestine (colon and rectum). Nearly two thirds of colorectal cancers occur in the rectum or sigmoid colon.
INCIDENCE/ PREVALENCE	Colorectal cancer is the third most common malignancy in the developed world. It accounts for about 20 000 deaths per year in the UK and 60 000 deaths per year in the USA. Although the incidence of and mortality from colorectal cancer have changed little over the past 40 years, recent evidence shows that the incidence of the disease is falling in both the UK and the USA.[1,2] Colon cancer affects almost equal proportions of men and women, most commonly between the ages of 60 and 80. Rectal cancer is more common in men.[1] In the UK, about a quarter of people with colorectal cancer present as emergencies with either intestinal obstruction or perforation.[3,4]
AETIOLOGY/ RISK FACTORS	The pathogenesis of colorectal cancer involves genetic and environmental factors. The most important environmental factor is probably diet.[5]
PROGNOSIS	Overall 5 year survival is about 50% and has not changed over the past 40 years. Evidence from USA and UK cancer registries shows that disease specific mortality is decreasing but reasons are unclear.[1,2] Surgery is undertaken with curative intent in over 80% of people, but about half suffer recurrence.
AIMS	To remove the tumour in order to prevent bowel obstruction or perforation; to avoid creating a permanent stoma by restoring intestinal continuity wherever technically possible; to prevent or minimise metastasis; to minimise adverse effects of treatment, and maximise quality of life.
OUTCOMES	Survival, proportion of patients with permanent stoma, incidence of local recurrence, rates of metastasis, adverse effects of treatment, quality of life.
METHODS	*Clinical Evidence* update search and appraisal May 2000, using key words: colorectal cancer, neoplasia, adjuvant chemotherapy, surgery, follow up, recurrence. All identified RCTs were reviewed.

QUESTION What are the effects of adjuvant chemotherapy?

RCTs have found that adjuvant systemic chemotherapy improves survival by at least 5% in people with Dukes' type B and C tumours. The evidence of benefit in people with Dukes' type B tumours is less clear. One recent, large multicentre trial found no effect of portal vein infusion adjuvant chemotherapy on 5 year survival. We found no good data on harmful effects.

Benefits: We found one systematic review (search date 1993), which identified 29 RCTs of adjuvant treatment in colorectal cancer (1673 people with Dukes' type C colon cancer and 695 with Dukes' type B or C rectal cancer).[6] The review reported a small but significant improvement in overall survival (OR for death with adjuvant versus no adjuvant treatment 0.91, 95% CI 0.83 to 0.99), which translated into an overall improvement in 5 year survival of 5% for people with colon cancer and 9% for people with rectal cancer. Twenty four of the 29 RCTs dated from before 1990. The data were less clear cut for Dukes' B than for Dukes' C type tumours, in part because of the smaller numbers of Dukes' type B tumours. A pooled analysis of three RCTs of adjuvant fluorouracil and folinic acid in colon cancer found a 10% survival advantage for Dukes' type C tumours at 3 years but no significant survival advantage for Dukes' type B tumours.[7]

Harms: We found little good evidence on the adverse effects of chemotherapy or on its impact on quality of life, partly because of the many different regimens used.[6] In the RCTs included in the systematic review, the incidence of severe adverse effects (stomatitis, diarrhoea, nausea, and leukopenia) with 5-fluorouracil and levamisole ranged from 10–30%, with life threatening toxicity occurring in around 5% of people. For every 10 people treated, up to three will experience an additional, severe adverse effect. However, three studies reported deaths related to chemotherapy in nearly 2% of people with advanced disease.

Comment: A much larger RCT of the effects of adjuvant chemotherapy in Dukes' type B tumours is now underway in the UK (D Kerr, personal communication, 1999).

QUESTION   What is the effect of preoperative radiotherapy for rectal cancer?

RCTs have found that, compared with surgery alone, preoperative radiotherapy significantly reduces the risk of local recurrence and can improve survival in some people with rectal cancer. About a third of the people have associated impairment of bowel function. One RCT found no significant survival benefit from short course preoperative radiotherapy compared with a longer course of postoperative radiotherapy.

Benefits: **Versus surgery alone:** We found no systematic review, but found one non-systematic review (published in 1999),[8] which identified 11 studies of preoperative radiotherapy versus surgery alone. The review did not pool data. Several RCTs found a significant reduction in the local recurrence rate, and a few found a survival advantage.[9–11] **Versus postoperative radiotherapy:** We found no systematic review. One RCT compared a short course of preoperative radiotherapy (25.5 Gy in 1 week) versus postoperative radiotherapy (60 Gy over 7–8 weeks) in people with Dukes' B or C rectal carcinoma. After 5 years, there was no significant difference between treatments for overall survival (P = 0.5), but preoperative radiotherapy significantly reduced local recurrence rates (13% with preoperative v 22% with postoperative treatment, P = 0.02).[12]

Harms: We found one systematic review (search date 1998) of morbidities associated with adjuvant radiotherapy.[13] **Versus surgery alone:** The review identified 19 RCTs of preoperative radiotherapy versus surgery alone (n = 5110). Preoperative radiotherapy was associated with significantly higher early postoperative morbidity and mortality compared with surgery alone. Early harms include diarrhoea, wound infections (20% with preoperative radiotherapy v 10% with surgery alone), bowel obstruction, cardiovascular problems, and pain. Analysis of data from 1027 people in two RCTs found that preoperative radiotherapy significantly increased the risk of venous thromboembolism, fracture of the hip, intestinal obstruction, postoperative fistulae, cardiovascular, and thrombotic events compared with surgery alone.[14] Increased bowel frequency and urgency impaired social life in around 30% of people after preoperative radiotherapy.[15] In patients with low rectal tumours, who underwent abdominoperineal excision, preoperative radiotherapy was associated with twice the rate of perineal wound breakdown compared with surgery alone (20% v 10%).[13] **Versus postoperative radiotherapy:** The systematic review[13] identified nine RCTs of postoperative radiotherapy. It found a greater risk of anastomotic complications (breakdown and stricture formation) after postoperative compared with preoperative radiotherapy.

Comment: The risk of local recurrence for T1 and T2 tumours is so low that preoperative radiotherapy is unlikely to provide much absolute benefit. There are unresolved issues about preoperative staging of rectal cancers and case selection for preoperative radiotherapy.

QUESTION What are the effects of routine follow up for colorectal cancer?

We found limited evidence that non-intensive surveillance (colonoscopy and computed tomography [CT] every 3–5 years) may be beneficial, but that more intensive, annual or biannual follow up confers no additional benefit. Whether the interval between follow up visits should be 3 or 5 years is uncertain. The potential harms of follow up are poorly understood. Limited evidence suggests that follow up is reassuring to most people.

Benefits: We found no systematic review. We found two RCTs. One, in 1418 people who had undergone removal of adenomatous polyps, compared follow up colonoscopy at 1 and 3 years versus 3 years only.[16] The proportion of participants in whom new polyps were detected was higher with more frequent follow up (42% v 32%; RR of detection compared with less frequent follow up 1.3, 95% CI 1.1 to 1.6). However, there was no significant difference in the proportion of detected polyps with advanced pathology (about 3% in both groups; RR 1.0, 95% CI 0.5 to 2.2). The other RCT, in 325 people who had undergone curative resection for newly diagnosed colorectal cancer (Dukes' type A, B, or C), compared standard versus intensive follow up. Standard follow up comprised clinical review (history, examination, liver function tests, carcinoembryonic antigen, and faecal occult blood testing) 3 monthly for 2 years, and thereafter 6 monthly for 5 years or until a major end point was reached. Intensive follow up comprised standard clinical review (as above) plus annual chest radiograph, CT scan of the liver, and colonoscopy. At 5 years' follow up there was no significant difference in survival between the two groups. Annual colonoscopy did not detect any asymptomatic local recurrences.[17]

Harms: Presymptomatic diagnosis of incurable recurrent disease may increase anxiety and reduce quality of life. Invasive tests such as colonoscopy also carry risks. No data on these outcomes were reported in the trials.

Comment: One RCT in 212 people being followed up after treatment for colorectal cancer found that 78% were "rather reassured" or "very reassured" by follow up. However, follow up had no effect on quality of life. Most trial participants said that they would still prefer follow up even if it did not lead to earlier detection of recurrence.[18] Current follow up regimens are haphazard in frequency and intensity. We found no evidence about whether follow up should be discontinued in elderly people (aged > 75 years), although many people with colorectal cancer fall into this age group. In the UK, people over the age of 75 years are not routinely considered for chemotherapy because of its potential toxicity. We found no firm evidence to comment on this policy. The role of carcino-embryonic antigen monitoring is also uncertain as 30% of colorectal cancers do not express this antigen.

QUESTION **What are the effects of total mesorectal excision for rectal cancer?**

We found no RCTs that evaluated total mesorectal excision for rectal cancer. Non-randomised studies suggest that it may reduce the rate of local recurrence.

Benefits: We found no systematic review or RCTs. We found several non-randomised studies (see table 1, p 252).[19–23]

Harms: With conventional anterior resection, some of the rectum is retained. The removal of the rectum in total mesorectal excision necessitates coloanal anastomosis, which increases stool frequency (median 4–5/day v 1–2/day with techniques leaving a rectal stump). Observational data found that resection also carries a higher incidence of anastomotic leakage (11–15% v 8–10%).[23] In order to reduce the incidence of anastomotic leakage, many surgeons routinely use a temporary defunctioning stoma after total mesorectal excision.[19]

Comment: Rectal cancer surgery is more technically demanding than colon cancer resection. An increasing volume of data (but no RCTs) suggest that surgical technique is especially important in resecting rectal cancer.

REFERENCES

1. *Mortality statistics, cause, England and Wales 1993.* OPCS dh22. London: HMSO, 1995.
2. Miller BA, Ries LA, Hankey BF, et al. *Cancer statistics review 1973–1989.* Rockville (MD): National Institutes of Health, National Cancer Institute. Report No: NIH-NCI 92–2789.
3. Mella J, Biffen A, Radcliffe AG, Stamatakis JD, Steele RJ. A population based on audit of colorectal cancer management in two United Kingdom health districts. *Br J Surg* 1997;84: 1731–1736.
4. Scholefield JH, Robinson MHE, Mangham C, Hardcastle JD. Screening for colorectal cancer reduces emergency admissions. *Eur J Surg Oncol* 1998;24:47–50.
5. Kune G, ed. *Causes and control of colorectal cancer: a model for cancer prevention.* Boston: Kluwer Academic Publishers, 1996.
6. Dube S, Heyen, F Jenicek M. Adjuvant chemotherapy in colorectal carcinoma. Results of a meta analysis. *Dis Colon Rectum* 1997;40:35–

41. Search date January 1959 to June 1993; primary source Medline.
7. International Multicenter Pooled Analysis of Colon Cancer Trials (IMPACT) Investigators. Efficacy of adjuvant fluouracil and folinic acid in colon cancer. *Lancet* 1995;348:939–944.
8. Wheeler JM, Warren BF, Jones AC, Mortensen NJ. Preoperative radiotherapy for rectal cancer: implications for surgeons, pathologists and radiologists. *Br J Surg* 1999;86:1108–1120. Search date not stated; primary source Medline (English language only).
9. Marsh P, James R, Schofield P. Adjuvant pre-opertive radiotherapy for locally advanced rectal carcinoma. Results from a propspective, randomised trial. *Dis Colon Rectum* 1994;37: 1205–1214.
10. Swedish Rectal Cancer Trial. Improved survival with pre-operative radiotherpay in resectable rectal cancer. *N Engl J Med* 1997;336;980–987.
11. Oates G, Stenning S, McAdam W, et al,

Randomised trial of surgery alone versus radiotherpay followed by surgery for potentially operable locally advanced rectal cancer. *Lancet* 1996;348:1605–1610.

12. Jansson-Frykholm G, GlimeliusB, Pahlman L. Preoperative or postoperative irradiation in adenocarcinoma of the rectum. Final treatment results of a randomised trial and an evaluation of late secondary effects. *Dis Colon Rectum* 1993; 36:564–572.

13. Ooi B, Tjandra J, Green M. Morbidities of adjuvant chemotherapy and radiotherapy for resectable rectal cancer: an overview. *Dis Colon and Rectum* 1999;42:403–418. Search date 1998; primary source Medline (English language only).

14. Holm T, Singnomklao T, Rutqvist LE, Cedermark B. Adjuvant preoperative radiotherapy in patients with rectal carcinoma. Adverse effects during long term follow-up of two trials. *Cancer* 1996;78:968–976.

15. Dahlberg M, Glimelius B, Graf W, Pahlman L. Preoperative irradiation affects functional results after surgery for rectal cancer: results from a randomised study. *Dis Colon Rectum* 1998;41: 543–549.

16. Winawer SJ, Zauber AG, O'Brien MJ, et al. Randomised comparison of surveillance intervals after colonoscopic removal of newly diagnosed adenomatous polyps: the national polyp study workgroup. *N Engl J Med* 1993;328:901–906.

17. Shoemaker D, Black R, Giles L, Toouli J. Yearly colonoscopy, liver CT and chest radiography do not influence 5 year survival of colorectal cancer patients. *Gastroenterology* 1998;114:7–14.

18. Stiggelbout AM, de Haes JCJM, Vree R, et al. Follow up of colorectal cancer patients: quality of life and attitudes towards follow up. *Br J Cancer* 1997;75:914–920.

19. McFarlane JK, Ryall RDH, Heald RJ. Mesorectal excision for rectal cancer. *Lancet* 1993;341:457–460.

20. Enker WE, Thaler HT, Cranor ML, Polyak T. Total mesorectal excision in the operative treatment of carcinoma of the rectum. *J Am Coll Surg* 1995; 181:335–346.

21. Singh S, Morgan MBF, Broughton M, Caffarey S, Topham C, Marks CG. A ten-year prospective audit of outcome of surgical treatment for colorectal carcinoma. *Br J Surg* 1995;82:1486–1490.

22. Arbman G, Nilsson E, Hallbook O, Sjodahl R. Local recurrence following total mesorectal excision for rectal cancer. *Br J Surg* 1996;83:375–379.

23. Karanja ND, Corder AP, Bearn P, Heald RJ. Leakage from stapled low anastomosis after total mesorectal excision for carcinoma of the rectum. *Br J Surg* 1994;81:1224–1226.

John Scholefield
Professor of Surgery
University Hospital
Nottingham
UK

Competing interests: None declared.

Digestive system disorders

TABLE 1 Effects of total mesorectal excision: results of non-randomised studies (see text, p 250).

Study	Duke's stage (number of patients)	Intervention	Recurrence at 5 years (95% CI)		RRR of death by 5 years (95% CI)	Incidence of anastomic leak (95% CI)
			Local	Overall		
McFarlane, et al.[19]	B (88)	TME	5% (0 to 7.5%)	18% (10 to 25%)	78% (68 to 88%)	11% clinical
	C (73)					6.4% radiological
Enker, et al.[20]	B (99) C (147)	TME	7.3%	23%	74%	NA
Singh, et al.[21]	A, B and C (158 in total)	TME	8%	24%	60%	10%
Arbman, et al.[22]	A (67) B (89) C (100)	TME Non-TME	6% at 1 year 14% at 1 year	NA	NA	8% (57% stoma rate) 9% (15% stoma rate)

TME, total mesorectal excision; NA not applicable.

David Katzka, Brendan Delaney, David Forman and Paul Moayyedi

Digestive system disorders

INTERVENTIONS

Key Messages

In people with non-erosive reflux disease

- One systematic review of RCTs that directly compared H_2 antagonists and proton pump inhibitors (PPIs) versus placebo has found both are more effective than placebo for symptom relief.

- One systematic review of RCTs that directly compared daily H_2 antagonists with PPIs has found PPIs are more effective for symptom relief.

- One RCT found PPIs are better than H_2 antagonists for maintaining remission.

- We found no evidence about surgical treatment for non-erosive disease.

In people with erosive oesophagitis

- One systematic review of indirect comparisons found that PPIs were more effective than H_2 antagonists at healing erosive oesophagitis, and that both were more effective than placebo. RCTs found no significant difference in rates of short term adverse events. We found no good data on long term risks of treatment or on possible long term benefits. One RCT found no evidence of a difference in relapse rates between PPIs and H_2 antagonists when used intermittently, although relief of symptoms was more rapid with PPIs.

- One RCT found no significant difference in effectiveness among different PPIs for people with erosive disease.
- We found no good evidence adequately comparing medical and surgical treatments in RCTs. One RCT found fundoplication to be significantly more effective than medical treatment, but it did not use PPIs, which might have increased the effectiveness of the medical treatment. We found no good comparative data on preventing relapse or complications.
- One RCT found that fundic mobilisation had no effect on postoperative symptoms or rates of cure, but increased rates of sliding hiatus hernia. One RCT found no difference in outcomes between total or partial fundoplication, other than increased flatulence with total fundoplication.

In people with gastro-oesophageal reflux complicated by erosive gastritis or Barrett's oesophagus

- We found no good evidence on the effects of treatment for gastro-oesophageal reflux in people with Barrett's oesophagus.

In people with extraoesophageal symptoms

- One systematic review did not find any evidence of an improvement in lung function in people with asthma treated for gastro-oesophageal reflux disease.

DEFINITION	Gastro-oesophageal reflux occurs when gastric contents enter the oesophagus because of transient or chronic relaxation of the lower oesophageal sphincter. Excessive reflux causes symptoms of gastro-oesophageal reflux disease (heartburn, acid taste in the mouth). It can be divided into non-erosive oesophagitis (predominant heartburn with a normal endoscopy, also termed "endoscopy negative reflux disease") and erosive oesophagitis (endoscopy shows inflammation and erosions).
INCIDENCE/ PREVALENCE	Gastro-oesophageal reflux disease is common. Weekly heartburn occurs in up to 20% of people questioned in population surveys. Up to 10% of these will have erosive disease.
AETIOLOGY/ RISK FACTORS	We found no evidence of clear predictive factors for gastro-oesophageal reflux disease.
PROGNOSIS	Gastro-oesophageal reflux disease is generally benign with little mortality. However, persistent symptoms can interfere with normal activities and cause considerable morbidity. Long term retrospective data (up to 22 years) suggest that in people with an initially normal endoscopy, endoscopy tends to remain normal.[1] A small subset of people develop strictures, Barrett's oesophagus, adenocarcinoma, or extraoesophageal manifestations (see table 1, p 265).[2]
AIMS	To relieve symptoms; to prevent complications in those with severe oesophagitis; to control extraoesophageal manifestations; to minimise adverse effects of treatment; to improve quality of life.
OUTCOMES	Frequency and severity of symptoms, degree of oesophagitis, prevalence and severity of extraoesophageal manifestations, incidence of stricture, adenocarcinoma. Symptoms do not correlate closely with the extent of oesophagitis. People with Barrett's oesophagus may have minimal symptoms, whereas people with severe symptoms may have no evidence of oesophagitis on endo-

scopy. Proxy outcomes include atrophic gastritis and Barrett's oesophagus, which some studies have found to be associated with adenocarcinoma.[3,4]

METHODS   *Clinical Evidence* update search and appraisal June 2000.

QUESTION   **What are the effects of treatment in non-erosive oesophagitis?**

OPTION   PROTON PUMP INHIBITORS VERSUS PLACEBO

One systematic review of RCTs has found PPIs to be more effective than placebo at relieving symptoms. We found no good evidence on recurrence.

Benefits: **Symptom relief:** We found one systematic review (search date 1999), which identified five RCTs evaluating the effect of PPIs in endoscopy negative reflux disease.[5] Meta-analysis of four trials with heartburn as an outcome found PPIs were significantly better than placebo (n = 1017; AR of still having heartburn 40% *v* 67%; RR 0.68, 95% CI 0.53 to 0.88). One subsequent RCT (n = 241) also found that PPI treatment was superior to placebo (complete resolution of heartburn during week 2: 41% *v* 5%, P < 0.001).[6] **Recurrence:** We found no placebo controlled trials with recurrence as an outcome.

Harms: See harms under erosive oesophagitis, p 257.

Comment: None.

OPTION   PROTON PUMP INHIBITORS VERSUS H$_2$ ANTAGONISTS

One systematic review found limited evidence that PPIs are more effective at relieving symptoms than H$_2$ antagonists. One RCT found limited evidence that PPIs are better at preventing recurrence than H2 antagonists.

Benefits: **Symptom relief:** We found one systematic review (search date 1999) comparing PPIs versus H2 antagonists.[5] This review identified two RCTs (n = 776) in endoscopy negative reflux disease. Meta-analysis found more people improved with PPIs but the difference was not significant for heartburn remission (AR of still having heartburn: 47% *v* 58%; RR 0.81, 95% CI 0.70 to 0.94). We found one subsequent RCT (n = 901), which compared lansoprazole 30 mg once daily versus lansoprazole 15 mg once daily versus ranitidine 150 mg twice daily for 8 weeks.[7] This trial found that people treated with PPIs had significantly lower heartburn scores (symptom free for at least 80% of treatment days: 37% with lansoprazole 15 mg, 35% with lansoprazole 30 mg, 23% with ranitidine, P < 0.05 for each lansoprazole group *v* ranitidine). The trials also found omeprazole was more likely than ranitidine to improve symptom and psychological wellbeing scores. **Recurrence:** We found one RCT in people in remission comparing omeprazole (n = 134) versus ranitidine (n = 129).[8] At 12 months, significantly more people were still in remission with omeprazole (68% *v* 39%, P < 0.0001).

Digestive system disorders

Harms: See harms of erosive oesophagitis, p 257.

Comment: None.

OPTION   H$_2$ ANTAGONISTS VERSUS PLACEBO

One systematic review of RCTs has found H$_2$ antagonists are more effective than placebo at relieving heartburn.

Benefits: **Symptom relief:** We found one systematic review comparing H$_2$ antagonists versus placebo (search date 1999, 2 RCTs, n = 514).[5] The review found H$_2$ antagonists were more likely than placebo to relieve heartburn (AR of still having heartburn 65% v 78%; RR 0.84, 95% CI 0.74 to 0.95). **Recurrence:** We found no systematic reviews or RCTs.

Harms: See harms of erosive oesophagitis, p 257.

Comment: None.

OPTION   SURGICAL TREATMENT

We found insufficient evidence on the effects of surgical treatment for non-erosive oesophagitis.

Benefits: We found no systematic review or RCTs comparing medical versus surgical treatment in people with non-erosive oesophagitis, nor any comparing different surgical techniques.

Harms: We found no good evidence.

Comment: Good long term trials are needed to compare laparoscopic fundoplication with PPIs, taking into account symptom relief, adherence, prevention of complications, and adverse effects of treatment.

QUESTION   What are the effects of treatments for erosive oesophagitis?

OPTION   PROTON PUMP INHIBITORS VERSUS PLACEBO

One systematic review of pooled results across treatment arms found PPIs had faster healing rates than placebo. RCTs found PPIs were better than placebo at preventing recurrence.

Benefits: **Healing:** One systematic review (published in 1997) identified 43 single and double blind RCTs in 7635 people which compared different drug treatments versus each other, versus placebo, or both (total of 95 study arms, treatment given for 2–12 weeks).[9] By pooling results across treatment arms, PPIs provided the fastest overall healing rate (11.7% healed per week, 95% CI 10.7% to 12.6%), four times faster than placebo (2.9%, 95% CI 2.4% to 3.4%). Doses of PPIs varied, not routinely exceeding 40 mg omeprazole or 30 mg lansoprazole. **Preventing recurrence:** One RCT found omeprazole was more effective than placebo at preventing relapse (n = 193). At 12 months, remission rates with omeprazole 20 mg daily were 74% (95% CI 62% to 86%), with omeprazole 10 mg daily 50%, (95% CI 34% to 66%), and with placebo 14%

(95% CI 2% to 26%).[10] One RCT in people who had already responded symptomatically to lansoprazole found lansoprazole was more effective than placebo at preventing relapse (n = 173; 12 months' remission rates 67% with lansoprazole 30 mg, 72% with lansoprazole 15 mg, 35% with placebo, CIs not reported.[11] **Preventing complications:** We found no good evidence.

Harms: **Short term adverse effects:** Rare adverse events of PPIs in people with gastro-oesophageal reflux disease include liver function test abnormalities, increased bowel bacterial counts, cytopenias, hypersensitivity reactions, and decreased (but not clinically important) vitamin B12 levels. **Long term adverse effects:** In two studies of chronic use of PPIs in the presence of *Helicobacter pylori*, infection has been linked to atrophic gastritis after 3–5 years.[12,13] Among people treated with omeprazole, none of whom had atrophic gastritis at baseline, atrophic gastritis developed in 18 of the 59 people infected with *H pylori* and two of the 46 people who were not infected.[12] A further study reported that out of 14 people with persistent *H pylori* infection, six developed mild to severe atrophy in 5 years.[13] Subgroup analysis from one RCT comparing long term omeprazole treatment with fundoplication found more people infected with *H pylori* who were treated with omeprazole developed gastric atrophy at 3 years' follow up but, the difference was not significant (8/31 [26%] v 3/31 [10%]; RR 2.6, 95% CI 0.8 to 6.1).[14]

Comment: The meta-analysis[9] did not compare groups as they were randomised, but compared one group from one trial with another group from another. This loses the benefits of randomisation since the groups being compared may not have had the same characteristics. The next issue of *Clinical Evidence* will consider the results from the individual trials. The clinical significance of atrophic gastritis is as a risk factor for gastric cancer, but there is debate about whether a clear definition of atrophic gastritis exists.[3–4]

OPTION   **PROTON PUMP INHIBITORS VERSUS H₂ ANTAGONISTS**

One systematic review of indirect comparative data found that PPIs were more likely than H₂ antagonists to heal erosive oesophagitis and prevent recurrence. RCTs found no significant difference in short term rates of adverse events. We found no good data on long term risks of treatment or on possible long term benefits. One RCT found no evidence of a difference in relapse rates between a PPI and H2 antagonist when used intermittently, although relief of symptoms was more rapid with PPIs.

Benefits: One systematic review (published in 1997) indirectly compared PPIs versus H₂ antagonists. It identified 43 single and double blind RCTs in 7635 people that compared different drug treatments versus each other, versus placebo, or both (total of 95 study arms, treatment given for 2–12 weeks).[9] **Healing:** By pooling results across treatment arms (omeprazole 20–80 mg daily, lansoprazole 30–60 mg daily, pantoprazole 40 mg daily, cimetidine 800–1600 mg daily, ranitidine 300–1200 mg daily, famotidine 40–80 mg daily, nizatidine 300–600 mg daily), the review found a higher healing rate by 12 weeks of erosive oesophagitis on endoscopic examination with PPIs (84% with PPIs, 95% CI 79% to 88%, v 52% with H_2 antagonists, 95% CI 47% to 57%). PPIs provided the fastest overall healing rate with 11.7% healed per week (95% CI 10.7% to 12.6%), twice as fast as H_2 antagonists (5.9% healed per week, 95% CI 5.5% to 6.3%). Two of the RCTs added a prokinetic agent to the H_2 antagonist, but results still strongly favoured the PPI.[15,16] One subsequent RCT (n = 133) also found that PPIs were more effective for healing (confirmed endoscopically after 4 weeks 79% v 42%, P < 0.001).[17] Doses of PPIs varied, not routinely exceeding 40 mg omeprazole or 30 mg lansoprazole. **Preventing recurrence:** We found no systematic review. We found three RCTs looking at recurrence rates. Two RCTs (one double blind and one single blind) compared omeprazole versus ranitidine (with or without cisapride) in people with endoscopically confirmed oesophagitis who had already received omeprazole for 4 weeks.[18,19] At 1 year, people treated with daily omeprazole were significantly less likely to relapse than those on ranitidine. In the first RCT, 159 people were randomised to either omeprazole 20 mg daily, omeprazole 20 mg on 3 consecutive days per week ("weekend omeprazole"), or ranitidine 150 mg twice daily. At 12 months, a significantly greater proportion of people treated with daily omeprazole remained in remission compared with daily ranitidine (ARR daily omeprazole v ranitidine 64%, 95% CI 50% to 78%). The trial found no significant difference between weekend omeprazole and daily ranitidine treatments (ARR weekend omeprazole v daily ranitidine 7%, 95% CI −11% to +25%).[18] In the second RCT, 175 people were randomised to omeprazole, ranitidine, or cisapride, alone and in various combinations. At 12 months, people on omeprazole were significantly more likely to be in remission than those on either ranitidine or cisapride alone (80% still in remission with omeprazole v 50% with ranitidine or cisapride, CIs not reported).[19] **Preventing complications:** We found no RCTs that examined possible longer term benefits of medical treatment. **Intermittent treatment:** We found one recent, multicentre, double blind RCT trial of intermittent, symptomatic treatment with omeprazole (10 mg or 20 mg) versus ranitidine (150 mg) over a 12 month period (n = 677).[20] The trial found that intermittent treatment with any of these regimens was moderately effective at controlling symptoms (40% had no relapse within 12 months; 93% had three or fewer relapses in the intermittent treatment phase), and that there was no significant difference between the three groups in terms of long term relapse rates. However, symptoms were controlled more rapidly by omeprazole than ranitidine (by the second week of symptom onset, proportion of people with symptom relief was 55% with 20 mg omeprazole, 40% with 10 mg omeprazole, and 26% with ranitidine). The trial did not compare intermittent treatment with maintenance treatment.

Harms:
Short term: The placebo controlled RCTs found similar rates of adverse effects with PPIs and H_2 antagonists. Most data on significant adverse effects come from case reports or uncontrolled trials. H_2 antagonists have been associated rarely with cytopenias, gynaecomastia, liver function test abnormalities, and hypersensitivity reactions. Rare adverse effects of PPIs in people with gastro-oesophageal reflux disease include liver function test abnormalities, increased small bowel bacterial counts, cytopenias, hypersensitivity

reactions, and decreased (but not clinically important) vitamin B12 levels. **Long term:** We found no RCTs with long term follow up on the safety of chronic use of H_2 antagonists. Chronic use of PPIs in the presence of *H pylori* infection has been linked in two studies to atrophic gastritis after 3–5 years.[12,13] Among people treated with omeprazole, none of whom had atrophic gastritis at baseline, atrophic gastritis developed in 18 out of 59 people infected with *H pylori* and two out of 46 people who were not infected, compared with no new cases of atrophic gastritis among 72 people treated with fundoplication (31 with *H Pylori* and 41 without).[12] One further study reported that out of 14 people with persistent *H pylori* infection, six developed mild to severe atrophy in 5 years.[13]

Comment: The meta-analysis did not compare groups as they were randomised, but compared one group from one trial with another group from another. This loses the benefits of randomisation since the groups being compared may have different characteristics. The next issue of *Clinical Evidence* will consider the results from the individual trials. The clinical significance of atrophic gastritis is as a risk factor for gastric cancer but there is debate whether a clear definition of atrophic gastritis exists.[3,4] Cisapride has recently been withdrawn in the UK and other countries because of associated mortality.

OPTION   **DIFFERENT PROTON PUMP INHIBITORS**

One RCT found no evidence of a difference between PPIs in healing erosive oesophagitis.

Benefits: **Healing:** We found no systematic review, but found one good multicentre, double blind RCT (225 people).[21] The trial found no significant difference in the proportion healed at 8 weeks by lansoprazole 30 mg versus 20 mg omeprazole in people with erosive oesophagitis (AR healing at 8 weeks 85% with lansoprazole, 87% with omeprazole; ARR 2%, 95% CI −6% to +14%; RRR 2%, 95% −7% to +16%). Relapse rates were not evaluated. Another double blind RCT (n = 202) compared 20 mg rabeprazole with 20 mg omeprazole and found no significant difference in healing of erosive and ulcerative oesophagitis at 4 weeks (81% v 81%) and at 8 weeks (92% rabeprazole v 94% omeprazole; ARR 2%, 95% CI −3% to +15%).[22] **Preventing recurrence:** We found no systematic review or RCTs that compared different maintenance treatments. **Preventing complications:** We found one small double blind RCT with three-arms (n = 30) in people who responded to omeprazole treatment.[23] All participants were treated with dilatation of the stenosis weekly and at the clinician's discretion. The trial compared omeprazole 20 mg twice daily versus lansoprazole 30 mg twice daily versus pantoprazole 40 mg twice daily. The trial found omeprazole was superior at maintaining remission (relapse rates 10%, 80%, 70%, omeprazole v other groups combined, P = 0.001).

Harms: See PPIs versus placebo, p 257.

Comment: None.

OPTION H₂ ANTAGONISTS VERSUS PLACEBO

One systematic review found indirect evidence that H$_2$ antagonists are more effective than placebo.

Benefits: **Healing:** One systematic review (published in 1997) indirectly compared H$_2$ antagonists versus placebo.[9] The review identified 43 single blind and double blind RCTs in 7635 people that compared different drug treatments versus each other, versus placebo, or both (total of 95 study arms, treatment given for 2–12 weeks). By pooling results across treatment arms, the review found that people in trials on H$_2$ antagonists had faster healing rates (5.9% healed per week, 95% CI 5.5% to 6.3%) than people in trials on placebo (2.9% healed per week, 95% CI 2.4% to 3.4%). **Preventing recurrence:** We found no systematic review. **Preventing complications:** We found no systematic review.

Harms: We found no RCTs examining the course of incompletely treated gastro-oesophageal reflux disease, nor any good data on the natural history of inflammatory oesophageal disease.[1] We also found no data on the level of gastric acid suppression needed to ensure adequate oesophageal healing. **Short term:** The RCTs with people on placebo found similar rates of adverse effects to the RCTs with people on H$_2$ antagonists. Most evidence about adverse effects is from case reports or uncontrolled trials. H$_2$ antagonists have been associated rarely with cytopenias, gynaecomastia, liver function test abnormalities, and hypersensitivity reactions. **Long term:** We found no controlled trials with long term follow up on the safety of chronic use of H$_2$ antagonists.

Comment: The meta-analysis did not compare groups as they were randomised, but compared one group from one trial with another group from another. This loses the benefits of randomisation since the groups being compared may have different characteristics. The next issue of *Clinical Evidence* will consider the results from the individual trials.

OPTION MEDICAL VERSUS SURGICAL TREATMENT

We found no RCTs that adequately compared medical and surgical treatments. One RCT found fundoplication to be significantly more effective than medical treatment, but it did not use PPIs, which would probably have increased the effectiveness of the medical treatment. We found preliminary data suggesting that PPIs and fundoplication are almost equally effective at healing. We found no good comparative data on preventing relapse or complications.

Benefits: We found no systematic review. **Healing:** We found one RCT (243 men and 4 women) comparing medical versus surgical treatment in people with complicated gastro-oesophageal reflux disease (defined as erosive oesophagitis, Barrett's oesophagus, stricture, or oesophageal ulcer).[24] The trial compared continuous medical treatment (antacids, ranitidine, metoclopramide, or sucralfate), medical treatment for symptoms only, and open fundoplication. Evaluation was performed at 6 weeks (n = 201), 1 year (n = 176), and 2 years (n = 106), using symptom score (range 74 [least severe] to

172 [most severe]) and grade of oesophagitis (range 1 [least severe] to 4 [most severe]). People receiving fundoplication had significantly better symptom scores (mean symptom score 78 with fundoplication v 88 with symptomatic medical treatment v 90 with continuous medical treatment; P value for improvement, surgery v either medical treatment < 0.003) and grade of oesophagitis (mean decrease in grade of oesophagitis 1.5 with fundoplication v 1.9 with symptomatic medical treatment v 2.2 with continuous medical treatment; P < 0.03). **Preventing relapse:** The trial did not evaluate relapse rates. Uncontrolled trials on the long term results of open fundoplication found that up to 90% of people continued to benefit 6–20 years after surgery in terms of relief of symptoms, reduced acid exposure on pH monitoring, and absence of inflammation on endoscopy.[25–27] **Preventing complications:** We found no good data.

Harms: **Medical treatment:** See PPIs versus placebo under harms, p 257. **Surgery:** The RCT found no operative deaths, but operative complications occurred in 15% and postoperative complications occurred in 18% of people.[24] Uncontrolled studies found that intraoperative complications included splenic trauma (0–4%), viscus perforation (1–2%), and, less commonly, abscess or inadvertent vagotomy. Immediate postoperative complications included pleural effusion, pulmonary embolism, or late abscess formation. Mortality related to surgery was usually less than 1%. Late adverse effects related to fundoplication included bloating, dysphagia, gastric herniation, or breakdown of the fundoplication. Up to 15% of people underwent reoperation.

Comment: Given the evidence that PPIs are more effective than H_2 antagonists for healing and maintenance of remission (see harms of proton pump inhibitors versus H_2 antagonists, p 255),[11,18,19,28] the use of only an H_2 antagonist in the RCT[24] may have biased the results in favour of fundoplication. Preliminary data from one RCT suggest similar efficacy when comparing fundoplication with omeprazole for people with erosive oesophagitis at 3 years' follow up.[29] Individual patient characteristics may direct the clinician towards medical or surgical treatment. Some people are refractory to PPIs[30] or have severe "mechanical" reflux requiring surgery. Some people may be high risk surgical candidates or have relative contraindications to reflux surgery (e.g. scleroderma, multiple previous laparotomies, or previous gastric surgery). Younger people may prefer surgery to lifelong drug treatment. We found no studies addressing these issues.

OPTION	DIFFERENT SURGICAL TECHNIQUES

One RCT found no difference in outcomes between total or partial fundoplication other than increased flatulence with total fundoplication. We found no RCTs comparing major kinds of surgical techniques. One RCT found no evidence that fundic mobilisation improved postoperative symptoms or rates of cure, but found that it increased rates of sliding hiatus hernia. One RCT found laparoscopic fundoplication was associated with more dysphagia than open surgery.

Benefits: **Total versus partial fundoplication:** We found one RCT comparing a total Nissen versus Toupet partial posterior fundoplication in

106 people with endoscopically proven gastro-oesophageal reflux.[31] The trial found no significant difference over a 3 year period in recurrent reflux symptoms or dysphagia between groups. **Fundic mobilisation:** We found one RCT of fundic mobilisation versus no mobilisation of Nissen fundoplication in 40 people undergoing surgery for confirmed gastro-oesophageal reflux.[32] It found no significant difference in recurrent reflux symptoms or oesophagitis between the two groups over a 3 year follow up period. We found no RCTs comparing techniques with Dor fundoplication or Hill gastroplasty. **Laparoscopic versus open surgery:** We found one RCT, which compared laparoscopic with open Nissen fundoplication in people with gastro-oesophageal reflux disease.[33] The trial found laparoscopic Nissen fundoplication was as effective as open surgery in controlling reflux symptoms but was associated with more dysphagia (7/46 with laparoscopic treatment v 0/57 with open treatment; P = 0.02), and the trial was discontinued at the interim analysis stage.

Harms: Individuals undergoing total fundoplication reported significantly more flatulence (P < 0.01).[31] Sliding hiatus hernia was significantly more common in those with fundic mobilisation (9/21 v 1/19; P = 0.02).[32]

Comment: None.

QUESTION **Does treatment for gastro-oesophageal reflux disease reduce the risk of progression of Barrett's oesophagus?**

We found no good evidence on the effects of treatment for gastro-oesophageal reflux in people with Barrett's oesophagus. One RCT found no significant difference in symptom control with omeprazole compared with ranitidine but it provided no clinical relevant outcomes on progression of Barrett's oesophagus.

Benefits: One double blind RCT randomised 68 people with Barrett's oesophagus to omeprazole 40 mg twice daily or ranitidine 150 mg twice daily.[34] Symptomatic control was better in the omeprazole arm, although this did not reach statistical significance. This was reflected in a significantly lower percentage of acid reflux after 3 months' treatment (0.1% v 9.4%, P < 0.001). The trial found a significant reduction in the area of Barrett's oesophagus in people allocated to omeprazole but the clinical significance of this finding is uncertain. Uncontrolled studies looking at the long term effect of cimetidine,[35] ranitidine,[35] or fundoplication[36] in people with Barrett's oesophagus found no significant effect. One uncontrolled study of PPIs found evidence of regression of Barrett's oesophagus,[37] but other uncontrolled studies found no evidence of regression.[38,39] None of these studies followed more than 27 people. Small, long term studies of the effects of fundoplication on Barrett's oesophagus found that effective fundoplication (defined by ambulatory pH monitoring, symptoms, and endoscopy) may lead to regression.[40,41]

Harms: We found no good evidence on harms of treatments for gastro-oesophageal reflux in people with Barrett's oesophagus. Small, long term studies of fundoplication suggest that after failed procedures there may be progression to dysplasia and carcinoma.[40,41]

Comment: Few centres see enough people with Barrett's oesophagus to perform long term RCTs. In addition, our poor understanding of the pathophysiology of Barrett's oesophagus means that we do not know what end point of treatment for gastro-oesophageal reflux (symptom relief, healing, elimination of acid reflux) may change the course of Barrett's metaplasia. It is also not clear whether progression can be measured endoscopically.[42,43] Only a long term, multicentre trial will be able to answer these questions.

QUESTION **Does treatment for gastro-oesophageal reflux alter outcome in people with extraoesophageal manifestations of gastro-oesophageal reflux disease?**

We found one systematic review which found no improvement in lung function in asthmatics treated for gastro-oesophageal reflux. We found no RCTs that looked at effects of treatment on other extraoesophageal manifestations (see table 1, p 265).

Benefits: **Asthma:** We found one systematic review of the effects of treatments in gastro-oesophageal reflux on asthma severity.[44] The review identified nine RCTs (3 of PPIs, 5 of H_2 antagonists, and one of long term conservative management). It found anti-reflux treatment did not consistently improve asthma symptoms, lung function, or the use of asthma medications compared with placebo. The reviewers concluded that there is no evidence that treating gastro-oesophageal reflux improves asthma symptoms, although they could not exclude the possibility that specific subgroups may benefit from this approach. **Other extraoesophageal manifestations:** We found no RCTs. One prospective open label cohort study of omeprazole in 182 people with chronic laryngitis and reflux found an improvement in symptoms.[45]

Harms: We found no good data on harms of treatment for gastro-oesophageal reflux specifically in people with extraoesophageal symptoms.

Comment: The link between extraoesophageal symptoms and gastro-oesophageal reflux is by association and it is often difficult to prove that gastro-oesophageal reflux is the primary cause. There was little standardisation in these trials with regard to treatments used or patient characteristics. Before good RCTs can be performed, further research must first identify clear criteria for reflux as the cause of these syndromes.

Substantive changes since last issue

PPIs versus H_2 antagonists One new systematic review and one subsequent RCT found PPIs are better than H_2 antagonists for symptom relief in non-erosive oesophagitis.[5,7]

PPIs versus H_2 antagonists One new RCT found that PPIs are more effective than H_2 antagonists for healing erosive oesophagitis.[14]

Omeprazole One small new RCT found omeprazole was superior to other PPIs for maintaining remission.[17]

Gastro-oesophageal reflux disease

Omeprazole Subgroup analysis from one RCT comparing omeprazole versus fundoplication found atrophic gastritis in 26% of the omeprazole group compared with 10% of the surgical group in *H pylori* positive people after 3 years' follow up. This difference was not significant.[23]

Laparoscopic Nissen fundoplication One RCT found laparoscopic Nissen fundoplication was as effective as open surgery in controlling reflux symptoms but was associated with more dysphagia.[33]

Omeprazole An RCT in people with Barrett's oesophagus found omeprazole insignificantly reduced symptoms compared with ranitidine.[34]

Asthmatics treated for gastro-oesophageal reflux One systematic review of RCTs found no evidence that treating gastro-oesophageal reflux improves asthma symptoms.[44]

REFERENCES

1. Isolauri J, Luostarinen M, Isolauri E, et al. The natural course of gastroesophageal reflux disease: 17–22 year follow-up of 60 patients. *Am J Gastroenterol* 1997;92:37–41.

2. Richter JE. Extraesophageal manifestations of gastroesophageal reflux disease. *Clin Perspectives* 1998;1:28–39.

3. Genta RM. Review article: gastric atrophy and atrophic gastritis – nebulous concepts in search of a definition. *Aliment Pharmacol Ther* 1998; 12(suppl 1):17–23.

4. Kokkola A, Haapianinen R, Laxen F, et al. Risk of gastric carcinoma in patients with mucosal dysplasia associated with atrophic gastritis: a follow up study. *J Clin Pathol* 1996;49:979–984.

5. Van Pinxteren B, Numans ME, Bonis PA, Lau J. Short-term treatment with proton pump inhibitors, H2-receptor antagonists and prokinetics for gastro-oesophageal reflux disease-like symptoms and endoscopy negative reflux disease. In: The Cochrane Library, Issue 2, 2000. Oxford: Update Software. Search date 1999.

6. Richter JE, Peura D, Benjamin SB, Joelsson B, Whipple J. Efficacy of omeprazole for the treatment of symptomatic acid reflux disease without esophagitis. *Arch Intern Med* 2000;160: 1810–1816.

7. Richter JE, Campbell DR, Kahrilas PJ, Huang B, Fludas C. Lansoprazole compared with ranitidine for the treatment of nonerosive gastroesophageal reflux disease. *Arch Intern Med* 2000;160:1803–1809.

8. Festen HPM, Shenk E, Tan G, et al. Omeprazole versus high-dose ranitidine in mild gastroesophageal reflux disease: short- and long-term treatment. *Am J Gastroenterol* 1999;94: 931–936.

9. Chiba N, DeGara CJ, Wilkinson JM, Hunt RH. Speed of healing and symptom relief in grade II to IV gastroesophageal reflux disease: a metaanalysis. *Gastroenterology* 1997;112:1798–1810. Search date July 1996; primary sources Medline and manual search of earlier issues of *Eur J Gastroenterol Hepatol*. Reference lists of retrieved articles searched.

10. Bate CM, Booth SN, Crowe JP, et al. Omeprazole 10 mg or 20 mg once daily in the prevention of recurrence of reflux oesophagitis. *Gut* 1995;36: 492–498.

11. Robinson M, Lanza F, Avner D, Haber M. Effective maintenance treatment of reflux esophagitis with low-dose lansoprazole: a randomized double blind placebo-controlled trial. *Ann Intern Med* 1996; 124:859–867.

12. Kuipers EJ, Lundell L, Klinkenberg-Knol EC, et al. Atrophic gastritis and *Helicobacter pylori* infection in patients with reflux esophagitis treated with omeprazole or fundoplication. *N Engl J Med* 1996; 334:1018–1022.

13. Eissele R, Brunner G, Simon B, Solcia E, Arnold R. Gastric mucosa during treatment with lansoprazole: *Helicobacter pylori* is a risk factor for argyrophil cell hyperplasia. *Gastroenterology* 1997;112:707–717.

14. Lundell L, Miettinen P, Myrvold HE, et al. Lack of effect of acid suppression therapy on gastric atrophy. *Gastroenterology* 1999;117:319–326.

15. Richter JE, Sabesin SM, Kogut DG, et al. Omeprazole versus ranitidine or ranitidine/metoclopramide in poorly responsive symptomatic gastroesophageal reflux disease. *Am J Gastroenterol* 1996;91:1766–1772.

16. Robinson M, Decktor DL, Maton PN, et al. Omeprazole is superior to ranitidine plus metoclopramide in the short-term treatment of erosive esophagitis. *Aliment Pharmacol Ther* 1993;7:67–73.

17. Jansen JB, Van Oene JC. Standard-dose lansoprazole is more effective than high-dose ranitidine in achieving endoscopic healing and symptom relief in patients with moderately severe reflux oesophagitis. *Aliment Pharmacol Ther* 1999; 13:1611–1620.

18. Dent J, Yeomans ND, Mackinnon M, et al. Omeprazole v ranitidine for prevention of relapse in reflux oesophagitis: a controlled double blind trial of their efficacy and safety. *Gut* 1994;35:590–598.

19. Vigneri S, Termini R, Leandro G, et al. A comparison of five maintenance therapies for reflux esophagitis. *N Engl J Med* 1995;333:1106–1110.

20. Bardhan KD, M ler-Lissner S, et al. Symptomatic gastro-oesophageal reflux disease: double-blind controlled study of intermittent treatment with omeprazole or ranitidine. *BMJ* 1999;318:502–507.

21. Hatlebakk JG, Berstad A, Carling L, et al. Lansoprazole versus omeprazole in short-term treatment of reflux oesophagitis. Results of a Scandinavian multicentre trial. *Scand J Gastroenterol* 1993;28:224–228.

22. Dekkers CP, Beker JA, Thjodleifsson B, et al. Double-blind, placebo-controlled comparison of rabeprazole 20 mg vs omeprazole 20 mg in the treatment of erosive or ulcerative gastro-oesophageal reflux disease. The European Rabeprazole Study Group. *Aliment Pharmacol Ther* 1999;13:49–50.

23. Jaspersen D, Diehl KL, Schoeppner H, Geyer P, Martens E. A comparison of omeprazole, lansoprazole and pantoprazole in the maintenance treatment of sever reflux oesophagitis. *Aliment Pharmacol Ther* 1998;12:49–52.

24. Spechler SJ. Comparison of medical and surgical therapy for complicated gastroesophageal reflux disease in veterans. *N Engl J Med* 1992;326: 786–792.

25. Martinez de Haro LF, Ortiz A, Parrilla P, et al. Long-term results of Nissen fundoplication in reflux esophagitis without strictures: clinical, endoscopic, and pH-metric evaluation. *Dig Dis Sci* 1992;37: 523–527.

26. Bjerkeset T, Edna T-H, Fjosne U. Long-term results after 'floppy' Nissen/Rosetti fundoplication for gastroesophageal reflux disease. *Scand J Gastroenterol* 1992;27:707–710.

27. Luostarinen M, Isolauri J, Laitinen J, et al. Fate of Nissen fundoplication after 20 years: a clinical, endoscopical, and functional analysis. *Gut* 1993; 34:1015–1020.

28. Klinkenberg-Knol EC, Festen HPM, Jansen JBMJ, et al. Long-term treatment with omeprazole for refractory reflux esophagitis: efficacy and safety. *Ann Intern Med* 1994;121:161–167.

29. Lundell L, Dalenback J, Hattlebakk J, et al. Omeprazole or antireflux surgery in the long term management of gastroesophageal reflux disease: results of a multicenter, randomized clinical trial. *Gastroenterology* 1998;114:A207.

30. Leite L, Johnston B, Just R, Castell DO. Persistent acid secretion during omeprazole therapy: a study of gastric acid profiles in patients demonstrating failure of omeprazole therapy. *Am J Gastroenterol* 1996;91:1527–1531.

31. Rydberg L, Ruth M, Abrahamsson H, Lundel L. Tailoring antireflux surgery: a randomized clinical trial. *World J Surg* 1999;23:612–618.

32. Luostarinen MES, Isolauri JO. Randomized trial to study the effect of fundic mobilization on long-term results of Nissen fundoplication. *Br J Surg* 1999;86:614–618.

33. Bais JE, Bartelsman JF, Bonjer HJ, et al. Laparoscopic or conventional Nissen fundoplication for gastro-oesophageal reflux disease: randomised clinical trial. *Lancet* 2000; 355:170–174.

34. Peters FTM, Ganesh S, Kuipers EJ, et al. Endoscopic regression of Barrett's oesophagus during omeprazole treatment: a randomised double blind study. *Gut* 1999;45:489–494.

35. Sampliner RE, Garewal HS, Fennerty MB, Aickin M. Lack of impact of therapy on extent of Barrett's esophagus in 67 patients. *Dig Dis Sci* 1990;35: 93–96.

36. Williamson WA, Ellis FH Jr, Gibb SP, Shahian DM, Aretz T. Effect of antireflux operation on Barrett's mucosa. *Ann Thorac Surg* 1990;49:537–542.

37. Gore S, Healey CJ, Sutton R, et al. Regression of columnar lined (Barrett's) esophagus with continuous omeprazole therapy. *Aliment Pharmacol Ther* 1993;7:623–628.

38. Sampliner RE. Effect of up to 3 years of high-dose lansoprazole on Barrett's esophagus. *Am J Gastroenterol* 1994;89:1844–1848.

39. Sharma P, Sampliner RE, Camargo E. Normalization of esophageal pH with high-dose proton pump inhibitor therapy does not result in regression of Barrett's esophagus. *Am J Gastroenterol* 1997;92:582–585.

40. Sagar PM, Ackroyd R, Hosie KB, et al. Regression and progression of Barrett's esophagus after antireflux surgery. *Br J Surg* 1995;82:806–810.

41. Csendes A, Braghetto I, Burdiles P, et al. Long-term results of classic antireflux surgery in 152 patients with Barrett's esophagus: clinical, radiologic, endoscopic, manometric and acid reflux test analysis before and late after operation. *Surgery* 1998;123:645–657.

42. Kim R, Baggott BB, Rose S, et al. Quantitative endoscopy: precise computerized measurement of metaplastic epithelial surface area in Barrett's esophagus. *Gastroenterology* 1995;108:360–366.

43. Sharma P, Morales TG, Bhattacharyya A, Garewal HS, Sampliner RE. Squamous islands in Barrett's esophagus: what lies underneath? *Am J Gastroenterol* 1998;93:332–335.

44. Gibson PG, Henry RL, Coughlan JL. Gastro-oesophageal reflux treatment for asthma in adults and children. In: The Cochrane Library, Issue 2, 2000. Oxford: Update Software. Search date not given; primary sources Cochrane Airways Group trials register; hand searched references.

45. Hanson DG, Kamel PL, Kahrilas PJ. Outcomes of anti-reflux therapy in the treatment of chronic laryngitis. *Ann Otol Rhinol Laryngol* 1995;104: 550–555.

David Katzka
Associate Professor
Hospital of the University of
Pennsylvania
Philadelphia
USA

Brendan Delaney
Senior Lecturer
University of Birmingham
Birmingham
UK

David Forman
Professor

Paul Moayyedi
Senior Lecturer

University of Leeds
Leeds
UK

Competing interests: PM has received lecture fees from AstraZeneca, and TAP-Abbott. DF has received lecture fees from AstraZeneca, Glaxo-Wellcome, Wyeth, and Takeda.

TABLE 1	**Extraoesophageal manifestations of gastro-oesophageal reflux disease (see text, p 254, p 263).**[2]		
Pulmonary	**Ear, nose, and throat**	**Other**	
Asthma, chronic bronchitis, aspiration pneumonia, sleep apnoea, atelectasis, interstitial pulmonary fibrosis	Chronic cough, hoarseness, enamel erosion, halitosis, pharyngitis, subglottic stenosis, vocal cord inflammation, granuloma, possible cancer	Non-cardiac chest pain, chronic hiccups, nausea	

Stomach cancer

Updated this issue

Peter McCulloch

INTERVENTIONS

Likely to be beneficial

Trade off between benefits and harms

Unknown effectiveness

Unlikely to be beneficial

To be covered in future issues of *Clinical Evidence*

Adjuvant radiotherapy

Adjuvant chemoradiotherapy

Endoscopic mucosal resection for early gastric cancer

Addition of bacterial and fungal extracts to adjuvant chemotherapy

Regional chemotherapy

See glossary, p 272

Key Messages

- Prospective and retrospective cohort studies have found a strong association between survival and complete excision of all tumour, with microscopic confirmation of clear resection margins.
- Retrospective cohort studies have found short survival and high perioperative mortality but improved quality of life in symptomatic people undergoing palliative gastrectomy.
- Two RCTs have found similar survival after total gastrectomy and subtotal gastrectomy in people with primary tumours in the distal stomach.
- Retrospective subgroup analysis of RCTs and prospective cohort studies has found increased morbidity and mortality from resection of additional organs (spleen and distal pancreas) versus no resection.
- Four RCTs have found no clear evidence of benefit or harm from extended lymph node dissection.
- Two systematic reviews of RCTs have found weak evidence of improved survival from adjuvant pre- or postoperative chemotherapy for stomach cancer.

© *Clinical Evidence* 2000;4:266–275.

DEFINITION	Stomach cancer is an adenocarcinoma arising in the stomach, including tumours arising at or just below the gastro-oesophageal junction (type 2 and 3 junctional tumours). Tumours are staged according to degree of invasion and spread (see table 1, p 275).
INCIDENCE/ PREVALENCE	The incidence of stomach cancer varies among countries and by sex (incidence per 100 000 population per year in Japanese men is around 80, Japanese women 30, British men 18, British women 10, white American men 11, white American women 7).[1] Incidence has declined dramatically in North America, Australia, and New Zealand since 1930, but decline in Europe has been slower.[2] In the USA, stomach cancer remains relatively common among particular ethnic groups, especially Japanese-Americans and some Hispanic groups. The incidence of cancer of the proximal stomach and gastro-oesophageal junction is rising rapidly in most Western countries; the reasons for this are poorly understood.[3,4]
AETIOLOGY/ RISK FACTORS	Distal stomach cancer is strongly associated with lifelong infection with *Helicobacter pylori* and poor dietary intake of antioxidant vitamins (A, C, E).[5,6] In Western Europe and North America, distal stomach cancer is associated with relative socioeconomic deprivation. Proximal cancer is strongly associated with smoking (OR around 4)[7] and is probably associated with gastro-oesophageal reflux, obesity, high fat intake, and medium to high socioeconomic status.[7]
PROGNOSIS	Invasive cancer (stages T_2–T_4) is fatal without surgery. Mean survival without treatment is less than 6 months from diagnosis.[8,9] Intramucosal or submucosal cancer (stage T_1) may progress slowly to invasive cancer over several years.[10] The prognosis after macroscopically and microscopically complete resection (R0) is related strongly to disease stage (see glossary, p 273), particularly penetration of the serosa (stage T_3) and lymph node involvement. Five year survival rates range from over 90% in intramucosal cancer to about 20% in people with stage T_3N_2 disease (see table 1, p 275). In the USA, over 50% of people recently diagnosed with stomach cancer have regional lymph node metastasis or involvement of adjacent organs. In Japan, the 5 year survival rate for advanced disease is reported to be around 50%, but the explanation of the difference remains unclear. Comparisons between Japanese and Western practice are confounded by factors such as age, fitness, and disease stage, as well as by tumour location because many Western series include gastro-oesophageal junction adenocarcinoma with a much lower survival after surgery.
AIMS	To prevent progression, extend survival, and relieve symptoms, with minimal adverse effects.
OUTCOMES	Survival, quality of life, adverse effects of treatment.
METHODS	*Clinical Evidence* update search and appraisal May 2000. Hand searches of conference proceedings and consultation with experts was also used to identify relevant studies.

OPTION   COMPLETE VERSUS INCOMPLETE TUMOUR RESECTION

Prospective and retrospective cohort studies have found a strong association between survival and complete excision of the primary tumour.

Benefits: **Surgery versus no surgery:** We found no systematic reviews or RCTs. We found two observational studies of surgery versus no surgery. People who did not undergo resection (generally those with the most advanced disease and highest comorbidity) had a near zero 5 year survival in all case series.[8,9] In people with similar stage, weight loss, and performance status, macroscopically incomplete tumour resection (palliative gastrectomy) was associated with twice the survival time of non-resection and with better quality of life due to relief of tumour symptoms.[11] **Positive versus clear microscopic resection margins:** We found no systematic reviews or RCTs that directly compared these options. Multivariate risk factor analysis of RCTs and retrospective cohort studies have found that failure to achieve microscopically clear resection margins was associated with a poor outcome independently of other indicators of tumour spread and behaviour.[12–14]

Harms: We found no systematic reviews or RCTs.

Comment: Current consensus is that improving long term survival is best achieved by complete resection of the primary tumour with microscopic confirmation of clear resection margins ("curative" gastrectomy).

OPTION   TOTAL VERSUS SUBTOTAL GASTRECTOMY FOR RESECTABLE DISTAL TUMOURS

Two RCTs have found similar survival after total and distal subtotal gastrectomy in people with primary tumours in the distal stomach.

Benefits: We found no systematic review but found two RCTs (n = 787) comparing total versus subtotal gastrectomy.[15–18] Neither RCT used blinded allocation. **Five year survival:** The larger RCT involved 648 people aged under 76 years with a resectable tumour and a macroscopic proximal margin of more than 6 cm.[17,18] All had regional lymphadenectomy (D2). There was no significant difference between the groups in the incidence of microscopic resection margin involvement (found in 15/315 [4.8%] with subtotal gastrectomy v 297/303 [2.0%] with total gastrectomy (see glossary, p 273); ARI 2.8%, 95% CI −0.1% to +9.6%) or in 5 year survival (Kaplan-Meier 5 year survival estimates 65% for subtotal v 62% for total gastrectomy; HR 0.89, 95% CI 0.68 to 1.17). Multivariate analysis found that after adjustment for covariates, the type of stomach surgery had no influence on survival (5 year HR 1.01, 95% CI 0.76 to 1.33). The other RCT studied 169 people with potentially curable distal stomach cancer. No difference was found in 5 year survival (48% in each group, CI not available). **Nutritional function**

and quality of life: These outcomes were better after distal subtotal gastrectomy than after total gastrectomy.[19-22]

Harms: **Postoperative morbidity:** Included intra-abdominal sepsis, chest infections, wound sepsis, and fistulae. The larger RCT found that subtotal gastrectomy reduced postoperative morbidity (29/320 [9%] for subtotal gastrectomy v 40/304 [13%] after total gastrectomy), and mean duration of hospital stay (13.8 days for subtotal v 15.4 days for total gastrectomy).[17,18] The other RCT found no significant differences in postoperative morbidity (25/76 [32%] for total gastrectomy v 32/93 [34%] for subtotal gastrectomy).[15,16]
Postoperative mortality: In the larger RCT, this was lower in the subtotal gastrectomy group, but not significantly so [1%] for subtotal v 7/304 [2%] for total). The other RCT found no significant differences in postoperative mortality (1/76 [1.3%] for total v 3/93 [3.2%] for subtotal gastrectomy). Nearly all non-randomised studies that we identified reported higher mortality after total gastrectomy compared with subtotal gastrectomy, but total gastrectomy tended to be performed on people with more extensive disease.

Comment: Infiltration of the proximal resection margin by microscopic tumour deposits is perceived as a problem in people with poorly differentiated "diffuse" cancer of the distal stomach undergoing distal subtotal gastrectomy. Some surgeons have therefore recommended total gastrectomy "de principe" (see glossary, p 273) for these tumours. The two RCTs have found similar survival after total and distal subtotal gastrectomy in people with primary tumours in the distal stomach. However, blinding of allocation was not performed in either RCT.[15-18] Both RCTs recruited otherwise fit people, which may explain the low postoperative mortality rates. The lack of any evidence of survival benefit, and the poorer nutritional and quality of life outcome, argue against total gastrectomy where subtotal distal gastrectomy (see glossary, p 273) is technically possible with an adequate margin.

OPTION	REMOVAL OF ADJACENT ORGANS

Retrospective analyses of removal of additional organs (spleen and distal pancreas) versus no removal have found increased morbidity and mortality.

Benefits: We found no systematic reviews and no RCTs that randomised people with stomach cancer to removal or no removal of adjacent organ.

Harms: Retrospective analyses of RCTs and cohort studies in which removal of the spleen and distal pancreas had been performed routinely during radical total gastrectomy (D2) (see table 2, p 275), and at the surgeon's discretion during non-radical total gastrectomy (D1) (see table 2, p 275), found that removal of the spleen or distal pancreas was associated with increased perioperative mortality (OR about 2) and no evidence of improved long term survival.[23,24]

Comment: Some advocates of radical surgery have suggested routine removal of the spleen and distal pancreas to ensure complete regional lymph node dissection during total gastrectomy. Current consensus is that removal of adjacent organs is justified only when necessary to ensure complete tumour removal, or when required because of trauma during surgery.

| OPTION | RADICAL VERSUS CONSERVATIVE LYMPHADENECTOMY |

Four RCTs have found no clear benefit from extended lymph node removal. The results may be affected by lack of experience with the extended dissection technique.

Benefits:

Regional (D2, D3) versus local lymphadenectomy (D1): We found no systematic review. Four RCTs (n = 711, 400, 55, and 43 people) compared radical removal of regional and local perigastric lymph nodes (see glossary, p 272) versus conservative removal of just the local lymph nodes.[25–28] There were no significant differences in overall 5 year survival. The largest trial reported 5 year survival rates of 45% after D1 resection and 47% after D2 resection (ARR 2%, 95% CI −5.6% to +9.6%).[28] The second largest trial reported non-significantly lower survival with radical removal (survival at 5 years 35% v 33%, HR 95% CI 0.87 to 1.39).[27] Subgroup analysis suggests a possible advantage for D2 resection in people with stage II and IIIA disease (corresponding to $T_1N_2M_0$, $T_2N_1M_0$, $T_3N_0M_0$, $T_2N_2M_0$, $T_3N_1M_0$, and $T_4N_0M_0$), particularly in people who did not have additional organ removal. **Para-aortic (D4) versus regional and local (D3, D2) lymphadenectomy:** We found one small RCT performed in Japan, which compared removal of local, regional, and para-aortic lymph nodes versus removal of only local and regional lymph nodes (see glossary, p 272) in 70 people with stomach cancer that had spread to the serosa or adjacent organs (T_3 or T_4).[29] This pilot study was too small to detect clinically important differences in survival.

Harms:

The four RCTs of regional and local versus local lymphadenectomy found increased perioperative mortality with the more extensive operation.[23–26] In the second largest trial, mortality was 13% with D2 resection versus 6% with D1 (P < 0.04).[24] In the largest trial, the difference in mortality nearly achieved significance (10% with D2 v 6% with D1, P = 0.06).[23] In both of these large trials, the excess mortality was associated closely with greater frequency of pancreatic and splenic removal with D2 resection.[23,24]

Comment:

One large prospective cohort study (1654 people with gastric cancer) found no benefit from D2 resection (defined within this study as over 25 lymph nodes removed; 300 people) versus D1 resection (25 or fewer nodes removed; 1096 people) in the entire cohort of people with gastric cancer after 10 years' follow up. A subgroup analysis found that there may be a beneficial effect of D2 versus D1 resection in the subgroup of people with stage II tumours (230 people; RR of long term survival 1.8, 95% CI 1.3 to 2.7).[30] Cohort studies comparing radical and conservative lymphadenectomy are affected by numerous biases, including selection bias owing to a recent tendency towards more radical treatment, patient differences (age, cancer stage, comorbidity), definition differences (in the meaning of "limited" and "extended"), and stage migration bias (see glossary, p 272). These biases make the interpretation of observational data difficult. The randomised trials were conducted by surgeons with limited prior experience and training in D2 resection, and may have been affected by both learning curve effects[31] and failure to apply the assigned treatment (contamination and non-compliance).[32] Differences in age, cancer stage, and comorbidity may explain why mortality for gastrectomy in Western countries remains high at 5–10%, compared with around 1% in many Japanese reports.[33]

QUESTION **What are the effects of adjuvant chemotherapy?**

Two systematic reviews of RCTs have found weak evidence of a beneficial effect of adjuvant chemotherapy (see glossary, p 272). The size of any benefit remains uncertain, but the treatment is frequently associated with morbidity, and can be associated with mortality. Modern regimens have not been evaluated fully in RCTs.

Benefits: **Adjuvant chemotherapy versus surgery alone:** We found two systematic reviews[34,35] and nine additional RCTs that compared adjuvant chemotherapy versus surgery alone. The first systematic review (search date 1991, 11 RCTs, 2096 people) found that adjuvant chemotherapy compared with surgery alone reduced the risk of death by the end of follow up, but the result was not significant (OR 0.88, 95% CI 0.78 to 1.08).[34] This review was criticised for involving trials that included people with known residual tumour after surgery, and trials that also included immunotherapy and intraperitoneal delivery of the adjuvant therapy. A subsequent update by the authors revised the meta-analysis (OR 0.82, 95% CI 0.68 to 0.97).[36] The second systematic review (search date 1999, 13 RCTs, 1990 people in non-Asian countries) excluded trials that included people with known residual tumour after surgery or that also included immunotherapy and intraperitoneal therapy.[35] The review found that adjuvant chemotherapy versus surgery alone reduced the risk of death slightly (AR 595/979 [61%] with chemotherapy v 660/1011 [65%] for controls; OR 0.80, 95% CI 0.66 to 0.97; RRR 6%, 95% CI 0% to 11%). We found eight Japanese trials that compared adjuvant chemotherapy versus surgery alone. In one of these trials, 579 people were randomised after curative gastrectomy for early cancer (stage T_1 and T_2) to either adjuvant chemotherapy (mitomycin, fluorouracil, uracil, and tegafur) or to no further treatment.[37] After a median follow up of 72 months, there was no significant difference in the death rate (47/288 [16%] with chemotherapy v 59/291 [20%] with no further treatment; OR 0.77, 95% CI 0.50 to 1.17). Of seven older studies published before 1985, only one found a significant benefit for chemotherapy.[38] This study included 120 people in three arms, and found a significant benefit for adjuvant mitomycin, cytarabine, and fluorouracil over both adjuvant mitomycin and surgery alone. However, a multi-institutional study of the same regimens with over 1200 patients failed to confirm this.[39] One recent small RCT (248 people thought to have stage II or stage III gastric cancer before surgery) found that surgery plus postoperative intraperitoneal chemotherapy versus surgery alone had no significant effect on 5 year survival (39% with surgery and chemotherapy v 29% with surgery only, P = 0.22).[40] Subgroup analysis found that in people with stage III gastric cancer adjuvant intraperitoneal chemotherapy may increase 5 year survival (49% v 18%). **Adjuvant chemotherapy in palliative care:** We found no systematic review, but found one RCT that compared no preoperative adjuvant treatment versus intravenous chemotherapy versus superselective intra-arterial chemotherapy in 386 consecutive people diagnosed with gastric cancer in a Ukrainian cancer centre who preoperatively were thought to have no liver or peritoneal metastases, no enlarged lymph nodes, and no locally advanced disease. All had surgery and 74 were then discovered to be inoperable. Subgroup analysis of these people found that compared with no adjuvant treatment, 1 year survival was significantly increased by selective intra-arterial chemotherapy but not by intravenous chemotherapy (11/20 survivors at 1 year with intra-arterial chemotherapy v 0/43 in the other groups; ARR 54%, 95% CI 5% to 95%; RR 47, 95% CI 5.3 to 82; NNT 2, 95% CI 1 to 20). The median survival was 91 days with no adjuvant treatment, 96 days with intravenous treatment, and 401 days with intra-arterial treatment.[41]

Harms: Two RCTs reported toxicity (mainly nausea and vomiting) in 53% of people.[42,43] Serious toxicity was usually due to cardiac or cumulative haematological problems; treatment related mortality was 1–2%. We found no definitive evidence from completed studies to justify the concern that preoperative chemotherapy increases postoperative morbidity or mortality.

Comment: The two systematic reviews included six RCTs in common. Only published trials were included. All included trials were reported in English. There was no evidence of publication bias. No statistical heterogeneity of effects was found, but a random effects meta-analysis was used, which may give a conservative estimate of the treatment effect. The observed significant effect might indicate a true effect or the impact of undetected biases. It is not known if certain subgroups respond more than others: a subgroup analysis in the second systematic review suggested an effect only in RCTs in which at least two thirds had node positive disease, but the power was insufficient to draw definite conclusions. Japanese adjuvant chemotherapy regimens often contain bacterial or fungal extracts. We found some evidence from one well designed RCT that addition of these substances to combined surgery and chemotherapy was associated with improved 5 year survival; this will be reviewed in a future issue.[44] The RCT of adjuvant chemotherapy in palliative care identified people before surgery who appeared to have no tumour spread, but who during surgery were found to have tumour spread. The analysis applies to only 19% of those randomised and may not generalise to all people with inoperable gastric cancer.

GLOSSARY

Adjuvant chemotherapy Treatment with cytotoxic drugs given in addition to surgery in an attempt to achieve cure.

Perigastric lymph nodes Lymph nodes that lie adjacent to the stomach.

Regional lymph nodes Lymph nodes that lie along the blood vessels that supply the stomach.

Stage migration bias Apparent increase in stage specific survival without influencing overall survival caused by recategorisation of the stage following removal of diseased lymph nodes.

Disease stage Surgical and microscopic assessment of the primary tumour. Microscopic spread to distant sites can be detected only by radical surgery, creating a potential bias (see glossary, p 272).

Subtotal distal gastrectomy Removal of lower part (usually two thirds or four fifths) of the stomach.

Super-radical extended lymphadenectomy A D4 lymph node dissection (see table 2, p 275) resection of additional organs, including pancreas, colon, kidney, and adrenal gland, to achieve full clearance of nodal disease.

Total gastrectomy Removal of the whole stomach.

Total gastrectomy "de principe" Total gastrectomy where it is not technically necessary to remove a distal tumour; this technique is used minimise the risk of resection line involvement or later second cancer of the gastric stump.

Substantive changes since last issue

Radical versus conservative lymphadenectomy One additional prospective cohort study found that D2 resection may be of benefit in stage II disease after 10 years' follow up.[30]

Adjuvant chemotherapy One additional RCT of surgery plus postoperative intra-peritoneal chemotherapy versus surgery alone found no significant effect on overall 5 year survival,[40] and one additional RCT of no preoperative adjuvant treatment versus intravenous chemotherapy versus superselective intra-arterial chemo-therapy in people with inoperable gastric cancer;[41] conclusions unchanged.

REFERENCES

1. Whelan SL, Parkin DM, Masuyer E, eds. *Trends in cancer incidence and mortality* (IARC scientific publication no. 102). Lyon: IARC Scientific Publications, 1993.
2. Cancer research campaign. *Factsheet 18*. London: Cancer Research Campaign, 1993.
3. Powell J, McConkey CC. Increasing incidence of adenocarcinoma of the gastric cardia and adjacent sites. *Br J Cancer* 1990;62:440–443.
4. Devesa SS, Blot WJ, Fraumeni JF Jr. Changing patterns in the incidence of esophageal and gastric carcinoma in the United States. *Cancer* 1998;83:2049–2053.
5. EUROGAST study group. An international association between *Helicobacter pylori* infection and gastric cancer. *Lancet* 1993;341:1359–1362.
6. Buiatti E, Palli D, Decarli A, et al. A case-control study of gastric cancer and diet in Italy. II Association with nutrients. *Int J Cancer* 1990;45:896–901.
7. Rios-Castellanos E, Sitas F. Shepherd NA, et al. Changing pattern of gastric cancer in Oxfordshire. *Gut* 1992;33:1312–1317.
8. Boddie AW Jr, McMurtrey MJ, Giacco GG, et al. Palliative total gastrectomy and oesophagogastrectomy: an evaluation. *Cancer* 1983;51:1195–2000.
9. McCulloch P. Should general surgeons treat gastric carcinoma? An audit of practice end results. *Br J Surg* 1994;81:417–420.
10. Kohli Y, Kawai K, Fujita S. Analytical studies of the growth of human gastric cancer. *J Clin Gastroenterol* 1981;3:129–133.
11. Haugstvedt T. Benefits of resection in palliative surgery. *Dig Surgery* 1994;11:121–125.
12. Maruyama K, Okabayashi K, Kinoshita T. Progress in gastric cancer surgery in Japan and its limits of radicality. *World J Surg* 1987;11:418–425.
13. Jakl RJ, Miholic J, Koller R, et al. Prognostic factors in adenocarcinoma of the cardia. *Am J Surg* 1995;169:316–319.
14. Allum WH, Hallissey MT, Kelly KA. Adjuvant chemotherapy in operable gastric cancer. 5 year follow-up of the first British Stomach Cancer Group trial. *Lancet* 1989;1:571–574.
15. Gouzi JL, Huguier M, Fagniez PL, et al. Gastrectomie totale contre gastrectomie partielle pour adeno-cancer de l'antre. Une etude francaise prospective controlee. *Ann Chir* 1989;43:356–360.
16. Gouzi JL, Huguier M, Fagniez PL, et al. Total versus subtotal gastrectomy for adenocarcinoma of the gastric antrum. A French prospective controlled study. *Ann Surg* 1989;209:162–166.
17. Bozzetti F, Marubini E, Bonfanti G, et al. for the Italian Gastrointestinal Tumor Study Group. *Ann Surg* 1997;226:613–620.
18. Bozzetti F, Marubini E, Bonfanti G, et al. for the Italian Gastrointestinal Tumor Study Group. Subtotal versus total gastrectomy for gastric cancer: five-year survival rates in a multicenter randomized Italian Trial. *Ann Surg* 1999;230:170–178.
19. Davies J, Johnston D, Sue-Ling H, et al. Total or subtotal gastrectomy for gastric carcinoma? A study of quality of life. *World J Surg* 1998;22:1048–1055.
20. Wu CW, Hsieh MC, Lo SS, et al. Quality of life of patients with gastric adenocarcinoma after curative gastrectomy. *World J Surg* 1997;21:777–782.
21. Svedlund J, Sullivan M, Liedman B, et al. Quality of life after gastrectomy for gastric carcinoma: controlled study of reconstructive procedures. *World J Surg* 1997;21:422–433.
22. Roder JD, Stein HJ, Eckel F, et al. Quality of life after total and subtotal gastrectomy for gastric carcinoma. *Dtsch Med Wochenschr* 1996;121:543–549.
23. Bonenkamp JJ, Songun I, Hermans J, et al. Randomised comparison of morbidity after D1 and

D2 dissection for gastric cancer in 996 Dutch patients. *Lancet* 1995;345:745–748.

24. Cuschieri A, Fayers P, Fielding J, et al. Postoperative morbidity and mortality after D1 and D2 resections for gastric cancer: preliminary results of the MRC randomised controlled surgical trial. *Lancet* 1996;347:995–999.

25. Dent DM, Madden MV, Price SK. Randomised comparison of R1 and R2 gastrectomy for gastric carcinoma. *Br J Surg* 1988;75:110–112.

26. Robertson CS, Chung SCS, Woods SDS, et al. A prospective randomised trial comparing R1 subtotal gastrectomy with R3 total gastrectomy for antral cancer. *Ann Surg* 1994;220:176–182.

27. Cuschieri A, Weedon S, Fielding J, et al. Patient survival after D1 and D2 resections for gastric cancer: long-term results of the MRC randomised surgical trial. *Br J Cancer* 1999;79:1522–1530.

28. Bonenkamp JJ, Hermans J, Sasako M, et al. Extended lymph-node dissection for gastric cancer. Dutch Gastric Cancer Group. *N Engl J Med* 1999; 340:908–914.

29. Maeta M, Yamashiro H, Saito H, et al. A prospective pilot study of extended (D3) and superextended para-aortic lymphadenectomy (D4) in patients with T3 or T4 gastric cancer managed by total gastrectomy. *Surgery* 1999;125:325–331.

30. Siewert JR, Bottcher K., Stein HJ, et al. Relevant prognostic factors in gastric cancer: ten-year results of the German Gastric Cancer Study. *Ann Surg* 1998;228:449–461.

31. Parikh D, Chagla L, Johnson M, et al. D2 gastrectomy: lessons from a prospective audit of the learning curve. *Br J Surg* 1996;83:1595–1599.

32. Bunt AMG, Hermans J, Boon MC, et al. Evaluation of the extent of lymphadenectomy in a randomised trial of Western versus Japanese style surgery in gastric cancer. *J Clin Oncol* 1994;12:417–422.

33. Bonenkamp JJ, van de Velde CJH, Kampschoer GHM, et al. A comparison of factors influencing the prognosis of Japanese, German and Dutch gastric cancer patients. *World J Surg* 1993;17:410–415.

34. Hermans J, Bonenkamp JJ, Ban MC, et al. Adjuvant therapy after curative resection for gastric cancer: a meta-analysis of randomised trials. *J Clin Oncol* 1993;11:1441–1447. Search date June 1991; primary sources Medline from 1980, and hand searched references.

35. Earle CC, Maroun JA. Adjuvant chemotherapy after curative resection for gastric cancer in non-Asian patients: revisiting a meta-analysis of randomised trials. *Eur J Cancer* 1999;35:1059–1064. Search date to January 1999; primary Sources Medline, CancerLit.

36. Hermans J, Bonenkamp H. In reply [letter]. *J Clin Oncol* 1994;12:879–880.

37. Nakajima T, Nashimoto A, Kitamura M, et al. Adjuvant mitomycin and fluorouracil followed by oral uracil plus tegafur in serosa-negative gastric cancer: a randomised trial. Gastric Cancer Surgical Study Group. *Lancet* 1999;354:273–277.

38. Nakajima T, Fukami A, Takagi K, et al. Adjuvant chemotherapy with mitomycin C and with a multi drug combination of mitomycin, fluoro-uracil and cytosine arabinoside, after curative resection of gastric cancer. *Jpn J Clin Oncol* 1990;10:187–194.

39. Imanaga H, Nakazato H. Results of surgery for gastric cancer, and effect of adjuvant Mitomycin C on cancer recurrence. *World J Surg* 1977;1:213–221.

40. Yu W, Whang I, Suh I, et al. Prospective randomized trial of early postoperative intraperitoneal chemotherapy as an adjuvant to resectable gastric cancer. *Ann Surg* 1998;228:347–354.

41. Shchepotin IB, Chorny V, Hanfelt J, et al. Palliative superselective intra-arterial chemotherapy for advanced nonresectable gastric cancer. *J Gastrointest Surg* 1999;3:426–431.

42. Coombes RC, Schein PS, Chilvers CE, et al. A randomised trial comparing adjuvant 5-fluoro-uracil, doxorubicin and mitomycin C with no treatment in operable gastric cancer. International Collaborative Cancer Group. *J Clin Oncol* 1990;8:1362–1369.

43. Hallissey MT, Dunn JA, Ward LC, et al. The second British Stomach Cancer Group trial of adjuvant radiotherapy or chemotherapy in advanced gastric cancer: 5 year follow-up. *Lancet* 1994;343:1309–1312.

44. Nakazato H, Koike A, Saji S, et al. Efficacy of immunochemotherapy as adjuvant treatment after curative resection of gastric cancer. Study Group of Immunochemotherapy with PSK for Gastric Cancer. *Lancet* 1994;343:1122–1126.

Peter McCulloch
Surgical Consultant
The Fazakerley Hospital
Liverpool
UK

Competing interests: None declared.

TABLE 1   **Staging of stomach cancer (see text, p 267).**

Stage	Description
T1	Involvement of mucosa +/− submucosa
T2	Involvement of muscularis propria
T3	Involvement of serosa but no spread to adjacent organs
T4	Involvement of adjacent organs
N0	No lymph node involvement
N1	Local (perigastric) nodes involved
N2	Regional nodes involved
N3	More distant intra-abdominal nodes involved
M0	No metastases
M1	Metastases

TABLE 2   **Different types of surgical resection for stomach cancer (see text, p 269).**

Rresection	Description
R0	Removal of all detectable tumour, with a margin of healthy tissue confirmed microscopically: synonymous with "curative" resection.
R1	Incomplete removal, with histological evidence of cancer at the resection margin.
R2	Incomplete removal, with macroscopically obvious remnants of the main tumour: synonymous with "palliative" resection.
D1	Removal of all or part of the stomach, together with local (perigastric) nodes.
D2	Removal of all or part of the stomach, together with local and regional nodes, which lie along the branches of the coeliac axis.
D3/D4	More radical lymph node resection, including removal of para-aortic nodes and nodes within the small bowel mesentery.

Middle ear pain and trauma during air travel

Updated this issue

Simon Janvrin

QUESTIONS

INTERVENTIONS

Likely to be beneficial

Unknown effectiveness

Key Messages

- We found limited evidence suggesting that oral decongestants may be effective in reducing ear pain and trauma during air travel in adults. One RCT found no evidence of benefit in children.
- We found insufficient evidence on the effects of topical decongestants in this setting.

DEFINITION	The effects of air travel on the middle ear can include tympanic membrane pain, vertigo, hearing loss, and perforation.
INCIDENCE/ PREVALENCE	The prevalence of symptoms depends on the altitude, type of aircraft, and characteristics of the passengers. One point prevalence study found that 20% of adult and 40% of child passengers had negative pressure in the middle ear after flight, and that 10% of adults and 22% of children had auroscopic evidence of damage to the tympanic membrane.[1] We found no data on the incidence of perforation, which seems to be extremely rare in commercial passengers.
AETIOLOGY/ RISK FACTORS	During aircraft descent, the pressure in the middle ear drops relative to that in the ear canal. A narrow, inflamed, or poorly functioning Eustachian tube impedes the necessary influx of air. As the pressure difference between the middle and outer ear increases, the tympanic membrane is pulled inward.
PROGNOSIS	In most people, symptoms resolve spontaneously. Experience in military aviation shows that most ear drum perforations will heal spontaneously.[2]
AIMS	To prevent ear pain and trauma during air travel.
OUTCOMES	Incidence and severity of pain and hearing loss; incidence of perforation of tympanic membrane.
METHODS	*Clinical Evidence* update search and appraisal May 2000.

QUESTION What are the effects of preventive interventions?

OPTION ORAL DECONGESTANTS

We found limited evidence from two RCTs suggesting that oral pseudoephedrine may reduce the incidence of pain and hearing loss during flight in passengers prone to symptoms. One RCT found no evidence of benefit in children.

Benefits: We found no systematic review. We found three RCTs. Two RCTs in adult passengers (n = 350) compared oral pseudoephedrine (120 mg given 30 minutes before flight) versus placebo.[3,4] All participants had a history of ear pain during air travel. Those with acute or chronic ear problems were excluded. A total of 272 passengers completed the post flight questionnaires. The incidence of symptoms in the combined treatment groups was 33% versus 64% in those receiving placebo (RR 0.51, 95% CI 0.31 to 0.84). The third RCT compared oral pseudoephedrine versus placebo in children up to the age of 6 years.[5] It found no difference in ear pain between people taking treatment versus placebo, at either take off or landing.

Harms: "Dry mouth or drowsiness" was reported by 7–15% of adult participants taking pseudoephedrine versus 2% on placebo.[3,4] In total, 60% of children taking pseudoephedrine were drowsy on take off compared with 13% taking placebo.[5]

Comment: None.

OPTION	TOPICAL NASAL DECONGESTANTS

We found insufficient evidence on the effects of topical decongestants in this setting.

Benefits: We found no systematic review. We found one RCT comparing oxymetazoline nasal spray versus placebo nasal spray in 83 participants during air travel.[3] It found no significant difference in reported ear pain between the two groups.

Harms: Nasal irritation was reported by 14% of people taking oxymetazoline. The rate in people taking placebo was not reported.

Comment: The RCT was too small to rule out an effect of topical decongestants.

REFERENCES

1. Stangerup S-E, Tjernstrom O, Klokke M, Harcourt J, Stokholm J. Point prevalence of barotitis in children and adults after flight, and the effect of autoinflation. *Aviat Space Environ Med* 1998;69: 45–49.
2. O'Reilly BJ. Otorhinolaryngology. In: Ernsting J, Nicholson AN, Rainford DJ, eds. *Aviation Medicine*. 3rd edition. Oxford: Butterworth-Heinemann, 1999:319–336.
3. Jones JS, Sheffield W, White LJ, Bloom MA. A double-blind comparison between oral pseudoephedrine and topical oxymetazoline in the prevention of barotrauma during air travel. *Am J Emerg Med* 1998;16:262–264.
4. Csortan E, Jones J, Haan M, Brown M. Efficacy of pseudoephedrine for the prevention of barotrauma during air travel. *Ann Emerg Med* 1994;23:1324–1327.
5. Buchanan BJ, Hoagland J, Fischer PR. Pseudoephedrine and air travel-associated ear pain in children. *Arch Pediatr Adolesc Med* 1999; 153:466–468.

Simon Janvrin
Former Senior Medical Officer
Civil Aviation Authority
West Sussex
UK

Competing interests: None declared.

Updated this issue

Ian Williamson

Ear, nose, and throat disorders

INTERVENTIONS

Key Messages

- We found insufficient evidence on the effects of strategies for preventing otitis media with effusion (OME).
- We found no clear answers from available evidence about the effects of pharmacological treatments.
- Two systematic reviews of RCTs and one non-systematic review found that antibiotics speed the resolution of OME, but are not effective in the long term. Adverse effects were reported frequently.
- We found insufficient evidence about sustained benefits from mechanical and surgical treatment.

DEFINITION OME or "glue ear", is characterised by fluid (serous or mucoid but not mucopurulent) in the middle ear. Children usually present with hearing loss and speech problems. In contrast to those with acute otitis media (see topic, p 165), children with OME do not suffer from acute ear pain, fever, or malaise. Hearing loss is usually mild and often identified when parents express concern about their child's behaviour, school performance, or language development.

INCIDENCE/ PREVALENCE At any time 5% of children aged 2–4 years have persistent (at least 3 months) bilateral hearing loss associated with OME. The prevalence declines considerably over age 6.[1] About 80% of children aged 10 years have been affected by OME at some time in the past. OME is the most common reason for referral for surgery in children in the UK. Middle ear effusions also occur infrequently in adults after upper respiratory tract infection or after air travel.

AETIOLOGY/ RISK FACTORS Aetiology is uncertain, but contributory factors include upper respiratory tract infection and narrow upper respiratory airways. Established risk factors include age at first onset, day care centre attendance, number of siblings, socioeconomic group, frequent upper respiratory tract infection, bottle feeding, and household smoking. Most factors are associated with about double the risk of developing OME.[2]

PROGNOSIS In 5% of preschool children, OME (identified by tympanometric screening) persists for a year.[3,4] One large study (n = 12 534) found that middle ear disease increased reported hearing difficulty at age 5 years (OR 1.44, 95% CI 1.18 to 1.76) and was associated with delayed language development in children up to age 10 years.[5]

AIMS To improve hearing and wellbeing; to avoid poor behavioural, speech and educational development; and to prevent recurrent earache and otitis media.

OUTCOMES Resolution of effusion (both speed and completeness) assessed by otoscopy, tympanometry, or global clinical assessment; hearing impairment, assessed by audiometry or tympanometry (although the positive predictive value of these tests has been reported as low as 49%);[6] developmental and behavioural tests; language and speech development; adverse effects of treatment. Hearing losses as small as 15 dB above the normal hearing threshold can be disabling in children. Patient centred outcomes in children with OME (e.g. disability or quality of life) need further development and evaluation.

METHODS *Clinical Evidence* update search and appraisal May 2000.

QUESTION What are the effects of preventive interventions?

OPTION AVOIDANCE OF MODIFIABLE RISK FACTORS

We found no RCTs that evaluated interventions to modify risk factors for OME, such as passive smoking and bottle feeding.

Benefits: We found no systematic review or RCTs of interventions aimed at modifying risk factors for OME.

Ear, nose, and throat disorders

Harms: We found insufficient data.

Comment: There is good epidemiological evidence that the risk of OME is increased by passive smoking,[7] bottle feeding,[8] low socioeconomic group, and exposure to a large number of other children.[8] Feasible preventive interventions may include strategies to reduce household smoking and encourage breast feeding.

| QUESTION | What are the effects of treatments? |

| OPTION | ANTIMICROBIAL DRUGS |

Two systematic reviews of RCTs and one subsequent non-systematic review have found that resolution of OME occurred faster with antibiotics versus placebo or no treatment. They found no significant effect on longer term outcomes. Adverse effects with antibiotics were frequent.

Benefits: We found two systematic reviews (search dates 1992 and 1993) and one subsequent non-systematic review.[6,9,10] Both systematic reviews found that OME resolves faster with antimicrobial drugs. **Short term outcomes:** The first review (search date 1992) identified 10 blinded RCTs in 1041 children with OME, which compared antimicrobial drugs (amoxicillin with or without clavulanate, cefaclor, erythromycin, sulphisoxazole, sulphamethoxazole, or trimethoprim) versus placebo or versus no treatment.[6] Treatment duration varied from 2–5 weeks. Follow up was from 10–60 days. At 1 month, resolution of effusion (assessed by pneumatic otoscopy, tympanometry, and audiometry) was significantly more likely with antimicrobial treatment (pooled ARR for non-resolution compared with placebo or no treatment 14%, 95% CI 4% to 24%; NNT 7). **Longer term outcomes:** The second systematic review of eight RCTs found no significant difference in presence of effusions between 6 weeks and 11 months after treatment (pooled ARR for presence of effusion compared with placebo 6%, 95% CI −3% to +14%).[9] This review also found no significant differences in effectiveness between antibiotics. A more recent meta-analysis based on eight RCTs (7 of 18 previously included RCTs and one newer RCT) compared antibiotics v placebo in OME (total n = 1292) and found no significant effect (cure rate 179/813 [22%] for antibiotics versus 85/479 [17%] for placebo; ARI of cure 4.3%, 95% CI −0.3% to +8%).[10]

Harms: The systematic reviews did not report rates of adverse events in children on placebo or no treatment. Adverse effects on antibiotics were frequent. For amoxicillin, diarrhoea was reported in 20–30% and rashes in 3–5% of children. For amoxicillin clavulanate, diarrhoea was reported in 9%, nausea and vomiting in 4%, and skin rashes and urticaria in 3% of children.[6,11] For antibiotics overall, nausea and vomiting, diarrhoea, or both were reported in 2–32% of children, and cutaneous reactions in less than 5%.[11] Adherence to long courses of antibiotics is poor. Prescribing antibiotics for minor illness encourages further consultations[12] and antibiotic resistance.[13]

Comment: In the third meta-analysis[10] the timing to outcomes was not clear.

| OPTION | STEROIDS |

Two systematic reviews of RCTs found no evidence of benefit from oral steroids in children with OME. We found no RCTs that adequately evaluated topical steroids.

Benefits: We found two systematic reviews (search dates 1990[14] and 1992[6]). **Oral steroids versus placebo:** The reviews identified three placebo controlled RCTs of oral steroids in 108 children with OME. Presence of effusion was assessed clinically by pneumatic otoscopy, tympanometry, and audiometry after 7–14 days of treatment. There was no significant difference in mean improvement at 2 weeks after treatment (AR of clearance compared with placebo 0.18, 95% CI –0.03 to +0.39). There were no available summary data beyond 6 weeks. **Added to antibiotic:** The systematic reviews identified four RCTs in 292 children comparing antibiotic plus oral steroids versus antibiotic alone. Time to measurement of results varied from 1 week to 2 months. There was no significant difference in clearance rates with combined treatment versus antibiotic alone (ARR for non-clearance versus antibiotic alone 0.25, 95% CI –0.01 to +0.5). **Topical steroids:** We found one RCT that compared intranasal beclomethasone with placebo as an adjunct to prophylactic antibiotics in 61 children with chronic middle ear infection.[15] It found significant improvement in middle ear pressure at 12 weeks (P < 0.05) and fewer effusions at 4 and 8 weeks (P < 0.05) in those treated with intranasal steroids and antibiotics, compared with either antibiotics alone or placebo spray.

Harms: Short courses of steroids can cause behavioural changes, increased appetite, and weight gain. Idiosyncratic reactions have been reported such as avascular necrosis of the femoral head and fatal varicella infections.

Comment: Small numbers and diverse clinical populations weaken the quality of the evidence.

| OPTION | ANTIHISTAMINES AND DECONGESTANTS |

One systematic review of RCTs found no benefit from antihistamines and decongestants versus placebo in children with OME.

Benefits: We found one systematic review (search date 1992, 4 placebo controlled RCTs, 1202 infants and older children).[6] Treatment lasted for 4 weeks. Meta-analysis found that combined antihistamine/decongestants had no significant effect on effusion clearance rate compared with placebo, as assessed by history, otoscopy, and tympanometry (difference in clearance rate –0.009, 95% CI –0.036 to +0.054).

Harms: Adverse effects of antihistamines include hyperactivity, insomnia, drowsiness, behavioural change, blood pressure variability, and seizures. Decongestant nose drops given for 3 weeks or more can lead to iatrogenic rhinitis.

Comment: The RCTs included clinically heterogeneous groups — for example, infants and older children — and selected individuals from ambulatory care or waiting lists. There were too few children with allergies for subgroup analysis.

OPTION	MUCOLYTICS

One systematic review of RCTs found that 1–3 month courses of mucolytics compared with placebo or no treatment had no significant effect on effusion resolution.

Benefits: We found one systematic review (search date 1993, 6 RCTs, 430 children) comparing S-carboxymethylcysteine, its lysine salt, or both, versus placebo or no treatment.[16] Treatment lasted for 15–90 days. Increased frequency of complete resolution with mucolytics did not quite reach significance (OR 2.25, 95% CI 0.97 to 5.22). Three small RCTs comparing another mucolytic, bromhexine, versus placebo in 155 children and 195 ears found conflicting results.

Harms: The review gave no information on adverse effects.[16] Reported adverse effects of S-carboxymethylcysteine include gastric irritation, nausea, and rashes.

Comment: The RCTs were heterogeneous in their clinical outcomes and treatment duration.

OPTION	AUTOINFLATION

One systematic review of RCTs found benefit from autoinflation using a nasal balloon, although some children may find autoinflation difficult. The value of other methods of autoinflation have not yet been adequately evaluated.

Benefits: We found one systematic review (search date not given, 6 RCTs) comparing autoinflation versus no treatment.[17] Improvement was variously defined as being effusion free, improved tympanogram, or improvement in hearing. The RCTs assessing different treatment effects had different results. However, three trials evaluating nasal balloons in 386 children found a homogeneous effect size. Children in the treatment group were more likely than controls to improve within 1 week to 3 months, using tympanometric and audiometric criteria (OR 1.85, 95% CI 1.22 to 2.8).[17]

Harms: No serious adverse effects have been reported.

Comment: The Eustachian tubes can be inflated by several methods, including blowing up a balloon through a plastic tube inserted into the nostril. In one RCT, 12% of children aged 3–10 years were unable to use the balloon.[17] The beneficial effects were noted when adherence was 70% or greater. The evidence is suboptimal because different methods were used, outcome assessments were not blinded, and follow up was short. Other methods of autoinflation (such as inflating a carnival blower through the nostril, or forcible exhalation through the nostrils, with closed mouth, into an anaesthetic mask with a flowmeter attachment) have not been adequately evaluated.

OPTION	SURGERY

One systematic review of heterogenous RCTs has found that surgery (insertion of grommets, adenoidectomy, or both) results in short term hearing gain. Grommets and adenoidectomy alone were of similar

effectiveness. A subsequent RCT found that grommets and adenoidectomy combined were more effective than adenotonsillectomy or grommets, either alone or combined. We found no good evidence of the effects of tonsillectomy.

Benefits: We found one systematic review of surgery in children with OME (search date 1992, 19 RCTs). Nine reported the data per child (n = 1508) and 10 reported data per ear (n = 1452). None were placebo controlled, although some used patients as their own controls.[18] Outcomes were mean change in audiometry, tympanometry, and clinical and otoscopic evidence of OME. The review concluded that evidence for the effectiveness of surgical interventions was still confused. **Grommets:** The review reported a mean 12 dB improvement in hearing after insertion of grommets (CI not available). However, the authors concluded that this was difficult to interpret clinically. **Grommets plus adenoidectomy:** The review found that adenoidectomy gave little additional benefit over grommets alone in terms of mean hearing gain, which varied from 1.1 to 2.6 dB. A subsequent RCT in 228 children compared adenotonsillectomy or adenoidectomy (analysed together) versus neither procedure.[19] All children had a grommet inserted into one ear. Outcomes were mean audiometric change and tympanometric and otoscopic clearance assessed over 6 months to 10 years after treatment. The trial found benefit in combining adenoidectomy with grommets. Median duration of glue ear assessed tympanometrically was reduced from 7.8 years without treatment to 4.9 years with grommets, 4 years with adenoidectomy, and 2.8 years with adenoidectomy and grommets combined. The difference between duration for adenoidectomy alone and grommets alone was not significant (P = 0.2) but all other comparisons were significant. **Tonsillectomy:** The review found no good RCTs of tonsillectomy alone in OME.

Harms: Otorrhoea occurred postoperatively in 13% of children after grommet insertion (AR 0.13, 95% CI 0.05 to 0.21) and persisted in 5% at 1 year.[20] The true incidence of persistent perforation beyond 1 year is not known. A systematic review of observational and experimental studies (search date 1998)[21] of the complications following grommet insertion found a reported prevalence of tympanosclerosis in 39–65% of ventilated ears as opposed to 0–10% of untreated ears. Partial atrophy was noted in 16–73% of ears treated, and in 5–31% of those untreated. Atelectasis ranged from 10–37% of ears treated as opposed to 1–20% untreated, and attic retraction between 10–52% and 29–40%, respectively. The average hearing loss associated with these abnormalities was less than 5 dB. **Adenoidectomy:** Deaths have been reported in 1/16 700–25 000 children when combined with tonsillectomy (no figures available for adenoidectomy alone), and postoperative haemorrhage in 0.5%.[22]

Comment: About half of children who have grommets inserted will undergo reinsertion within 5 years.[23] Resolution after surgery takes longer in younger children and in those whose parents smoke, irrespective of treatment.[19]

Substantive changes since last issue

Harms from surgery New systematic review of complications following grommet insertion.[21]

REFERENCES

1. Williamson IG, Dunleavey J, Bain J, Robinson D. The natural history of otitis media with effusion: a three year study of the incidence and prevalence of abnormal tympanograms in four SW Hampshire infant and first schools. *J Laryngol Otol* 1994;108: 930–934.

2. Haggard M, Hughes E. *Objectives, values and methods of screening children's hearing – a review of the literature*. London: HMSO, 1991.

3. Zeilhuis GA, Rach GH, Broek PV. Screening for otitis media with effusion in pre-school children. *Lancet* 1989;1:311–314.

4. Fiellau-Nikolajsen M. Tympanometry in three year old children: prevalence and spontaneous course of MEE. *Ann Otol Rhinol Laryngol* 1980;89(suppl 68):233–237.

5. Bennett KE, Haggard MP. Behaviour and cognitive outcomes in middle ear disease. *Arch Dis Child* 1999;80:28–35.

6. Stool SE, Berg SO, Berman S, et al. Otitis media with effusion in young children: clinical practice guideline number 12. AHCPR Publication 94–0622. Rockville, Maryland: Agency for Health Care Policy and Research, Public Health Service, United States Department of Health and Human Services, July, 1994. Search date 1992; primary sources online database of National Library of Medicine; 10 specialised bibliographic databases.

7. Strachan DP, Cook DG. Health effects of passive smoking. 4. Passive smoking, middle ear disease and adenotonsillectomy in children. *Thorax* 1998; 53:50–56. Search date 1997; primary sources Medline; Embase.

8. Paradise JL, Rockette HE, Colborn DK, et al. Otitis media in 2253 Pittsburgh area infants: prevalence and risk factors during the first two years of life. *Pediatrics* 1997;99:318–333.

9. Williams RL, Chalmers TC, Strange KC, Chalmers FT, Bowlin SJ. Use of antibiotics in preventing recurrent acute otitis media and in treating otitis media with effusion: a meta-analytic attempt to resolve the brouhaha. *JAMA* 1993;270:1344–1351. Search date 1966 to 1993; primary source Medline.

10. Cantekin EI, Linder TE. Aggressive and ineffective therapy for otitis media. *Otol Rhinol Laryngol Nova* 1998;8:136–147.

11. Computerised clinical information system. Denver, Colorado: Micromedex Inc, June 1993.

12. Little P, Gould C, Williamson I, Warner G. Gantley M, Kinmonth AL. Reattendance and complications in a randomised trial of prescribing strategies for sore throat: the medicalising effect of prescribing antibiotics. *BMJ* 1997;315:350–352.

13. Anonymous. Antimicrobial resistance is a major threat to public health (Editorial). *BMJ* 1998;317: 609–610.

14. Rosenfield RM, Mandel EM, Bluestone CD. Systemic steroids for otitis media with effusion in children. *Arch Otolaryngol Head Neck Surg* 1991; 117:984–989. Search date 1990; primary sources not provided.

15. Tracy TM, Demain JG, Hoffman KM, Goetz DW. Intranasal beclomethasone as an adjunct to treatment of chronic middle ear effusion. *Ann Allergy Asthma Immunol* 1998;80:198–206.

16. Pignataro O, Pignataro LD, Gallus G, Calori G, Cordaro CI. Otitis media with effusion and S-carboxymethylcysteine and/or its lysine salt: a critical overview. *Int J Pediatr Otorhinolaryngol* 1996;35:231–241. Search date 1993; primary sources Medline; Embase; Biosis.

17. Reidpath DD, Glasziou PP, Del Mar C. Systematic review of autoinflation for treatment of glue ear in children. *BMJ* 1999;318:1177–1178. Search date not given. Primary sources Medline; Cochrane Library and Pharmaceutical company database.

18. University of York. Centre for Reviews and Dissemination. 1992. The treatment of persistent glue ear in children. *Effective Health Care* 1(4). Search date 1992; primary sources BIDS; Medline; Embase.

19. Maw R, Bawden R. Spontaneous resolution of severe chronic glue ear in children and the effect of adenoidectomy, tonsillectomy, and insertion of ventilation tubes. *BMJ* 1993;306:756–760.

20. Mclelland CA. Incidence of complications from tympanostomy tubes. *Arch Otolaryngol* 1980;106: 97–99.

21. Schilder AG. Assessment of complications of the conditions and of the treatment of otitis media with effusion. *Int J Pediatr Otolaryngol* 1999;49: 247–251. Search date 1998; primary sources not stated.

22. Yardley MP. Tonsillectomy, adenoidectomy and adenotonsillectomy; are they safe day case procedures. *J Laryngol Otol* 1992;106:299–300.

23. Maw AR. Development of tympanosclerosis in children with otitis media with effusion and ventilation tubes. *J Laryngol Otol* 1991;105:614–617.

Ian Williamson
Senior Lecturer in Primary Medical Care
Southampton University
Southampton
UK

Competing interests: None declared.

Recurrent tonsillitis

Updated this issue

Martin Burton

QUESTIONS
Effects of tonsillectomy in severe tonsillitis in children and adults . . .287

INTERVENTIONS

Unknown effectiveness

Tonsillectomy versus
   antibiotics 287

To be covered in future issues of
Clinical Evidence
Intermittent antibiotics
Long term antibiotics

Key Messages

- We found no RCTs evaluating tonsillectomy in adults, and we found inconclusive evidence from RCTs in children.

DEFINITION	Tonsillitis is infection of the parenchyma of the palatine tonsils. It is only one cause of "sore throat," which may be caused by infection of other pharyngeal tissues. Severe tonsillitis has been defined as seven episodes in the preceding year, five episodes per year in the preceding 2 years, or three per year in the preceding 3 years.[1]
INCIDENCE/ PREVALENCE	Recurrent sore throat has an incidence in general practice in the UK of 100 per 1000 population per year.[2] Acute tonsillitis is more common in childhood.
AETIOLOGY/ RISK FACTORS	Common bacterial pathogens include β haemolytic and other streptococci. The part played by viruses is uncertain.
PROGNOSIS	We found no good data on the natural history of tonsillitis or recurrent sore throat in children or adults. Participants in RCTs who were randomised to medical treatment (courses of antibiotics as required) have shown a tendency towards improvement over time.[1,3]
AIMS	To abolish tonsillitis; to reduce the frequency and severity of throat infections; to improve general wellbeing, behaviour, and educational achievement, with minimal adverse effects.
OUTCOMES	Number and severity of episodes of tonsillitis or sore throat; requirement for antibiotics and analgesics; time off work or school; behaviour, school performance, general wellbeing; morbidity and mortality of surgery, and adverse effects of drugs.
METHODS	We searched Medline and Embase up to 1997 for RCTs and controlled clinical trials using the key words tonsillitis, tonsillectomy, and tonsil. *Clinical Evidence* update search and appraisal May 2000.

QUESTION   Is tonsillectomy effective in severe tonsillitis in children and adults?

OPTION   TONSILLECTOMY VERSUS ANTIBIOTICS

Limited evidence from one RCT suggests that tonsillectomy may benefit some children with severe tonsillitis. We found no good evidence on tonsillectomy in adults. We found that many important outcome measures have not been considered.

Benefits: We found two systematic reviews (search dates 1997 and 1998).[4,5] **Children:** Both reviews identified the same two RCTs as being the only ones that met quality inclusion criteria.[1,3] The smaller RCT involved 91 children who fulfilled stringent diagnostic criteria for "severe tonsillitis" (see definition above).[1] The children were randomised to tonsillectomy alone (n = 27), adenotonsillectomy (n = 16), or intermittent courses of antibiotics as needed (n = 48). Some children (n = 16) were withdrawn from the non-surgical group by their parents and had surgery, and children who developed infections after surgery received antibiotics as necessary for each episode of infection. Secondary outcome measures such as time off school were also considered. The authors concluded that children undergoing tonsillectomy experienced significantly fewer throat infections than those on antibiotics, amounting to an average of three fewer throat infections in the first 2 years, but by the third year the difference was no longer significant. The larger RCT, in 246 "less severely affected children" is published only in abstract form.[3] Some children in this study also underwent adenoidectomy. The limited data available provide no evidence of a difference between surgical and medical treatment. The second review concluded that it was not possible to determine the effectiveness of tonsillectomy from these RCTs.[5] **Adults:** The reviews found no RCTs that evaluated tonsillectomy in adults with recurrent tonsillitis or sore throats.

Harms:

The risks of tonsillectomy include those associated with general anaesthesia and those specific to the procedure. The overall complication rate in the smaller RCT was 14%[1] (all were "readily managed or self limiting") compared with 2.3–7.8% in one Scottish tonsillectomy audit.[6] Haemorrhage, either primary (in the immediate postoperative period) or secondary, occurred in 4% of children studied in the larger RCT[3] and fewer than 1% of children in the Scottish tonsillectomy audit.[6] Potentially harmful effects of non-surgical treatment are principally those associated with antibiotic usage. In the smaller RCT,[1] erythematous rashes occurred in 4% of children in the non-surgical group while taking penicillin.

Comment:

In the smaller RCT,[1] there were significant baseline differences between groups before treatment, and the authors pooled the results of tonsillectomy and adenotonsillectomy, making it impossible to assess the effectiveness of tonsillectomy alone. Tonsillectomy is one of the most frequently performed surgical procedures in the UK, particularly in children, and accounts for about 20% of all operations performed by otolaryngologists.[6] We found no RCT that found improved general wellbeing, development, or behaviour—despite suggestions that these are influenced by tonsillectomy.[6] Adenoidectomy is now only performed with tonsillectomy when there is a specific indication to remove the adenoids as well as the tonsils.

REFERENCES

1. Paradise JL, Bluestone CD, Bachman RZ, et al. Efficacy of tonsillectomy for recurrent throat infection in severely affected children. *N Engl J Med* 1984;310:674–683.
2. Shvartzman P. Careful prescribing is beneficial. *BMJ* 1994;309:1101–1102.
3. Paradise JL, Bluestone CD, Rogers KD, et al. Comparative efficacy of tonsillectomy for recurrent throat infection in more versus less severely affected children [abstract]. *Pediatric Res* 1992; 31:126A.
4. Marshall T. A review of tonsillectomy for recurrent throat infection. *Br J Gen Pract* 1998;48:1331–

1335. Search date 1997; primary sources Cochrane Library; Medline.
5. Burton MJ, Towler B, Glasziou P. Tonsillectomy versus non-surgical treatment for chronic/recurrent acute tonsillitis. In: The Cochrane Library, Issue 4, 1999. Oxford: Update Software. Search date 1998; primary sources Medline; Embase; Cochrane Controlled Trials Register and hand searched references..
6. Blair RL, McKerrow WS, Carter NW, Fenton A. The Scottish tonsillectomy audit. *J Laryngol Otol* 1996; 110(suppl 20):1–25.

Martin Burton
Consultant Otolaryngologist
Department of Otolaryngology
Radcliffe Infirmary NHS Trust
Oxford
UK

Competing interests: None declared.

New topic

Martin Burton and Elizabeth Mogg

Ear, nose, and throat disorders

INTERVENTIONS

*Although many practitioners consider these to be standard treatments, we found no RCTs regarding the benefits or harms of these interventions.
See glossary, p 292

Key Messages

- We found no good evidence about mechanical methods of removing ear wax.
- One small RCT found that wax softeners were better than no treatment at completely removing ear wax without syringing.

DEFINITION	Ear wax is normal and becomes a problem only if it produces deafness, pain, or other aural symptoms. Ear wax may also need to be removed if it prevents inspection of the ear drum. The term "impacted" is used in different ways, and may merely imply the coexistence of wax obscuring the ear drum with symptoms in that ear.[1,2]
INCIDENCE/ PREVALENCE	A survey found that 289 Scottish general practitioners each saw an average of nine people a month requesting removal of ear wax.[1]
AETIOLOGY/ RISK FACTORS	Factors that prevent the normal extrusion of wax from the ear canal (e.g. wearing a hearing aid, using cotton buds) increase the chance of ear wax accumulating.
PROGNOSIS	Most ear wax emerges from the external canal spontaneously. Without impaction or adherence to the drum, there is likely to be minimal, if any, hearing loss. One survey of 21 unselected outpatients with completely obstructing wax found that the average improvement in hearing following syringing was 5.5 dB (95% CI 0.6 to 10.5 dB).[1]
AIMS	To relieve symptoms or to allow examination by completely removing impacted wax or obstructing wax; to soften impacted wax to ease mechanical removal.
OUTCOMES	Proportion of people (or ears) with relief of hearing loss or discomfort; total removal of wax; proportion of people requiring further intervention to improve symptoms; ease of mechanical removal measured, for example, by the volume of water used to accomplish successful syringing.
METHODS	*Clinical Evidence* search and appraisal March 2000.

QUESTION What are the effects of methods to remove ear wax?

OPTION WAX SOFTENERS

One RCT found limited evidence that using a wax softener for 5 days increases the chance of an ear being cleared of wax compared with no treatment. One third of untreated ears cleared in the same period. Nine RCTs found no consistent evidence that any one type of wax softener was superior to the others.

Benefits: We found no systematic review. **Versus placebo:** We found one RCT in 113 people with impacted wax (see glossary, p 292) in one or both ears.[2] The ears were randomly allocated to treatment by the nursing staff with sterile water, sodium bicarbonate, a proprietary softening agent (arachis oil/chlorobutanol/p-dichlorobenzene), or no treatment. Active treatment allocation was double blind. The participants were recruited in a hospital for the elderly. People already using ear drops, and people with known pathology of the ear canal or ear drum, were excluded. Of those recruited, 13 left hospital and three died before completing the trial. Analysis of the remaining 97 people (155 ears) found that the risk of persisting impaction at the end of the trial was reduced by any active form of treatment compared with no treatment (AR of persistent impaction: 26/38 [68%] ears with no treatment; 55/117 [47%] with any active treatment; ARR 21%, 95% CI 3% to 35%; RRR 31%, 95% CI 6% to 75%; NNT 5, 95% CI 3 to 34). **Versus other wax softeners:** We found nine RCTs reported in seven publications comparing wax softeners (see table 1, p 293).[1–8] Three of these rather than randomisation used alternate allocation, and an additional four did not state their methods of randomisation. The trials were conducted in a variety of settings. They varied in size from 35 people to 286 ears. The commonest outcomes were a subjective assessment of the amount of wax remaining, the need for syringing, or the perceived ease, the result of syringing, or both. The RCTs found no consistent evidence that any one type of wax softener was clinically superior to any other.

Harms: Six RCTs did not report complications or adverse effects. Two found single cases of irritation, itch, or buzzing.[3,4] One study found that 16% (17/106) using either arachis oil/chlorobutanol/p-dichlorobenzene or a proprietary agent whose composition was not stated (Otocerol) reported adverse effects, including pain or irritation, giddiness, and dislike of the smell of the wax softener.[6]

Comment: We found no good evidence about the optimal duration of treatment. Most trials did not use rigorous methods of randomisation. Many trials were sponsored by companies that manufactured only one of the products being tested, but the possibility of publication bias has not been assessed. The inclusion criteria for the RCTs were not always clear: many stated that the participants had impacted wax without defining how this was assessed. The RCT that included a no-treatment group found that 32% of ears with impacted wax showed spontaneous resolution after 5 days.[2]

| OPTION | MECHANICAL METHODS |

We found no good evidence concerning the benefits or harms of mechanical removal of wax.

Benefits: We found no systematic review and no RCTs comparing mechanical methods intended to remove ear wax with no treatment or alternative treatment.

Harms: A survey found that 38% of 274 general practitioners performing ear syringing reported complications, including otitis externa, perforation of the tympanic membrane, damage to the skin of the external canal, tinnitus, pain, and vertigo.[1] We found no study of the incidence of these complications. People may experience dizziness when wax is removed by suction.

Comment: There is consensus that syringing is effective, and that training can reduce complications, but we found no evidence establishing these points. Other mechanical techniques include manual removal under direct vision, with or without a microscope, using suction, probes, or forceps. These methods require specific training and access to appropriate equipment.

Wax in ear

GLOSSARY

Obstructing wax Wax that obscures direct vision of the ear drum.

Impacted wax Wax that has accumulated in the ear canal, completely obstructing the lumen. In practice, many RCTs define impaction as the presence of symptoms associated with obstructing wax.

REFERENCES

1. Sharp JF, Wilson JA, Ross L, Barr-Hamilton RM. Ear wax removal: a survey of current practice. *BMJ* 1990;301:1251–1252.
2. Keane EM, Wilson H, McGrane D, Coakley D, Walsh JB. Use of solvents to disperse ear wax. *Br J Clin Pract* 1995;49:7–12.
3. Dummer DS, Sutherland IA, Murray JA. A single-blind, randomized study to compare the efficacy of two ear drop preparations ('Andax' and 'Cerumol') in the softening of ear wax. *Curr med Res Opin* 1992;13:26–30.
4. Lyndon S, Roy P, Grillage MG, Miller AJ. A comparison of the efficacy of two ear drop preparations ('Aurax' and 'Earex') in the softening and removal of impacted ear wax. *Curr Med Res Opin* 1992;13:21–25.
5. Fahmy S, Whitefield M. Multicentre clinical trial of Exterol as a cerumenolytic. *Br J Clin Pract* 1982; 36:197–204.
6. Jaffe G, Grimshaw J. A multicentric clinical trial comparing Otocerol with Cerumol as cerumenolytics. *J Int Med Res* 1978;6:241–244.
7. Amjad AH, Scheer AA. Clinical evaluation of cerumenolytic agents. *Eye Ear Nose Throat Mon* 1975;54:76–77.
8. Chaput de Saintonge DM, Johnstone CI. A clinical comparison of triethanolamine polypeptide oleate-condensate ear drops with olive oil for the removal of impacted wax. *Br J Clin Pract* 1973;27:454–455.

Martin Burton
Consultant Otolaryngologist

Elizabeth Mogg
Senior House Officer

The Radcliffe Infirmary
Oxford
UK

Competing interests: None declared.

TABLE 1 Effects of wax softeners: results of comparative RCTs (see text, p 291).

Reference	Wax softener	Administration	Selection characteristic; setting	Number of people (ears)	Randomisation; blind	Outcome	Results	Adverse effects
2	(a) Arachis oil Chlorobutanol P-dichlorobenzene Sodium bicarbonate (in glycerol) (b) Sterile water (c) Nothing	4 drops twice a day for 5 days	Impacted ear(s); hospital	113 recruited; 97 completed (155)	Double blind (active treatments)	Residual wax; 3 tiered clinical rating scale	Treatment better than no treatment; no difference between agents	None
3	(a) Ethyleneoxide-polyoxypropylene glycol Choline salicylate (b) Arachis oil Chlorobutanol P-dichlorobenzene		Impacted or hardened wax; general practice	50 (100)	Not stated; single blind	Wax amount, colour and consistency; objective hearing; global impression of efficiency	No difference	Two irritation with (a); one itch, one buzzing with (b)
4	(a) Ethyleneoxide-polyoxypropylene glycol Choline salicylate (b) Arachis oil Almond oil Rectified camphor oil	Drops to fill ear twice a day for 4 days	Symptoms requiring wax softener; general practice	36 (72)	Not stated; not blind	Need for syringing; ease of syringing; global impression of efficiency	(a) better than (b); easy removal: 37/38 v 19/30	One irritation with (b); one disliked smell

TABLE 1 continued

5	(a) 5% urea hydrogen peroxide in glycerol (b) Glycerol	5–10 drops twice a day for a week	Ear wax problems; ENT dept	40 (80)	Alternation; double blind	Need for syringing; ease of syringing	(a) better than glycerol; success: 35/40 v 20/40	None
5	(a) 5% urea hydrogen peroxide in glycerol (b) Arachis oil Chlorobutanol P-dichlorobenzene	5–10 drops twice a day for a week	Ear wax problems; ENT dept	50 (100)	Alternation; double blind	Need for syringing; ease of syringing	(a) better than (b); success: 47/50 v 24/50	None
5	(a) 5% urea hydrogen peroxide in glycerol (b) Arachis oil Chlorobutanol P-dichlorobenzene	5–10 drops twice a day for a week	Ear wax problems; general practice	160 (286)	Alternation; double blind	Need for syringing; ease of syringing	(a) better than (b); success: 146/157 v 93/129	None
6	(a) Otocerol (b) Arachis oil Chlorobutanol P-dichlorobenzene	Three consecutive nights	For whom a wax softener would normally be prescribed; general practice	106 (not stated)	Random allocation; double blind	3 tiered clinical rating scale	No difference overall; (38/53 v 33/53)	Pain; irritation; giddiness; smell (Otocero; 7/53) (Cerumol; 10/53)
7	(a) Triethanolamine polypeptide oleate condensate (b) Carbamide peroxide	One dose 30 minutes before syringing	Hard or impacted wax; setting unclear	80 (not stated)	Random allocation; double blind	Result of syringing; 4 tiered clincal rating scale	(a) better than (b), but (b) normally used as multiple installations	None
8	(a) Triethanolamine polypeptide oleate condensate (b) Olive oil	One dose 20 minutes before syringing	Impacted wax suitable for syringing; hospital outpatient dept	67 (number of patients not stated)	Random order; double blind	3 tiered clinical rating scale	No difference overall (20/32 v 21/35); (a) needed less water	None

ENT, ear, nose, and throat.

Updated this issue

Ronald Sigal

Endocrine disorders

INTERVENTIONS

Key Messages

- Diabetes mellitus increases the risk of cardiovascular disease. Cardiovascular risk factors in people with diabetes include conventional risk factors (age, prior cardiovascular disease, cigarette smoking, hypertension, dyslipidaemia, sedentary lifestyle, family history of premature cardiovascular disease) and more diabetes specific risk factors (elevated urinary protein excretion, poor glycaemic control).

RCTs have found that:

- Antihypertensive treatment in people with diabetes reduces cardiovascular events.

- Aggressive control with target diastolic blood pressures of ≤ 80 mmHg reduces cardiovascular morbidity and mortality compared with less tight control.

- Statins and fibrates are effective in primary and secondary prevention of cardiovascular disease in people with diabetes and dyslipidaemia.

- Aspirin is effective in primary and secondary prevention of cardiovascular disease in people with diabetes.

- Aggressive control of blood glucose with insulin and oral agents, or both, does not increase the risk of cardiovascular disease, and may decrease this risk.

- An angiotensin converting enzyme (ACE) inhibitor reduced subsequent cardiovascular events and overall mortality in people with diabetes over age 55 with additional cardiac risk factors and/or previously diagnosed coronary vascular disease (CVD).

- Coronary artery bypass grafting reduces the death rate more than percutaneous transluminal coronary angioplasty in people with diabetes and multivessel coronary artery disease.

■ The combination of stent and glycoprotein IIb/IIIa inhibition in people with diabetes undergoing percutaneous coronary revascularisation reduces restenosis rates and serious morbidity.

DEFINITION **Diabetes mellitus:** See aetiology under glycaemic control in diabetes, p 320. **Cardiovascular disease:** Atherosclerotic disease of the heart and/or the coronary, cerebral, or peripheral vessels leading to clinical events such as acute myocardial infarction, congestive heart failure, sudden cardiac death, stroke, gangrene, and/or need for revascularisation procedures.

INCIDENCE/ Diabetes mellitus is a major risk factor for cardiovascular disease. In
PREVALENCE the USA, 60–75% of people with diabetes die from cardiovascular causes.[1] The annual incidence of cardiovascular disease is increased two- to threefold in diabetic men and three- to fourfold in diabetic women after adjusting for age and other cardiac risk factors.[2] About 45% of middle aged and older white people with diabetes have evidence of coronary artery disease, compared with about 25% of people without diabetes in the same populations.[2] In a population based cohort study of 1059 diabetic and 1373 non-diabetic Finnish adults aged 45–64 years, the 7 year risk of myocardial infarction was as high in adults with diabetes without previous cardiac disease as it was in people without diabetes with previous cardiac disease.[3]

AETIOLOGY/ Conventional risk factors for cardiovascular disease contribute to
RISK FACTORS increasing its relative risk in people with diabetes to about the same extent as in those without diabetes, and are reviewed elsewhere in this volume (see aetiology under primary prevention, p 51). The absolute risk of cardiovascular disease is the same in diabetic women as in diabetic men. Cardiovascular risk factors relatively specific to people with diabetes include longer duration of diabetes during adulthood (the years of exposure to diabetes before age 20 add little to risk of cardiovascular disease);[4] raised blood glucose concentrations (reflected in fasting blood glucose or HbA1c); and microalbuminuria (albuminuria 30–299 mg/24 hours)). People with diabetes and microalbuminuria have about two to three times the coronary morbidity and mortality of people with normal levels of urinary albumin and a similar duration of diabetes.[5,6] The relative risk of major cardiac events associated with clinical proteinuria is about threefold in type 2 diabetes[7] and ninefold in type 1 diabetes,[4,8,9] compared with individuals with the same type of diabetes having normal albumin excretion.

PROGNOSIS Diabetes mellitus increases the risk of mortality or serious morbidity after a coronary event about 1.5 to 3 fold.[2,3,10,11] This excess risk is only partly accounted for by the greater prevalence of other cardiac risk factors in people with diabetes. In a systematic review the presence of "stress hyperglycaemia" in diabetic patients on admission to hospital for myocardial infarction (MI) was associated with a relative risk for in-hospital mortality of 1.7 (95% CI 1.2 to 2.4) compared with diabetic patients with lower glucose levels on admission for MI.[12]

AIMS To reduce mortality and morbidity from cardiovascular disease, with minimum adverse effects.

OUTCOMES	Incidence of fatal or non-fatal acute myocardial infarction (AMI); congestive heart failure; sudden cardiac death; coronary revascularisation; stroke; gangrene; angiographic evidence of coronary, cerebral vascular, or peripheral arterial stenosis.
METHODS	*Clinical Evidence* update search and appraisal May 2000. We searched for systematic reviews and RCTs with at least 10 confirmed clinical cardiovascular events among people with diabetes. Studies reporting only intermediate end points (e.g. regression of plaque on angiography, lipid changes) were not considered. When a good systematic review was available, only additional RCTs published after the date of search for the systematic review were included.

QUESTION **What are the effects of screening for high cardiovascular risk?**

We found no good evidence.

Benefits:	We found no systematic review and no large RCTs of screening people with diabetes for cardiovascular risk.
Harms:	We found inadequate data.
Comment:	Screening for conventional risk factors as well as regular determination of HbA1c (up to quarterly), lipid profile, and urinary albumin excretion will identify people at high risk.[13,14] Consensus opinion recommends screening for cardiovascular disease with exercise stress testing in previously sedentary adults with diabetes who are planning to undertake vigorous exercise programmes.[13,15] We found no evidence that such testing prevents cardiac events.

QUESTION **Which interventions improve cardiovascular outcomes in people with diabetes?**

OPTION SMOKING CESSATION

Observational studies have found that cigarette smoking is associated with increased cardiovascular death in people with diabetes. In non-diabetic people, smoking cessation has been found to be associated with reduced risk.

Benefits:	We found no systematic review. Cohort studies have found that cigarette smoking increased the incidence of cardiovascular death in diabetic people up to fourfold depending on the amount smoked- (see smoking cessation in people at high risk under secondary prevention of ischaemic cardiac events, p 83).[16]
Harms:	None known.
Comment:	We found little published literature on smoking cessation specifically in people with diabetes. However, such people are likely to benefit from smoking cessation at least as much as people who do not have diabetes, but have other risk factors for cardiovascular events (see smoking cessation under secondary prevention of ischaemic cardiac events, p 83).

| OPTION | ANTIHYPERTENSIVE TREATMENT |

One systematic review of RCTs has found that angiotensin converting enzyme (ACE) inhibitors, diuretics, and β blockers are effective for primary prevention of cardiovascular events in people with diabetes. We found no clear evidence that any of these three classes of drug is more effective than another. However, one large trial found that an alpha blocker increased the risk of congestive heart failure compared with chlorthalidone, and the alpha blocker arm of that study was therefore stopped. Two large trials found excess cardiovascular morbidity with long acting dihydropyridine calcium channel blockers compared with ACE inhibitors, but another trial in elderly diabetic people found that aggressive therapy beginning with a long acting dihydropyridine reduced cardiovascular morbidity compared with placebo. The review found that setting lower target blood pressures reduces cardiovascular events, and that ,β blockers and ACE inhibitors reduce the risk of major cardiovascular events in people with diabetes and a previous AMI. One large RCT found that an ACE inhibitor reduced subsequent cardiovascular events and overall mortality in people with diabetes aged over 55 with additional cardiac risk factors and/or previously diagnosed coronary vascular disease (CVD). No class of medication had significant adverse effects on metabolism or quality of life at the doses used in the trials reviewed.

Benefits: One systematic review of antihypertensive treatment in diabetes (published in 1997) analysed individual patient data for 5823 people with diabetes within 14 RCTs. The trials also enrolled people without diabetes.[17] **Primary prevention:** (see table 1, p 309). The systematic review identified two primary prevention studies, including 1355 people with diabetes who received either active treatment (stepped care beginning with a diuretic) or less active treatment (either placebo[18] or referral to usual care in the community[19]). Cardiovascular morbidity and mortality were significantly reduced with active treatment (OR for morbidity and mortality 0.64, 95% CI 0.50 to 0.82; for overall mortality 0.85, 95% CI 0.62 to 1.17). The absolute risk of major cardiovascular events was high (AR 27% with control and 19% with active treatment during a 5 year period). Thirteen middle aged and older adults with diabetes would have to be treated for 5 years to prevent one major cardiovascular event. In the first RCT, 4695 people (495 with diabetes) aged ≥ 60 years with blood pressure 165–220/< 95 mmHg were randomised to active treatment (beginning with nitrendipine) or placebo and followed for a median of 2 years.[20] Active treatment reduced all cardiovascular events (AR 13/252 [5.2%] for active treatment) 31/240 [12.9%] for controls; ARR 8%, 95% CI 3% to 10%; RRR 60%, 95% CI 25% to 79%; NNT 13, 95% CI 10 to 31) but had no significant effect on overall mortality (AR 16/252 for active treatment, 26/240 for controls; ARR 4.5%, 95% CI −0.7% to +7.4%; RRR 4%, 95% CI −6% to +68%). In the second RCT 10 985 participants aged 25–66 years with diastolic blood pressure > 100 mmHg were randomised to captopril 50 mg daily (including 309 people with diabetes) or conventional treatment with diuretics or β blockers (including 263 people with diabetes) for a mean of 6.1 years.[21] In people with diabetes, it found that captopril reduced the combined risk of fatal and non-fatal myocardial infarction, stroke, and other fatal cardiovascular events compared with conventional treatment (RR for combined end point 0.59, 95% CI 0.38 to 0.91; RR for overall mortality 0.59, 95% CI 0.31 to 0.96; AR and NNT not available).

Primary and secondary prevention: We found one RCT (3577 diabetic people in a total study population of 9541, aged ≥55 years, with at least one of the following risk factors: diagnosed CVD, current smoker, hypercholesterolaemia, hypertension or microalbuminuria) comparing ramipril 10 mg or placebo and vitamin E or placebo over 4.5 years in a 2x2 factorial design (see table 3, p 313).[22] Compared with placebo, ramipril reduced the rate of major cardiovascular events (CVD death, MI or stroke 277/1808 with ramipril v 351/1769 with placebo; RRR 0.25, 95% CI 0.12 to 0.36; ARR 4.5%, 95% CI 2% to 7%; NNT 22 older people with diabetes and additional risk factors treated for 4.5 years to prevent one major cardiovascular event, 95% CI 14 to 43), and death from any cause (196/1808 v 248/1769; RRR 24%, 95% CI 8 % to 37%; ARR 3.2%, 95% CI 1% to 5.3%; NNT 32, 95% CI 19 to 98). The relative effect of ramipril was present in all patient subgroups regardless of hypertensive status, microalbuminuria, type of diabetes, and nature of diabetes treatment (diet, oral agents, or insulin). Vitamin E treatment had no effect on morbidity or mortality.[22] In another randomised trial,[23] men and women aged 55 years or older with hypertension and either previous CVD or at least one additional CVD risk factor were randomised to receive chlorthalidone, doxazosin, amlodipine or lisinopril. After 3.3 years of follow up there was no difference between doxasosin and chlorthalidone in the primary outcome (fatal coronary heart disease (CHD) or non-fatal MI), but the doxazosin arm was terminated because of an excess risk of combined CVD events (coronary heart disease death, non-fatal MI, stroke, revascularisation procedures, angina, congestive heart failure, and peripheral vascular disease) compared with chlorthalidone (OR 1.24, 95% CI 1.12 to 1.38, for 3183 people with diabetes randomised to doxazosin compared with 5481 randomised to chlorthalidone; number of events in people with diabetes unspecified). **Secondary prevention:** (see table 2, p 311). The systematic review included seven trials of secondary prevention with follow up of at least 1 year, including 2564 people with diabetes.[17] The review found that both ACE inhibitors and β blockers reduced the risk of subsequent cardiac events in people with diabetes with previous MI, with or without hypertension; there were reductions in all causes of mortality (OR from six trials with 2402 people: 0.82, 95% CI 0.69 to 0.99) and cardiovascular morbidity and mortality (OR from two trials with 654 people: 0.82, 95% CI 0.60 to 1.13). Five other trials of secondary prevention in 1904 people with diabetes had follow up of less than 1 year and found all causes of mortality reduced (OR 0.64, 95% CI 0.50 to 0.83), and cardiovascular morbidity and mortality reduced (OR from three trials with 1612 people: 0.68, 95% CI 0.43 to 1.05). **Target blood pressure:** We found several recent trials with large numbers of participants with diabetes (see table 1, p 309 and table 2, p 311). In two large RCTs, tighter control of blood pressure reduced the risk of major cardiovascular events.[24–26] In one, people with diabetes who were randomised to target diastolic blood pressure ≤80 mmHg had half the risk of major cardiovascular events compared with their counterparts randomised to target blood pressure ≤90 mmHg.[26] In the other large RCT, people with hypertension and type 2 diabetes randomised to tight blood pressure control (< 150/< 85 mmHg) with atenolol (n = 358) or captopril (n = 400) had reduced incidence of "any diabetes related end point" deaths (primarily cardiovascular deaths), stroke, and microvascular disease.[24,25]

Harms: In one RCT, people in the atenolol group gained weight compared with people taking catopril (3.4 ± 8.0 kg weight gain with atenolol, v 1.6 ± 9.1 kg weight gain with captopril, P = 0.02).[25] Over the first 4 years of the trial, people allocated to atenolol had higher mean HbA1c (7.5% ±1.4% v 7.0 ±1.4%, P = 0.0044), but there was no difference between groups over the subsequent 4 years. There was no difference between atenolol and captopril in rates of hypoglycaemia, lipid concentrations, tolerability, blood pressure lowering, or prevention of disease events. Two trials compared a long acting dihydropyridine calcium antagonist with an ACE inhibitor in people with type 2 diabetes.[27,28] In both trials, the two classes of drug were equally effective in lowering blood pressure, but calcium channel blockers were associated with a two- to fivefold greater risk of a major cardiovascular event compared with ACE inhibitor. However, in one other RCT, in which all groups received the long acting calcium antagonist felodipine, cardiovascular morbidity and mortality were relatively low.[26] In a further RCT, the long acting calcium antagonist nitrendipine reduced cardiovascular morbidity and mortality compared with placebo.[20] More people allocated to ramipril than to placebo withdrew because of cough (7% v 2%). This was the only adverse effect occurring more frequently in the ACE inhibitor recipients than in controls.[22]

Comment: There is good evidence that, in the absence of contraindications, an ACE inhibitor decreases cardiovascular events and death rates in older people with diabetes with existing cardiovascular disease or at least one additional cardiac risk factor. Although it is clear that aggressive lowering of blood pressure in diabetic people with hypertension reduces cardiovascular morbidity and mortality, it is not clear whether any one major class of antihypertensive medication is superior to others.

OPTION LIPID LOWERING AGENTS

Subgroup analyses of data from people with diabetes enrolled into large trials of statins and fibrates have found that these are effective in primary and secondary prevention of AMI.

Benefits: **Primary prevention:** We found no systematic review. Three large RCTs with significant numbers of diabetic participants have compared lipid lowering agents with placebo (see table 1, p 309). In the first, men aged 45–73 years and postmenopausal women aged 55–73 years were randomised to diet plus lovastatin 20–40 mg/day or diet plus placebo, and followed for a mean of 5.2 years.[29] Only people with total cholesterol 4.65–6.82 mmol/l, LDL-C 3.36–4.91 mmol/l, HDL-C ≤1.16 mmol/l (men) or ≤1.22 mmol/l (women), and triglycerides ≤4.52 mmol/l were included in the trial. In the second RCT, 4081 Finnish men aged 40–55 years were randomised to gemfibrozil 600 mg twice daily or placebo and followed up for 5 years. Required baseline lipid concentrations (total minus HDL-C) were ≥5.2 mmol/l; participants were not excluded on the basis of triglyceride level.[30] In the third RCT, 164 men and women with type 2 diabetes aged 35–65 years were randomised to bezafibrate versus placebo for 3 years.[31] Required baseline lipids included one or more of the following: total cholesterol 5.2 to 8.0 mmol/l, serum triglyceride 1.8–8.0 mmol/l, HDL-C ≤1.1 mmol/l, or total-to-HDL C ratio ≥4.7. **Secondary prevention:** We found no systematic review but found four RCTs involving people with diabetes (see table 2, p 311). One RCT (in 4444 men and women aged 35–70 years with previous MI or angina pectoris, total cholesterol concentrations of 5.5–8.0 mmol/l, and triglycerides ≤2.5 mmol/l) compared simvastatin versus placebo over a median of 5.4 years.[32] Simvastatin dosage was initially 20 mg daily, with blinded dosage titration up to 40 mg daily, according to cholesterol response during the first 6–18 weeks. The relative risk of main end points in people with diabetes treated with simvastatin were as follows: total mortality 0.57 (95% CI 0.30 to 1.08), major cardiovascular events 0.45 (95% CI 0.27 to 0.74), and any atherosclerotic event 0.63 (95% CI 0.43 to 0.92).[22] The second RCT (4159 men and women aged 21–75 years, 3–20 months after MI and with total cholesterol < 6.2 mmol/l, triglycerides < 3.92 mmol/l, and LDL-C 3.0–4.5 mmol/l) compared pravastatin 40 mg/day with placebo over a median of 5 years.[33] Among the participants with diabetes, the relative risk of major coronary events (death from coronary disease, non-fatal MI, coronary artery bypass grafting [CABG], or percutaneous transluminal coronary angioplasty [PTCA]) was 0.75 (95% CI 0.57 to 1.0). The third RCT, (9014 men and women aged 31–75 with AMI or unstable angina, plasma total cholesterol 4.0–7.0 mmol/l, and plasma triglycerides < 5.0 mmol/l) compared pravastatin 40 mg daily with placebo for a mean of 6.1 years.[34] Among the 782 participants with diabetes, the relative risk of CHD death or non-fatal AMI was 0.84 (95% CI 0.59 to 1.10). The fourth RCT (2531 men aged < 74 with previous CVD (MI, angina, revascularisation, or angiographically documented coronary stenosis), (HDL-C ≤ 1.0 mmol/l, LDL-C ≤ 3.6 mmol/l and triglycerides ≤ 3.4 mmol/l) compared gemfibrozil 1200 mg daily with placebo for a median of 5.1 years.[35] Among the 627 participants with diabetes, the relative risk of CHD death or non-fatal MI was 0.76 (95% CI 0.57 to 1.0).

Harms: None reported.

Comment: Most published clinical trials with sufficient statistical power to detect effects on cardiovascular events have enrolled comparatively small numbers of diabetic participants or excluded them altogether. The available evidence is therefore based almost entirely on subgroup analyses of larger trials. Several large ongoing trials are evaluating the effects of fibrates in people with diabetes.

OPTION BLOOD GLUCOSE CONTROL

In most cohort studies, higher average concentrations of blood glucose in people with diabetes were associated with a higher incidence of cardiovascular disease. RCTs provide modest support for glucose lowering with insulin, sulphonylureas, or metformin in primary prevention of cardiovascular disease, and strong support for intensive insulin treatment after AMI.

Benefits:

Primary prevention: (see table 1, p 309). We found no systematic review. In people with diabetes, higher average levels of blood glucose are associated with higher incidence of cardiovascular disease. We found two RCTs. Both found that intensive hypoglycaemic treatment reduced the risks of microvascular diabetic complications in both type 1 and type 2 diabetes, although neither trial found that intensive glycaemic control significantly reduced cardiovascular risk.[36,37] In the first trial, 1441 people with type 1 diabetes aged 13–39 years and free of cardiovascular disease, hypertension, hypercholesterolaemia, and obesity at baseline, were randomly assigned to conventional or intensive diabetes treatment and followed for a mean of 6.5 years. Major macrovascular events were almost twice as frequent in the conventionally treated group (40 events) as in the intensive treatment group (23 events), although the differences were not significant (ARR 2.2%; RRR 0.41, 95% CI −0.10 to +0.68). In the second trial, 3867 people aged 25–65 years (median 54 years) with type 2 diabetes that was inadequately controlled on diet alone, were randomised to conventional treatment (diet only, n = 1138, drugs added only if needed to keep fasting glucose < 15.0 mmol/l), intensive treatment with a sulphonylurea (n = 1573), or insulin (n = 1156). People who were ≥ 120% of ideal body weight were randomised to conventional treatment (n = 411), metformin (n = 342), sulphonylureas (n = 542), or insulin (n = 409). Intensive treatment beginning with a sulphonylurea or insulin improved glycaemic control (HbA1c 7.9% with conventional treatment compared with 7% with intensive treatment). Compared with conventional treatment, intensive treatment reduced diabetes related end points (RRR 12%, 95% CI 1% to 20%; NNT 39 for 5 years to prevent one additional diabetes related end point) and the risk of AMI (ARs 14.7/1000 patient years for intensive, 17.4/1000 patient years for conventional; RRR 16%, 95% CI 0% to 29%). Risks of stroke and amputation did not differ significantly among groups.[36] **Secondary prevention:** (see table 2, p 311). We found no systematic review but found two RCTs. One small RCT (153 men with type 2 diabetes, mean age 60 years, many of whom had previous cardiovascular events) compared standard insulin (once daily) with intensive treatment with a stepped plan designed to achieve near normal blood sugar levels.[38] After 27 months, the rate of new cardiovascular events was not significantly different between the groups (24/75 32% with intensive therapy v 16/80 20% with standard insulin; RR 1.6, 95% 0.92 to 2.5). In the second trial, 620 people (mean age 68 years, 63% men, 84% type 2) with random blood glucose ≥ 11 mmol/l were randomised within 24 hours of an AMI to either standard treatment or intensive insulin treatment.[39,40] The intensive insulin group received an insulin glucose infusion for 24 hours followed by subcutaneous insulin four times daily for at least 3 months. The standard treatment group received insulin only when it was clinically indicated. HbA1c fell significantly with intensive insulin treatment (fall of 1.1% with intensive treatment v 0.4% with standard treatment at 3 months and 0.9% v 0.4% at 12 months). Intensive treatment lowered mortality (ARs 19% v 26% at 1 year and 33% v 44% at a mean of 3.4 years; RRR 28%, 95% CI 8% to 45%; NNT 9 treated for 3.4 years to prevent one additional premature death). The absolute reduction in the risk of mortality was particularly striking in people who were not previously taking insulin and had no more than one of the following risk factors before the AMI that preceded randomisation: age ≥ 70 years, history of previous AMI, history of congestive heart failure, current treatment with digitalis. In this low risk subgroup, the ARR was 15% (NNT 7 for 3.4 years).

Harms:
Sulphonylureas and insulin, but not metformin, increased the risks of weight gain and hypoglycaemia. On an intention to treat basis, the proportions of people per year with severe hypoglycaemic episodes were 0.7%, 1.2%, 1%, 2%, and 0.6% for conventional, chlorpropamide, glibenclamide, insulin, and metformin groups. These frequencies of hypoglycaemia were much lower than those observed with intensive treatment in people with type 1 diabetes in the first primary prevention RCT.[41,42] Two RCTs found no evidence that any specific treatment (insulin, sulphonylurea, or metformin) increased overall risk of cardiovascular disease.[36,37]

Comment:
The role of intensive glucose lowering in primary prevention of cardiovascular events remains unclear. However, such treatment clearly reduces the risk of microvascular disease and does not increase the risk of cardiovascular disease. The potential of the second and larger primary prevention RCT to demonstrate an effect of tighter glycaemic control was limited by the small difference achieved in median HbA1c between intensive and conventional treatment. In contrast, in the first primary prevention trial, a larger 1.9% difference in median HbA1c was achieved between groups, but the young age of the participants and consequent low incidence of cardiovascular events limited the power of the study to detect an effect of treatment on incidence of cardiovascular disease.[41,42] The small study of insulin in type 2 diabetes[38] included men with a high baseline risk of cardiovascular events and achieved a 2.1% difference in HbA1c. The RCT was small and the observed difference between groups could have arisen by chance. The design of the trial of intensive versus standard glycaemic control following AMI does not distinguish whether the early insulin infusion or the later intensive subcutaneous insulin treatment was the more important determinant of improved survival in the intensively treated group. The larger primary prevention trial found no evidence that oral hypoglycaemics increase cardiovascular mortality,[36,37] but the possibility that oral hypoglycaemics may be harmful after AMI cannot be ruled out.

| OPTION | ASPIRIN |

Very large clinical trials of primary and mixed primary and secondary prevention, and a systematic review of secondary prevention, support a cardioprotective role for aspirin.

Benefits: **Primary prevention:** In the only large primary prevention trial comparing aspirin with placebo and reporting data on people with diabetes, 22 701 US male physicians aged 40–85 years were randomly assigned to aspirin 325 mg every other day or placebo, and followed up for an average of 5 years.[43] The trial found that, after 5 years, among the 533 physicians with diabetes, aspirin reduced the risk of AMI compared with placebo (AMI occurred in 11/275 [4%] with aspirin and 26/258 [10.1%] with placebo; RR of AMI with aspirin v placebo 0.39, 95% CI 0.20 to 0.79; NNT 16, 95% CI 12 to 47 to prevent one MI). A second trial comparing aspirin with placebo did not specify the number of people with diabetes, although it did report that aspirin reduced AMI to a similar degree in the subgroup of people with diabetes and in the overall trial population (RRR about 15%).[26] **Primary and early secondary prevention:** The largest RCT of aspirin prophylaxis in people with diabetes involved 3711 diabetic men and women (30% with type 1 diabetes, 48% with prior cardiovascular disease).[44] It compared aspirin (650 mg/day) with placebo and followed the participants for a mean of 5 years. It found a non-significant reduction in overall mortality in those treated with aspirin (RR 0.91, 95% CI 0.75 to 1.11). AMI occurred in 289 people (16%) in the aspirin group and 336 (18%) in the placebo group (ARR 2%, 95% CI 0.1% to 4.9%). Fifty people would need to be treated for 5 years with aspirin 650 mg/day to prevent one additional AMI. **Secondary prevention:** We found one systematic review, which analysed 145 clinical trials of antiplatelet treatment (primarily aspirin) published before March 1990.[45] Results for people with diabetes are included in table 2 (see table 2, p 311).

Harms: In the large trial comparing aspirin versus placebo for primary and secondary prevention, fatal or non-fatal stroke occurred in 5% on aspirin and 4.2% on placebo (P = NS).[44] There was no significant increase with aspirin in the risks of vitreous, retinal, gastrointestinal, or cerebral haemorrhage. In the systematic review, doses of aspirin ranged from 75–1500 mg/day. Most trials used 75–325 mg/day of aspirin. Doses higher than 325 mg/day increased the risk of haemorrhagic adverse effects without improving preventive efficacy. No difference in efficacy or adverse effects was found in the dose range 75–325 mg.[45]

Comment: We found insufficient evidence to define precisely which people with diabetes should be treated with aspirin. The risk of cardiovascular disease is very low before age 30; most white diabetic adults aged over 30 are at increased risk of cardiovascular disease. Widely accepted contraindications to aspirin treatment include aspirin allergy, bleeding tendency, anticoagulant treatment, recent gastrointestinal bleeding, and clinically active liver disease.[13,46]

OPTION   TREATING PROTEINURIA

Elevated urinary protein excretion is a risk factor for cardiovascular disease. One large RCT found that an ACE inhibitor reduced cardiovascular risk compared with placebo in people with or without microalbuminuria.

Benefits: We found no good evidence.

Harms: We found no good evidence.

Comment: One large RCT found that the ACE inhibitor ramipril, which reduces urinary protein excretion, also reduced cardiovascular morbidity and mortality in older diabetic people with other cardiac risk factors.[22] However, the cardioprotective effect was present to the same extent in people with or without microalbuminuria.

OPTION   CORONARY ARTERY BYPASS GRAFT VERSUS PERCUTANEOUS TRANSLUMINAL CORONARY ANGIOPLASTY

One RCT has found that coronary artery bypass grafting (CABG) reduces the death rate more than percutaneous transluminal coronary angioplasty (PTCA) in people with diabetes and multivessel coronary artery disease.

Benefits: We found no systematic review but found one RCT (1829 people with two or three vessel coronary disease, 353 with diabetes; mean age 62 years) comparing CABG with PTCA, without stenting or glycoprotein IIb/IIIa blockade [47] (see table 2, p 311). After a mean 7.7 years of follow up, fewer diabetic people assigned to CABG than PTCA died or suffered Q-wave MI (85/170 [50%] with PTCA v 60/173 [34.7%] with CABG; ARR 15%, 95% CI 5 to 26%; RRR 31%, 95% CI 11 to 46%, NNT 7, 95% CI 4 to 20). This survival benefit was confined to those receiving at least one internal mammary graft.

Harms: In the RCT, in-hospital mortality among people with diabetes was 1.2% after CABG versus 0.6% after PTCA. Myocardial infarction during the initial hospitalisation was three times more common after CABG than after PTCA (5.8% v 1.8%). None of these differences was significant.

Comment: Adjunctive therapies (heparin or abciximab) were not used in the RCT.

OPTION   GLYCOPROTEIN IIB/IIIA INHIBITORS AND INTRACORONARY STENTING (AS ADJUNCT TO PERCUTANEOUS CORONARY REVASCULARISATION)

Two RCTs found that the combination of stent and glycoprotein IIb/IIIa inhibition (abciximab) reduces restenosis rates and serious morbidity in people with diabetes undergoing percutaneous coronary angioplasty.

Benefits: We found no systematic review but found two RCTs (see table 2, p 311).[48–50,51] The first RCT (2792 people, 638 with diabetes; mean age 61 years; 38% female; all undergoing PTCA or directional atherectomy without stenting) compared placebo plus standard dose heparin versus abciximab plus standard dose heparin versus abciximab plus low dose heparin. Abciximab was given as a bolus plus 12 hour infusion. The primary indications for intervention were unstable angina (51%), stable ischaemia (33%), and recent myocardial infarction (16%). A total of 44% had a prior coronary intervention, 56% had multivessel disease, and 74% a history of hypertension. Compared with placebo, abciximab reduced the combined end point of death or myocardial infarction in both standard dose and low dose heparin arms (at 30 days by over 60% and at 6 months by over 50%). Abciximab reduced the rate of restenosis in people without diabetes (hazard ratio 0.78) but not in people with diabetes. The second RCT (2401 people, 491 with diabetes; mean age 60 years; 29% female; 69% hypertensive, 30% recent smokers, 48% prior MI, 10% prior CABG) compared stent plus placebo (n = 173) versus stent plus abciximab (n = 162) versus balloon angioplasty plus abciximab (n = 156). At 12 months, death or large MI occurred in 13.9% of those receiving stent and placebo, 8.3% with PTCA and abciximab and 4.9% with stent and abciximab. Subsequent revascularisation rates following stent and abciximab (13.7%) were much lower than those following stent and placebo (22.4%) or PTCA and abciximab (25.3%).[49,50,51] For both outcomes, the difference between the stent plus abciximab group and the other two groups was significant. We found an analysis of individual patient results of these two trials and a third, earlier trial.[52] In the 1462 diabetic patients, abciximab reduced overall mortality (26/540 [4.8%] to 21/844 [2.5%], ARR 2.3%, 95% CI 0.2% to 4.4%; NNT 43, 95% CI 23 to 421).

Harms: There was slightly more bleeding in patients given abciximab than given placebo (4.3% v 3.0% for major bleeding; 6.9% v 6.3% for minor bleeding; 0% v 0.17% for intracranial haemorrhage). None of these differences was statistically significant.[53]

Comment: For people with diabetes undergoing percutaneous procedures, the combination of stent and glycoprotein IIb/IIIa inhibition reduces restenosis rates and serious morbidity. It is unclear whether these adjunctive therapies would reduce morbidity, mortality, and restenosis associated with percutaneous revascularisation procedures to the levels seen with CABG. There was imbalance of the baseline characteristics among the study groups of the second RCT.[49] However, in a multivariate analysis, the treatment effects remained after adjusting for baseline differences.

Substantive changes since last issue

Lipid lower agent/secondary prevention New RCT; evidence of effectiveness of a fibrate in people with diabetes.[35]

Antihypertensive treatment New RCT; alpha-blocker arm discontinued because of increased risk of congestive heart failure compared with chlorthalidone.[23]

CABG versus PTCA Updated follow up of RCT; conclusion unchanged.[43]

Stent + GP IIb/IIIa inhibitors Updated follow up of RCT; conclusion unchanged.[51]

Stent + GP IIb/IIIa inhibitors New meta-analysis; abciximab reduced mortality compared with placebo.[53]

REFERENCES

1. Geiss LS, Herman WH, Smith PJ. Mortality in non-insulin-dependent diabetes. In: Harris MI, ed. *Diabetes in America*. 2nd ed. Bethesda, MD: National Institutes of Health, 1995:233–255.
2. Wingard DL, Barrett-Connor E. Heart disease and diabetes. In: Harris MI, ed. *Diabetes in America*. 2nd ed. Bethesda, MD: National Institutes of Health, 1995:429–448.
3. Haffner SM, Lehto S, Ronnemaa T, et al. Mortality from coronary heart disease in subjects with type 2 diabetes and in nondiabetic subjects with and without prior myocardial infarction. *N Engl J Med* 1998;339:229–234.
4. Krolewski AS, Warram JH, Freire MB. Epidemiology of late diabetic complications. A basis for the

development and evaluation of preventive programs. *Endocrinol Metab Clin North Am* 1996; 25:217–242.
5. Messent JW, Elliott TG, Hill RD, et al. Prognostic significance of microalbuminuria in insulin-dependent diabetes mellitus: a twenty-three year follow-up study. *Kidney Int* 1992;41:836–839.
6. Dinneen SF, Gerstein HC. The association of microalbuminuria and mortality in non-insulin-dependent diabetes mellitus: a systematic overview of the literature. *Arch Intern Med* 1997; 157:1413–1418. Search date 1995; primary sources Medline 1966 to 1994; Scisearch; hand-searching of bibliographies.
7. Valmadrid CT, Klein R, Moss S E, Klein BE. The

risk of cardiovascular disease mortality associated with microalbuminuria and gross proteinuria in persons with older-onset diabetes mellitus. *Arch Intern Med* 2000;160:1093–1100.

8. Borch Johnsen K, Andersen PK, Deckert T. The effect of proteinuria on relative mortality in type 1 (insulin-dependent) diabetes mellitus. *Diabetologia* 1985;28:590–596.

9. Warram JH, Laffel LM, Ganda OP, et al. Coronary artery disease is the major determinant of excess mortality in patients with insulin-dependent diabetes mellitus and persistent proteinuria. *J Am Soc Nephrol* 1992;3(suppl 4):104–110.

10. Behar S, Boyko V, Reicher-Reiss H, et al. Ten-year survival after acute myocardial infarction: comparison of patients with and without diabetes. SPRINT Study Group. Secondary Prevention Reinfarction Israeli Nifedipine Trial. *Am Heart J* 1997;133:290–296.

11. Mak KH, Moliterno DJ, Granger CB, et al. Influence of diabetes mellitus on clinical outcome in the thrombolytic era of acute myocardial infarction. GUSTO-I Investigators. Global Utilization of Streptokinase and Tissue Plasminogen Activator for Occluded Coronary Arteries. *J Am Coll Cardiol* 1997;30:171–179.

12. Capes SE, Hunt D, Malmberg K, Gerstein HC. Stress hyperglycaemia and increased risk of death after myocardial infarction in patients with and without diabetes: a systematic overview. *Lancet* 2000;355:773–778. Search date 1998; primary sources Medline, Science Citation Index and hand searches of bibliographies of relevant articles and contact with experts in the field.

13. Meltzer S, Leiter L, Daneman D, et al. Clinical practice guidelines for the management of diabetes in Canada. *Can Med Assoc J* 1998; 159(suppl 8):1–29.

14. American Diabetes Association. Clinical practice recommendations 2000. *Diabetes Care* 2000;23(suppl 1):1–116.

15. American Diabetes Association. Diabetes mellitus and exercise. *Diabetes Care* 2000;23(suppl 1):50–54.

16. Stamler J, Vaccaro O, Neaton JD, et al. Diabetes, other risk factors, and 12-year mortality for men screened in the Multiple Risk Factor Intervention Trial. *Diabetes Care* 1993;16:434.

17. Fuller J, Stevens LK, Chaturvedi N, et al. Antihypertensive therapy in diabetes mellitus. In: The Cochrane Library, Issue 4, 1999. Search date not given; primary sources Medline; Embase; and hand searches of specialty journals in cardiovascular disease, stroke, renal disease, and hypertension.

18. Curb JD, Pressel SL, Cutler JA, et al. Effect of diuretic-based antihypertensive treatment on cardiovascular disease risk in older diabetic patients with isolated systolic hypertension. Systolic Hypertension in the Elderly Program Cooperative Research Group. *JAMA* 1996;276: 1886–1892.

19. Davis BR, Langford HG, Blaufox MD, et al. The association of postural changes in systolic blood pressure and mortality in persons with hypertension: the Hypertension Detection and Follow-up Program experience. *Circulation* 1987; 75:340–346.

20. Tuomilehto J, Rastenyte D, Birkenh ger WH, et al. Effects of calcium-channel blockade in older patients with diabetes and systolic hypertension. *N Engl J Med* 1999;340:677–684.

21. Hansson L, Lindholm LH, Niskanen L, et al. Effect of angiotensin-converting enzyme inhibition compared with conventional therapy on cardiovascular morbidity and mortality in hypertension: the Captopril Prevention Project (CAPPP) randomised trial. *Lancet* 1999;353:611–616.

22. Heart Outcomes Prevention Evaluation (HOPE) Study Investigators. Effects of ramipril on cardiovascular and microvascular outcomes in people with diabetes mellitus: results of the HOPE study and the MICRO-HOPE substudy. *Lancet* 2000;355:253–259.

23. ALLHAT Collaborative Research Group. Major cardiovascular events in hypertensive patients randomised to doxazosin vs chlorthalidone: the antihypertensive and lipid-lowering treatment to prevent heart attack trial (ALLHAT). *JAMA* 2000; 283:1967–1975.

24. UK Prospective Diabetes Study Group. Tight blood pressure control and risk of macrovascular and microvascular complications in type 2 diabetes: UKPDS 38. *BMJ* 1998;317:703–713.

25. UK Prospective Diabetes Study Group. Efficacy of atenolol and captopril in reducing risk of macrovascular and microvascular complications in type 2 diabetes: UKPDS 39. *BMJ* 1998;317:713–720.

26. Hansson L, Zanchetti A, Carruthers SG, et al. Effects of intensive blood-pressure lowering and low-dose aspirin in patients with hypertension: principal results of the Hypertension Optimal Treatment (HOT) randomised trial. *Lancet* 1998; 351:1755–1762.

27. Estacio RO, Jeffers BW, Hiatt WR, et al. The effect of nisoldipine as compared with enalapril on cardiovascular events in patients with non-insulin-dependent diabetes and hypertension. *N Engl J Med* 1998;338:645–652.

28. Tatti P, Pahor M, Byington RP, et al. Outcome results of the Fosinopril versus Amlodipine Cardiovascular Events randomised Trial (FACET) in patients with hypertension and NIDDM. *Diabetes Care* 1998;21:597–603.

29. Downs JR, Clearfield M, Weis S, et al. Primary prevention of acute coronary events with lovastatin in men and women with average cholesterol levels: results of AFCAPS/TexCAPS. Air Force/Texas Coronary Atherosclerosis Prevention Study. *JAMA* 1998;279:1615–1622.

30. Koskinen P, Manttari M, Manninen V, et al. Coronary heart disease incidence in NIDDM patients in the Helsinki Heart Study. *Diabetes Care* 1992;15:820–825.

31. Elkeles RS, Diamond JR, Poulter C, et al. Cardiovascular outcomes in type 2 diabetes. A double-blind placebo-controlled study of bezafibrate: the St Mary's, Ealing, Northwick Park Diabetes Cardiovascular Disease Prevention (SENDCAP) Study. *Diabetes Care* 1998;21:641–648.

32. Pyorala K, Pedersen TR, Kjekshus J, et al. Cholesterol lowering with simvastatin improves prognosis of diabetic patients with coronary heart disease. A subgroup analysis of the Scandinavian Simvastatin Survival Study (4S). *Diabetes Care* 1997;20:614–620.

33. Sacks FM, Pfeffer MA, Moye LA, et al. The effect of pravastatin on coronary events after myocardial infarction in patients with average cholesterol levels. Cholesterol and Recurrent Events Trial investigators. *N Engl J Med* 1996;335:1001–1009.

34. The Long-term Intervention with Pravastatin in Ischemic Disease (LIPID) Study Program. Prevention of cardiovascular events and death with pravastatin in patients with coronary heart disease and a broad range of initial cholesterol levels. *N Engl J Med* 1998;339:1349–1357.

35. Rubins HB, Robins SJ, Collins D, et al. Gemfibrozil for the secondary prevention of coronary heart disease in men with low levels of high-density

lipoprotein cholesterol. Veterans Affairs High-Density Lipoprotein Cholesterol Intervention Trial Study Group. *N Engl J Med* 1999;341:410–418.

36. UK Prospective Diabetes Study Group. Intensive blood-glucose control with sulphonylureas or insulin compared with conventional treatment and risk of complications in patients with type 2 diabetes (UKPDS 33). *Lancet* 1998;352:837–853.

37. UK Prospective Diabetes Study Group. Effect of intensive blood-glucose control with metformin on complications in overweight patients with type 2 diabetes (UKPDS 34). *Lancet* 1998;352:854–865.

38. Abraira C, Colwell J, Nuttall F, et al. Cardiovascular events and correlates in the Veterans Affairs Diabetes Feasibility Trial: Veterans Affairs Cooperative Study on glycemic control and complications in type II diabetes. *Arch Intern Med* 1997;157:181–188.

39. Malmberg K, Ryden L, Efendic S, et al. Randomised trial of insulin-glucose infusion followed by subcutaneous insulin treatment in diabetic patients with acute myocardial infarction (DIGAMI study): effects on mortality at 1 year. *J Am Coll Cardiol* 1995;26:57–65.

40. Malmberg K. Prospective randomised study of intensive insulin treatment on long term survival after acute myocardial infarction in patients with diabetes mellitus. DIGAMI (Diabetes Mellitus, Insulin Glucose Infusion in Acute Myocardial Infarction) Study Group. *BMJ* 1997;314:1512–1515.

41. DCCT Research Group. The effect of intensive treatment of diabetes on the development and progression of long-term complications in insulin-dependent diabetes mellitus. *N Engl J Med* 1993;329:977–986.

42. DCCT Research Group. Effect of intensive diabetes management on macrovascular events and risk factors in the Diabetes Control and Complications Trial. *Am J Cardiol* 1995;75:894–903.

43. Steering Committee of the Physicians' Health Study Research Group. Final report on the aspirin component of the ongoing Physicians' Health Study. *N Engl J Med* 1989;321:129–135.

44. ETDRS Investigators. Aspirin effects on mortality and morbidity in patients with diabetes mellitus. *JAMA* 1992;268:1292–1300.

45. Collaborative overview of randomised trials of antiplatelet therapy–I: Prevention of death, myocardial infarction, and stroke by prolonged antiplatelet therapy in various categories of patients. Antiplatelet Trialists' Collaboration. *BMJ* 1994;308:81–106. Search date March 1990; primary sources Medline; Current Contents; manual searches of journals; reference lists from clinical trial and review articles; inquiry among colleagues, and manufacturers of antiplatelet agents for unpublished studies.

46. American Diabetes Association. Aspirin therapy in diabetes. *Diabetes Care* 1997;20:1772–1773.

47. The BARI Investigators. Seven-year outcome in the Bypass Angioplasty Revascularization Investigation (BARI) by treatment and diabetic status. *J Am Coll Cardiol* 2000;35:1122–1129.

48. Kleiman NS, Lincoff AM, Kereiakes DJ, et al. Diabetes mellitus, glycoprotein IIb/IIIa blockade, and heparin: evidence for a complex interaction in a multicenter trial. EPILOG Investigators. *Circulation* 1998;97:1912–1920.

49. Marso SP, Lincoff AM, Ellis SG, et al. Optimizing the percutaneous interventional outcomes for patients with diabetes mellitus: results of the EPISTENT (Evaluation of platelet IIb/IIIa inhibitor for stenting trial) diabetic substudy. *Circulation* 1999;100:2477–2484.

50. The EPISTENT Investigators. Randomised placebo-controlled and balloon-angioplasty-controlled trial to assess safety of coronary stenting with use of platelet glycoprotein- IIb/IIIa blockade. The EPISTENT Investigators. Evaluation of platelet IIb/IIIa inhibitor for stenting. *Lancet* 1998;352:87–92.

51. Topol EJ, Mark DB, Lincoff AM, et al. Outcomes at 1 year and economic implications of platelet glycoprotein IIb/IIIa blockade in patients undergoing coronary stenting: results from a multicentre randomised trial. EPISTENT Investigators. Evaluation of Platelet IIb/IIIa Inhibitor for Stenting (published erratum appears in *Lancet* 2000 Mar 25;355:1104). *Lancet* 1999;354:2019–2024.

52. The EPIC Investigation. Use of a monoclonal antibody directed against the platelet glycoprotein IIb/IIIa receptor in high-risk coronary angioplasty. *N Engl J Med* 1994;330:956–961.

53. Bhatt DL, Marso SP, Lincoff AM, Wolski KE, Ellis SG, Topol EJ. Abciximab reduces mortality in diabetics following percutaneous coronary intervention. *J Am Coll Cardiol* 2000;35:922–928.

Ronald Sigal

Assistant Professor of Medicine
University of Ottawa
Ottawa
Canada

Competing interests: RS has been reimbursed by Bristol Myers Squibb, manufacturer of Pravastatin, for attending a conference and has received speaker's fees from Eli Lilly and Novo-Nordisk (manufacturers of insulin).

TABLE 1 Primary prevention of cardiovascular events in people with diabetes: evidence from systematic reviews and randomised trials (see text, pp 298, 300, 302).

Type of intervention	Study	Study type	Duration (years)	Outcome	Events / Sample size (%)*		NNT	95% CI for NNT
					Intervention group	Control group		
Antihypertensive medication								
	Cochrane meta-analysis: diabetes and hypertension[17]	SR	5	CVD mortality and morbidity	121/647 (18.7%)	188/708 (26.6%)	13	9 to 28
	UKPDS Hypertension Study[24,25]	RCT	8.4	AMI (fatal or non-fatal)	107/758 (14.1%)	83/390 (21.3%)	14	9 to 35
	"Tight" target BP (≤150/ ≤85) with captopril or atenolol v "less tight" target (≤180/ ≤105)			Stroke	38/758 (5.0%)	34/390 (8.7%)	27	18 to 116
				Peripheral vascular events	8/758 (1.1%)	8/390 (2.1%)	–	–
	HOT[26]	RCT	3.8	AMI (fatal or non-fatal), stroke (fatal or non-fatal) or other cardiovascular death	22/499 (4.4%) Target diastolic BP 80 mm Hg	45/501 (9.0%) Target diastolic BP 90 mm Hg	22	16 to 57
	Felodipine and ACE-inhibitor, or β blocker, with 3 distinct target BPs							
	FACET[28]	RCT	2.9	AMI, stroke, or admission to hospital for angina	14/189 (7.4%) Fosinopril	27/191 (14%) Amlodipine	15	10 to 199
	Fosinopril v amlodipine							
	ABCD[27]	RCT	5	AMI (fatal or non-fatal)	5/235 (2.1%) Enalapril	25/235 (11%) Nisoldipine	12	10 to 19
	Enalapril v nisoldipine							

TABLE 1 Continued

							13	10 to 31
Syst-Eur[20]	Nitrendipine; enalapril ± hydrochlorothiazide (20 mm Hg BP lowering) v placebo	RCT	2	MI, CHF, or sudden cardiac death	13/252 (5.2%)	31/240 (12.9%)	13	10 to 31
Lipid-lowering								
AFCAPS/TexCAPS[29]	Lovastatin	RCT	5	MI, unstable angina, or sudden cardiac death	4/84 (4.8%)	6/71 (8.5%)	27	NS
SENDCAP[31]	Bezafibrate	RCT	3	MI or new ischaemic changes on ECG	5/64 (7.8%)	16/64 (25.0%)	6	5 to 20
Helsinki[30]	Gemfibrozil	RCT	5	MI or cardiac death	2/59 (3.4%)	8/76 (10.5%)	14	NS
Blood glucose control								
DCCT[41,42]	Intensive insulin therapy in Type 1 diabetes	RCT	6.5	Major macrovascular events**	23/711 (3.2%)	40/730 (5.5%)	45	28 to 728
UKPDS[36]	Intensive therapy with insulin and/or sulphyoaylurea v conventional therapy	RCT	5	MI (fatal or non-fatal)	387/2729 (14.2%)	186/1138 (16.3%)	46	NS
UKPDS[37]	Intensive therapy with metformin v conventional therapy	RCT	5	MI (fatal or non-fatal)	39/342 (11.4%)	73/411 (17.8%)	16	10 to 71
Aspirin								
Physicians' Health Study[43]	Aspirin	RCT	5	MI (fatal or non-fatal)	11/275 (4.0%)	26/258 (10.1%)	16	12 to 47
ETDRS (mixed primary & secondary prevention)[44]	Aspirin	RCT	5	MI (fatal or non-fatal)	289/1856 (15.6%)	336/1855 (18.1%)	39	21 to 716

*Diabetic patients only **Combined MI (fatal or non-fatal), sudden cardiac death, revascularisation procedure, angina with coronary artery disease confirmed by angiography or by noninvasive testing, stroke, lower limb amputation, peripheral arterial events requiring revascularisation, claudication with angiographic evidence of peripheral vascular disease. AMI, acute myocardial infarction; CHF chronic heart failure; CVD, cardiovascular disease; MI, myocardial infarction; NNT, number needed to treat; RCT, randomised controlled trials; SR, systematic review.

TABLE 2 Secondary prevention of cardiovascular events in people with diabetes: evidence from systematic reviews and randomised trials (see text, pp 301, 302, 304, 305).

Type of intervention	Study	Interventions	Study Type	Duration (years)	Outcome	Events / Sample size (%)*		NNT	95% CI for NNT
						Intervention group	Control group		
Antihypertensive medication									
	Cochrane review: long-term secondary prevention[17]	Various antihypertensive medications	SR	≥ 1 year	CVD mortality and morbidity	130/316 (41.1%)	157/338 (46.4%)	19	NS
	Cochrane review: short-term secondary prevention[17]	Various antihypertensive medications	SR	< 1 year	CVD mortality and morbidity	8/245 (3.3%)	21/288 (7.3%)	25	17 to 1145
Lipid-lowering									
	4S[32]	Simvastatin	RCT	5.4 years	CHD death or non-fatal MI	24/105 (22.9%)	44/97 (45.4%)	5	3 to 10
	CARE[33]	Pravastatin	RCT	5 years	Coronary disease death, non-fatal MI, or revascularisation	81/282 (28.7%)	112/304 (36.8%)	12	7 to 194
	LIPID[34]	Pravastatin	RCT	6.1 years	CHD death or non-fatal MI	76/396 (19.2%)	88/386 (22.8%)	28	NS
	Veterans[35]	Gemfibrozil	RCT	5.1	CHD death or non-fatal MI	88/309 (28.5%)	116/318 (36.5%)	13	7 to 144
Blood glucose control									
	DIGAMI[39,40]	Insulin infusion followed by intensive insulin therapy v usual care	RCT	3.4 years	Overall mortality	102/306 (33.3%)	138/314 (43.9%)	9	6 to 33

TABLE 2 Continued

							NNT	
Aspirin								
Antiplatelet trialists[45]	Aspirin v placebo	SR	Median 2 years	CVD mortality and morbidity	415/2248 (18.5%)	502/2254 (22.3%)	26	17 to 66
Revascularization								
BARI[47]	CABG v PTCA	RCT	7.7	Death or non-fatal q wave MI	CABG 60/173 (34.7%)	PTCA 85/170 (50%)	7	4 to 21
Glycoprotein IIb/IIIa blockers								
ERIC/EPILOG/ EPISTENT[53]	Abciximab v control	Pooled	1	Overall death rate	26/540 (4.8%)	21/844 (2.5%)	43	23 to 422
ERIC/EPILOG/ EPISTENT[53]	Abciximab v control	Pooled	1	Death or non-fatal MI	185/540 (34.3%)	246/844 (29.1%)	20	9 to 1423

*Diabetic patients only. CABG, coronary artery bypass grafting; CHD, coronary heart disease; CVD, cardiovascular disease; MI, myocardial infarction; NNT, number needed to treat; PTCA, percutaneous transluminal coronary angioplasty; RCT, randomised controlled trials; SR, systematic review.

TABLE 3 Mixed primary and secondary prevention of cardiovascular events in people with diabetes (see text, p 300).

Type of intervention	Interventions	Study type	Duration (years)	Outcome	Events/Sample size (%) (diabetic patients only)		NNT	95% CI for NNT
					Intervention group	Control group		
Mixed primary and secondary prevention[22]								
	Ramipril 10 mg daily	RCT	4.5	Myocardial infarction, stroke or cardiovascular death	277/1808 (15%)	351/1769 (20%)	22	14 to 49
Antihypertensive medication[22]								
	Ramipril 10 mg daily	RCT	4.5	Overall mortality	196/1808 (11%)	240/1769 (14%)	32	19 to 83

Endocrine disorders

Foot ulcers in diabetes

Updated this issue

Derek Hunt and Hertzel Gerstein

INTERVENTIONS

Key Messages

- One RCT has found that screening and referral to a footcare clinic for people with diabetes who are at high risk of developing foot ulcers reduces the risk of foot ulcers and major amputation.

- We found limited evidence from one RCT that total contact casting improves the healing of chronic, non-infected diabetic foot ulcers.

- One systematic review of RCTs found that topical growth factors may improve the rate of healing of chronic, non-infected foot ulcers.

- We found limited evidence from two small RCTs that systemic hyperbaric oxygen reduces the absolute risk of foot amputation in people with severe infected foot ulcers.

- We found limited evidence from one non-randomised trial that therapeutic footwear decreases the recurrence of foot ulceration.

- We found limited evidence from one non-randomised trial that patient education, provided after acute foot complications, decreases the risks of ulcer recurrence and major amputation.

DEFINITION	Diabetic foot ulceration refers to full thickness penetration of the dermis of the foot in a person with diabetes. Non-traumatic lower limb amputation refers to the surgical removal of all or part of the lower extremity. Minor amputations involve partial removal of a foot, including toe or forefoot resections. Major amputations refer to above or below knee amputations.
INCIDENCE/ PREVALENCE	The annual incidence of foot ulcers among people with diabetes is 2.5–10.7%, and the annual incidence of amputation is 0.25–1.8%.[1–8]
AETIOLOGY/ RISK FACTORS	Risk factors for foot ulcers and amputation include duration of diabetes, poor glycaemic control, and the presence of microvascular complications (retinopathy, nephropathy, and neuropathy). The strongest predictors, however, are altered foot sensation and previous foot ulcer.[1–8]
PROGNOSIS	People with diabetes are at risk of developing complications in the lower extremities. These include foot ulcers, infections, and vascular insufficiency. Amputation of a lower extremity is indicated if complications are severe or do not improve with appropriate treatment. As well as affecting quality of life, these complications contribute significantly to the healthcare costs associated with diabetes. For people with healed diabetic foot ulcers, the 5 year cumulative rate of ulcer recurrence is 66% and of amputation is 12%.[9]
AIMS	To prevent diabetic foot complications, including ulcers and amputations, and to improve ulcer healing and prevent amputations where ulcers already exist, with minimum adverse effects.
OUTCOMES	Rates of development or recurrence of foot ulcers or major foot lesions; rate of amputation; time ulcers take to heal, or the proportion healed in a given period; rates of hospital admission; rates of foot infection; adverse effects of treatment.
METHODS	*Clinical Evidence* update search and appraisal May 2000.

QUESTION What are the effects of preventive interventions?

OPTION SCREENING AND REFERRAL TO FOOTCARE CLINIC

One RCT has found that screening for altered sensation and absent pedal pulses followed by referral to footcare clinics (for education, footwear, and podiatry) reduces the risk of foot ulcers and major amputation.

Benefits: We found one systematic review (search date 1998), which identified one RCT.[10] The RCT (n = 2001 people attending a general diabetes clinic) compared usual care versus a diabetes screening and protection programme. People in the intervention group were screened for deficits in pedal pulses, light touch, and vibration sensation. People with persistent abnormal findings were referred to the diabetic foot clinic if they had a history of foot ulcer, were found to have a low ankle-brachial index (< 0.75), or were noted to have foot deformities. The clinic provided podiatry and protective shoes as well as education regarding foot care. Follow up 2 years after enrolment found that the number of people who had undergone major amputation was only one in the intervention group and 12 in the control group (RRR 92%; ARR 1.1%, 95% CI 0.4% to 1.9%; NNT 91, 95% CI 53 to 250).

Harms: No harms were reported.

Comment: None.

OPTION TOTAL CONTACT CASTING

Limited evidence from one small RCT suggests that total contact casting compared with traditional dressing changes increases the likelihood and speed of healing of chronic, non-infected diabetic foot ulcers. Total contact casting has not been directly compared with the use of topical growth factors.

Benefits: We found one systematic review (search date 1998), which identified one RCT.[11] This compared total contact casting versus traditional dressing changes in 40 people with diabetes and plantar foot ulcers but free of signs of infection or gangrene. All participants were told to minimise weight bearing during treatment. Casts were applied by an experienced physical therapist, changed after 5–7 days, and then every 2–3 weeks until healing occurred. Control participants were provided with accommodative footwear and crutches or a walker. They were instructed to complete wet to dry dressing changes 2–3 times daily. Ulcer healing occurred in 91% of people treated with total contact casting and 32% of people in the control group (absolute difference 59%, 95% CI 31% to 87%; NNT 2, 95% CI 1 to 3). Healing was quicker in people treated with total contact casting than controls (a mean of 42 days v 65 days). Five control participants were admitted to hospital because of infection, and two required amputation. No participants in the total contact casting group required hospital admission.

Harms: In the RCT, 3 of 21 people treated with total contact casting developed fungal infections that required topical treatment. These events did not prevent continued casting.

Comment: Total contact casting is the application of a layer of plaster over the foot and lower leg designed to distribute pressure evenly over the entire plantar aspect of the foot to reduce exposure of plantar ulcers to pressure, even when the patient is walking. Soft tissue infections and osteomyelitis are contraindications to total contact casting. Other methods aimed at decreasing the pressure applied to plantar ulcers during walking, such as removable cast walkers, half shoes, healing sandals, and felted foam, have not been evaluated in RCTs.

OPTION CULTURED HUMAN DERMIS AND TOPICAL GROWTH FACTORS

One systematic review found that cultured human dermis and topical growth factors may improve the rate of healing of chronic, non-infected foot ulcers. These therapeutic interventions have not been directly compared with total contact casting.

Benefits: We found one systematic review (search date 1998), which identified two unblinded RCTs of cultured human dermis and six double blind RCTs of four different topical growth factors.[11] These compared topical application of cultured human dermis or a growth factor versus placebo in people attending hospital outpatient clinics with diabetic foot ulcers who were free of signs of infection or severe vascular compromise. All received wound debridement and were encouraged to avoid weight bearing on the affected limb. For cultured human dermis, one RCT (n = 50) found that treatment with neonatal cultured fibroblasts (weekly for 8 weeks) increased healing rates (AR of non-healing 50% v 92% for placebo; RRR 46%; ARR 42%, 95% CI 5% to 80%; NNT 2, 95% CI 1 to 20). The second RCT (n = 281) of cultured human dermis found a non-significant effect on healing rate (AR non-healing 61% v 68% with control; RRR 10%; ARR 7%, 95% CI −6% to +20%). The systematic review identified six RCTs of topical growth factors. One RCT (n = 65) found that treatment with an arginine-glycine-aspartic (RGD) acid matrix twice weekly for up to 10 weeks increased healing rates (AR non-healing 65% v 92% with placebo; RRR 29%; ARR 27%, 95% CI 6% to 48%; NNT 4, 95% CI 2 to 15). One RCT (n = 118) found that treatment with platelet derived growth factors (30 µg/g once daily for up to 20 weeks) increased healing rates (AR non-healing 52% v 75% with placebo; RRR 31%; ARR 23%, 95% CI 5% to 41%; NNT 5, 95% CI 2 to 19). A second RCT (n = 382) found that treatment with platelet derived growth factors (100 µg/g once daily for up to 20 weeks) increased healing rates (AR non-healing 50% v 65% with placebo; RRR 23%; ARR 15%, 95% CI 2% to 28%; NNT 7, 95% CI 4 to 42). This second RCT found no benefit with platelet derived growth factors 30 µg/g once daily for up to 20 weeks compared with placebo (AR non-healing 64% v 65% with placebo). Two RCTs evaluated CT-102, a growth factor derived from thrombin-induced human platelets, applied twice weekly. One small RCT (n = 13) found no significant effect on healing rates (AR non-healing 29% v 83% with placebo; RRR 66%; ARR 55%, 95% CI −2% to +81%). The second, larger RCT (n = 81) of CT-102 found a significant difference in healing rates (AR of non-healing 20% v 71% with placebo; RRR 72%; ARR 51%, 95% CI 19% to 84%; NNT 2, 95% CI 1 to 5). One small RCT in 17 people found no benefit from recombinant platelet-derived growth factor versus control treatment.

Harms: Adverse events, when reported, were no more common in the intervention arms than in the control arms.

Comment: These therapeutic agents are not yet widely available and may be expensive. There has been little long term follow up of people treated with these growth factors.

| OPTION | SYSTEMIC HYPERBARIC OXYGEN |

Two small RCTs have found that, compared with routine care, systemic hyperbaric oxygen reduces the absolute risk of foot amputation in people with severe infected foot ulcers.

Benefits: We found one systematic review (search date 1998),[11] and one additional RCT.[12] The review identified one RCT in 70 people with severe infected diabetic foot ulcers and compared usual care (aggressive debridement, broad spectrum intravenous antibiotics, revascularisation if indicated, and optimised glycaemic control) versus usual care plus daily 90 minute sessions of systemic hyperbaric oxygen at 2.2–2.5 atmospheres.[13] Participants either had full thickness gangrene or abscess or a large infected ulcer that had not healed after 30 days. After 10 weeks, rates of major amputation were significantly lower in the intervention group (8.6% v 33% in the control group; RRR 74%, 95% CI 16% to 92%; ARR 24%, 95% CI 4% to 45%; NNT 5, 95% CI 2 to 23). The additional RCT in 30 people with chronic infected foot ulcers compared usual treatment (including debridement, intravenous antibiotics, and optimised glycaemic control) versus usual treatment plus four treatments with hyperbaric oxygen over 2 weeks. It found no significant reduction of the risk of major amputation in the intervention group (ARR 33%, 95% CI –1.6% to +68%).[12]

Harms: In the larger RCT, two people developed symptoms of barotraumatic otitis, but this did not interrupt treatment.[13]

Comment: None.

OPTION   APPROPRIATE FOOTWEAR

Limited evidence from one non-randomised trial suggests that therapeutic footwear, made according to the Towey guidelines, decreases recurrence of ulceration.

Benefits: We found one systematic review (search date 1998), which identified one non-randomised controlled trial.[10] Sixty nine people with a previous diabetic foot ulcer were alternately allocated to either an intervention group, in which people received therapeutic shoes, or to a control group, in which people continued to wear their ordinary shoes. Therapeutic shoes were manufactured according to the Towey guidelines (super depth to fit customised insoles and toe deformities and made with soft thermoformable leather along with semirocker soles) and fitted with custom moulded insoles. All participants received information on foot care and footwear. After 1 year, it found a significant reduction of ulcer recurrence with intervention versus control (AR 27% with intervention v 58% with control; RRR 53%; ARR 31%, 95% CI 7% to 55%; NNT 4, 95% CI 2 to 14).

Harms: The trial did not report any adverse effects associated with therapeutic shoes.

Comment: Alternate allocation leaves open the possibility of bias from non-comparability of the two treatment groups.

OPTION   EDUCATION

Limited evidence from one non-randomised trial suggests that patient education provided after the management of acute foot complications decreases ulcer recurrences and major amputations.

Benefits: We found one systematic review (search date 1998), which identified one non-randomised controlled trial.[11] The RCT (227 people who presented with foot infection, ulcer, or for assistance following a previous amputation) allocated people according to their social security number and evaluated the effect of providing a single, 1 hour educational class on diabetic foot complications and important components of foot care. Surgical treatment was provided for all people when necessary. Follow up at 2 years found that allocation to the educational session significantly reduced ulcer recurrences (AR 14.7% for control group v 4.5% for education; RRR 69%; ARR 10%, 95% CI 4% to 16%; NNT 10, 95% CI 6 to 26) and major amputation (AR 10.2% v 2.8%; RRR 72%; ARR 7%, 95% CI 2% to 13%; NNT 14, 95% CI 8 to 50).

Harms: None reported.

Comment: Allocation by social security number may introduce biases and could create non-comparable groups.

REFERENCES

1. Rith-Najarian SJ, Stolusky T, Gohdes DM. Identifying diabetic patients at high risk for lower-extremity amputation in a primary health care setting. *Diabetes Care* 1992;15:1386–1389.
2. Veves A, Murray HJ, Young MJ, et al. The risk of foot ulceration in diabetic patients with high foot pressure: a prospective study. *Diabetologia* 1992;35:660–663.
3. Young MJ, Breddy JL, Veves A, et al. The prediction of diabetic neuropathic foot ulceration using vibration perception thresholds: a prospective study. *Diabetes Care* 1994;7:557–560.
4. Humphrey ARG, Dowse GK, Thoma K, et al. Diabetes and nontraumatic lower extremity amputations. Incidence, risk factors, and prevention: a 12 year follow-up study in Nauru. *Diabetes Care* 1996;19:710–714.
5. Lee JS, Lu M, Lee VS, et al. Lower-extremity amputation: incidence, risk factors, and mortality in the Oklahoma Indian diabetes study. *Diabetes* 1993;42:876–882.
6. Lehto S, Ronnemaa T, Pyorala K, et al.. Risk factors predicting lower extremity amputations in patients with NIDDM. *Diabetes Care* 1996;19:607–612.
7. Moss SE, Klein R, Klein B. Long-term incidence of lower-extremity amputations in a diabetic population. *Arch Fam Med* 1996;5:391–398.
8. Nelson RG, Gohdes DM, Everhart JE, et al. Lower-extremity amputations in NIDDM: 12 year follow-up study in Pima Indians. *Diabetes Care* 1988;11:8–16.
9. Apelqvist J, Larsson J, Agardh CD. Long-term prognosis for diabetic patients with foot ulcers. *J Intern Med* 1993;233:485–491.
10. Mason J, O'Keeffe C, McIntosh A, et al. A systematic review of foot ulcer in patients with type 2 diabetes mellitus. I: prevention. *Diabet Med* 1999;16:801–812. Search date 1998; primary sources Cochrane Trials Register 1983 to 1998; Medline 1983 to 1998; Embase 1983 to 1998; Cinahl 1983 to 1998; Healthstar 1983 to 1998; Psyclit 1983 to 1998; Science Citation 1983 to 1998; Social Science Citation 1983 to 1998; Index to Scientific and Technical Conference Proceedings (ISI) 1983 to 1998; HMIC database 1983 to 1988 and SIGLE 1983 to 1998.
11. Mason J, O'Keeffe C, Hutchinson A, et al. A systematic review of foot ulcer in patients with type 2 diabetes mellitus. II: treatment. *Diabet Med* 1999;16:889–909. Search date 1998; primary sources Cochrane Trials Register 1983 to 1998; Medline 1983 to 1998; Embase 1983 to 1998; Cinahl 1983 to 1998; Healthstar 1983 to 1998; Psyclit 1983 to 1998; Science Citation 1983 to 1998; Social Science Citation 1983 to 1998; Index to Scientific and Technical Conference Proceedings (ISI) 1983 to 1998; HMIC database 1983 to 1988 and SIGLE 1983 to 1998.
12. Doctor N, Pandya S, Supe A. Hyperbaric oxygen therapy in diabetic foot. *J Postgrad Med* 1992;38:112–114.
13. Faglia E, Favales F, Aldeghi A, et al. Adjunctive systemic hyperbaric oxygen therapy in treatment of severe prevalently ischemic diabetic foot ulcer. *Diabetes Care* 1996;19:1338–1343.

Dereck Hunt
Clinical Scholar

Hertzel Gerstein
Associate Professor of Medicine

McMaster University
Hamilton, Ontario
Canada

Competing interests: None declared.

Endocrine disorders

Glycaemic control in diabetes

Last updated Issue 3

William Herman

QUESTIONS
Effects of intensive versus conventional glycaemic control 322
Optimum target blood glucose 325

INTERVENTIONS	
Beneficial	**Trade off between benefits and harms**
Intensive control of hyperglycaemia in people aged 13–75 years 322	Intensive control of hyperglycaemia in people with frequent severe hypoglycaemia. 322

Key Messages

- We found strong evidence from one systematic review and three large subsequent RCTs that intensive compared with conventional treatment reduces the development and progression of microvascular and neuropathic complications in both type 1 and type 2 diabetes. A second systematic review of RCTs has found that intensive treatment is associated with a small reduction in cardiovascular risk.

- We found no evidence that intensive treatment causes adverse cardiovascular outcomes. RCTs have found that intensive treatment is associated with hypoglycaemia and weight gain without adverse impact on neuropsychological function or quality of life.

- Large RCTs have found that diabetic complications increase with HbA1c concentrations above the non-diabetic range.

DEFINITION Diabetes mellitus is a group of disorders characterised by hyper glycaemia (definitions vary slightly, one current North American definition is fasting plasma glucose ≥ 7.0 mmol/l, or ≥ 11.1 mmol/l 2 hours after a 75 g oral glucose load, on two or more occasions). Intensive treatment is designed to achieve blood glucose values as close to the non-diabetic range as possible. The essential components of such treatment are education, counselling, monitoring, self management, and pharmacological treatment with insulin or oral antidiabetic agents to achieve specific glycaemic goals.

INCIDENCE/ PREVALENCE Diabetes is diagnosed in around 5% of adults aged 20 years or over in the USA.[1] A further 2.7% have undiagnosed diabetes on the basis of fasting glucose. The prevalence is similar in men and women, but diabetes is more common in some ethnic groups. The prevalence in people aged 40–74 years has increased over the past decade.

AETIOLOGY/ RISK FACTORS Diabetes results from deficient insulin secretion, decreased insulin action, or both. Many processes can be involved, from autoimmune destruction of the β cells of the pancreas to incompletely understood abnormalities that result in resistance to insulin action. Genetic factors are involved in both mechanisms. In type 1 diabetes there is an absolute deficiency of insulin. In type 2 diabetes, insulin resistance and an inability of the pancreas to compensate are involved. Hyperglycaemia without clinical symptoms but sufficient to cause tissue damage can be present for many years before diagnosis.

PROGNOSIS Severe hyperglycaemia causes numerous symptoms, including polyuria, polydipsia, weight loss, and blurred vision. Acute, life threatening consequences of diabetes are hyperglycaemia with ketoacidosis or the non-ketotic hyperosmolar syndrome. There is increased susceptibility to certain infections. Long term complications of diabetes include retinopathy (with potential loss of vision), nephropathy (leading to renal failure), peripheral neuropathy (increased risk of foot ulcers, amputation, and Charcot joints), autonomic neuropathy (cardiovascular, gastrointestinal, and genitourinary dysfunction), and greatly increased risk of atheroma affecting large vessels (macrovascular complications of stroke, myocardial infarction, or peripheral vascular disease). The physical, emotional, and social impact of diabetes and demands of intensive treatment can also create problems for people with diabetes and their families. One systematic review (search date 1998) of observational studies in people with type 2 diabetes found a positive association between increased blood glucose concentration and mortality.[2] It found no minimum threshold level.

AIMS To slow development and progression of the microvascular, neuropathic, and cardiovascular complications of diabetes, while minimising adverse effects of treatment (hypoglycaemia and weight gain) and maximising quality of life.

OUTCOMES Quality of life; short term burden of treatment; long term clinical complications; risks and benefits of treatment. Both the development of complications in people who have previously been free of them, and the progression of complications, are used as outcomes. Scales of severity are used to detect disease progression (e.g. 19

step scales of diabetic retinopathy; normoalbuminuria, microalbuminuria, and albuminuria for nephropathy; absence or presence of clinical neuropathy).

METHODS We searched Medline and Embase in October 1999 for systematic reviews and subsequent RCTs assessing the impact of control of blood glucose in people with diabetes that measured clinical outcomes of the type described above. *Clinical Evidence* update search and appraisal May 2000.

QUESTION What are the effects of intensive versus conventional glycaemic control?

One systematic review of sixteen RCTs and three subsequent RCTs in people with type 1 and type 2 diabetes have found that intensive treatment compared with conventional treatment reduces development and progression of microvascular and neuropathic complications. A second systematic review of six RCTs in people with type 1 diabetes, and two additional RCTs in people with type 2 diabetes, have found no evidence that intensive treatment increases adverse cardiovascular outcomes. Intensive treatment reduced the number of macrovascular events but had no significant effect on the number of people that developed macrovascular disease. Intensive treatment is associated with hypoglycaemia and weight gain, but does not seem to affect neuropsychological function or quality of life adversely.

Benefits: **Microvascular and neuropathic complications:** We found one systematic review (search date 1991)[3] and three subsequent long term RCTs[4,6,7] (one in type 1 diabetes and two in type 2 diabetes) that assessed the impact of intensive compared with conventional treatment on microvascular and neuropathic complications. The systematic review of 16 small RCTs in type 1 diabetes provided follow up ranging from 8–60 months.[3] One subsequent RCT studied 1441 people with type 1 diabetes over 6.5 years (about half had no retinopathy and half had mild retinopathy at baseline).[4] A further follow up study 4 years after the end of the trial (all participants offered intensive treatment) found a narrowing of the difference in median HbA1c concentrations but that the reduction in the risk of progression of retinopathy and nephropathy was maintained.[5] The proportion of people with worsening retinopathy and nephropathy was significantly lower for those who had received intensive treatment. The second RCT studied 110 people with insulin treated type 2 diabetes over 6 years.[6] The third RCT compared a conventional dietary treatment policy with two different intensive treatment policies based on sulfonylurea and insulin (3867 people with newly diagnosed type 2 diabetes; age 25–65 years; fasting plasma glucose 6.1–15.0 mmol/l after 3 months dietary therapy; no symptoms of hyperglycaemia; follow up 10 years). HbA1c rose steadily in both groups. Intensive treatment was associated with a significant reduction in any diabetes related end point (40.9 *v* 46.0 events/1000 person years; RRR 12%, 95% CI 1% to 21%), but no evidence was found of an effect on diabetes related deaths (10.4 *v* 11.5 deaths/1000 person years; RRR 10%, 95% CI −11% to +27%) or all cause mortality (17.9 *v* 18.9 deaths/1000 person years; RRR 6%, 95% CI −10% to +20%). Secondary analysis found that intensive treatment was associated with a significant reduction in microvascular end points (8.6 v 11.4/1000 person years; RRR 25%, 95% CI 7% to 40%) compared with conventional treatment (see table 1, p 327)[7] The systematic review and all the subsequent RCTs found that the relative risks of retinopathy, nephropathy, and neuropathy were all significantly reduced. **Cardiovascular outcomes:** We found one systematic review, which included six RCTs comparing intensive insulin treatment versus conventional treatment on cardiovascular outcomes in type 1 diabetes (1731 people; follow up 2–8 years).[8] Intensive insulin treatment decreased the number of macrovascular events (OR 0.55, 95% CI 0.35 to 0.88), but had no significant affect on the number of people developing macrovascular disease (OR 0.72, 95% CI 0.44 to 1.17) or on macrovascular mortality (OR 0.91, 95% CI 0.31 to 2.65). We found two additional RCTs in people with type 2 diabetes.[6,7] In the first RCT the number of major cerebrovascular, cardiovascular, and peripheral vascular events in the intensive treatment group was half that of the conventional treatment group (0.6 v 1.3 events/100 person years), but the event rate in this small trial was low and the results were not significant.[6] In the second RCT, intensive treatment versus conventional treatment was associated with a non–significant reduction in the risk of myocardial infarction (AR 387/2729 [14%] with intensive treatment v 186/1138 [16%] with conventional treatment; RRR 13%, 95% CI –2% to +27%), a non-significant increase in the risk of stroke (AR 148/2729 [5.4%] v [55/1138 [4.8%]; RRI 12%, 95% CI –17% to +51%), and a non-significant reduction in the risk of amputation or death from peripheral vascular disease (AR 29/2729 [1.1%] v 18/1138 [1.6%]; RRR 33%, 95% CI –20% to +63%).[7]

Harms: **Hypoglycaemia:** We found one systematic review (search date 1996), which identified 14 RCTs in type 1 diabetes with at least 6 months' follow up and monitoring of glycaemia by glycosylated haemoglobin (2067 people; follow up 0.5 to 7.5 years).[9] The median incidence of severe hypoglycaemia was 7.9 episodes/100 person years among intensively treated people and 4.6 episodes/100 person years among conventionally treated people (OR 3.0, 95% CI 2.5 to 3.6). The risk of severe hypoglycaemia was associated with the degree of glycosylated haemoglobin lowering in the intensive treatment groups (P = 0.005). We found three RCTs in type 2 diabetes where the rates of hypoglycaemia were lower.[6,7] In the first RCT (n = 110) there was no significant difference between groups.[6] In the second RCT (3867 people) the rates of major hypoglycaemic episodes per year were 0.7% with conventional treatment, 1.0% with chlorpropamide, 1.4% with glibenclamide, and 1.8% with insulin. People in the intensive treatment group had significantly more hypoglycaemic episodes than those in the conventional group (P < 0.0001).[7] In the third RCT (1704 overweight people) major hypoglycaemic episodes occurred in 0.6% of overweight people in the metformin treated group.[10] **Weight gain:** Four RCTs found more weight increase with intensive treatment than with standard treatment.[4,6,7,11] One RCT found weight remained stable in people with type 1 diabetes in the conventional treatment group, but body mass index increased by 5.8% in the intensive treatment group (95% CI not presented, P < 0.01).[11] In the second RCT

(1441 people with type 2 diabetes) intensive treatment was associated with a 33% increase in the relative risk of developing a body weight more than 120% above the ideal (12.7 cases per 100 person years with intensive treatment v 9.3 cases per 100 person years with conventional treatment). At 5 years, people treated intensively gained 4.6 kg more than people treated conventionally (CI not presented for weight data).[4] In the third RCT, the increase in body mass index from baseline to 6 years was not significant in either group (intensive treatment group 20.5 to 21.2 kg/m^2, conventional treatment group 20.3 to 21.9 kg/m^2).[6] In the fourth RCT, weight gain at 10 years was significantly higher in people with type 2 diabetes in the intensive treatment group compared with people in the conventional treatment group (mean 2.9 kg) (P < 0.001), and people assigned insulin had a greater gain in weight (4.0 kg) than those assigned chlorpropamide (2.6 kg) or glibenclamide (1.7 kg).[7] We found one systematic review (search date 1996, 10 RCTs)[12] and one subsequent RCT[10] that compared metformin and sulfonylurea. Meta-analysis in the review found that sulfonylurea was associated with an increase in weight from baseline and metformin with a decrease (difference 2.9 kg, 95% CI 1.1 to 4.4 kg). In the subsequent RCT, overweight participants randomly assigned to intensive blood glucose control with metformin had a similar change in body weight to the conventional treatment group, and less increase in mean body weight than people receiving intensive treatment with sulfonylureas or insulin.[10] **Neuropsychological impairment:** We found no systematic review on neuropsychological impairment, but found two RCTs. One RCT (102 people) that compared intensified with standard treatment in people with type 1 diabetes. It found no cognitive impairment associated with hypoglycaemia after 3 years.[13,14] The second RCT found that intensive treatment did not affect neuropsychological performance.[15] In addition, people who had repeated episodes of hypoglycaemia did not perform differently from people who did not have repeated episodes.[16] **Quality of life:** We found two RCTs that reported quality of life in people undergoing intensive versus conventional treatment. One RCT (1441 people) found that intensive treatment did not reduce quality of life in people with type 1 diabetes.[17] Severe hypoglycaemia was not consistently associated with a subsequent increase in distress caused by symptoms or decline in the quality of life. In the primary prevention intensive treatment group, however, repeated severe hypoglycaemia (three or more events resulting in coma or seizure) tended to increase the risk of distress caused by symptoms. The second large RCT, in people with type 2 diabetes, assessed disease specific (2431 people) and generic measures (3104 people) of quality of life (QoL) in two large cross sectional samples at 8 and 11 years after randomisation, and disease specific QoL in a small cohort of participants (374 people) at 6 months and annually thereafter for 6 years.[18] The cross sectional studies found that treatments had no significant effect on QoL scores for mood, cognitive mistakes, symptoms, work satisfaction, or general health. The longitudinal study also found no significant difference in QoL scores for the specific domains assessed (other than showing marginally more symptoms in patients allocated to conventional than to intensive treatment). In the cross sectional studies, people who had macrovascular or microvascular complications in the last year had worse QoL than people without complications. People treated with insulin who had two or more hypoglycaemic episodes during the previous year reported more tension, more overall mood disturbance, and less work satisfaction as measured by the disease specific questionnaire than those with no hypoglycaemic attacks (after adjusting for age, time from randomisation, systolic blood pressure, HbA1c, and sex). It was unclear, however, whether frequent hypoglycaemic episodes affected QoL, or whether people with certain personality traits or symptoms simply reported increased numbers of hypoglycaemic attacks. The authors concluded that in people with type 2 diabetes, complications affected QoL, but interventions that reduced the risk of complications did not affect QoL.

Comment: None.

<hr>

QUESTION **What is the optimum target blood glucose?**

Large RCTs in people with type 1 and type 2 diabetes have found that risk of development or progression of complications increases progressively as glycosylated haemoglobin increases above the non-diabetic range.

Benefits: We found no systematic review but found two large RCTs.[18,19] One large RCT in people with type II diabetes found that, as concentrations of glycosylated haemoglobin were reduced, the relative risk of complications fell but the risk of hypoglycaemia increased.[18] The other RCT in people with type I diabetes also found that lower glycosylated haemoglobin was associated with a lower risk of complications.[19]

Harms: Both RCTs found that hypoglycaemia was increased by intensive treatment.[18,19]

Comment: It is difficult to weigh the benefit of reduced complications against the harm of increased hypoglycaemia. The balance between benefits and harms of intensive treatment in type 1 diabetes may be less favourable in children under 13 years or in older adults, and in people with repeated severe hypoglycaemia or unawareness of hypoglycaemia. Similarly, the balance between benefits and harms of intensive treatment in type 2 diabetes may be less favourable in people over 65 years or in those with longstanding diabetes. The benefit of intensive treatment is limited by the complications of advanced diabetes (such as blindness, end stage renal disease or cardiovascular disease), major comorbidity, and reduced life expectancy. The risk of intensive treatment is increased by a history of severe hypoglycaemia or unawareness of hypoglycaemia, advanced autonomic neuropathy, or cardiovascular disease, and impaired ability to detect or treat hypoglycaemia (such as altered mental state, immobility, or lack of social support). For people likely to have limited benefit or increased risk with intensive treatment, less intensive goals for glycaemic management should be negotiated, reflecting the individual's self determined goals of care and willingness to make lifestyle modifications.

REFERENCES

1. Harris MI, Flegal KM, Cowie CC, et al. Prevalence of diabetes, impaired fasting glucose, and impaired glucose tolerance in US adults: the third national health and nutrition examination survey, 1988–1994. *Diabetes Care* 1998;2:518–524.
2. Groeneveld Y, Petri H, Hermans J, et al. Relationship between blood glucose level and mortality in type 2 diabetes mellitus: a systematic review. *Diabet Med* 1999;16:2–13.
3. Wang PH, Lau J, Chalmers TC. Meta-analysis of effects of intensive blood glucose control on late complications of type I diabetes. *Lancet* 1993; 341:1306–1309. Search date 1991; primary sources Medline 1966 to December 1991.
4. The Diabetes Control and Complications Trial Research Group. The effect of intensive treatment of diabetes on the development and progression of long-term complications of insulin-dependent diabetes mellitus. *N Engl J Med* 1993;329:977–986.
5. The DCCT/Epidemiology of Diabetes Interventions and Complications Research Group. Retinopathy and nephropathy in patients with type 1 diabetes four years after a trial of intensive therapy. *N Engl J Med* 2000;342:381–389.
6. Ohkubo Y, Kishikawa H, Arake E, et al. Intensive insulin therapy prevents the progression of diabetic microvascular complications in Japanese patients with non-insulin-dependent diabetes mellitus: a randomized prospective 6-year study. *Diabetes Res Clin Pract* 1995;28:103–117.
7. UK Prospective Diabetes Study Group. Intensive blood-glucose control with sulphonylureas or insulin compared with conventional treatment and risk of complications in patients with type 2 diabetes. *Lancet* 1998;352:837–853.
8. Lawson ML, Gerstein HC, Tsui E, et al. Effect of intensive therapy on early macrovascular disease in young individuals with type 1 diabetes. *Diabetes Care* 1999;22:B35–B39. Search date 1996; primary sources Medline, Citation Index, reference lists, and personal files.
9. Egger M, Smith GD, Stettler C, et al. Risk of adverse effects of intensified treatment in insulin-dependent diabetes mellitus: a meta-analysis. *Diabet Med* 1997;14:919–928. Search date not given; primary sources Medline, reference lists, and specialist journals.
10. UK Prospective Diabetes Study Group. Effect of intensive blood-glucose control with metformin on complications in overweight patients with type 2 diabetes. *Lancet* 1998;352:854–865.
11. Reichard P, Berglund B, Britz A, et al. Intensified conventional insulin treatment retards the microvascular complications of insulin-dependent diabetes mellitus (IDDM): the Stockholm diabetes intervention study (SDIS) after 5 years. *J Int Med* 1991;30:101–108.
12. Johansen K. Efficacy of metformin in the treatment of NIDDM. *Diabetes Care* 1999;22:33–37. Search date January 1996; primary sources current list of medical literature 1957 to 1959; Index Medicus 1959 to 1965; Medline 1966 to January 1966; Embase 1989 to January 1996 and hand searched references.
13. Reichard P, Nilsson BY, Rosenqvist U. The effect of long-term intensified insulin treatment on the development of microvascular complications of diabetes mellitus. *N Engl J Med* 1993;29:304–309.
14. Reichard P, Berglund A, Britz A, et al. Hypoglycaemic episodes during intensified insulin treatment: increased frequency but no effect on cognitive function. *J Int Med* 1991;229:9–16.
15. The Diabetes Control and Complications Trial Research Group. Effects of intensive diabetes therapy on neuropsychological function in adults in the diabetes control and complications trial. *Ann Intern Med* 1996;124:379–388.
16. Austin EJ, Deary IJ. Effects of repeated hypoglycaemia on cognitive function. A psychometrically validated reanalysis of the diabetes control and complications trial data. *Diabetes Care* 1999;22:1273–1277.
17. The Diabetes Control and Complications Trial Research Group. Influence of intensive diabetes treatment on quality-of-life outcomes in the diabetes control and complications trial. *Diabetes Care* 1996;19:195–203.
18. UK Prospective Diabetes Study Group. Quality of life in type 2 diabetic patients is affected by complications but not by intensive policies to improve blood glucose or blood pressure control (UKPDS 37). *Diabetes Care* 1999;22:1125–1136.
19. The Diabetes Control and Complications Trial Research Group. The absence of a glycaemic threshold for the development of long-term complications: the perspective of the diabetes control and complications trial. *Diabetes* 1996; 45:1289–1298.

William Herman
Professor of Internal Medicine and Epidemiology
University of Michigan Medical Center
Ann Arbor, Michigan
USA

Competing interests: None declared.

TABLE 1 Risk (odds ratio) for development or progression of microvascular, nephropathic, and neuropathic complications with intensive versus conventional treatment. Odds ratio (OR), number needed to treat (NNT), and confidence intervals (CI) were all calculated from data in papers (see text, p 323).

	Systematic Review[3]	DCCT[4]	Kumamoto[6]	UKPDS[7]
Studies	16 RCTs	RCT	RCT	RCT
Number of participants	–	1441	110	3867
Type of diabetes	Type 1	Type 1	Type 2	Type 2*
Follow up	8 to 60 months	6.5 years	6 years	10 years
Change in HbA1c	1.4%	2.0%	2.0%	0.9%
Progression of retinopathy				
OR (95% CI)	0.49 (0.28 to 0.85)	0.39 (0.28 to 0.55)	0.25 (0.09 to 0.65)	0.66 (0.48 to 0.92)
NNT (95% CI) over duration of study	–	5 (4 to 7)	4 (3 to 11)	10 (6 to 50)
Development of retinopathy				
OR (95% CI)	–	0.22 (0.14 to 0.36)	–	–
NNT (95% CI) over duration of study	–	6 (5 to 7)	–	–
Development or progression of nephropathy				
OR (95% CI)	0.34 (0.20 to 0.58)	0.50 (0.39 to 0.63)	0.26 (0.09 to 0.76)	0.54 (0.25 to 1.18)
NNT (95% CI) over duration of study	–	7 (6 to 11)	5 (4 to 19)	–
Development or progression of neuropathy				
OR (95% CI)	–	0.36 (0.24 to 0.54)	–	0.42 (0.23 to 0.78)
NNT (95% CI) over duration of study	–	13 (11 to 18)	–	5 (3 to 16)

*All participants had fasting plasma glucose > 6.0 mmol/L on two occasions: 93% had fasting plasma glucose ≥ 7.0 mmol/L (American Diabetic Association criterion) and 86% had fasting plasma glucose ≥ 7.8 mmol/L (WHO criterion).

Endocrine disorders

New topic

Polly Hitchcock Noël, David Arterburn and Cynthia Mulrow

Key Messages

Centrally acting agents

- Small RCTs have found limited evidence that phenylpropanolamine, phentermine, mazindol, and diethlyproprion result in modest weight loss in people more than 15% overweight, when compared with placebo, over short periods of follow up. Weight regain has been reported with discontinuation of treatment and longer treatment periods. We found no long term evidence on weight regain or adverse effects of continued treatment.

- A systematic review of dexfenfluramine and small RCTs of fenfluramine found modest reductions in weight at 6 and 12 months in people more than 20% overweight, when compared with placebo. Dexfenfluramine and the combination of fenfluramine with phentermine have been associated with valvar heart disease.

- Two RCTs found limited and conflicting evidence comparing the selective serotonergic reuptake inhibitor fluoxetine with placebo.

- RCTs have found limited evidence that sibutramine can increase weight loss compared with placebo in healthy adults with a body mass index (BMI) (see glossary, p 333) between 27–40 kg/m^2. Effects are not sustained over time or when the medication is discontinued. We found no evidence on long term safety.

Orlistat

- A systematic review of RCTs found orlistat plus a low calorie diet has a modest effect on body weight compared with placebo plus diet in people with a BMI between 28–47 kg/m^2. We found no evidence on weight regain after stopping treatment, and no evidence of long term safety.

DEFINITION	Obesity is a chronic condition characterised by an excess of body fat. It is most often defined by the body mass index (BMI), a mathematical formula that is highly correlated with body fat. BMI is weight in kilograms divided by height in metres squared (kg/m^2). In the USA and the UK, people with BMIs between 25–30 kg/m^2 are categorised as overweight, and those with BMIs above 30 kg/m^2 are categorised as obese.[1]
INCIDENCE/ PREVALENCE	Obesity has increased steadily in certain countries since 1900. In England, in 1994, it was estimated that 13% of men and 16% of women were obese.[1,2] In the past decade alone, the prevalence of obesity in the USA has increased from 12.0% in 1991 to 17.9% in 1998.[3]
AETIOLOGY/ RISK FACTORS	The aetiology of obesity includes both genetic and environmental factors. Obesity may also be induced by drugs (e.g. high dose glucocorticoids) or be secondary to a variety of neuroendocrine disorders such as Cushing's syndrome and polycystic ovary syndrome.[4]
PROGNOSIS	Obesity is a risk factor for several chronic diseases, including hypertension, dyslipidaemia, diabetes, cardiovascular disease, sleep apnoea, osteoarthritis, and some cancers.[1] The relation between increasing body weight and mortality is curvilinear, with mortality increasing in people with low body weight. Whether this is caused by increased mortality risk at low body weights or by unintentional weight loss is not clear.[5] Data from five prospective cohort studies and 1991 national statistics suggest that the number of annual deaths attributable to obesity among US adults is approximately 280 000.[6]
AIMS	To achieve realistic gradual weight loss and prevent the morbidity and mortality associated with obesity, without undue adverse effects.
OUTCOMES	We found no studies which used the primary outcomes of functional morbidity or mortality. Proxy measures include mean weight loss (kg), number of people losing 5% or more of baseline body weight, and maintaining weight loss.
METHODS	*Clinical Evidence* search and appraisal June 2000.

<hr>

QUESTION **What are the effects of drug treatments in adults?**

OPTION CENTRALLY ACTING DRUGS

Limited evidence from small RCTs suggests that phenylpropanolamine, phentermine, mazindol, and diethylproprion result in modest weight loss in people more than 15% overweight, when compared with placebo, over short periods of follow up. Weight regain has been reported with discontinuation of treatment and longer treatment periods. We found no evidence about weight regain and adverse effects of continued treatment. A systematic review of dexfenfluramine and small RCTs of fenfluramine found that modest reductions in weight occur at 6 and 12 months in people more than 20% overweight, when compared with placebo. Dexfenfluramine and the combination of fenfluramine with phentermine have been associated with valvar heart disease. Two RCTs

Endocrine disorders

found limited and conflicting evidence comparing fluoxetine with placebo. Limited evidence from six RCTs suggests that sibutramine can increase weight loss compared with placebo in healthy adults with BMI (see glossary, p 333) between 27–40 kg/m². The weight loss was not sustained over time or after stopping treatment. We found no evidence on long term safety.

Benefits: We found no systematic review or RCTs examining effects of centrally acting drugs on functional morbidity and mortality. **Phenylpropanolamine:** We found one non-systematic meta-analysis of seven trials that examined the effect of phenylpropanolamine alone on the weight of 643 obese people (BMI not given). It found that, compared with placebo, phenylpropanolamine (dose not specified) produced an additional weight loss of 0.21 kg/week at 4 weeks. At the end of these trials (duration not specified), there was an additional weight loss of 0.14 kg/week compared with placebo.[7] **Phentermine:** We found one RCT in 108 people who were more than 20% overweight. It found that phentermine 30 mg/day reduced weight more than placebo at 9 months (−12.2 kg with phentermine v −4.8 kg with placebo; mean difference −7.4 kg, 95% CI −11.2 to −4.6 kg). All groups were placed on a diet of 1000 kcal/day.[8] **Phentermine plus fenfluramine:** See below. **Mazindol:** We found one RCT in 65 people who were more than 15% overweight. It found that mazindol 3 mg/day reduced weight more than placebo at 3 months (−6.4 kg with mazindol v −2.6 kg with placebo; mean difference −3.8 kg, 95% CI not reported, P < 0.001). Weight loss was not sustained when treatment was discontinued.[9] **Diethylproprion:** We found two small RCTs with conflicting results. The first included 20 people who were 15–20% overweight and found that diethylproprion 75 mg/day reduced weight more than placebo at 6 months (−11.6 kg with diethylproprion v −2.5 kg with placebo; mean difference −9.1 kg, 95% CI not reported). Both groups were placed on a "strict diet".[10] The second trial included 32 people with mean weight 13 kg above ideal body weight. It found no significant difference in weight loss between diethylproprion 75 mg/day and placebo at 12 months (−8.9 kg with diethylproprion v −10.5 kg with placebo; mean difference +1.6 kg, 95% CI not reported). Both groups were placed on a "low carbohydrate diet".[11] **Dexfenfluramine:** One systematic review (search date December 1995, 5 RCTs) found that dexfenfluramine 30–120 mg/day reduced weight more than placebo after 1 year of treatment. The review pooled data from four trials in a total of 634 adults who were at least 20% overweight. The mean difference in weight at 1 year for dexfenfluramine versus placebo was −2.6 kg (95% CI −3.8 to −1.3 kg). All participants were also prescribed a calorie restricted diet.[2] **Fenfluramine:** Two RCTs with 45 and 134 people who were more than 15% overweight found no significant difference between fenfluramine alone, fenfluramine with behavioural therapy, and behavioural therapy or diet alone (results not pooled).[12,13] **Fenfluramine plus phentermine:** One RCT with 121 people who were 30–80% overweight found that a combination of phentermine 15 mg/day and fenfluramine 60 mg/day reduced weight more than placebo at 6 months (−14.3 kg with phentermine/fenfluramine v −4.6 kg with placebo; mean difference −9.7 kg, 95% CI −12.0 to −7.4 kg). The trial found that weight loss ceased at 18 weeks of treatment; weight regain was noted after 60 weeks of treatment.[14] **Fluoxetine:** Three systematic reviews found two RCTs of at least 1 year's duration evaluating the selective serotonin reuptake inhibitor, fluoxetine[2,15,16] One RCT with 458 people (mean BMI 35 kg/m^2) found no significant difference in weight loss between fluoxetine 60 mg/day and placebo at 1 year (−1.4 kg with fluoxetine v −1.2 kg with placebo; mean difference −0.2 kg, 95% CI not reported).[17] The second small trial, in 19 people with diabetes and BMI greater than 30 kg/m^2, found that fluoxetine 60 mg/day reduced weight more than placebo at 12 months (−4.3 kg with fluoxetine v +1.5 kg with placebo; mean difference −5.8 kg, 95% CI not reported).[18] **Sibutramine:** We found one systematic review (search date 1998), which identified six placebo controlled RCTs examining effects of sibutramine on weight loss.[19] Participants were adults aged 18–65 years with BMIs between 27 and 40 kg/m^2.[19] The studies generally excluded participants with comorbidity, described the participants as healthy, or did not specify participants' health status. In three of the six trials, both sibutramine and placebo groups received cointerventions such as diet or calorie restriction, behaviour modification, or exercise.[20–22] A fourth trial placed participants on a diet of 220–800 kcal/day 4 weeks before randomisation.[23] Four trials were of 8–24 weeks and two were 12 months long. Although no quantitative summary was reported, the largest trial (1 024 people) found that sibutramine 30 mg/day reduced weight more than placebo at 24 weeks (mean weight loss 6.5 kg with sibutramine v 0.9 kg with placebo, P < 0.001, 95% CI not reported); the percentage of people losing 5% or more of body weight at 24 weeks was 63% with sibutramine v 13% with placebo (P < 0.001, 95% CI not reported).[20] Mean weight changes for the two 12 month trials ranged from 4.4–5.2 kg for people on 15 mg of sibutramine versus maximal weight losses of 1.6 kg with placebo.[23,24] In both trials, weight loss stabilised after 6 months of sibutramine. Weight regain of up to 25% of previously lost weight was observed within 1–6 weeks of stopping medication in three of the trials.[20–22]

Harms: **Phenylpropanolamine, phentermine, mazindol, and diethlyproprion:** Adverse effects include headache, tachycardia, dry mouth, nausea, diarrhoea, dizziness, and insomnia.[25] Mazindol was associated with more headache, dry mouth, and nausea than placebo.[9] A review of 142 case reports of severe adverse effects associated with phenylpropanolamine reported cases of intracranial haemorrhage, acute psychotic reactions, hypertensive episodes, seizures, cardiac arrhythmia, and deaths. The frequency of adverse effects with these agents is not clear.[25] **Dexfenfluramine and fenfluramine:** These agents have been associated with valvar heart disease and primary pulmonary hypertension,[26,27] and are no longer marketed.[28] A 25 centre retrospective cohort study in 1473 people found prevalence rates and relative risk of aortic regurgitation of 8.9% with dexfenfluramine (RR 2.18, 95% CI 1.32 to 3.59) and 13.7% with phentermine/fenfluramine (RR 3.34, 95% CI 2.09 to 5.35), compared with 4.1% with no treatment.[29] A prospective study in 1072 participants found no greater risk of valvar heart disease in people taking dexfenfluramine less than 3 months than in those taking placebo (sustained release dexfenfluramine RR 1.6, 95% CI 0.8 to 3.4, regular dexfenfluramine RR 1.4, 95% CI 0.7 to

3.0, when compared with placebo).[30] A case control study in 95 people with primary pulmonary hypertension and 355 matched controls found a history of fenfluramine use was associated with increased risk of primary pulmonary hypertension (OR 6.3, 95% CI 3.0 to 13.2). The odds ratio was higher among people who had taken fenfluramine in the past year (OR 10.1, 95% CI 3.4 to 29.9), and among individuals treated for more than 3 months (OR 23.1, 95% CI, 6.9 to 77.7).[31] **Fluoxetine:** One RCT comparing fluoxetine versus placebo for obesity reported more frequent gastrointestinal symptoms, sleep disturbance, sweating, tremor, amnesia, and thirst in the active treatment groups (frequency of events not provided).[17] One systematic review of antidepressant treatment found that selective serotonin reuptake inhibitors were associated with a 10–15% incidence of anxiety, diarrhoea, dry mouth, headache, and nausea.[32] **Sibutramine:** Common adverse effects were headache, dry mouth, anorexia, constipation, insomnia, rhinitis, and pharyngitis occurring in 10–30% of people taking sibutramine versus 8–19% of people on placebo (significance of difference not reported).[19] Mean increases in blood pressure (1–3 mm Hg) and heart rate (4–5 beats/minute) have been reported in people taking sibutramine at doses of 5–20 mg/day.[19]

Comment: **Phenylpropanolamine, phentermine, mazindol, and diethlyproprion:** The few trials that we identified were small, with short duration of follow up and high withdrawal rates. **Sibutramine:** Sibutramine has generally been compared against placebo in combination with one or more of the following elements: behaviour modification, physical activity, or diet, and compared to combinations of placebo and the same elements.

OPTION   ORLISTAT

One systematic review of RCTs has found that orlistat combined with a low calorie diet modestly increases weight loss in adults with obesity, compared with placebo plus diet. We found no evidence on weight gain following discontinuation, or on long term adverse effects.

Benefits: We found no systematic reviews or RCTs examining effects of orlistat on functional morbidity and mortality. We found one systematic review (search date 1999), which identified seven RCTs examining effects of orlistat on weight loss.[33] Trials lasted between 1 and 2 years, in 4188 adults with BMIs between 28–47 kg/m^2. Meta-analysis of five of the trials found that orlistat combined with a low calorie diet (below 1500 kcal/day) increased weight loss more than placebo plus diet after 1 year (mean weight loss 6.1 kg with orlistat 120 mg three times daily v 2.6 kg with placebo, P < 0.001, 95% CI not reported).[34] A greater proportion of the participants lost 10% or more of their initial weight in the orlistat groups than in the placebo groups at 12 months (20.2% v 8.3%, P < 0.001). In a 1 year trial in 322 people with type II diabetes (included in the review but not the meta-analysis), 30.2% of the orlistat plus diet group and 13.2% of the placebo plus diet group lost 5% or more of their initial body weight.[35] We found two subsequent multicentre trials (placebo controlled, double blind, 796 people[36] and 783 people[37]) whose results were consistent with the earlier systematic review. Generally healthy obese adults (BMI 28 to 44 kg/m^2) were randomised to placebo or orlistat (60 or 120 mg) three times a day for 2 years after a 4 week placebo and reduced energy diet run-in, which 54 /796 and 161/783 participants did not complete. Participants in both trials followed a reduced energy diet for the first year and a weight maintenance diet for the second year. People taking orlistat were significantly more likely to lose 10% or more of initial body weight compared with those taking placebo at the end of the first year (28.6–38.2% with orlistat 60 mg v 11.3–18.6% with placebo) and to maintain this weight loss after 2 years (28.2–33.0% with orlistat 60 mg v 6.6–18.6% with placebo). One of the trials reported significantly improved "quality of life" on orlistat compared with placebo, but this consisted of reduced obesity specific distress and treatment satisfaction.[37]

Harms: Common adverse effects included oily spotting from the rectum, flatulence, and faecal urgency in 22–27% of people taking orlistat versus 1–7% of people taking placebo.[33]

Comment: People in six of the seven trials in the systematic review were selected for participation after losing weight on a preliminary low calorie diet with placebo for 4–5 weeks before randomisation.[33]

GLOSSARY

Body mass index (BMI) is expressed as weight in kilograms divided by height in metres squared (kg/m^2). In the USA individuals with BMIs between 25–30 kg/m^2 are considered overweight; those with BMIs above 30 kg/m^2 are considered obese.[1]

REFERENCES

1. National Institutes of Health. *Clinical guidelines on the identification, evaluation, and treatment of overweight and obesity in adults: the Evidence Report.* Bethesda, Maryland: US Department of Health and Human Services, 1998.

2. University of York, NHS Centre for Reviews and Dissemination. A systematic review of the interventions for the prevention and treatment of obesity, and the maintenance of weight loss. York, England: NHS Centre for Reviews and Dissemination; 1997. Search date 1995; primary sources Medline, Embase, Bids, Dare, Psychlit, bibliographies of review articles, and contributions from peer reviewers.

3. Mokdad AH, Serdula MK, Dietz WH, Bowman BA, Marks JS, Koplan JP. The spread of the obesity epidemic in the United States 1991–1998. *JAMA* 1999;282:1519–1522.

4. Bray GA. Obesity: etiology. *UpToDate* [serial on CD-ROM] 2000;8(1). Available from UpToDate, Inc, Wellesley, Massachusetts, USA.

5. Bray GA. Obesity: Overview of therapy for obesity. *UpToDate* [serial on CD-ROM] 2000;8(1). Available from UpToDate, Inc, Wellesley, Massachusetts, USA.

6. Allison DB, Fontaine KR, Manson JE, Stevens J, Vanitallie TB. Annual deaths attributable to obesity in the United States. *JAMA* 1999;282:1530–1538.

7. Greenway FL. Clinical studies with phenylpropanolamine: a metaanalysis. *Am J Clin Nutr* 1992;55(suppl 1):203–205.

8. Munro JF, MacCuish AC, Wilson EM, et al. Comparison of continuous and intermittent anorectic therapy in obesity. *BMJ* 1968;1:352–354.

9. Vernace BJ. Controlled comparative investigation of mazindol, D-amphetamine, and placebo. *Obesity Bariatric Med* 1974;3:124–129.

10. McKay RHG. Long-term use of diethylproprion in obesity. *Curr Med Res Opin* 1973;1:489–493.

11. Silverstone JT, Solomon T. The long-term management of obesity in general practice. *Br J Clin Pract* 1965;19:395–398.

12. Ost LG, Gotestam KG. Behavioral and pharmacological treatments for obesity: an experimental comparison. *Addict Behav* 1976;1:331–338.

13. Stunkard AJ, Craighead LW, O'Brien R. Controlled trial of behavior therapy, pharmacotherapy, and their combination in the treatment of obesity. *Lancet* 1980;2:1045–1047.

14. Weintraub M. Long term weight control study: the National Heart, Lung, and Blood Institute funded multimodal intervention study. *Clin Pharmacol Ther* 1992;51:581–646.

15. Douketis JD, Feightner JW, Attia J, et al. Periodic health examination, 1999 update: 1. Detection, prevention and treatment of obesity. Canadian Task Force on Preventive Health Care. *Can Med Assoc J* 1999;160:513–525. Search date 1998; primary sources Medline, bibliographies of review articles, and *Current Content* listings.

16. National Task Force on the Prevention and Treatment of Obesity. Long-term pharmacotherapy in the management of obesity. *JAMA* 1996;276:1907–1915. Search date 1996; primary sources Medline and manual search of bibliographies.

17. Goldstein DJ, Rampey AH Jr, Enas GG, et al. Fluoxetine: a randomized clinical trial in the treatment of obesity. *Int J Obes* 1994;18:129–135.

18. O'Kane M, Wiles PG, Wales JK. Fluoxetine in the treatment of obese type II diabetic patients. *Diabet Med* 1994;11:105–110.

19. Luque CA, Rey JA. Sibutramine: a serotonin-norepinephrine reuptake-inhibitor for the treatment of obesity. *Ann Pharmacother* 1999;33: 968–978. Search date 1998; primary sources Medline, Embase, manual search, and reference lists of relevant articles.

20. Bray GA, Blackburn GL, Ferguson JM, et al. Sibutramine produces dose-related weight loss. *Obes Res* 1999;7:189–198.

21. Hanotin C, Thomas F, Jones SP, Leutenegger E, Drouin P. Efficacy and tolerability of sibutramine in obese patients: a dose-ranging study. *Int J Obes Relat Metab Disord* 1998;22:32–38.

22. Weintraub M, Rubio A, Golik A, Byrne L, Scheinbaum ML. Sibutramine in weight control: a dose-ranging, efficacy study. *Clin Pharmacol Ther* 1991;50:330–337.

23. Apfelbaum M, Vague P, Ziegler O, Hanotin C, Thomas F, Leutnegger E. Long-term maintenance of weight loss after a very-low calorie diet: a randomized blinded trial of the efficacy and tolerability of sibutramine. *Am J Med* 1999;106: 179–184.

24. Jones SP, Smith IG, Kelly F, Gray JA. Long-term weight loss with sibutramine [abstract]. *Int J Obes Relat Metab Disord* 1995;19(suppl 2):S41.

25. Lake CR, Gallant S, Masson E, Miller P. Adverse drug effects attributed to phenylpropanolamine: a review of 142 case reports. *Am J Med* 1990;89: 195–208.

26. Poston WS, Foreyt, JP. Scientific and legal issues in fenfluramine/dexfenfluramine litigation. *J Texas Med* 2000;96:48–56.

27. Connolly HM, Crary JL, McGoon MD, et al. Valvular heart disease associated with fenfluramine-phentermine. *N Engl J Med* 1997;337:581–588.

28. Scheen AJ, Lefebvre PJ. Pharmacological treatment of obesity: present status. *Intl J Obes Relat Metab Disord.* 1999;23(suppl 1):47–53.

29. Gardin JM, Schumacher D, Constantine G, et al. Valvular abnormalities and cardiovascular status following exposure to dexfenfluramine and phentermine/fenfluramine. *JAMA* 2000;283:703–709.

30. Weissman NJ, Tighe JF, Gottdiener JS, Gwynne JT. An assessment of heart-valve abnormalities in obese patients taking dexfenfluramine, sustained-release dexfenfluramine, or placebo. Sustained release dexfenfluramine study group. *N Engl J Med* 1998;339:725–732.

31. Abenhaim L, Moride Y, Brenot F, et al. Appetite-suppressant drugs and the risk of primary pulmonary hypertension. International primary pulmonary hypertension study group. *N Engl J Med* 1996;335:609–616.

32. Mulrow CD, Williams JW Jr, Trivedi M, et al. Treatment of depression – newer pharmacotherapies. *Psychopharmacol Bull* 1998; 34:409–795. Search date 1998; primary sources the Cochrane and collaboration depression, anxiety and neurosis (CCDAN) Review Group's registry, and bibliographies of trial and review articles.

33. Anonymous. Orlistat: no hurry. *Can Fam Physician* 1999;45:2331–2351. Primary sources and search dates Medline (1999), Embase (1998), Reactions (1998), Cochrane (1999); international journals, the Prescribe Library, and clinical pharmacology reference texts were also searched. Data were also obtained from the Produits Roche, the European Medicines Evaluation Agency, and Food and Drug Administration committees.

34. European Agency for the Evaluation of Medicinal Products. *Committee for proprietary medicinal products. European public assessment report (EPAR) – Xenical*. London: European Agency for the Evaluation of Medicinal Products, 1998.

35. Hollander PA, Elbein SC, Hirsch IR, et al. Role of orlistat in the treatment of obese patients with type 2 diabetes: a 1-year randomized double-blind study. *Diabetes Care* 1998;21:1288–1294.

36. Hauptman J, Lucas C, Boldrin MN, Collins H, Segal KR. Orlistat in the long-term treatment of obesity in primary care settings. *Arch Fam Med* 2000;9:160–167.

37. R ssner S, Sj strom L, Noack R, Meinders AE, Noseda G. Weight loss, weight maintenance, and improved cardiovascular risk factors after 2 years treatment with orlistat for obesity. *Obes Res* 2000; 8:49–61.

Polly Hitchcock Noël
Associate Director
VERDICT, a VA HSR&D Center of
Excellence, South Texas Veterans
Health Care System, US Department
of Veterans Affairs
San Antonio, Texas
USA

David Arterburn
Senior Resident
University of Texas, Health Science
Center at San Antonio
San Antonio
USA

Cynthia Mulrow
Professor of Medicine
University of Texas Health Science
Center
San Antonio, Texas
USA
Competing interests: None declared.

The views expressed in this article are those of the authors and do not necessarily represent the views of the US Department of Veterans Affairs.

Updated this issue

Kimble Matos, André Curi and Carlos Pavesio

QUESTIONS

INTERVENTIONS

Likely to be beneficial

Unknown effectiveness

To be covered in future issues of
Clinical Evidence
Mydriatics
Subconjunctival steroid injection
Oral steroids
Slow taper of drug treatment
Treatment of chronic iridocyclitis

See glossary, p 338

Key Messages

- Available RCTs were too small to prove or exclude clinically important differences between steroid eye drops and placebo or between steroid and non-steroidal eye drops. The limited evidence suggests that steroid eye drops are more effective than non-steroidal eye drops.

DEFINITION Anterior uveitis is inflammation of the uveal tract and includes iritis and iridocyclitis. It can be classified according to its clinical course into acute or chronic uveitis, or according to its clinical appearance into granulomatous or non-granulomatous uveitis. Acute anterior uveitis is characterised by an extremely painful red eye, often associated with photophobia and occasionally decreased visual acuity. Chronic uveitis is defined as inflammation lasting more than 6 weeks. It is usually asymptomatic, but many people have mild symptoms during exacerbations.

INCIDENCE/ PREVALENCE Acute anterior uveitis is rare, with an annual incidence of 12/100 000 population.[1] It is common in Finland (annual incidence 22.6/100 000, prevalence 68.7/100 000), probably owing to genetic factors such as the high frequency of HLA-B27.[2] It occurs equally in both sexes and less than 10% of cases occur before the age of 20.[2,3]

AETIOLOGY/ RISK FACTORS Between 60% and 80% of cases of anterior uveitis are classified as idiopathic. The range of systemic disorders associated with anterior uveitis are ankylosing spondylitis, Reiter's syndrome, juvenile chronic arthritis, Kawasaki syndrome, infectious uveitis, Behçet's syndrome, inflammatory bowel disease, interstitial nephritis, sarcoidosis, multiple sclerosis, Wegener's granulomatosis, Vogt-Koyanagi-Harada syndrome, and masquerade syndromes (see glossary, p 338). Acute anterior uveitis also occurs in association with HLA-B27 not linked to any systemic disease, and it may be the first manifestation of eye disorders such as Fuchs' iridocyclitis, Posner-Schlossman syndrome, Schwartz syndrome, postsurgical inflammation, and drug or hypersensitivity reactions.[2,3]

PROGNOSIS Acute anterior uveitis is often self limiting, but we found no data on how often it resolves spontaneously, in which people, or over what time period. Complications include posterior synechiae (see glossary, p 338), cataract, glaucoma, and chronic uveitis. In a study of 154 people (232 eyes) with acute anterior uveitis (119 people HLA-B27 positive), visual acuity was better than 20/60 in 209 eyes (90%), and 20/60 or worse in 23 people and 23 eyes (10%), with 11 eyes (5%) having legal blindness (visual acuity worse than 20/200). In people with impaired visual acuity, 19/23 had cataract and four had secondary glaucoma and complications of surgery. HLA-B27 status made no significant difference to the rate of complications or to visual outcome.[4]

AIMS To reduce inflammation; to relieve pain; and to prevent complications and loss of visual acuity, with minimal adverse effects.

OUTCOMES Degree of inflammation, using scores that register cell counts and flare in the anterior chamber; keratic precipitates; ciliary flush; severity of symptoms (photophobia and pain).

METHODS *Clinical Evidence* update search and appraisal May 2000. We found no relevant systematic reviews. Large, well designed RCTs are needed to provide adequate evidence about the effectiveness of interventions, because of the small expected differences in outcomes with different treatments, the self limiting nature of some types of anterior uveitis, and the variation in severity of clinical manifestations.

OPTION   TOPICAL STEROID TREATMENTS

Available RCTs were too small to either confirm or exclude clinically important differences between steroid eye drops and placebo or between steroid and non-steroidal eye drops. They suggest that steroid eye drops are more effective and faster acting than non-steroidal eye drops. Limited evidence suggests that new topical steroids such as rimexolone may be as effective as prednisolone but with less risk of raised intraocular pressure.

Benefits: We found no systematic review. **Versus placebo:** We found one double blind RCT comparing betamethasone phosphate 1%, clobetasone butyrate 0.1%, and placebo in 60 people with acute unilateral, non-granulomatous anterior uveitis. Twelve participants were lost to follow up. Participants received two drops every 2 hours, atropine 1% twice daily, and acetazolamide when necessary in cases of secondary glaucoma, and were followed up for 3 weeks. There was no significant difference between the three groups, but the trial included too few people to exclude a clinically important effect.[5] **Versus each other:** We found two RCTs comparing prednisolone 1% with new topical steroids, rimexolone 1% and loteprednol etabonate 0.5%. The rimexolone trial in people with acute uveitis, recurrent iridocyclitis or chronic uveitis (divided into two studies with n = 183 randomised and n = 93 randomised) found no significant difference in cell and flare scores between groups, except at day 28 in the larger study when prednisolone 1% was associated with greater improvement in flare score.[6] Of the loteprednol trials (also divided into two studies, 245 people with acute anterior uveitis), the larger study (n = 175) found that prednisolone acetate was associated with a significantly higher rate of resolution by the final visit at 28 days of treatment (72% v 87%; P = 0.015). The smaller study found more people achieved resolution with prednisolone acetate by 42 days of treatment but the difference was not significant.[7] **Versus topical non-steroidal treatments:** See topical non-steroidal treatments, p 338.

Harms: Adverse effects of topical eye drops include local irritation, hyperaemia, oedema, and blurred vision. Rarely, topical eye drops have been associated with glaucoma, cataract, and herpes simplex keratitis. In the trials reported above, adverse events were generally mild, resolved without treatment, and did not result in permanent harms. In one of the trials comparing loteprednol etabonate with prednisolone acetate, four people were withdrawn because of adverse effects: cystoid macular oedema and ocular symptoms in the loteprednol group, and interstitial keratitis and increase in age related macular degeneration in the prednisolone group.[7] **Raised intraocular pressure:** Clinically significant increases in intraocular pressure (defined as > 10 mmHg from baseline) were found more frequently with prednisolone than with the new steroids (prednisolone v rimexolone[6] 11 v 6 and 8 v 1; prednisolone v loteprednol[7] 1 v 0 and 6 v 1).

Comment: Topical steroids have been standard treatment for acute anterior uveitis since the early 1950s, especially for people with acute and severe uveitis. The placebo controlled trial was too small to rule out a clinically important effect of topical steroids.[5] We are not aware of any further trials under way or planned.

OPTION   **TOPICAL NON-STEROIDAL TREATMENTS**

Available RCTs were too small to either confirm or exclude clinically important differences between non-steroid eye drops and placebo or between non-steroidal eye drops and steroid eye drops. Limited evidence suggests that non-steroidal eye drops are less effective and slower acting than steroid eye drops.

Benefits: **Versus topical steroids.** We found two RCTs. The first (71 people with acute unilateral idiopathic non-granulomatous uveitis) compared prednisolone disodium phosphate 0.5%, betamethasone disodium phosphate 0.1%, and tolmetin sodium dihydrate 5%.[8] Participants were asked to instil one drop every 2 hours during the waking period, and all received atropine 1% once daily. Clinical cure was reported in 68% on prednisolone disodium phosphate, 90% on betamethasone disodium phosphate, and 57% on tolmetin (no measure of significance reported); 11 people were excluded from statistical analysis. The second RCT (49 people with acute anterior non-granulomatous uveitis) compared dexamethasone 0.1% versus indomethacin 1% eye drops administered 6 times daily.[9] Most participants (equal numbers in each group) also received atropine drops 3 times a day. After 7 days of treatment the inflammatory score was significantly lower in the group receiving dexamethasone. By day 14, there was no significant difference between groups. **Versus topical steroids and placebo:** We found one RCT (100 people with acute unilateral idiopathic non-granulomatous anterior uveitis) comparing prednisolone 0.5%, tolmetin 5%, and sterile saline 0.9% (placebo). Participants were asked to instil drops every 2 hours during the waking period and also atropine 1% once daily. Six people were excluded from the study. There was no significant difference between groups in cure rates (47% with tolmetin, 53% with saline, and 69% with prednisolone), but the prednisolone treated group had the highest percentage of patients cured at all stages in the trial.[10]

Harms: See topical steroid treatments, p 337.

Comment: None.

GLOSSARY

Masquerade syndromes Comprise a group of disorders that occur with intra-ocular inflammation and are often misdiagnosed as a chronic idiopathic uveitis.
Posterior synechiae Adhesions between the iris and the lens capsule.

REFERENCES

1. Darrel RW, Wagner HP, Kurland CT. Epidemiology of uveitis: incidence and prevalence in a small urban community. *Arch Ophthalmol* 1962;68:501–514.

2. Paivonsalo-Hietanen-T, Tuominen-J, Vaahtoranta-Lehtonen-H, Saari-KM. Incidence and prevalence of different uveitis entities in Finland. *Acta Ophthalmol Scand* 1997;75:76–81.

3. Rosenbaum JT. Uveitis. An internist's view. *Arch Intern Med* 1989;149;1173–1176.

4. Linssen A, Meenken C. Outcomes of HLA-B27-Positive and HLA-B27-Negative acute anterior uveitis. *Am J Ophthalmol* 1995;120:351–361.

5. Dunne JA, Travers JP. Topical steroids in anterior uveitis. *Trans Ophthal Soc UK* 1979;99:481–484.

6. Foster CS, Alter G, Raymond DeBarge L, et al. Efficacy and safety of rimexolone 1% ophthalmic suspension vs prednisolone acetate in the treatment of uveitis. *Am J Ophthalmol* 1996 122: 171–182.

7. The Loteprednol Etabonate US Uveitis Study Group. Controlled evaluation of loteprednol etabonate and prednisolone acetate in the treatment of acute anterior uveitis. *Am J Ophthalmol* 1999;127:537–544.

8. Dunne JA, Jacobs N, Morrison A, Gilbert DJ. Efficacy in anterior uveitis of two known steroids and topical tolmetin. *Br J Ophthalmol* 1985;69: 120–125.

9. Sand BB, Krogh E. Topical indometacin, a prostaglandin inhibitor, in acute anterior uveitis. A controlled clinical trial of non-steroid versus steroid anti-inflammatory treatment. *Acta Ophthalmol* 1991;69:145–148.

10. Young BJ, Cunninghan WF, Akingbehin T: Double-masked controlled clinical trial of 5% tolmetin versus 0.5% prednisolone versus 0.9% saline in acute endogenous nongranulomatous anterior uveitis. *Br J Ophthalmol* 1982;66:389–391.

Kimble Matos
Research Fellow

André Curi
Clinical Research Fellow

Carlos Pavesio
Consultant Ophthalmic Surgeon

Moorfields Eye Hospital
London
UK

Competing interests: None declared.

Age related macular degeneration

Updated this issue

Jennifer Arnold and Shirley Sarks

INTERVENTIONS

Key Messages

- Four large RCTs have found that laser photocoagulation decreases the rate of severe visual loss and preserves contrast sensitivity in selected people with exudative age related macular degeneration (AMD): those with well demarcated lesions on fluorescein angiography. Choroidal neovascularisation recurs within 2 years in about half of patients. Photocoagulation may reduce visual acuity initially.

- Three RCTs found no evidence of an effect of external beam radiation on moderate visual loss in people with exudative AMD within 1 year. We found insufficient evidence on long term efficacy or safety, but one RCT found no evidence of an association with cataract formation at 1 year.

- We found insufficient evidence on the effects of submacular surgery.

- One large multicentre RCT found no evidence of benefit from subcutaneous interferon α-2a, and found evidence of serious ocular and systemic adverse effects.

- One large multicentre RCT found that photodynamic treatment with verteporfin reduced the risk of moderate and severe vision loss in selected people with exudative AMD (those with predominantly classic lesions on fluorescein angiography) who constitute about 10–30% of people with exudative AMD).

- Overall, we found no evidence that the main treatment options are of benefit to most people with exudative AMD.

DEFINITION Age related macular degeneration (AMD) is the late stage of age related maculopathy. AMD has two forms: atrophic (or dry) AMD, characterised by geographic atrophy; and exudative (or wet) AMD, characterised by choroidal neovascularisation, which eventually causes a disciform scar.

INCIDENCE/ PREVALENCE AMD is the commonest cause of blind registration in industrialised countries. Atrophic AMD is more common than the more sight threatening exudative AMD, affecting about 85% of people with AMD.[3] End stage (blinding) AMD is found in about 1.7% of all people aged over 50, and incidence rises with age (0.7% to 1.4% in people aged 65–75, 11.0% to 18.5% in people aged over 85).[4–6]

AETIOLOGY/ RISK FACTORS Age is the strongest risk factor. Ocular risk factors for the development of exudative AMD include the presence of soft drusen, macular pigmentary change, and choroidal neovascularisation in the other eye. Systemic risk factors are hypertension, smoking, and positive family history.[7,8] The role of diet and exposure to ultraviolet light is suspected but unproved.

PROGNOSIS AMD impairs central vision, which is required for reading, driving, face recognition, and all fine visual tasks. **Atrophic AMD** progresses slowly over many years, and time to legal blindness (visual acuity < 20/200) is highly variable (usually about 5–10 years).[9,10] **Exudative AMD** is more threatening to vision; 90% of people with severe visual loss due to AMD have the exudative type. It usually manifests with a sudden worsening and distortion of central vision. It progresses rapidly (typically over weeks or months) until scarring is complete and no further vision is lost, at which point legal blindness has usually been reached. Most people (estimates vary from 60–90%) with exudative AMD progress to legal blindness and develop a central defect (scotoma) in the visual field.[11–14] Peripheral vision is preserved, allowing the person to mobilise and be independent. The ability to read with visual aids depends on the size and density of the central scotoma and the degree to which the person retains sensitivity to contrast. Once exudative AMD has developed in one eye, the other eye is at high risk (cumulative estimated incidence: 10%, 28%, and 42% at 1, 3, and 5 years).[7]

AIMS To minimise loss of visual acuity and central vision; to preserve the ability to read with or without visual aids; to optimise quality of life; to minimise adverse effects of treatment.

OUTCOMES Visual acuity, rates of legal blindness, contrast sensitivity, quality of life, appearance of retina on fluorescein angiography, rate of adverse effects of treatment. Visual acuity is measured using special eye charts, usually the Early Treatment of Diabetic Retinopathy Study (ETDRS) chart, although many studies do not specify which chart was used. Stable vision is usually defined as loss of two lines or less on the ETDRS chart. Moderate and severe visual loss is defined as a loss of greater than three and six lines respectively, which corresponds to a doubling and quadrupling of the vision angle. Loss of vision to legal blindness (< 20/200) is also used as an outcome. A reading of 20/200 (or 6/60 in metric) on the Snellen chart means that a person can see at 20 yards (or 6 meters) what a normally sighted person can see at 200 yards (or 60 metres).

METHODS *Clinical Evidence* update search and appraisal May 2000.

Eye disorders

OPTION   THERMAL LASER PHOTOCOAGULATION

Four large RCTs have found that laser photocoagulation decreases the rate of severe visual loss and preserves contrast sensitivity in selected people with exudative AMD (those with well demarcated lesions). Choroidal neovascularisation recurs within 2 years in about half of those treated. Photocoagulation may reduce visual acuity initially.

Benefits: We found no systematic review. **Versus no treatment:** We found four large unblinded multicentre RCTs comparing laser photocoagulation versus no treatment (see table 1, p 349) in a selected population.[11–17] We also found four smaller RCTs that included a wider range of people.[18–21] All four of the large trials found that treatment conferred clinically and statistically significant benefit, in terms of reduced risk of severe visual loss (defined as loss of six or more lines on the special eye chart), which persisted beyond 3 years. Participants differed in terms of the position of the choroidal neovascularisation (see glossary, p 346) on the retina, whether far, near, or under the centre of fixation (extrafoveal,[11,13] juxtafoveal,[14,15] or subfoveal,[12,16,17]). In the study of extrafoveal choroidal neovascularisation, the treatment was beneficial despite the fact that 19% of eyes randomised to observation later received laser.[11,13] Re-analysis of people with juxtafoveal choroidal neovascularisation found that benefit was limited to those with pure classic lesions (no occult element) on fluorescein angiography (52% of randomised eyes), who were more than twice as likely to avoid developing severe visual loss compared with people receiving no treatment (OR 2.2, 95% CI 1.4 to 3.4 at 3 years). The two trials in people with subfoveal choroidal neovascularisation found benefit from treatment despite an immediate loss of vision in the treated groups (average three lines on the special eye chart).[12] At 5 years after treatment, rates of recurrence of choroidal neovascularisation ranged from 39% to 76%, with most occurring within 2 years. Of the four smaller RCTs, one found that fovea sparing laser photocoagulation preserved visual acuity compared with no treatment.[18] The other three found that scatter (non-confluent) laser was no better than no treatment in occult choroidal neovascularisation.[19–21] However, the trials were too small to rule out a beneficial effect. **Different wavelengths:** We found three large multicentre RCTs that compared two wavelengths of laser (krypton red or argon green) for photocoagulation of choroidal neovascularisation in AMD.[22,23] All found no significant difference in outcome. **Effects in people with choroidal neovascularisation identified by indocyanine green angiography:** We found no RCTs. Uncontrolled case series have reported good outcomes in selected people.

Harms: Laser destroys new vessels and surrounding retina, and the resultant scar causes a corresponding defect in the central visual field. If the laser is applied to subfoveal lesions, or if the laser burn spreads to the fovea, visual acuity will be impaired; two of the RCTs described immediate loss of visual acuity (an average loss of three lines on the special eye chart).[12,17] We found no evidence of other adverse effects.

Comment: The benefits of laser photocoagulation depend on accurate, complete treatment, requiring high quality angiography and trained, experienced practitioners.[11–17] The risk of immediate loss of visual acuity with laser photocoagulation may limit its acceptability.

OPTION   RADIOTHERAPY

Three RCTs found no evidence of an effect of external beam radiation on the risk of moderate visual loss in people with exudative AMD within 1 year. We found insufficient evidence on long term safety, but one RCT found no evidence of an association with cataract formation at 1 year.

Benefits: We found no systematic review. **External beam radiation:** We found three RCTs. The first trial, a large multicentre double blind RCT, compared external beam radiation (16 Gy in 2 Gy fractions) delivered to the macula versus no treatment in 205 people with new subfoveal choroidal neovascularisation.[24] The control group received 'sham' radiation treatment (8 fractions of 0 Gy). At 12 months, 51.1% of treated people and 52.6% of controls had moderate visual loss, defined as loss of three or more lines on a special eye chart (P = 0.88). No treatment benefit was detected for subgroups of patients classified into classic and occult lesions on the basis of fluorescein angiographic appearance. The second trial, a small, single blind RCT compared external beam radiation (24 Gy in 6 Gy fractions) delivered to the macula versus no treatment in 74 people with new subfoveal choroidal neovascularisation.[25] At 12 months, there was no significant difference between treated and untreated people in terms of their risk of moderate or severe visual loss (defined as losses of three or six lines on the special eye chart): the absolute risk of moderate visual loss was reduced by 20% with treatment, but the confidence interval spanned zero (AR −20%, 95% CI −44% to +4%). The third RCT was a small single blind randomised pilot study comparing single fraction external beam radiation of 7.5 Gy against no treatment in 27 people.[26] No treatment benefit was detected over a mean follow up of 17 months (range 7–32 months). **Other techniques:** We found conflicting and inconclusive evidence from non-randomised pilot studies using proton beam and scleral plaque (local) radiotherapy in a variety of dosing and timing schedules.

Harms: All RCTs reported no adverse effects after 12 months. Uncontrolled pilot studies suggest that the main risks using current dosing and delivery techniques are cataract (2/41 people in one series)[27] and transient keratoconjunctivitis with epiphora (10/75 in one series).[28] However, the large multicentre RCT found no significant difference in cataract formation between treated and untreated people at 12 months (10% treated v 16% control) or dry eye symptoms (40% treated v 45% control).[24] Doses of up to 25 Gy delivered in daily fractions of 2 Gy or less, are generally claimed not to cause damage to the retina or optic nerve. However, radiotherapy is potentially toxic to the retina, optic nerve, lens, and lacrimal system, with toxic effects sometimes manifesting 2 years after treatment.[29] A two centre case series of people treated with external beam radiation reported an abnormal choroidal vascular growth pattern associated with macular bleeding and exudation and marked loss of visual acuity.[30] This change was detected in 12.6% of 95, and 7.1% of 98 people, 3–12 months after radiotherapy, and may explain the lack of treatment benefit.

Comment: One multicentre RCT of radiation for AMD is under way (U Chakravarthy, personal communication, 1999). Trials with less than 2 years' follow up may miss important adverse effects.

OPTION SUBMACULAR SURGERY

We found insufficient evidence on the effects of submacular surgery. Rates of recurrent choroidal neovascularisation are high, and there is a clinically significant risk of ocular complications resulting in visual loss and further surgical intervention.

Benefits: We found no systematic review. **Versus no treatment:** We found no RCTs. **Versus laser photocoagulation.** We found one pilot RCT (n = 70) comparing submacular surgery (see glossary, p 346) versus laser photocoagulation for recurrent subfoveal choroidal neovascularisation (S Bressler, Macular Society Meeting, San Francisco, personal communication, 1999). It found no significant difference between the two treatment groups. **Versus alternative surgical techniques:** We found one RCT on 80 eyes with exudative AMD comparing surgery plus subretinal injection of tissue plasminogen activator, versus surgery plus subretinal injection of a control solution.[31] The trial found no significant difference in visual or anatomic outcome.

Harms: Submacular surgery can have effects that threaten vision or require further surgical intervention. However, we found no good data on the frequency of adverse events. The largest case series of people with age-related and non-age related macular degeneration reported cataract formation (in up to 40%), retinal detachment (5–8%), recurrent new vessel formation (18–35% within 12 months), and macular complications (haemorrhage and pucker; no rates given).[32]

Comment: Most evidence for submacular surgery currently comes from small uncontrolled case series (< 50 people with AMD) with short follow up, often including people with other types of macular degeneration. These found that few people with AMD experienced improved vision with surgery.[29,32] Comparing results is difficult because of evolving surgical techniques, changes in outcome measures, and variations in follow up. A large non-blinded RCT is currently recruiting and will compare standardised surgical technique versus no treatment in new and haemorrhagic choroidal neovascularisation in people with AMD (S Bressler, personal communication, 1999). Other surgical techniques are being developed in volunteers, including macular translocation and retinal pigment epithelial transplantation, but these have yet to be formally evaluated.

OPTION SUBCUTANEOUS INTERFERON α-2A

One large RCT found no evidence of benefit from subcutaneous interferon α-2a (an antiangiogenesis drug) and found evidence of serious ocular and systemic adverse effects.

Benefits: We found no systematic review. We found one multicentre, double blind RCT on 481 people with subfoveal choroidal neovascularisation due to AMD.[32] This compared three doses of subcutaneous interferon α-2a (1.5, 3, and 6 mIU given three times a week for 1 year) versus placebo. At 52 weeks, treatment at all doses was associated with a higher risk of losing at least three lines of vision on the Snellen chart compared with placebo (AR 50% v 38%, ARI 12%, 95% CI 0% to 23%). No benefit was found for secondary end points or in subgroups of patients.

Harms: Adverse effects of interferon α-2a were common and potentially severe in this and other poorer quality RCTs. These included fatigue and influenza like symptoms, as well as gastrointestinal, and central and peripheral nervous system effects. Although at least one adverse event was reported in 86% of people taking placebo, the proportion of people on active treatment who suffered adverse effects increased with dose, as did the severity of adverse effects. Up to 5% of treated people experienced interferon α-2a induced retinopathy.[33]

Comment: There is widespread interest in safe effective antiangiogenesis drugs for prophylaxis in exudative AMD. Several drugs are currently under preclinical and early phase clinical study. RCTs are currently investigating thalidomide with and without concurrent laser photocoagulation, and intravitreal triamcinolone.

OPTION	PHOTODYNAMIC TREATMENT

One large multicentre RCT found that photodynamic treatment with verteporfin reduced the risk of moderate and severe vision loss in selected people with exudative AMD (those with predominantly classic lesions on fluorescein angiography. The trial found no evidence that photodynamic therapy is beneficial for people with evidence of occult neovascularisation.

Benefits: We found one systematic review (updated in 2000), which identified one high quality placebo controlled RCT.[34] It included one multicentre, double blind RCT of photodynamic treatment (see glossary, p 346) in 609 people with new and recurrent subfoveal choroidal neovascularisation due to AMD. The intervention was a two stage procedure: infusion of verteporfin (see glossary, p 346) followed by phototherapy with activating laser light. The control group received infusion of sugar water followed by phototherapy. Twice as many participants were randomised to verteporfin. Treatments were repeated if necessary every 3 months. Outcomes were moderate and severe loss of visual acuity (defined as loss of 15 and 30 letters — about 3 and 6 lines) on a special eye chart; a change in contrast sensitivity and fluorescein angiographic appearance. At each follow up visit (up to 12 months), all outcome measures were clinically and statistically significantly better in the treatment than in the control group. At the 12 month follow up visit, 61% of treated people versus 46% of controls had lost less than 15 letters of vision (RR 0.72, 95% CI 0.61 to 0.86). Subgroup analysis found that this benefit was greater for people with predominantly classic choroidal neovascularisation lesions (67% treated v 39% control; RR 0.54,

95% CI 0.41 to 0.71), and was most marked for pure classic lesions (77% treated *v* 27% control; RR 0.34, 95% CI 0.22 to 0.51). This last finding was based on only 143 eyes. No treatment benefit for visual acuity was seen in the group without predominantly classic lesions. The systematic review calculated numbers needed to treat, to prevent one person losing three or more lines of vision, as 6.7 (95% CI 4.3 to 14.3) for the entire study population. This fell to 2 (95% CI 1.6 to 3.3) for eyes with pure classic lesions.

Harms: Verteporfin is a photosensitive dye and care must be taken to avoid tissue extravasation during infusion, and exposure to bright sunlight for 24 hours after treatment. The treatment was well tolerated but was more likely than the control intervention to cause a transient decrease in vision (18% treated *v* 12% control); injection site reactions (13% treated *v* 3% control); photosensitivity (3% treated *v* 0% control); and infusion related low back pain (2% *v* 0% control).

Comment: The study found no common short term adverse effects of treatment. However, the possibility of rare but severe adverse events remains. The RCT is ongoing and will report outcomes at 24 months' follow up. A further multicentre double blind RCT is underway which compares photodynamic treatment with verteporfin in a wider range of people with exudative AMD.

GLOSSARY

Age related maculopathy Degenerative disease of the macula (centre of the retina) classified as early (marked by drusen and pigmentary change, and usually associated with normal vision) and late, when it is known as age related macular degeneration (AMD).

Choroidal neovascularisation (CNV) New vessels in the choroid, classified on the basis of fluorescein angiography: in terms of its position in relation to the fovea — extrafoveal, juxtafoveal, or subfoveal; in terms of its appearance — classic (well defined) or occult (poorly defined); and in terms of its borders — well demarcated or poorly demarcated.

Legal blindness Visual acuity < 20/200.

Photodynamic treatment A two step procedure of intravenous infusion of a photosensitive dye followed by application of a non-thermal laser which activates the dye. The treatment aims to cause selective closure of the choroidal new vessels.

Submacular surgery Removal of haemorrhage and/or choroidal neovascularisation after vitrectomy.

Verteporfin A photosensitive dye used in photodynamic treatment.

Substantive changes since last issue

Photodynamic therapy New systematic review included; no change in conclusions.[34]

REFERENCES

1. The International ARM Epidemiological Study Group. An international classification and grading system for age-related maculopathy and age-related macular degeneration. *Surv Ophthalmol* 1995;39:367–374.
2. Macular Photocoagulation Study Group. Subfoveal neovascular lesions in age-related macular degeneration: Guidelines for evaluation and treatment in the Macular Photocoagulation Study. *Arch Ophthalmol* 1991;109:1242–1257.
3. Bressler SB, Bressler NM, Fine SL. Age-related macular degeneration. *Surv Ophthalmol* 1988;32: 375–413.
4. Klein R, Klein BEK, Linton KLP. Prevalence of age-related maculopathy: the Beaver Dam Eye Study. *Ophthalmology* 1992;99:933–943.
5. Vingerling JR, Dielemans I, Hofman A, et al. The prevalence of age-related maculopathy in the Rotterdam study. *Ophthalmology* 1995;102:205–210.
6. Mitchell P, Smith W, Attebo K, et al. Prevalence of age-related maculopathy in Australia. The Blue Mountains Eye Study. *Ophthalmology* 1995;102: 1450–1640.
7. Macular Photocoagulation Study Group. Risk factors for choroidal neovascularisation in the second eye of patients with juxtafoveal or subfoveal choroidal neovascularisation secondary to age-related macular degeneration. *Arch Ophthalmol* 1997;115:741–747.
8. Pieramici DJ, Bressler SB. Age-related macular degeneration and risk factors for the development of choroidal neovascularization in the fellow eye. *Curr Opin Ophthalmol* 1998;9:38–46.
9. Maguire P, Vine AK. Geographic atrophy of the retinal pigment epithelium. *Am J Ophthalmol* 1986;102:621–625.
10. Sarks JP, Sarks SH, Killingsworth M. Evolution of geographic atrophy of the retinal pigment epithelium. *Eye* 1988;2:552–577.
11. Macular Photocoagulation Study Group. Argon laser photocoagulation for neovascular maculopathy: Five-year results from randomized clinical trials. *Arch Ophthalmol* 1991;109:1109–1114.
12. Macular Photocoagulation Study Group. Laser photocoagulation of subfoveal neovascular lesions of age-related macular degeneration: updated findings from two clinical trials. *Arch Ophthalmol* 1993;111:1200–1209.
13. Macular Photocoagulation Study Group. Argon laser photocoagulation for neovascular maculopathy. Three-year results from randomized clinical trials. *Arch Ophthalmol* 1986;104:694–701.
14. Macular Photocoagulation Study Group. Laser photocoagulation for juxtafoveal choroidal neovascularisation. Five-year results from randomized clinical trials. *Arch Ophthalmol* 1994; 112:500–509.
15. Macular Photocoagulation Study Group. Occult choroidal neovascularization. Influence on visual outcome in patients with age-related macular degeneration. *Arch Ophthalmol* 1996;114:400–412.
16. Macular Photocoagulation Study Group. Persistent and recurrent neovascularization after laser photocoagulation for subfoveal choroidal neovascularization of age-related macular degeneration. *Arch Ophthalmol* 1994;112:489–499.
17. Macular Photocoagulation Study Group. Visual outcome after laser photocoagulation for subfoveal choroidal neovascularization secondary to age-related macular degeneration. The influence of initial lesion size and initial visual acuity. *Arch Ophthalmol* 1994;112:480–488.
18. Coscas G, Soubrane G, Ramahefasolo C, et al. Perifoveal laser treatment for subfoveal choroidal new vessels in age-related macular degeneration. Results of a randomized clinical trial. *Arch Ophthalmol* 1991;109:1258–1265.
19. Bressler NM, Maguire MG, Murphy PL, et al. Macular scatter ("grid") laser treatment of poorly demarcated subfoveal choroidal neovascularisation in age-related macular degeneration. Results of a randomised pilot trial. *Arch Ophthalmol* 1996;114:1456–1464.
20. Arnold J, Algan M, Soubrane G, et al. Indirect scatter laser photocoagulation to subfoveal choroidal neovascularization in age-related macular degeneration. *Graefes Arch Clin Exp Ophthalmol* 1997;235:208–216.
21. Barondes MJ, Pagliarini S, Chisholm IH, et al. Controlled trial of laser photocoagulation of pigment epithelial detachments in the elderly: 4 year review. *Br J Ophthalmol* 1992;76:5–7.
22. Macular Photocoagulation Study Group. Evaluation of argon green vs krypton red laser for photocoagulation of subfoveal choroidal neovascularisation in the Macular Photocoagulation Study. *Arch Ophthalmol* 1994; 112:1176–1184.
23. Willan AR, Cruess AF, Ballantyne M. Argon green vs krypton red laser photocoagulation for extrafoveal choroidal neovascularization secondary to age-related macular degeneration: 3-year results of a multicentre randomized trial. *Can J Ophthalmol* 1996;31:11–17.
24. The Radiation Therapy for age-related macular degeneration (RAD) study group. A prospective randomized double-masked trial on radiation therapy for neovascular age-related macular degeneration (RAD) study. *Ophthalmology* 1999; 106:2239–2247.
25. Bergink GJ, Hoyng CB, van der Maazen RW, et al. A randomized controlled clinical trial on the efficacy of radiation therapy in the control of subfoveal choroidal neovascularization in age-related macular degeneration: radiation versus observation. *Graefes Arch Clin Exp Ophthalmol* 1998;236:321–325.
26. Char DH, Irvine AI, Posner MD, et al. Randomized trial of radiation for age-related macular degeneration. *Am J Ophthalmol* 1999;127:574–578.
27. Hart PM, Chakravarthy U, MacKenzie G, et al. Teletherapy for subfoveal choroidal neovascularisation of age-related macular degeneration: results of follow up in a non-randomised study. *Br J Ophthalmol* 1996;80: 1046–1050.
28. Finger PT, Berson A, Sherr D, et al. Radiation therapy for subretinal neovascularization. *Ophthalmology* 1996;103:878–889.
29. Ciulla TA, Danis RP, Harris A. Age-related macular degeneration: A review of experimental treatments. *Surv Ophthalmol* 1998;43:134–146.
30. Spaide RF, Leys A, Herrmann-Delemazure B, et al. Radiation-associated choroidal neovasculopathy. *Ophthalmology* 1999;106:2254–2260.
31. Lewis H, Van der Brug MS. Tissue plasminogen activator-assisted surgical excision of subfoveal choroidal neovascularization in age-related macular degeneration: a randomized, double-masked trial. *Ophthalmology* 1997;104:1847–1851.
32. Thomas MA, Dickinson JD, Melberg NS, et al. Visual results after surgical removal of subfoveal

choroidal neovascular membranes. *Ophthalmology* 1994;101:1384–1396.

33. Pharmacological Therapy for Macular Degeneration Study Group. Interferon alfa-2a is ineffective for patients with choroidal neovascularization secondary to age-related macular degeneration: results of a prospective randomized placebo-controlled clinical trial. *Arch Ophthalmol* 1997;115:865–872.

34. Wormald R, Evans J, Smeeth L. Photodynamic therapy for neovascular age-related macular degeneration. In: The Cochrane Library, Issue 2, 2000. Oxford: Update Software. Search date December 1999; primary sources Cochrane Controlled Trials Register; Cochrane Eyes and Vision Group Register; Medline; Embase; Science Citation Index; experts and hand searched references.

Jennifer Arnold
Consultant Ophthalmologist
Aberdeen Royal Hospitals NHS Trust
Aberdeen
UK

Shirley Sarks
Honorary Senior Research Associate
Prince of Wales Medical Research
Institute
Randwick, NSW
Australia

Competing interests: JA was a clinical investigator in the study of photodynamic treatment using verteporfin, funded by CIBA Vision/QLT; has been supported by CIBA Vision for attendance at conferences and symposia; and holds shares in QLT.

TABLE 1 Laser photocoagulation of choroidal neovascularisation (CNV) versus observation in exudative AMD. Results of Macular Photocoagulation Study Group RCTs (see text, p 342).[11-17,19]

Site of CNV (type of laser)	Number of eyes	Severe visual loss (6 or more lines)	Vision level treated v control	Rate of recurrence in treated eyes
Extrafoveal CNV (argon blue-green)[11,13]	236	RR 1.5 at 6 months to 5 years; P = 0.001	33% v 22% ≥ 20/40 at 3 years	54% at 5 years
Juxtafoveal CNV (krypton red)[14,15]	496	RR 1.2 at 6 months to 5 years; P = 0.04	13% v 7% ≥ 20/40 at 3 years	76% at 5 years (classic CNV only)
New subfoveal CNV (argon green or krypton)[12,16,17,19]	373	20% treated v 37% control at 2 years; P < 0.01	12% v 11% > 20/200 at 4 years	44% at 3 years
Recurrent subfoveal CNV (argon green or krypton)[12,16,19]	206	9% treated v 28% control at 2 years; P = 0.03	25% v 12% > 20/200 at 3 years	39% at 3 years

CNV; choroidal neovascularisation.

Updated this issue

Christine Chung and Elisabeth Cohen

INTERVENTIONS

Beneficial

Topical antibiotics
(fluoroquinolones, polymyxin combinations, aminoglycosides, fusidic acid) 351, 352

Trade off between benefits and harms

Topical chloramphenicol. 352

To be covered in future issues of *Clinical Evidence*

Propamidine isethionate ("Golden Eye")
Systemic antibiotics
Gonococcal conjunctivitis/ gonococcal ophthalmia neonatorum
Conjunctivitis in contact lens wearers

Key Messages

- Bacterial conjunctivitis is usually self limiting.

- In people with suspected bacterial conjunctivitis, one systematic review found limited evidence from one RCT that topical norfloxacin was associated with a significantly higher rate of clinical and microbiological improvement than placebo. Comparative RCTs found no significant difference between different topical antibiotics in rates of clinical or microbiological cure.

- In people with bacterial conjunctivitis proved on culture, RCTs found faster clinical and microbiological improvement with topical ciprofloxacin and ofloxacin than with placebo. Ofloxacin was associated with reduced relapse rate compared with placebo. Comparative RCTs found no significant difference between topical lomefloxacin and ciprofloxacin in clinical and microbiological cure rates. One RCT found fusidic acid to be superior to chloramphenicol.

- Chloramphenicol is the only topical antibiotic possibly associated with serious systemic adverse effects (aplastic anaemia), but we found no good evidence about the magnitude of this risk for chloramphenicol versus other topical antibiotics.

- We found no trials that examined the potential growth of resistant organisms from the use of antibiotics in bacterial conjunctivitis.

DEFINITION Conjunctivitis is any inflammation of the conjunctiva, generally characterised by irritation, itching, foreign body sensation, and tearing or discharge. Bacterial conjunctivitis may usually be distinguished from other types of conjunctivitis by the presence of a yellow–white mucopurulent discharge. There is also usually a papillary reaction (small bumps with fibrovascular cores on the palpebral conjunctiva, appearing grossly as a fine velvety surface). Bacterial conjunctivitis is usually unilateral, as opposed to viral conjunctivitis which often starts in one eye and spreads to the other. This review covers only non-gonococcal bacterial conjunctivitis.

INCIDENCE/ PREVALENCE We found no good evidence on the incidence or prevalence of bacterial conjunctivitis.

AETIOLOGY/ RISK FACTORS Conjunctivitis may be infectious (caused by bacteria or viruses) or allergic. In adults, bacterial conjunctivitis is less common than viral conjunctivitis, although estimates vary widely (viral conjunctivitis has been reported to account for 8–75% of acute conjunctivitis).[1–3] Staphylococcus species are the most common bacterial pathogens, followed by *Streptococcus pneumoniae* and *Haemophilus influenzae*.[4,5] In children, bacterial conjunctivitis is more common than viral, and is mainly caused by *H influenzae, S pneumoniae*, and *Moraxella catarrhalis*.[6,7]

PROGNOSIS Most bacterial conjunctivitis is self limiting. One systematic review of RCTs (updated in April 1999) reported clinical cure or significant improvement on placebo within 2–5 days in 64% of people (99% CI 54% to 73%).[8] Some organisms cause corneal or systemic complications, or both; otitis may develop in 25% of children with *H influenzae* conjunctivitis,[9] and systemic meningitis may complicate primary meningococcal conjunctivitis in 18% of people.[10] Conjunctivitis in children is more likely to be bacterial than viral, warranting heightened awareness of possible systemic complications.

AIMS To achieve rapid cure of inflammation, and to prevent complications, with minimum adverse effects of treatment.

OUTCOMES Time to cure or improvement. **Clinical signs/symptoms:** hyperaemia, discharge, papillae, follicles, chemosis, itching, pain, photophobia. Most studies used a numbered scale to grade signs and symptoms. Some studies also included evaluation by investigators and patients regarding success of treatment. **Culture results:** proxy outcomes usually expressed as the number of colonies, sometimes with reference to a threshold level. Results were often classified into categories such as eradication, reduction, persistence, and proliferation.

METHODS *Clinical Evidence* update search and appraisal May 2000. All identified systematic reviews and subsequent RCTs were reviewed.

QUESTION What are the effects of empirical treatment with topical antibiotics in adults and children with suspected bacterial conjunctivitis?

One systematic review found limited evidence from one RCT that topical norfloxacin was associated with a significantly higher rate of clinical and

microbiological improvement than placebo. Comparative RCTs found no significant difference between different topical antibiotics in rates of clinical or microbiological cure.

Benefits: **Versus placebo:** We found one systematic review (updated in 1999), which identified one RCT comparing topical norfloxacin (143 adults) versus placebo (141 adults); 50% of participants were culture positive.[8] The review found significantly higher rates of clinical and microbiological cure or improvement at 5 days with norfloxacin (88%, 95% CI 81% to 93% v 72%, 95% CI 63% to 79%; P < 0.01). **Versus each other:** We found no systematic review. We found 19 comparative RCTs in adults and children. These found no significant difference between different topical antibiotics in rates of clinical or microbiological cure (see table on website; www.clinica-levidence.org). Six of the RCTs (evaluating lomefloxacin, fusidic acid, rifamycin, chloramphenicol, and tobramycin) included grading by patients of effectiveness and tolerability. No significant differences were found.[11–16]

Harms: The placebo controlled RCT reported minor adverse events in 4.2% of people using norfloxacin and 7.1% using placebo (no statistical analysis available).[5] Placebo contained higher proportions of benzalkonium chloride (0.01% v 0.0025% in the norfloxacin solution). One non-systematic review described complications of topical antibiotics.[17] These included four reported cases of idiosyncratic aplastic anaemia associated with topical chloramphenicol and three cases of Stevens–Johnson syndrome associated with topical sulphonamides, but the review gave no figures on the number of people using these drugs.

Comment: The placebo controlled RCT did not address the effect of using topical antibiotics on antibiotic resistance, which would be of interest given the self limiting nature of the disease.[5] None of the trials specified their methods for selecting participants. The findings may not be generaliseable to primary care populations. Most trials included children as well as adults, and the ratio of children to adults was usually not specified. The comparisons of lomefloxacin versus chloramphenicol and fusidic acid, and the comparison of norfloxacin versus fusidic acid, were single blind. Lomefloxacin and fusidic acid are not available in the USA, and chloramphenicol is rarely used in the USA because of reports of idiosyncratic aplastic anaemia.

QUESTION What are the effects of topical antibiotics in adults and children with culture positive conjunctivitis?

RCTs in people with bacterial conjunctivitis proved on culture found faster clinical and microbiological improvement with ciprofloxacin, ofloxacin, or polymyxin–bacitracin than with placebo. Ofloxacin was associated with reduced relapse rates. Comparative RCTs found no significant difference between tobramycin and ciprofloxacin or between trimethoprim–polymyxin B, and sulfacetamide in clinical and microbiological cure rates. One RCT found greater clinical efficacy and less microbiological resistance with fusidic acid than chloramphenicol.

Benefits: **Versus placebo:** We found one systematic review (updated in 1999), which identified three placebo controlled RCTs evaluating polymyxin–bacitracin, ciprofloxacin, and ofloxacin in bacterial conjunctivitis proved by culture. The review identified no trials of gentamicin that included only culture proved conjunctivitis.[8] One RCT was in children (n = 84).[18] It found that in culture proved *H influenzae* and *S pneumoniae* bacterial conjunctivitis, there was a higher clinical cure rate at days 3–5 with polymyxin–bacitracin than placebo, although by days 8–10 the difference was not significant (62% *v* 28% at days 3–5, P < 0.02; 91% *v* 72% at days 8–10, P > 0.05). The microbiological cure rate was significantly higher with antibiotics both at days 3–5 and days 8–10. When systemic antibiotics were given for concurrent problems, there was no significant difference between groups, but the numbers were too small to rule out a clinically important effect (see table on website; http://www.clinicalevidence.org). Two other trials identified in the review did not specify the age of participants. One did not evaluate clinical outcome but found significantly greater microbiological improvement at day 3 in people treated with ciprofloxacin (n = 177).[19] One RCT was published as an abstract only; it found significantly greater clinical and microbiological improvement at day 2 in people treated with ofloxacin (n = 132, 64% *v* 22% improved at day 2, P < 0.001). It also found a lower relapse rate in people treated with ofloxacin 2 days after treatment stopped.[20] A fourth was published in Japanese and was not reviewed.[21] **Versus each other:** We found no systematic review which met our quality criteria. We found one RCT that did not specify the age of participants, three RCTs in children only, and one small RCT in children and adults. The RCT that did not specify age found no significant difference in microbiological eradication or improvement between ciprofloxacin (n = 140) and tobramycin (n = 111); eradication or improvement occurred in 94.3% *v* 91.9% (P > 0.5, no CI available).[19] Clinical cure was not evaluated. Of the three RCTs in children, two found no significant difference in clinical or overall microbiological efficacy between ciprofloxacin and tobramycin (n = 70 *v* 71, eradication 90% *v* 84%, P = 0.29; cure 87% *v* 90%, P = 0.6) or between trimethoprim–polymyxin B, gentamicin, and sulfacetamide (n = 53 *v* 57 *v* 46, eradication 83% *v* 68% *v* 72%, P > 0.1; cure 84% *v* 88% *v* 89%, P > 0.1).[22–23] The third (non-blinded) RCT found more clinical efficacy and less microbiological resistance with fusidic acid than chloramphenicol (n = 114 *v* 25, cure 85% *v* 48%, P < 0.0001; resistance 16% *v* 55%, statistical analysis not provided).[24] The RCT in children and adults (ratio not specified) found no difference between lomefloxacin and ofloxacin (n = 40, resolution of symptoms and signs at day 7: 88% *v* 75%, P < 0.08).[25]

Harms: Of the 116 children initially enrolled in the first RCT described above, one was excluded because of possible allergic reaction to the ointment; the other exclusions were unrelated to adverse effects[18] In RCTs that included people with both culture proved and suspected bacterial conjunctivitis, minor adverse events were reported with antibiotics: burning, bitter taste, pruritus, or punctate epithelial erosions (35% with tobramycin *v* 20% with ciprofloxacin; no statistical detail available from abstract),[26] bad taste (20% with norfloxacin v 6% with fusidic acid),[27] stinging (50% with norfloxacin v 37% with fusidic acid)[27] and burning (33% with gentamicin v 20% with lomefloxacin).[13]

Comment: None of the RCTs addressed the effect on antibiotic resistance of using topical antibiotics in bacterial conjunctivitis, which would be of interest given the self limiting nature of the disease. Furthermore, they did not report on patient oriented outcomes or look at rates of reinfection.

Substantive changes since last issue

Empirical treatment with topical antibiotics in adults and children with suspected bacterial conjunctivitis: versus each other One new RCT; conclusions unchanged.[16]

Topical antibiotics in adults and children with culture positive conjunctivitis One new RCT; conclusions unchanged.[25]

REFERENCES

1. Wishart PK, James C, Wishart MS, Darougar S. Prevalence of acute conjunctivitis caused by chlamydia, adenovirus, and herpes simplex virus in an ophthalmic casualty department. Br J Ophthalmol 1984;68:653–655.

2. Fitch CP, Rapoza PA, Owens S, et al. Epidemiology and diagnosis of acute conjunctivitis at an inner-city hospital. Ophthalmology 1989;96:1215–1220.

3. Woodland RM, Darougar S, Thaker U, et al. Causes of conjunctivitis and keratoconjunctivitis in Karachi, Pakistan. Trans R Soc Trop Med Hygiene 1992;86:317–320.

4. Seal DV, Barrett SP, McGill JI. Aetiology and treatment of acute bacterial infection of the external eye. Br J Ophthalmol 1982;66:357–360.

5. Miller IM, Wittreich J, Vogel R, Cook TJ, for the Norfloxacin-Placebo Ocular Study Group. The safety and efficacy of topical norfloxacin compared with placebo in the treatment of acute bacterial conjunctivitis. Eur J Ophthalmol 1992;2:58–66.

6. Gigliotti F, Williams WT, Hayden FG, et al. Etiology of acute conjunctivitis in children. J Pediatr 1981; 98:531–536.

7. Weiss A, Brinser JH, Nazar-Stewart V. Acute conjunctivitis in childhood. J Pediatr 1993;122: 10–14.

8. Sheikh A, Hurwitz B, Cave J. Antibiotics for acute bacterial conjunctivitis. In: The Cochrane Library, Issue 4, 1999. Oxford: Update Software. Updated April 1999, search date September 1998 primary sources Cochrane Controlled Trial Register 1998 issue, Medline 1994 to September 1998, bibliographies of identified trials, Science Citation Index, and personal contacts with investigators and pharmaceutical companies.

9. Bodor FF. Conjunctivitis-otitis media syndrome: more than meets the eye. Contemp Pediatr 1989; 6:55–60.

10. Barquet N, Gasser I, Domingo P, et al. Primary meningococcal conjunctivitis: report of 21 patients and review. Rev Infect Dis 1990;12:838–847.

11. Kettenmeyer A, Jauch A, Boscher M, et al. A double-blind double-dummy multicenter equivalence study comparing topical lomefloxacin 0.3% twice daily with norfloxacin 0.3% four times daily in the treatment of acute bacterial conjunctivitis. J Clin Res 1998;1:75–86.

12. Agius-Fernandez A, Patterson A, Fsadni M, et al. Topical lomefloxacin versus topical chloramphenicol in the treatment of acute bacterial conjunctivitis. Clin Drug Invest 1998;15: 263–269.

13. Montero J, Casado A, Perea E, et al. A double-blind double-dummy comparison of topical lomefloxacin 0.3% twice daily with topical gentamicin 0.3% four times daily in the treatment of acute bacterial conjunctivitis. J Clin Res 1998; 1:29–39.

14. Adenis JP, Arrata M, Gastaud P, et al. Etude randomisee multicentrique acide fusidique gel ophtalmique et rifamycine collyre dans les conjonctivites aigues. J Fr Ophtalmol 1989;12: 317–322.

15. Huerva V, Ascaso FJ, Latre B, et al. Tolerancia y eficacia de la tobramicina topica vs cloranfenicol en el tratamiento de las conjunctivitis bacterianas. Ciencia Pharmaceutica 1991;1:221–224.

16. Gallenga PE, Lobefalo L, Colangelo L, et al. Topical lomefloxacin 0.3% twice daily versus tobramycin 0.3% in acute bacterial conjunctivitis: a multicenter double-blind phase III study. Ophthalmologica 1999;213:250–257.

17. Stern GA, Killingsworth DW. Complications of topical antimicrobial agents. Int Ophthalmol Clin 1989;29:137–142.

18. Gigliotti G, Hendley JO, Morgan J, et al. Efficacy of topical antibiotic therapy in acute conjunctivitis in children. J Pediatr 1984;104:623–626.

19. Leibowitz HM. Antibacterial effectiveness of ciprofloxacin 0.3% ophthalmic solution in the treatment of bacterial conjunctivitis. Am J Ophthalmol 1991;112:29S–33S.

20. Ofloxacin Study Group III. A placebo-controlled clinical study of the fluoroquinolone ofloxacin in patients with external infection. Invest Ophthalmol Vis Sci 1990;31:572.

21. Mitsui Y, Matsuda H, Miyajima T, et al. Therapeutic effects of ofloxacin eye drops (DE-055) on external infection of the eye: multicentral double blind test. J Rev Clin Ophthalmol 1986;80:1813–1828.

22. Gross RD, Hoffman RO, Lindsay RN. A comparison of ciprofloxacin and tobramycin in bacterial conjunctivitis is children. Clin Pediatr 1997;36: 435–444.

23. Lohr JA, Austin RD, Grossman M, et al. Comparison of three topical antimicrobials for acute bacterial conjunctivitis. Pediatr Infect Dis J 1988;7:626–629.

24. Van Bijsterveld OP, el Batawi Y, Sobhi FS, et al. Fusidic acid in infections of the external eye. Infection 1987;15:16–19.

25. Tabbara KF, El-Sheik HF, Monowarul Islam SM, Hammouda E. Treatment of acute bacterial conjunctivitis with topical lomefloxacin 0.3%

compared to topical ofloxacin 0.3%. *Eur J Ophthalmol* 1999; 9:269–275.

26. Alves MR, Kara JN. Evaluation of the clinical and microbiological efficacy of 0.3% ciprofloxacin drops and 0.3% tobramycin drops in the treatment of acute bacterial conjunctivitis. *Revista Brasiliera de Oftalmol* 1993;52:371–377.

27. Wall AR, Sinclair N, Adenis JP. Comparison of Fucithalmic (fusidic acid viscous eye drops 1%) and Noroxin (norfloxacin ophthalmic solution 0.3%) in the treatment of bacterial conjunctivitis. J *Clin Res* 1998;1:316–325.

28. The Trimethoprim-Polymyxin B Sulphate Ophthalmic Ointment Study Group. Trimethoprim-polymyxin B sulphate ophthalmic ointment versus chloramphenicol ophthalmic ointment in the treatment of bacterial conjunctivitis—a review of four clinical studies. J *Antimicrob Chemother* 1989;23:261–266.

29. Behrens-Baumann W, Quentin CD, Gibson JR, et al. Trimethoprim-polymyxin B sulphate ophthalmic ointment in the treatment of bacterial conjunctivitis: a double-blind study versus chloramphenicol ophthalmic ointment. *Curr Med Res Opin* 1988;11:227–231.

30. van-Rensburg SF, Gibson JR, Harvey SG, Burke CA. Trimethoprim-polymyxin ophthalmic solution versus chloramphenicol ophthalmic solution in the treatment of bacterial conjunctivitis. *Pharmatherapeutica* 1982;3:274–277.

31. Gibson JR. Trimethoprim-polymyxin B ophthalmic solution in the treatment of presumptive bacterial conjunctivitis—a multicentre trial of its efficacy versus neomycin-polymyxin B-gramicidin and chloramphenicol ophthalmic solutions. J *Antimicrob Chemother* 1983;11:217–221.

32. Genee E, Schlechtweg C, Bauerreiss P, Gibson JR. Trimethoprim-polymyxin eye drops versus neomycin-polymyxin-gramicidin eye drops in the treatment of presumptive bacterial conjunctivitis—a double-blind study. *Ophthalmologica* 1982;184:92–96.

33. Malminiemi K, Kari O, Latvala M-L, et al. Topical lomefloxacin twice daily compared with fucidic acid in acute bacterial conjunctivitis. *Acta Ophthalmol Scand* 1996;74:280–284.

34. Carr WD. Comparison of Fucithalmic (fusidic acid viscous eye drops 1%) and Chloromycetin Redidrops (chloramphenicol eye drops 0.5%) in the treatment of acute bacterial conjunctivitis. J *Clin Res* 1998;1:403–411.

35. Horven I. Acute conjunctivitis. A comparison of fusidic acid viscous eye drops and chloramphenicol. *Acta Ophthalmol* 1993;71:165–168.

36. Hvidberg J. Fusidic acid in acute conjunctivitis. Single-blind, randomized comparison of fusidic acid and chloramphenicol viscous eye drops. *Acta Ophthalmol* 1987;65:43–47.

37. Uchida Y. Clinical efficacy of topical lomefloxacin (NY-198) in bacterial infections of the external eye. *Folia Ophthalmologica* 1991;42:59–70.

38. References 28 to 37 relate to the table, which appears on the clinical evidence website: www.clinicalevidence.org.

Christine Chung
Cornea Fellow

Elisabeth Cohen
Director

Cornea Service, Wills Eye Hospital
Jefferson Medical College
Philadelphia
USA

Competing interests: None declared.

Updated this issue

Colm O'Brien and Jeremy Diamond

QUESTIONS

INTERVENTIONS

Likely to be beneficial

To be covered in future issues of *Clinical Evidence*

Treating ocular hypertension in
  people without established
  glaucoma
Early detection of glaucoma
  (opportunistic case finding,
  population screening)

Key Messages

- RCTs have found that topical medical treatments reduce raised intraocular pressure in people with primary open angle glaucoma, but their protective effect on visual fields is uncertain.

- We found limited evidence suggesting that laser trabeculoplasty and surgical trabeculectomy provide greater protection of visual fields than medical treatment. However, trabeculectomy is associated with morbidity, including cataract formation and loss of visual acuity.

- One RCT found that reducing intraocular pressure slowed progression of visual field loss in normal pressure glaucoma.

DEFINITION	Glaucoma constitutes a group of diseases characterised by progressive optic neuropathy. It is generally bilateral though asymmetric. The different forms of glaucoma share features of optic nerve cupping and pallor, and peripheral visual field loss. The most common forms are primary open angle glaucoma (where the level of intraocular pressure is greater than the upper limit of the normal 21 mmHg) and low tension or normal pressure glaucoma (intraocular pressure < 22 mmHg).
INCIDENCE/ PREVALENCE	Glaucoma is found in 1–2% of white people aged over 40, rising to 5% at 70 years. Primary open angle glaucoma accounts for two thirds and normal pressure glaucoma for up to a quarter of those affected.[1,2] In black people, glaucoma is more prevalent, presents earlier with higher pressures, is more difficult to control, and results in more blindness.[1] Glaucoma blindness is responsible for 8% of new blind registrations in the UK.[3]
AETIOLOGY/ RISK FACTORS	The major risk factor for developing primary open angle glaucoma is raised intraocular pressure. Lesser risk factors include family history, myopia, and ethnic origin. Additional risk factors for normal pressure glaucoma include peripheral vascular diseases such as Raynaud's syndrome.
PROGNOSIS	People often fail to recognise peripheral field loss, and consequently 20% of people with glaucoma have advanced field loss at diagnosis.[4] As the disease progresses, people with glaucoma have difficulty moving from a bright room to a darker room and judging steps and kerbs. Blindness results from gross loss of visual field or loss of central vision. The rate of progression is probably dictated by the level of intraocular pressure.[5] Once early field defects have appeared, and where the intraocular pressure is greater than 30 mmHg, untreated people may lose the remainder of the visual field in 3 years or less.[5] Progression of visual field loss is often slower in normal pressure glaucoma.
AIMS	To prevent progression of visual field loss.
OUTCOMES	Visual acuity; visual fields; optic disc cupping and intraocular pressure are intermediate outcomes.
METHODS	*Clinical Evidence* update search and appraisal May 2000.

QUESTION **What are the effects of treatments for established primary open angle glaucoma?**

OPTION **TOPICAL MEDICAL TREATMENT**

RCTs have found that topical medical treatment reduces intraocular pressure compared with placebo, but the few trials with long term follow up found no benefit in terms of protection against loss of visual field.

Benefits: We found one systematic review (search date 1991), which identified 102 RCTs in people with primary open angle glaucoma.[6] Comparative trials (n = 86) were excluded from the review. **Intraocular pressure:** Pooled analysis of the 16 placebo controlled trials found a significant reduction in mean intraocular pressure of 4.9 mmHg (95% CI 2.5 to 7.3 mmHg). **Visual field loss:** Data on long term visual field change were available in only three RCTs (302 participants). Pooled data did not show a significant protective effect of medical treatment (OR for any worsening of visual field loss 0.75, 95% CI 0.42 to 1.35). We found no substantial RCTs published since the systematic review.

Harms: Systemic adverse effects of topical treatments are uncommon but may be serious, including exacerbation of chronic obstructive airways disease after use of non-selective topical β blockers. Non-selective topical β blockers can also cause systemic hypotension and reduction in resting heart rate and are contraindicated in people with cardiac failure.[7]

Comment: It was not possible to identify the types of participants or topical treatments from the published report.[6] Four RCTs sponsored by the US National Institutes of Health are under way: the early manifest glaucoma study, the ocular hypertension treatment study, the collaborative initial glaucoma treatment study, and the advanced glaucoma intervention study.

OPTION **LASER TRABECULOPLASTY**

One RCT found greater long term improvement in intraocular pressure and visual fields from laser trabeculoplasty plus medical treatment than from medical treatment alone.

Benefits: We found no systematic review. We found one RCT in 203 participants selected from 271 people with newly diagnosed primary open angle glaucoma. This compared initial laser trabeculoplasty followed by medical treatment versus medical treatment alone.[8] After a mean follow up of 7 years those treated initially with laser surgery had a 1.2 mmHg greater reduction in intraocular pressure (P = 0.001), a 0.6 dB greater improvement in visual field (P < 0.001), and significantly less deterioration in optic disc appearance (P = 0.005) compared with those given medical treatment only.

Harms: Adverse effects of laser trabeculoplasty are mild and include a transient rise in intraocular pressure (> 5 mmHg in 91 of 271 participants) and formation of peripheral anterior synechiae (in 93 of 271 participants).[8]

Comment: This was a multicentre trial with multiple observers.[8] The report does not state whether the observers were blind to the intervention.

OPTION **SURGICAL TRABECULECTOMY**

Two RCTs found that early surgical trabeculectomy offered greater protection of visual fields than medical treatment. However, surgical drainage is associated with a reduction in central visual activity. One RCT found that initial surgical trabeculectomy followed by laser trabeculoplasty conferred greater benefit than initial laser trabeculoplasty followed by surgical trabeculectomy, but that response depended on ethnic origin.

Benefits: We found no systematic review. **Versus medical treatment:** We found two RCTs. One RCT compared trabeculectomy (followed by medical treatment when indicated) versus medical treatment (followed by trabeculectomy when medical treatment failed) in 116 people with newly diagnosed primary open angle glaucoma.[9] The authors concluded that after a mean follow up of 4.6 years there was no significant difference in visual acuity between the groups, but the medical treatment group had significantly greater loss of visual field. The second RCT randomised 186 people with glaucoma to receive laser, medication, or early trabeculectomy surgery.[10] After 5 years major deterioration in visual fields was found in participants on medical and laser treatment but not in those receiving surgery. There was no difference in visual acuity between the three groups after 5 years. **Versus initial laser trabeculoplasty:** One RCT compared surgical trabeculectomy versus laser trabeculoplasty as initial treatment in 776 eyes with advanced glaucoma (451 African–American, 325 white). Initial trabeculectomy was followed by laser trabeculoplasty and repeat trabeculectomy as required; initial laser trabeculoplasty was followed by trabeculectomy as required. Outcome measures included loss of visual field (progressive glaucoma) and loss of central vision (progressive cataract). Overall, initial surgical trabeculectomy was associated with the greatest reduction in intraocular pressure. The response to treatment differed according to ethnic origin. In black patients, vision (both field and acuity) was best preserved in the group receiving initial laser trabeculoplasty, and this benefit continued for 7 years. In white patients, the greater protection of visual fields switched after 1 year of follow up to the group receiving initial surgical trabeculectomy.[11]

Harms: Surgical trabeculectomy is associated with a reduction in central vision. In one study, 83% of participants lost two lines of Snellen visual acuity.[12]

Comment: It was not possible to extract numerical data from either report.

QUESTION **What are the effects of lowering intraocular pressure in people with normal pressure glaucoma?**

One RCT found that reducing intraocular pressure slowed progression of visual field loss in normal pressure glaucoma.

Benefits: We found no systematic review. We found one RCT (144 eyes in 140 people with normal pressure glaucoma). This compared a treatment to reduce pressure by 30% (with drugs or surgical drainage, or both, 61 eyes) versus no treatment (79 eyes). Progression of visual field loss was defined in terms of deepening of an existing scotoma, a new or expanded "threat to fixation," or a fresh scotoma in a previously normal part of the visual field. Optic disc changes were photographed and independently assessed by two ophthalmologists. Progression occurred in seven (12%) of the treated eyes and 28 (35%) of the control eyes (P < 0.0001). By using survival analysis, mean time from baseline to progression was 2688 days for the treated group and 1695 days for the control group.[13] A companion paper suggests that the favourable effect of pressure lowering is evident only when the cataract inducing effect of drainage surgery is removed and, moreover, that not all cases of normal pressure glaucoma progress when untreated (40% at 5 years).[14]

Harms: There was a significantly higher rate of cataract formation in the treated group than in the control group (34 cataracts reported, 23 [38%] in the treatment group and 11 [14%] in the control group, P = 0.001); the excess risk was confined to those treated surgically (P = 0.0001).

Comment: None.

REFERENCES

1. Sommer A, Tielsch JM, Katz J, et al. Relationship between intraocular pressure and primary open angle glaucoma among white and black Americans. *Arch Ophthalmol* 1991;109:1090–1095.

2. Coffey M, Reidy A, Wormald R, Xian WX, Wright L, Courtney P. The prevalence of glaucoma in the west of Ireland. *Br J Ophthalmol* 1993;77:17–21.

3. Government Statistical Service. *Causes of blindness and partial sight amongst adults.* London: HMSO, 1988.

4. Sheldrick JH, Ng C, Austin DJ, Rosenthal AR. An analysis of referral routes and diagnostic accuracy in cases of suspected glaucoma. *Ophthalmic Epidemiol* 1994;1:31–38.

5. Jay JL, Murdoch JR. The rates of visual field loss in untreated primary open angle glaucoma. *Br J Ophthalmol* 1993;77:176–178.

6. Rossetti L, Marchetti I, Orzalesi N, Scorpiglione N, Torri V, Liberati A. Randomised clinical trials on medical treatment of glaucoma: are they appropriate to guide clinical practice? *Arch Ophthalmol* 1993;111:96–103. Search date 1991; primary source Medline 1975 to 1991.

7. Diamond JP. Systemic adverse effects of topical ophthalmic agents: implications for older patients. *Drugs Aging* 1997;11:352–360.

8. Glaucoma Laser Trial Group. The glaucoma laser trial (GLT) and glaucoma laser trial follow-up study: Results. *Am J Ophthalmol* 1995;120:718–731.

9. Jay JL, Allan D. The benefit of early trabeculectomy versus conventional management in primary open angle glaucoma relative to severity of disease. *Eye* 1989;3:528–535.

10. Migdal C, Gregory W, Hitchins R, Kolker AE. Long-term functional outcome after early surgery compared with laser and medicine in open angle glaucoma. *Ophthalmology* 1994;101:1651–1657.

11. The Advanced Glaucoma Intervention Study (AGIS): 4. Comparison of treatment outcomes within race. Seven year results. *Ophthalmology* 1998;105:1146–1164.

12. Costas UP, Smith M, Spaeth GL, Gondham S, Markovitz B. Loss of vision after trabeculectomy. *Ophthalmology* 1993;100:599–612.

13. Anonymous. Comparison of glaucomatous progression between untreated patients with normal-tension glaucoma and patients with therapeutically reduced intraocular pressure. *Am J Ophthalmol* 1998;126:487–497.

14. Anonymous. The effectiveness of intraocular pressure reduction in the treatment of normal-tension glaucoma. *Am J Ophthalmol* 1998;126:498–505.

Colm O'Brien
Consultant Ophthalmic Surgeon
Mater Hospital
Dublin
Republic of Ireland

Jeremy Diamond
Consultant Ophthalmic Surgeon
Bristol Eye Hospital
Bristol
UK

Competing interests: None declared.

QUESTIONS

INTERVENTIONS

Key Messages

Prevention of scarring trachoma by reducing active trachoma

- One RCT has found that promotion of face washing versus no promotion significantly reduces the rate of severe trachoma. It found no significant reduction of the overall rate of trachoma but the study was too small to rule out a clinically important effect.
- In a single pilot study for an RCT, the number of new cases of trachoma was reduced by fly control using insecticide versus no intervention.
- One unpublished systematic review found limited evidence from small RCTs that antibiotics may reduce active trachoma compared with placebo at 3 and 12 months follow up. The same review found limited evidence from three RCTs that oral azithromycin may reduce active trachoma compared with topical tetracycline after 3 months. These RCTs were small or of unusual design, and at 12 months the difference between treatments disappeared.

Treatment of scarring trachoma

- In people with trichiasis who have six or more lashes in contact with the globe, we found limited evidence from two RCTs that bilamellar tarsal rotation may relieve entropion and trichiasis more often than tarsal advance and rotation.
- In people with trichiasis who have five lashes or fewer in contact with the globe, one RCT found that tarsal rotation relieved entropion and trichiasis more often than electrolysis or cryoablation. In these trials, one experienced surgeon performed most of the operations.

DEFINITION Active trachoma is chronic inflammation of the conjunctiva caused by infection with *Chlamydia trachomatis*. The World Health Organization (WHO) classification for acute trachoma defines mild trachoma (grade TF) as the presence of five or more follicles in the upper tarsal conjunctiva of at least 0.5 mm diameter. Severe trachoma (grade TI) is defined as pronounced inflammatory thickening of the upper tarsal conjunctiva that obscures more than half of the normal deep vessels. Repeated infection causes scarring trachoma, in which the upper eyelid is shortened and distorted (entropion), and the lashes abrade the eye (trichiasis). Blindness results from corneal opacification, which is related to the degree of entropion/trichiasis.

INCIDENCE/ PREVALENCE Trachoma is the world's leading cause of preventable blindness and is second only to cataract as an overall cause of blindness.[1] Globally, active trachoma affects an estimated 150 million people, most of them children. About 5.5 million people are blind or at risk of blindness as a consequence of trachoma. Trachoma is a disease of poverty regardless of geographical regions. Scarring trachoma is prevalent in large regions of Africa, the Middle East, South-West Asia, the Indian subcontinent, and Aboriginal communities in Australia, and there are small focuses in Central and South America.[1] In areas where trachoma is constantly present at high prevalence, active disease is found in more than 50% of preschool children and may have a prevalence of 60–90%.[2] As many as 75% of women and 50% of men over the age of 45 may show signs of scarring disease.[3] The prevalence of active trachoma decreases with increasing age, with less than 5% of adults showing signs of active disease.[2] Although similar rates of active disease are observed in male and female children, the later sequelae of trichiasis, entropion, and corneal opacification are more common in women than men.[2]

AETIOLOGY/ RISK FACTORS Active trachoma is associated with young age and where there is close contact between people. Discharge from the eyes and nose may be a source of further reinfection.[4] Sharing a bedroom with someone who has active trachoma is a risk factor for infection.[5] Facial contact with flies is held to be associated with active trachoma, but studies reporting this relationship had weak methods.[6]

PROGNOSIS Corneal damage from trachoma is caused by multiple processes. Scarring may cause an inadequate tear film, and a dry eye may be more susceptible to damage from inturned lashes, leading to corneal opacification. The prevalence of scarring and consequent blindness increases with age and is most commonly seen in older adults.[7]

AIMS To prevent active trachoma; to reduce the rate of progression to scarring; and to relieve entropion and trichiasis in people with scarring trachoma, with minimal side effects of treatment.

OUTCOMES Rates of active trachoma; clinical signs of active trachoma using the WHO grading scale; laboratory evidence of *Chlamydia trachomatis* infection; eyelid position; and degree of entropion/trichiasis.

METHODS *Clinical Evidence* search and appraisal March 2000.

QUESTION What are the effects of interventions to prevent scarring trachoma by reducing active trachoma?

OPTION PUBLIC HEALTH INTERVENTIONS

One RCT has found that promotion of face washing compared with no advice significantly reduces the rate of severe trachoma. It found no significant reduction of the overall rate of trachoma, but the study was not powered to exclude a clinically important effect. One small RCT found that the number of new cases of trachoma was reduced by fly control using insecticide compared with no intervention.

Benefits: **Promotion of face washing:** We found no systematic review but found one RCT that randomised six villages to either promotion of face washing plus 30 days of daily topical tetracycline ointment or 30 days of daily topical tetracycline ointment only.[8] It found that, in 1417 children aged 1–7 years, promotion of face washing increased the likelihood of children having a clean face on at least two of three follow up visits, but the result was not significant (OR for having a clean face with intervention v control 1.6, 95% CI 0.94 to 2.74). After 1 year, promotion of face washing plus topical tetracycline compared with topical tetracycline reduced the risk of severe trachoma (OR for severe trachoma 0.62, 95% CI 0.40 to 0.97), but the reduction was not significant for all grades of trachoma (OR for mild and severe trachoma 0.81, 95% CI 0.42 to 1.59). When all participants from intervention and control villages were pooled, children who had a sustained clean face were less likely to have active trachoma than those who ever had a dirty face (OR 0.58, 95% CI 0.47 to 0.72). **Fly control using insecticide:** We found no systematic review and no completed RCTs. We found one pilot study for an RCT comparing spraying of deltamethrin for 3 months compared with no intervention in two pairs of villages.[6] One pair received the intervention or none in the wet season, one pair received the intervention or none in the dry season. There were a total of 191 children under 10 years in the control villages and 223 children in the intervention villages. The number of new cases of trachoma (WHO classification) at 3 months was 75% lower in the children living in the intervention villages than in the comparison group (RR 0.25, 95% CI 0.09 to 0.64).

Harms: None were identified.

Comment: The cluster randomisation used in both RCTs limits the power to detect differences between groups, and makes difficult interpretation of the results for individual children.[8]

OPTION ANTIBIOTICS

One unpublished systematic review has found limited evidence from low powered RCTs that antibiotics reduce active trachoma at 3 and 12 months compared with no treatment. The same review found limited evidence from three RCTs that oral azithromycin may reduce active trachoma compared with topical tetracycline after 3 months. These RCTs were low powered or of unusual design and at 12 months the difference between treatments disappeared.

Benefits: **Versus placebo or no treatment:** We found one unpublished systematic review (search date 1999).[9] It identified eight RCTs that compared topical and oral antibiotics with no treatment, placebo, or a monthly vitamin tablet in people with active trachoma. All reported outcomes at 3 months. Five trials reported outcomes at 12 months (999 people in the treatment group, 76% completed the study; 832 people in the control group, 71% completed the study) (see table 1, p 367). The review found that antibiotics reduced active trachoma at 3 months (OR for active trachoma based on clinical assessment, antibiotics v control 0.43, 95% CI 0.35 to 0.52) and at 12 months (OR 0.47, 95% CI 0.38 to 0.60). It also found that antibiotics reduced *Chlamydia trachomatis* infection rates based on bacteriological testing compared with control at 12 months (1 RCT; OR 0.27 95% CI 0.11 to 0.67). At 3 months the infection rate was also reduced but not significantly (3 RCTs; OR for infection, antibiotic v control 0.63, 95% CI 0.38 to 1.05). **Oral versus topical antibiotics:** We found one unpublished systematic review of three RCTs comparing rates of active trachoma and bacteriological infection following oral azithromycin or topical tetracycline (see table 2, p 368).[9] All trials had problems with methods that limit the results (see comment below). At 3 months, oral azithromycin compared with topical tetracycline reduced active trachoma (3 RCTs, n = 6226; OR 0.82, 95% CI 0.71 to 0.94) and infection rates (OR 0.49, 95% CI 0.39 to 0.62). At 12 months, the review found no significant difference between treatments for active trachoma (1 RCT, n = 5573; OR 0.88, 95% CI 0.77 to 1.01), but found that oral azithromycin reduced bacteriologically defined infection compared with topical tetracycline (OR 0.70, 95% CI 0.57 to 0.87).

Harms: None were reported.

Comment: **Versus placebo or no treatment:** The trials were undertaken in various settings; most were in children attending boarding schools. Several unusual study designs were used, for example family based treatment. The trials were all of moderate or poor quality and many had no intention to treat analysis. Antibiotic treatments included topical and oral doses. **Oral versus topical treatment:** Two of the RCTs were small (total n = 224) and low powered. The third trial compared mass treatment, in which people were treated irrespective of disease status, and were randomly allocated by village (cluster randomisation). Correlation analysis found some similarity between individuals within a cluster, so limiting the validity of results. We found no evidence about the development of bacterial resistance.

QUESTION   **Effects of surgical treatments for scarring trachoma (entropion and trichiasis)**

We found no good evidence on the effects of surgery to improve visual acuity in people with scarring trachoma. In people with trichiasis who have six or more lashes in contact with the globe, we found limited evidence from two RCTs that bilamellar tarsal rotation may relieve entropion and trichiasis more often than tarsal advance and rotation. In people with trichiasis who have five lashes or fewer in contact with the globe, one RCT found that tarsal rotation relieves entropion and trichiasis more often than electrolysis or cryoablation. In these trials, one experienced surgeon performed most of the operations.

Benefits: We found no systematic review but found two RCTs comparing surgical interventions for entropion and trichiasis.[10,11] In both trials, one experienced surgeon performed most of the operations. Both trials defined operative success as no lashes in contact with the globe in primary position of gaze, and complete lid closure with gentle voluntary effort. **Major trichiasis:** See glossary, p 366. The first trial compared five surgical techniques (bilamellar tarsal rotation, eversion splinting, tarsal advance, tarsal grooving, and tarsal advance and rotation (see glossary, p 366) in 165 Omani villagers with major trichiasis (as defined for these trials). There were a total of 165 eyelids.[10] The trial found very limited evidence that bilamellar tarsal rotation was more successful than other surgical treatments. However, analysis was not by intention to treat, and the power of the trial was very low. The second RCT compared tarsal rotation with tarsal advance and rotation in Omani villagers with major trichiasis (total of 200 eyelids).[11] It found that bilamellar tarsal rotation was more successful than tarsal advance and rotation, after 25 months' follow up (HR for failure following tarsal advance and rotation v bilamellar tarsal rotation 3.1, 95% CI 1.9 to 5.2). **Minor trichiasis:** See glossary, p 366. The second RCT compared tarsal rotation versus cryoablation versus electrolysis in people with minor trichiasis (as defined for this trial) (total of 172 eyelids).[11] It found that tarsal rotation was more successful than the other treatments after 25 months' follow up (HR of failure, electrolysis v tarsal rotation 6.1, 95% CI 2.9 to 12.8; HR of failure, cryoablation v tarsal rotation 7.5, 95% CI 3.6 to 15.4).

Harms: Adverse outcomes of interventions were corneal exposure, ulceration, phthisis bulbi (see glossary, p 366), and severe recurrent trichiasis.[10,12] In these two trials, major trichiasis and defective closure after surgical procedures for scarring trachoma were more common after eversion splinting, tarsal advance, and tarsal grooving than after bilamellar tarsal rotation and tarsal advance and rotation. Cryoablation of the eyelashes can cause necrosis of the lid margin, corneal ulcers, and in the RCT in which cryoablation was used[11] it was the only procedure associated with onset of phthisis (2 cases out of 57). Further details of harms are summarised in a table on the online version of *Clinical Evidence* cure (see table on website; www.clinicalevidence.org).

Comment: The pragmatic definitions of major and minor trichiasis are limited to use in these trials. The first RCT was very low powered, and was not analysed by intention to treat.[10] In both RCTs, one experienced operator performed most of the surgery. The evidence of both benefits and harms may not be applicable to different operators, or where the quality of surgical equipment does not match those in the trials.

GLOSSARY

Bilamellar tarsal rotation The upper lid is cut full thickness horizontally in a line parallel and 3 mm from the eyelid margin and running from just lateral to the lacrimal punctum to the lateral canthus. Everting sutures are then placed through all layers of the lid to prevent the margin from turning inwards.

Eversion splinting The lid margin is split posterior to the lashes, the eversion of the anterior section is maintained by sutures tied over a roll of paraffin gauze.

Tarsal advance The lid margin is split posterior to the lashes. The skin, lashes, and orbicularis are freed from the tarsal plate and retracted away from the cornea and are sutured back on to the tarsal plate leaving a bare area of tarsus to act as the lid margin.

Tarsal grooving A wedge of skin, orbicularis, and tarsus is removed parallel to the lid margin. Sutures through all layers act to evert the lid margin.

Tarsal advance and rotation The upper lid is everted over a speculum. The tarsal plate is fractured parallel to and 3 mm from the lid margin. In this operation the skin and orbicularis are not cut. The short portion of tarsal plate attached to the lid margin is then rotated through 180 degrees and sutured into place to form the new lid margin.

Major trichiasis Lid closure complete; six or more lashes in contact with eyeball.

Minor trichiasis Lid closure complete; one to five lashes in contact with eyeball.

Phthisis bulbi A disorganised, shrunken eye which has no perception of light.

REFERENCES

1. Thylefors B, Negrel AD, Pararajasegaram R, et al.. Global data on blindness. *Bull World Health Organ* 1995;73:115–121.
2. West SK, Munoz B, Turner VM, et al. The epidemiology of trachoma in central Tanzania. *Int J Epidemiol* 1991;20:1088–1092.
3. Courtright P, Sheppard J, Schachter J, et al. Trachoma and blindness in the Nile Delta: current patterns and projections for the future in the rural Egyptian population. *Br J Ophthalmol* 1989;73: 536–540.
4. Bobo L, Munoz B, Viscidi R, et al. Diagnosis of *Chlamydia trachomatis* eye infection in Tanzania by polymerase chain reaction/enzyme immunoassay. *Lancet* 1991;338:847–850.
5. Bailey R, Osmond C, Mabey DCW, et al. Analysis of the household pattern of trachoma in a Gambian village using a Monte Carlo simulation procedure. *Int J Epidemiol* 1989;18:944–951.
6. Emerson PM, Lindsay SW, Walraven GE, et al. Effect of fly control on trachoma and diarrhoea. *Lancet* 1999;353:1401–1403.
7. Munoz B, West SK. The forgotten cause of blindness. *Epidemiol Rev* 1997;19:205–217.
8. West S, Munoz B, Lynch M, et al. Impact of facewashing on trachoma in Kongwa, Tanzania. *Lancet* 1995;345:155–158.
9. Mabey D, Fraser-Hurt N. Antibiotics for trachoma (Protocol for a Cochrane Review). In: The Cochrane Library, Issue 2, 2000. Oxford: Update software. Search date 1999; primary sources Medline, Embase, Cinalh, Science Citation Index, and personal contacts.
10. Reacher MH, Huber MJE, Canagaratnam R, et al. A trial of surgery for trichiasis of the upper lid from trachoma. *Br J Ophthalmol* 1990;74:109–113.
11. Reacher MH, Munoz B, Alghassany A, et al. A controlled trial of surgery for trachomatous trichiasis of the upper lid. *Arch Ophthalmol* 1992; 110:667–674.
12. Reacher MH, Taylor HR. The management of trachomatous trichiasis. *Rev Int Trach Pathol Ocul Trop Subtrop Sante Publique* 1990;67:233–262.
13. Attiah MA, el Kohly AM. Clinical assessment of the comparative effect of terramycin and GS 2989 in the mass treatment of trachoma. *Rev Int Trach Pathol Ocul Trop Subtrop Sante Publique* 1973; 50:11–20.
14. Darougar S, Jones BR, Viswalingam N, et al. Family-based suppressive intermittent therapy of hyperendemic trachoma with topical oxytetracycline or oral doxycycline. *Br J Ophthalmol* 1980;64:291–295.
15. Dawson CR, Hanna L, Wood TR, et al. Controlled trials with trisulphapyrimidines in the treatment of chronic trachoma. *J Infect Dis* 1969;119:581–590.
16. Foster SO, Powers DK, Thygeson P. Trachoma therapy: a controlled study. *Am J Ophthalmol* 1966;61:451–455.
17. Hoshiwara I, Ostler HB, Hanna L, et al. Doxycycline treatment of chronic trachoma. *JAMA* 1973;224:220–223.
18. Shukla BR, Nema HV, Mathur JS, et al. Gantrisin and madribon in trachoma. *Br J Ophthalmol* 1966;50:218–221.
19. Tabbara KF, Summanen P, Taylor PB, et al. Minocycline effects in patients with active trachoma. *Int Ophthalmol* 1988;12:59–63.
20. Woolridge RL, Cheng KH, Chang IH, et al. Failure of trachoma treatment with ophthalmic antibiotics and systemic sulphonamides used alone or in combination with trachoma vaccine. *Am J Ophthalmol* 1967;63(suppl):1577–1586.
21. Dawson CR, Schachter J, Sallam S, et al. A comparison of oral azithromycin with topical oxytetracycline/polymyxin for the treatment of trachoma in children. *Clin Infect Dis* 1997;24: 363–368.
22. Schachter J, West SK, Mabey D, et al. Azithromycin in control of trachoma. *Lancet* 1999; 354:630–635.
23. Tabbara KF, Abu el Asrar A, al Omar O, et al. Single-dose azithromycin in the treatment of trachoma. A randomized, controlled study. *Ophthalmology* 1996;103:842–846.

Denise Mabey
Guy's and St Thomas' Hospital Trust
London
UK

Nicole Fraser-Hurt
Epiconsult Ltd.
Nhlangano
Swaziland
Competing interests: None declared.

TABLE 1 Interventions to prevent scarring trachoma by reducing active trachoma: results of randomised controlled trials of antibiotics compared with no treatment placebo, or a monthly vitamin tablet in people with active trachoma (see text, p 364).

Study	Treatment	Route	Dose	Duration	Comparison
13	Tetracycline derivative GS2989	Topical	0.25%	Once every school day for 11 weeks	No treatment
13	Terramycin	Topical	Not stated	Once every school day for 11 weeks	No treatment
14	Oxytetracycline	Topical	1%	Twice daily for 7 consecutive days every month for 12 months	Vitamin pills, orally, 1 dose per month for 12 months
14	Doxycycline	Oral	5 mg/kg	1 dose per month for 12 months	Vitamin pills, orally, 1 dose per month for 12 months
15	Trisulfapyrimidine	Oral	3.5 g/day	3 daily during 3 consecutive weeks	Lactose, orally, 3 daily for 3 consecutive weeks
15	Trisulfapyrimidine	Oral	3.5 g/day	3 daily during 3 consecutive weeks	Lactose, orally, 3 daily for 3 consecutive weeks
16	Sulfametopyridazine	Oral	0.5 g	Once daily for 5 consecutive days every week for 3 weeks	No treatment
16	Tetracycline	Topical	1%	3 times daily on 5 consecutive days every week for 6 weeks	No treatment
17	Doxycycline	Oral	2.5–4.0 mg/kg	Once daily for 5 consecutive days every week up to 28 doses in 40 days	Placebo once daily for 5 consecutive days every week up to 28 doses in 40 days
18	Sulfafurazole + Sulfadimetoxine	Topical + oral	15%/100 mg/kg	Twice daily for 5 consecutive days every month for 5 months/bi-weekly for 5 months	No treatment
18	Sulfadimethoxine	Oral	100 mg/kg	Twice weekly or weekly dose for 5 months	No treatment
18	Sulfafurazole	Topical	15%	Twice daily for 5 consecutive days every month for 5 months	No treatment
19	Minocycline	Oral	100 mg	Once daily on 5 consecutive days every week for 5 weeks	Placebo topically twice daily on 5 consecutive days every week for 5 weeks
19	Tetracycline	Topical	1%	Twice daily on 5 consecutive days every week for 5 weeks	Placebo topically twice daily on 5 consecutive days every week for 5 weeks
20	Tetracycline	Topical	1%	Twice daily for 6 consecutive days per week for 6 weeks	No treatment

Bd, to be taken twice a day; Qds, to be taken four times a day.

TABLE 2 Interventions to prevent scarring trachoma by reducing active trachoma: results of RCTs comparing rates of active trachoma and bacteriological infection following oral azithromycin or topical tetracycline (see text, p 364).

Study	Treatment	Dose	Duration	Comparison	Dose/duration
21	Azithromycin orally	20 mg/kg	1 dose, or 3 times 1 dose at weekly intervals, or 6 times 1 dose at 28 day intervals	1% topical oxytet/polymyxin + oral placebo	Ointment once daily for 5 consecutive days monthly for six months
22	Azithromycin orally	20 mg/kg up to 1 g	Once a week for 3 weeks	1% topical oxytetracycline	Once daily for 6 weeks
	Women of childbearing age erythromycin	500 mg bds or 250 mg qds	14 days		
23	Azithromycin orally	20 mg/kg	1 dose	1% topical tetracycline	Twice daily for 5 consecutive days per week for 6 weeks

Updated this issue

Piero Olliaro

QUESTIONS

Treating toxoplasmosis in pregnancy 371

INTERVENTIONS

Unknown effectiveness
Spiramycin and other antiparasitic
  drugs 371

To be covered in future issues of
Clinical Evidence
Pregnancy termination
Screening

Key Messages

- We found insufficient evidence to determine the effects on mother or baby of current antiparasitic treatment for women who seroconvert during pregnancy.

DEFINITION Toxoplasmosis is caused by the parasite *Toxoplasma gondii*. Infection is asymptomatic or unremarkable in immunocompetent individuals but leads to a lifelong antibody response. During pregnancy, toxoplasmosis can be transmitted across the placenta and cause intrauterine death, neonatal growth retardation, mental retardation, ocular defects, and blindness in later life. Congenital toxoplasmosis (confirmed infection of the fetus or newborn) can present at birth, either as subclinical disease, which may evolve with neurological or ophthalmological disease later in life, or as a disease of varying severity, ranging from mild ocular damage to severe mental retardation.

INCIDENCE/ PREVALENCE We found few prospective population surveys of toxoplasma seroprevalence. Reported rates vary across and within countries, as well as over time. The risk of primary infection is highest in young people, including young women during pregnancy. We found no cohort studies describing annual seroconversion rates in women of childbearing age nor incidence of primary infection. One systematic review identified 15 studies that reported rates of seroconversion ranging from 2.4–16/1000 in Europe and from 2–6/1000 in the USA.[1] France began screening for congenital toxoplasmosis in 1978, and during the period 1980–1995 the seroconversion rate during pregnancy was 4–5/1000.[2]

AETIOLOGY/ RISK FACTORS Toxoplasma infection is usually acquired by ingesting either sporocysts (from unwashed fruit or vegetables contaminated by cat faeces) or tissue cysts (from raw or undercooked meat). The risk of contracting toxoplasma infection varies with eating habits, contact with cats and other pets, and occupational exposure. Infection can also be acquired congenitally.

PROGNOSIS One systematic review of studies conducted from 1983–1996 found no population based prospective studies of the natural history of toxoplasma infection during pregnancy.[1] One systematic review reported nine controlled, non-randomised studies and found that untreated toxoplasmosis acquired during pregnancy was associated with infection rates in children of between 10–100%.[3] We found two European studies that correlated gestation at time of seroconversion with risk of transmission and severity of disease at birth.[4,5] Risk of transmission increased with gestational age at maternal seroconversion, reaching 70–90% for infections acquired after 30 weeks' gestation. In contrast, the risk of the infected infant developing clinical disease was highest when infection occurred early in pregnancy. The highest risk of early signs of disease (including chorioretinitis and hydrocephaly) was about 10%, and occurred with infection between 24 and 30 weeks' gestation.[5] Infants with untreated congenital toxoplasmosis and generalised neurological abnormalities at birth develop mental retardation, growth retardation, blindness or visual defects, seizures, and spasticity. Children with untreated subclinical infection at birth may develop cognitive and motor deficits and visual defects or blindness up to the age of 20. One case-control study in 845 school children in Brazil found mental retardation and retinochoroiditis to be significantly associated with positive toxoplasma serology (population attributable risk 6–9%).[6]

AIMS	To prevent fetal transmission, congenital infection, ocular defects, and mental retardation in neonates and in later life, with minimum adverse effects.
OUTCOMES	Incidence of spontaneous abortion, fetal infection, and overt neonatal disease (mental retardation and ocular defects); serological positivity in the newborn; adverse effects of treatment.
METHODS	*Clinical Evidence* update search and appraisal May 2000.

QUESTION **What are the effects on mother and baby of antiparasitic treatment in women found to be seropositive for toxoplasma during pregnancy?**

We found no reliable evidence on the effects of treating women who seroconvert during pregnancy.

Benefits: We found two systematic reviews (search dates 1998). The first identified no RCTs.[3] The second review identified nine small cohort studies comparing treatments (spiramycin alone, pyrimethamine-sulphonamides, or a combination of the two treatments) versus no treatment.[7] One study of case series of women treated with spiramycin or spiramycin plus pyrimethamine/sulphonamide found no evidence of difference in outcomes (fetal infection, overt neonatal disease) associated with treatment.[8] Comparing data from these studies was difficult because of different follow up periods.

Harms: Spiramycin and pyrimethamine-sulphonamides are reportedly well tolerated and non-teratogenic.[9] Sulpha drugs are known to carry a risk of kernicterus in the newborn and should be avoided if possible in the third trimester; there is also a risk of bone marrow suppression, which can be reduced through concomitant use of folinic acid.[9]

Comment: We found the quality of evidence to be poor, so we are uncertain whether antiparasitic drugs are more beneficial than harmful. Studies included in the systematic review were small, groups were not directly comparable, only two studies provided information about the control group, congenital infection was common in the treatment groups, and treatment was associated with reduced transmission in only 5/9 of the included studies.[7] One decision analysis on screening for and treating intrauterine toxoplasma infection has suggested a theoretical risk that treatment may save the pregnancy without preventing infection in the neonate, leading to a net increase in congenital cases.[10] Drug regimens of cotrimoxazole (trimethoprim plus sulphamethoxazole), atovaquone, or fluoroquinolones that are either used or are being tested for secondary prophylaxis of toxoplasmosis in immunocompromised people (particularly those with HIV infection) have not been studied in pregnancy because their reproductive toxicity has not been properly documented. Finally, optimal duration of follow up is not established, although the longer the children are observed, the higher the incidence of sequelae.

Infectious diseases

REFERENCES

1. Eskild A, Oxman A, Magnus P, et al. Screening for toxoplasmosis in pregnancy: what is the evidence of reducing a health problem? *J Med Screen* 1996;3:188–194. Search date February 1996; primary sources Medline 1983 to February 1996; Cochrane Pregnancy and Childbirth Database and hand searched references.

2. Carme B, Tirard-Fleury V. Toxoplasmosis among pregnant women in France: Seroprevalence, seroconversion and knowledge levels. Trends 1965–1995. *Med Malad Infect* 1996;26:431–436.

3. Wallon M, Liou C, Garner P, et al. Congenital toxoplasmosis: systematic review of evidence of efficacy of treatment in pregnancy. *BMJ* 1999; 318:1511–1514. Search date 1997; primary sources Medline, Embase, Pascal, Biological Abstracts, and personal communications.

4. Foulon W, Villena I, Stray-Pedersen B, et al. Treatment of toxoplasmosis during pregnancy: a multicenter study of impact on fetal transmission and children's sequelae at age 1 year. *Am J Obstet Gynecol* 1999;180:410–415.

5. Dunn D, Wallon M, Peyron F, et al. Mother-to-child transmission of toxoplasmosis: risk estimates for clinical counselling. *Lancet* 1999;353:1829–1833.

6. Caiaffa WT, Chiari CA, Figueiredo AR, et al. Toxoplasmosis and mental retardation–report of a case-control study. *Mem Inst Oswaldo Cruz* 1993; 88:253–261.

7. Peyron F, Wallon M, Liou C, et al. Treatments for toxoplasmosis in pregnancy. In: The Cochrane Library, Issue 2, 2000. Oxford: Update Software. Search date 1997; primary sources Medline, Embase, Pascal, Biological Abstracts and the Cochrane Controlled Trials Register.

8. Vergani P, Ghidini A, Ceruti P, et al. Congenital toxoplasmosis: efficacy of maternal treatment with spiramycin alone. *Am J Reprod Immunol* 1998; 39:335–340.

9. Garland SM, O'Reilly MA. The risks and benefits of antimicrobial therapy in pregnancy. *Drug Saf* 1995;13:188–205.

10. Bader TJ, Macones GA, Asch DA. Prenatal screening for toxoplasmosis. *Obstet Gynecol* 1997; 90:457–464.

Piero Olliaro
Scientist/Manager
UNDP/World Bank/WHO Special
Programme for Research and Training in
Tropical Diseases, CDS/CRD
World Health Organization
Geneva
Switzerland

Competing interests: None declared.

Updated and expanded this issue

Guy de Bruyn

INTERVENTIONS

Key Messages

- RCTs have found that empirically treating travellers' diarrhoea with antibiotics reduces the length of illness by 1–2 days.
- In community acquired diarrhoea, RCTs have found that ciprofloxacin reduces the duration of diarrhoea by 1–2 days. Trials of other antibiotics have found no evidence of benefit or have not reported time to cure.
- RCTs found that treatment prolonged excretion of organisms and was associated with the development of resistant organisms.
- One small RCT found no significant difference in the volume or duration of diarrhoea between rehydration intravenously or by nasogastric tube.
- Small RCTs found that amino acid oral rehydration solutions (ORS) compared with standard ORS reduced the total volume and duration of diarrhoea. ORS where bicarbonate was replaced with chloride or citrate were of similar effectiveness as standard ORS.
- Three RCTs found a small and inconsistent effect of reduced osmolarity ORS compared with standard ORS.
- One systematic review found that rice based ORS compared with standard ORS reduced the 24 hour stool volume.

DEFINITION Diarrhoea is defined as watery or liquid stools, usually with an increase in stool weight above 200 g per day and an increase in daily stool frequency.

INCIDENCE/ PREVALENCE An estimated 4000 million cases of diarrhoea occurred worldwide in 1996, resulting in 2.5 million deaths.[1] In developing countries, diarrhoea is reported to cause more deaths in children aged under 5 years than any other condition.[1] In the USA, which has a low incidence, the estimated incidence for infectious intestinal disease is 0.44 episodes per person per year, or one episode per person every 2.3 years, resulting in about one consultation with a doctor per person every 28 years.[2] The epidemiology of travellers' diarrhoea (in people who have crossed a national boundary) is not well understood. Incidence is higher in travellers visiting developing countries but varies widely by location and season of travel.[3]

AETIOLOGY/ RISK FACTORS The cause depends on geographic location, standards of food hygiene, sanitation, water supply, and season. The commonly identified causes of sporadic diarrhoea in adults in developed countries include *Campylobacter*, *Salmonella*, *Shigella*, *Escherichia coli*, *Yersinia*, protozoa, and viruses. No pathogens are identified in over half of patients. In returning travellers, about 80% of episodes are caused by bacteria, such as enterotoxigenic *E coli*, *Salmonella*, *Shigella*, *Campylobacter*, *Vibrio*, enteroadherent *E coli*, *Yersinia*, and *Aeromonas*.

PROGNOSIS Few studies have examined which factors predict poor outcome in adults. In developed countries, death from infectious diarrhoea is rare although serious complications causing admission to hospital sometimes occur, such as severe dehydration and renal failure. Elderly people and those in long term care have an increased risk of death.[4]

AIMS To reduce the infectious period, length of illness, risk of dehydration, risk of transmission to others, and rates of severe illness; to prevent complications and death.

OUTCOMES Time from start of treatment to last loose stool; number of loose stools per day; stool volume; duration of diarrhoea; relief of cramps, nausea, and vomiting; rate of hospital admission; incidence of vomiting; incidence of severe illness; time to first formed stool; duration of excretion of organisms; and presence of bacterial resistance.

METHODS *Clinical Evidence* update search and appraisal May 2000. Trial quality was assessed on allocation concealment and inclusion of all randomised participants. Trials were excluded if they did not meet epidemiological quality criteria. Most trial participants had moderate to severe diarrhoea, usually defined as acute diarrhoea lasting less than a week, more than three loose stools in 24 hours or more than two in 8 hours, and symptoms of an enteric illness such as nausea, vomiting, and cramps.

QUESTION What are the effects of empirical antibiotic treatment in travellers' diarrhoea?

RCTs have found that empirical treatment with antibiotics shortens illness duration in adults with diarrhoea acquired overseas. Treatment was associated in some people with prolonged presence of bacterial pathogens in the stool and development of resistant strains.

Benefits: We found no systematic review. We found 15 RCTs in a total of 2251 travellers comparing empirical use of one or more antibiotics with placebo.[5-19] Eight trials evaluated quinolones, four evaluated co-trimoxazole, and one evaluated each of trimethoprim, aztreonam, bicozamycin, pivmecillinam, and rifaximin.[5-19] Seven trials studied US students aged over 18 years visiting Guadalajara, Mexico, during summer months. The other eight were in different locations. Entry criteria varied among trials and treatment duration ranged from a single dose to 5 days. All trials found reduced duration of diarrhoea ranging from 1 to 2.5 days, but confidence intervals were not available from published data in seven of the trials (see table 1, p 380). The largest trial, in which 70% of the 598 participants had a history of recent travel, found a 1 day improvement in the median duration of diarrhoea, from 4 to 3 days (no CI available).[5]

Harms: Adverse effects varied by agent, with incidence in the trials ranging from 1.7% to 18%.[7,11] Commonly reported harms were gastrointestinal symptoms (cramps, nausea, anorexia), dermatological symptoms (rash), and respiratory symptoms (cough, sore throat). In the largest trial, people with salmonella infection treated with norfloxacin had significantly prolonged excretion of *Salmonella* in stool compared with those given placebo (median time to clearance of *Salmonella* from stool 50 days in the norfloxacin group compared with 23 days in the placebo group).[5] In addition, six of nine *Campylobacter* isolates obtained after treatment had developed resistance to norfloxacin. One small trial reported that four of eight participants treated with ciprofloxacin developed resistant isolates at 48 hours (difference from placebo group 50%, 95% CI 15% to 85%).[7] One trial reported continued excretion of *Shigella* in three people treated with co-trimoxazole. Two of these isolates were resistant to the drug. The participants were clinically well. Other trials did not find increased resistance after antibiotic treatment or did not report it.[8]

Comment: Studies were generally well conducted. All but one were double blinded. Participant blinding through use of identical placebo was used and well described in 10 of the studies, and probably adequate in the remaining five although not as clearly stated.[18] However, only one study reported using an appropriate statistical method for analysing time to event outcomes.[15] Several trials reported surrogate end points, such as change in faecal consistency, rather than the primary outcome of interest.[12,18,19]

QUESTION What are the effects of empirical antibiotic treatment in community acquired diarrhoea?

RCTs have found that ciprofloxacin reduces duration of diarrhoea developed in the community by 1–2 days. Trials of other empirical treatments with antibiotics either found no effect or did not report data on time to cure.

Benefits: We found no systematic review. We found nine RCTs in eight reports (1760 people) comparing one or more antibiotics with placebo (see table 2, p 381).[20–27] Trials were conducted in 12 sites in 11 countries. Four trials were conducted in developed countries, and the others took place in developing countries. The largest study included 332 adults in hospital in a multicentre trial of fleroxacin.[20] Eight trials evaluated quinolones, four evaluated co-trimoxazole, and one evaluated cloquinol.[20–27] Entry criteria varied between trials, and treatment duration ranged from a single dose to 5 days. Three trials found that antibiotics reduced illness duration or decreased number of liquid stools at 48 hours, while five found no benefit in reducing illness duration.[20–24,26,27] One trial found reduced duration for ciprofloxacin but not for co-trimoxazole.[25]

Harms: Adverse effects varied by agent. In one RCT of lomefloxacin, 33% of treated people reported adverse effects compared with 2.7% in the placebo group (ARI 31%, 95% CI 17% to 46%). Two were withdrawn from the trial after developing anaphylactoid reactions.[23] In the same trial, 18% of treated people developed isolates resistant to lomefloxacin.[23] In the multicentre trial of ciprofloxacin and co-trimoxazole, five people with *Campylobacter* isolated from stool (two treated with ciprofloxacin and three treated with co-trimoxazole) developed isolates resistant to the treatment antibiotic.[25] In the largest trial, three deaths occurred (two people treated with fleroxacin and one person who received placebo). Two of the deaths occurred from hypovolaemic shock (one with fleroxacin, one with placebo).[20]

Comment: The main pathogenic organisms found in each study varied and may partly explain variations in effect. Reported outcomes varied between trials, which precludes direct comparisons or summaries of treatment effect.

QUESTION What are the effects of oral rehydration for severe diarrhoea? New

We found no direct studies of oral rehydration compared with placebo or no treatment. Numerous RCTs compared one type of rehydration with another. One small RCT found no difference in duration or volume of diarrhoea following rehydration intravenously or by nasogastric tube. Two RCTs found that amino acid oral rehydration solutions (ORS) compared with standard ORS (see glossary, p 378) reduced the total volume and duration of diarrhoea. One small RCT found no significant effect of replacing bicarbonate with chloride, and three RCTs found no effect of replacing bicarbonate with citrate. Three RCTs found a small and inconsistent effect of reduced osmolarity ORS compared with standard ORS. One systematic review found that rice based ORS compared with standard ORS reduced the 24 hour stool volume.

Benefits: Results of the studies are summarised in table 3—see table on website http://www.clinicalevidence.org. **No rehydration:** We found no systematic review or RCTs. Such studies would be unethical. **Intravenous rehydration:** We found no systematic review. We found one small RCT (20 adults with cholera and severe dehydration) of enteral rehydration via nasogastric tube compared with intravenous rehydration.[28] Both groups received initial intravenous fluids. The RCT found no significant difference in the total duration of diarrhoea (44 hours v 37 hours; difference 7 hours; 95% CI −6 to +20 hours), total volume of stool passed (8.2 litres v 11 litres; difference −2.8 litres; 95% CI −8 to +3 litres), or duration of *Vibrio* excretion (1.1 day v 1.4 day; difference 0.3 day; 95% CI 0 to +1 day). **Amino acid ORS:** We found no systematic review. We found three RCTs.[29–31] In the two RCTs where intravenous rehydration was given, the amino acid ORS compared with the standard ORS reduced the total duration of diarrhoea and the total volume of stool.[29,30] **Bicarbonate free ORS:** We found no systematic review. We found one small RCT (60 people with cholera and severe dehydration) which compared standard ORS plus bicarbonate with an otherwise identical ORS in which the bicarbonate was replaced with chloride.[32] It found no significant difference in total stool output or duration of diarrhoea. **Citrate ORS:** We found no systematic review. We found three RCTs (n = 367).[33–35] None of the trials found a significant difference between citrate and standard/bicarbonate ORS in the duration or volume of diarrhoea. **Reduced osmolarity ORS:** We found no systematic review. We found three RCTs.[36–38] They found a small and inconsistent effect on total volume of stool and duration of diarrhoea. **Rice based ORS:** We found one systematic review (22 RCTs, search date June 1998) in people with cholera and non-cholera diarrhoea.[39] It found that in adults and children with cholera, rice based ORS compared with standard ORS reduced the 24 hour stool volume in adults (4 RCTs; WMD −51.1 ml/kg, 95% CI −65.9 to −35.3 ml/kg) and in children (5 RCTs; WMD −67.4, 95% CI −94.3 to −41.0). One RCT found that both rice based ORS, and low sodium rice based ORS reduced stool output compared with standard ORS (4 litres for rice based ORS v 5 litres for standard ORS, P < 0.02; 3 litres for low sodium rice based ORS v 5 litres for standard ORS, P < 0.05).[38]

Harms: **Versus amino acid ORS:** One trial reported no episodes of hypernatraemia or hyponatraemia in people taking a modified ORS or standard ORS.[31] **Citrate versus bicarbonate ORS:** One trial reported that more people taking citrate ORS had an unpleasant taste than those taking bicarbonate ORS (29% v 13%).[34] In another trial 2/115 people taking an effervescent citrate ORS had an unpleasant taste (data not reported for bicarbonate ORS).[35] **Versus reduced osmolarity ORS:** Reduced osmolarity ORS significantly increased the risk of non-symptomatic hyponatraemia (OR 2.1, 95% CI 1.1 to 4.1).[36] No one developed symptomatic hyponatraemia in trials reporting this outcome.[36,37]

Comment: All participants with cholera received antibiotic therapy in addition to fluid therapy. Oral tetracycline or doxycycline were widely used, and were initiated at varying intervals after the start of oral fluid therapy. Response to ORS in people with cholera may not be comparable to those with less severe forms of diarrhoea.

Infectious diseases

GLOSSARY

Standard oral rehydration solution (ORS) A solution that includes citrate 10 mmol/l, glucose 111 mmol/l, and has an osmolarity of 311 mosm/l.

REFERENCES

1. The World Health Report 1997. Geneva: World Health Organization, 1997:14–22.
2. Garthwright WE, Archer DL, Kvenberg JE. Estimates of incidence and costs of intestinal infectious diseases in the United States. *Public Health Rep* 1988;103:107–115.
3. Cartwright RY, Chahed M. Foodborne diseases in travellers. *World Health Stat Q* 1997;50:102–110.
4. Lew JF, Glass RI, Gangarosa RE, et al. Diarrheal deaths in the United States 1979 through 1987. *JAMA* 1991;265:3280–3284.
5. Wistrom J, Jertborn M, Ekwall E, et al. Empiric treatment of acute diarrheal disease with norfloxacin: a randomized, placebo-controlled study. Swedish Study Group. *Ann Intern Med* 1992;117:202–208.
6. Ericsson CD, Johnson PC, DuPont HL, et al. Ciprofloxacin or trimethoprim-sulfamethoxazole as initial therapy for travelers' diarrhea: a placebo-controlled, randomized trial. *Ann Intern Med* 1987; 106:216–220.
7. Wistrom J, Gentry LO, Palmgren AC, et al. Ecological effects of short-term ciprofloxacin treatment of travellers' diarrhoea. *J Antimicrob Chemother* 1992;30:693–706.
8. Wistrom J, Jertborn M, Hedstrom SA, et al. Short-term self-treatment of travellers' diarrhoea with norfloxacin: a placebo-controlled study. *J Antimicrob Chemother* 1989;23:905–913.
9. DuPont HL, Ericsson CD, Mathewson JJ, et al. Five versus three days of ofloxacin for traveler's diarrhea: a placebo-controlled study. *Antimicrob Agents Chemother* 1992;36:87–91.
10. Mattila L, Peltola H, Siitonen A, et al. Short-term treatment of traveler's diarrhea with norfloxacin: a double-blind, placebo-controlled study during two seasons. *Clin Infect Dis* 1993;17:779–782.
11. Salam I, Katelaris P, Leigh-Smith S, et al. Randomised trial of single-dose ciprofloxacin for travellers' diarrhoea. *Lancet* 1994;344:1537–1539.
12. Steffen R, Jori R, DuPont HL, et al. Efficacy and toxicity of fleroxacin in the treatment of traveler's diarrhea. *Am J Med* 1993;94(3A):S182–186.
13. DuPont HL, Reves RR, Galindo E, et al. Treatment of travelers' diarrhea with trimethoprim/sulfamethoxazole and with trimethoprim alone. *N Engl J Med* 1982;307:841–844.
14. Ericsson CD, Johnson PC, DuPont HL, et al. Role of a novel antidiarrheal agent, BW942C, alone or in combination with trimethoprim-sulfamethoxazole in the treatment of traveler's diarrhea. *Antimicrob Agents Chemother* 1986;29:1040–1046.
15. Ericsson CD, DuPont HL, Mathewson JJ, et al. Treatment of traveler's diarrhea with sulfamethoxazole and trimethoprim and loperamide. *JAMA* 1990; 263:257–261.
16. DuPont HL, Ericsson CD, Mathewson JJ, et al. Oral aztreonam, a poorly absorbed yet effective therapy for bacterial diarrhea in US travellers to Mexico. *JAMA* 1992;267:1932–1935.
17. Ericsson CD, DuPont HL, Sullivan P, et al. Bicozamycin, a poorly absorbable antibiotic, effectively treats travellers' diarrhoea. *Ann Intern Med* 1983;98:20–25.
18. Christensen OE, Tuxen KK, Menday P. Treatment of travellers' diarrhoea with pivmecillinam. *J Antimicrob Chemother* 1988;22:570–571.
19. Vinci M, Gatto A, Giglio A, et al. Double-blind clinical trial on infectious diarrhoea therapy: rifaximin versus placebo. *Curr Ther Res* 1984;36:92–99.
20. Butler T, Lolekha S, Rasidi C, et al. Treatment of acute bacterial diarrhea: a multicenter international trial comparing placebo with fleroxacin given as a single dose or once daily for 3 days. *Am J Med* 1993;94(3A):187–194.
21. De la Cabada FJ, DuPont HL, Gyr K, et al. Antimicrobial therapy of bacterial diarrhea in adult residents of Mexico–lack of an effect. *Digestion* 1992;53:134–141.
22. Lolekha S, Patanacharoen S, Thanangkul B, et al. Norfloxacin versus co-trimoxazole in the treatment of acute bacterial diarrhoea: a placebo controlled study. *Scand J Infect Dis* 1988;56(suppl):35–45.
23. Ellis-Pegler RB, Hyman LK, Ingram RJ, et al. A placebo controlled evaluation of lomefloxacin in the treatment of bacterial diarrhoea in the community. *J Antimicrob Chemother* 1995;36:259–263.
24. Pichler HE, Diridl G, Stickler K, et al. Clinical efficacy of ciprofloxacin compared with placebo in bacterial diarrhea. *Am J Med* 1987;82(suppl 4A):329–332.
25. Goodman LJ, Trenholme GM, Kaplan RL, et al. Empiric antimicrobial therapy of domestically acquired acute diarrhea in urban adults. *Arch Intern Med* 1990;150:541–546.
26. Noguerado A, Garcia-Polo I, Isasia T, et al. Early single dose therapy with ofloxacin for empirical treatment of acute gastroenteritis: a randomised, placebo-controlled double-blind clinical trial. *J Antimicrob Chemother* 1995;36:665–672.
27. Dryden MS, Gabb RJ, Wright SK. Empirical treatment of severe acute community-acquired gastroenteritis with ciprofloxacin. *Clin Infect Dis* 1996;22:1019–1025.
28. Pierce NF, Sack RB, Mitra RC, et al. Replacement of water and electrolyte losses in cholera by an oral glucose-electrolyte solution. *Ann Intern Med* 1969;70:1173–1181.
29. Nalin DR, Cash RA, Rahman M, Yunus MD. Effect of glycine and glucose on sodium and water absorption in patients with cholera. *Gut* 1970;11:768–772.
30. Patra FC, Sack DA, Islam A, Alam AN, Mazumder RN. Oral rehydration formula containing alanine and glucose for treatment of diarrhoea: a controlled trial. *BMJ* 1989;298:1353–1356.
31. Khin-Maung-U, Myo-Khin, Nyunt-Nyunt-Wai, Tin-U. Comparison of glucose/electrolyte and maltodextrin/glycine/glycyl-glycine/electrolyte oral rehydration solutions in cholera and watery diarrhoea in adults. *Ann Trop Med Parasitol* 1991; 85:645–650.
32. Sarker SA, Mahalanabis D. The presence of bicarbonate in oral rehydration solution does not influence fluid absorption in cholera. *Scand J Gastroenterol* 1995;30:242–245.
33. Mazumder RN, Nath SK, Ashraf H, Patra FC, Alam AN. Oral rehydration solution containing trisodium citrate for treating severe diarrhoea: controlled clinical trial. *BMJ* 1991;302:88–89.
34. Hoffman SL, Moechtar MA, Simanjuntak CH, et al. Rehydration and maintenance therapy of cholera patients in Jakarta: citrate-based versus bicarbonate-based oral rehydration salt solution. *J Infect Dis* 1985;152:1159–1165.

35. Ahmed SM, Islam MR, Butler T. Effective treatment of diarrhoeal dehydration with an oral rehydration solution containing citrate. *Scand J Infect Dis* 1986;18:65–70.

36. Alam NH, Majumder RN, Fuchs GJ, et al. Efficacy and safety of oral rehydration solution with reduced osmolarity in adults with cholera: a randomised double-blind clinical trial. *Lancet* 1999;354:296–299.

37. Faruque ASG, Mahalanabis D, Hamadani JD, Zetterstrom R. Reduced osmolarity oral rehydration salt in cholera. *Scand J Infect Dis* 1996;28:87–90.

38. Bhattacharya MK, Bhattacharya SK, Dutta D, et al. Efficacy of oral hyposmolar glucose-based and rice-based oral rehydration salt solutions in the treatment of cholera in adults. *Scand J Gastroenterol* 1998;33:159–163.

39. Fontaine O, Gore SM, Pierce NF. Rice-based oral rehydration solution for treating diarrhoea. In: The Cochrane Library, Issue 2, 2000. Oxford: Update Software. Search date 1998; primary sources Medline, Embase, Lilacs, Cochrane Controlled Trials Register, Cochrane Infectious Diseases Group.

Guy de Bruyn
Resident in Internal Medicine
Baylor College of Medicine
Houston, Texas
USA

Competing interests: None declared.

TABLE 1 Effects of empirical antibiotic treatment of travellers' diarrhoea: results of placebo controlled RCTs (see text, p 375).[5-11,13-17]

Intervention	Total number of participants	Mean duration of diarrhoea from start of treatment		Difference between means (95% CI)*
		Placebo group	Intervention group	
Ofloxacin 300 mg bid for 3 days[9]	232	56 h	28 h	−28 h (−40.5 h to −15.5 h)
Ofloxacin 300 mg bid for 5 days[9]	232	56 h	39 h	−17 h (−31.2 h to +2.8 h)
Ciprofloxacin 500 mg single dose[11]	83	53.5 h	24.8 h	−28.7 h (−40.2 h to −17.2 h)
Bicozamycin 500 mg qid for 5 days[17]	148	63.7 h	28.2 h	−35.5 h (−48.1 h to −22.9 h)
Norfloxacin 400 mg bid for 5 days[5]	511	4 days†	3 days†	NA
Ciprofloxacin 500 mg bid for 5 days[6]	181	81 h	29 h	−52 h
Cotrimoxazole 160/800 mg bid for 5 days[6]	181	81 h	20 h	−61 h
Ciprofloxacin 250 mg bid for 3 days[7]	15	60 h	26 h	−34 h
Norfloxacin 400 mg bid for 3 days[8]	94	4.4 days	3.2 days	−1.2 days
Norfloxacin 400 mg bid for 3 days[10]	106	3.3 days	1.2 days	−2.1 days
Cotrimoxazole 160/800 mg bid for 5 days[13]	110	92.8 h	29.2 h	−63.6 h
Trimethoprim 200 mg bid for 5 days[13]	110	92.8 h	30.7 h	−62.1 h
Cotrimoxazole 160/800 mg bid for 3 days[14]	134	59 h	24 h	−35 h
Cotrimoxazole 320/1600 mg single dose[15]	227	58 h	28 h	−30 h
Cotrimoxazole 160/800 mg bid for 3 days[15]	227	58 h	36 h	−22 h
Aztreonam 100 mg tid for 5 days[16]	191	84 h	44 h	−40 h

*If available from published data; †median duration of post-treatment diarrhoea; bid, twice daily; h, hours; NA, not available from published data; qid, four times daily; tid, three times daily.

TABLE 2 Effects of empirical antibiotic treatment of community acquired diarrhoea: results of placebo controlled RCTs (see text, p 376).[21,23-27]

Intervention	Total number of participants	Mean duration of diarrhoea from start of treatment		Difference between means (95% CI)*
		Placebo group	Intervention group	
Lomefloxacin 400 mg daily for 5 days[23]	84	3.2 days	4.4 days	1.2 days (0.1 day to 2.5 days)
Ofloxacin 400 mg single dose[26]	117	3.4 days	2.5 days	−0.9 days (−1.8 days to 0.0 days)
Cotrimoxazole 800/160 mg bid for 3 days[21]	287	30.2 h	24.4 h	−5.8 h
Cloquinol 250 mg tid for 3 days[21]	287	30.2 h	25.5 h	−4.7 h
Enoxacin 400 mg bid for 5 days[21]	137	44.9 h	38.9 h	−6 h
Cotrimoxazole 160/800 mg bid for 5 days[21]	137	44.9 h	42.3 h	−2.6 h
Ciprofloxacin 500 mg bid for 5 days[24]	162	2.9 days	1.5 days	1.4 days
Ciprofloxacin 500 mg bid for 5 days[25]	173	3.4 days	2.4 days	1 day
Cotrimoxazole 160/800 mg bid for 5 days[25]	173	3.4 days	NA	NA
Ciprofloxacin 500 mg bid for 5 days[27]	85	4.6 days	2.2 days	−2.4 days

*If available from published data; bid, twice daily; h, hours; NA, not available from published data; tid, three times daily.

Updated this issue

David Wilkinson, Andrew Phillips and Margaret Johnson

Key Messages

Prevention

- One RCT found that effective treatment of symptomatic sexually transmitted diseases (STDs) reduced the incidence of HIV infection.

- One RCT found no evidence of benefit from presumptive, mass treatment for STDs.

- We found limited evidence suggesting that improving STD prevention and treatment services, and targeting them at high risk groups such as sex workers, reduces the incidence of HIV infection.

- We found limited evidence suggesting that postexposure prophylaxis with zidovudine may reduce the risk of HIV infection. Evidence from other settings suggests that combining several antiretroviral drugs is likely to be more effective than zidovudine alone.

Treatment

- Two large RCTs have found that triple therapy (combining two nucleoside analogue drugs and a protease inhibitor) halves the risk of AIDS and death over about 1 year compared with double therapy.

- Large RCTs have found no evidence that the overall risk of serious adverse effects is significantly greater on triple than on double therapy. Triple therapy is likely to reduce the risk of drug resistance compared with double therapy.

- Early trials of zidovudine monotherapy have so far found no evidence that treatment is more effective if started early, while the person is asymptomatic, than if it is delayed until early signs of disease occur. We found no RCTs evaluating delayed versus early treatment with two or three drug regimens.

DEFINITION HIV infection refers to infection with the human immunodeficiency virus type 1 or type 2. Clinically, this is characterised by a variable period (average around 8–10 years) of asymptomatic infection, followed by repeated episodes of illness of varying and increasing severity as immune function deteriorates. The type of illness varies greatly by country, availability of specific treatment for HIV, and prophylaxis for opportunistic infections.

INCIDENCE/ PREVALENCE Worldwide estimates suggest that, by December 1999, around 50 million people had been infected with HIV, about 16 million people had died as a result, and about 16 000 new HIV infections were occurring each day.[1] About 90% of HIV infections occur in the developing world.[1] Occupationally acquired HIV infection in health-care workers has been documented in 95 definite and 191 possible cases, although this is likely to be an underestimate.[2]

AETIOLOGY/ RISK FACTORS The major risk factor for transmission of HIV is unprotected hetero-sexual or homosexual intercourse. Other risk factors include needle-stick injury and blood transfusion. An HIV infected woman may also transmit the virus to her baby. This has been reported in 15–30% of pregnant women with HIV infection. Not everyone who is exposed to HIV will become infected, although risk increases if exposure is repeated, at high dose, or through blood. There is at least a 2–5-fold increased risk of HIV infection among people with STDs.[3]

PROGNOSIS Without treatment, about half of people infected with HIV will become ill and die from AIDS over about 10 years.

AIMS To reduce transmission of HIV; to prevent or delay the onset of AIDS, as manifested by opportunistic infections and cancers; to increase survival; to minimise loss of quality of life caused by inconvenience of current regimens and adverse effects of interventions.

OUTCOMES Incidence of HIV infection, new AIDS diseases, and adverse events; mortality; quality of life.

METHODS *Clinical Evidence* update search and appraisal May 2000. In addition, we contacted experts in the field, and reviewed abstract books and CDs for conferences held since 1995. Trials were included if they were designed to detect differences in clinical end points. We have included data on single and two drug antiretroviral regimens because the evidence may be useful in countries where three drug treatment is not currently widely available.

QUESTION What are the effects of preventive interventions?

OPTION EARLY DETECTION AND TREATMENT OF STDS

One RCT found that effective treatment of symptomatic STDs reduced the incidence of HIV infection.

Benefits: We found no systematic review. One trial randomised 12 communities in Tanzania (about 12 000 people) to intervention or no intervention. Intervention consisted of providing effective drugs for STDs and healthcare workers trained in STD case management.[4] Intervention notably reduced the risk of acquiring HIV over 2 years (RRR 42%, 95% CI 21% to 58%).

Harms: Syndromic case management (treating people for the most likely causes of their symptoms and signs) may result in wrong or unnecessary treatment. The RCT gave no information on this.[4]

Comment: There is a clear biological mechanism for the synergistic effect of STDs on HIV transmission, and for STD control as an HIV control strategy. The inflammation associated with STDs increases HIV shedding in genital secretions, and treating STDs reduces this inflammation.[5] Syndromic management of STDs is more commonly used in developing countries. In developed countries, a microbiological diagnosis is usually made, allowing specific treatment. The trial, randomised by the community and analysed by the individual, uses regression analysis in an attempt to overcome the associated cluster bias, but it is unclear if this is successful.

OPTION   **PRESUMPTIVE STD TREATMENT**

One RCT found no evidence of benefit from presumptive, mass treatment for STDs.

Benefits: We found no systematic review. One RCT randomised 10 communities in Uganda (about 12 000 people) to intervention or no intervention.[6] Intervention consisted of treating all adults with several drugs for STDs every 10 months. Although prevalence of some STDs fell in intervention communities, there was no significant difference in the incidence of HIV between intervention and control communities over 20 months of follow up (incidence of HIV in both groups about 1.5 per 100 person years; RR intervention *v* control 0.97, 95% CI 0.81 to 1.16).[6]

Harms: Mass treatment means that many uninfected people will be unnecessarily treated for STDs, exposing them to risks of adverse drug reactions and drug resistance. The RCT gave no information on these.

Comment: The trial's negative finding has several possible explanations other than ineffectiveness of the intervention: a high incidence of symptomatic STDs between rounds of mass treatment; a low population attributable risk for treatable STDs; or intense exposure to HIV. The trial, randomised by the community and analysed by the individual, uses regression analysis in an attempt to overcome the associated cluster bias, but it is unclear if this is successful. As many as 80% of STDs are unrecognised or asymptomatic.[7]

OPTION   **IMPROVING AND TARGETING PREVENTIVE SERVICES**

One observational study found that improving STD prevention and treatment services and targeting them at high risk groups, such as sex workers, reduced the incidence of HIV infection.

Benefits: We found no systematic review and no RCTs. One observational study in 531 sex workers in Zaire found that the incidence of HIV infection fell from 11.7% to 4.4% (P = 0.003) over 3 years following promotion of condoms, improvement of STD treatment services, and monthly screening of women for STDs.[8]

Harms: None reported.

Comment: This non-randomised study is subject to selection bias and confounding. For example, over time the number of uninfected sex workers, and therefore the pool of people susceptible to infection, will fall, which may partly explain the fall in HIV incidence.

QUESTION What are the effects of postexposure prophylaxis in healthcare workers?

One case control study found that, in people exposed to HIV, those who went on to become infected were less likely to have received postexposure prophylaxis with zidovudine. Evidence from other settings suggests that combined treatment with several antiretroviral drugs is likely to be more effective than treatment with zidovudine alone.

Benefits: We found no systematic review or RCTs. **Zidovudine alone:** One case control study from the USA and France evaluated outcomes in 31 health workers who acquired HIV infection after occupational exposure, and outcomes in 679 controls who did not acquire HIV infection despite occupational exposure.[9] This study included people followed up for at least 6 months after exposure. HIV infection was less likely in people who received postexposure prophylaxis compared with those who did not (reduction in OR by 81%, 95% CI 43% to 94%). It found that that the risk of seroconversion increased with severity of exposure; for example, a penetrating injury with a hollow, bloody needle carried the greatest risk.[9] **Zidovudine plus other antiretroviral drugs:** We found no studies of postexposure prophylaxis using combinations of antiretroviral drugs.

Harms: Short term toxicity (including fatigue, nausea, and vomiting) and gastrointestinal discomfort have been reported by 50–75% of people taking zidovudine and caused 30% to discontinue postexposure prophylaxis.[10] Treatment studies suggest that frequency of adverse effects is higher in people taking a combination of antiretroviral drugs (reported in 50–90%), which may reduce adherence to postexposure prophylaxis (24–36% discontinued). The risk of drug interactions is also increased. Severe adverse effects, including hepatitis and pancytopenia, have been reported in people taking combination postexposure prophylaxis, but the incidence is not known.

Comment: Case control studies are considered sufficient because experimental studies are hard to justify ethically, and are logistically difficult because of the low rate of seroconversion in those exposed. A summary of 25 studies (22 seroconversions in 6955 exposed people) found that the risk of HIV transmission after percutaneous exposure was 0.32% (95% CI 0.18% to 0.45%) and the risk after mucocutaneous exposure was 0.03% (95% CI 0.006% to 0.19%).[2]

Indirect evidence for postexposure prophylaxis comes from animal studies[9] and from a placebo controlled RCT of zidovudine in pregnant women, which found reduced frequency of mother to child HIV transmission, presumed to be caused in part by postexposure prophylaxis.[11] Combinations of two, three, or more antiretroviral drugs are more effective than single drug regimens in suppressing viral replication. There is also an unquantified risk that zidovudine alone may not prevent transmission of zidovudine resistant strains of HIV. This constitutes the rationale for combining antiretroviral drugs for postexposure prophylaxis.

QUESTION   **What are the effects of different antiretroviral treatment regimens?**

OPTION   TWO DRUG VERSUS ONE DRUG ANTIRETROVIRAL REGIMENS

Large RCTs, with an average follow up of 3.5 years, have found that two drug regimens (zidovudine plus another nucleoside analogue drug) reduce the risk of new AIDS defining illnesses and death compared with zidovudine alone. Adverse events were more common with two drug regimens.

Benefits: We found one systematic review (search date not given), which identified six RCTs (n = 7700) comparing zidovudine/didanosine or zidovudine/zalcitabine versus zidovudine alone.[12] Participants entered the trials with various stages of infection and were followed for an average of 29 months, during which time 2904 progressed and 1850 died. The combined drug regimens were associated with both delayed progression (RR with addition of didanosine 0.74, 95% CI 0.67 to 0.82; RR with addition of zalcitabine 0.86, 95% CI 0.78 to 0.94), and death versus single drug treatment (RR with addition of didanosine 0.72, 95% CI 0.64 to 0.82; RR with addition of zalcitabine 0.87, 95% CI 0.77 to 0.98). After 3 years, the estimated percentages of people who were alive and without a new AIDS event were 53% for zidovudine plus didanosine, 49% for zidovudine plus zalcitabine, and 44% for zidovudine alone; the percentages alive were 68%, 63%, and 59%. One trial of zalcitabine plus saquinavir (a protease inhibitor) found significantly fewer cases of clinical disease or death compared with either drug as monotherapy (n = 940; RR 0.51, 95% CI 0.36 to 0.72).[13] Another large trial found that, in people with low CD4 positive T cell counts (25–250/mm^3), adding lamivudine (a nucleoside analogue) to regimens containing zidovudine (zidovudine alone in 62%, zidovudine plus didanosine or zalcitabine in the rest) significantly reduced the risk of AIDS or death over about a year (HR 0.42, 95% CI 0.32 to 0.57).[14]

Harms: Adverse effects such as anaemia and neutropenia were common in all groups in these trials. Up to a third of participants experienced a serious adverse event, with the highest rates in those with lower CD4 counts. Adverse events led to cessation of blind treatment in about a third of participants. The addition of didanosine to zidovudine increased the risk compared to zidovudine alone of nausea, (RR 1.8, 95% CI 1.1 to 2.9), abdominal pain (RR 1.6, 95% CI 1.0

Infectious diseases

to 2.7), and pancreatitis (RR 4.6, 95% CI 1.0 to 22.0). Addition of zalcitabine increased the risk of neuropathy (RR 2.2, 95% CI 1.4 to 3.6).[12] Addition of lamivudine did not significantly increase the rate of adverse events.[14]

Comment: Two drug regimens, using two nucleoside analogue reverse transcriptase inhibitors, allow substantial residual viral replication in an environment where drug resistant variants have selective advantage. Resistance to these drugs (as measured *in vitro*) tends to develop over several months to years. The relevance of this is not fully understood but resistance to drugs tends to be associated with poorer virological response to the drug and to others of the same class.[15,16]

OPTION THREE DRUG REGIMENS CONTAINING PROTEASE INHIBITOR VERSUS TWO DRUG REGIMENS

Two RCTs have found that using a protease inhibitor with two nucleoside analogue drugs halves the risk of new AIDS diseases or death over about 1 year compared with two nucleoside analogue drugs alone. The risk of serious adverse effects was not significantly increased over this time period.

Benefits: We found no systematic review. We found two large RCTs with less than 2 years' follow up. The first RCT compared zidovudine/lamivudine versus zidovudine/lamivudine/indinavir in people who had previously been treated with zidovudine (CD4 counts < 200/mm³).[17] It found a significant difference in rates of AIDS or death in favour of triple therapy (RR 0.50, 95% CI 0.33 to 0.76; ARR 5%). The second RCT, published only in abstract form, compared zidovudine/zalcitabine/saquinavir with zidovudine/zalcitabine and zidovudine/saquinavir in people with CD4 counts of 50–350/mm³, who had no previous experience of zidovudine (H-J Stellbrink, Sixth European Conference on Clinical Aspects and Treatment of HIV Infection, Hamburg, 1997). It also found greater benefit with triple therapy (RR of AIDS or death 0.5, P = 0.0001). This RCT found that health related quality of life did not change significantly over 48 weeks for those in the triple therapy group (change from baseline −0.4 points for physical health summary and +1.4 for mental health summary); a deterioration occurred in both dual therapy groups (−2.5 and +0.1, respectively, for zalcitabine + saquinavir and −2.2 and +0.3, respectively, for zidovudine + saquinidine).[18]

Harms: In the first RCT, about a fifth of participants in both groups experienced serious adverse events.[17] The most common were non-specific discomfort, malaise, fever, headache, nausea, and vomiting. The addition of indinavir reduced the risk of neutropenia (5% v 15%; P < 0.001) but increased the risk of hyperbilirubinaemia (6% v 1%; P < 0.001) and renal colic/nephrolithiasis (4% v 1%; P = 0.001).

Comment: Longer term follow up of patients taking protease inhibitors has found abnormal fat distribution, hyperglycaemia, and raised triglyceride and cholesterol concentrations. The clinical significance of these changes is uncertain. Many drugs interact with protease inhibitors because of inhibition of cytochrome P450.

OPTION   EARLY VERSUS DEFERRED ANTIRETROVIRAL TREATMENT

RCTs have compared early with delayed antiretroviral treatment, but these were all started when zidovudine was the only drug available. Overall, no evidence of differences in risk of AIDS or death was found with extended follow up. We found no RCTs exploring this question with two or three drug regimens.

Benefits:
We found one systematic review (search date not given), which identified nine RCTs (n = 7722) comparing treating people with asymptomatic infection immediately at the time of randomisation with deferring treatment until the occurrence of early signs of disease.[12] Participants were mainly those with initial CD4 counts > 200/mm^3. The review, and two other published meta-analyses,[19,20] found that early initiation of zidovudine reduced rates of AIDS and death in the short term, but that the beneficial effects decreased over time. Symptomatic people benefited more than asymptomatic people. Analysis of data from trials based at the UK Medical Research Council Clinical Trials Unit found no significant difference in risk of AIDS and death up to and over 6 years follow up (RR 1.02, 95% CI 0.91 to 1.15).[21] At 6 years, overall survival was 64% with immediate and 65% with deferred zidovudine (RR 1.04, 95% CI 0.94 to 1.15).[12]

Harms:
The larger meta-analysis[20] presented pooled toxicity data in terms of events per 100 patient years. In asymptomatic people, early treatment conferred a significant but small increase in the risk of anaemia (RR of haemoglobin < 8.0 g/dl, early v deferred treatment 2.1, 95% CI 1.1 to 4.1; AR 0.4 events per 100 person years). There was also a small increase in risk of neutropenia with early treatment (AR 1.1 events per 100 person years; P = 0.07). In symptomatic people, the excess incidence of severe anaemia probably reflected the high doses of zidovudine (1200–1500 mg/day; RR of severe anaemia, high v low dose 3.6, 95% CI 1.3 to 10). The authors advised that the toxicity results should be interpreted cautiously, as the data varied considerably.

Comment:
No new trials on this question are ongoing. This is probably because, with three drug regimens, rates of AIDS and death are currently low and treatment is known to be beneficial up to and over a 2 year period (see option, p 387). Most feel sufficiently certain about when to start treatment — based on data on HIV pathogenesis, resistance, immune regeneration with treatment, and long term adverse effects — and so would not consider randomisation to immediate versus deferred treatment. Decisions on when to initiate multidrug treatment are currently based on our understanding of how HIV induces immune damage, the capacity for immune regeneration while on treatment, the toxicity and inconvenience of treatment, and the risk of resistance, rather than on results of RCTs.

REFERENCES

1. United Nations AIDS website: http://www.unaids.org.
2. Public Health Laboratory Services. Occupational transmission of HIV. Summary of published reports. London: PHLS, December 1997.
3. Centres for Disease Control and Prevention. HIV prevention through early detection and treatment of other sexually transmitted diseases – Unites States. MMWR Morb Mortal Wkly Rep 1998;47: RR12.
4. Grosskurth H, Mosha F, Todd J, et al. Impact of improved treatment of sexually transmitted diseases on HIV infection in rural Tanzania: randomised controlled trial. Lancet 1995;346: 530–536.
5. Cohen MS, Hoffman IF, Royce RA, et al. Reduction of concentration of HIV-1 in semen after treatment of urethritis: implications for prevention of sexual transmission of HIV-1. Lancet 1997;349:1868–1873.
6. Wawer MJ, Sewankambo NK, Serwadda D, et al. Control of sexually transmitted diseases for AIDS prevention in Uganda: a randomised community trial. Lancet 1999;353:525–535.
7. Wilkinson D, Abdool Karim SS, Harrison A, et al. Unrecognised sexually transmitted infections in rural South African women: a hidden epidemic. Bull World Health Organ 1999;77:22–28.
8. Laga M, Alary M, Nzila N, et al. Condom promotion, sexually transmitted diseases treatment, and declining incidence of HIV-1 infection in female Zairian sex workers. Lancet 1994;344:246–248.
9. Centers for Disease Control and Prevention. Public health service guidelines for the management of health-care worker exposures to HIV and recommendations for post exposure prophylaxis. MMWR Morb Mortal Wkly Rep 1998;47:RR7.
10. Cardo DM, Culver DH, Ciesielski CA, et al. Case-control study of HIV seroconversion in health care workers after percutaneous exposure. N Engl J Med 1997;337:1485–1490.
11. Connor EM, Sperling RS, Gelber R, et al. Reduction of maternal–infant transmission of human immunodeficiency virus type 1 with zidovudine treatment: paediatric AIDS clinical trials group protocol 076 study group. N Engl J Med 1994;331:1173–1180.
12. HIV Trialists' Collaborative Group. Zidovudine, didanosine, and zalcitabine in the treatment of HIV infection: meta-analyses of the randomised evidence. Lancet 1999;353:2014–2015. Search date not given; primary sources Medline; investigators and pharmaceutical companies; and hand search of conference proceedings.
13. Haubrich R, Lalezari J, Follansbee SE, et al. Improved survival and reduced clinical progression in HIV-infected patients with advanced disease treated with saquinavir plus zalcitabine. Antivir Ther 1998;3:33–42.
14. CAESAR Co-ordinating Committee. Randomized trial of addition of lamivudine or lamivudine plus loviride to zidovudine-containing regimens for patients with HIV-1 infection: the CAESAR trial. Lancet 1997;349:1413–1421.
15. D'Aquila RT, Johnson VA, Welles SL, et al. Zidovudine resistance and HIV-1 disease progression during antiretroviral therapy. Ann Intern Med 1995;122:401–408.
16. De Gruttola V, Dix L, D'Aquila R, et al. The relationship between baseline HIV drug resistance and response to antiretroviral therapy: re-analysis of retrospective and prospective studies using a standardized data analysis plan. Antivir Ther 2000; 5:41–48
17. Hammer SM, Squires KE, Hughes MD, et al. A controlled trial of two nucleoside analogues plus indinavir in persons with HIV infection and CD4 cell counts of 200/mm3 or less. N Engl J Med 1997;337:725–733.
18. Revick DA, Moyle G, Stellbrink HJ, Barker C. Quality of life outcomes of combination zalcitabine–zidovudine, saquinavir–zidovudine, and saquinavir–zalcitabine–zidovudine therapy for HIV-infected adults with CD4 cell counts between 50 and 350/mm3. AIDS 1999;13:851–858.
19. Egger M, Neaton JD, Phillips AN, Davey Smith G. Concorde trial of immediate versus deferred zidovudine [letter]. Lancet 1994;343:1355.
20. Ioannidis JP, Cappelleri JC, Lau J, et al. Early or deferred zidovudine therapy in HIV-infected patients without an AIDS-defining illness: a meta-analysis. Ann Intern Med 1995;122:856–866. Search date 1994; primary sources Medline, AIDSLine, AIDSTrials, AIDSDrugs, CHEMID, and hand search of current contents and international conferences on AIDS.
21. Joint Concorde and Opal Coordinating Committee. Long-term follow-up of randomized trials of immediate versus deferred zidovudine in symptom-free HIV infection. AIDS 1998;12:1259–1265.

David Wilkinson
Professor
South Australian Centre for Rural and Remote Health University of Adelaide and University of South Australia
Whyalla
Australia

Andrew Phillips
Professor
Royal Free Centre for HIV Medicine and Department of Primary Care and Population Sciences, Royal Free and University College Medical School
London
UK

Margaret Johnson
Consultant in HIV Medicine
Royal Free Hospital
London
UK

Competing interests: DW, none declared. AP has received reimbursement for attending and speaking at symposia, funds for research and members of staff, and fees for consulting from various pharmaceutical companies producing antiretroviral drugs, including Glaxo Wellcome, Bristol Myers Squibb, Roche, and Dupont.

Malaria: prevention in travellers

Updated this issue

Ashley Croft

Key Messages

Non-drug preventive interventions

- One systematic review in residents of an endemic malaria area has found that nets treated with insecticide reduce the number of mild episodes of malaria and reduce child mortality.

- One RCT found that wraps and top sheets treated with insecticide reduce the number of episodes of malaria.

- Three other interventions have been evaluated in observational studies that used malarial illness as an outcome: air conditioning, wearing trousers and long sleeved shirts (both found to reduce the incidence of malaria), and aerosol insecticides (for which no evidence of an effect was found).

- Several other interventions have been found, mainly in observational studies, to reduce the risk of being bitten. These include insecticide treated clothing, electric fans, mosquito coils, vaporising mats, smoke, insect repellent soap, and topical DEET.

Drug prophylaxis

- Single RCTs in soldiers found doxycycline and mefloquine to be effective. We found insufficient evidence on the effects of other antimalarial drugs.

- We found little good evidence on the adverse effects of antimalarial drugs, particularly mefloquine. Observational studies have associated DEET and doxycycline with severe adverse effects in children.

Vaccines

- We found insufficient evidence on the effects of antimalarial vaccines in travellers.

DEFINITION   Malaria is caused by a protozoan infection of red blood cells with one of four species of the genus Plasmodium: *P falciparum*, *P vivax*, *P ovale*, and *P malariae*.[1] Clinically, malaria may present in different ways, but is usually characterised by fever (which may be swinging), tachycardia, rigors, and sweating. Anaemia, hepatosplenomegaly, cerebral involvement, renal failure, and shock may occur.

INCIDENCE/   Each year there are 300–500 million clinical cases of malaria.
PREVALENCE   About 40% of the world's population is at risk of acquiring the disease.[2,3] Each year 25–30 million people from non-tropical countries visit malaria endemic areas, of whom 10 000–30 000 contract malaria.[4,5] Most RCTs of malaria prevention have been carried out on western travellers and soldiers. The results of these trials may not be generalisable to people such as refugees and migrants, who are likely to differ in their health status and their susceptibility to disease and adverse drug reactions.

AETIOLOGY/   Malaria is mainly a rural disease, requiring nearby standing water. It
RISK FACTORS is transmitted by bites of infected female anopheline mosquitoes, mainly at dusk and during the night.[1,6–8] In cities, mosquito bites are usually from female culicene mosquitoes, which are not vectors of malaria.[9] Malaria is resurgent in most tropical countries and risk to travellers is increasing.[10]

PROGNOSIS   Ninety per cent of travellers who contract malaria do not become ill until after they return home.[5] "Imported malaria" is easily treated if diagnosed promptly, and follows a serious course in only about 12% of people.[11,12] The most severe form of the disease is cerebral malaria, with a case fatality rate in adult travellers of 2–6%, mainly because of delays in diagnosis.[13,14]

AIMS   To reduce the risk of infection; to prevent illness and death.

OUTCOMES   Rates of malarial illness and death, and adverse effects of treatment. Proxy measures include numbers of mosquito bites and numbers of mosquitoes in indoor areas. We found limited evidence linking numbers of mosquito bites and risk of malaria.[15]

METHODS   *Clinical Evidence* update search and appraisal May 2000. We reviewed all identified systematic reviews and RCTs.

Malaria: prevention in travellers

| QUESTION | What are the effects of non-drug preventive interventions in adult travellers? |

| OPTION | AEROSOL INSECTICIDES |

We found insufficient evidence on the effects of aerosol insecticides in travellers.

Benefits: We found no systematic review or RCTs. We found one questionnaire based survey of 89 617 European tourists returning from East Africa, which found no evidence that commercially available personal aerosol insecticides alone significantly reduced the incidence of malaria (P = 0.55).[16]

Harms: We found no reports of adverse effects.

Comment: None.

| OPTION | BIOLOGICAL CONTROL MEASURES |

We found no good evidence for the effectiveness of biological control measures in preventing malaria, nor evidence of harm.

Benefits: We found no systematic review or RCTs. Observational studies based on mosquito counts have found no evidence that growing the citrosa plant and encouraging natural predation of insects by erecting bird or bat houses reduce bites to humans from infected anopheline mosquitoes.[17]

Harms: We found no evidence of harm.

Comment: The only known way to reduce mosquitoes naturally is to eliminate sources of standing water, such as tree stump holes, discarded tyres, cans, and bottles.[17]

| OPTION | AIR CONDITIONING AND ELECTRIC FANS |

One large observational study in travellers found that air conditioning reduced the incidence of malaria. One small observational study found that electric fans reduced numbers of mosquitoes in indoor spaces.

Benefits: We found no systematic review or RCTs. One questionnaire based survey of 89 617 European tourists returning from East Africa found that sleeping in an air conditioned room significantly reduced the incidence of malaria (P = 0.04).[16] One observational study of various antimosquito interventions in six experimental huts in Pakistan villages found that fans significantly reduced catches of culicene mosquitoes (P < 0.05) but did not significantly reduce catches of blood fed anopheline mosquitoes.[18]

Harms: We found no evidence of harm.

Comment: These studies support the finding that mosquitoes are reluctant to fly in windy conditions.[19]

OPTION   INSECT BUZZERS AND ELECTROCUTERS

We found no evidence for the effectiveness of insect electrocuters and ultrasonic buzzers in preventing malaria.

Benefits: We found no systematic review and no RCTs with malarial illness as an outcome. Observational studies have found no evidence that insect electrocuters and ultrasonic buzzers reduce bites to humans from infected anopheline mosquitoes.[20,21]

Harms: We found no evidence of harm.

Comment: See comment under biological control measures, p 392.

OPTION   MOSQUITO COILS AND VAPORISING MATS

One RCT of coils and one observational study of pyrethroid vaporising mats found that these devices reduced numbers of mosquitoes in indoor spaces.

Benefits: We found no systematic review and no RCTs that used malarial illness as an outcome. We found one RCT in 18 houses in Malaysia of various mosquito coil formulations that found coils reduced populations of culicene mosquitoes by 75%.[22] One observational study of pyrethroid vaporising mats in six experimental huts in a Pakistan village setting found that the mats reduced total catches of blood fed anopheline mosquitoes by 56%.[17]

Harms: We found no evidence of harms.

Comment: None.

OPTION   SMOKE

One controlled trial found that smoke acted as a cheap and effective means of repelling mosquitoes during the evening.

Benefits: We found no systematic review and no RCTs that used malarial illness as an outcome. One controlled trial, in which five small fires were tended on five successive evenings in a village in Papua New Guinea, found a smoke specific and species specific effect from different types of smoke. Catches of one anopheline species were reduced by 84% through burning betelnut (95% CI 62% to 94%), by 69% through burning ginger (95% CI 25% to 87%), and by 66% through burning coconut husks (95% CI 17% to 86%).[23]

Harms: There may be an irritant and toxic effect of smoke on the eyes and respiratory system, but this effect was not quantified.[23]

Comment: None.

OPTION   INSECTICIDE TREATED NETS

One systematic review of RCTs has found that insecticide treated nets prevent malaria and reduce overall mortality.

Benefits: We found a systematic review (search date not given), which identified 18 RCTs in malaria endemic settings (non-traveller participants).[24] It found that nets sprayed or impregnated with permethrin reduced the number of mild episodes of malaria (ARR 39%, 95% CI 27% to 48%) and child mortality (RR of death compared with no nets or untreated nets 0.83, 95% CI 0.77 to 0.90; NNT 180).

Harms: Permethrin is an odourless synthetic pyrethroid with low toxicity in mammals.[17,25] It is poorly absorbed by the skin and rapidly inactivated by ester hydrolysis.[26]

Comment: Permethrin remains active for about 4 months.[6]

OPTION   INSECTICIDE TREATED CLOTHING

One RCT has found that insecticide treated wraps and top sheets significantly reduce the risk of contracting malaria.

Benefits: We found no systematic review.One RCT in 102 refugee households in north-western Pakistan found a significantly lower unadjusted relative risk for falciparum malaria (RR 0.56, 95% CI 0.41 to 0.78) in participants using permethrin-treated wraps and top sheets, compared with placebo.[27]

Harms: **Permethrin:** See harms of insecticide treated nets above. **DEET:** See harms of topical insect repellents, p 395.

Comment: None.

OPTION   LIFESTYLE CHANGE

One observational study in travellers found that wearing trousers and long sleeved shirts prevented malaria.

Benefits: We found no systematic review or RCTs. **Clothing:** We found one questionnaire survey of 89 617 European tourists returning from East Africa, which found that wearing long sleeved shirts and trousers significantly reduced the incidence of malaria (P = 0.02).[16] **Other lifestyle changes:** We found no studies (see comment below).

Harms: None.

Comment: Lifestyle change implies not travelling to malaria endemic regions during the rainy season (when most malaria transmission occurs), and not going out of doors in the evening or at night. Travellers who take day trips from a malaria free city to a malarious region may be at minimal risk if they return to the city before dusk.[28] It would seem sensible to wear long sleeved shirts and trousers at dusk, and to wear light rather than dark colours, as insects prefer landing on dark surfaces.[9,28]

OPTION   TOPICAL INSECT REPELLENTS

One RCT found that an insect repellent soap reduced insect bites. No RCTs have examined whether topical insect repellents prevent malaria. One very small crossover RCT found that DEET preparations protect against mosquito bites.

Infectious diseases

Benefits: We found no systematic review and no RCTs using malarial illness as an outcome. One small RCT (8 people in a Colombian forest setting) compared repellent soap (20% DEET and 0.5% permethrin) with placebo soap and found repellent soap reduced the numbers of sandfly bites at 4 and 8 hours (P < 0.05).[29] One small crossover RCT (n = 4) involving successive random exposure to *Aedes aegyptii* mosquitos compared six different controlled release preparations of DEET. It found that all gave at least 95% protection against mosquito bites.[30] **Combined with insecticide treated clothing:** See insecticide treated clothing, p 395.

Harms: We found a case series of systemic toxic reactions (confusion, irritability, insomnia) in US national park employees after repeated and prolonged use of DEET.[31] We found 14 case reports of contact urticaria and of irritant contact dermatitis (mostly in soldiers) as a result of DEET.[16] The antecubital fossa seems especially at risk if DEET is left on overnight.[32] DEET may be harmful to children under 8 years if applied in excessive amounts (see antimalarial interventions in children, p 398). It also attacks certain plastics, such as spectacle frames.[33]

Comment: DEET is a broad spectrum repellent effective against mosquitoes, biting flies, chiggers, fleas, and tics,[17] which has been used for 40 years. Although most authorities would recommend the use of topical repellents in malaria endemic areas, the only evidence comes from small RCTs with non-clinical outcomes. Larger RCTs are needed to compare DEET with other topical repellents and placebo in preventing malaria.

> **QUESTION** What are the effects of drug prophylaxis in adult travellers?

> **OPTION** CHLOROQUINE

We found insufficient evidence on the effects of chloroquine prophylaxis in travellers.

Benefits: We found no systematic review. We found one RCT comparing chloroquine with sulfadoxine plus pyrimethamine in 173 Austrian industrial workers based in Nigeria.[34] It found no evidence of a difference in the incidence of malaria.

Harms: We found no large cohort studies in travellers. In one RCT, the commonest reported symptom with chloroquine was insomnia, occurring in 3% of people.[34] Retrospective, questionnaire surveys suggest that severe adverse effects are rare at prophylactic dosages.[35]

Comment: Most drug trials have been in soldiers, and the trial results may not be generalisable to tourists or business travellers.[36,37] Alcohol consumption, other medication, and comorbidities can modify the effects of antimalarial drugs.[38,39]

> **OPTION** CHLOROQUINE PLUS PROGUANIL

RCTs found no evidence that chloroquine plus proguanil is more effective than proguanil alone or than chloroquine plus other antimalarial drugs.

Benefits: We found no systematic review. We found two RCTs in travellers. One open label RCT in Scandinavian travellers to East Africa found no significant difference in rates of *P falciparum* infection between groups (4 *v* 3 cases of *P falciparum* malaria in 384 and 383 travellers using chloroquine plus proguanil *v* chloroquine and sulfadoxine plus pyrimethamine).[40] **Versus proguanil alone:** The second RCT in Dutch travellers to Africa found no significant difference in incidence of *P falciparum* malaria with chloroquine plus proguanil compared with proguanil alone (risk per 100 person months: cholorquine 300 mg weekly plus proguanil 200 mg daily 2.8, 95% CI 0.9 to 10.1; proguanil 200 mg daily 6.0, 95% CI 2.6 to 14.0).[41]

Harms: In one RCT in Scandinavian travellers, adverse effects associated with chloroquine plus proguanil were nausea (3%), diarrhoea (2%), and dizziness (1%).[34] One cohort study in 470 British soldiers in Belize found that the risk of mouth ulcers almost doubled with chloroquine plus proguanil compared with proguanil alone (RR 1.9, P = 0.025).[42]

Comment: The rates of confirmed *P falciparum* infection in both trials were small and so a clinically significant effect cannot be excluded.

OPTION   DOXYCYCLINE

One RCT in soldiers found doxycycline to be effective. Short term adverse effects, including skin reactions and nausea and vomiting, were reported in up to 40% of people with malaria. We found no evidence on long term safety.

Benefits: We found no systematic review. One RCT (136 Indonesian soldiers) found that doxycycline reduced the risk of malaria when compared to placebo (AR 1/67 [2%] with doxycycline *v* 53/69 [77%] with placebo; ARR 75%, 95% CI 62% to 84%; RRR 98%, 95% CI 86% to 99.7%; NNT 1, 95% CI 1 to 2).[43] One RCT (300 Indonesian adults with limited immunity) found 96.3% protective efficacy relative to placebo against falciparum malaria (95% CI 85.4% to 99.6%), and 98% protective efficacy relative to placebo against vivax malaria (95% CI 88% to 99.9%).[44]

Harms: In one RCT in soldiers, commonly reported adverse effects were unspecified dermatological problems (33%), cough (31%), and headache (16%).[43] One questionnaire survey (383 returned Australian travellers) found that 40% reported nausea or vomiting, 12% reported diarrhoea, and 9% of female travellers reported vaginitis.[45] Evidence from case reports suggests that, in sunny conditions, up to 50% of travellers using doxycycline may experience photoallergic skin rash.[46]

Comment: Trials in soldiers may not be generalisable to other travellers. The first trial is a three arm parallel RCT. It compared mefloquine (n = 68) doxycycline (n = 67) and placebo (n = 69). Only the comparison of docycycline and placebo is included here.[42]

OPTION   MEFLOQUINE

One systematic review of RCTs has found that mefloquine is effective in preventing malaria. We found no good evidence that reliably attributes serious adverse reactions to mefloquine.

Benefits: We found one systematic review, which identified five RCTs in travellers (all soldiers).[47] Only one, a placebo controlled trial in 137 Indonesian soldiers, assessed the protective efficacy of mefloquine in a malaria endemic setting.[43] It found that in an area of drug resistance, mefloquine had a protective efficacy of 100% (95% CI 93% to 100%) in preventing malaria.

Harms: The review found no significant difference in the rate of withdrawals from mefloquine compared with other drug treatments.[47] Commonly reported adverse effects associated with mefloquine were headache (16%), insomnia (15%), and fatigue (8%).[47] Retrospective questionnaire surveys in tourists and business travellers found that sleep disturbance and psychosis were common.[48,49] One review of 74 dermatological case reports found that up to 30% of mefloquine users developed a maculopapular rash, and 4–10% had pruritus.[50] Nine cohort studies in tourists found that women tolerated mefloquine less well than men.[45,48,49,51–56] One retrospective questionnaire survey of 93 668 European travellers to East Africa found that elderly travellers tolerated mefloquine better than younger travellers ($P < 0.05$).[57] There is evidence from nonrandomised studies that mefloquine is a potentially harmful drug for tourists and business travellers and requires more careful evaluation through an RCT in these groups.[47]

Comment: Trials in soldiers may not be generalisable to other travellers. The trial is a three arm parallel RCT. It compared mefloquine (n = 68) doxycycline (n = 67) and placebo (n = 69). Only the comparison of mefloquine and placebo is included here.[43]

OPTION **OTHER ANTIMALARIAL DRUGS**

We found insufficient evidence on the effects of other antimalarial drugs in travellers.

Benefits: We found no systematic review. **Sulfadoxine plus pyrimethamine:** One open label RCT in 767 Scandinavian travellers to East Africa found no significant difference in rates of falciparum malaria between a combination of chloroquine plus sulfadoxine/pyrimethamine compared with chloroquine plus proguanil.[40] **Amodiaquine:** We found no RCTs in travellers. **Atovaquone plus proguanil:** We found no RCTs in travellers. **Pyrimethamine plus dapsone:** We found no RCTs in travellers. One RCT in Thai soldiers comparing pyrimethamine/dapsone with proguanil/dapsone found no significant differences in *P falciparum* infection rates over 40 days.[58]

Harms: **Sulfadoxine plus pyrimethamine:** One retrospective cohort study in 182 300 American travellers taking prophylactic sulfadoxine plus pyrimethamine reported severe cutaneous reactions (erythema multiforme, Stevens-Johnson syndrome, toxic epidermal necrolysis) in 1/5000–8000 users, with a mortality of about 1 per 11 000–25 000 users.[59] **Amodiaquine:** One retrospective cohort study in 10 000 British travellers taking prophylactic amodiaquine reported severe neutropenia in about 1/2000 users.[60] We found 28 case reports describing liver damage or hepatitis in travellers who had taken amodiaquine to treat or prevent malaria.[61–66] **Atovaquone**

plus proguanil: We found no evidence of adverse effects in travellers. **Pyrimethamine plus dapsone:** One RCT in Thai soldiers found that fewer than 2% reported any drug related symptoms from pyrimethamine plus dapsone.[67] One retrospective cohort study in 15 000 Swedish travellers taking pyrimethamine plus dapsone reported agranulocytosis in about 1/2000 users.[59]

Comment: None.

> **QUESTION** What are the effects of antimalarial vaccines in travellers?

We found insufficient evidence on the effects of antimalarial vaccines in travellers.

Benefits: We found no systematic review or RCTs of antimalarial vaccines in travellers.

Harms: In all but one of the trials of SPf66, fewer than 10% of recipients reported a systemic reaction (fever, headache, gastric symptoms, muscle pain, dizziness), and fewer than 35% reported a local reaction (inflammation, nodules, pain, erythema, pruritis, induration, injection site warmth).[68] The remaining trial found a larger proportion of local cutaneous reactions, although these resolved within 24 hours with symptomatic treatment. It also reported higher systemic reaction rates after vaccination (11–16%), although rates after placebo were also higher (10–13%). Surveillance was also more intense than in the other trials.

Comment: One systematic review (search date September 1998) identified 12 RCTs in residents of malaria endemic areas. It found that only the SPf66 vaccine reduced first attacks of *P falciparum* malaria (OR 0.80, 95% CI 0.71 to 0.90).[68]

> **QUESTION** What are the effects of antimalarial interventions in child travellers, pregnant women travellers, and airline pilots?

> **OPTION** IN CHILDREN

We found insufficient evidence on the effects of antimalarial interventions in child travellers. Case reports in young children have found serious adverse effects with DEET when used excessively, and with doxycycline. It is not clear which topical insect repellents are safe in children.

Benefits: We found no systematic review or RCTs evaluating antimalarial interventions in child travellers.

Harms: We found little evidence in child travellers. **DEET:** We found 13 case reports of encephalopathic toxicity in children aged under 8 years after excessive use of topical insect repellents containing DEET.[69,70] **Doxycycline:** Case reports have found that doxycycline inhibits bone growth and discolours teeth in children aged under 12 years.[9,35] **Mefloquine:** Three RCTs of mefloquine treatment found that children tolerate higher doses of this drug than adults.[71–73]

Comment: Infants and young children have thinner skin and greater surface area to mass ratio.[74] Some authors advise that ethylhexanediol should be used as a topical insect repellent in preference to DEET in children aged 1–8 years, and that in infants, only plant based topical repellents such as citronella oil are safe.[75] However, we found insufficient evidence about the effects of these alternative repellents.

OPTION   IN PREGNANT WOMEN

We found insufficient evidence on the effects of antimalarial interventions in pregnant women travellers. It is unclear which topical insect repellents are safe in pregnancy. One RCT found chloroquine to be safe in pregnancy, although it was too low powered to rule out rare adverse effects. The safety of mefloquine in pregnancy has not been established.

Benefits: We found no systematic review or RCTs of antimalarial interventions in pregnant women travellers. **Insecticide treated nets:** We found one RCT of permethrin treated nets in 341 pregnant women living in Thailand.[75] It found that treated nets reduced the incidence of malaria in pregnancy from 56% to 33% (RR 1.67, 95% CI 1.07 to 2.61).[76] **Drugs:** We found one systematic review (search date not given), which identified 15 RCTs of antimalarial drugs in pregnancy, all in residents of malaria endemic settings.[77] It found no significant difference in the number of perinatal deaths or preterm births. However, it found fewer episodes of fever during the first pregnancy (OR 0.36, 95% CI 0.15 to 0.86) and higher birth weight in the infant (OR 0.53, 95% CI 0.32 to 0.81).[77]

Harms: We found little evidence relating to pregnant women travellers. **Insecticide treated nets:** The trial of permethrin treated nets in Thailand found no evidence of toxic effects to mother or fetus.[76] **Topical insect repellents:** Some, but not all, animal studies have found that DEET crosses the placental barrier.[78] Animal studies of reproductive effects of DEET are conflicting.[79,80] We found one case report indicating an adverse fetal outcome (mental retardation, impaired sensorimotor coordination, craniofacial dysmorphology) in a child whose mother had applied DEET daily throughout her pregnancy.[81] **Chloroquine:** One RCT in 1464 long term residents of Burkina Faso found no adverse effects in pregnant women.[82] **Doxycycline:** Case reports have found that doxycycline taken in pregnancy or while breastfeeding may damage fetal or infant bones or teeth.[9,35] **Mefloquine:** One placebo controlled RCT in 339 long term Thai residents found more reports of dizziness with mefloquine (28% v 14%, P < 0.005) but no other significant adverse effects on the mother, the pregnancy, or on infant survival or development over 2 years of follow up.[83]

Comment: Pregnant women are relatively immunosuppressed and are at greater risk of malaria than non-pregnant women.[84] Contracting malaria significantly increases the likelihood of losing the fetus.[79] Because of a theoretical risk of mutagenicity from DEET, some authors advise that only plant based topical insect repellents such as citronella oil are safe in pregnancy.[75] However, we found insufficient evidence on the effects of this alternative repellent. Mefloquine is secreted in small quantities in breast milk, but it is believed that levels are too low to harm infants.[35]

OPTION   IN AIRLINE PILOTS

We found insufficient evidence about the effects of antimalarial drugs in airline pilots.

Benefits: We found no systematic review or RCTs.

Harms: **Doxycycline:** One retrospective questionnaire survey of 28 Israeli pilots found that 39% experienced adverse effects from doxycycline (abdominal pain 7/28, fatigue 5/28).[85] **Mefloquine:** One placebo controlled RCT in 23 trainee commercial pilots found no evidence that mefloquine significantly affected flying performance (mean total number of errors recorded by the instrument coordination analyser 12.6 with mefloquine v 11.7 with placebo).[86] One retrospective questionnaire survey of 15 Israeli non-aviator aircrew found that 13% experienced adverse effects from mefloquine (dizziness, nausea, and abdominal pain in 2/15, abdominal discomfort in 1/15).[85]

Comment: None.

Substantive changes since last issue

Insecticide treated clothing One new RCT found that permethrin treated wraps and top sheets reduced episodes of malaria.[27]

Topical insect repellent One small cross over RCT found all DEET formulations equally effective at preventing mosquito bites.[39]

Mefloquine Two new cohort studies on the harms of mefloquine; conclusions unaltered.[14,56]

REFERENCES

1. White NJ. Malaria. In: Cook GC, ed. *Manson's tropical diseases.* 20th ed. London: WB Saunders, 1996:1087–1164.
2. World Health Organization. *The world health report 1997. Conquering suffering, enriching humanity.* Geneva: WHO Office of Information, 1997.
3. Murphy GS, Oldfield EC. Falciparum malaria. *Infect Dis Clin North Am* 1996;10:747–755.
4. Kain KC, Keystone JS. Malaria in travelers. Epidemiology, disease and prevention. *Infect Dis Clin North Am* 1998;12:267–284.
5. World Health Organization. *International Travel and Health.* Geneva: WHO, 1999.
6. Winstanley P. Malaria: treatment. *J R Coll Physicians Lond* 1998;32:203–207.
7. Baudon D, Martet G. Paludisme et voyageurs: protection et information [in French]. *Med Trop (Mars)* 1997;57:497–500.
8. *Health information for international travel, 1996–97.* Atlanta: US Department of Health and Human Services, Public Health Service, Centers for Disease Control and Prevention, National Center for Infectious Diseases, Division of Quarantine; 1997 HHS Publication No 95:8280.
9. Bradley DJ, Warhurst DC. Guidelines for the prevention of malaria in travellers from the United Kingdom. *Commun Dis Rep CDR Rev* 1997;Sep 19;7:R137–152.
10. Krogstad DJ. Malaria as a reemerging disease. *Epidemiol Rev* 1996;18:77–89.
11. Olsen VV. Principielle overvejelser vedrørende malariaprofylakse. *Ugeskr Læger* 1998;160: 2410–2411.
12. Miller SA, Bergman BP, Croft AM. Epidemiology of malaria in the British Army from 1982–1986. *J R Army Med Corps* 1999;145:20–22.
13. Murphy GS, Oldfield EC. Falciparum malaria. *Infect Dis Clin North Am* 1996;10:747–775.
14. Dolmans WMV, van der Kaay HJ, Leentvaar-Kuijpers A, et al. Malariaprofylaxe: adviezen wederom aangepast. *Ned Tijdschr Geneeskd* 1996;140:892–893.
15. Beier JC, Oster CN, Onyango FK, et al. *Plasmodium falciparum* incidence relative to entomological inoculation rates at a site proposed for testing malaria vaccines in western Kenya. *Am J Trop Med Hyg* 1994;50:529–536.
16. Schoepke A, Steffen R, Gratz N. Effectiveness of personal protection measures against mosquito bites for malaria prophylaxis in travelers. *J Travel Med* 1998;128:931–940.
17. Fradin MS. Mosquitoes and mosquito repellents: a clinician's guide. *Ann Intern Med* 1998;128:931–940.
18. Hewitt SE, Farhan M, Urhaman H, et al. Self-protection from malaria vectors in Pakistan: an evaluation of popular existing methods and appropriate new techniques in Afghan refugee communities. *Ann Trop Med Parasitol* 1996;90: 337–344.
19. Service MW. *Mosquito ecology: field sampling*

methods. 2nd ed. London: Chapman and Hall, 1993.

20. Nasci RS, Harris CW, Porter CK. Failure of an insect electrocuting device to reduce mosquito biting. *Mosquito News* 1983;43:180–183.

21. Lewis DJ, Fairchild WL, Leprince DJ. Evaluation of an electronic mosquito repeller. *Can Entomol* 1982;114:699–702.

22. Yap HH, Tan HT, Yahaya AM, et al. Field efficacy of mosquito coil formulations containing d-allethrin and d-transallethrin against indoor mosquitoes especially *Culex quinquefasciatus* Say. *Southeast Asian J Trop Med Public Health* 1990;21:558–563.

23. Vernéde R, van Meer MMM, Aplers MP. Smoke as a form of personal protection against mosquitos, a field study in Papua New Guinea. *Southeast Asian J Trop Med Public Health* 1994;25:771–775.

24. Lengeler C. Insecticide treated bednets and curtains for preventing malaria. In: The *Cochrane Library*, Issue 4, 1999. Oxford: Update software. Search date not given; primary sources Cochrane Infectious Diseases Group Trial Register; Medline; Embase; reference lists; hand search of relevant journals, funding agents and manufacturers.

25. Carnevale P, Mouchet J. La protection individuelle contre les insectes vecteurs [in French]. *Med Trop (Mars)* 1997;57:505–510.

26. Anonymous. Insect repellents [letter]. *Med Lett Drugs Ther* 1989;31:45–47.

27. Rowland M, Durrani N, Hewitt S, et al. Permethrin-treated *chaddars* and top-sheets: appropriate technology for protection against malaria in Afghanistan and other complex emergencies. *Trans R Soc Trop Med Hyg* 1999;93:465–472.

28. Juckett G. Malaria prevention in travelers. *Am Fam Physician* 1999;59:2523–2530.

29. Alexander B, Cadena H, Usma MC, et al. Laboratory and field evaluations of a repellent soap containing diethyl toluamide (DEET) and permethrin against phlebotomine sand flies (Diptera: Psychodidae) in Valle del Cauca, Colombia. *Am J Trop Med Hyg* 1995;52:169–173.

30. Gupta RK, Rutledge LC. Laboratory evaluation of controlled-release repellent formulations on human volunteers under three climatic regimens. *J Am Mosq Control Assoc* 1989;5:52–55.

31. McConnell R, Fidler AT, Chrislip D. Everglades National Park health hazard evaluation report. Cincinatti, Ohio: US Department of Health and Human Services, Public Health Service, 1986. NIOSH Health Hazard evaluation Report No. HETA-83-085–1757.

32. Lamberg SI, Mulrennan JA. Bullous reaction to diethyl toluamide (DEET) resembling a blistering insect eruption. *Arch Dermatol* 1969;100:582–586.

33. Curtis CF, Townson H. Malaria: existing methods of vector control and molecular entomology. *Br Med Bull* 1998;54:311–325.

34. Stemberger H, Leimer R, Widermann G. Tolerability of long-term prophylaxis with Fansidar: a randomized double-blind study in Nigeria. *Acta Trop* 1984;41:391–399.

35. Petersen E. Malariaprofylakse. *Ugeskr Læger* 1997;159:2723–2730.

36. Croft A, Garner P. Mefloquine to prevent malaria: a systematic review of trials. *BMJ* 1997;315:1412–1416.

37. Anonymous. Mefloquine and malaria prophylaxis [letter]. *Drug Ther Bull* 1998;36:20–22.

38. Gherardin T. Mefloquine as malaria prophylaxis. *Aust Fam Physician* 1999;28:310.

39. Schlagenhauf P. Mefloquine for malaria chemoprophylaxis 1992–1998: a review. *J Travel Med* 1999;6:122–133.

40. Fogh S, Schapira A, Bygbjerg IC, et al. Malaria chemoprophylaxis in travellers to east Africa: a comparative prospective study of chloroquine plus proguanil with chloroquine plus sulfadoxine-pyrimethamine. *BMJ* 1988;296:820–822.

41. Wetsteyn JCFM, de Geus A. Comparison of three regimens for malaria prophylaxis in travellers to east, central, and southern Africa. *BMJ* 1993;307:1041–1043.

42. Drysdale SF, Phillips-Howard PA, Behrens RH. Proguanil, chloroquine, and mouth ulcers. *Lancet* 1990;335:164.

43. Ohrt C, Richie TL, Widjaja H, et al. Mefloquine compared with doxycycline for the prophylaxis of malaria in Indonesian soldiers. A randomized, double-blind, placebo-controlled trial. *Ann Intern Med* 1997;126:963–972.

44. Taylor WR, Richie TL, Fryauff DJ, et al. Malaria prophylaxis using azithromycin: a double-blind, placebo-controlled trial in Irian Jaya, Indonesia. *Clin Infect Dis* 1999;28:74–81.

45. Phillips MA, Kass RB. User acceptability patterns for mefloquine and doxycycline malaria chemoprophylaxis. *J Travel Med* 1996;3:40–45. Search date May 2000; primary sources Medline; Embase; LILACS; Cochrane Infections Diseases Group Register; The Cochrane Library Issue 2 2000; Science Citation Index; hand searched references; drug manufacturers; hand searched conference proceedings.

46. Leutscher PDC. Malariaprofylakse. *Ugeskr Læger* 1997;159:4866–4867.

47. Croft AMJ, Garner P. Mefloquine for preventing malaria in non-immune adult travellers. In: The *Cochrane Library*, Issue 3, 2000. Oxford: Update software.

48. Barrett PJ, Emmins PD, Clarke PD, Bradley DJ. Comparison of adverse events associated with use of mefloquine and combinations of chloroquine and proguanil as antimalarial prophylaxis: postal and telephone survey of travellers. *BMJ* 1996;313:525–528.

49. Weinke T, Trautmann M, Held T, et al. Neuropsychiatric side effects after the use of mefloquine. *Am J Trop Med Hyg* 1991;45:86–91.

50. Smith HR, Croft AM, Black MM. Dermatological adverse effects with the antimalarial drug mefloquine: a review of 74 published case reports. *Clin Exp Dermatol* 1999;24:249–254.

51. Bem L, Kerr L, Stuerchler D. Mefloquine prophylaxis: an overview of spontaneous reports of severe psychiatric reactions and convulsions. *J Trop Med Hyg* 1992;95:167–169.

52. Huzly D, Schönfeld C, Beurle W, et al. Malaria chemoprophylaxis in German tourists: a prospective study on compliance and adverse reactions. *J Travel Med* 1996;3:148–155.

53. Schlagenhauf P, Steffen R, Lobel H, et al. Mefloquine tolerability during chemoprophylaxis: focus on adverse event assessments, stereochemistry and compliance. *Trop Med Int Health* 1996;1:485–494.

54. Handschin JC, Wall M, Steffen R, et al. Tolerability and effectiveness of malaria chemoprophylaxis with mefloquine or chloroquine with or without co-medication. *J Travel Med* 1997;4:121–127.

55. van Riemsdijk MM, van der Klauw MM, van Heest JAC, et al. Neuro-psychiatric effects of antimalarials. *Eur J Clin Pharmacol* 1997;52:1–6.

56. Micheo C, Arias C, Rovira A. Adverse effects and compliance with mefloquine or chloroquine + proguanil malaria chemoprophylaxis. Proceedings of the Second European Conference on Travel Medicine; 2000 Mar 29–31; Venice, Italy. Venice: Fondazione Cini, 2000.

57. Mittelholzer ML, Wall M, Steffen R, et al. Malaria prophylaxis in different age groups. *J Travel Med* 1996;4:219–223.

58. Shanks GD, Edstein MD, Suriyamongkol V, et al. Malaria chemoprophylaxis using proguanil / dapsone combinations on the Thai-Cambodian border. *Am J Trop Med Hyg* 1992;46:643–648.

59. Miller KD, Lobel HO, Satriale RF, et al. Severe cutaneous reactions among American travelers using pyrimethamine-sulfadoxine for malaria prophylaxis. *Am J Trop Med Hyg* 1986;35:451–458.

60. Hatton CSR, Peto TEA, Bunch C, et al. Frequency of severe neutropenia associated with amodiaquine prophylaxis against malaria. *Lancet* 1986;1:411–414.

61. Neftel K, Woodtly W, Schmid M, et al. Amodiaquine induced agranulocytosis and liver damage. *BMJ* 1986;292:721–723.

62. Larrey D, Castot A, Pessayre D, et al. Amodiaquine-induced hepatitis. A report of seven cases. *Ann Intern Med* 1986;104:801–803.

63. Woodtli W, Vonmoos P, Siegrist P, et al. Amodiaquin-induzierte hepatitis mit leukopenie. *Schweiz Med Wochenschr* 1986;116:966–968.

64. Bernuau J, Larrey D, Campillo B, et al. Amodiaquine-induced fulminant hepatitis. *J Hepatol* 1988;6:109–112.

65. Charmot G, Goujon C. Hépatites mineures pouvant être dues à l'amodiaquine. *Bull Soc Pathol Exot* 1987;80:266–270.

66. Raymond JM, Dumas F, Baldit C, et al. Fatal acute hepatitis due to amodiaquine. *J Clin Gastroenterol* 1989;11:602–603.

67. Shanks GD, Edstein MD, Suriyamongkol V, et al. Malaria chemoprophylaxis using proguanil / dapsone combinations on the Thai-Cambodian border. *Am J Trop Med Hyg* 1992;46:643–648.

68. Graves P, Gelbland H. Vaccines for preventing malaria. In: The Cochrane Library, Issue 4, 1999. Oxford: Update software. Search date September 1998; primary sources Cochrane Infectious Diseases Group Trials Register; Cochrane Controlled Trials Register; Medline; Embase; reference lists; organisations and researchers in the field.

69. Osimitz TG, Murphy JV. Neurological effects associated with use of the insect repellent N,N-diethyl-m-toluamide (DEET). *J Toxicol Clin Toxicol* 1997;35:435–441.

70. de Garbino JP, Laborde A. Toxicity of an insect repellent: N,N-diethyl-m-toluamide. *Vet Hum Toxicol* 1983;25:422–423.

71. Smithuis FM, van Woensel JBM, Nordlander E, et al. Comparison of two mefloquine regimens for treatment of *Plasmodium falciparum* malaria on the northeastern Thai-Cambodian border. *Antimicrob Agents Chemother* 1993;37:1977–1981.

72. ter Kuile FO, Dolan G, Nosten F, et al. Halofantrine versus mefloquine in treatment of multidrug-resistant falciparum malaria. *Lancet* 1993;341:1044–1049.

73. Luxemburger C, Price RN, Nosten F, et al. Mefloquine in infants and young children. *Ann Trop Paediatr* 1996;16:281–286.

74. Are insect repellents safe? [editorial] *Lancet* 1988;2:610–611.

75. Bouchaud O, Longuet C, Coulaud JP. Prophylaxie du paludisme. *Rev Prat* 1998;48:279–286.

76. Dolan G, ter Kuile FO, Jacoutot V, et al. Bed nets for the prevention of malaria and anaemia in pregnancy. *Trans R Soc Trop Med Hyg* 1993;87:620–626.

77. Garner P, G Imezoglu AM. Prevention versus treatment for malaria in pregnant women. In: The Cochrane Library, Issue 4, 1999. Oxford: Update software. Search date not given; primary sources Cochrane Infectious Diseases Group trials register; Cochrane Controlled Trials' Register Isssue 1; Medline 1966 to 1999; Embase 1974 to 1999; researchers; and hand searched references.

78. Blomquist L, Thorsell W. Distribution and fate of the insect repellent 14C-N, N-diethyl-m-toluamide in the animal body. II. Distribution and excretion after cutaneous application. *Acta Pharmacol Toxicol (Copenh)* 1977;41:235–243.

79. Osimitz TG, Grothaus RH. The present safety assessment of DEET. *J Am Mosq Control Assoc* 1995;11:274–278.

80. Samuel BU, Barry M. The pregnant traveler. *Infect Dis Clin North Am* 1998;12:325–354.

81. Schaefer C, Peters PW. Intrauterine diethyltoluamide exposure and fetal outcome. *Reprod Toxicol* 1992;6:175–176.

82. Cot M, Roisin A, Barro D, et al. Effect of chloroquine chemoprophylaxis during pregnancy on birth weight: results of a randomized trial. *Am J Trop Med Hyg* 1992;46:21–27.83.

83. Nosten F, ter Kuile F, Maelankiri L, et al. Mefloquine prophylaxis prevents malaria during pregnancy: a double-blind, placebo-controlled study. *J Infect Dis* 1994;169:595–603.

84. Suh KN, Keystone JS. Malaria prophylaxis in pregnancy and children. *Infect Dis Clin Pract* 1996;5:541–546.

85. Shamiss A, Atar E, Zohar L, Cain Y. Mefloquine versus doxycycline for malaria prophylaxis in intermittent exposure of Israeli Air Force aircrew in Rwanda. *Aviat Space Environ Med* 1996;67:872–873.

86. Schlagenhauf P, Lobel H, Steffen R, et al. Tolerance of mefloquine by Swissair trainee pilots. *Am J Trop Med Hyg* 1997;56:235–240.

Ashley Croft
Consultant in Public Health Medicine
Ministry of Defence
London
UK

Competing interests: None declared.

Updated this issue

C Hart

QUESTIONS

INTERVENTIONS

Likely to be beneficial

Prophylactic antibiotics in
  contacts 404

Unknown effectiveness

Antibiotics for throat carriage
  (reduce carriage but unknown
  effect on risk of disease) . . .405

To be covered in future issues of
Clinical Evidence

Vaccines (monovalent/multivalent,
  polysaccharide alone, or
  conjugate)

Empirical treatment of suspected
  meningococcal disease

Treatment of meningococcal
  disease

Key Messages

- We found no randomised evidence about the effects of prophylactic antibiotics on the incidence of meningococcal disease among contacts. Observational data suggest that antibiotics reduce the risk of disease. We found no good evidence to address the question of which contacts should be treated.

- RCTs have found that antibiotics reduce throat carriage of the meningococcus. We found no evidence that eradicating throat carriage reduces the risk of meningococcal disease.

Meningococcal disease

DEFINITION Meningococcal disease is any clinical condition caused by *Neisseria meningitidis* (the meningococcus) groups A, B, C, or other serogroups. These conditions include purulent conjunctivitis, septic arthritis, meningitis, and septicaemia with or without meningitis.

INCIDENCE/ PREVALENCE Meningococcal disease is sporadic in temperate countries, and is most commonly caused by group B or C meningococci. The incidence in the UK varies from 2–8 cases per 100 000 people per year,[1] and in the USA from 0.6–1.5/100 000 population.[2] Occasional outbreaks occur among close family contacts, secondary school pupils, and students living in halls of residence. Sub-Saharan Africa has regular epidemics due to serogroup A, particularly in countries lying between Gambia in the west and Ethiopia in the east (the "meningitis belt"), where incidence during epidemics reaches 500/100 000.[3]

AETIOLOGY/ RISK FACTORS Meningococcus infects healthy people and is transmitted by close contact, probably by exchange of upper respiratory tract secretions (see table 1, p 408). Risk of transmission is greatest in the first week of contact.[7] Risk factors include crowding and exposure to cigarette smoke.[13] Children younger than 2 years have the highest incidence, with a second peak between ages 15–24. There is currently an increased incidence of meningococcal disease among university students, especially among those in their first term and living in catered accommodation,[14] although we found no accurate numerical estimate of risk from close contact in, for example, halls of residence. Close contacts of an index case have a much higher risk of infection than people in the general population.[7,10,11] The risk of epidemic spread is higher with group A and C meningococci than with group B meningococci.[4-6,8] It is not known what makes a meningococcus virulent, but certain clones tend to predominate at different times and in different groups. Carriage of meningococcus in the throat has been reported in 10–15% of people; recent acquisition of a virulent meningococcus is more likely to be associated with invasive disease.

PROGNOSIS Mortality is highest in infants and adolescents, and is related to disease presentation: case fatality rates are 19–25% in septicaemia, 10–12% in meningitis plus septicaemia, and less than 1% in meningitis alone.[15-17]

AIMS To prevent disease in contacts.

OUTCOMES Rates of infection; rates of eradication of throat carriage; adverse effects of treatment.

METHODS The author searched Medline and BIDS in December 1998, and drew from a collection of references from the pre-electronic data era. All studies were considered for inclusion. *Clinical Evidence* update search and appraisal May 2000.

QUESTION **What are the effects of prophylactic antibiotics on risk of disease in people exposed to someone with meningococcal disease?**

We found no randomised evidence on the effects of prophylactic antibiotics on the incidence of meningococcal disease among contacts.

Observational studies suggest that antibiotics reduce the risk of disease. We found no good evidence to address the question of which contacts should be treated.

Benefits: We found no systematic review and no RCTs examining the effect of prophylactic antibiotics in people who have been in contact with someone with meningococcal disease. **Rifampicin:** We found only anecdotal data. **Penicillin:** We found one retrospective study whose results cannot be generalised beyond the sample tested.[18] **Sulfadiazine:** One observational cohort study of soldiers in temporary troop camps in the 1940s compared the incidence of meningococcal disease in camps where sulfadiazine was given to everyone after a meningococcal outbreak, versus incidence in camps where no prophylaxis was given. The study reported a higher incidence of meningococcal disease in soldiers not given prophylaxis (approximate figures 17/9500 v 2/7000 over 8 weeks).[19]

Harms: **Rifampicin:** No excess adverse effects compared with placebo were found in RCTs on throat carriage of meningococcal disease.[20,21] However, rifampicin is known to turn urine and contact lenses orange and to induce hepatic microsomal enzymes, potentially rendering oral contraception ineffective. Rifampicin prophylaxis may be associated with emergence of resistant strains.[22] **Sulfadiazine:** One in 10 soldiers experienced minor adverse events, including headache, dizziness, tinnitus, and nausea.[19]

Comment: RCTs addressing this question are unlikely to be performed, because the intervention has few associated risks whereas meningitis has high associated risks. RCTs would also need to be large to find a difference in incidence of meningococcal disease. In the sulfadiazine cohort study, the two infected people in the treatment group only became infected after leaving the camp.[19]

QUESTION What are the effects of antibiotics in people with throat carriage of meningococcal disease?

RCTs have found that antibiotics reduce throat carriage of meningococcus. We found no evidence that eradicating throat carriage reduces the risk of meningococcal disease.

Benefits: We found no systematic review. **Incidence of disease:** We found no RCTs or observational studies examining whether eradicating throat carriage of meningococcus reduces the risk of meningococcal disease. **Throat carriage:** We found five placebo controlled RCTs examining the effect of antibiotics on carriage of meningococcus in the throat (see table 2, p 409).[20–21,23–25] All trials reported that antibiotics (rifampicin, minocycline, or ciprofloxacin) achieved high rates of eradication (ranging from 90–97%), except one trial of rifampicin in students with heavy growth on culture, where the rate of eradication was 73%. Eradication rates on placebo ranged from 9–29%. We found seven RCTs comparing different antibiotic regimens (see table 3, p 410).[26–32] Three RCTs found no significant difference between rifampicin and either minocycline, ciprofloxacin, or intramuscular ceftriaxone.[27,30,32] A fourth trial randomised households to different treatments and found that intramuscular ceftriaxone achieved higher eradication rates than rifampicin.[29]

However, confidence in this result is reduced by its cluster randomisation design. In another trial, oral azithromycin proved as effective as rifampicin in eradicating meningococcal throat carriage.[31]

Harms: **Minocycline:** One RCT reported adverse effects (one or more of nausea, anorexia, dizziness, and abdominal cramps) in 36% of participants.[23] **Rifampicin:** See harms of postexposure antibiotic prophylaxis, p 404. **Ciprofloxacin:** Trials of single dose prophylactic regimens reported no more adverse effects than comparators or placebo.[24,25,30] Ciprofloxacin is contraindicated in pregnancy and in children because animal studies have indicated a possibility of articular cartilage damage in developing joints.[33] **Ceftriaxone:** Two trials of ceftriaxone found no significant adverse effects.[29,30] In one trial, 12% of participants complained of headache.[29] Ceftriaxone is given as a single intramuscular injection. **Azithromycin:** No serious or moderate adverse effects were reported, but nausea, abdominal pain, and headache of short duration were reported equally in the azithromycin and rifampicin treated groups.[31]

Comment: Eradication of meningococcal throat carriage is a well accepted surrogate for prevention of meningococcal disease. It is unlikely that any RCT will be conducted on the efficacy of prophylactic antibiotics in preventing secondary community acquired meningococcal disease in household contacts, because the number of participants required would be large.

Substantive changes since last issue

Antibiotics for throat carriage New RCT.[32]

REFERENCES

1. http://www.phls.co.uk/facts/meni.htm. Disease Facts: Meningococcal Disease.
2. Centers for Disease Control. Summary of notifiable diseases United States, 1997. *Morbid Mortal Wkly Rtn* 1998;46:1–87.
3. Hart CA, Cuevas LE. Meningococcal disease in Africa. *Ann Trop Med Parasitol* 1997;91:777–785.
4. French MR. Epidemiological study of 383 cases of meningococcus meningitis in the city of Milwaukee, 1927–1928 and 1929. *Am J Public Health* 1931;21:130–137.
5. Pizzi M. A severe epidemic of meningococcus meningitis in 1941–1942, Chile. *Am J Public Health* 1944;34:231–239.
6. Lee WW. Epidemic meningitis in Indianapolis 1929–1930. *J Prev Med* 1931;5:203–210.
7. De Wals P, Herthoge L, Borlée-Grimée I, et al. Meningococcal disease in Belgium. Secondary attack rate among household, day-care nursery and pre-elementary school contacts. *J Infect* 1981;3(suppl 1):53–61.
8. Kaiser AB, Hennekens CH, Saslaw MS, Hayes PS, Bennett JV. Seroepidemiology and chemoprophylaxis of disease due to sulphonamide resistant *Neisseria meningitidis* in a civilian population. *J Infect Dis* 1974;130:217–221.
9. Zangwill KM, Schuchat A, Riedo FX, et al. School-based clusters of meningococcal disease in the United States. *JAMA* 1997;277:389–395.
10. The Meningococcal Disease Surveillance Group. Meningococcal disease secondary attack rate and chemoprophylaxis in the United States. *JAMA* 1976;235:261–265.
11. Olcen P, Kjellander J, Danielson D, Linquist BC. Epidemiology of *Neisseria meningitidis*: prevalence

and symptoms from the upper respiratory tract in family members to patients with meningococcal disease. *Scand J Infect Dis* 1981;13:105–109.
12. Hudson, PJ, Vogt PL, Heun EM, et al. Evidence for school transmission of *Neisseria meningitidis* during a Vermont outbreak. *Pediatr Infect Dis* 1986;5:213–217.
13. Stanwell-Smith RE, Stuart JM, Hughes AO, et al. Smoking, the environment and meningococcal disease: a case control study. *Epidemiol Infect* 1994;112:315–328.
14. Communicable Disease Surveillance Centre. Meningococcal disease in university students. *Commun Dis Rep CDR Wkly* 1998;8:49.
15. Andersen BM. Mortality in meningococcal infections. *Scand J Infect Dis* 1978;10:277–282.
16. Thomson APJ, Sills JA, Hart CA. Validation of the Glasgow meningococcal septicaemia prognostic score: a 10 year retrospective survey. *Crit Care Med* 1991;19:26–30.
17. Riordan FAI, Marzouk O, Thomson APJ, Sills JA, Hart CA. The changing presentation of meningococcal disease. *Eur J Pediatr* 1995;154: 472–474.
18. Hoiby EA, Moe PJ, Lystad A, Froholm LO, Bovre K. Phenoxymethyl-penicillin treatment of household contacts of meningococcal disease patients. *Antonie Van Leeuwenhoek* 1986;52:255–257.
19. Kuhns DW, Nelson CT, Feldman HA, Kuhns LR. The prophylactic value of sulfadiazine in the control of meningococcic meningitis. *JAMA* 1943;123:335–339.
20. Deal WB, Sanders E. Efficacy of rifampicin in treatment of meningococcal carriers. *N Engl J Med* 1969;281:641–645.
21. Eickhoff TC. In vitro and in vivo studies of

resistance to rifampicin in meningococci. *J Infect Dis* 1971;123:414–420.

22. Weidmer CE, Dunkel TB, Pettyjohn FS, Smith CD, Leibowitz A. Effectiveness of rifampin in eradicating the meningococcal carrier state in a relatively closed population: emergence of resistant strains. *J Infect Dis* 1971;124:172–178.

23. Devine LF, Johnson DP, Hagerman CR, Pierce WE, Rhode SL, Peckinpaugh RO. The effect of minocycline on meningococcal nasopharyngeal carrier state in naval personnel. *Am J Epidemiol* 1971;93:337–345.

24. Renkonen OV, Sivonen A, Visakorpi R. Effect of ciproflaxacin on carrier rate of *Neisseria meningitidis* in army recruits in Finland. *Antimicrob Agents Chemother* 1987;31:962–963.

25. Dworzack DL, Sanders CC, Horowitz EA, et al. Evaluation of single dose ciprofloxacin in the eradication of *Neisseria meningitidis* from nasopharyngeal carriers. *Antimicrob Agents Chemother* 1988;32:1740–1741.

26. Artenstein MS, Lamson TH, Evans JR. Attempted prophylaxis against meningococcal infection using intramuscular penicillin. *Mil Med* 1967;132:1009–1011.

27. Guttler RB, Counts GW, Avent CK, Beaty HN. Effect of rifampicin and minocycline on meningococcal carrier rates. *J Infect Dis* 1971;124:199–205.

28. Blakebrough IS, Gilles HM. The effect of rifampicin on meningococcal carriage in family contacts in northern Nigeria. *J Infect* 1980;2:137–143.

29. Schwartz B, Al-Tobaiqi A, Al-Ruwais A, et al. Comparative efficacy of ceftriaxone and rifampicin in eradicating pharyngeal carriage of Group A *Neisseria meningitidis*. *Lancet* 1988;i:1239–1242.

30. Cuevas LE, Kazembe P, Mughogho GK, Tillotson GS, Hart CA. Eradication of nasopharyngeal carriage of *Neisseria meningitidis* in children and adults in rural Africa: A comparison of ciprofloxacin and rifampicin. *J Infect Dis* 1995;171:728–731.

31. Girgis N, Sultan Y, Frenck RW Jr, et al. Azithromycin compared with rifampin for eradication of masopharyngeal colonization by *Neisseria meningitidis*. *Pediatr Infect Dis J* 1998; 17:816–819.

32. Simmons G, Jones N, Calder L. Equivalence of ceftriaxone and rifampicin in eliminating nasopharyngeal carriage of serogroup B *Neisseria meningitidis*. *J Antimicrob Chemother* 2000;45:909–911.

33. Schulter G. Ciproflozacin: a review of its potential toxicologic effects. *Am J Med* 1987(suppl 4A):38–46.

C Hart
Professor
Department of Medical Microbiology and Genitourinary Medicine
University of Liverpool
Liverpool
UK

Competing interests: None declared.

TABLE 1 Risk of infection among contacts (see text, p 404).

Group of Meningococcus	Setting	Risk
A	Household contacts in Milwaukee, USA[4]	AR 1100/100 000; RR not possible to estimate.
	General population in Santiago province, Chile. Household contacts[5]	Attack rate in general population 23–261.6/100 000 (1941 and 1942). Attack rate in household contacts 250/100 000 (2.5%) over both years.
	General population in Indianapolis, USA[6]	AR 4500/100 000; RR not possible to estimate.
B	Household contacts in Belgium[7]	RR 1245*
	Nursery schools[7]	RR 23*
	Day care centres[7]	RR 76*
C	Household contacts from two lower socioeconomic groups Dade County, Florida, USA[8]	Attack rate in two communities 13/100 000 population. Attack rate in household contacts 5/85 (582/100 000)
Unspecified	School based clusters in USA. Predominant meningococcal types: 13 Clusters of Gp C, 7 Gp B, 1 Gp Y, 1 GpC/W135 (impossible to distinguish)[9]	RR 2.3*
	Household contacts from several states in USA, meningococcus types B and C predominantly[10]	RR 500–800*
	Household contact in Norway. Meningococcus types A, B and C predominantly[11]	RR up to 4000*
	Schools. Predominant meningococcus type C[12]	OR 14.1 (95% CI 1.6 to 127)

*Compared with the risk in the general population.

TABLE 2 Effect of antibiotics on throat carriage: results of placebo controlled RCTs (see text, p 405).

Antibiotic	Group of Meningococcus	Participants	Treatment (%)	Placebo (%)	RR (95% CI)
				Eradication	
Rifampicin (oral)[20]	B, X, Z	30 students with heavy growth on culture	11/15 (73)	2/15 (13)	5.5 (1.46 to 20.7)
Rifampicin (oral)[21]	B, C, Y, Z29 E, W 135, NT	76 airforce recruits	36/38* (95)	3/22** (14)	6.95 (5.77 to 8.12)
Minocycline (oral)[23]	Predominantly Y (63%)	149 naval recruits	37/41 (90)†	14/48 (29)‡	3.09 (2.55 to 3.63)
Ciprofloxacin (oral)[24]	Non-groupable (61%), B (17.5%)	120 army recruits in Finland	54/56 (97) 5 second samples missing	7/53 (13) 6 second samples missing or not a carrier	7.3 (6.52 to 8.08)
Ciprofloxacin (oral)[25]	B (41%), Z (33%)	46 healthy volunteers	22/23 (96) (one did not adhere to treatment)	2/22 (9)	10.52 (8.91 to 12.1)

*9 lost to follow up. †37 either did not have meningococci prior to therapy or did not provide a full set of cultures. **7 lost to follow up. ‡23 either did not have meningococci prior to therapy or did not provide a full set of cultures.

TABLE 3 Effects of antibiotics on throat carriage: results of comparative RCTs (see text, p 405).

Antibiotic	Group of meningococcus	Participants	Rate of eradication (%)	RR (95% CI)
Penicillin (im)[26]	C (49%), B (33%), NG (17%)	Adults	41/118 (35)	No data
Erythromycin (oral)[26]	C	Adults	0/7 (0)	No data
Rifampicin (oral)[27]	B + C (31%), NG (69%)	Adults	43/51 (84)	0.89 (0.76 to 1.02)
Minocycline (oral)[27]	B + C (31%), NG (69%)	Adults	36/38 (95)	No data
Rifampicin (oral)[27]	A	Children	37/48 (77)	No data
Sulfadimidine (oral)[28]	A	Children	0/34 (0)	No data
Ceftriaxone (im)[29]	A	Adults and children	66/68 (97)	1.29 (1.10 to 1.49)
Rifampicin (oral)[29]	A	Adults and children	27/36 (75)	No data
Ceftriaxone (im)[30]	A	Adults and children	39/41 (95)	No data
Ciprofloxacin (oral)[30]	A	Adults and children	70/79 (89)	No data
Rifampicin (oral)[30]	A	Adults and children	85/88 (97)	No data
Azithromycin (oral)[31]	B (63%), A (37%)	Adults	56/60 (93)	No data
Rifampicin (oral)[31]	B (63%), A (37%)	Adults	56/59 (95)	No data
Ceftriaxone (im)[32]	B (54%), other serogroups (46%)	Adults and children	97/100 (97)	No data
Rifampicin (oral)[32]	B (51%), other serogroups (49%)	Adults and children	78/82 (95.1)	No data

Im, intramuscular.

Infectious diseases

INTERVENTIONS

Beneficial

TMP/SMX (for PCP and toxoplasmosis). 414

Atovaquone, (no difference from dapsone, aerosolised pentamidine for PCP, in people intolerant of TMP/SMX). 415

Tuberculosis prophylaxis versus placebo. 416

Aciclovir (for HSV and VZV) . . .421

Likely to be beneficial

Azithromycin (for PCP) 416

Azithromycin (for MAC) 418

Clarithromycin (for MAC) 418

Clarithromycin plus ethambutol (for MAC in people with previous MAC) 419

Itraconazole (for *Penicillium marneffei* and cryptococcal meningitis) 423

Stopping prophylaxis for PCP and toxoplasmosis in people with CD4 > 200/mm^3 on HAART .423

Stopping prophylaxis for MAC in people with CD4 > 100/mm^3 on HAART 424

Trade off between benefits and harms

Isoniazid tuberculosis prophylaxis for 6–12 months versus combination therapy for 2 months (similar benefits, fewer harms). 417

Rifabutin plus either clarithromycin or azithromycin (for MAC) . . .419

Oral ganciclovir (in people with severe CD4 depletion) 420

Fluconazole or itraconazole (invasive fungal disease). . . .422

Unknown effectiveness

Famciclovir (for recurrent HSV) .421

Itraconazole (for histoplasmosis) 423

Stopping prophylaxis for CMV in people with CD4 > 100/mm^3 on HAART 424

Likely to be beneficial

Clofazimine or high dose clarithromycin (for MAC in people with previous MAC) 419

Valaciclovir (CMV) 421

To be covered in future issues of
Clinical Evidence

Pentamidine versus placebo for prevention of PCP

Opportunistic infections, treatment

Immune reconstitution related syndromes (see glossary, p 425)

Covered elsewhere in this issue

Different antiretroviral regimens (see HIV infection, p 382)

See glossary, p 425

Key Messages

- Systematic reviews have found that TMP/SMX is more effective than pentamidine or placebo at reducing the incidence of *Pneumocystis carinii* pneumonia (PCP) or toxoplasmosis.

- One systematic review found no significant difference between high and low dose TMP/SMX for PCP, although adverse effects were more common with the higher dose.

- Systematic reviews have found that TMP/SMX compared with dapsone/pyrimethamine reduces the incidence of PCP, but does not reduce the incidence of toxoplasmosis.

- Two systematic reviews of RCTs have found that antituberculosis prophylaxis reduces the rate of tuberculosis and death in the short term in people who are human immunodeficiency virus (HIV) and tuberculin skin test positive. We found insufficient evidence about the long term effects on rates of tuberculosis and death. The reviews found no evidence of benefit in people who are HIV positive but tuberculin skin test negative.

- We found evidence from RCTs that
  - Dapsone or aerosolised pentamidine have similar effectiveness to atovaquone at preventing PCP in TMP/SMX intolerant people.
  - Azithromycin, either alone or in combination with rifabutin, reduces the risk of PCP compared with rifabutin alone in people receiving standard PCP prophylaxis.
  - Regimens using combinations of tuberculosis drugs for 2–3 months have similar effectiveness as those using isoniazid alone for 6–12 months. One RCT found that adverse reactions causing cessation of treatment are more common with multidrug regimens.
  - Azithromycin and clarithromycin reduce the incidence of *Mycobacterium avium* complex (MAC) more than placebo.
  - Clarithromycin alone, and clarithromycin plus rifabutin, both reduce the incidence of MAC compared with rifabutin alone. Azithromycin plus rifabutin reduce the incidence of MAC compared with azithromycin alone.
  - Clarithromycin plus ethambutol, with or without rifabutin, reduces the incidence of MAC in people with previous MAC disease. Clofazimine and high dose clarithromycin are associated with increased mortality.
  - Oral ganciclovir may reduce the incidence of cytomegalovirus (CMV) in people with severe CD4 depletion compared with placebo, but one RCT found important side effects.
  - Valaciclovir reduces the incidence of CMV more than aciclovir, but is associated with increased mortality. One systematic review found that aciclovir did not reduce the incidence of CMV compared with placebo, but significantly reduced herpes simplex virus (HSV) and varicella zoster virus (VZV) infection and overall mortality in people at different stages of HIV infection.
  - Famciclovir compared with placebo reduces the rate of HSV shedding, but we found insufficient evidence on the effect of famciclovir on HSV recurrence.
  - Fluconazole and itraconazole reduce the incidence of invasive fungal infections compared with placebo in people with advanced HIV disease. Fluconazole reduces the incidence of invasive fungal disease and mucocutaneous candidiasis more than clotrimazole. There was no significant difference between high and low dose fluconazole.

- Itraconazole reduces the incidence of relapse of *Penicillium marneffei* infection, and is more effective than fluconazole in reducing the relapse of cryptococcal meningitis.
- In people with adequate increases in CD4 cell count while on potent antiretroviral therapy, stopping prophylaxis does not increase the incidence of PCP, toxoplasmosis, or MAC disease.
- We found insufficient evidence on the effects of stopping maintenance therapy for CMV retinitis or other end organ disease.

DEFINITION   Opportunistic infections are intercurrent infections that occur in people infected with HIV. Prophylaxis aims to avoid either the first occurrence of these infections (primary prophylaxis) or their recurrence (secondary prophylaxis, maintenance therapy). This review includes *Pneumocystis carinii* pneumonia (PCP), *Toxoplasma gondii* encephalitis, *Mycobacterium tuberculosis*, *Mycobacterium avium* complex (MAC) disease, cytomegalovirus (CMV) disease (most often retinitis), infections from other herpes viruses (herpes simplex virus [HSV] and varicella zoster virus [VZV]), and invasive fungal disease (*Cryptococcus neoformans*, *Histoplasma capsulatum* and Penicillium marneffei).

AETIOLOGY/   Opportunistic infections are caused by a wide array of pathogens
RISK FACTORS and result from immune defects induced by HIV. The risk of developing opportunistic infections increases dramatically with progressive impairment of the immune system. Each opportunistic infection has a different threshold of immune impairment, beyond which the risk increases substantially.[1] Opportunistic pathogens may infect the immunocompromised host *de novo*, but usually they are simply reactivations of latent pathogens in such hosts.

PROGNOSIS   Prognosis depends on the type of opportunistic infection. Even with treatment they may cause serious morbidity and mortality. Most deaths due to HIV infection are caused by opportunistic infections.

AIMS   To prevent the occurrence and relapse of opportunistic infections; to discontinue unnecessary prophylaxis; to minimise adverse effects of prophylaxis, and loss of quality of life.

OUTCOMES   First occurrence and relapse of opportunistic infections and adverse effects of treatments. We have not considered neoplastic diseases associated with specific opportunistic infections.

METHODS   *Clinical Evidence* search and appraisal March 2000. We also reviewed abstract books/CDs for the following conferences held between 1995 and early 2000: European Clinical AIDS, HIV Drug Therapy, Interscience Conferences on Antimicrobial Agents and Chemotherapy, National Conferences on Human Retroviruses and Opportunistic Infections, North American Retrovirus and Opportunistic Infection (Washington/Chicago, USA), and World AIDS Conference. We placed emphasis on systematic reviews and RCTs published after 1993. We considered observational evidence if no RCTs were available or if it covered a broader spectrum than randomised evidence.

QUESTION | What are the effects of prophylaxis for PCP and toxoplasmosis?

John Ioannidis

OPTION | TMP/SMX

Systematic reviews have found that TMP/SMX is more effective than pentamidine or placebo at reducing the incidence of PCP or toxoplasmosis. Two systematic reviews found that TMP/SMX compared with dapsone (with or without pyrimethamine) reduced the incidence of PCP, but found no difference in the incidence of toxoplasmosis. One systematic review and one subsequent RCT found no significant difference between high and low dose TMP/SMX for PCP prophylaxis, although adverse effects were more common with the higher dose.

Benefits:
TMP/SMX versus placebo: We found one systematic review (39 RCTs, search date 1995) in people with either CD4 < 200/mm^3, or a prior history of PCP, of prophylaxis for PCP (39 RCTs, n = 6583), and toxoplasmosis (15 RCTs, n = 3641).[2] People with oropharyngeal candidiasis were often also considered for prophylaxis. Overall, it found that prophylaxis with TMP/SMX reduced the incidence of PCP more than placebo (RR 0.32, 95% CI 0.23 to 0.46). There were no placebo controlled data on the incidence of toxoplasmosis. One subsequent RCT (n = 545) in sub-Saharan Africa compared TMP/SMX against placebo in 545 people with symptomatic disease (2nd or 3rd clinical stage disease in the WHO staging system (see glossary, p 425) regardless of CD4 cell count.[3] It found no significant difference in incidence of PCP or toxoplasmosis. **TMP/SMX versus pentamidine:** We found two systematic reviews.[2,4] The first review (search date 1995) found that TMP/SMX was significantly more effective at preventing PCP than aerosolised pentamidine (RR 0.58, 95% CI 0.45 to 0.75).[2] The second (22 RCTs, search date 1995) found similar results.[4] TMP/SMX was also more effective than aerosolised pentamidine at preventing toxoplasmosis.[4] **TMP/SMX versus dapsone (with or without pyrimethamine):** The first systematic review found that TMP/SMX compared with dapsone (with or without pyrimethamine) reduced the incidence of PCP, but the result did not reach significance (RR 0.61, 95% CI 0.34 to 1.10).[2] The second review found that TMP/SMX was significantly more effective in preventing PCP than dapsone/pyrimethamine (RR 0.49, 95% CI 0.26 to 0.92).[4] It found no significant difference between TMP/SMX and dapsone/pyrimethamine in preventing toxoplasmosis (RR 1.17, 95% CI 0.68 to 2.04). **High versus low dose TMP/SMX:** The first systematic review found no significant difference between lower dose TMP/SMX 160/800 mg three times weekly or 80/400 mg daily, and higher dose TMP/SMX, 160/800 mg daily (failure rate per 100 person years was 1.6, 95% CI 0.9 to 2.5 with lower dose v 0.5, 95% CI 0% to 2.9% with higher dose).[2] A subsequent RCT (n = 2625) also found no significant difference in the rate of PCP infection in people receiving daily compared with thrice weekly TMP/SMX 160/800 mg (3.5 v 4.1 per 100 person years; P = 0.16).[5]

Harms: One systematic review found that adverse effects (predominantly rash, fever, and haematological side effects) severe enough to lead to discontinuation within 1 year occurred in more people taking higher doses of TMP/SMX than taking lower doses (25% v 15%).[2] The RCT comparing high dose with low dose TMP/SMX found that discontinuation due to adverse effects was significantly more common in people taking high doses of TMP/SMX (RR 2.14; P < 0.001).[5] Adverse effects occurred in more people taking high doses than low doses of dapsone (29% v 12%).[2] The RCT in sub-Saharan Africa found that people on TMP/SMX were less likely to suffer a serious event (death or hospital admission, irrespective of the cause) than those on placebo regardless of their initial CD4 cell count (84 v 124; hazard ratio 0.57, 95% CI 0.43 to 0.75; P < 0.001). Moderate neutropenia occurred more frequently with TMP/SMX (neutropenia AR 62/271 [23%] with TMP/SMX versus 26/244 [10%] with placebo; RR 2.1, 95% 1.4 to 3.3; NNH 8, 95% CI 5 to 14).[3] Two RCTs (abstract only; largest n = 377) found that gradual initiation of TMP/SMX may improve tolerance of the regimen.[6,7] Two RCTs (n = 238, n = 50) found no significant benefit from acetylcysteine in preventing TMP/SMX hypersensitivity reactions in HIV infected people.[8,9] Bronchospasm occurred in 2.5% of people taking aerosolised pentamidine 300 mg monthly.[2]

Comment: **Concomitant coverage for toxoplasmosis:** Standard TMP/SMX prophylaxis or dapsone should offer adequate coverage for toxoplasmosis. Pentamidine has no intrinsic activity against *T gondii*. Toxoplasmosis risk is probably clinically meaningful only with CD4 < 100/mm^3 and positive toxoplasma serology.[1] **Role of HAART:** We found more than 50 RCTs on the prophylaxis of PCP and/or toxoplasmosis, but their results should be interpreted with caution since they were conducted mostly before the advent and widespread use of highly active antiretroviral regimens. Although this is unlikely to affect the comparative results, HAART has resulted in a large decrease in the rate of PCP, toxoplasmosis and other opportunistic infections. Therefore, the absolute benefits of these prophylactic regimens are probably smaller when used with HAART. **Prophylaxis in Africa:** Beneficial effects of TMP/SMX in Africa are mostly due to coverage for bacterial infections rather than PCP.

OPTION	ATOVAQUONE IN TMP/SMX INTOLERANT PEOPLE

RCTs found no significant difference between atovaquone, dapsone, or aerosolised pentamidine in preventing PCP. None of the interventions were compared to placebo.

Benefits: We found no systematic review. **Versus placebo:** We found no RCTs. **Versus dapsone:** One RCT in 1057 people, of whom 298 had a history of PCP, found no significant difference between atovaquone (1500 mg daily) compared with dapsone (100 mg daily) in people intolerant of TMP/SMX (15.7 v 18.4 cases of PCP per 100 person years; P = 0.20).[10] **Versus pentamidine:** One RCT in 549 people intolerant of TMP/SMX compared high dose with low dose atovaquone (1500 mg daily v 750 mg daily) with monthly aerosolised pentamidine (300 mg). It found no significant difference between the groups in the incidence of PCP (26% v 22% v

17%) or mortality (20% *v* 13% *v* 18%) after a median follow up of 11.3 months.[11]

Harms: The RCT comparing atovaquone with dapsone found that the overall risk of stopping treatment owing to adverse effects was similar in the two arms (RR 0.94, 95% CI 0.74 to 1.19).[10] Atovaquone was stopped more frequently than dapsone in people who were receiving dapsone at baseline (RR 3.78, 95% CI 2.37 to 6.01; P < 0.001), and less frequently in people not receiving dapsone at baseline (RR 0.42, 95% CI 0.30 to 0.58; P < 0.001).

Comment: See role of HAART in comment under TMP/SMX, p 415.

OPTION   AZITHROMYCIN

One RCT found that azithromycin, either alone or in combination with rifabutin, reduced the risk of PCP compared with rifabutin alone in people receiving standard PCP prophylaxis.

Benefits: We found no systematic review. **Versus placebo:** We found no RCTs. **Versus other drugs:** We found one RCT (n = 693), which compared azithromycin, rifabutin, and both drugs in combination, in people who were already receiving standard PCP prophylaxis. It found that azithromycin, either alone or in combination with rifabutin, reduced the risk of developing PCP by 45% when compared with rifabutin alone (P = 0.008).[12]

Harms: Gastrointestinal side effects are common with azithromycin, but they are usually mild and do not lead to stopping treatment. The addition of rifabutin significantly increased the risk of stopping treatment (RR 1.67; P = 0.03).[13]

Comment: See role of HAART in comment under TMP/SMX, p 415. The low incidence of PCP infection in people taking HAART means that the benefit of prophylaxis is smaller.

QUESTION   What are the effects of antituberculosis prophylaxis in people with HIV infection?

Margaret Johnson, Andrew Phillips, and David Wilkinson

OPTION   ANTITUBERCULOSIS PROPHYLACTIC REGIMENS VERSUS PLACEBO

Two systematic reviews of RCTs have found that in people who are HIV and tuberculin skin test positive antituberculosis prophylaxis reduces frequency of tuberculosis in the short term. Long term effects on rates of tuberculosis and death are unknown. The reviews found no evidence of benefit in people who are HIV positive but tuberculin skin test negative.

Benefits: We found two systematic reviews; one (updated in 1999)[14] identified six well conducted RCTs in 4652 HIV positive adults from Haiti, Kenya, USA, Zambia, and Uganda. All compared isoniazid (6–12 months) or combination therapy (3 months) with placebo. Mean follow up was 2–3 years, and the main outcomes, stratified by tuberculin skin test positivity, were tuberculosis (either microbiological or clinical) and death. Among tuberculin skin test positive adults, antituberculosis prophylaxis significantly reduced the incidence of tuberculosis (RR compared with placebo 0.24, 95% CI 0.14 to 0.40) and was associated with a trend towards reducing the risk of death (RR compared with placebo 0.77, 95% CI 0.58 to 1.03). Among tuberculin skin test negative adults, there was no significant difference in risk of tuberculosis (RR compared with placebo 0.87, 95% CI 0.56 to 1.36) or death (RR compared with placebo 1.07, 95% CI 0.88 to 1.30). The second review included seven trials comprising 4529 participants and compared isoniazid with placebo only. Among tuberculin skin test positive participants the incidence of tuberculosis was significantly reduced (RR compared with placebo 0.40, 95% CI 0.24 to 0.65), but this was not so among tuberculin skin test negative participants (RR compared with placebo 0.84, 95% CI 0.54 to 1.30). There was no evidence of any impact on mortality in this review.[15]

Harms: Data on adverse drug reactions were not always stratified by tuberculin skin test positivity. In the first review there was a significant increase in adverse drug reactions requiring cessation of treatment on isoniazid compared with placebo (RR 1.75, 95% CI 1.23 to 2.47).[14] In the second review, the estimated RR was 1.36 (95% CI 1.00 to 1.86).[15]

Comment: Without prophylaxis, people who are HIV and tuberculin skin test positive have a 50% or more lifetime risk of developing tuberculosis, compared with a 10% lifetime risk in people who are HIV positive but tuberculin skin test negative.[16] Clinical features of tuberculosis may be atypical in people with HIV infection, and diagnosis may be more difficult, disease progression more rapid, and outcome worse.

OPTION	DIFFERENT ANTITUBERCULOSIS PROPHYLACTIC REGIMENS

RCTs have found no evidence of a difference in effectiveness between regimens using combinations of tuberculosis drugs for 2–3 months and those using isoniazid alone for 6–12 months. Adverse reactions causing cessation of treatment are more common with multidrug regimens.

Benefits: We found no systematic review. We found four published RCTs. Three compared isoniazid with rifampicin/pyrazinamide in people who were HIV and tuberculin skin test positive (n = 750, n = 1583, and n = 393).[17–19] All found no significant difference in rates of tuberculosis. The fourth RCT included 1564 HIV and tuberculin skin test positive people from Uganda.[20] It found that the risk of tuberculosis was reduced with isoniazid alone (RR compared with placebo 0.33, 95% CI 0.14 to 0.77), and with isoniazid and rifampicin combined (RR compared with placebo 0.40, 95% CI 0.18 to 0.86), and showed a trend towards reduction with isoniazid, rifampicin, and pyrazinamide combined (RR compared with placebo 0.51, 95% CI 0.24 to 1.08).

Harms: The proportion of people discontinuing treatment increased with the number of drugs given: isoniazid 0.6%, isoniazid plus rifampicin 2.3%, and all three drugs 5.6%.[20]

Comment: There is concern about emergence of rifampicin resistance if this drug is used in antituberculosis prophylaxis, although we found no reports of this. On the other hand, there is a theoretical risk that widespread, unsupervised use of isoniazid alone could promote resistance to this drug, although there is no evidence that this has happened. We found no adequate comparison of the long term effects of single drug compared with combination drug antituberculosis prophylaxis.

QUESTION What are the effects of prophylaxis for disseminated MAC disease for people without previous MAC disease?

John Ioannidis

OPTION AZITHROMYCIN

One RCT found that azithromycin reduced the incidence of MAC more than placebo.

Benefits: We found no systematic review. One RCT (174 people with AIDS and CD4 < 100/mm^3) found that azithromycin reduced the incidence of MAC more than placebo (10.6% v 24.7%; P = 0.004).[21]

Harms: Gastrointestinal side effects were more likely with azithromycin than with placebo (71/90 [79%] v 25/91 [28%]), but they were rarely severe enough to cause discontinuation of treatment (8% v 2.3% in the two arms; P = 0.14).[21]

Comment: Prospective cohort studies have found that the risk of disseminated MAC disease increases substantially with a lower CD4 count and is clinically important only for CD4 < 50/mm^3.[1] **Role of HAART:** Most of the RCTs of MAC prophylaxis were conducted before the widespread use of HAART. HAART reduces the absolute risk of MAC infection. The absolute risk reduction of prophylactic regimens may be smaller when used in people treated with HAART.

OPTION CLARITHROMYCIN

One RCT found that clarithromycin reduced the incidence of MAC compared with placebo.

Benefits: We found one systematic review of prophylaxis and treatment of MAC (search date 1997).[22] It identified one RCT in 682 people with advanced AIDS, which found that clarithromycin compared with placebo significantly reduced the incidence of MAC (6% v 16%; hazard ratio 0.31; 95% CI 0.18 to 0.53). It found no significant difference in the death rate (32% v 41%; hazard ratio 0.75; P = 0.026).[23]

Harms: Adverse effects led to discontinuation of treatment in more people taking clarithromycin than placebo (8% v 6%; P = 0.45). More people taking clarithromycin suffered taste perversion (11% v 2%) or rectal disorders (8% v 3%).[23]

Comment: Prospective cohort studies found that the risk of disseminated MAC disease increased substantially with a lower CD4 count and was clinically important only for CD4 < 50/mm^3.[1] See role of HAART in comment under azithromycin, p 416.

OPTION	COMBINATION THERAPY

RCTs have found that clarithromycin alone, and clarithromycin plus rifabutin, both reduce the incidence of MAC compared with rifabutin alone. Azithromycin plus rifabutin reduced the incidence of MAC compared with azithromycin alone.

Benefits:
Clarithromycin plus rifabutin: We found no systematic review. One RCT in 1178 people with AIDS compared rifabutin with clarithromycin, and rifabutin with clarithromycin and rifabutin combined.[24] It found that the risk of MAC was significantly reduced in the clarithromycin alone group (RRR 44% for clarithromycin v rifabutin; P = 0.005) and the combination group when compared with rifabutin alone (RRR 57% for combination v rifabutin; P = 0.0003). There was no significant difference in the risk of MAC between the combination and clarithromycin arms (P = 0.36). **Azithromycin plus rifabutin:** We found one systematic review of prophylaxis and treatment of MAC (search date 1997).[22] It identified one RCT (n = 693), found the combination of azithromycin and rifabutin was more effective than azithromycin alone (1 year incidence of MAC: 15.3% with rifabutin, 7.6% for azithromycin, 2.8% for rifabutin plus azithromycin: P = 0.008 for rifabutin v azithromycin, P = 0.03 for combination v azithromycin).[13]

Harms:
In one RCT, dose limiting toxicity was more likely with azithromycin plus rifabutin than with azithromycin alone (hazard ratio 1.67; P = 0.03).[13] In another RCT adverse events occurred in 31% of people receiving the combination of clarithromycin and rifabutin compared with 16% on clarithromycin alone and 18% on rifabutin alone (P < 0.001).[24] Uveitis occurred in 42 people: 33 were on clarithromycin plus rifabutin, seven were on rifabutin alone, and two were on clarithromycin alone. **Uveitis:** We found one systematic review in 54 people with rifabutin associated uveitis (search date December 1996).[25] It found that uveitis was dose dependent. It occurred from 2 weeks to more than 7 months after initiation of rifabutin therapy, and was more likely in people taking rifabutin and clarithromycin. In most cases uveitis resolved 1–2 months after discontinuation of rifabutin.

Comment:
Prospective cohort studies have found that the risk of disseminated MAC disease increased substantially with a lower CD4 count and was clinically important only for CD4 < 50/mm^3.[1] Clarithromycin may inhibit rifabutin metabolism; rifabutin may decrease levels of delavirdine and saquinavir. See role of HAART in comment under azithromycin, p 416.

QUESTION	What are the effects of prophylaxis for disseminated MAC disease for people with previous MAC disease?

John Ioannidis

OPTION	COMBINATION THERAPY

RCTs found that clarithromycin and ethambutol, with or without rifabutin, reduced the incidence of MAC. Clofazimine and high dose clarithromycin were associated with increased mortality.

Benefits: We found no systematic review but found four RCTs. The first RCT in 95 people found that the combination of clarithromycin (1000 mg daily), clofazimine and ethambutol was associated with significantly fewer relapses of MAC than the combination of clarithromycin plus clofazimine without ethambutol (68% relapsed in three-drug regimen v 12% in two-drug regimen at 36 weeks; P = 0.004).[26] The second RCT (n = 106) found that the addition of clofazimine to clarithromycin and ethambutol did not improve clinical response and was associated with higher mortality.[27] The third RCT (n = 144) found that the combination of clarithromycin, rifabutin, and ethambutol reduced the relapse rate of MAC compared with clarithromycin plus clofazimine.[28] The fourth RCT found no difference in survival between people taking clarithromycin plus ethambutol and people taking clarithromycin plus ethambutol plus rifabutin.[29]

Harms: The second RCT, which added clofazimine to clarithromycin plus rifabutin, found a higher mortality in the clofazimine arm (62% with clofazimine v 38% without clofazimine; P = 0.012).[27] High doses of clarithromycin (1000 mg twice daily)[30,31] and clofazimine[27] were associated with increased mortality. One RCT of clarithromycin 500 mg bd compared with 1000 mg bd found that after a median follow up of 4.5 months, more people died with the higher dose (17/40 [43%] with 1000 mg bd v 10/45 [22%] with 500 mg bd; ARI 20%, 95% CI 0.2% to 33%; NNH 5, 95% CI 3 to 470).[30] A similar difference was seen in another RCT (n = 154).[31] Combinations of drugs may lead to increased toxicity. Optic neuropathy may occur with ethambutol, but has not been reported in RCTs in people with HIV where the dose and symptoms were carefully monitored.

Comment: The observed increased mortality associated with high doses of clarithromycin and clofazimine has led to avoidance of these drugs.

QUESTION | **What are the effects of prophylaxis for CMV, HSV and VZV?**

John Ioannidis

OPTION | **GANCICLOVIR**

One RCT found that oral ganciclovir reduced the incidence of CMV in people with severe CD4 depletion compared with placebo. It found that 25% of people who did not develop CMV developed severe neutropenia. A subsequent RCT found no significant differences.

Benefits: We found no systematic review. **Versus placebo:** We found two RCTs. The first RCT in 725 people with a median CD4 count of 22/mm^3 found that oral ganciclovir halved the incidence of CMV compared with placebo (event rate 16% v 30%; P = 0.001).[32] The second RCT in 994 HIV-1 infected people with CD4 < 100/mm^3 and CMV seropositivity found no difference in the rate of CMV in people taking oral ganciclovir compared with placebo (event rates 13.1 v 14.6 per 100 person years; hazard ratio 0.92, 95% CI 0.65 to 1.27).[33] Both RCTs found no significant difference in overall mortality.

Harms: In the first RCT, 25% of people who did not develop CMV developed severe neutropenia (and were then treated with granulocyte colony stimulating factor).[32]

Comment: Differences in the results of RCTs may have arisen by chance or protocol variability; for example, no baseline ophthalmologic examinations were performed in the second trial.[33] The low incidence of CMV disease in people taking HAART, and the high rates of adverse events, means that the clinical value of oral ganciclovir in people who have not had active CMV disease is unclear.

OPTION **ACICLOVIR AND VALACICLOVIR**

A systematic review found that aciclovir did not reduce the incidence of CMV compared with placebo, but significantly reduced HSV and VZV infection and overall mortality in people at different clinical stages of HIV infection. One RCT found that valaciclovir reduced the incidence of CMV more than aciclovir, but was associated with increased mortality.

Benefits: We found one systematic review of individual data (8 RCTs, search date not stated) in people with asymptomatic HIV infection to full-blown AIDS. It found no difference in protection against CMV disease between aciclovir compared with no therapy or placebo. However, aciclovir significantly reduced overall mortality (RR 0.81; P = 0.04), HSV, and VZV infections (P < 0.001 for both).[34] One RCT in 1227 CMV seropositive people with CD4 < 100/mm^3 compared valaciclovir, high dose aciclovir, and low dose aciclovir. It found increased mortality in the valaciclovir group, which did not reach statistical significance (P = 0.06).[35] The CMV rate was lower in the valaciclovir group than the aciclovir groups (11.7% v 17.5%; P = 0.03).

Harms: In the RCT, toxicity and early medication discontinuations were significantly more frequent in the valaciclovir arm (1 year discontinuation rate: 51% for valaciclovir v 46% for high dose aciclovir v 41% for low dose aciclovir).[35]

Comment: The survival benefit with aciclovir is unclear. The absolute risk reduction may be higher in people who have frequent HSV or VZV infections.

OPTION **FAMCICLOVIR**

One small RCT found that famciclovir compared with placebo reduced the rate of viral shedding, but provided insufficient evidence on the effect of famciclovir on HSV recurrence.

Benefits: We found no systematic review. One small crossover placebo controlled RCT (n = 48) found that famciclovir suppressed HSV in people with frequent recurrences (HSV was isolated in 9/1071 famciclovir days v 122/1114 placebo days; P < 0.001).[36] Breakthrough reactivations on famciclovir were shortlived and often asymptomatic.

Harms: Famciclovir was well tolerated, and the incidence of adverse effects was similar in both groups.

Comment: The conclusions of this study are difficult to interpret. The randomisation process allocated participants to groups, but the intention to treat analysis involved the number of days with symptoms rather than the number of participants who improved. There was no assessment of statistical significance of clinical outcomes. The trials' completer analysis is impeded by a high dropout rate.

> **QUESTION** What are the effects of prophylaxis for invasive fungal disease in people without previous fungal disease?

John Ioannidis

> **OPTION** AZOLES

RCTs have found that both fluconazole and itraconazole reduce the incidence of invasive fungal infections compared with placebo in people with advanced HIV disease. One RCT found that fluconazole reduced the incidence of invasive fungal disease and mucocutaneous candidiasis more than clotrimazole. One RCT found no difference between high and low dose fluconazole.

Benefits: We found no systematic review. **Fluconazole versus placebo:** One RCT in 323 women with CD4 $\leq 300/mm^3$ found that fluconazole was more effective in reducing the incidence of candidiasis than placebo (44% v 58% suffered at least one episode of candidiasis; RR 0.56, 95% CI 0.41 to 0.77).[37] **Itraconazole versus placebo:** One RCT in 295 people with advanced HIV disease found that itraconazole reduced the incidence of invasive fungal infections (6 v 19; P = 0.0007).[38] It found no significant effect on recurrent or refractory candidiasis.[39] **High dose versus low dose fluconazole:** One RCT (n = 636) compared fluconazole 200 mg daily with 400 mg once weekly and found no difference in the rate of invasive fungal infections over a follow up of 74 weeks (7.7% v 5.5%; ARR 2.2%, 95% CI −1.7% to +6.%). However the incidence of thrush was twice as common in people taking the weekly dose.[40] **Fluconazole versus clotrimazole:** One RCT found that fluconazole reduced the incidence of invasive fungal disease and mucocutaneous candidal infections compared with clotrimazole (4.1% v 10.9%; relative hazard 3.3, 95% CI 1.5 to 7.6).[39] None of the above RCTs found any difference in mortality.

Harms: Congenital anomalies have occurred in a few children born to mothers receiving fluconazole. Itraconazole is embryotoxic and teratogenic in animals. Azoles may interact with antiretroviral regimens.[41] Azole drugs inhibit the metabolism of terfenadine, astemizole, or cisapride. Theoretically they may increase the risk of sudden death due to ventricular tachycardia.

Comment: Azoles effectively reduce invasive fungal disease. Any absolute benefit is probably even lower in people treated with HAART. Lack of evidence of any survival benefit, potential for complex drug interactions with current antiretroviral regimens, and potential for developing resistant fungal isolates, means that there is doubt about routine anti-fungal prophylaxis in HIV infected people without previous invasive fungal disease.

QUESTION | What are the effects of prophylaxis for invasive fungal disease in people with previous fungal disease?

John Ioannidis

OPTION | AZOLES

One RCT found that itraconazole reduced the incidence of relapse of Penicillium marneffei (see glossary, p 425) infection. One RCT found itraconazole was more effective in reducing the relapse of cryptococcal meningitis compared with fluconazole.

Benefits: We found no systematic review. **Itraconazole versus placebo:** One RCT in 71 people with AIDS in Asia found that itraconazole reduced the relapse of *Penicillium marneffei* infection compared with placebo (0/36 [0%] v 20/35 [57%] relapsed within 1 year; P < 0.001).[42] **Itraconazole versus fluconazole:** One RCT in 108 people with HIV infection found that itraconazole reduced relapses of successfully treated cryptococcal meningitis more than fluconazole (13/57 [23%] v 2/51 [4%]; ARR 19%, 95% CI 6.2 to 31.7; RR 0.17, 95% CI 0.04 to 0.71; NNT 5, 95% CI 3 to 16).[43] The trial was stopped early, because of the higher rate of relapse with fluconazole.

Harms: In the second RCT, discontinuation of itraconazole occurred in two people because of skin rashes, one due to severe anaemia and one due to gastrointestinal effects compared with none taking fluconazole.[43]

Comment: In addition to these studies, one open label uncontrolled study (n = 44) found that itraconazole may be effective in preventing the relapse of histoplasmosis.[44] Recurrent infection is common in people with previous *C neoformans, H capsulatum,* and *Penicillium marneffei* infections. Maintenance for life may be needed in the presence of immune impairment.

QUESTION | What are the effects of discontinuing prophylaxis against opportunistic pathogens in people on HAART?

John Ioannidis

OPTION | DISCONTINUATION OF PROPHYLAXIS FOR PCP AND TOXOPLASMOSIS IN PEOPLE WITH CD4 > 200/MM^3 ON HAART

Two unblinded RCTs found that discontinuation of prophylaxis did not increase the incidence of PCP or toxoplasmosis.

Benefits: We found no systematic review. We found two unblinded RCTs. The first RCT (abstract only) in 332 people with a satisfactory response to HAART (CD4 > 200/mm^3 and viral load < 5000 copies/mm3 for > 3 months) compared discontinuation with continuation of PCP prophylaxis.[45] It found no PCP episodes in either group over a mean follow up of 6.6 months. The second RCT, in 302 people with a satisfactory response to HAART, compared discontinuation with continuation of toxoplasma prophylaxis.[46] It found no episodes of toxoplasmic encephalitis in either group over a median of 10 months. A new trial related to discontinuation of primary prophylaxis for Pneumocystis carinii pneumonia and toxoplasmic encephlitis in human immunodeficiencey virus type I-infected people has been recently published and will be considered in future issues.[47]

Harms: The trials found no direct harms from discontinuing prophylaxis.

Comment: We found a number of retrospective and prospective cohort studies (see table 1, p 429).[48–56] They all found that discontinuation of prophylaxis was safe in people with adequate response to antiretroviral therapy and appropriate recovery of the CD4 cell count. The risk of PCP may increase again in people who do not respond to antiretroviral therapy. We found no direct evidence on the effects of different HAART regimens on the risk of PCP or toxoplasmosis. Antiretroviral regimens with different mechanisms of action may have different clinical effects on opportunistic infections and HIV disease progression, despite inducing satisfactory suppression of HIV-1 replication and adequate CD4 responses. Also, CD4 cell count is an incomplete marker of immune reconstitution. It is theoretically conceivable that people with the same CD4 count may have different immune deficits regarding control of PCP and other opportunistic pathogens. An extensive amount of research is being conducted on other parameters of immune reconstitution, but the clinical implications are uncertain at present.

OPTION DISCONTINUATION OF PROPHYLAXIS FOR MAC DISEASE IN PEOPLE WITH CD4 > 100/MM^3 ON HAART

One RCT found that discontinuation of prophylaxis for MAC disease did not increase the incidence of MAC disease.

Benefits: We found no systematic review. We found one RCT in 520 people without previous MAC disease, with CD4 > 100/mm^3 in response to HAART, which compared azithromycin with placebo.[57] There were no episodes of confirmed MAC disease in either group over a median follow up of 12 months.

Harms: Adverse effects leading to discontinuation of therapy were more common with azithromycin than with placebo (7.4% v 1.1%; $P = 0.002$).

Comment: It is not clear whether different antiretroviral regimens may have different clinical effects on opportunistic infections and the need for specific prophylaxis.

OPTION DISCONTINUATION OF MAINTENANCE THERAPY FOR CMV IN PEOPLE WITH A CD4 > 100/MM^3 ON HAART

We found insufficient evidence on the effects of discontinuation of maintenance therapy for CMV retinitis or other end organ disease.

Benefits: We found no systematic review or RCTs.

Harms: WE found no evidence from systematic reviews or RCTs.

Comment: We found several small case series (see table 2, p 429).[58–64] No cases of CMV retinitis reactivation or progression were recorded in the six studies with average follow up less than 1 year. The study with longer follow up (mean 14.5 months) found five relapses among 17 participants who withdrew from maintenance; all of them occurred after the CD4 cell count had dropped again to below 50/mm^3 (8 days to 10 months after this event).[59] In one observational series 12/14 participants had evidence of immune reconstitution retinitis even before starting withdrawal of prophylaxis.[58] Worsening uveitis was associated with a substantial vision loss (> 3 lines) in three participants. It is difficult to conduct an RCT of adequate sample size to exclude modest differences in relapse rates. The observational evidence suggests that withdrawal of CMV maintenance therapy may be considered in selected people in whom CMV disease is in remission, CD4 > 100mm^3, and HIV replication remains suppressed. We found no clear data on whether quantification of CMV viraemia should be considered in the decision to withdraw from maintenance. One small case series found that relapses were associated with a drop in the CD4 cell count.[59] However, we found no randomised or other reliable data of when CMV maintenance therapy should be reinstituted.

GLOSSARY

Immune reconstitution related syndromes are due to excess inflammation when the immune system is recovering on antiretroviral therapy.

Penicillium marneffei infection is a common opportunistic infection in Southeast Asia.

The WHO staging system for HIV infection and disease consists of a "clinical axis" which is represented by a sequential list of clinical conditions believed to have prognostic significance, which subdivides the course of HIV infection into four clinical stages; and a "laboratory axis" which subdivides each clinical stage into three strata according to CD4 cell count or total lymphocyte count.

REFERENCES

1. Gallant JE, Moore RD, Chaisson RE. Prophylaxis for opportunistic infections in patients with HIV infection. *Ann Intern Med* 1994;120:932–44.

2. Ioannidis JPA, Cappelleri JC, Skolnik PR, Lau J, Sacks HS. A meta-analysis of the relative efficacy and toxicity of *Pneumocystis carinii* prophylactic regimens. *Arch Intern Med* 1996;156:177–88. search date to late 1995; primary sources MEDLINE and conference abstracts.

3. Anglaret X, Chene G, Attia A, et al. Early chemoprophylaxis with trimethroprim-sulphamethoxazole for HIV-1-infected adults in Abidjan, cote d'Ivoire: a randomized trial. *Lancet* 1999;353:1463–1468.

4. Bucher HC, Griffith L, Guyatt GH, Opravil M. Meta-analysis of prophylactic treatments against *Pneumocystis carinii* pneumonia and toxoplasma encephalitis in HIV-infected patients. *J Acquir Immune Defic Syndr Hum Retrovirol* 1997;15: 104–114.

5. El-Sadr W, Luskin-Hawk R, Yurik TM, et al. A randomized trial of daily and thrice weekly trimethoprim-sulfamethoxazole for the prevention of *Pneumocystis carinii* pneumonia in HIV-infected individuals. *Clin Infect Dis* 1999;29:775–783.

6. Leoung G, Stanford J, Giordano M, et al. A randomized, double-blind trial of TMP/SMX dose escalation v direct challenge in HIV+ persons at risk for PCP and with prior treatment-limiting rash

or fever. In: Abstracts of the 37th Interscience Conference on Antimicrobial Agents and Chemotherapy. Washington, DC: American Society for Microbiology, 1997. Abstract no. LB10.

7. Para MF, Dolin M, Frame P, et al for the ACTG 268 Study Team. ACTG 268 Trial – gradual initiation of trimethoprim/sulfamethoxazole (T/S) as primary prophylaxis for *Pneumocystis carinii* pneumonia (PCP). In: Program and abstracts: 4th Conference on Retroviruses and Opportunistic Infections. Alexandria, Virginia: Westover Management Group, 1997. Abstract no. 2.

8. Walmsley SL, Khorasheh S, Singer J, Djurdjev O. A randomized trial of N-acetylcysteine for prevention of trimethoprim-sulfamehtoxazole hypersensitivity reactions in *Pneumocystis carinii* pneumonia prophylaxis (CTN057). Canadian HIV Trials Network 057 Study Group. *J Acquir Immune Defic Syndr Hum Retrovirol* 1998;19:498–505.

9. Akerlund B, Tynell E, Bratt G, Bielenstein M, Lidman C. N-acetylcysteine treatment and the risk of toxic reactions to trimethoprim-sulphamethoxazole in primary *Pneumocystis carinii* prophylaxis in HIV-infected patients. *J Infect* 1997; 35:143–147.

10. El Sadr WM, Murphy RL, Yurik TM, et al. Atovaquone compared with dapsone for the prevention of *Pneumocystis carinii* pneumonia in patients with HIV infection who cannot tolerate

trimethoprim, sulfonamides, or both. Community Programs for clinical Research on AIDS and the AIDS Clinical Trials Group. *N Engl J Med* 1998; 339:1889–1895.

11. Chan C, Montaner J, Lefebre EA, et al. Atovaquone suspension compared with aerosolized pentamidine for prevention of *Pneumocystis carinii* in human immunodeficiency virus-infected subjects intolerant of trimethoprim or sulfonamides. *J Infect Dis* 1999;180:369–376.

12. Dunne MW, Bozzette S, McCutchan JA, et al. Efficacy of azithromycin in prevention of *Pneumocystis carinii* pneumonia: a randomized trial. California Collaborative Treatment Group. *Lancet* 1999;354:891–895.

13. Havlir DV, Dube MP, Sattler FR, et al. Prophylaxis against disseminated *Mycobacterium avium* complex with weekly azithromycin, daily rifabutin, or both. California Collaborative Treatment Group. *N Engl J Med* 1996;335:392–398.

14. Wilkinson D. Drugs for preventing tuberculosis in HIV infected persons. In: The Cochrane Library, Issue 4, 1999. Oxford: Update software. Search date July/August 1998; primary sources Cochrane Infectious Diseases Group Trials Register; Cochrane Controlled Trials Register Issue 3, 1998; Medline 1982 to 1998, Embase 1980 to 1998, and hand searched references.

15. Bucher HC, Griffith LE, Guyatt GH, et al. Isoniazid prophylaxis for tuberculosis in HIV infection: a meta-analysis of randomised controlled trials. *AIDS* 1999;13:501–507. Search date not given; primary sources Medline, Embase, CAB Health, Biosis, Health Star, IDIS Drug File, DHSS-Data, Medical Toxicology and Health, Drug Information, AIDSLINE, AIDSTRIAL, AIDSDRUG, Cochrane Controlled Trials Register, hand search references, and conference proceedings.

16. Selwyn PA, Hartel D, Lewis VA, et al. A prospective study of the risk of tuberculosis among intravenous drug users with human immunodeficiency virus infection. *N Engl J Med* 1989;320:545–550.

17. Halsey NA, Coberly JS, Desmormeaux J, et al. Randomised trial of isoniazid versus rifampicin and pyrazinamide for prevention of tuberculosis in HIV-1 infection. *Lancet* 1998;351:786–792.

18. Mwinga A, Hosp M, Godfrey-Fausset P, et al. Twice weekly tuberculosis preventive therapy in HIV infection in Zambia. *AIDS* 1998;12:2447–2457.

19. Gordin F, Chaisson RE, Matts JP, et al. Rifampin and Pyrazinamide vs Isoniazid for Prevention of Tuberculosis in HIV-Infected Persons: An International Randomized Trial. *JAMA* 2000;283: 1445–1450.

20. Whalen CC, Johson JL, Okwera A, et al. A trial of threee regimens to prevent tuberculosis in Ugandan adults with the human immunodeficiency virus. *N Engl J Med* 1997;337:801–808.

21. Oldfield EC, Fessel WJ, Dunne MW, et al. Once weekly azithromycin therapy for prevention of *Mycobacterium avium* complex infection in patients with AIDS: a randomized, double-blind, placebo-controlled multicenter trial. *Clin Infect Dis* 1998;26:611–619.

22. Faris MA, Raasch RH, Hopfer RL, Butts JD. Treatment and prophylaxis of disseminated *Mycobacterium avium* complex in HIV-infected individuals. *Ann Pharmacother* 1998;32:564–573. Search date 1997; primary sources Medline 1966 to 1997, Aidsline 1980 to 1997.

23. Pierce M, Crampton S, Henry D, et al. A randomized trial of clarithromycin as prophylaxis against disseminated *Mycobacterium avium* complex infection in patients with advanced immunodeficiency syndrome. *N Engl J Med* 1996; 335:384–391.

24. Benson CA, Williams PL, Cohn DL, et al. Clarithromycin or rifabutin alone or in combination for primary prophylaxis of *Mycobacterium avium* complex disease in patients with AIDS: a randomized, double-blind, placebo-controlled trial. *J Infect Dis* 2000;181:1289–1297.

25. Tseng AL, Walmsley SL. Rifabutin-associated uveitis. *Ann Pharmacother* 1995;29:1149–1155.

26. Dube MP, Sattler FR, Torriani FJ, et al. A randomized evaluation of ethambutol for prevention of relapse and drug resistance during treatment of *Mycobacterium avium* complex bacteremia with clarithromycin-based combination therapy. *J Infect Dis* 1997;176:1225–1232.

27. Chaisson RE, Keiser P, Pierce M, et al. Clarithromycin and ethambutol with or without clofazimine for the treatment of bacteremic *Mycobacterium avium* complex disease in patients with HIV infection. *AIDS* 1997;11:311–317.

28. May T, Brel F, Beuscart C, et al. Comparison of combination therapy regimens for the treatment of human immunodeficiency virus-infected patients with disseminated bacteremia due to *Mycobacterium avium*. ANRS Trial 033 Curavium Group. Agence Nationale de Reserche sur le Sida. *Clin Infect Dis* 1997;25:621–629.

29. Gordin F, Sullam P, Shafran S, et al. A placebo-controlled trial of rifabutin added to a regimen of clarithromycin and ethambutol in the treatment of *M. avium* complex bacteremia. *Clin Infect Dis* 1999;28:1080–1085.

30. Cohn DL, Fisher EJ, Peng GT, et al. A prospective randomized trial of four three-drug regimens in the treatment of disseminated *Mycobacterium avium* complex disease in AIDS patients: excess mortality associated with high-dose clarithromycin. Terry Beirn Programs for Clinical Research on AIDS. *Clin Infect Dis* 1999;29:125–133.

31. Chaisson RE, Benson CA, Dube MP, et al. Clarithromycin therapy for bacteremic *Mycobacterium avium* complex disease: a randomized, double-blind, dose-ranging study in patients with AIDS. *Ann Intern Med* 1994;121: 905–911.

32. Spector SA, McKinley GF, Lalezari JP, et al. Oral ganciclovir for the prevention of cytomegalovirus disease in persons with AIDS. Roche Cooperative Oral Ganciclovir Study Group. *N Engl J Med* 1996; 334:1491–1497.

33. Brosgart CL, Louis TA, Hillman DW, et al. A randomized, placebo-controlled trial of the safety and efficacy of oral ganciclovir for prophylaxis of cytomegalovirus disease in HIV-infected individuals. Terry Beirn Community Programs for Clinical Research on AIDS. *AIDS* 1998;12:269–277.

34. Ioannidis JPA, Collier AC, Cooper DA, et al. Clinical efficacy of high-dose acyclovir in patients with human immunodeficiency virus infection: a meta-analysis of randomized individual patient data. *J Infect Dis* 1998;178:349–359. Search date not stated; primary sources Medline; abstract searching from major meetings; trial directories; and communication with experts, investigators of the identified trials, and industry researchers.

35. Feinberg JE, Hurwitz S, Cooper D, et al. A randomized, double-blind trial of valaciclovir prophylaxis for cytomegalovirus disease in patients with advanced human immunodeficiency virus infection. AIDS Clinical Trials Group Protocol 204/ Glaxo Wellcome 123–014 International CMV Prophylaxis Study Group. *J Infect Dis* 1998;177: 48–56.

36. Schacker T, Hu HL, Koelle DM, et al. Famciclovir for the suppression of symptomatic and asymptomatic herpes simplex virus reactivation in HIV-infected persons: a double-blind, placebo-

controlled trial. *Ann Intern Med* 1998;128:21–28.

37. Schuman P, Capps L, Peng G, et al. Weekly fluconazole for the prevention of mucosal candidiasis in women with HIV infection: a randomized, double-blind, placebo-controlled trial. *Ann Intern Med* 1997;126:689–696.

38. McKinsey DS, Wheat LJ, Cloud GA, et al. Itraconazole prophylaxis for fungal infections in patients with advanced human immunodeficiency virus infection: randomized, placebo-controlled, double-blind study. National Institute of Allergy and Infectious diseases Mycoses Study Group. *Clin Infect Dis* 1999;28:1049–1056.

39. Powderly WG, Finkelstein DM, Feinberg J, et al. A randomized trial comparing fluconazole with clotrimazole troches for the prevention of fungal infections in patients with advanced human immunodeficiency virus infection. *N Engl J Med* 1995;332:700–705.

40. Havlir DV, Dube MP, McCutchan JA, et al. Prophylaxis with weekly versus daily fluconazole for fungal infections in patients with AIDS. *Clin Infect Dis* 1998;27:253–256.

41. Tseng AL, Foisy MM. Management of drug interactions in patients with HIV. *Ann Pharmacother* 1997;31:1040–1058.

42. Supparatpinyo K, Perriens J, Nelson KE, Sirisanthana T. A controlled trial of itraconazole to prevent relapse of *Penicillium marneffei* infection in patients with the human immunodeficiency virus. *New Engl J Med* 1998;339:1739–1743.

43. Saag MS, Cloud GA, Graybill JR, et al. A comparison of itraconazole versus fluconazole as maintenance therapy for AIDS-associated cryptococcal meningitis. *Clin Infect Dis* 1999;28: 291–296.

44. Wheat J, Hafner R, Wulfsohn M, et al. Prevention of relapse of histoplasmosis with itraconazole in patients with the acquired immunodeficiency syndrome. *Ann Intern Med* 1993;118:610–616.

45. Lopez JC, Pena JM, Miro JM, Podzamczer D, and the GESIDA 04/98 study group. Discontinuation of PCP prophylaxis (PRO) is safe in HIV-infected patients (PTS) with immunological recovery with HAART. Preliminary results of an open, randomized and multicentric clinical trial (GESIDA 04/98). In: Abstracts of the 6th Conference on Retroviruses and Opportunistic Infections, Alexandria, Virginia: Foundation for Retrovirology and Human Health, 1999. Abstract no. LB7.

46. Mussinin C, Pezzotti P, Govoni A, Borghi V, Antinori A, D'Arminio Monforte A, De Luca A, Mongiardo N, Cerri MC, Chiodo F,Conica E, Bonazzi L, Moroni M, Ortona L, Esposito R, Cossarizza A, De Rienzo B. Discontinuation of primary prophylaxis for Pneumocystis carinii pneumonia and toxoplasmic encephalitis in human immunodeficiency virus type I-infected patients: the changes in opportunistic prphylaxis study. *J Infect Dis* 2000; 181:1635–42.

47. Miro JM, Lopez JC, Podzamcer D, et al, and the GESIDA 04/98B study group. Discontinuation of toxoplasmic encephalitis prophylaxis is safe in HIV-1 and T. gondii co-infected patients after immunological recovery with HAART. Preliminary results of the GESIDA 04/98-B study. In: Abstracts of the 7th Conference on Retroviruses and Opportunistic Infections, Alexandria, Virginia: Foundation for Retrovirology and Human Health. Abstract no. 230.

48. Koletar SL, Heald AE, Murphy RL, et al. Discontinuing primary and secondary PCP prophylaxis in patients who have increased CD4 counts in response to antiretroviral therapy: preliminary results – ACTG 888. In: Abstracts of the 7th Conference on Retroviruses and Opportunistic Infections, Alexandria, Virginia:

Foundation for Retrovirology and Human Health. Abstract no. 243.

49. Lederberger B, Mocroft A, Reiss P, et al. Is it safe to discontinue secondary prophylaxis for PCP in HIV-infected patients treated with HAART: results from eight prospective European cohorts. In: Abstracts of the 7th Conference on Retroviruses and Opportunistic Infections, Alexandria, Virginia: Foundation for Retrovirology and Human Health. Abstract no. LB5.

50. Yangco BG, Von Bargen JC, Moorman AC, Holmberg SD. Discontinuation of chemoprophylaxis against *Pneumocystis carinii* pneumonia in patients with HIV infection. HIV outpatient study (HOPS) investigators. *Ann Intern Med* 2000;132:201–205.

51. Kirk O, Lundgren JD, Pedersen C, Nielsen H, Gerstoft J. Can chemoprophylaxis against opportunistic infections be discontinued after an increase in CD4 cells induced by highly active antiretroviral therapy? *AIDS* 1999;13:1647–1651.

52. Furrer H, Egger M, Opravil M, et al. Discontinuation of primary prophylaxis against *Pneumocystis carinii* pneumonia in HIV-1 infected adults treated with combination antiretroviral therapy. Swiss HIV cohort Study. *N Engl J Med* 1999;340:1301–1306.

53. Furrer H, Opravil M, Rossi M, et al. The Swiss StopCox study: is it safe to discontinue PCP prophylaxis in patients with detectable viremia, low nadir CD4 count or T. gondii seropositivity? In: Abstracts of the 7th Conference on Retroviruses and Opportunistic Infections, Alexandria, Virginia: Foundation for Retrovirology and Human Health. Abstract no. 244.

54. Weverling GJ, Mocroft A, Lederberger B, et al. Discontinuation of *Pneumocystis carinii* pneumonia prophylaxis after start of highly active antiretroviral therapy in HIV-1 infection. EuroSIDA Study Group. *Lancet* 1999;353:1293–1298.

55. Schneider MM, Borleffs JC, Stolk RP, Jaspers CA, Hoepelman AI. Discontinuation of prophylaxis for *Pneumocystis carinii* pneumonia in HIV-1-infected patients treated with highly active antiretroviral therapy. *Lancet* 1999;353:201–203.

56. Garcia Vazquez E, de Gorgolas Hernandez M, Garcia Delgado R, Fernandez Guerrero ML. Withdrawal of *Pneumocystis carinii* pneumonia prophylaxis in patients receiving efficacious combined antiretroviral treatment. Study of 85 cases. *Med Clin (Barc)* 1999;113:89–90.

57. El-Sadr WM, Burman WJ, Grant LB, et al. Discontinuation of prophylaxis for *Mycobacterium avium* complex disease in HIV-infected patients who have a response to antiretroviral therapy. *N Engl J Med* 2000;342:1085–1092.

58. Whitcup SM, Fortin E, Lindblad AS, et al. Discontinuation of anticytomegalovirus therapy in patients with HIV infection and cytomegalovirus retinitis. *JAMA* 1999;282:1633–1637.

59. Torriani FJ, Freeman WR, MacDonald JC, et al. CMV retinitis recurs after stopping treatment in virological and immunological failure of potent antiretroviral therapy. *AIDS* 2000;14:173–180.

60. Postelmans L, Gerald M, Sommereijns B, Caspers-Velu L. Discontinuation of maintenance therapy for CMV retinitis in AIDS patients on highly active antiretroviral therapy. *Ocul Immunol Inflamm* 1999;7:199–203.

61. Jabs DA, Bolton SG, Dunn JP, Palestine AG. Discontinuing anticytomegalovirus therapy in patients with immune reconstitution after combination therapy. *Am J Opthalmol* 1998;126: 817–822.

62. Vrabec TR, Baldassano VF, Whitcup SM. Discontinuation of maintenance therapy in

patients with quiescent cytomegalovirus retinitis and elevated CD4+ counts. *Ophthalmology* 1998; 105:1259–1264.

63. McDonald JC, Torriani FJ, Morse LS, Karavellas MP, Reed JB, Freeman WR. Lack of reactivation of cytomegalovirus (CMV) retinitis after stopping CMV maintenance therapy in AIDS patients with sustained elevations in CD4 T cells in response to highly active antiretroviral therapy. *J Infect Dis* 1998;177:1182–1187.

64. Tural C, Romeu J, Sirera G, et al. Long-lasting remission of cytomegalovirus retinitis without maintenance therapy in human immunodeficiency virus-infected patients. *J Infect Dis* 1998;177: 1080–1083.

John Ioannidis
Chairman
Department of Hygiene and Epidemiology, University of Ioannina School of Medicine
Ioannina
Greece

Margaret Johnson
Consultant in HIV Medicine
Royal Free Hospital
London
UK

Andrew Phillips
Professor
Royal Free Centre for HIV Medicine and Department of Primary Care and Population Sciences, Royal Free and University College Medical School
London
UK

David Wilkinson
Professor
South Australian Centre for Rural and Remote Health University of Adelaide and University of South Australia
Whyalla
Australia

Competing interests: None declared.

TABLE 1	Observational studies of discontinuation of PCP prophylaxis (see text, p 424).			
Author	Criteria for discontinuation	Participants (prior PCP)	Person (years)	PCP events
Koletar[48]	CD4 > 200 sustained	269 (125)	186	0
Lederberger*[49]	CD4 277–371 (8 cohorts)	246 (246)	236	0
Yangco[50]	CD4 > 200 sustained	146 (0)	221	0
Kirk[51]	Increased CD4 for ≥ 6 months	219 (26)	174	1
Furrer[52,53]	CD4 > 200 and >14% for ≥ 12 weeks	381 (0)	473	1
Weverling[54]	CD4 274 median	378 (59)	247	0
Schneider[55]	CD4 > 200 twice, 1 month apart	78 (16)	83	0
Vazquez[56]	CD4 > 200	85 (6)	84	0

Studies with at least 80 person years of follow up are included in the table.*Combined analysis from eight cohorts of prophylaxis discontinuations among people with previous PCP; it may include prophylaxis discontinuations from Schneider et al,[55] Weverling et al,[54] and Kirk et al.[50] CD4 count is measured in cells/mm^3. PCP, Pneumocystis carinii pneumonia.

TABLE 2	Observational studies of discontinuation of CMV maintenance therapy in people with previous CMV disease (see text, p 425).		
Author	Criteria for discontinuation	Participants	Follow up (months)	Relapses
Torriani*[59]	CD4 > 70	17	14.5 (mean)	5
Postelmans[60]	CD4 ≥ 75	8	8 (median)	0
Whitcup[58]	CD4 > 150	14	16.4 (mean)	0
Jabs[61]	CD4 297 median	15	8 (median)	0
Vrabec[62]	CD4 > 100	8	11.4 (mean)	0
McDonald*[63]	(183 median)	11	5 (median)	0
Tural[64]	CD4 > 150, VL < 200/ml −ve CMV by PCR	7	9 (median)	0

Studies with more than five people are included. CD4 count is measured in cells/mm^3; CMV, cytomegalovirus; PCR, polymerase chain reaction; VL, viral load (HIV-1 RNA in plasma).*McDonald et al is an early report of the same study followed by the Torriani et al report. All relapses in the latter report occurred in people who had already experienced a decrease of CD4 to < 50 cells/mm^3.

Postherpetic neuralgia

Last updated Issue 3

John Yaphe and Tim Lancaster

INTERVENTIONS

Key Messages

Preventing postherpetic neuralgia

- One systematic review of five RCTs has found that daily aciclovir reduces the relative risk of postherpetic pain at 6 months by about 50% compared with placebo. One RCT found that famciclovir significantly reduced pain duration after acute herpes zoster. Another RCT found that valaciclovir was associated with slightly decreased prevalence of postherpetic neuralgia compared with aciclovir. Another RCT found no advantage of netivudine over aciclovir.

- One systematic review of RCTs found idoxuridine to be associated with short term pain relief in acute herpes zoster but no evidence that it reduced the risk of postherpetic neuralgia.

- We found conflicting evidence from RCTs about the effects of corticosteroids alone on postherpetic neuralgia. We found limited evidence that high dose steroids added to antiviral agents may speed healing of acute herpes zoster, but we found no evidence that it reduces the risk of postherpetic neuralgia.

- One small RCT found that amitriptyline started during the acute episode was associated with a non-significantly reduced postherpetic neuralgia prevalence at 6 months.

- We found insufficient evidence on the effects of other drug treatments in acute herpes zoster.

Treating established postherpetic neuralgia

- One systematic review of RCTs has found that tricyclic antidepressants are associated with pain relief from postherpetic neuralgia.

- RCTs have found that topical counterirritants such as capsaicin are associated with relief of postherpetic neuralgia but can also cause painful skin reactions.

- One small RCT of lignocaine patches found short term pain relief in postherpetic neuralgia.

- One RCT found that gabapentin relieved postherpetic neuralgia.

- One crossover RCT found oral oxycodone to be associated with relief from postherpetic neuralgia. One small RCT found that epidural morphine was poorly tolerated and of little benefit. One RCT of dextromethorphan found no evidence of benefit.

DEFINITION	Postherpetic neuralgia is pain that sometimes follows resolution of acute herpes zoster and healing of the zoster rash. It can be severe, accompanied by itching, and follows the distribution of the original infection. Herpes zoster is an acute infection caused by activation of latent varicella zoster virus (human herpes virus 3) in people who have been rendered partially immune by a previous attack of chickenpox. Herpes zoster infects the sensory ganglia and their areas of innervation. It is characterised by pain along the distribution of the affected nerve and crops of clustered vesicles over the area.
INCIDENCE/ PREVALENCE	In a UK general practice survey of 321 cases, the annual incidence of herpes zoster was 3.4/1000.[1] Incidence varied with age. Herpes zoster was relatively uncommon in people under the age of 50 years (< 2/1000 per year) but rose to 5–7/1000 per year in people aged 50–79, and 11/1000 in people aged 80 years or older. In a population based study of 590 cases in Rochester, Minnesota, USA, the overall incidence was lower (1.5/1000) but with similar increases in incidence with age.[2] Prevalence of postherpetic neuralgia depends on when it is measured after acute infection, for which there is no agreed time point.
AETIOLOGY/ RISK FACTORS	The main risk factor for postherpetic neuralgia is increasing age. In a UK general practice study (involving 3600–3800 people) there was little risk in those under the age of 50 years, but postherpetic neuralgia developed in over 20% of people aged 60–65 and in 34% aged over 80.[1] No other risk factor has been found to predict consistently which people with herpes zoster will experience continued pain.
PROGNOSIS	About 2% of people in the UK general practice survey had pain for more than 5 years.[1] Prevalence of pain falls as time elapses after the initial episode. Among 183 people aged over 60 years in the placebo arm of a UK trial, the prevalence of pain was 61% at 1 month, 24% at 3 months, and 13% at 6 months after the acute infection.[3] In a more recent RCT, the prevalence of postherpetic pain at 6 months was 35% in 72 people over 60 years old in the placebo arm.[4]
AIMS	To prevent or reduce postherpetic neuralgia by intervention during acute attack; to reduce the severity and duration of established postherpetic neuralgia with minimal adverse effects of treatment.

Postherpetic neuralgia

OUTCOMES   Prevalence of persistent pain 6 months after resolution of acute infection and healing of rash. We did not consider short term outcomes such as rash healing or pain reduction during the acute episode. It is difficult to assess the clinical significance of reported changes in "average pain". We therefore present data as dichotomous outcomes where possible (pain absent or greatly reduced, or pain persistent).

METHODS   Our initial search was part of two systematic reviews of RCTs of treatments for acute herpes zoster and postherpetic neuralgia based on comprehensive searches of published and unpublished studies to 1993.[5,6] The details of the searches are described in the published reports. This search was updated by a *Clinical Evidence* search and appraisal from 1993 to November 1999. Where meta-analytic estimates from systematic reviews were available, these were taken to be the most reliable estimates of treatment effectiveness. In studies, the most common time point chosen for assessing the prevalence of persistent pain was 6 months, which we use in this review unless otherwise specified.

QUESTION   What are the effects of interventions during an acute attack of herpes zoster aimed at preventing postherpetic neuralgia?

OPTION   ORAL ANTIVIRAL AGENTS (ACICLOVIR, FAMCICLOVIR, VALACICLOVIR, NETIVUDINE)

One systematic review of five RCTs has found that daily aciclovir reduces the relative risk of postherpetic pain at 6 months by about 50% compared with placebo. One RCT found that famciclovir significantly reduced pain duration after acute herpes zoster. Another RCT found that valaciclovir was associated with slightly decreased prevalence of postherpetic neuralgia compared with aciclovir. Another RCT found no advantage of netivudine over aciclovir.

Benefits: **Aciclovir versus placebo:** We found two systematic reviews. The first review (search date 1993) pooled estimates from eight placebo controlled RCTs of aciclovir in both inpatient and general practice settings (n = 932). It found no significant pain reduction from aciclovir at 6 months (OR 0.70, 95% CI 0.47 to 1.06).[5] A more recent systematic review (search date 1997) identified five placebo controlled RCTs (n = 792) of oral aciclovir, including one not published at the time of the earlier systematic review. Taking a minimum of 4 g aciclovir daily for at least 7 days was associated with a significant reduction in prevalence of postherpetic neuralgia at 6 months (OR for presence of pain 0.54, 95% CI 0.36 to 0.81; ARR 0.16; NNT 7, 95% CI not available).[7] **Famciclovir versus placebo:** We found no systematic review. One multicentre RCT of famciclovir (2 doses) in immunocompetent adults (age > 18 years) defined duration of postherpetic neuralgia as time to pain resolution.[8] The trial reported a significant reduction in duration of pain after acute herpes zoster on both doses of famciclovir compared with placebo (median duration of pain with 500 mg [n = 138] 63 days, with 750 mg [n = 135] 61 days, with placebo [n = 146] 119 days). **Aciclovir versus other antivirals:** We found no systematic review. One RCT (n = 1141) compared valaciclovir (a precursor of aciclovir) given three times daily for 7 or 14 days versus 7 days of aciclovir.[9] When the results from the two valaciclovir regimens were combined, those treated with valaciclovir had a lower prevalence of pain at 6 months (RRR 8%; ARR 6%, 95% CI 1% to 11%; NNT 16, 95% CI 9 to 100). A second, double blind RCT of netivudine versus aciclovir (n = 511) found no difference in effectiveness between the two.[10] **Addition of amitriptyline:** We found no systematic review or RCTs.

Harms: The most common adverse effects reported with aciclovir were headache and nausea. In placebo controlled trials, these effects occurred with similar frequency with treatment and placebo (headache 37% v 43%, nausea 13% v 14%). There were no major adverse events reported in the RCTs included in the systematic review.[5] In the RCTs, famciclovir, valaciclovir, and netivudine had similar safety profiles to aciclovir.[8–10]

Comment: Adherence to treatment may be better with the newer antiviral drugs because they are given one to three times daily compared with five times daily for aciclovir. We found no evidence on adherence. Subsequent to our search we identified one systematic review, which will be considered in the next issue of *Clinical Evidence*.[11]

OPTION	TOPICAL ANTIVIRAL AGENTS (IDOXURIDINE) FOR RELIEF OF ACUTE PAIN ONLY

One systematic review of RCTs found idoxuridine to be associated with short term pain relief in acute herpes zoster and no evidence that it reduced the risk of postherpetic neuralgia.

Benefits: We found one systematic review (search date 1993), which identified three RCTs including 242 participants in total.[5] Two found treatment during acute attack to be associated with significant pain relief at 1 month but not at 6 months. However, pooled results were not reported because of heterogeneity and poor quality of the trials. The other RCT compared topical idoxuridine versus oral aciclovir. It found idoxuridine to be associated with greater pain relief at 1 month (OR 0.41, 95% CI 0.15 to 1.11) but no significant difference in prevalence of pain at 6 months (RR 0.38, 95% CI 0.13 to 1.00).[12]

Harms: We found no reports of significant adverse effects from idoxuridine. Application beneath dressings may be cumbersome.

Comment: Subsequent to our search we identified another systematic review, which will be considered in the next issue of *Clinical Evidence*.[11]

OPTION	CORTICOSTEROIDS

We found conflicting evidence from RCTs about the effects of corticosteroids alone on postherpetic neuralgia. We found limited evidence that high dose steroids added to antiviral agents may speed healing of acute herpes zoster, but we found no evidence that it reduces the risk of postherpetic neuralgia.

Benefits: **Corticosteroids alone:** We found one systematic review (search date 1993), which was conducted before antiviral agents were available. It included RCTs of corticosteroids with conflicting results and concluded that it was not possible to assess the effect of corticosteroids.[5] **Corticosteroids plus aciclovir:** We found no systematic review. We found two recent RCTs. One (n = 400) randomised people into four active treatment groups: 7 days of aciclovir (n = 101); 7 days of aciclovir and 21 days of prednisolone (n = 99); 21 days of aciclovir (n = 101); or 21 days of aciclovir plus prednisolone (n = 99).[13] There were no significant differences in relief of posterpetic neuralgia between groups. The second RCT (n = 208) had a factorial design, randomising participants to 21 days of aciclovir plus prednisone (60 mg initially, tapered over 3 weeks), prednisone plus placebo, aciclovir plus placebo, or two placebos. Although there was evidence of short term benefit from prednisone, there was no significant effect of prednisone on pain prevalence at 6 months after disease onset.[14]

Harms: It is feared that corticosteroids might cause dissemination of herpes zoster. This effect was not reported in the RCT of prednisolone.[5] In the aciclovir plus prednisone trial, two people receiving prednisone plus aciclovir placebo and one receiving aciclovir plus prednisone placebo developed cutaneous dissemination of lesions.[14]

Comment: Subsequent to our search we identified one systematic review, which will be considered in the next issue of *Clinical Evidence*.[11]

OPTION TRICYCLIC ANTIDEPRESSANTS (AMITRIPTYLINE)

One small RCT found that amitriptyline started during the acute episode was associated with a non-significantly reduced prevalence of posterpetic neuralgia at 6 months.

Benefits: We found no systematic review. We found one double blind, placebo controlled RCT of amitriptyline 25 mg taken within 48 hours of rash onset and continued for 90 days in 72 people aged over 60 years.[4] Amitriptyline was associated with a non significantly reduced prevalence of posterpetic neuralgia at 6 months (RRR 0.55; ARR 0.19, 95% CI −0.003 to +0.39).

Harms: The RCT did not report adverse effects.[4] In another RCT, amitriptyline was associated with adverse anticholinergic effects such as dry mouth, sedation, and urinary difficulties.[5]

Comment: Interpretation of the RCT is complicated because practitioners were allowed to decide whether an antiviral agent was prescribed as well as amitriptyline.[4]

OPTION OTHER DRUG TREATMENTS

We found insufficient evidence on the effects of other drug treatments in acute herpes zoster.

Benefits: We found one systematic review (search date 1993), which identified small, single RCTs of adenosine monophosphate, amantadine, and levodopa.[5] These trials reported some short term benefit in treating herpes zoster. No benefit was found in small studies of cimetidine and isoprinosine.[5]

Harms: We found no evidence.

Comment: Subsequent to our search we identified one systematic review, which will be considered in the next issue of *Clinical Evidence*.[11]

QUESTION What are the effects of interventions after the rash has healed to relieve established postherpetic neuralgia?

OPTION TRICYCLIC ANTIDEPRESSANTS

One systematic review of RCTs has found that tricyclic antidepressants are associated with pain relief from postherpetic neuralgia.

Benefits: We found one systematic review (search date 1993, 3 RCTs, n = 216).[6] Two trials compared amitriptyline with placebo, and the third compared desipramine with placebo. In pooled analysis, taking tricyclic antidepressants for 3–6 weeks was significantly associated with pain relief from postherpetic neuralgia at the end of the treatment period (OR for complete or large reduction in pain at end of treatment period 0.15, 95% CI 0.08 to 0.27).

Harms: Tricyclic antidepressants are associated with anticholinergic adverse effects. In one trial, dry mouth (38%), sedation (38%), and urinary difficulties (21%) were the most common adverse effects.[15] Syncope and heart block were encountered in one person in a trial of desipramine in people with postherpetic neuralgia.[16]

Comment: The adverse effects of tricyclic antidepressants are dose related. They may therefore be less pronounced when used to treat postherpetic neuralgia, because relatively low doses are used compared with doses for treating depression.

OPTION TOPICAL COUNTERIRRITANTS

RCTs have found that topical counterirritants such as capsaicin are associated with relief of postherpetic neuralgia but can also cause painful skin reactions.

Benefits: We found one systematic review (search date 1993), which identified two placebo controlled RCTs of capsaicin. Pooled analysis found capsaicin to be associated with pain relief (total n = 205; OR for complete or greatly reduced pain 0.29, 95% CI 0.16 to 0.54).[5]

Harms: Reported local skin reactions included burning, stinging, and erythema. These effects tended to subside with time and frequency of use.[17]

Comment: The difficulty in blinding studies with capsaicin because of skin burning may have caused overestimation of its benefit.

OPTION TOPICAL ANAESTHESIA

One small RCT of lignocaine patches found short term pain relief in postherpetic neuralgia.

Benefits: We found no systematic review. We found one small, placebo controlled RCT of lignocaine patches (n = 35). Active patches were associated with reduced average pain scores on a visual analogue scale over 12 hours.[18]

Harms: No systemic adverse effects were noted with lignocaine patches, and systemic absorption as determined by blood concentrations was minimal.[18]

Comment: None.

OPTION   GABAPENTIN

One RCT found that gabapentin relieved postherpetic neuralgia.

Benefits: We found no systematic review. We found one multicentre, double blind, placebo controlled RCT of the anticonvulsant drug gabapentin (n = 229) in people who remained on tricyclic antidepressants or opiates during the trial.[19] At the end of the 8 week treatment period, gabapentin was associated with a significant reduction in reported pain (much or moderately reduced: RRR 0.27; ARR 0.20, 95% CI 0.08 to 0.30; NNT 5, 95% CI 3 to 13).

Harms: Gabapentin was associated with somnolence, dizziness, ataxia, and peripheral oedema more frequently than placebo in one trial. However, rates of withdrawal from treatment were not significantly different between the two groups.[19]

Comment: None.

OPTION   NARCOTIC ANALGESICS

One crossover RCT found oral oxycodone to be associated with relief from postherpetic neuralgia. One small RCT found that epidural morphine was poorly tolerated and of little benefit. One RCT of the non-opioid dextromethorphan found no evidence of benefit.

Benefits: We found no systematic review. We found one double blind, placebo controlled, crossover RCT of oxycodone (4 weeks on each treatment, n = 50). Oxycodone was associated with significant pain reduction on a visual analogue scale, but these data could not be converted into a dichotomous outcome. However, the authors reported that 67% of people had a masked preference for oxycodone compared with 11% for placebo.[20] In a small, single blinded, placebo controlled RCT, epidural morphine led to pain reduction of more than 50% in two of 11 people, but this could not be sustained beyond 36 hours; six other people could not tolerate the treatment because of adverse effects.[21] A third, small, double blind, crossover placebo controlled RCT (n = 18) found no evidence of pain relief from 6 weeks' treatment with dextromethorphan (a codeine analogue).[22]

Harms: Oxycodone was reported to produce adverse effects such as constipation, nausea, and sedation with greater frequency than placebo (76% v 49%; RR 1.4, 95% CI 0.5 to 3.4).[19] Epidural morphine produced intolerable opioid effects in 7/8 people treated.[21] High dose dextromethorphan produced sedation and ataxia, causing treatment cessation in 5/18 participants.[22]

Comment: None.

REFERENCES

1. Hope-Simpson RE. Postherpetic neuralgia. *J R Coll Gen Pract* 1975;25:571–575.
2. Ragozzino MW, Melton J III, Kurland LT, et al. Population based study of herpes zoster and its sequelae. *Medicine* 1982;61:310–316.
3. Mckendrick MW, McGill JI, Wood MJ. Lack of effect of aciclovir on postherpetic neuralgia. *BMJ* 1989;298:431.
4. Bowsher D. The effects of pre-emptive treatment of postherpetic neuralgia with amitriptyline: a randomised, double-blind, placebo-controlled trial. *J Pain Symptom Manage* 1997;13:327–331.
5. Lancaster T, Silagy C, Gray S. Primary care management of acute herpes zoster: systematic review of evidence from randomised controlled trials. *Br J Gen Pract* 1995;45:39–45. Search date 1966 to 1993; primary sources Medline, handsearched primary care journals, references from books; specialists and manufacturers of drugs in identified trials for published and unpublished data.
6. Volmink J, Lancaster T, Gray S, et al. Treatments for postherpetic neuralgia–a systematic review of randomised controlled trials. *Fam Pract* 1996;13: 84–91. Search date December 1993; primary sources Datastar software system for Medline and Embase.
7. Jackson JL, Gibbons R, Meyer G, et al. The effect of treating herpes zoster with oral aciclovir in preventing postherpetic neuralgia. A meta-analysis. *Arch Intern Med* 1997;157:909–912. Search date 1966 to 1996; primary sources Medline, National Institute of Health database of funded studies, Cochrane registered central database.
8. Tyring S, Barbarash RA, Nahlik JE, et al. Famciclovir for the treatment of acute herpes zoster: effects on acute disease and postherpetic neuralgia. A randomised, double-blind, placebo-controlled trial. Collaborative famciclovir herpes zoster study group. *Ann Intern Med* 1995;123: 89–96.
9. Beutner KR, Friedman DJ, Forszpaniak C, et al. Valaciclovir compared with aciclovir for improved therapy for herpes zoster in immunocompetent adults. *Antimicrob Agents Chemother* 1995;39: 1546–1553.
10. Soltz-Szots J, Tyring S, Andersen PL, et al. A randomised controlled trial of aciclovir versus netivudine for treatment of herpes zoster. International zoster study group. *J Antimicrob Chemother* 1998;41:549–556.
11. Alper BS, Lewis R. Does treatment of acute herpes zoster prevent or shorten postherpetic neuralgia? A systematic review of the literature. *J Fam Pract* 2000;49:255–264. Search date December 1998; primary sources Medline 1966 to December 1998; Cochrane Controlled Trials Register 1998 issue 4; hand searched reference lists and ads-based searches.
12. Aliaga A, Armijo M, Camacho F, et al. A topical solution of 40% idoxuridine in dimethyl sulfoxide compared to oral aciclovir in the treatment of herpes zoster. A double-blind multicenter clinical trial [in Spanish]. *Med Clin (Barc)* 1992;98:245–249.
13. Wood MJ, Johnson RW, McKendrick MW, et al. A randomised trial of aciclovir for 7 days or 21 days with and without prednisolone for treatment of acute herpes zoster. *N Engl J Med* 1994;330: 896–900.
14. Whitley RJ, Weiss H, Gnann JW Jr, et al. Aciclovir with and without prednisone for the treatment of herpes zoster. A randomized, placebo-controlled trial. The National Institute of Allergy and Infectious Diseases Collaborative Antiviral Study Group. *Ann Intern Med* 1996;125:376–383.
15. Max MB, Schafer SC, Culnane M, et al. Amitriptyline, but not lorazepam, relieves postherpetic neuralgia. *Neurology* 1988;38: 1427–1432.
16. Kishore-Kumar R, Max MB, Schafer SC, et al. Desipramine relieves postherpetic neuralgia. *Clin Pharmacol Ther* 1990;47:305–312.
17. Bernstein JE, Korman NJ, Bickers DR, et al. Topical capsaicin treatment of chronic postherpetic neuralgia. *J Am Acad Dermatol* 1989; 21:265–270.
18. Rowbotham MC, Davies PS, Verkempinck C, et al. Lidocaine patch: double-blind controlled study of a new treatment method for postherpetic neuralgia. *Pain* 1996;65:39–44.
19. Rowbotham M, Harden N, Stacey B, et al. Gabapentin for the treatment of postherpetic neuralgia: a randomised controlled trial. *JAMA* 1998;280:1837–1842.
20. Watson CP, Babul N. Efficacy of oxycodone in neuropathic pain: a randomised trial in postherpetic neuralgia. *Neurology* 1998;50: 1837–1841.
21. Watt JW, Wiles JR, Bowsher DR. Epidural morphine for postherpetic neuralgia. *Anaesthesia* 1996;51: 647–651.
22. Nelson KA, Park KM, Robinovitz E, et al. High-dose oral dextromethorphan versus placebo in painful diabetic neuropathy and postherpetic neuralgia. *Neurology* 1997;48:1212–1218.

John Yaphe
Department of Family Medicine Rabin
Medical Centre
Petach, Tikvah
Israel

Tim Lancaster
Reader in General Practice
Department of Primary Health Care
University of Oxford
Oxford
UK

Competing interests: None declared.

Updated this issue

Alison Holmes and Paul Garner

INTERVENTIONS

Key Messages

Treating newly diagnosed tuberculosis

■ RCTs found no evidence of a difference in relapse rates between standard short
course (6 months) and longer term (8–9 months) chemotherapy in people with
pulmonary tuberculosis. RCTs suggest that taking pyrazinamide in the first 2
months speeds up sputum clearance, but that there is conflicting evidence
relating to its effect on relapse rates.

- We found limited evidence from one RCT of no significant difference between daily and thrice weekly short course regimens.
- One systematic review of RCTs found evidence that reducing treatment from 6 to 4 months results in higher relapse rates.
- We found no good evidence comparing regimens containing quinolones versus existing regimens.

Treating multidrug resistant tuberculosis

- We found no good evidence comparing different drug regimens for multidrug resistant tuberculosis.

Improving adherence and reattendance

- We found limited evidence suggesting that adherence to treatment may be improved by cash incentives, and health education by a nurse.
- We found insufficient evidence on the effects of training of health staff (health education by a doctor, prompts, direct patient observations, or sanctions) on adherence to treatment.
- Limited evidence from RCTs suggests that prompts and contracts may increase reattendance for Mantoux test reading.

DEFINITION	Tuberculosis is caused by *Mycobacterium tuberculosis* and can affect many organs. Specific symptoms relate to site of infection and are generally accompanied by fever, sweats, and weight loss.
INCIDENCE/ PREVALENCE	About a third of the world's population is infected with *M tuberculosis*. The organism kills more people than any other infectious agent. The World Health Organization estimates that 95% of cases are in developing countries, and that 25% of avoidable deaths in developing countries are caused by tuberculosis.[1]
AETIOLOGY/ RISK FACTORS	Social factors include poverty, overcrowding, homelessness, and inadequate health services. Medical factors include HIV and immunosuppression.
PROGNOSIS	Prognosis varies widely and depends on treatment.[2]
AIMS	To cure tuberculosis; eliminate risk of relapse; reduce infectivity; avoid emergence of drug resistance; and prevent death.
OUTCOMES	*M tuberculosis* in sputum (smear examination and culture), symptoms, weight, and relapse rates.
METHODS	*Clinical Evidence* update search and appraisal May 2000. Search terms: tuberculosis, pulmonary; isoniazid, pyrazinamide, rifampicin. We included all Cochrane systematic reviews and studies that were randomised or used alternate allocation, had over 300 people, and had at least 1 year follow up after completion of treatment.

QUESTION What are the effects of different drug regimens in people with newly diagnosed pulmonary tuberculosis?

OPTION SHORT COURSE CHEMOTHERAPY (6 MONTHS)

RCTs found no evidence of a difference in relapse rates between standard short course (6 months) and longer term (8–9 months) chemotherapy in people with pulmonary tuberculosis. RCTs suggest that

Infectious diseases

use of pyrazinamide in the first 2 months speeds up sputum clearance, but the evidence relating to its effect on relapse rates is conflicting.

Benefits: We found no systematic review. **Versus longer courses:** Two RCTs (published in the mid 1980s), compared 6 versus 8 or 9 months' chemotherapy in a total of 1295 people with untreated, culture/smear positive pulmonary tuberculosis.[3,4] Participants were followed up for at least 1 year after treatment was completed. The trials were performed in the UK and in East and Central Africa, and used different combinations of isoniazid, rifampicin, ethambutol, streptomycin, and pyrazinamide for initial (first 2 months) and continuation treatment. Overall, there was no significant difference between short course and longer regimens. **Different short course regimens:** One trial found no difference between regimens using ethambutol or streptomycin as the fourth drug in the initial phase.[4] A 6 month regimen using rifampicin and isoniazid throughout was highly effective (relapse rate 2%) and significantly better than isoniazid alone in the 4 month continuation phase (relapse rate 9%). When use of isoniazid alone was prolonged in a 6 month continuation phase, the relapse rate was not significantly better than with 4 months' continuation.[3] **Pyrazinamide:** One RCT found that sputum conversion was faster with regimens containing pyrazinamide for the first 2 months, but there was no significant difference in relapse rates at 3 years' follow up.[4] A second RCT compared four different 6 month regimens and found that bacterial relapse in the 12 months after chemotherapy was higher for those not receiving pyrazinamide (12/160 v 8/625).[5] A third RCT (n = 497) of ongoing pyrazinamide found that relapse at 18 months was more likely in those not receiving pyrazinamide, but the difference was not significant (3.1% v 1%).[6]

Harms: In the largest trial, possible adverse reactions were reported in 24/851 people (3%), with six requiring modification of treatment.[3] Two people in the trial developed jaundice, one of whom died. **Pyrazinamide:** Adding pyrazinamide did not increase the incidence of hepatitis (4% with and without pyrazinamide).[4] However, mild adverse effects were more common, including arthralgia, skin rashes, flu like symptoms, mild gastrointestinal disturbance, vestibular disturbance, peripheral neuropathy, and confusion. Arthralgia was the most common adverse effect, reported in about 0.7% of people on pyrazinamide, but was mild and never required modification of treatment.[3,4]

Comment: In people treated previously the organisms may have acquired drug resistance, so short course chemotherapy may not be effective.

OPTION   INTERMITTENT SHORT COURSE CHEMOTHERAPY

We found no evidence of a significant difference between daily and thrice weekly short course regimens, but the limited data available do not exclude a clinically important difference.

Benefits: We found one systematic review (search date 1999, 1 RCT) comparing thrice weekly (n = 199) versus daily (n = 200) chemotherapy for 6 months in people with newly diagnosed pulmonary tuberculosis.[7] One month after treatment was completed, there was no significant difference in rates of bacteriological cure (defined as negative sputum culture, 99.9% v 100%) or relapse (5/186 people v 1/192 people; RR 4.0, 95% CI 0.7 to 24.1). At least 12 cohort studies have found cure rates of 80–100% with thrice weekly regimens taken over 6–9 months.[7]

Harms: Intermittent treatment has the potential to contribute to drug resistance, but this was not shown in the studies.[7]

Comment: The trial was too small to exclude a clinically significant difference between the dosing regimens.

OPTION   CHEMOTHERAPY FOR LESS THAN 6 MONTHS

Limited evidence from one systematic review of RCTs suggests that reducing duration of treatment to less than 6 months results in significantly higher relapse rates.

Benefits: We found one systematic review (search date January 1999), which identified seven RCTs published between 1979 and 1989 of outpatients with newly diagnosed pulmonary tuberculosis.[8] The trials included 2248 people in India, Hong Kong, Singapore, and Germany, and compared a variety of shorter (minimum 2 months) and longer (maximum 12 months) drug regimens. Relapse rates were consistently higher after the shorter duration treatments. One trial found that people given a 2 month regimen were less likely to change or discontinue drugs than those given a 12 month regimen. The event rates were small but the difference was significant (6/299 v 17/299; RR 0.35; RRR 0.65, 95% CI 0.12 to 0.86).[8]

Harms: There was little difference in adverse events or toxicity in the review.

Comment: The treatments were given under ideal conditions. In clinical practice, relapse rates with shorter regimens are likely to be worse.

OPTION   REGIMENS CONTAINING QUINOLONES

We found insufficient evidence on regimens containing quinolones.

Benefits: We found no systematic review. We found two RCTs.[9,10] One RCT (n = 200) from Tanzania found that many more people relapsed following a regimen containing ciprofloxacin, but the difference was not significant (RR of relapse at 6 months 16, 95% CI 0.94 to 278).[9] A relatively low dosage of ciprofloxacin was used (750 mg daily).

Harms: None reported.[10]

Comment: Quinolones have good bactericidal activity *in vitro*. Some of the newer quinolones have enhanced antimycobacterial activity compared with ciprofloxacin.

QUESTION   What are the effects of different drug regimens in people with multidrug resistant tuberculosis?

We found insufficient evidence comparing different drug regimens for multidrug resistant tuberculosis. We found no systematic review and no RCTs comparing different regimens in people with multidrug resistant

tuberculosis. We found insufficient data. Current clinical practice in multidrug resistant tuberculosis is to include at least three drugs to which the particular strain of tuberculosis is sensitive, using as many bactericidal agents as possible. People are directly observed and managed by a specialised clinician.

QUESTION   Which interventions improve adherence to treatment?

OPTION   STAFF TRAINING

We found insufficient evidence on the effects of training of health staff on adherence to treatment.

Benefits: We found one systematic review (search date 1999), which identified one poorly randomised RCT (see comment below).[11] The trial compared intensive staff supervision versus routine supervision at centres in Korea performing tuberculosis extension activities. Centres were paired and randomised, and supervision was carried out by senior doctors. Higher completion rates were achieved with intensive supervision (RR 1.2, CIs not estimated because of cluster design).

Harms: None reported.

Comment: The trial used cluster randomisation and there were insufficient data to adjust for this.

OPTION   PROMPTS

We found no good evidence.

Benefits: We found one systematic review (search date 1999), which found no RCTs of prompts to return for treatment.

Harms: None.

Comment: None.

OPTION   DEFAULTER ACTIONS

A systematic review of two RCTS has found that intensive action for defaulters improves completion of treatment.

Benefits: We found one systematic review (search date 1999), which identified two RCTs, both conducted in India.[11] The first RCT found that up to four home visits to defaulters improved completion of treatment compared with routine policy of a reminder letter followed by one home visit (RR 1.32, 95% CI 1.02 to 1.71). In the second study, up to two reminder letters improved completion of treatment (RR 1.21, 95% CI 1.05 to 1.39), even in people who were illiterate.

Harms: None reported.

Comment: None.

OPTION CASH INCENTIVES

A systematic review of two RCTs has found that cash incentives improve adherence among people living in deprived circumstances.

Benefits: We found one systematic review (search date 1999), which identified two RCTs, both conducted in the USA.[11] One, in homeless men, found that money ($5) improved attendance at the first appointment (RR 1.6, 95% CI 1.3 to 2.0). The other, in migrants, found that combining cash ($10) with health education improved attendance compared with usual care (RR 2.4, 95% CI 1.5 to 3.7).

Harms: None measured.

Comment: None.

OPTION HEALTH EDUCATION

One RCT found that health education by a nurse improved treatment completion, with no evidence of benefit from health education by a doctor. One RCT in drug users found no significant effect of health education.

Benefits: We found one systematic review (search date 1999), which identified two RCTs, both conducted in the USA.[11] One trial compared three methods of health education versus an educational leaflet. Health education consisted of telephoning by a nurse, visiting by a nurse, or consultation by the clinic doctor. The trial found that, compared with the leaflet, treatment completion was significantly increased by the nurse phone call (75/80 v 55/77; RR 1.31; relative benefit increase 31%, 95% CI 15% to 47%) and by the nurse visit (75/79 v 55/77; RR 1.33; relative benefit increase 33%, 95% CI 17% to 49%). However, consultation by the clinic doctor was not significantly better than the education leaflet (64/82 v 55/77; RR 1.09; relative benefit increase 9%, 95% CI −10% to +28%). The second trial in drug users found that 5–10 minutes of health education had no effect on whether people kept a scheduled appointment (RR 1.04, 95% CI 0.70 to 1.54).

Harms: None measured.

Comment: Education is often part of a package of care that includes prompts and incentives, which makes it difficult to evaluate the independent effects of education.

OPTION SANCTIONS

We found insufficient evidence on the effects of sanctions for failure to adhere to treatment.

Benefits: We found one systematic review (search date 1999), which identified no RCTs of sanctions.[11]

Harms: The use of sanctions may be ethically dubious.

Comment: In New York, the "locked hospital" was thought to have given credibility to the Department of Health's strategy for curing some patients.[12]

OPTION COMMUNITY HEALTH WORKERS

One RCT found that health advisors recruited from the community increased attendance for treatment.

Benefits: We found one systematic review (search date1999), which identified one RCT in homeless people.[11] It found evidence that health advisors recruited from the community helped people keep their appointments (62/83 attended v 42/79; RR 1.41, 95% CI 1.1 to 1.79).

Harms: None reported.

Comment: None.

OPTION DIRECT PATIENT OBSERVATION

We found limited evidence from two RCTs on the effects of direct observation on treatment adherence.

Benefits: We found one systematic review (search date 1999)[11] and one subsequent RCT.[13] The review identified one RCT (n = 216) conducted in South Africa that compared direct observation of people as they took their drugs versus self administered treatment at home. It found no significant difference between the two strategies, although overall adherence in the study was low.[14] The subsequent RCT (n = 836) conducted in Thailand compared self treatment with direct observation (either from health centre staff, community members or a family member). It found that direct observation versus self treatment improved treatment completion (347/414 [84%] v 320/422 [76%]; RR 1.11, 95% CI 1.04 to 1.16; NNT 13, 95% CI 8 to 36) and cure rate (RR 1.64, 95% CI 1.17 to 2.3).[13]

Harms: Potential harms include reduced co-operation between patient and doctor, removal of individual responsibility, detriment to long term sustainability of antituberculosis programmes, and increased burden on health services to the detriment of care for other diseases. None of these have been adequately investigated.

Comment: Numerous observational studies have evaluated interventions described as directly observed treatment, but all were packages of interventions that included specific investment in antituberculosis programmes, such as strengthened drug supplies, improved microscopy services, and numerous incentives, sanctions and other co-interventions that were likely to influence adherence.[15,16]

QUESTION Which interventions improve reattendance for Mantoux test reading?

OPTION PROMPTS AND CONTRACTS TO IMPROVE REATTENDANCE FOR MANTOUX TEST READING

One RCT found that routine prompts improved reattendance for Mantoux test reading. One RCT found that verbal or written commitments improved reattendance for Mantoux screening.

Benefits: **Prompts:** We found one systematic review (search date 1999), which identified one RCT in 701 healthy people.[11] The trial compared an automatic telephone message prompt to return for Mantoux reading versus no prompt. People were slightly more likely to return in the intervention group (93% v 88%; RR 1.05, 95% CI 1.0 to 1.10). **Contracts:** We found no systematic review. One RCT in healthy students in the USA found that, compared with no commitment, reattendance for Mantoux reading was improved by verbal commitments (RR 1.1, 95% CI 1.03 to 1.18) and by written commitments (RR 1.12, 95% CI 1.05 to 1.19).[11]

Harms: None reported.

Comment: None.

Substantive changes since last issue

Direct observation New RCT.[13]

REFERENCES

1. Global Tuberculosis Programme. *Treatment of tuberculosis.* Geneva: World Health Organization, 1997:WHO/TB/97.220.

2. Enarson D, Rouillon A. Epidemiological basis of tuberculosis control. In: Davis PD, ed. *Clinical tuberculosis.* 2nd ed. London: Chapman and Hall Medical, 1998.

3. East and Central African/British Medical Research Council Fifth Collaborative Study. Controlled clinical trial of 4 short–course regimens of chemotherapy (three 6-month and one 8-month) for pulmonary tuberculosis. *Tubercle* 1983;64: 153–166.

4. British Thoracic Society. A controlled trial of 6 months chemotherapy in pulmonary tuberculosis, final report: results during the 36 months after the end of chemotherapy and beyond. *Br J Dis Chest* 1984;78:330–336.

5. Hong Kong Chest Service/British Medical Research Council. Controlled trial of four thrice weekly regimens and a daily regimen given for 6 months for pulmonary tuberculosis. *Lancet* 1981;1:171–174.

6. Farga V, Valenzuela M, et al. Short-term chemotherapy of tuberculosis with 5-month regimens with and without pyrazinamide in the second phase (TA-82) [in Spanish]. *Rev Med Chil* 1986;114:701–705.

7. Mwandumba HC, Squire SB. Fully intermittent dosing with drugs for tuberculosis. In: The Cochrane Library. Issue 1, 2000. Oxford: Update Software. Search date January 1999; primary sources Cochrane Infectious Diseases Group Trials Register; Cochrane Controlled Trials Register; Medline 1996 to 1999; Embase 1988–1999; reference lists of article; researchers contacted for unpublished trials.

8. Gelband H. Regimens of less than six months treatment for TB. In: The Cochrane Library. Issue 1, 2000. Oxford: Update Software. Search date 1999; primary sources Medline 1966 to 1999;

   Cochrane Parasitic Diseases Trials Register; contact with researchers, and hand searched references.

9. Kennedy N, Berger L, Curran J, et al. Randomized controlled trial of a drug regimen that includes ciprofloxacin for the treatment of pulmonary tuberculosis. *Clin Infect Dis* 1996;22:827–833.

10. Kennedy N, Fox R, Uiso L, Ngowi FI, Gillespie SH. Safety profile of ciprofloxacin during long-term therapy for pulmonary tuberculosis. *J Antimicrob Chemother* 1993;32:897–902.

11. Volmink J, Garner P. Interventions for prompting adherence to tuberculosis treatment. In: The Cochrane Library. Issue 1, 2000. Oxford: Update Software. Search date 1999; primary sources Medline 1966 to September 1999; Embase January to July 1999; Cochrane Controlled Trials Register 1998, Issue 3; Cochrane Collaboration Effective Professional Practice (CCEPP) Registry Trials to 14 October 1996; LILACS to 1998; hand searched journals, references, and contact with authors.

12. Fujiwara PI, Larkin C, Frieden TR. Directly observed therapy in New York history, implementation, results and challenges. *Tuberculosis* 1997;18: 135–148.

13. Kamolratanakul P, Sawert H, Lertmaharit S, et al. Randomized controlled trial of directly observed treatment (DOT) for patients with pulmonary tuberculosis in Thailand. *Trans R Soc Trop Med Hyg* 1999;93:552–557.

14. Zwarenstein M, Schoeman JH, Vundule C, Lombard C, Tatley M. Randomised controlled trial of self-supervised and directly observed treatment of tuberculosis. *Lancet* 1998;352:1340–1343.

15. Garner P. What makes DOT work? *Lancet* 1998; 352:1326.

16. Volmink J, Matchaba P, Garner P. Directly observed therapy and treatment adherence. *Lancet* 2000; 355:1345–1350.

Alison Holmes
Senior Lecturer
Hammersmith Hospital Imperial
College
London
UK

Paul Garner
Senior Lecturer
Liverpool School of Tropical Medicine
Liverpool
UK
Competing interests: None declared.

Kidney disorders

Updated this issue

John Kellum and Martine Leblanc

INTERVENTIONS

To be covered in future issues of
Clinical Evidence
Prevention of acute renal failure
Growth factors
Atrial natriuretic factor and
urodilatin
Calcium channel blockers
Norepinephrine
Adenosine antagonists
Antibodies against adhesion
molecules
Antioxidants
Nutritional management

* We found no good evidence for
role in treatment, but found good
evidence refuting role for
prevention of ARF. This will be
discussed in subsequent issues
of *Clinical Evidence*.
See glossary, p 451

Key Messages

- One systematic review found insufficient evidence from small observational studies to compare continuous and intermittent renal replacement.
- Limited evidence from RCTs suggests that, compared with non-biocompatible membranes, biocompatible membranes reduce mortality in critically ill people with acute renal failure (ARF).
- We found insufficient evidence from low powered RCTs on the effects of diuretics in critically ill people with ARF.
- We found no good evidence on the effects of dopamine, bolus versus continuous loop diuretics, or combined albumin and diuretics in critically ill people with ARF.

DEFINITION Acute renal failure (ARF) is characterised by abrupt and sustained decline in glomerular filtration rate,[1] which leads to accumulation of urea and other chemicals in the blood. There is no clear consensus on a biochemical definition,[2] but most studies define it as a serum creatinine of 2–3 mg/dl (200–250 µmol/l), an elevation of more than 0.5 mg/dl (45 µmol/l) over a baseline creatinine below 2 mg/dl (170 µmol/l), or a twofold increase of baseline creatinine. "Severe" ARF has been defined as a serum concentration of creatinine above 5.5 mg/dl (500 µmol/l) or as requiring renal replacement therapy. ARF is usually classified according to the location of the predominant primary pathology (prerenal, intrarenal, and postrenal failure — see glossary, p 451). People who are critically ill are those who are unstable and at imminent risk of death, which usually implies that they are people who need to be, or have been admitted to, the intensive care unit (ICU).

INCIDENCE/ PREVALENCE Two prospective observational studies (2576 people) have found that established ARF affects nearly 5% of patients in hospital and as many as 15% of critically ill people depending on the definitions used.[3,4]

AETIOLOGY/ RISK FACTORS Prerenal (or functional ARF) is caused by reduced blood flow to the kidney that can result from renal artery disease, systemic hypotension, or maldistribution of blood flow. Intrarenal ARF is caused by parenchymal injury, most commonly acute tubular necrosis, but also interstitial nephritis, embolic disease, glomerulonephritis, vasculitis, or small vessel disease. Postrenal or obstructive ARF is caused by urinary tract obstruction. Observational studies, in several hundred people from Europe, North America, and West Africa, found that 40–80% of people with ARF had a prerenal cause, 10–50% an intrarenal cause, and the remainder (< 10%) a postrenal cause.[5–9] In people who are critically ill, the commonest type of renal dysfunction is prerenal,[5,10] although ARF in this context is usually part of a multiorgan or multisystem failure, and most frequently due to acute tubular necrosis resulting from ischaemic or nephrotoxic injury, or both.[11,12] Well recognised risk factors for ARF include hypovolaemia, hypotension, sepsis, pre-existing renal, hepatic or cardiac dysfunction, diabetes mellitus, and drugs such as aminoglycosides, amphotericin B, immunosuppressive agents, non-steroidal anti-inflammatory drugs, angiotensin converting enzyme inhibitors, and intravenous contrast media.

PROGNOSIS One retrospective study in 1347 people with ARF found that mortality was less than 15% in people with isolated ARF.[13] One recent prospective study in over 700 people found that, in people with ARF, overall mortality and the need for dialysis was higher in ICU than in a non-ICU setting, despite no significant difference between the groups in mean maximal serum creatinine (need for dialysis 71% in ICU v 18%, P < 0.001; mortality 72% in ICU v 32%, P = 0.001).[14]

AIMS To prevent death; to prevent complications of ARF (volume overload, acid base disturbance, and electrolyte abnormalities); and to prevent the need for chronic dialysis, with minimum adverse effects.

OUTCOMES	Rate of death; rate of renal recovery; adverse effects of treatment. Extent of naturesis is a proxy outcome.
METHODS	*Clinical Evidence* update search and appraisal May 2000. Search terms: kidney failure acute/epidemiology, aetiology, therapy; diuretics; dopamine; haemodialysis membranes; albumin/therapeutic uses. We identified additional studies from the bibliographies of review articles and from personal files.

QUESTION   **What are effects of treatments for critically ill people with acute renal failure?**

OPTION   CONTINUOUS VERSUS INTERMITTENT RENAL REPLACEMENT THERAPY

One systematic review found insufficient evidence to compare continuous renal replacement therapy (CRRT) versus intermittent renal replacement therapy (IRRT) in this setting.

Benefits:	We found no RCTs.
Harms:	We found no good studies comparing the adverse effects of CRRT and IRRT. Heparin is often used with CRRT, and this can have adverse effects (see thromboembolism, p 144).[15]
Comment:	We found one systematic review (search date 1986 to 1994), which found 15 observational, mostly small retrospective and prospective studies in a total of 1173 people.[16] Eleven of these studies reported mortality. The review found no overall evidence of a significant difference in survival to hospital discharge between patients treated with CRRT and IRRT (survival to discharge 31% with CRRT *v* 26% with IRRT; RR CRRT *v* IRRT 1.07, 95% CI 0.99 to 1.16; P = 0.10; calculated by authors using the Mantel–Haenzel method and the true sample of 1006 people after correction for double counting). Biocompatible membranes were used in CRRT more than in IRRT; this could confound results. An important RCT (425 people) has been published since the current *Clinical Evidence* search.[17] This RCT found a significant decrease in mortality (from 59% to 43%) when the dose of renal replacement therapy was increased. Detailed review of this study, and any others that are relevant, will be included in Issue 5 of *Clinical Evidence*.

OPTION   BIOCOMPATIBLE VERSUS NON-BIOCOMPATIBLE DIALYSIS MEMBRANES

We found limited evidence from three out of four RCTs that biocompatible membranes (see glossary, p 451) may reduce mortality in critically ill people with ARF, compared with non-biocompatible membranes.

| Benefits: | We found no systematic review, but found four RCTs (n = 491)[18–22] comparing biocompatible (synthetic) versus non-biocompatible (cellulose based) dialysis membranes in critically ill people with all cause ARF; despite being described as randomised, two of the studies had important methodological problems. The first trial, in which membrane assignment was made in alternating order,[19] found that when recruitment from the original sample of 72 people |

with ARF[18] was extended to 153,[19] there was a significant difference in survival to discharge (57% with biocompatible membranes v 46% with non-biocompatible; 72 people; P = 0.03) and recovery of renal function (64% v 43%, P = 0.001).[18,19] This study found that mortality due to sepsis (by time of discharge) was lower with biocompatible membranes (12% v 46%; P = 0.016).[18] The second RCT (52 people) found a better survival rate with biocompatible membranes (62% v 35%; P = 0.05) and a higher incidence of renal recovery at time of discharge with biocompatible membranes (62% v 37%, P < 0.05).[20] The third RCT (180 people) found 60% survival with biocompatible membranes versus 58% with bio-incompatible membranes (OR 1.07, 95% CI 0.54 to 2.11; P = 0.87), and identical rates of recovery of renal function between groups (57%).[21] This study, however, was not analysed by intention to treat, and 12% of people were excluded after randomisation. It was funded by makers of bio-incompatible membranes. A recent study (106 people) compared two types of synthetic membranes to a semi-synthetic cellulose based membrane, and found no significant difference in survival at 80 days.[22]

Harms: Severe anaphylactoid reactions in people taking angiotensin converting enzyme inhibitors have been reported occasionally with certain synthetic biocompatible membranes (exact frequency unknown).

Comment: One prospective observational cohort study in 2410 people with chronic renal failure found a 25% relative increase in mortality in people using non-biocompatible (cellulose based) versus biocompatible (synthetic) membranes (P < 0.001).[23] The ability of the membrane to cause immune activation depends on the structure of the material used.[24] We found no evidence that the results comparing synthetic and cellulose based materials can be extrapolated to highly substituted cellulose based ("semi-biocompatible") membranes.

OPTION   DOPAMINE

We found insufficient evidence on the effects of dopamine in critically ill people with ARF.

Benefits: We found no good prospective studies.

Harms: Dopamine has recognised adverse effects. We found no data on actual incidence/prevalence of harms in this setting.

Comment: We found good evidence refuting the use of dopamine in the prevention of ARF; this will be addressed in a future issue of *Clinical Evidence*.

Kidney disorders

OPTION DIURETICS

Two small RCTs found that diuretics versus placebo had no significant effect on renal recovery, the number of days spent on dialysis, and mortality. The study lacked power to exclude a clinically important effect, and included people from a non-ICU setting.

Benefits: We found no systematic review, but found two RCTs (66 and 58 people) comparing intravenous furosemide with placebo in people with oliguric ARF of various causes. Some people were being cared for in the ICU, and some were not (exact numbers not reported).[25,26] In the second study, all people received one dose of furosemide 1 g and were then randomised to continued treatment or placebo. Neither RCT found significant differences in renal recovery (first RCT: 22/23 [58%] with furosemide v 22/23 [67%] with placebo; ARR 9%, 95% CI −12% to +33%;[25] second RCT: 10/28 [36%] with furosemide v 12/28 [43%] with placebo; ARR 7%, 95% −19% to +27%)[26] or mortality, although the studies lacked power to exclude a clinically important effect of diuretics on these outcomes.

Harms: Ototoxicity can occur with high dose loop diuretics. No adverse effects were reported in the first trial.[25] Deafness occurred in two people in the second trial; both were randomised to furosemide. Hearing loss was permanent in one of these people.[26] Diuretics may reduce renal perfusion and add a prerenal component to the renal failure, but the frequency of this event is uncertain.[27]

Comment: We found good evidence refuting the use of diuretics in the prevention of ARF; this will be addressed in a future issue of *Clinical Evidence*.

OPTION CONTINUOUS INFUSION VERSUS BOLUS INJECTION OF LOOP DIURETICS

We found insufficient evidence to compare continuous versus bolus injection of loop diuretics.

Benefits: We found no systematic review, and no RCTs in critically ill people with ARF.

Harms: One small, crossover RCT in eight people with acute deterioration of chronic renal failure (mean creatinine clearance 0.28 ml/s) found that fewer people experienced myalgia when treated with continuous infusion than with bolus dosing of bumetanide (3/8 people had myalgias with bolus dosing, none with continuous infusion).[28]

Comment: The small crossover trial found that continuous infusion resulted in a net increase in sodium excretion over a 24 hour period (mean increase in naturesis 48 mmol/day, 95% CI 16 to 60 mmol/day, P = 0.01).

OPTION	INTRAVENOUS ALBUMIN SUPPLEMENTATION PLUS DIURETICS

We found insufficient evidence on the effects of adding intravenous albumin to diuretic treatment in critically ill people with ARF.

Benefits: We found no systematic review. One RCT of nine people with nephrotic syndrome (crossover study) compared furosemide alone versus furosemide plus albumin versus albumin alone.[29] This small trial measured urinary volume and sodium excretion. Furosemide was superior to albumin alone, and furosemide plus albumin resulted in the greatest diuresis/nateuresis. The clinical meaning of this finding is unclear.

Harms: We found insufficient evidence in people with ARF. One systematic review of 30 RCTs (1419 people, most without ARF) found that albumin increased the risk of death in unselected critically ill people (mortality 14% with albumin v 8% with control; RR 1.68, CI 1.26 to 2.23). All of the included trials were small and combined highly heterogeneous populations.[30]

Comment: None.

GLOSSARY

Biocompatibility This refers to the tendency of artificial materials to induce an inflammatory response. The response may be humoral (including complement) or cellular. Materials are classified as biocompatible if they are less likely to induce an immune response or induce a less severe response compared with bio-incompatible materials. We found no standards by which this comparison can be made. Biocompatible dialysis membranes are made from synthetic materials whereas bio-incompatible membranes are cellulose based.

Intrarenal ARF Caused by parenchymal injury, most commonly acute tubular necrosis, but also interstitial nephritis, embolic disease, glomerulonephritis, vasculitis, or small vessel disease.

Postrenal (obstructive) ARF Caused by urinary tract obstruction.

Prerenal (functional) ARF Caused by renal hypoperfusion, secondary to renal artery disease, systemic hypotension, or maldistribution of blood flow.

REFERENCES

1. Nissenson AR. Acute renal failure: definition and pathogenesis. Kidney Int Suppl 1998;66:7–10.
2. Bellomo R, Ronco C. The changing pattern of severe acute renal failure. Nephrology 1991;2:602–610.
3. Hou SH, Bushinsky DA, Wish JB, Cohen JJ, Harrington JT. Hospital-acquired renal insufficiency: a prospective study. Am J Med 1983;74:243–248.
4. Brivet FG, Kleinknecht DJ, Loirat P, Landais PJM on behalf of the French Study Group on Acute Renal Failure. Acute renal failure in intensive care units-causes, outcomes and prognostic factors of hospital mortality: a prospective multicenter study. Crit Care Med 1996;24:192–198.
5. Thadhani R, Pascual M, Bonventre JV. Acute renal failure. N Engl J Med 1996;334:1448–1460.
6. Kleinknecht D. Epidemiology in acute renal failure in France today. In: Biari D, Neild G, eds. Acute renal failure in intensive therapy unit. Berlin: Springer-Verlag;1990:13–21.
7. Coar D. Obstructive nephropathy. Del Med J 1991;63:743–749.
8. Kaufman J, Dhakal M, Patel B, Hamburger R.

Community acquired acute renal failure. Am J Kidney Dis 1991;17:191–198.
9. Bamgboye EL, Mabayoje MO, Odutala TA, Mabadeje AF. Acute renal failure at the Lagos University Teaching Hospital. Ren Fail 1993;15:77–80.
10. Cantarovich F, Bodin L. Functional acute renal failure. In: Cantarovich F, Rangoonwala B, Verho M, eds. Progress in acute renal failure 1998. Paris: Hoechst Marion Roussel; 1998:55–65.
11. Brezis M, Rosen S. Hypoxia of the renal medulla. Its implication for disease. N Engl J Med 1995;332:647–655.
12. Bonventre JV. Mechanisms of ischemic acute renal failure. Kidney Int 1993;43:1160–1178.
13. Turney JH, Marshall DH, Brownjohn AM, Ellis CM, Parsons FM. The evolution of acute renal failure, 1956–1988. QJM 1990;74:83–104.
14. Liano F, Junco E, Pascual J, Madero R, Verde E. The spectrum of acute renal failure in the intensive care unit compared to that seen in other settings. The Madrid Acute Renal Failure Study Group. Kidney Int Suppl 1998;53:16–24.
15. Ronco C. Continuous renal replacement therapies

for the treatment of acute renal failure in intensive care patients. *Clin Nephrol* 1993;40:187–198.

16. Jakob SM, Frey FJ, Uehlinger DE. Does continuous renal replacement therapy favourably influence the outcome of the patients? *Nephrol Dial Transplant* 1996;11:1250–1255. Search date 1986–1994; primary sources not available.

17. Ronco C, Bellomo R, Homel P, et al. Effects of different doses in continuous veno-venous haemofiltration on outcomes of acute renal failure: a prospective randomised trial. *Lancet* 2000;356:26–30.

18. Hakim RM, Wingard RL, Parker RA. Effect of the dialysis membrane in the treatment of patients with acute renal failure. *N Engl J Med* 1994;331:1338–1342.

19. Himmelfarb J, Tolkoff RN, Chandran P, Parker RA, Wingard RL, Hakim RM. A multicenter comparison of dialysis membranes in the treatment of acute renal failure requiring dialysis. *J Am Soc Nephrol* 1998;9:257–266.

20. Schiffl H, Lang SM, Konig A, Strasser T, Haider MC, Held E. Biocompatible membranes in acute renal failure: prospective case-controlled study. *Lancet* 1994;344:570–572.

21. Jorres A, Gahl GM, Dobis C, et al. Haemodialysis-membrane biocompatibility and mortality of patients with dialysis-dependent acute renal failure: a prospective randomised multicentre trial. International Multicentre Study Group. *Lancet* 1999;354:1337–1341.

22. Gastaldello K, Melot C, Kahn RJ, Vanherweghem JL, Vincent JL, Tielemans C. Comparison of cellulose diacetate and polysulfone membranes in the outcome of acute renal failure. A prospective randomized study. *Nephrol Dial Transplant* 2000;15:224–230.

23. Hakim RM, Held PJ, Stannard DC, et al. Effect of the dialysis membrane on mortality of chronic hemodialysis patients. *Kidney Int* 1996;50:566–570.

24. Kellum JA. Primum non nocere and the meaning of modern critical care. *Curr Opin Critical Care* 1998;4:400–405.

25. Kleinknecht D, Ganeval D, Gonzales-Duque LA, Fermanian J. Furosemide in acute oliguric renal failure. A controlled trial. *Nephron* 1976;17:51–58.

26. Brown CB, Ogg CS, Cameron JS. High dose furosemide in acute renal failure: a controlled trial. *Clin Nephrol* 1981;15:90–96.

27. Kellum JA. Use of diuretics in the acute care setting. *Kidney Int* 1998;53(suppl 66):67–70.

28. Rudy DW, Voelker JR, Greene PK, et al. Loop diuretics for chronic renal insufficiency: a continuous infusion is more efficacious than bolus therapy. *Ann Intern Med* 1991;115:360–366.

29. Fliser D, Zurbruggen I, Mutschler E, et al. Coadministration of albumin and furosemide in patients with the nephrotic syndrome. *Kidney Int* 1999;55:629–634.

30. The Albumin Reviewers. Human albumin solution for resuscitation and volume expansion in critically ill patients. In: *The Cochrane Library*, Issue 1, 2000. Oxford: Update Software. Search date 1998; primary sources The Cochrane Injuries Group Register; Cochrane Library; Medline; Embase; BIDS Index to Scientific and Technical Proceedings; and hand searched references.

John Kellum
Associate Professor of Anesthesiology/Critical Care Medicine and Medicine
University of Pittsburgh
Pittsburgh
USA

Martine Leblanc
Assistant Professor of Nephrology and Critical Care
Maisonneuve-Rosemont Hospital
University of Montreal
Montreal
Canada

Competing interests: JK has been paid by Gambro Healthcare Inc. for lecturing and running educational programmes on acute renal failure.

Updated and expanded this issue

Michael Barry and Claus Roehrborn

QUESTIONS

INTERVENTIONS

Key Messages

- One systematic review of RCTs has found that α blockers are more effective than placebo for improving lower urinary tract symptoms in men with benign prostatic hyperplasia. RCTs have found that 5α reductase inhibitors also reduce symptoms compared with placebo. Two RCTs found that α blockers were more effective than 5α reductase inhibitors for reducing symptoms. We found no direct comparisons of these drugs with surgical treatment.

- One RCT found evidence that transurethral resection (TURP) was more effective than watchful waiting for improving symptoms and reducing complications, and found no evidence that it was associated with an increase in the risk of erectile dysfunction or incontinence.

- TURP has not yet been adequately compared with medical treatments or with newer, less invasive techniques.

- RCTs have found that transurethral microwave thermotherapy (TUMT) is more effective than sham treatment at reducing symptoms. Weaker data provide no evidence of any difference in short term symptom relief between TURP and TUMT, but one RCT found evidence that TURP was more effective than transurethral needle ablation (TUNA) in men with benign prostatic hyperplasia.

- One systematic review found that self rated improvement was better in men taking saw palmetto compared with placebo. It found no difference in symptom scores between saw palmetto and finasteride.

Benign prostatic hyperplasia

DEFINITION	Benign prostatic hyperplasia (BPH) is a histologically defined process. Clinically, it is characterised by lower urinary tract symptoms (urinary frequency, urgency, a weak and intermittent stream, needing to strain, a sense of incomplete emptying, and nocturia) and can lead to complications, including acute urinary retention.
INCIDENCE/ PREVALENCE	Estimates of the prevalence of symptomatic BPH range from 10–30% for men in their early 70s, depending on how BPH is defined.[1]
AETIOLOGY/ RISK FACTORS	The mechanisms by which BPH causes symptoms and complications are poorly understood, although bladder outlet obstruction is an important factor.[2] The best documented risk factors are increasing age and functioning testes.[3]
PROGNOSIS	Community, as well as practice based studies, suggest that men with lower urinary tract symptoms can expect slow progression over time.[4,5] However, symptoms can wax and wane without treatment. In men with symptoms of BPH, rates of acute urinary retention necessitating surgery range from 1–2% per year.[5–7]
AIMS	To reduce or alleviate lower urinary tract symptoms, to prevent complications, and to minimise adverse effects of treatment.
OUTCOMES	Burden of lower urinary tract symptoms; rates of acute urinary retention and prostatectomy; rates of adverse effects of treatment. Symptoms are measured using the validated International Prostate Symptom Score (IPSS), which includes seven questions quantifying symptoms on an overall scale from 0–35, with higher scores representing more frequent symptoms.[8] Older studies used a variety of symptom assessment instruments, which makes comparisons difficult.
METHODS	This review was originally based on ongoing Medline searches and prospective journal hand searches by the Patient Outcomes Research Team for Prostatic Diseases (Agency for Health Care Policy and Research grant number HS0837). *Clinical Evidence* update search and appraisal May 2000.

QUESTION **What are the effects of medical treatments?**

OPTION α BLOCKERS

One systematic review of RCTs has found that α blockers are more effective than placebo for improving lower urinary tract symptoms in men with a diagnosis of benign prostate hyperplasia (BPH). Two RCTs found that α blockers were more effective in improving symptoms than 5α reductase inhibitors. We found no direct comparison of α blockers with surgical treatment.

Benefits:	**Versus placebo:** We found one recent systematic review (search date 1998, 21 placebo controlled RCTs).[9] All trials found a greater improvement in symptoms with α blockers than with placebo (results presented graphically; significance not stated). The largest RCT compared terazosin at doses of up to 10 mg daily for 1 year versus placebo in 2084 men with BPH. Treatment achieved a significantly greater mean improvement in International Prostate

Symptom Score (IPSS) (−7.6 points from baseline with terazosin v −3.7 with placebo; mean change, terazosin v placebo −3.9 points, 95% CI −5.5 points to −3.3 points).[10] We found insufficient evidence on the effect of α blockers on complications of BPH. One small RCT found sustained release alfazosin (5 mg bd) for 48 hours increased the success rate of catheter removal after acute retention from 5% to 29% (NNT 4).[11] **Versus each other:** The systematic review[9] identified three head to head comparisons which reported clinical outcomes, and we found one subsequent RCT.[12] The largest trial (n = 256) compared tamsulosin versus alfuzosin.[11] The second trial compared alfuzosin versus prazosin (n = 103), and the third trial compared tamsulosin versus terazosin (total n = 98). The trials found no significant difference in symptom score among α blockers. The subsequent RCT (n = 212) found that tamsulosin improved total IPSS compared with terazosin (9.7% change from baseline with tamsulosin v 8.5% with terazosin, P < 0.05).[12] **Versus 5 α reductase inhibitors:** We found no systematic review. We found two RCTs. One RCT compared finasteride versus an α blocker or both treatments in 1229 men with a diagnosis of BPH.[13] Terazosin was associated with a greater reduction in symptoms regardless of prostate size than finasteride. The difference in mean IPSS scores at 1 year was 2.9 points. There was no difference between treatment with both agents versus terazosin alone. A second trial compared alfuzosin versus finasteride versus combination therapy over 6 months. Again, alfuzosin versus finasteride resulted in a significant decrease in mean IPSS scores from baseline, and there was no difference between combination therapy and a blocker alone.[14] **Versus TUMT:** See TUMT, p 458.

Harms: The systematic review found that withdrawals because of adverse events were similar for alfuzosin, tamsulosin (0.4 mg dose), and placebo (results presented graphically; significance not stated).[9] However, a higher withdrawal rate was found with doxazosin, terazosin, and tamsulosin (0.8 mg dose). There was little observable difference between the number of men experiencing dizziness with alfuzosin or tamsulosin compared with placebo (results presented graphically; significance not stated). However, more men experienced dizziness after terazosin and doxazosin than placebo (results were presented graphically; significance not stated). One large RCT included in the systematic review compared tamsulosin versus a less selective α blocker, alfuzosin. It found that adverse effects were similar. Dizziness was seen in 7%, asthenia in 2%, and postural hypotension in 2%.[9] One RCT from China compared low dose terazosin (2 mg daily) and tamsulosin (0.2 mg daily). It found dizziness (32% v 10%) and hypotension limiting therapy (9% v 1%) were more common with terazosin.[12] Both selective and less selective α blockers may be associated with abnormal ejaculation: the risk of abnormal ejaculation was higher with tamulosin than placebo (4.5% v 1%) but similar with tamsulosin versus alfuzosin (0.8% v 0%).[15] **Versus 5α reductase inhibitors:** In the trial comparing terazosin versus finasteride, dizziness was seen in about 25% of men on terazosin, generalised weakness in 15%, rhinitis in 8%, and postural hypotension in 8%, whereas sexual dysfunction was more common in men taking finasteride.[13]

Benign prostatic hyperplasia

Comment: Men with severe symptoms can expect the largest absolute fall in their symptom scores with medical treatment.[10,16] Prazosin, alfuzosin, terazosin and doxasosin lower blood pressure and may be used to treat both hypertension and BPH.[17]

OPTION   **5α REDUCTASE INHIBITORS**

RCTs have found that 5α reductase inhibitors are more effective than placebo for improving lower urinary tract symptoms and reducing complications in men with BPH, especially in men with larger prostates. Two RCTs found that 5α reductase inhibitors were less effective at improving symptoms than α blockers. We found no direct comparison with surgical treatment.

Benefits: We found no systematic review. **Versus placebo:** We found two non-systematic reviews[18,19] and two subsequent RCTs.[7,20] One meta-analysis (not a systematic review, published in 1996) combined the results of six RCTs of finasteride.[18] Treatment compared with placebo was associated with a significantly greater reduction in symptom scores (difference in symptom score −0.9 points, 95% CI −1.2 to −0.6 [range of score 0–30 points]). The benefit over placebo was greatest in men with larger prostates (≥ 40 g). The second meta-analysis (not a systematic review, published in 1997) combined the results of three placebo controlled RCTs of finasteride.[18] Treatment reduced the 2 year risk of acute urinary retention requiring catheterisation from 2.7% to 1.1% (NNT 62), of progression to prostatectomy from 6.5% to 4.2% (NNT 44), and of either event from 7.5% to 4.9% (NNT 38). One subsequent RCT compared finasteride 5 mg daily versus placebo in 3040 men with enlarged prostates and symptoms of BPH.[7] After 4 years of treatment, finasteride compared with placebo significantly reduced symptoms (difference in symptom score −1.6 points, range of score 0–34 points, 95% CI −2.5 to −0.7). Finasteride versus placebo significantly reduced the risk of acute urinary retention (6.6% v 2.8%; NNT 26, 95% CI 22 to 38), prostatectomy (8.3% v 4.2%; NNT 24, 95% CI 19 to 37), and of the risk of either event (13.2% v 6.6%; NNT 15, 95% CI 12 to 20). There was a greater effect among men with higher concentrations of prostate specific antigen (PSA) at baseline (3.3–12.0 ng/ml), reflecting larger prostates (risk of either acute urinary retention or of needing prostatectomy was 19.9% with placebo v 8.3% with finasteride; NNT 8, 95% CI 7 to 11).[21] The second subsequent RCT found that after 4 years, finasteride versus placebo produced a larger fall in IPSS score. The fall was greater for men with PSA greater than 1.3 ng/ml than with men with PSAs ≤ 1.3 ng/ml.[20] **Versus α blockers:** See α blockers, p 454. We found two RCTs. Neither trial selected men on the basis prostate size.[13,14]

Harms: The most common adverse events associated with finasteride in the first year were decreased libido (6%), impotence (8%), and decreased ejaculate (4%). After the first year of treatment, adverse effects were less common.[7] Although finasteride reduced concentrations of prostate specific antigen by an average of 50% (individual responses were highly variable), its use for up to 4 years did not change the rate of detection of prostate cancer compared with placebo.[7] **Versus α blockers:** See α blockers, p 454.

Comment: The meta-analysis of finasteride's impact on symptoms at 1–2 years found that finasteride was significantly more effective in men with larger prostates.[18] However, the absolute difference in mean decrease of symptom score from baseline between men with the smallest and largest prostates was only about one point. The relative effectiveness of finasteride versus placebo also seemed higher in men with slightly raised PSA,[20] and it is assumed that the higher PSA is a proxy for a larger prostate.

QUESTION What are the effects of surgical treatments?

OPTION TRANSURETHRAL RESECTION (TURP)

We found limited evidence from one RCT that TURP is more effective than watchful waiting for improving symptoms and reducing complications, and does not increase the risk of erectile dysfunction or incontinence. We found no good long term comparisons of TURP with medical treatments or with newer, less invasive techniques such as transurethral incision, laser ablation, and electrovaporisation.

Benefits: We found no recently updated systematic review of RCTs. **Versus watchful waiting:** We found one RCT that compared TURP versus watchful waiting in 556 men with moderate symptoms of BPH.[22] More men receiving TURP compared with watchful waiting improved (90% v 39%), and had reduced symptoms. After 5 years, the treatment failure rate was 21% with TURP versus 10% with watchful waiting (NNT9, 95% CI 7 to 17), and 36% of men assigned to watchful waiting had crossed over to surgery.[23] Treatment failure was defined as death, acute urinary retention, high residual urine volume, renal azotaemia, bladder stones, persistent incontinence, or a high symptom score. The major categories of treatment failure reduced by TURP were acute urinary retention, development of a large bladder residual (> 350 ml), and deterioration to a severe symptom level. **Versus less invasive techniques:** Numerous small RCTs have shown similar symptomatic outcomes with TURP and with transurethral incision of the prostate (TUIP) in men with smaller prostates. In the trial with the longest follow up, symptomatic outcomes were similar up to 6 years for TURP and TUIP in 120 men with resectable weights estimated to be less than 20 g.[24] Long term durability of symptom relief and effect on the incidence of complications of BPH have not yet been adequately evaluated. Two recently reported trials of older laser techniques versus TURP found higher surgical retreatment rates after laser (38% v 16% at 5 years with a side firing laser),[25] (18% v 9% at 3 years with a contact laser).[26] Several small short term RCTs (maximum 2 years) found either no difference between TURP and laser ablation or electrovaporisation[27–35] or that TURP achieved better symptom relief. **Versus TUMT and TUNA:** See TUMT, p 458.

Harms: Analysis of administrative data found that mortality in the 30 days after TURP for BPH ranged from 0.4% for men aged 65–69 years to 1.9% for men aged 80–84 years, and has been falling in recent years.[36] In one review of observational studies, TURP for BPH was associated with immediate surgical complications in 12% of cases, bleeding requiring intervention in 2%, erectile dysfunction in 14%, retrograde ejaculation in 74%, and incontinence in about 5%.[37–39] Analysis of claims data found a reoperation rate, implying need for retreatment, of about 1% per year.[36] However, in the only comparative trial, men randomised to prostatectomy did not seem to have a greater rate of erectile dysfunction or incontinence than men assigned to watchful waiting.[22,23] Laser prostatectomy and electrovaporisation require less hospital time and may cause fewer short term adverse effects and less bleeding than TURP.[27–32,40,41]

Comment: Rapid changes in techniques and few controlled trials with adequate follow up make comparisons between TURP and newer surgical techniques difficult.

OPTION   TRANSURETHRAL MICROWAVE THERMOTHERAPY (TUMT)

RCTs have found that TUMT is more effective than sham treatment at reducing symptoms of BPH. We found conflicting evidence about whether TUMT provides as effective short term symptom relief as TURP. One RCT found limited evidence that TUMT was more effective than α blockers over 6 months.

Benefits: We found no systematic review. **Versus sham treatment:** Several small to medium sized RCTs compared TUMT versus sham treatment. In the largest trial (n = 220), the IPSS fell from 23.6 at baseline to 12.7 points with active treatment after 6 months, a decrease of 5.0 points more than the decrease with sham treatment. The difference between active and sham treatments at 6 months was significant ($P < 0.05$).[42] **Versus TURP:** Two small trials with follow up to 2.5 years found no difference in symptom relief between TUMT and TURP.[43,44] A third trial found significantly better symptomatic outcomes with TURP.[45] **Versus α blockers:** One small trial randomised 103 men to TUMT or terazosin (up to 10 mg daily) and found significantly better improvement in IPSS after TUMT at 6 months.[45]

Harms: Adverse events associated with TUMT varied among trials, but included the need for catheterisation for more than a week (8% with TUMT v 2% with sham treatment),[46] persistent irritative symptoms (22% v 8%),[40] haematuria (14% v 1%),[45] and sexual dysfunction (mostly haematospermia and other ejaculatory abnormalities, 29% v 1%).[43] In one trial, retrograde ejaculation seemed substantially less common after TUMT (27%) than TURP (74%).[44]

Comment: TUMT uses heat generated by a microwave antennae in the urethra to coagulate prostate tissue at a single outpatient session. The long term effects of TUMT have not been adequately evaluated in controlled studies.

OPTION   TRANSURETHRAL NEEDLE ABLATION (TUNA)

We found limited evidence from one RCT that TURP is more effective than TUNA in men with BPH, although TUNA caused fewer adverse effects.

Benefits: We found no systematic review. **Versus TURP:** We found one RCT in 121 men compared TUNA versus TURP.[47] It found that the mean

IPSS fell from 24.7 to 11.1 points at 1 year with TUNA, 2.4 points less than the decrease following TURP. Benefit at 1 year was significantly greater with TURP than TUNA (IPPS 11.1 with TUNA *v* 8.3 with TURP, P = 0.04).

Harms: Compared with TURP, TUNA was associated with less retrograde ejaculation (38% *v* 0%) and bleeding (100% *v* 32%).[47]

Comment: TUNA uses radiofrequency energy via two intraprostatic electrodes to generate heat to coagulate prostate tissue, again in the outpatient setting. Anaesthesia requirements vary in reported studies. The long term effects of treatment have not been adequately evaluated.

QUESTION What are the effects of non-medical treatments? New

OPTION SAW PALMETTO PLANT EXTRACTS

One systematic review found that self rated improvement was better in men taking saw palmetto compared with placebo. It found no difference in symptom scores between saw palmetto and finasteride.

Benefits: We found one systematic and one non-systematic review. The systematic review (18 RCTs) included all saw palmetto preparations;[48] the non-systematic review (11 RCTs) included only one pure saw palmetto preparation (Permixon).[49] **Versus placebo:** The systematic review found that patient rated improvement was better in people taking saw palmetto compared with placebo (6 RCTs, RR 1.7, 95% CI 1.2 to 2.4). It found no significant difference in nocturia in men receiving saw palmetto compared with placebo (10 RCTs, WMD of 0.76 episodes per night, 95% CI 0.32 to 1.21). The non-systematic review focused only on nocturia and found similar results.[49] **Versus finasteride:** The systematic review found similar symptom scores with saw palmetto and finasteride.[48]

Harms: In the systematic review, withdrawal rates were significantly higher with saw palmetto versus placebo (9% *v* 7%, P = 0.02), and lower versus finasteride (9% *v* 11%, P = 0.87). Risks of erectile dysfunction were similar with saw palmetto versus placebo (1.1% *v* 0.7%, P = 0.58), but significantly lower versus finasteride (1.1% *v* 4.9%, P < 0.001).[48]

Comment: The RCTs were of limited duration and few used a validated symptom score. Different preparations, which may not be equivalent, are available directly to consumers without prescription in many countries.

Substantive changes since last issue

α **Blockers versus placebo** New RCT.[11]
α **Blockers versus each other** New RCT.[12]
α **Blockers, harms** Two new RCTs.[12,15]
α **Reductase inhibitors versus placebo** New RCT.[20]
TURP versus less invasive techniques Five new RCTs.[25,26,33–35]

Benign prostatic hyperplasia

REFERENCES

1. Bosch JL, Hop WC, Kirkels WJ, Schroder FH. Natural history of benign prostatic hyperplasia: appropriate case definition and estimation of its prevalence in the community. Urology 1995; 46(suppl A):34–40.

2. Barry MJc, Adolfsson J, Batista JE, et al. Committee 6: measuring the symptoms and health impact of benign prostatic hyperplasia and its treatments. In: Denis L, Griffiths K, Khoury S, et al, eds. Fourth International Consultation on BPH, Proceedings. Plymouth, UK: Health Publication Ltd, 1998:265–321.

3. Oishi K, Boyle P, Barry MJ, et al. Committee 1: Epidemiology and natural history of benign prostatic hyperplasia. In: Denis L, Griffiths K, Khoury S, et al, eds. Fourth International Consultation on BPH, Proceedings. Plymouth, UK: Health Publication Ltd, 1998:23–59.

4. Jacobsen SJ, Girman CJ, Guess HA, Rhodes T, Oesterling JE, Lieber MM. Natural history of prostatism: longitudinal changes in voiding symptoms in community dwelling men. J Urol 1996;155:595–600.

5. Barry MJ, Fowler FJ, Bin L, Pitts JC, Harris CJ, Mulley AG. The natural history of patients with benign prostatic hyperplasia as diagnosed by North American urologists. J Urol 1997;157:10–15.

6. Jacobsen S, Jacobson D, Girman C, et al. Natural history of prostatism: risk factors for acute urinary retention. J Urol 1997;158:481–487.

7. McConnell J, Bruskewitz R, Walsh P, et al. The effect of finasteride on the risk of acute urinary retention and the need for surgical treatment among men with benign prostatic hyperplasia. N Engl J Med 1998;338:557–563.

8. Barry MJ, Fowler FJ Jr, O' Leary MP, et al. The American Urological Association symptom index for benign prostatic hyperplasia. J Urol 1992;148:1549–1557.

9. Djavan B, Marberger M. A meta-analysis on the efficacy and tolerability of α1–adrenoceptor antagonists in patients with lower urinary tract symptoms suggestive of benign prostatic obstruction. Eur Urol 1999;36:1–13. Search date October 1998; primary source Medline.

10. Roehrborn CG, Oesterling JE, Auerbach S, et al. The Hytrin community assessment trial study: a one–year study of terazosin versus placebo in the treatment of men with symptomatic benign prostatic hyperplasia. Urology 1996;47:159–168.

11. McNeil SA, Daruwala PD, Mitchell IDC, Shearer MG, Hargreave TB. Sustained-release alfuzosin and trial without catheter after acute urinary retention: a prospective placebo-controlled trial. BJU Int 1999;84:622–627.

12. Na YJ, Guo YL, Gu F-L, et al. Clinical comparison of selective and non-selective alpha 1A-adreno receptor antagonists for bladder outlet obstruction associated with benign prostatic hyperplasia: studies on tamsulosin and terazosin in Chinese patients. J Med 1998;29:289–303.

13. Lepor H, Williford WO, Barry MJ, et al. The efficacy of terazosin, finasteride, or both in benign prostatic hyperplasia. Veterans' Affairs cooperative studies benign prostatic hyperplasia study group. N Engl J Med 1996;335:533–539.

14. Debruyne FMJ, Jardin A, Colloi D, et al. Sustained-release alfuzosin, finasteride and the combination of both in the treatment of benign prostatic hyperplasia. Eur Urol 1998;34:169–175.

15. Hofner K, Claes H, De Reijke TM, et al. Tamsulosin 0.4 mg once daily: effect on sexual function in patients with lower urinary tract symptoms suggestive of benign prostatic obstruction. Eur Urol 1999;36:335–341.

16. Mobley D, Dias N, Levenstein M. Effects of doxazosin in patients with mild, intermediate, and severe benign prostatic hyperplasia. Clin Ther 1998;20:101–109.

17. Kaplan S, Kaplan N. Alpha–blockade: monotherapy for hypertension and benign prostatic hyperplasia. Urology 1996;48:541–550.

18. Boyle P, Gould AL, Roehrborn CG. Prostate volume predicts outcome of treatment of benign prostatic hyperplasia with finasteride: meta-analysis of randomized clinical trials. Urology 1996;48:398–405.

19. Andersen J, Nickel J, Marshall V, Schulman C, Boyle P. Finasteride significantly reduces acute urinary retention and need for surgery in patients with symptomatic benign prostatic hyperplasia. Urology 1997;49:839–845.

20. Roehrborn CG, Boyle P, Bergner D, et al. Serum prostate specific antigen and prostate volume predict long-term changes in symptoms and flow rate: results of a four-year, randomised trial comparing finasteride and placebo. Urology 1999: 54:663–669

21. Roehrborn CG, McConnell JD, Lieber M, et al. Serum prostate-specific antigen concentration is a powerful predictor of acute urinary retention and the need for surgery in men with clinical benign prostatic hypoplasia. Urology 1999;53:473–480.

22. Wasson J, Reda D, Bruskewitz R, et al. A comparison of transurethral surgery with watchful waiting for moderate symptoms of benign prostatic hyperplasia. N Engl J Med 1995;332:75–79.

23. Flanigan RC, Reda DC, Wasson JH, Anderson RJ, Abdellatif M, Bruskewitz RC. Five year outcome of surgical resection and watchful waiting for men with moderately symptomatic benign prostatic hyperplasia: a Department of Veterans' Affairs cooperative study. J Urol 1998;160:12–17.

24. Riehmann M, Knes JM, Heisey D, Madsen PO, Bruskewitz RC. Transurethral resection versus incision of the prostate: a randomized, prospective study. Urology 1995;45:768–775.

25. McAllister WJ, Absalom MJ, Mir K, et al. Does endoscopic laser ablation of the prostate stand the test of time? Five-year results test results from a multicentre randomised controlled trial of endoscopic laser ablation against transurethral resection of the prostate. BJU Int 2000;85:437–439.

26. Keoghane SR, Lawrence KC, Gray AM, et al. A double-blind randomized controlled trial and economic evaluation of transurethral resection vs contact laser vaporization for benign prostatic enlargement: a 3-year follow-up. BJU Int 2000; 85:74–78

27. Shokeir A, Al-Sisi H, Farage Y, El-Maaboud M, Saeed M, Mutabagani H. Transurethral prostatectomy: a prospective randomized study of conventional resection and electrovaporisation in benign prostatic hyperplasia. Br J Urol 1997;80:570–574.

28. Kaplan S, Laor E, Fatal M, Te A. Transurethral resection of the prostate versus transurethral electrovaporization of the prostate: a blinded, prospective comparative study with 1-year follow up. J Urol 1998;159:454–458.

29. Kupeli S, Baltaci S, Aytac S, Yulmaz E, Budak M. A prospective randomized study of transurethral resection of the prostate and transurethral vaporization of the prostate as a therapeutic alternative in the management of men with BPH. Eur Urol 1998;34:15–18.

30. Hammadeh MY, Madaan S, Singh M, Philp T. Two

year follow-up of a prospective randomised trial of electrovaporization versus resection of prostate. *Eur Urol* 1998;34:188–192.

31. Gallucci M, Puppo P, Perachino M, et al. Transurethral electrovaporization of the prostate vs. Transurethral resection. *Eur Urol* 1998;33: 359–364.

32. Kupeli S, Yalcinkaya F, Topaloglu H, Karabacak O, Gunlusoy B, Unal S. Efficacy of transurethral electrovaporization of the prostate with respect to transurethral resection. *J Endourol* 1998;12:591–594.

33. Tuhkaren K, Heino A, Ala-Opas M. Contact laser prostatectomy compared to TURP in prostatic hyperplasia smaller than 40 ml. *Scand J Urol Nephrol* 1999;33:31–34.

34. Carter A, Sells H, Speakman M, Ewings P, MacDonagh R, O'Boyle P. A prospective randomized controlled trial of hybrid laser treatment or transurethral resection of the prostate, with a 1-year follow-up. *BJU Int* 1999; 83:254–259.

35. Shingleton WB, Terrell F, Renfoe DL, Kolski JM, Fowler JE. A randomised prospective study of laser ablation of the prostate versus transurethral resection of the prostate in men with benign prostatic hyperplasia. *Urology* 1999;54:1017–1021.

36. Lu-Yao GL, Barry MJ, Chang CH, Wasson JH, Wennberg JE, and the Prostate PORT. Transurethral resection of the prostate among Medicare beneficiaries in the United States: time trends and outcomes. *Urology* 1994;44:692–698.

37. McConnell JD, Barry MJ, Bruskewitz RC, et al. Direct treatment outcomes–complications. Benign prostatic hyperplasia: diagnosis and treatment. Clinical Practice Guideline, Number 8. Rockville, Maryland: Agency for Health Care Policy and Research, Public Health Service, US Department of Health and Human Services, 1994:91–98.

38. McConnell JD, Barry MJ, Bruskewitz RC, et al. Direct treatment outcomes – sexual dysfunction. Benign prostatic hyperplasia: diagnosis and treatment. Clinical Practice Guideline, Number 8. Rockville, Maryland: Agency for Health Care Policy and Research, Public Health Service, US Department of Health and Human Services, 1994: 99–103.

39. McConnell JD, Barry MJ, Bruskewitz RC, et al. Direct treatment outcomes – urinary incontinence. Benign prostatic hyperplasia: diagnosis and treatment. Clinical Practice Guideline, Number 8. Rockville, Maryland: Agency for Health Care Policy and Research, Public Health Service, US Department of Health and Human Services, 1994: 105–106.

40. Cowles RS III, Kabalin JN, Childs S, et al. A prospective randomized comparison of transurethral resection to visual laser ablation of the prostate for the treatment of benign prostatic hyperplasia. *Urology* 1995;46:155–160.

41. Kabalin JN, Gill HS, Bite G, Wolfe V. Comparative study of laser versus electrocautery prostatic resection: 18-month followup with complex urodynamic assessment. *J Urol* 1995;153:94–97.

42. Roehrborn C, Preminger G, Newhall P, et al. Microwave thermotherapy for benign prostatic hyperplasia with the Dornier Urowave: results of a randomized, double-blind, multicenter, sham-controlled trial. *Urology* 1998;51:19–28.

43. Ahmed M, Bell T, Lawrence WT, Ward JP, Watson GM. Transurethral microwave thermotherapy (Prostatron version 2.5) compared with transurethral resection of the prostate for the treatment of benign prostatic hyperplasia: a randomized, controlled, parallel study. *Br J Urol* 1997;79:181–185.

44. Francisca EA, D'Ancona FC, Meuleman EJ, Debruyne FM, DeLaRosette JJ. Sexual function following high energy microwave thermotherapy: results of a randomized controlled study comparing transurethral microwave thermotherapy to transurethral prostatic resection. *J Urol* 1999; 161:486–490.

45. Djavan B, Roehrborn CG, Shariat S, Ghawidel K, Marberger M. Prospective randomized comparison of high energy transurethral microwave thermotherapy versus alpha blocker treatment of patients with benign prostatic hyperplasia. *J Urol* 1999;161:139–143.

46. Larson T, Blute M, Bruskewitz R, Mayer R, Ugarte R, Utz W. A high–efficiency microwave thermoablation system for the treatment of benign prostatic hyperplasia: results of a randomized, sham–controlled, prospective, double-blind, multicenter clinical trial. *Urology* 1998;51:731–742.

47. Bruskewitz R, Issa M, Roehrborn C, et al. A prospective, randomized 1-year clinical trial comparing transurethral needle ablation to transurethral resection of the prostate for the treatment of symptomatic benign prostatic hyperplasia. *J Urol* 1998;159:1588–1594.

48. Wilt T, Ishani A, Stark G, Mac Donald R, Mulrow C, and Lau J. Serenoa repens for benign prostatic hyperplasia. In: The Cochrane Library, Issue 2, 2000. Oxford: Update Software. Search date 1997; primary sources Medline, Embase, Phytodok, The Cochrane library.

49. Boyle P, Robertson C, Lowe F, Roehrborn C. Meta-analysis of clinical trials of Permixon in the treatment of benign prostatic hyperplasia. *Urology* 2000;55:533–539.

Michael Barry
General Medicine Unit, Massachusetts
General Hospital
Boston, Massachusetts
USA

Claus Roehrborn
Associate Professor
Department of Urology, The University of
Texas, Southwestern Medical Center
Dallas, Texas
USA

Competing interests: None declared.

Chronic prostatitis

Updated this issue

Jeffry Stern and Anthony Schaeffer

Men's health

QUESTIONS

INTERVENTIONS

Key Messages

In men with chronic bacterial prostatitis

- Antimicrobial drugs have not been adequately evaluated. Retrospective cohort studies report cure rates of 0%–90% depending on the drug used and the duration of treatment.

- We found no good evidence that local injection of antimicrobial agents is more effective than oral or parenteral antimicrobial treatment.

- Limited evidence from one RCT suggests that adding α blockers to antimicrobial treatment may improve outcome and reduce recurrence.

- We found that transurethral resection and radical prostatectomy have not yet been adequately evaluated.

In men with chronic abacterial prostatitis

- Limited evidence from one RCT suggests that α blockers may improve symptoms.

- Limited evidence from one RCT suggests that transurethral microwave thermotherapy may improve symptoms; we found no evidence on cure or recurrence rate.

- Allopurinol thermotherapy, prostatic massage, Sitz baths, and biofeedback have not yet been adequately evaluated.

DEFINITION	**Chronic bacterial prostatitis** is characterised by a positive culture of expressed prostatic secretions. It can be symptomatic (recurrent urinary tract infection, suprapubic, lower back, or perineal pain), asymptomatic, or associated with minimal urgency, frequency, and dysuria. **Chronic abacterial prostatitis** is characterised by pelvic or perineal pain, often associated with urinary urgency, nocturia, weak urinary stream, frequency, dysuria, hesitancy, dribbling after micturition, interrupted flow, and inflammation (white cells) in prostatic secretions. Symptoms can also include suprapubic, scrotal, testicular, penile, or lower back pain or discomfort, known as prostodynia in the absence of inflammation in prostatic secretions.
INCIDENCE/ PREVALENCE	One community based study estimated that 9% of men have a diagnosis of chronic prostatitis at any one time.[1] Another study found that, of men with genitourinary symptoms, 8% presenting to urologists and 1% presenting to primary care physicians are diagnosed with chronic prostatitis.[2] Most cases of chronic prostatitis are abacterial. Acute bacterial prostatitis, while easy to diagnose and treat, is rare.
AETIOLOGY/ RISK FACTORS	Organisms commonly implicated in bacterial prostatitis include *Escherichia coli*, other Gram negative *Enterobacteriaciae*, occasionally *Pseudomonas* species, and rarely Gram positive enterococci. The cause of abacterial prostatitis is unclear, but autoimmunity may be involved.[3]
PROGNOSIS	One recent study found that chronic abacterial prostatitis had an impact on quality of life similar to that from angina, Crohn's disease, or a previous myocardial infarction.[4]
AIMS	To relieve symptoms and eliminate infection where present, with minimum adverse effects.
OUTCOMES	Symptom improvement (symptom scores, bother scores); quality of life; urodynamics; rates of bacteriological cure (clearance of previously documented organisms from prostatic secretions).
METHODS	We searched Medline up to July 1998. A full update *Clinical Evidence* search and appraisal was performed in May 2000. No systematic reviews were identified. We reviewed all relevant RCTs identified.

QUESTION	**What are the effects of treatments for chronic bacterial prostatitis?**

OPTION	ORAL ANTIMICROBIAL DRUGS

We found that oral antimicrobial drugs have not been adequately evaluated in men with chronic bacterial prostatitis. Retrospective cohort studies report cure rates (clearing prostatic secretions of previously documented organisms) of 0%–90% depending on the drug used and the duration of treatment. Limited evidence from retrospective studies suggests that quinolones may be more effective than trimethoprim-sulfamethoxazole (TMP-SMZ).

Benefits: We found no systematic review and no RCTs. **TMP-SMZ:** One non-systematic review identified 10 retrospective cohort studies in

Chronic prostatitis

135 men with bacteriologically confirmed prostatitis treated with TMP-SMZ 160 mg/800 mg twice daily for 10–140 days.[5] The studies reported bacteriological cure rates of 0%–67%. Over 30% of men were cured when treated for at least 90 days. **Quinolones:** One review summarised three retrospective cohort studies in 106 men treated with norfloxacin 400 mg twice daily for 10, 28, and 174 days.[6] The studies reported cure rates of 64%–88%. We also found six retrospective cohort studies in 141 men treated with ciprofloxacin 250–500 mg twice daily for 14–259 days, with cure rates of 60%–75%. **Amoxicillin/clavulanic acid and clindamycin:** One cohort study included 50 men who were resistant to empirical treatment with quinolone. The expressed prostatic secretions from 24 of these men exhibited high colony counts of Gram positive and Gram negative anaerobic bacteria, either alone (18 men) or in combination with aerobic bacteria (6 men). After treatment with either amoxicillin/clavulanic acid or clindamycin for 3–6 weeks, all patients had a decrease or total elimination of symptoms, and no anaerobic bacteria were detected in prostatic secretions.[7]

Harms: The studies of TMP-SMZ did not report adverse effects. In the other studies, toxicity from quinolones was rare. Late relapse (6–12 months after treatment) was common.

Comment: Higher cure rates with quinolones may be explained by greater penetration into the prostate.[8] We reviewed only studies that used standard methods to localise infection to the prostate.[9]

OPTION   LOCAL INJECTION OF ANTIMICROBIALS

We found no good evidence that local injection of antimicrobial agents is more effective than oral or parenteral antimicrobial treatment.

Benefits: We found no systematic review and no RCTs. One small cohort study of 24 men with refractory chronic bacterial prostatitis found that eradication of infection was eventually achieved after an unstated period in 15 men with 160 mg gentamicin plus 3 g cefazolin injected directly into the prostate via the perineum.[10]

Harms: Although not reported in this study, infection is a potential risk of this invasive procedure.

Comment: None.

OPTION   α BLOCKERS

We found limited evidence from one RCT suggesting that adding α blockers to antimicrobial treatment may improve outcome and reduce recurrence in men with chronic bacterial prostatitis.

Benefits: We found no systematic review. We found one RCT of α blockers (either 1–2 mg terazosin daily or 2.5 mg terazosin daily or 2.5 mg alfuzosin once or twice daily) in 270 men with bacterial or abacterial prostatitis or prostadynia.[11] Antimicrobials were given to all men with positive culture of expressed prostatic secretions and to half of those with inflammatory expressed prostatic secretions. Of men with bacterial prostatitis, those given α blockers and antimicrobials had significantly higher rates of clinical improvement and significantly lower rates of recurrence (assessed by culture of expressed prostatic secretions) compared with those given antimicrobials alone (P = 0.019, no RR or CI given).

Harms: No adverse effects of α blockers were reported in this study.[11]

Comment: None.

OPTION   TRANSURETHRAL RESECTION

We found insufficient evidence on the effects of transurethral resection of the prostate in men with chronic bacterial prostatitis.

Benefits: We found no systematic review, RCTs, or prospective cohort studies.

Harms: One trial in men with benign prostatic hypertrophy found no difference in the incidence of impotence or urinary incontinence with transurethral resection or watchful waiting.[12]

Comment: One retrospective cohort study reported 40%–50% cure rates in 50 men with chronic prostatitis treated with transurethral resection. However, proof of bacterial prostatitis was not shown in many cases.[13]

OPTION   RADICAL PROSTATECTOMY

Radical prostatectomy is associated with impotence, stress incontinence, and complications of open surgery. We found that its use in men with chronic prostatitis has not been adequately evaluated.

Benefits: We found no RCTs. We found one report of radical prostatectomy in two young men whose refractory bacterial prostatitis caused relapsing haemolytic crises.[14]

Harms: Radical prostatectomy can cause impotence (9–75% depending upon age)[15] and varying degrees of urinary stress incontinence (8%).[16] Other potential harms include those associated with any open surgery.

Comment: None.

QUESTION   What are the effects of treatments for chronic abacterial prostatitis?

OPTION   α BLOCKERS

Limited evidence from one RCT suggests that α blockers may relieve symptoms in men with abacterial prostatitis.

Benefits: We found no systematic review. We found one RCT of α blockers (either 1–2 mg terazosin daily or 2.5 mg terazosin daily or 2.5 mg alfuzosin once or twice daily) in 270 men with bacterial or abacterial prostatitis or prostadynia.[11] Antimicrobials were given to all men with positive culture of expressed prostatic secretions and to half of those with inflammatory expressed prostatic secretions. Of men with abacterial prostatitis, those given α blockers had significantly lower rates of symptomatic recurrence compared with those given either no treatment or antimicrobials (P < 0.001, no RR or CI given).

Harms: No adverse effects of α blockers were reported.[11]

Comment: None.

OPTION   TRANSURETHRAL MICROWAVE THERMOTHERAPY

We found insufficient evidence on the effects of thermotherapy in abacterial prostatitis for cure or recurrence rate. One small RCT found that it relieved symptoms compared with sham treatment.

Benefits: We found no systematic review. We found one small double blind RCT comparing transurethral microwave thermotherapy versus sham treatment in 20 men.[17] Outcomes were assessed using a symptom severity index and symptom frequency questionnaire. Seven of 10 men in the treatment group improved significantly over a mean of 21 months' follow up, compared with one of the 10 men in the sham group (no CI or P value reported).

Harms: Four men complained of transient (resolved in 3 weeks) adverse reactions, including haematuria (2 men), urinary tract infection, impotence, urinary retention, urinary incontinence, and premature ejaculation (each occurring in one man).[17]

Comment: The trial measured changes in clinical symptoms to determine efficacy. Thermotherapy caused persistent elevation of leukocytes in the prostatic fluid, which could indicate tissue damage.

OPTION   ALLOPURINOL

We found no good evidence on the effects of allopurinol in men with chronic abacterial prostatitis.

Benefits: We found one systemic review,[18] which identified one RCT. Fifty four men were initially enrolled in the study and divided into three groups: treatment with 600 mg allopurinol daily, treatment with 300 mg allopurinol daily, and placebo. Thirty four men completed the study, which lasted 240 days. The trial found that there was a significant effect of allopurinol on urate concentration in expressed prostatic secretion; men in treatment groups had a far lower ratio of urate to creatinine in their expressed prostatic secretions than did the placebo group. Moreover, the "degree of discomfort" score was lower among the allopurinol groups than the placebo group (P = 0.019).

Harms: No men receiving allopurinol reported any significant adverse effects.

Comment: From the data presented, it is not clear that the decreases in urate concentration in expressed prostatic secretion led directly to symptom relief. The symptom score was not validated.[18]

OPTION   OTHER INTERVENTIONS

We found that prostatic massage, Sitz baths, and biofeedback (training the patient to contract and relax the pelvic floor muscles to interrupt the myofascial pain attacks) have not yet been formally evaluated in men with chronic abacterial prostatitis.

Benefits: We found no systematic review or RCTs.

Harms: Insufficient data.

Comment: None.

REFERENCES

1. Roberts RO, Lieber MM, Rhodes T, et al. Prevalence of a physician-assigned diagnosis of prostatitis: the Olmsted County study of urinary symptoms and health status among men. *Urology* 1998;51:578–584.
2. Collins MM, Stafford, RS, O'Leary MP, Barry MJ. How common is prostatitis? A national survey of physician visits. *J Urol* 1998;159:1224–1228.
3. Alexander RB, Brady F, Ponniah S. Autoimmune prostatitis: evidence of T cell reactivity with normal prostatic proteins. *Urology* 1997;50:893–899.
4. Wenninger K, Heiman JR, Rothman I, Berghuis JP, Berger RE. Sickness impact of chronic nonbacterial prostatitis and its correlates. *J Urol* 1996;155:965–968.
5. Hanus PM, Danzinger LH. Treatment of chronic bacterial prostatitis. *Clin Pharm* 1984;3:49–55.
6. Naber KG, Sorgel F, Kees F, et al. Norfloxacin concentration in prostatic adenoma tissue (patients) and in prostatic fluid in patients and volunteers. 15th International Congress of Chemotherapy, Landsberg. In: Weidner N, Madsen PO, Schiefer HG, eds. Prostatitis: etiopathology, diagnosis and therapy. New York: Springer Verlag, 1987.
7. Szoke I, Torok L, Dosa E, et al. The possible role of anaerobic bacteria in chronic prostatitis. *Int J Androl* 1998;21:163–168.
8. Cox CE. Ofloxacin in the management of complicated urinary tract infections, including prostatitis. *Am J Med* 1980;87(suppl 6c):61–68.
9. Meares EM, Stamey TA. Bacteriologic localization patterns in bacterial prostatitis and urethritis. *Invest Urol* 1968;5:492–518.
10. Baret L, Leonare A. Chronic bacterial prostatitis: 10 years of experience with local antibiotics. *J Urol* 1998;140:755–757.
11. Barbalias GA, Nikiforidis G, Liatsikos EN. Alpha-blockers for the treatment of chronic prostatitis in combination with antibiotics. *J Urol* 1998;159:883–887.
12. Wasson JH, Reda DJ, Bruskewitz RC, et al. A comparison of transurethral surgery with watchful waiting for moderate symptoms of benign prostatic hyperplasia. *N Engl J Med* 1995;332:75–79.
13. Smart CJ, Jenkins JD, Lloyd RS. The painful prostate. *Br J Urol* 1975;47:861–869.
14. Davis BE, Weigel JW. Adenocarcinoma of the prostate discovered in 2 young patients following total prostatovesiculectomy for refractory prostatitis. *J Urol* 1990;144:744–745.
15. Quinlan DM, Epstein JI, Carter BS, Walsh PC. Sexual function following radical prostatectomy: influence of preservation of neurovascular bundles. *J Urol* 1991;145:998–1002.
16. Steiner MS, Morton RA, Walsh PC. Impact of radical prostatectomy on urinary continence. *J Urol* 1991;145:512–515.
17. Nickel J, Sorensen R. Transurethral microwave thermotherapy for nonbacterial prostatitis: a randomized double-blind sham controlled study using new prostatitis specific assessment questionnaires. *J Urol* 1996;155:1950–1955.
18. Persson B, Ronquist G, Ekblom M. Ameliorative effect of allopurinol on nonbacterial prostatitis: a parallel double-blind controlled study. *J Urol* 1996;155:961–964.

Jeffrey Stern

Anthony Schaeffer

Northwestern University Medical School
Chicago
USA

Competing interests: AS has been reimbursed by Ortho McNeil for attending and speaking at several conferences. He has also received consulting fees from Bayer Corp. and Johnson and Johnson.

Men's health

Updated and expanded this issue

Michael O'Leary

Key Messages

- We found good evidence from well conducted RCTs that yohimbine and sildenafil are effective and well tolerated compared with placebo. We found no trials comparing one directly with the other. Limited evidence from indirect comparison of data from placebo controlled trials suggests that yohimbine may be less effective but safer.

- Small RCTs found no evidence that L-arginine or trazodone were more effective than placebo, although the trials were not adequately powered to rule out a clinically important difference.

- RCTs have found that prostaglandin E1 (alprostadil) is effective in about 30–80% of men, and more effective when administered by intracavernosal injection than intraurethrally. For both methods, adherence to treatment in the long term is poor. One small RCT found that topical prostaglandin E1 was significantly more effective than placebo, but sequential allocation of men to each group may mean that groups were not comparable.

- Neither vacuum devices nor penile prostheses have been adequately evaluated in RCTs.

DEFINITION	Erectile dysfunction has largely replaced the term "impotence." It is defined as the persistent inability to obtain or maintain sufficient rigidity of the penis to allow satisfactory sexual performance.
INCIDENCE/ PREVALENCE	There is little good epidemiological information, but current normative data suggest that age is the variable most strongly associated with erectile dysfunction, and that up to 30 million men in the USA may be affected.[1] Even among men in their 40s, nearly 40% report at least occasional difficulty obtaining or maintaining erection, whereas this approaches 70% in 70 year olds.
AETIOLOGY/ RISK FACTORS	It is now believed that about 80% of cases of erectile dysfunction have an organic cause, the rest being psychogenic in origin. Erectile problems fall into three categories: failure to initiate; failure to fill, caused by insufficient arterial inflow into the penis to allow engorgement and tumescence, owing to vascular insufficiency; and failure to store, owing to veno-occlusive dysfunction.
PROGNOSIS	In erectile dysfunction of organic cause, treatment is almost always symptomatic. We found no good data on prognosis in untreated organic erectile dysfunction.
AIMS	To restore satisfactory erections with minimal adverse effects.
OUTCOMES	Patient and partner self reports of satisfaction and sexual function; objective tests of penile rigidity; adverse effects of treatment.
METHODS	*Clinical Evidence* update search and appraisal May 2000. All identified systematic reviews and RCTs were reviewed.

QUESTION   What are the effects of treatments?

OPTION   YOHIMBINE

RCTs have found that yohimbine is effective compared with placebo. Yohimbine has not yet been compared directly with other oral or local treatments. Mild, transient adverse effects are reported in up to a third of men.

Benefits: We found one systematic review (search date 1997, 7 RCTs, 11–100 men with erectile dysfunction (defined variously as organic, psychogenic, and of unknown cause) comparing the α blocker, yohimbine, versus placebo.[2] Duration of treatment ranged from 2–10 weeks, and outcomes varied from self reported improvement in sexual function to objective tests of penile rigidity. The RCTs found positive responses in 34–73% of men on yohimbine compared with 9–28% on placebo (OR for positive response with treatment compared with placebo 3.85, 95% CI 2.22 to 6.67). One subsequent placebo controlled, crossover trial (n = 22, randomisation not mentioned) found no evidence that yohimbine (single daily dose 100 mg for 30 days) significantly promoted erections more than placebo.[3]

Harms: Adverse events were reported in 10–30% of men receiving yohimbine and were generally mild, including agitation, anxiety, headache, mild increase in blood pressure, increased urinary output and gastrointestinal upset. In at least one study, however, no men discontinued treatment.[3]

Comment: The end points in some of these trials were subjective and of questionable validity.

OPTION	SILDENAFIL

RCTs have found that sildenafil is effective compared with placebo and well tolerated in men with and without diabetes. It has not yet been compared directly with other treatments for erectile dysfunction. Mild transient adverse effects are reported in up to a fifth of men, and deaths have been reported in men on concomitant treatment with oral nitrates. Long term safety is unknown.

Benefits: We found no systematic review. We found six RCTs. **In men with any cause of erectile dysfunction:** Three RCTs evaluated sildenafil in 1496 men with erectile dysfunction from a variety of causes. All three trials found that sildenafil improved outcomes compared with placebo.[4-6] The largest trial comparing sildenafil versus placebo (n = 861, age 20–87 years) involved two different evaluations in men with 3–5 years of erectile dysfunction from all causes.[4] In the first evaluation, 532 men were randomised to receive either placebo or 25 mg, 50 mg, or 100 mg sildenafil about 1 hour before planned sexual activity, but not more than once per day, for 24 weeks. In the second, 329 different men were randomised to placebo or sildenafil in an escalating dose up to 100 mg for 12 weeks, followed by open label treatment for a further 32 weeks. More men taking sildenafil had successful attempts at sexual intercourse than those on placebo (69% v 22%, P < 0.001; CI values not quoted in report). Efficacy increased with increasing dose and did not vary according to the cause of erectile dysfunction. **In men with diabetes:** One double blind multicentre RCT in 268 men with erectile dysfunction and diabetes found that sildenafil significantly improved erections over placebo at 12 weeks (AR 56% v 10%; ARR 46%, 95% CI 30% to 62%; RR 5.5, 95% CI 3.9 to 7.0; NNT 2, 95% CI 2 to 3).[7] **In men with spinal cord injury:** We found two RCTs. The first compared sildenafil with placebo in 26 men with spinal cord injury (T6 through L5). It found that sildenafil significantly improved erections (9/12 in treatment group v 1/14 in placebo group, P = 0.0043). At 28 days, significantly more men in the treatment group reported improvements in quality of sex life (P = 0.0012) and wished to continue treatment (P = 0.018).[8] The second trial was a double blind two way crossover comparison of oral sildenafil versus placebo in 111 men with erectile dysfunction secondary to spinal trauma. It found that sildenafil improved sexual intercourse more than placebo (80% reported improved sexual intercourse with sildenafil v 10% with placebo).[6]

Harms: In the first trial, headache, flushing, and dyspepsia were reported in 6–18% of men taking sildenafil.[3,4] In the trial in men with diabetes, cardiovascular events were comparable between the two groups with comparable cardiovascular adverse events (3% sildenafil v 5% placebo).[7] None of the men with spinal cord injury in the third trial discontinued treatment.[8] Another article reported specifically on adverse effects of sildenafil. It summarised results from a series of double blind placebo controlled RCTs in a total of 4274 men aged 19–87 years with erectile dysfunction due to a range of causes for more than 6 months and a mean of 5 years. All men were treated for up to 6 months, and 2199 received open label treatment for up to a further year. Headache, flushing, and dyspepsia were reported in 7–16% of men taking sildenafil compared with 1–4% taking placebo. Similar proportions in both groups discontinued treatment (about 2.4%). An important contraindication to prescribing sildenafil is concomitant use of oral nitrates. This combination results in precipitous hypotension. To date, about 60 deaths have been reported to the US Food and Drug Administration in men who had been given prescriptions for sildenafil. However, it is not known whether any were directly attributable to the drug. Long term (> 1 year) safety of sildenafil is unknown.

Comment: None.

OPTION   L-ARGININE   New

One small RCT found no evidence that L-arginine improved sexual function compared with placebo, although the trial was inadequately powered to rule out a clinically important difference.

Benefits: We found no systematic review. We found one small double blind RCT comparing high dose L-arginine (5 g per day given orally) versus placebo in 50 men with erectile dysfunction.[10] The trial found no evidence of a significant difference in sexual function between L-arginine and placebo, although the power of the study was not adequate to rule out a clinically important difference (sexual function improved in 9/29 men with L-arginine v 2/17 with placebo, P = NS, four men not included in analysis).

Harms: The trial reported decreases in systolic or diastolic blood pressure, or both, although this caused no systemic effects and required no drug interruptions. The trial found some "fluctuation in heart rate," which was described as clinically insignificant. Nausea, vomiting, diarrhoea, headache, flushing, and numbness have been reported after the administration of L-arginine, although none of the men in this study reported any such complaints.

Comment: None.

OPTION   TRAZODONE

One small RCT found no evidence that trazodone was more effective than placebo in men with erectile dysfunction, although the trial was inadequately powered to rule out a clinically important effect.

Benefits: We found no systematic review. One small two way, crossover RCT (washout period 3 weeks) compared trazodone versus placebo in 48 men with erectile dysfunction.[11] Men were treated with either trazodone 50 mg or placebo at bedtime for 3 months. The trial found no evidence that trazodone improved erections or libido (improved erections reported by 19% v 24% receiving placebo, P < 0.50; improved libido reported by 35% v 20% with placebo, P < 0.36).

Harms: The trial reported drowsiness (31% of men), dry mouth (1%), and fatigue (19%, comparative rates for trazodone v placebo not available).

Comment: None.

Erectile dysfunction

OPTION   INTRAURETHRAL PROSTAGLANDIN E1

RCTs have found that intraurethral administration of prostaglandin E1 (alprostadil) leads to satisfactory erection in about 40% of men. About a third of men suffered penile ache, which caused many to discontinue treatment. Intraurethral prostaglandin E1 has not yet been directly compared with either intracavernosal or oral drug treatment.

Benefits: We found no systematic review. One double blind RCT began by testing the response to intraurethral alprostadil in 1511 men aged 27–88 years who had erectile dysfunction of organic cause for at least 3 months. In clinic testing, 66% had erections sufficient for intercourse. These men (n = 996) were randomised to intraurethral alprostadil or placebo for use at home.[12] Over 3 months, those given alprostadil were more likely to report having successful sexual intercourse (64.9% v 18.6% on placebo, P < 0.001) and at least one orgasm (63.6% v 23.6% on placebo, P < 0.001). Subsequent RCTs, published only in abstract form, found slightly lower efficacies of 30–48% on alprostadil.

Harms: The most common adverse effect was mild to moderate penile ache, occurring in about a third of men.[12] This caused many men to discontinue treatment. We found no reports of priapism, penile fibrosis, or other serious adverse events.

Comment: The trial preselected men who had a good response to alprostadil before randomisation. This limits the generaliseability of results.

OPTION   INTRACAVERNOSAL PROSTAGLANDIN E1

RCTs have found that intracavernosal injection of prostaglandin E1 (alprostadil) leads to satisfactory erection in about 80% of men, but long term adherence is poor. Intracavernosal prostaglandin E1 has not yet been directly compared with either intraurethral or oral drug treatment.

Benefits: We found no systematic review. The largest study was a multicentre trial in 1128 men aged 20–79 years with all causes of erectile dysfunction.[13] Heavy smokers and men with uncontrolled hypertension or diabetes were excluded. Nearly 300 men were randomly assigned to double blind doses of placebo or 2.5 g, 5 g, 10 g, or 20 g of alprostadil. Injections were given, and outcome was assessed by an investigator or research nurse. None of the 59 men who received placebo had a response. There were significant differences in response between all doses versus placebo, and a significant dose response relationship. The remaining 884 men, including 52 who had taken part in the dose response study, were enrolled in a single blind, dose escalation study (201 men) and an uncontrolled open label flexible dose study to assess efficacy, safety, and feasibility of self injection at home (683 men). Of the 13 762 injections for which men recorded their response, nearly 90% were followed by satisfactory sexual activity. **Versus vacuum devices:** One crossover RCT compared intracavernosal self injections versus vacuum devices in 50 men with erectile dysfunction, 44 of whom completed the study.[14] Outcome was assessed by a questionnaire to men and their partners after 15 uses for each device, and couples were followed for 18–24 months. There was no significant difference in the ability to achieve an erection suitable for intercourse. However, the ability to attain orgasm was significantly better with injection (P < 0.05). On a scale of 1 to 10, overall satisfaction was significantly better when using injections, both for men (6.5 v 5.4, P < 0.05) and partners (6.5 v 5.1, P < 0.05). Younger men (< 60 years) and those with shorter duration of erectile dysfunction (< 12 months) favoured injections (P < 0.05).

Harms: Penile pain was reported by half of the men in the study of efficacy and safety of alprostadil injection, and priapism (prolonged erection for > 4 hours) by 1%.[13] There was no significant difference in the frequency of adverse events between vacuum devices and injections.[14]

Comment: Most men can be taught to inject themselves using small gauge needles. In the RCT comparing injections and vacuum devices, 80% of the 44 couples who completed the study were still using one or other treatment after 18–24 months.[14]

OPTION **TOPICAL PROSTAGLANDIN E1** New

One small, single blind RCT found that topical prostaglandin E1 was significantly more effective than placebo, but sequential allocation of men to each group may mean that groups were not comparable.

Benefits: We found no systematic review. We found one single blind trial in 48 men with erectile dysfunction due to organic, psychogenic, or mixed causes that compared topical prostaglandin E1 versus placebo.[15] Men were assigned in sequential order to either 0.5 mg, 1 mg, or 2.5 mg prostaglandin gel (n = 36), or placebo (n = 12). One dose of prostaglandin or placebo gel was applied to the glans and shaft of the penis and washed off after 3 hours. Significantly more men achieved an erection sufficient for intercourse with any dose of prostaglandin E1 versus placebo (25/36 [69%] with prostaglandin E1 v 2/12 [17%] with placebo; ARI 53%, 95% CI 13% to 76%; RR 4.2, 95% CI 1.8 to 5.5; NNT 2, 95% CI 1 to 8).

Harms: Men receiving prostaglandin were significantly more likely to have skin irritation than those on placebo (100% on 0.5 mg dose v 67%, no P value provided). Irritation was more severe with prostaglandin than with placebo (measured by mean irritation score ranging from 0–2; 1.75 with 0.5 mg dose v 0.67 with placebo, P < 0.0013).[15]

Comment: Allocation of men to each group was sequential and may mean that the groups were not comparable; the characteristics of each group were not reported. The study was too small to exclude a clinically important effect of dose on effectiveness.

OPTION **VACUUM DEVICES**

Vacuum devices have not been adequately evaluated in RCTs. One small RCT found that they were as effective as intracavernosal prostaglandin E1 injections.

Benefits: We found no systematic review. **Versus intracavernosal injections:** See benefits of intracavernosal prostaglandin E1, p 472.

Men's health

Harms: Insufficient data.

Comment: Vacuum devices may be less popular with patients than injections because only the distal portion of the penis becomes firm, but they are presumed to be safe.[14]

OPTION **PENILE PROSTHESES**

Penile prostheses have not been formally evaluated in RCTs. They are usually considered only after less invasive treatments have failed.

Benefits: We found no RCTs. Anecdotal evidence suggests that patient satisfaction may be high, but we found no good studies.

Harms: One recent study found the morbidity of penile prostheses to be 9% (surgical revision 7%, mechanical failure 2.5%). Infection rates were between 2% and 7%.[16]

Comment: None.

REFERENCES

1. Feldman HA, Goldstein I, Dimitrios GH, Krane RJ, McKinlay JB. Impotence and its medical and psychosocial correlates: results of the Massachusetts male aging study. *J Urol* 1994; 151:54–61.
2. Ernst E, Pittler MH. Yohimbine for erectile dysfunction: a systemic review and meta-analysis of randomized clinical trials. *J Urol* 1998;159: 433–436. Search date 1997; primary sources Medline 1966 to 1997; Embase 1974 to 1997; Cochrane Library, Issue 4, 1999; and hand searched references.
3. Teloken C, Rhoden EL, Sogari P, Dambros M, Souto CA. Therapeutic effects of high dose yohimbine hydrochloride on organic erectile dysfunction. *J Urol* 1998;159:122–124.
4. Goldstein I, Lue TF, Harin PN, Rosen RC, Steers WD, Wicker PA, for the Sildenafil Study Group. Oral sildenafil in the treatment of erectile dysfunction. *N Engl J Med* 1998;338:1397–1404.
5. Montorsi F, McDermott PED, Morgan R, et al: Efficacy and safety of fixed dose oral sildenafil in the treatment of erectile dysfunction of various etiologies. *Urology* 1999;53:1011–1018.
6. Dinsmore WW, Hodges M, Hargreaves C, et al. Sildenafil citrate in erectile dysfunction: near normalization in men with broad spectrum erectile dysfunction compared with age-matched healthy control subjects. *Urology* 1999;53:800–805.
7. Rendell MS, Rajfer J, Wicker PA, Smith MD. Sildenafil for treatment of erectile dysfunction in men with diabetes: A randomized controlled trial. *JAMA* 1999;281:421–426.
8. Derry FA, Dinsmore WW, Fraser M, et al. Efficacy and safety of oral sildenafil in men with erectile dysfunction caused by spinal cord injury. *Neurology* 1998;51:1629–1633.
9. A, Gingell C, Collins M, Wicker PA, Osterloh IH. Clinical safety of oral sildenafil citrate (Viagra) in the treatment of erectile dysfunction. *Int J Impot Res* 1998;10:69–74.
10. Chen J, Wollman Y, Chernichovsky T, et al: Effect of oral administration of high-dose nitric oxide donor L-Arginine in men with organic erectile dysfunction: results of a double-blind randomized placebo-controlled study. *BJU Int* 1999;83:269–273.
11. Costabile RA, Spevak M. Oral trazodone is not effective therapy for erectile dysfunction: a double blind placebo-controlled trial. *J Urol* 1999;161: 1819–1822.
12. Padma-Nathan H, Hellstrom WJ, Kaiser FE, et al, for the Medicated Urethral System for Erection (MUSE) Study Group. Treatment of men with erectile dysfunction with transurethral alprostadil. *N Engl J Med* 1997;336:1–7.
13. PGE1 Study Group. Prospective, multicenter trials of efficacy and safety of intracavernosal alprostadil (prostaglandin E1) sterile powder in men with erectile dysfunction. *N Engl J Med* 1996;334: 873–877.
14. Soderdahl DW, Thrasher JB, Hansberry KL, et al. Intracavernosal drug induced erection therapy vs external vacuum device in the treatment of erectile dysfunction. *Br J Urol* 1997;79:952–957.
15. McVary KT, Polepalle S, Riggi S, Pelham RW. Topical prostaglandin E1 SEPA gel for the treatment of erectile dysfunction. *J Urol* 1999; 162:726–730.
16. Goldstein I, Newman L, Baum N, et al. Safety and efficacy outcome of Mentor α 1 inflatable penile prosthesis implantation for impotence treatment. *J Urol* 1997;157:833–839.

Michael O'Leary
Associate Professor of Surgery
Harvard Medical School
Boston
USA

Competing interests: The author has received honoraria from Pfizer for educational programs on sildenafil, and has received research support to study this agent.

Last updated Issue 3

Matthew Smith, Philip Kantoff and James Talcott

QUESTIONS

INTERVENTIONS

METASTATIC PROSTATE CANCER

Likely to be beneficial

Unknown effectiveness

Likely to be ineffective or harmful

ANDROGEN INDEPENDENT METASTATIC DISEASE

Likely to be beneficial

Unknown effectiveness

Key Messages

In men with metastatic prostate cancer

- We found limited data from RCTs suggesting that androgen deprivation reduced mortality.
- One systematic review of RCTs has found that androgen deprivation improves symptoms and objective signs of disease in most men but found no evidence of a difference between different methods of androgen deprivation (orchiectomy, diethylstilboestrol, luteinising hormone releasing hormone [LHRH] agonists).
- Systematic reviews of RCTs have found no clear evidence of benefit from adding androgen blockade to androgen deprivation compared with androgen deprivation alone.
- RCTs have found no evidence that deferring androgen deprivation until disease progression is apparent reduces survival compared with immediate treatment for metastatic disease. In the absence of surveillance, deferred androgen deprivation results in higher rates of complications. Immediate androgen deprivation may improve survival in men with advanced prostate cancer but no evidence of bone metastases.
- We found no trials that evaluated the long term effects of intermittent androgen deprivation on mortality, morbidity, or quality of life.

In men with symptomatic androgen independent prostate cancer

- RCTs have found that chemotherapy has palliative benefit but found no evidence that it prolongs survival.

Prostate cancer: metastatic

- One systematic review of trials comparing different schedules of external beam radiation found that pain was reduced in some men. We found no comparison of external beam radiation with other palliative treatments.
- We found limited evidence suggesting that radionuclides with selective bone localisation decrease pain in some men.
- We found insufficient evidence to evaluate bisphosphonates.

DEFINITION	See non-metastatic prostate cancer, p 483. Androgen independent metastatic disease is defined as disease that progresses despite androgen deprivation.
INCIDENCE/ PREVALENCE	See non-metastatic prostate cancer, p 483.
AETIOLOGY/ RISK FACTORS	See non-metastatic prostate cancer, p 483.
PROGNOSIS	Prostate cancer metastasises predominantly to bone. Metastatic prostate cancer can result in pain, weakness, paralysis, and death.
AIMS	To prevent premature death and disability, to control symptoms and maximise quality of life, and to minimise adverse effects of treatment.
OUTCOMES	Survival, response in terms of symptoms and signs, quality of life, adverse effects of treatment.
METHODS	*Clinical Evidence* search December 1999.

QUESTION What are the effects of treatment in men with metastatic prostate cancer?

OPTION ANDROGEN DEPRIVATION

We found limited evidence from RCTs suggesting that androgen deprivation reduces mortality in men with metastatic prostate cancer. One systematic review of RCTs has found that androgen deprivation improves symptoms and objective signs of disease in most men, but it found no evidence of a difference in effectiveness between different methods of androgen deprivation (orchiectomy, diethylstilboestrol, LHRH agonists).

Benefits: **Versus no initial treatment:** We found no systematic review and no recent RCTs. Three RCTs performed between 1959 and 1975 compared androgen deprivation (diethylstilboestrol, orchiectomy, or oestrogens) versus no initial treatment in about 4000 men with all stages of prostate cancer. They found no difference in overall survival. Reanalysis of updated data from these RCTs found a modest survival advantage with androgen deprivation.[1] The report did not provide statistical details. **Different types of androgen deprivation:** We found one systematic review (search date not given), which identified 25 RCTs comparing different types of androgen deprivation (orchiectomy, diethylstilboestrol, LHRH agonist) in men with metastatic disease.[2] Disease related symptoms and objective criteria, including radiographic findings and laboratory tests, improved in most men (symptomatic and objective response seen in 22% to 90% of people). There were no significant differences in response rates, time to progression, or survival. For all forms of androgen deprivation, duration of response was 12–18 months, and overall survival was 24–36 months.

Harms: All forms of androgen deprivation are known to be associated with vasomotor flushing, loss of libido, gynaecomastia, weight gain, osteoporosis, and loss of muscle mass; we found insufficient prospective frequency data for these adverse effects. **Diethylstilboestrol** is associated with an increased risk of cardiovascular events, gastric irritation, and allergic reactions, and for these reasons is not routinely used. **Orchiectomy** has cosmetic and potential psychological consequences. **LHRH agonists** may cause an initial clinical flare owing to transient increases in androgen levels.

Comment: The high cardiovascular event rate with high dose diethylstilboestrol in the early RCTs[1] may have masked any survival benefit of androgen deprivation.

OPTION **COMBINED ANDROGEN BLOCKADE (ANDROGEN DEPRIVATION AND ANTIANDROGEN)**

Evidence from systematic reviews of RCTs is conflicting. The largest review found no clear evidence of additional benefit from combined androgen blockade (androgen deprivation plus an antiandrogen) compared with androgen deprivation alone.

Benefits: We found three systematic reviews. The largest (search date not given) identified 22 RCTs with 3283 deaths in 5710 men, most of whom had stage D2 disease (see table 1 in non-metastatic prostate cancer, p 483).[3] Individual patient data were obtained. Interventions were androgen deprivation (orchiectomy or LHRH agonist) with or without an antiandrogen. The review found no clear significant difference in 5 year survival among treatments (AR of dying within 5 years with androgen deprivation alone 77.2% compared with 73.8% with combined blockade; RR 0.96, 95% CI 0.93 to 1.00). Four of the 22 RCTs used cyproterone acetate, a steroidal antiandrogen with intrinsic androgenic activity and lower antiandrogenic activity than non-steroidal antiandrogens. Exclusion of these four studies did not alter the results. One smaller systematic review (search date not given) identified nine RCTs comparing androgen deprivation (orchiectomy or LHRH agonist) with or without non-steroidal antiandrogens.[4] Combined androgen blockade improved overall survival (RR of death compared with androgen deprivation alone 0.78, 95% CI 0.67 to 0.90). Another review (search date not given) identified nine RCTs (4128 men with advanced prostate cancer) comparing androgen deprivation (orchiectomy or LHRH agonist) with or without antiandrogen (flutamide).[5] It found no clear evidence that combined androgen blockade improved overall survival (RR of death compared with androgen deprivation alone 0.90, 95% CI 0.79 to 1.00).

Harms: Combined androgen blockade using flutamide, a non-steroidal antiandrogen, is associated with significantly higher rates of diarrhoea (6.3% v 2.7%, P = 0.002) and anaemia (8.5% v 5.4%, P = 0.024) than androgen deprivation alone.[6]

Comment: An updated meta-analysis has recently been published and will be included in the next issue of *Clinical Evidence*.[3]

| OPTION | IMMEDIATE VERSUS DEFERRED ANDROGEN DEPRIVATION |

In men with metastatic disease, RCTs have found no survival benefit from immediate treatment compared with deferring androgen deprivation until disease progression becomes apparent. However, without surveillance, deferred androgen deprivation results in higher rates of complications. Immediate androgen deprivation may improve survival in men with locally advanced prostate cancer but no evidence of bone metastases.

Benefits: We found no systematic review. We found two RCTs in 2841 men with stage C and D prostate cancer (see table 1 in non-metastatic prostate cancer, p 492), comparing immediate versus deferred androgen deprivation (orchiectomy or LHRH antagonist). Immediate androgen deprivation was initiated at diagnosis of prostate cancer; deferred androgen deprivation was initiated at the time of clinical disease progression. One of these RCTs had no formal surveillance requirements or criteria for starting androgen deprivation in the deferred treatment group.[6] It included 938 men with stage C (locally advanced) and D (asymptomatic metastatic) disease. It found a reduction in disease related mortality with immediate treatment (62% of deaths were from prostate cancer compared with 71% in the deferred treatment arm, P = 0.001), but this was limited to men with stage C disease.[6] Immediate androgen suppression almost halved the risk of major complications such as pathological fractures (AR 2.3% with immediate treatment v 4.5% with deferred treatment), spinal cord compression (AR 1.9% v 4.9%), ureteric obstruction (AR 7% v 11.8%), and extraskeletal metastases (AR 7.9% v 11.8%). The report did not provide confidence intervals nor make clear the time interval over which outcomes were recorded, although this seemed to be at least 10 years. Again, the lower incidence of complications was more apparent in men with stage C disease. The other RCT had rigorous surveillance requirements and formal criteria for starting androgen deprivation in the deferred treatment group. In men with distant metastases at study entry, there was no significant difference in overall survival. Of the men with stage C disease, 14% in the immediate treatment group died from prostate cancer compared with 17.5% assigned to delayed treatment.[1]

Harms: We found no good data on adverse effects of androgen deprivation in men with metastatic prostate cancer.

Comment: The high rate of complications in the deferred treatment group in the first RCT suggests that men with advanced prostate cancer in whom hormonal treatment is deferred require careful surveillance for disease progression. About 10% of men assigned to deferred hormonal treatment were not treated until they developed a pathological fracture or spinal cord compression.[7] The other RCT found no significant difference in rates of complication between immediate and deferred treatment.[1]

OPTION   **INTERMITTENT VERSUS CONTINUOUS ANDROGEN DEPRIVATION**

OPTION   INTERMITTENT VERSUS CONTINUOUS ANDROGEN DEPRIVATION

We found insufficient evidence on the effects of intermittent androgen deprivation in men with metastatic prostate cancer.

Benefits: We found no systematic review and no RCTs evaluating the long term effects of intermittent androgen deprivation on mortality, morbidity, or quality of life.

Harms: Insufficient data.

Comment: None.

QUESTION   **Are there any effective treatments for men with symptomatic androgen independent metastatic disease?**

OPTION   CHEMOTHERAPY

RCTs have found that chemotherapy decreases pain and prolongs palliation in some men with symptomatic androgen independent prostate cancer. We found no evidence that chemotherapy prolongs survival.

Benefits: We found no systematic review. We found three RCTs, all using crossover designs, only one of which has been published in full. This compared mitoxantrone plus prednisone versus prednisone alone in 161 men with symptomatic androgen independent metastatic prostate cancer.[8] It found that men receiving chemotherapy were more likely to experience pain reduction (29% with chemotherapy plus steroids *v* 12% with steroids alone, P = 0.01), enjoyed longer palliation (43 *v* 18 weeks, P < 0.0001), and showed improvements in quality of life. There was no difference in overall survival. Two other RCTs are published only in abstract form. One compared mitoxantrone plus prednisone versus prednisone alone in 242 men. Pain and analgesic use were reduced after chemotherapy.[9] The other compared suramin plus hydrocortisone versus hydrocortisone alone in 458 men.[10] Chemotherapy improved pain and duration of palliation.

Harms: The RCTs reported no treatment related deaths. There were nine episodes of febrile neutropenia (World Health Organization grade 3 or 4) among 130 men treated with 796 courses of mitoxantrone. Five men experienced cardiac arrhythmias or decreased left ventricular ejection fraction, including two who developed congestive heart failure.[8]

Comment: The crossover design of these RCTs precludes reliable conclusions about the effect of chemotherapy on survival, because men who died while in one arm of the study were not available for evaluation in the other.

OPTION   EXTERNAL BEAM RADIATION

One systematic review has found no evidence of a difference in survival benefit between external beam radiation, strontium-89, or both

treatments combined. However, strontium-89 seems to reduce the number of new pain sites. One systematic review of RCTs comparing different radiation schedules has found that external beam radiation provides effective pain relief in some men. We found no comparisons of external beam radiation with other palliative treatments.

Benefits: **Versus other palliative treatments:** We found no systematic reviews or RCTs. **Versus or as an adjunct to radionuclides:** We found one systematic review (search date not given), which identified two RCTs in men with prostate cancer and symptomatic bone metastases.[11] The first compared strontium-89 versus placebo in 126 men who had received external beam radiation. It found no significant difference in median survival (27 v 34 weeks) or symptom relief (clinical response rate 80% v 60%). However, strontium-89 significantly reduced the number of new pain sites ($P < 0.02$), and the requirement for analgesia (17% stopped taking analgesics with radionuclide v 2% on placebo, $P < 0.05$) and subsequent radiotherapy (median time to radiotherapy 35 weeks v 20 weeks on placebo, $P = 0.06$). The second RCT compared external beam radiation versus strontium-89 in 305 men. Strontium-89 was associated with significantly fewer new sites of pain ($P < 0.05$), and reduced need for additional radiotherapy ($P < 0.04$). Effect on survival was not reported. **Different schedules and doses:** We found one systematic review (search date 1994), which identified nine RCTs in 1486 men with symptomatic bone metastases from a variety of malignancies. The trials compared different radiation treatment fractionation schedules and doses of external beam radiation.[12] There were minimal differences in effectiveness between different fractionation schedules and doses. External beam radiation produced greater than 50% pain relief in 42% of men and complete pain relief in 27%.

Harms: External beam radiation was associated with a 10% higher rate of gastrointestinal adverse effects.[11] Thrombocytopenia occurred twice as often with strontium-89 (6.9% v 3.4% with external beam radiation) and 3% of men receiving strontium-89 developed leukopenia.[11] There was no significant difference between treatment schedules and doses in rates of nausea, vomiting, or diarrhoea.[12]

Comment: The systematic review of different radiation treatment schedules provides no direct information on effectiveness of external beam radiation in men with bone metastasis, since all participants in the trials received radiation treatment.[12]

OPTION **RADIONUCLIDE TREATMENT**

We found limited evidence from one RCT that radionuclides with selective bone localisation may reduce pain in men with symptomatic bone metastases. One systematic review of RCTs found no difference in survival between radionuclides and external beam radiation, and no effect of radionuclides on survival. However, radionuclides seem to reduce the number of new pain sites.

Benefits: **Versus placebo:** We found no systematic review. We found one RCT comparing rhenium-186 with placebo in nine men with prostate cancer and symptomatic bone metastases.[13] Treatment with rhenium-186 resulted in significantly better pain control than placebo (no RR or CI reported). **Versus or as an adjunct to external beam radiation:** See external beam radiation, p 0.[11]

Harms: Strontium-89 resulted in thrombocytopenia (WHO grade 3 or 4) in 7–33% of men, and leukopenia (WHO grade 3 or 4) in 3–12%.[11,13] Other radionuclides with selective bone localisation have similar rates of haematological toxicity.

Comment: None.

OPTION	BISPHOSPHONATES

We found insufficient evidence on the effects of bisphosphonates in men with prostate cancer.

Benefits: One systematic review (search date not given) identified two RCTs in 156 men with prostate cancer and symptomatic bone metastases.[14] The trials found no significant reduction in bone pain with bisphosphonates. Both RCTs were flawed. One did not use a pain scale. The other evaluated etidronate, a bisphosphonate that is pharmacologically unsuitable for treating bone metastases.

Harms: The systematic review identified a total of 18 RCTs of bisphosphonates in men with bone metastases from a variety of cancers.[14] No RCT reported major toxicity. Treatment with pamidronate was associated with increased frequency of anterior uveitis and episcleritis.

Comment: None.

REFERENCES

1. Byar DP, Corle DK. Hormone therapy for prostate cancer: results of the Veterans Administration cooperative urologic research group studies. *NCI Monogr* 1988;7:165–170.
2. Robson M, Dawson N. How is androgen-dependent metastatic prostate cancer best treated? *Hematol Oncol Clin North Am* 1996;10: 727–747. Search date not given; primary sources not given.
3. Prostate Cancer Clinical Trialists' Collaborative Group. Maximum androgen blockade in advanced prostate cancer: an overview of the randomized trials. *Lancet* 2000;355:1491–1498. Search date not given; primary sources computerised literature search, proceedings of congresses, contacts with authors, trial groups and pharmaceutical industry.
4. Caubet JF, Tosteson TD, Dong EW, et al. Maximum androgen blockade in advanced prostate cancer: a meta-analysis of published randomized controlled trials using nonsteroidal antiandrogens. *Urology* 1997;49:71–78. Search date not given; primary sources Medline, CancerLit, Current Contents 1994–1995, reference lists, contact with authors.
5. Bennett CL, Tosteson TD, Schmitt B, et al. Maximum androgen-blockade with medical or surgical castration in advanced prostate cancer: a meta-analysis of published randomized controlled trials and 4128 patients using flutamide. *Prostate Cancer Prostat Dis* 1999;24–28. Search date not given; primary sources not given.
6. Eisenberger MA, Blumenstein BA, Crawford ED, et al. Bilateral orchiectomy with or without flutamide for metastatic prostate cancer. *N Engl J Med* 1998;339:1036–1042.
7. Medical Research Council Prostate Cancer Working Party Investigators Group. Immediate versus deferred treatment for advanced prostatic cancer: initial results of the Medical Research Council trial. *Br J Urol* 1997;79:235–246.
8. Tannock IF, Osoba D, Stockler MR, et al. Chemotherapy with mitoxantrone plus prednisone or prednisone alone for symptomatic hormone-resistant prostate cancer: a Canadian randomized trial with palliative end points. *J Clin Oncol* 1996; 14:1756–1764.
9. Kantoff PW, Halabi S, Conaway M, et al. Hydrocortisone with or without mitoxantrone in men with hormone-refractory prostate cancer: results of the Cancer and Leukemia Group B 9182 Study. *J Clin Oncol* 1999;17:2506–2513.
10. Small EJ, Marshall E, Reyno L, et al. Superiority of suramin + hydrocortisone over placebo + hydrocortisone: results of a multicenter double-blind phase III study in patients with hormone refractory prostate cancer [abstract]. *Proc Am Soc Clin Oncol* 1998;17:1187.
11. McQuay HJ, Carroll D, Moore RA. Radiotherapy for painful bone metastases: a systematic review. *Clin Oncol (R Coll Radiol)* 1997;9:150–154. Search date not given; primary sources Medline 1966 to March 1996, The Oxford Pain Relief database 1950–1994, Embase, The Cochrane Library, and reference lists.
12. Robinson RG, Preston DF, Schiefelbein M, et al. Strontium 89 therapy for the palliation of pain due to osseous metastases. *JAMA* 1995;274:420–424. Search date December 1994; primary source Medline.
13. Maxon HR, Schroder LE, Hertzberg VS, et al. Rhenium-186(Sn)HEDP for treatment of painful osseous metastases: results of a double-blind

crossover comparison with placebo. *J Nucl Med* 1991;32:1877–1881.

14. Bloomfield DJ. Should bisphosphonates be part of the standard therapy of patients with multiple myeloma or bone metastases from other cancers?
An evidence-based review. *J Clin Oncol* 1998;16: 1218–1225. Search date not given; primary sources Medline from 1976, hand search of major cancer journals, reference lists, and contact with experts.

Matthew Smith
Instructor in Medicine
Massachusetts General Hospital

Philip Kantoff
Director
Lank Center for Genitourinary Oncology
Dana Farber Cancer Institute

James Talcott
Assistant Professor of Medicine
Harvard Medical School
Boston
USA

Competing interests: None declared.

Updated and expanded this issue

Timothy Wilt and Michael Brawer

INTERVENTIONS

Key Messages

In men with clinically localised disease

- We found no clear evidence for the superiority of any one treatment, including androgen deprivation. Limited evidence from one RCT suggests that radical prostatectomy may reduce recurrence compared with radiation treatment.

- Limited data from RCTs provide no evidence that radical prostatectomy or external beam radiation improve survival or reduce the risk of metastatic disease or need for palliative treatment compared with watchful waiting.

- We found no RCTs comparing external beam radiation, brachytherapy, and cryosurgery versus watchful waiting.

- We found no RCTs examining whether androgen deprivation should be offered to asymptomatic men in whom raised concentrations of prostate specific antigen (PSA) are detected after primary treatment or during watchful waiting.

In men with locally advanced disease

■ We found limited evidence from RCTs suggesting that treatment with androgen deprivation from time of diagnosis (compared with deferral to disease progression) improves survival and reduces the risk of major complications.

■ One RCT has found that immediate antiandrogen treatment after radical prostatectomy and pelvic lymphadenectomy reduces mortality compared with radical prostatectomy and deferred androgen suppression in men with node–positive prostate cancer and local node metastasis.

■ One systematic review has found that adding androgen deprivation to radiation treatment improves survival compared with radiation alone. A subsequent RCT found no difference in overall survival or disease control after orchiectomy, whether or not it was combined with radiotherapy.

■ We found no good evidence that radiation alone improves survival.

DEFINITION Prostatic cancer is staged according to two systems: the tumour, node, metastasis (TNM) classification system and the American Urologic Staging system (see table 1, p 492). Non-metastatic prostate cancer can be divided into clinically localised disease and advanced disease.

INCIDENCE/ PREVALENCE Prostate cancer is the most common non-dermatological malignancy worldwide and the second commonest cause of cancer death in men in the USA.[1] There were an estimated 180 400 new cases and 31 900 deaths in the USA in 2000.[2] For a 50 year old man with a life expectancy of 25 years, the lifetime risk of microscopic prostate cancer is about 42%, the risk of clinically evident prostate cancer is 10%, and that of fatal prostate cancer is 3%.[3]

AETIOLOGY/ RISK FACTORS Risk factors include age, family history of prostate cancer, black race, and possibly higher dietary fat and calcium intake.

PROGNOSIS The chance that men with well to moderately differentiated, palpable, clinically localised prostate cancer will remain free of symptomatic progression is 70% at 5 years and 40% at 10 years.[4] The risk of symptomatic disease progression is higher in men with poorly differentiated prostate cancer.[5] One retrospective analysis of a large surgical series in men with clinically localised prostate cancer found that the median time from the increase in PSA concentration to the development of metastatic disease was 8 years. Time to PSA progression, PSA doubling time, and Gleason score (see glossary, p 491) were predictive of the probability and time to development of metastatic disease. Once men developed metastatic disease, the median actuarial time to death was 5 years.[6] Morbidity from local or regional disease progression includes haematuria, bladder obstruction, and lower extremity oedema. In the USA, population based studies found that rates of death from prostate cancer have declined by only about 1/100 000 men since 1992, despite widespread testing for PSA and increased rates of radical prostatectomy and radiotherapy.[7,8] Regions of the USA with the greatest decreases in mortality are those with the lowest rates of testing for PSA and treatment with radical prostatectomy or radiation.[8] Countries with low rates of testing and treatment do not have consistently higher age adjusted rates of death from prostate cancer than countries with high rates of testing and treatment such as the USA.

AIMS	To prevent premature death and disability while minimising adverse effects of treatment.
OUTCOMES	Survival; time to progression; response in terms of symptoms and signs; quality of life; adverse effects of treatment. Where clinical outcomes are not available, surrogate outcome have been used (PSA concentration; Gleason score for histological grade.
METHODS	We searched the Cochrane Library and Medline to May 2000 for systematic reviews and RCTs, using the search strategy of the Department of Veterans' Affairs Coordinating Centre for the Cochrane Review Group on Prostatic Diseases.

QUESTION **What are the effects of treatment in men with clinically localised prostate cancer?**

OPTION **WATCHFUL WAITING**

Limited data from RCTs suggest that watchful waiting provides similar length of life in men with clinically localised prostate cancer compared with other management strategies. We found no information from RCTs on quality of life.

Benefits: We found no recent systematic reviews, but found one overview that did not itemise the studies included (search date 1993,165 articles),[1] and one non-systematic decision analysis (search date not given, published 1993).[9] We found two more recent, large cohort studies, which found that, in men managed with watchful waiting, 15 years disease specific survival was 80%, ranging from 95% for well differentiated to 30% for poorly differentiated cancers.[10,11] **Versus early androgen deprivation:** We found no RCTs. **Versus radical prostatectomy:** See glossary, p 491. We found one RCT (see benefits of radical prostatectomy, p 486).[12]

Harms: Watchful waiting may avoid the risks of surgery but does not remove a cancer that is potentially curable that may progress to cause death and disability. However, we found insufficient evidence to comment on whether early intervention reduces the risk of disease specific death and disability compared with watchful waiting.

Comment: There is about a 10 year lead time between the detection of cancers by raised PSA concentrations and detection by digital rectal examination or the development of symptoms. This means that outcomes are likely to be similar in men with palpable tumours who are followed for 15 years and men whose tumours are detected because of raised PSA concentrations who are followed for 25 years (lead time bias).

OPTION **RADICAL PROSTATECTOMY**

Limited data from one RCT provided no evidence that radical prostatectomy may not improve survival compared with watchful waiting. Radical prostatectomy may reduce the risk of metastases compared with external beam radiation. Radical prostatectomy carries the risks of major surgery and of sexual and urinary dysfunction.

Prostate cancer: non-metastatic

Benefits: We found no recent systematic reviews. **Versus watchful waiting:** One RCT compared radical prostatectomy versus watchful waiting in 142 men with clinically localised prostate cancer. After a median follow up of 23 years (range 19–27 years), it found no difference in survival between the two groups (median survival 10.6 years with prostatectomy v 8 years with watchful waiting, no 95% CI quoted).[12] **Versus external beam radiation:** One RCT compared radical prostatectomy versus external beam radiation in 97 men with clinically localised prostate cancer. Men receiving radiation had an increased risk of metastases (4 "treatment failures" with prostatectomy v 17 with radiation).[13]

Harms: Fatal complications have been reported in 0.5–1% of men treated with radical prostatectomy and may exceed 2% in men aged 75 years and older.[14] Nearly 8% of men older than 65 years suffered major cardiopulmonary complications within 30 days of operation. The incidence of other adverse effects of surgery was over 80% for sexual dysfunction, 30% for urinary incontinence requiring pads or clamps to control wetness, 18% for urethral stricture, 3% for total urinary incontinence, 5% for faecal incontinence, and 1% for bowel injury requiring surgical repair.[1,15–17]

Comment: Both RCTs of radical prostatectomy took place before the advent of tests for PSA and were too small to rule out a clinically important difference between groups. Radical prostatectomy may benefit selected groups of men with localised prostate cancer, particularly younger men with higher grade tumours, but the studies did not look for this effect. The available data suggest that in most men the benefits in quality adjusted life expectancy are at best small and sensitive to patients' preferences.[9] No differences have been found in the general health related quality of life among non-randomised groups treated with radical prostatectomy, radiation, or watchful waiting.[18] Two ongoing trials are comparing radical prostatectomy versus watchful waiting.[19,20]

OPTION   **EXTERNAL BEAM RADIATION**

We found limited evidence from one small RCT that, compared with radical prostatectomy, external beam radiation increased the risk of metastases in men with clinically localised prostate cancer. External beam radiation has not been compared directly with watchful waiting. One RCT found that conformal radiation therapy (see glossary, p 491) reduces rates of radiation proctitis and rectal bleeding compared with conventional radiotherapy. We found no evidence of a difference in survival between conventional and conformal radiation therapy.

Benefits: **Versus watchful waiting:** We found no RCTs. **Versus radical prostatectomy:** We found one RCT (see benefits of radical prostatectomy above).[13] **Conformal versus conventional radiotherapy:** One RCT in 225 men with non-metastatic prostate cancer (T1-T4, N0 or M0) compared conformal versus conventional radiotherapy.[21] Primary outcomes were adverse effects (see harms). It did not report on survival, but found no significant difference in tumour control (by PSA level) between treatments after a median follow up of 3.6 years.

Harms: The RCT of radiotherapy versus radical prostatectomy made no mention of adverse effects.[13] One survey of men treated with external beam radiation reported that 7% wore pads to control wetness, 23–32% were impotent, and 10% reported problems with bowel dysfunction.[22] Treatment related mortality is less than 0.5%.[1] External beam radiation requires that men return for daily outpatient treatment for up to 6 weeks. **Conventional versus conformal radiotherapy:** The RCT found that significantly fewer men treated with conformal radiation developed radiation induced proctitis and rectal bleeding. It found no differences between groups for adverse effects on the bladder.[21]

Comment: Up to 30% of men with clinically localised prostate cancer treated with radiotherapy still have positive biopsies 2–3 years after treatment.[23] One retrospective, non-randomised, multicentre pooled analysis found 5 year estimates of overall survival, disease specific survival, and freedom from biochemical failure (as defined by raised PSA) to be 85%, 95%, and 66%. Estimated 5 year rates of no biochemical recurrence according to PSA concentrations before treatment and Gleason histological scores ranged from 81% for pretreatment PSA < 10 ng/ml to 29% for PSA ≥ 20 ng/ml, and a Gleason score from 7 to 10.[24]

OPTION   BRACHYTHERAPY

One systematic review found no direct evidence from RCTs that brachytherapy (see glossary, p 491) improves length or quality of life in men with clinically localised prostate cancer.

Benefits: We found one systematic review (published in 1997), which identified no RCTs comparing brachytherapy alone or in combination with other treatments (androgen deprivation or radiation).[25]

Harms: Complications reported in case series include urinary retention (6–8%), incontinence (13–18%), cystitis/urethritis (4–7%), proctitis (6–14%), and impotence (6–50%).[26] Long term outcomes from a representative national sampling of men have not been reported.

Comment: One retrospective cohort study (1872 men) found that, in low risk men (see table 1, p 492) (stage T1c, stage T2a, PSA concentration ≤ 10 ng/ml, and Gleason score ≤ 6) the chance of a high PSA concentration at 5 years was similar whether they were treated with radiation or brachytherapy implant (with or without preceding androgen deprivation) or with radical prostatectomy. Men at intermediate or high risk (Gleason score > 6 or PSA > 10 ng/ml) were more likely to have high PSA concentration at 5 years with brachytherapy than with radical prostatectomy (RR of high PSA in men at intermediate risk 3.1, 95% CI 1.5 to 6.1; RR in men at high risk 3.0, 95% CI 1.8 to 5.0).[27] The study used proxy outcomes (PSA concentrations) rather than clinical outcomes. RCTs comparing brachytherapy versus radical prostatectomy are planned.

OPTION   CRYOSURGERY

We found no direct evidence from RCTs that cryosurgery improves length or quality of life in men with clinically localised prostate cancer.

Benefits: We found no systematic review or RCTs.

Harms: Complications reported in case series include impotence (65%), transient scrotal oedema (10%), sloughed urethral tissue (3%), urethral stricture (1%), incontinence, urethrorectal fistula, and prostatic abscess (1%).[28]

Comment: One ongoing trial is comparing cryosurgery with radiation.

OPTION   ANDROGEN DEPRIVATION

We found no direct evidence from RCTs that primary treatment with early androgen deprivation in the absence of symptoms improves length or quality of life in men with clinically localised prostate cancer.

Benefits: We found no systematic review or RCTs.

Harms: See harms of androgen deprivation for the treatment of men with locally advanced prostate cancer, p 489.

Comment: None.

QUESTION   In men who have received primary treatment and remain asymptomatic, should androgen deprivation be offered when raised concentrations of PSA are detected?

We found insufficient evidence on the effects of initiating androgen suppression when PSA rises or persists after primary treatment.

Benefits: We found one systematic review, which identified no RCTs.[29]

Harms: See harms of androgen deprivation for the treatment of men with locally advanced prostate cancer, p 489.

Comment: In the USA, clinicians often monitor blood concentrations of PSA and offer androgen suppression when these rise. Consequently, more men with persistent disease are considered for androgen suppression and treatment initiated earlier in the natural course of the disease. RCTs are needed to evaluate the effectiveness of this approach and of intermittent treatment, where androgen suppression is initiated when PSA rises after primary treatment and discontinued when the antigen concentrations return to nadir.[29]

QUESTION   What are the effects of treatment in men with locally advanced prostate cancer?

OPTION   ANDROGEN DEPRIVATION

RCTs have found limited evidence that, in men with locally advanced disease, androgen deprivation initiated at diagnosis reduces complications and may improve survival.

Benefits: **Versus no initial treatment:** We found no recent RCTs. Three RCTs performed between 1960 and 1975 compared androgen deprivation (stilboestrol, orchiectomy, or oestrogens) versus no initial treatment in about 4000 men with all stages of prostate cancer. They found no difference in overall survival. Reanalysis of updated data from these RCTs provided tentative evidence of a modest survival advantage with androgen deprivation.[30] **Immediate (initiated at diagnosis) versus deferred androgen deprivation:** We found one systematic review, which identified three RCTs (n = 2143), two of which were conducted in the 1960s.[29] None had a uniform protocol for initiating deferred treatment, so deferred treatment in these trials reflects the varied practices of the treating clinicians. Men in the deferred hormonal therapy group were not closely monitored with PSA testing. The systematic review found no significant survival difference at 5 years between immediate compared with deferred androgen deprivation (HR 0.91, 95% CI 0.81 to 1.03).[30] The more recent trial, which included 938 men with stage C (locally advanced) and D (asymptomatic metastatic) disease, reported a survival benefit from immediate treatment (62% of deaths were from prostate cancer compared with 71% in the deferred treatment arm, P < 0.001). The survival benefit was limited to men with stage C disease.[31] Immediate androgen deprivation almost halved the risk of major complications, such as pathological fractures (AR 2.3% v 4.5% with deferred treatment), spinal cord compression (AR 1.9% v 4.9%), ureteric obstruction (AR 7% v 11.8%), and extraskeletal metastases (AR 7.9% v 11.8%). The report did not quote CIs, nor make clear the time interval over which outcomes were recorded, though this seemed to be at least 10 years. The lower incidence of complications was more apparent in men presenting with stage C disease.

Harms: Adverse events were not well reported in the review. Earlier initiation of androgen deprivation means longer exposure to adverse effects, which include osteoporosis, weight gain, hot flushes (10–60%), loss of muscle mass, gynaecomastia (5–10%), impotence (10–30%), and loss of libido (5–30%).[29] These adverse effects are particularly important in the treatment of men with long life expectancy or younger men with lower grade cancers.

Comment: The RCTs conducted in the 1960s[29] included men who were older and had more advanced cancers than those in the more recent RCT.[31] RCTs are needed to evaluate the effectiveness of androgen deprivation before surgery when disease extends beyond the capsule.

OPTION **EXTERNAL BEAM RADIATION IN ADDITION TO ANDROGEN DEPRIVATION**

Androgen deprivation improves survival in men with locally advanced disease treated with radiotherapy. One RCT found no difference in overall survival or local disease control after orchiectomy, whether or not it was combined with radiotherapy.

Benefits: **External beam radiation versus or in addition to androgen deprivation:** We found one systematic review,[29] and one additional RCT.[32] The review (4 RCTs, 1565 men) compared early versus deferred androgen deprivation in men receiving external beam radiation.[29] Early androgen deprivation was initiated at the same time as radiation treatment for locally advanced, or asymptomatic but clinically evident metastatic prostate cancer, and continued until the development of hormone refractory disease. The deferred group received radiation treatment alone, with androgen deprivation initiated only in those in whom the disease progressed. The systematic review found that early androgen deprivation improved overall 5 year survival compared with deferred treatment (percentage surviving at 5 years 76.5% v 68.2%; ARR 8.3%; HR 0.63, 95% CI 0.48 to 0.83; NNT at 5 years 12).[29] The additional RCT compared orchiectomy alone versus radiotherapy alone, versus radiotherapy in addition to orchiectomy in 277 men with advanced localised prostate cancer (T2-T4, M0, with and without nodal disease).[32] It found no significant differences between the three treatment groups for overall survival or need for further treatment for local disease progression (data presented as a diagram, no P value given).

Harms: The review reported adverse effects of androgen deprivation.[29] In the additional RCT, adverse effects attributable to radiotherapy included bowel symptoms (19%), urinary symptoms excluding transient frequency (8%), bowel and urinary complications (1%), rectal bleeding necessitating blood transfusion (2%), and radiation proctitis (1%), which was a contributory factor in the two patients that died. After orchiectomy, hot flushes (15%) were the predominant adverse effect.

Comment: We found no evidence from RCTs about the effectiveness of external beam radiation alone versus no treatment in men with locally advanced prostate cancer.

OPTION | **ANDROGEN DEPRIVATION PLUS RADICAL PROSTATECTOMY AND PELVIC LYMPHADENECTOMY** New

One RCT has found that immediate androgen deprivation after radical prostatectomy and pelvic lymphadenectomy improves survival and reduces the risk of recurrence in men with node-positive prostate cancer compared with radical prostatectomy, pelvic lymphadenectomy, and deferred androgen deprivation.

Benefits: **Radical prostatectomy and pelvic lymphadenectomy plus androgen deprivation:** We found one RCT (98 men after radical prostatectomy and pelvic lymphadenectomy for nodal metastases) of immediate androgen deprivation (with either goserelin or bilateral orchiectomy) versus androgen deprivation deferred until disease progression.[33] It found that antiandrogens decreased mortality in the long term (median follow up 7.1 years, mortality 7/47 [14.9%] with antiandrogen v 18/51 [35.3%] with watchful waiting, ARR 20.4%, P < 0.01) and resulted in a higher proportion of men with undetectable PSA (P < 0.001).

Harms: The RCT found that, compared with deferred androgen deprivation, immediate androgen deprivation caused more haematological effects (15% v 4%), gastrointestinal effects (25% v 6%), nonspecific genitourinary effects (48% v 12%), hot flushes (56% v 0%), and weight gain (18% v 2%).

Comment: None.

GLOSSARY

Brachytherapy Radiotherapy, where the source of ionising radiation is applied by permanently inserting many radioactive implants directly into the prostate gland.

Gleason score A number from 1–10 with 1 being the most well differentiated and 10 being the most poorly differentiated.

Radical prostatectomy Surgical removal of the prostate with its capsule, seminal vesicles, ductus deferens, some pelvic fasciae, and sometimes pelvic lymph nodes; performed via either the retropubic or the perineal route.

Conformal radiation therapy 3D radiotherapy planning systems and methods to match the radiation treatment to irregular tumour volumes.

Substantive changes since last issue

External beam radiation: Conformal versus conventional radiotherapy New RCT.[21]

External beam radiation versus or in addition to androgen deprivation New RCT.[32]

REFERENCES

1. Middleton RG, Thompson IM, Austenfeld MS, et al. Prostate cancer clinical guidelines panel summary report on the management of clinically localized prostate cancer. *J Urol* 1995;154:2144–2148. Search date December 1993; primary source Medline 1966 to December 1993.
2. Landis SH, Murray T, Bolden S, et al. Cancer statistics. *CA Cancer J Clin* 2000;50:12–13.
3. Whitmore WF. Localized prostatic cancer: management and detection issues. *Lancet* 1994; 343:1263–1267.
4. Adolfsson J, Steineck G, Hedund P. Deferred treatment of clinically localized low-grade prostate cancer: actual 10-year and projected 15-year follow-up of the Karolinska series. *Urology* 1997; 50:722–726.
5. Johansson J-E, Holmberg L, Johansson S, et al. Fifteen-year survival in prostate cancer: prospective, population-based study in Sweden. *JAMA* 1997;277:467–471.
6. Pound CR, Partin AW, Eisenberger MA, et al. Natural history of progression after PSA elevation following radical prostatectomy. *JAMA* 1999;281: 1591–1597.
7. Brawley OW. Prostate carcinoma incidence and patient mortality. *Cancer* 1997;80:1857–1863.
8. Wingo PA, Ries LAG, Rosenberg HM, et al. Cancer incidence and mortality, 1973–1995. *Cancer* 1998;82:1197–1207.
9. Fleming C, Wasson J, Albertsen PC, et al. A decision analysis of alternative strategies for clinically localized prostate cancer. *JAMA* 1993; 269:2650–2658.
10. Albertsen PC, Hanley JA, Gleason DF, Barry MJ. Competing risk analysis of men aged 55 to 74 years at diagnosis managed conservatively for clinically localized prostate cancer. *JAMA* 1998; 280:975–980.
11. Lu-Yao GL, Yao S. Population-based study of long-term survival in patients with clinically localised prostate cancer. *Lancet* 1997;349:906–910.
12. Iversen P, Madsen PO, Corle DK. Radical prostatectomy versus expectant treatment for early carcinoma of the prostate: 23 year follow-up of a prospective randomized study. *Scand J Urol Nephrol* Suppl 1995;172(suppl):65–72.
13. Paulsen DF, Lin GH, Hinshaw W, et al. The uro-oncology group: radical surgery versus radiotherapy for adenocarcinoma of the prostate. *J Urol* 1982;128:502–504.
14. Lu-Yao GL, McLerran D, Wasson JH. An assessment of radical prostatectomy: time trends, geographic variation, and outcomes. *JAMA* 1993; 269:2633–2636.
15. Anonymous. Screening for prostate cancer. *Ann Intern Med* 1997;126:480–484.
16. Fowler FJ, Barry MJ, Lu-Yao G, et al. Patient-reported complications and follow-up treatment after radical prostatectomy: the national Medicare experience 1988–1990 (updated June 1993). *Urology* 1993;42:622–629.
17. Bishoff JT, Motley G, Optenberg SA, et al. Incidence of fecal and urinary incontinence following radical perineal and retropubic prostatectomy in a national population. *J Urol* 1998;160:454–458.
18. Litwin MS, Hays RD, Fink A, et al. Quality-of-life outcomes in men treated for localized prostate cancer. *JAMA* 1995;273:129–135.
19. Wilt TJ, Brawer MK. The prostate cancer intervention versus observation trial. *Oncology* 1997;11:1133–1139.
20. Norlen BJ. Swedish randomized trial of radical prostatectomy versus watchful waiting. *Can J Oncol* 1994;4(suppl 1):38–42.
21. Dearnaley DP, Khoo VS, Norman AR, et al. Comparison of radiation side-effects of conformal and conventional radiotherapy in prostate cancer: a randomized trial. *Lancet* 1999;353:267–272.
22. Fowler FJ, Barry MJ, Lu-Yao G, et al. Outcomes of external beam radiation therapy for prostate cancer: a study of Medicare beneficiaries in three surveillance, epidemiology, and end results areas. *J Clin Oncol* 1996;14:2258–2265.
23. Crook J, Perry G, Robertson S, Esche B. Routine prostate biopsies: results for 225 patients. *Urology* 1995;45:624–632.
24. Shipley WU, Thames HD, Sandler HM, et al. Radiation therapy for clinically localized prostate cancer. A multi-institutional pooled analysis. *JAMA* 1999;281:1598–1604.
25. Brachytherapy for prostate cancer. Tec assessment program. *Blue Cross Blue Shield Assoc* 1997;12:1–27. Primary sources Medline; 1980–May 1997; Current Contents; bibliographies; and abstracts of proceedings of scientific meetings. Talcott JA, Clark JC, Stark P, Nadir B, Ragde N. Long term complications of brachytherapy for early prostate cancer: A survey of treated patients. American Society of Clinical Oncology Annual Meeting 1999; Abstract 1196.
26. D'Amico AV, Whittington R, Malkowicz SB, et al. Biochemical outcome after radical prostatectomy, external beam radiation therapy, or interstitial

radiation therapy for clinically localized prostate cancer. *JAMA* 1998;280:969–974.

27. Talcott JA, Clark JC, Stark P, Nadir B, Ragde N. long term complications of brachytherapy for early prostate cancer. A survey of treated patients. American Society of Clinical Oncology Annual Meeting 1999; Abstract 1196.

28. Littrup PJ, Mody A, Sparschu RA. Prostate cryosurgery complications. *Semin Int Radiol* 1994; 11:226–230.

29. Agency for Health Care Policy and Research. Relative effectiveness and cost-effectiveness of methods of androgen suppression in the treatment of advanced prostatic cancer. Summary. Rockville, MD: Agency for Health Care Policy and Research, 1999. (Evidence Report/Technology Assessment: No 4.) http://www.ahcpr.gov/clinic/prossumm.htm. Search date 1998; primary sources Medline; Cancerlit; Embase; Current Contents on Diskette, and Cochrane Library.

30. Byar DP, Corle DK. Hormone treatment for prostate cancer: results of the Veterans' Administration cooperative urologic research group studies. *NCI Monograph* 1988;7:165–170.

31. The Medical Research Council Prostate Cancer Working Party Investigators Group. Immediate versus deferred treatment for advanced prostatic cancer: initial results of the Medical Research Council trial. *Br J Urol* 1997;79:235–246.

32. Fellows GJ, Clark PB, Beynon, LL, et al. Treatment of advanced localised prostatic cancer by orchiectomy, radiotherapy, or combined treatment. *Br J Urol* 1992:70;304–309.

33. Messing EM, Manola J, Sarodsy M, Wilding G, Crawford ED, Trump D. Immediate hormonal therapy compared with observation after radical prostatectomy and pelvic lymphadenectomy in men with node-positive prostate cancer. *N Engl J Med* 1999;341:1781–1789.

Timothy Wilt
Associate Professor of Medicine
VA Coordinating Center for the
Cochrane Review Group in Prostate
Diseases and Urologic Malignancies
Center for Chronic Diseases Outcomes
Research
Minneapolis VA Hospital
Minneapolis
USA

Michael Brawer
Director
Northwest Prostate Institute
Seattle
USA
Competing interests: None declared.

TABLE 1	Prostatic cancer staging systems (see text, p 487).

Tumour, node, metastasis (TNM) classification system

Tumour	
T0	Clinically unsuspected
T1	Clinically inapparent (not palpable or visible by imaging)
T2	Tumour confined within prostate
T3	Tumour outside capsule or extension into vesicle
T4	Tumour fixed to other tissue
Nodes	
N0	No evidence of involvement of regional nodes
N1	Involvement of regional node
Metastases	
M0	No evidence of distant metastases
M1	Evidence of distant metastases

American urologic staging system

Stage A	No palpable tumour
Stage B	Tumour confined to the prostate gland
Stage C	Extracapsular extension
Stage D	Metastatic prostate cancer
Stage D1	Pelvic lymph node metastases
Stage D2	Distant metastases

INTERVENTIONS

Key Messages

- Most RCTs used proxy outcome measures such as cognitive function, rather than clinical outcomes likely to be important to people with Alzheimer's disease and their carers, such as quality of life.
- Systematic reviews of RCTs have found:
  - Improved cognitive function and global clinical state with donepezil 10 mg compared with placebo. Treatment is well tolerated.
  - Improved cognitive function with rivastigmine 6–12 mg; possibly less effective than donepezil. Nausea is common.
  - No evidence that tacrine improves cognitive function or behaviour. In trials, tacrine is associated with hepatotoxicity.
  - Reduced anxiety with short term treatment with thioridazine, but no evidence of an effect on clinical global state. A link between thioridazine and cardiac arrhythmias has been suggested.
  - Improved cognitive function, behaviour, and mood with selegiline compared with placebo, but no evidence of an effect on clinical global state; treatment is well tolerated with no serious adverse events.
  - Improved cognitive function with ginkgo biloba. Treatment is well tolerated.
- One small RCT found no benefit from diclofenac compared with placebo.
- One systematic review of small RCTs found that reality orientation is associated with improved cognitive function and behaviour compared with no treatment.
- We found insufficient evidence on the effects of reminisence therapy.

Alzheimer's disease

DEFINITION	**Dementia** is characterised by global impairment of cerebral function with preservation of clear consciousness. It usually results in loss of memory (initially of recent events), loss of executive function (such as the ability to make decisions or sequence complex tasks), and changes in personality. **Alzheimer's disease** is characterised by an insidious onset and slow deterioration, and may be diagnosed after other systemic and neurological causes of dementia have been excluded clinically and by laboratory investigation.
INCIDENCE/ PREVALENCE	About 5% of people aged over 65 years and 20% of people aged over 80 years have some form of dementia.[1] Dementia is rare before the age of 60. The most common type of dementia is Alzheimer's disease, accounting for about 60% of cases in the UK.[2] The rest comprise mainly vascular dementia, mixed vascular and Alzheimer's disease, and cortical Lewy body dementia.[3]
AETIOLOGY/ RISK FACTORS	The cause of Alzheimer's disease is poorly understood. A key pathological process is thought to be a defect in amyloid precursor protein leading to deposition of abnormal amyloid in the central nervous system.[4] Most cases of the relatively rare condition of early onset dementia (before age 60) show autosomal dominance. Later onset dementia sometimes clusters in families. Vascular dementia is related to cardiovascular risk factors, such as smoking, hypertension, and diabetes.
PROGNOSIS	Alzheimer's disease usually has an insidious onset when it is often difficult to diagnose. There is inexorable reduction in cerebral function over time, with an average life expectancy after diagnosis of 7–10 years.[3] Behavioural problems, depression, and psychosis occur in most people at some stage.[5,6] Eventually, most people with dementia find it difficult to perform simple tasks without help.
AIMS	To improve cognitive function (memory, orientation, attention, and concentration); to reduce behavioural problems (wandering and aggression); to improve quality of life, with minimum adverse effects of treatment.
OUTCOMES	Quality of life both of the person with dementia and their carer (rarely used in clinical trials). Comprehensive scales of cognitive function such as the Alzheimer's disease assessment scale cognitive subscale (ADAS-cog, where lower scores signify improving function)[7] are more sensitive than briefer scales such as the mini-mental status examination (MMSE),[8] but both are proxy measures that may not reflect outcomes important to people with dementia or their careers. A seven point change in the ADAS-cog may be regarded as clinically significant. Overall condition is reflected in scales such as global clinical state. One measure of global state is the clinician interview-based impression of change with caregiver input (CIBIC-Plus) scale. Psychiatric symptoms are assessed using scales such as the dementia mood assessment scale (DMAS) and the brief psychiatric rating scale (BPRS) (both of which use lower scores to signify improved symptoms). Other outcomes include time to institutionalisation or death.
METHODS	*Clinical Evidence* update search and appraisal May 2000. All relevant systematic reviews and RCTs were reviewed.

QUESTION   **What are the effects of drug treatments?**

OPTION   CHOLINESTERASE INHIBITORS

One systematic review of RCTs has found evidence that donepezil is well tolerated and is better than placebo in improving cognitive function and global clinical state. One systematic review of RCTs has found no evidence of benefit from tacrine in terms of improved cognitive function or behaviour. Tacrine has also been associated with hepatotoxicity. One large RCT found that rivastigmine is associated with improved cognitive function in older people with Alzheimer's disease but that nausea was common. We found no evidence that any of the drugs significantly improved quality of life.

Benefits: **Donepezil:** We found one systematic review (search date 2000), which identified three placebo controlled RCTs evaluating cholinesterase inhibitors.[9] The trials included 1102 people with mild or moderate Alzheimer's disease. The review found that donepezil 10 mg was associated with improved cognitive function, measured by the ADAS-cog score (WMD −3.01, 95% CI −3.92 to −2.09; 5 mg: WMD −2.61, 95% CI −3.45 to −1.78) and improved global clinical state (OR 0.38, 95% CI 0.26 to 0.56). There was no evidence of an effect on self rated quality of life. One 24 week double blind RCT included in the systematic review, comparing 10 mg donezepil with placebo in 473 people with mild to moderate Alzheimer's disease, found that the NNT was 4 for a four point improvement in ADAS-cog and 6 for a seven point improvement.[10] We found one subsequent 30 week RCT (818 people with Alzheimer's) comparing donepezil 10 mg versus donepezil 5 mg versus placebo. It found improved global state to be associated with both donepezil treatments (NNT 10, 95% CI 6 to 25 with donepezil 10 mg v placebo for a three point improvement in CIBIC score). It found no evidence of a difference in quality of life.[11] **Tacrine:** We found one systematic review (search date November 1998), which identified five placebo controlled RCTs in 1434 people.[12] Various dosages of tacrine were given for 1–39 weeks. The review found no significant difference in overall clinical improvement (OR 0.87, 95% CI 0.61 to 1.23), a significant (but probably clinically insignificant) improvement in cognition (WMD in ADAS-cog −0.22, 95% CI −0.32 to −0.12), and no significant difference in MMSE (SMD 0.14, 95% CI −0.02 to +0.3). There was no evidence of improved behaviour (SMD in behavioural disturbance on the non-cognitive subscale of ADAS −0.04, 95% CI −0.52 to +0.43). **Rivastigmine:** We found one systematic review, which identified seven RCTs (search date 1999).[13] Two of the trials, accounting for 1379 people (49% of all trial people for this drug), remain unpublished and the data were not made available to the reviewers. The review found an NNT of 20 (95 % CI 13 to 50) for a four point change in the ADAS-cog for 6–12 mg rivastigmine compared with placebo. There was no significant difference between 1–4 mg rivastigmine and placebo. One multicentre, placebo controlled RCT evaluated rivastigmine 6–12 mg for 24 weeks in 725 people with probable Alzheimer's disease.[14] It found that significantly more people had a four point improvement in the ADAS-cog score with rivastigmine than with placebo (57/242 [24%] v 39/238

[16%] NNT 13 95% CI 7 to 113). The trial found no significant difference between low dose rivastigmine 1–4 mg and placebo for these outcomes.

Harms:
Donepezil was well tolerated in the trials. The main adverse effects reported were mild and transient nausea, vomiting, and diarrhoea. No hepatotoxicity was reported. More people withdrew from the donepezil 10 mg group than the placebo group (69/315 v 43/315, OR 1.79, 95% CI 1.19 to 2.70), although withdrawal rates for donepezil 5 mg versus placebo were similar (12.6% v 14.9%).[9]
Tacrine: Withdrawals were common and related to dosage. Inconsistencies in reporting make it hard to give an overall withdrawal figure. Two studies where this was possible (812 people) gave an odds ratio for withdrawal of 5.7 (95% CI 4.1 to 7.9). In one high dose study, 72% of people taking tacrine 160 mg withdrew.[15] Reversible hepatotoxicity was reported in about half of participants. Diarrhoea, anorexia, and abdominal pain were also common.
Rivastigmine: One trial reported no serious adverse effects.[14] However, 33% of people taking the high dose withdrew. The most commonly reported adverse effects were nausea (50%), vomiting (34%), dizziness (20%), headache (19%), and diarrhoea (17%).[12]

Comment:
The trials all used proxy outcomes (cognitive scores) rather than outcomes likely to be important to people with Alzheimer's disease and their carers. All trials of donepezil used reliable methods, but participants were highly selected and may not be representative. Quality of life of carers was not assessed.[9] The quality of tacrine trials was generally poor. The longest RCT lasted 30 weeks[15] and doses varied considerably between trials. Although the NNT was higher than that for donepezil, rivastigmine is the only cholinesterase inhibitor we found to have been studied in a routine clinical (pragmatic) setting.[14] Data on 49% of all people in the phase II/III trials of rivastigmine have not been reported. As a consequence there may have been an overestimation of the reported treatment effect in the meta-analysis. A significant issue with dementia trials is the way missing data are managed. Many trials show much higher dropout rates (30% or more) at doses where the drug is effective than in the placebo arm. Missing data are often managed using last observation carried forward (LOCF) in these studies. In dementing people, the likely trend over the course of the trial will be to get worse. If people drop out of the trial, relatively better scores are carried forward to end point than if the person completed. If more people drop out of the intervention arm, an artificially better score, compared with the placebo arm, will result.

OPTION **THIORIDAZINE**

One systematic review of RCTs has found that short term treatment with thioridazine reduces anxiety but found no evidence of an effect on clinical global state. We found only limited data on adverse effects.

Benefits:
We found one systematic review (updated 1998, 7 RCTs). Six trials were of 3–4 weeks' duration and one lasted 8 weeks; of the seven, two were placebo controlled.[16] The review found evidence that thioridazine reduced symptoms of anxiety (v placebo OR 4.91, 95%

CI 3.12 to 7.50; *v* diazepam OR 1.8, 95% CI 1.04 to 3.10) but did not significantly affect clinical global state (*v* placebo OR 1.58, 95% CI 0.42 to 5.96).

Harms: The trials included in the review did not report adverse events systematically.[16] Adverse effects were no more common with thioridazine than with placebo (OR 0.41, 95% CI 0.09 to 1.86) or diazepam (OR 0.84, 95% CI 0.25 to 2.82). One trial included in the review (60 people) found that people taking thioridazine were less alert than people taking chlormethiazole (OR for alertness 0.31, 95% CI 0.11 to 0.89) and less likely to be continent of urine (OR 0.24, 95% CI 0.07 to 0.69). A link between thioridazine and cardiac arrhythmias has been suggested.[17]

Comment: The dose of thioridazine varied from 10–200 mg. Doses of comparator drugs also varied. The review identified 51 studies.[16] However, all but seven were excluded because of poor quality methods or lack of usable data. All trials were of short duration.

OPTION   SELEGILINE

One systematic review of RCTs has found that selegiline is better than placebo at improving cognitive function, behavioural disturbance, and mood in people with Alzheimer's disease. It found no evidence of an effect on clinical global state. Selegiline was well tolerated with no serious adverse events.

Benefits: We found one systematic review (search date 2000), which identified 15 RCTs comparing selegiline versus placebo (average n = 50, typical duration of treatment 3 months).[18] Analysis of pooled data found that selegiline improved several outcome measures: cognitive function scores (as measured by several parameters, SMD −0.56, 95% CI −0.88 to −0.24); mood score (DMAS), SMD −1.14, 95% CI −2.11 to −0.18); and behavioural symptom score (BPRS, SMD −0.53, 95% CI −0.94 to −0.12). However, the review found no evidence of an effect on global rating scales (SMD −0.11, 95% CI −0.49 to +0.27).

Harms: Withdrawal rates were low and, except in one study, no significant difference was found between groups.[19] The trials reported no major adverse events.

Comment: The trials all used proxy outcomes (cognitive function) rather than clinical outcomes likely to be important to people with Alzheimer's disease and their carers.

OPTION   GINKGO BILOBA

One systematic review of RCTs found good evidence that ginkgo biloba improves cognitive function and is well tolerated.

Benefits: One systematic review (search date 2000) identified nine double blind RCTs in people with Alzheimer's disease, vascular or mixed Alzheimer/vascular dementia.[20] Most of these trials were of short duration and used different entry criteria, outcomes, and dosage. Eight of these found that ginkgo biloba was superior to placebo for a variety of outcomes. The largest and longest trial (52 weeks; 309

people, of which 236 had Alzheimer's disease) found treatment in people with Alzheimer's disease to be significantly associated with improved ADAS-cog score (−1.7, 95% CI −3.2 to −0.2), GERRI (care giver assessed improvement, −0.19, 95% CI −0.28 to −0.08), but not in mean clinician's global impression of change (0, 95% CI −0.2 to +0.2).[20] The trial suffered from high withdrawal rate (137 withdrew); completer analysis for people with Alzheimer's disease or vascular dementia yielded the number needed to treat for a four point change in ADAS-cog at 8 (95% CI, 5 to 50).

Harms: The largest trial reported adverse events in 31% with ginkgo biloba versus 31% with placebo.[21] No specific pattern of adverse events was reported.

Comment: In the UK ginkgo biloba is currently classified as a foodstuff, and can be purchased freely. Manufacturers of ginkgo biloba sponsored all trials identified in the review. The high withdrawal rate of the longer RCT cited above weakens its conclusions, although the authors did conduct completer and intention-to-treat analysis.[21]

OPTION   NON-STEROIDAL ANTI-INFLAMMATORY DRUGS   New

One small RCT found no benefit from diclofenac compared with placebo.

Benefits: We found no systematic review. We found one RCT comparing diclofenac plus misoprostol versus placebo for 25 weeks (41 people).[22] No significant differences were found between the groups, although for most outcome measures there was a trend to improvement in the NSAID arm, including ADAS-cog scores (mean difference 1.14, 95% CI −2.9 to +5.2) and clinician global impression of change (0.24, 95% CI −0.26 to 0.74).

Harms: Twelve (50%) participants in the treatment arm withdrew by week 25, compared with two in the placebo group. No serious drug related adverse events were reported[22]

Comment: Inflammatory processes may play a part in the pathogenesis of Alzheimer's disease. However, despite the considerable interest in the putative role of NSAIDs, there is poor evidence at present to support the use of these drugs in Alzheimer's disease.

QUESTION   What are the effects of non-drug treatments?

OPTION   REMINISCENCE THERAPY

We found insufficient evidence on the effects of reminiscence therapy (see glossary, p 499) in people with dementia.

Benefits: We found one systematic review of reminiscence therapy (search date 1998), which identified two trials. Analysis of pooled data was compromised by poor trial methods and diverse outcomes.[23]

Harms: We found no evidence.

Comment: None.

OPTION	REALITY ORIENTATION

One systematic review of small RCTs found that reality orientation (see glossary below) was associated with improved cognitive function and behaviour compared with no treatment. We found no data on adverse events.

Benefits: We found one systematic review (search date 1997, 6 RCTs, 125 people).[24] These compared reality orientation versus no treatment, using different measures of cognition. The review found that reality orientation improved cognitive function score (SMD −0.59, 95% CI −0.95 to −0.22) and behavioural symptom score (SMD −0.66, 95% CI −1.27 to −0.05).

Harms: The trials gave no information on adverse effects.[24]

Comment: The trials did not use standardised interventions or outcomes, and the review did not pool the data.[24]

GLOSSARY

Reality orientation Involves presenting information that is designed to reorient a person in time, place, or person. It may range in intensity from a board giving details of the day, date, and season, to staff reorienting a patient at each contact.

Reminiscence therapy Involves encouraging people to talk about the past in order to enable past experiences to be brought into consciousness. It relies on remote memory, which is relatively well preserved in mild to moderate dementia.

Substantive changes since last issue

Cholinesterase inhibitors New systematic review found that rivastigmine improved cognitive function more than placebo in Alzheimer's disease.[13]

REFERENCES

1. Livingston G. The scale of the problem. In Burns A, Levy R, eds. *Dementia*. 1st ed. London: Chapman and Hall, 1994:21–35.
2. Panisset M, Stern Y, Gauthier S, eds. *Clinical diagnosis and management of Alzheimer's disease*, 1st ed. London: Dunitz, 1996:129–139.
3. McKeith I. The differential diagnosis of dementia. In: Burns A, Levy R, eds. *Dementia*. 1st ed. London: Chapman and Hall, 1994:39–57.
4. Hardy J. Molecular classification of Alzheimer's disease. *Lancet* 1991;i:1342–1343.
5. Eastwood R, Reisberg, B. Mood and behaviour. In: Panisset M, Stern Y, Gauthier S, eds. *Clinical diagnosis and management of Alzheimer's disease*, 1st ed. London: Dunitz, 1996:175–189.
6. Absher JR, Cummings JL. Cognitive and noncognitive aspects of dementia syndromes. In: Burns A, Levy R, eds. *Dementia*. 1st ed. London: Chapman and Hall, 1994:59–76.
7. Rosen WG, Mohs RC, Davis KL. A new rating scale for Alzheimer's disease. *Am J Psychiatry* 1984; 141:1356–1364.
8. Folstein MF, Folstein SE, McHugh PR. Mini Mental State: a practical method for grading the cognitive state of patients for the clinician. *J Psychiatr Res* 1975;12:189–198.
9. Birks JS, Melzer D. Donepezil for mild and moderate Alzheimer's disease. In: The Cochrane Library, Issue 2, 2000. Oxford: Update Software. Search date 1998; primary sources Cochrane Dementia and Cognitive Impairment Group Register of Clinical Trials, Medline, PsychLit, Embase and general contact with members of the Donepezil Study Group and Eisai Inc.
10. Rogers SL, Farlow MR, Doody RS, et al. A 24-week double blind placebo controlled trial of donepezil in patients with Alzheimer's disease. *Neurology* 1998;50:136–145.
11. Burns A, Rossor M, Gauthier S, et al. The effects of donezepil in Alzheimer's disease – results from a multinational trial. *Dementia Geriatr Disord* 1999;10:237–244.
12. Qizilbash N, Birks J, Lopez Arrieta J, et al. Tacrine in Alzheimer's disease. In: The Cochrane Library, Issue 2, 2000. Oxford: Update Software. Search date November 1998; primary sources Cochrane Dementia Group Register of Clinical Trials.
13. Birks, J Iakovidou V, Tsolaki, M. Rivastigmine for Alzheimer's disease. In: The Cochrane Library, Issue 2, 2000. Oxford: Update Software. Search date 1999; primary sources Cochrane Controlled Trials Register, Cochrane Dementia Group Register of Clinical Trials, Medline, Embase, Psychlit, Cinahl, and hand searches of geriatric and dementia journals and conference abstracts.
14. Rosler M, Anand R, Cicin-Sain A. Efficacy and safety of rivastigmine in patients with Alzheimer's disease: international randomised controlled trial. *BMJ* 1999;318:633–640.
15. Knapp MJ, Knopman DS, Soloman PR, et al. A 30-week randomized controlled trial of high-dose tacrine in patients with Alzheimer's disease. *JAMA* 1994;271:985–991.
16. Kirchner V, Kelly C, Harvey R. Thioridazine for dementia. In: The Cochrane Library, Issue 2, 2000. Oxford: Update Software. Search date not given, amended August 1998; primary sources

Medline, Embase, Psychlit, Cinahl, Cochrane Group Register of Clinical Trials, and Novartis, the pharmaceutical company that develops and markets thioridazine was approached and asked to release any published or unpublished data they had on file.

17. Reilly JG, Ayis SA, Ferrier IN, et al. QT interval abnormalities and pychotropic drug therapy in psychiatric patients. Lancet 2000;355:1048–1052.

18. Birks J, Flicker L. Selegiline for Alzheimer's disease. In: The Cochrane Library, Issue 4, 1999. Oxford: Update Software. Search date not given, review amended August 1998; primary sources Cochrane Dementia and Cognitive Impairment Group Register of Clinical Trials.

19. Freedman M, Rewilak D, Xerri T, et al. L deprenyl in Alzheimer's disease. Cognitive and behavioural effects. Neurology 1998;50:660–668.

20. Ernst E, Pittler MH. Ginkgo biloba for dementia. Clin Drug Invest 1999;17:301–308. Search date 1998; primary sources Medline, Embase, Biosis, Cochrane Register of Controlled Clinical Trials, hand searches of bibliographies, and contact with manufacturers.

21. Le Bars P, Katz MM, Berman N, Itil T, Freedman A, Schatzberg. A placebo-controlled, double-blind, randomised trial of an extract of ginkgo biloba for dementia. JAMA 1997;278:1327–1332.

22. Scharf S, Mander A, Ugoni A, Vajda F, Christophidis N. A double-blind, placebo-controlled trial of diclofenac/misoprostol in Alzheimer's disease. Neurology 1999;53:197–201.

23. Spector A Orrell M. Reminiscence therapy for dementia. In: The Cochrane Library, Issue 4, 1999. Oxford: Update Software. Search date 1998; primary sources Cochrane Controlled Trials Register, Medline, Psychlit, Embase, Omni, Bids, Dissertation Abstracts International, Sigle, and reference lists of relevant articles, relevant internet sites, and hand searching of specialist journals.

24. Spector A, Orrell M, Davies S, et al. Reality orientation for dementia. In: The Cochrane Library, Issue 2, 2000. Oxford: Update Software. Search date 1997; primary sources Medline, Psychlit, Embase, Cochrane Database of Systematic Reviews, Omni, Bids, Dissertation Abstracts International, Sigle, plus Internet searching of HealthWeb, Mental Health Infosources, American Psychiatric Association, Internet Mental Health, Mental Health Net, NHS Confederation, and hand searching of specialist journals.

James Warner
Senior Lecturer/Consultant in Old Age Psychiatry
Imperial College School of Medicine
London
UK

Rob Butler
Lecturer in Old Age Psychiatry
Imperial College School of Medicine
London
UK

Competing interests: JW has been reimbursed by Novartis, the manufacturer of rivastigmine, for conference attendance. RB, none declared.

Updated and expanded this issue

Christopher Gale and Mark Oakley-Browne

INTERVENTIONS

Key Messages

Cognitive therapy

- Two systematic reviews of RCTs have found that cognitive therapy, with a combination of behavioural interventions such as exposure to anxiogenic circumstances, relaxation, and cognitive restructuring, is more effective than remaining on the waiting list, anxiety management training alone, or nondirective therapy. We found no evidence of adverse effects.

Applied relaxation

- One systematic review of RCTs comparing psychological treatments for generalised anxiety disorder has not established or excluded a clinically important difference in the effects of applied relaxation and cognitive therapy.

Benzodiazepines

- Two systematic reviews of RCTs have found that, compared with placebo, benzodiazepines are an effective and rapid treatment for generalised anxiety disorder (GAD). They increase the risk of dependence, sedation, industrial accidents and road traffic accidents. They have been associated with neonatal and infant morbidity when used late in pregnancy or while breast feeding. One RCT found no significant difference in the effects of slow release alprazolam and bromazepam.

Buspirone

- One systematic review has found that buspirone is effective in GAD. Limited evidence from RCTs found no significant difference in benefits between busipirone, benzodiazepines or antidepressants. Buspirone had slower onset than benzodiazepines but fewer adverse effects.

Antidepressants

■ RCTs have found that imipramine, trazodone, venlafaxine, and paroxetine are effective treatments for GAD. One trial found that paroxetine was more effective than a benzodiazepine. Adverse effects of antidepressants include sedation, confusion, and falls.

Antipsychotic drugs

■ One RCT in people with GAD found that trifluoperazine reduced anxiety more than placebo, but caused more adverse effects.

β Blockers

■ We found that β blockers have not been adequately evaluated in GAD.

DEFINITION Generalised anxiety disorder (GAD) is defined as excessive worry and tension, on most days, for at least 6 months, together with the following symptoms and signs: increased motor tension (fatigability, trembling, restlessness, muscle tension); autonomic hyperactivity (shortness of breath, rapid heart rate, dry mouth, cold hands, and dizziness) but not panic attacks; and increased vigilance and scanning (feeling keyed up, increased startling, impaired concentration). One non-systematic review of epidemiological and clinical studies found marked reduction of quality of life and psychosocial functioning in people with anxiety disorder (including generalised anxiety disorder).[1] Significant impairment was also found in people with mild forms of anxiety disorders.[1]

INCIDENCE/ PREVALENCE Assessment of the incidence and prevalence of GAD is difficult. There is a high rate of comorbidity with other anxiety disorders and depressive disorders.[2] The reliability of the measures used in epidemiological studies is unsatisfactory.[3] One US study, which used the criteria of the Diagnostic and Statistical Manual of Mental Disorders, third edition, revised (DSM-III-R), has estimated that one in every 20 people will develop GAD at some time during their lives.[4] One recent non-systematic review found that the incidence of GAD in men is only half the incidence in women.[5] One non-systematic review of seven studies found reduced prevalence of anxiety disorders in older people.[6]

AETIOLOGY/ RISK FACTORS One small community study found that GAD was associated with an increase in the number of minor stressors, independent of demographic factors.[7] People with GAD complain of more somatic symptoms and respond in a rigid, stereotyped manner if placed under physiological stress. Autonomic function is similar to that of control populations, but muscle tension is increased.[8] One non-systematic review (five observational studies) of psychological sequelae to civilian trauma found rates of GAD reported in four of the five studies were increased significantly compared with a control population (rate ratio 3.3, 95% CI 2.0 to 5.5).[9]

PROGNOSIS GAD is a long term condition. It often begins before or during young adulthood and can be a lifelong problem. Spontaneous remission is rare.[4]

AIMS To reduce anxiety; to minimise disruption of day to day functioning; and to improve quality of life, with minimum adverse effects.

OUTCOMES   Severity of symptoms and effects on quality of life, as measured by symptom scores, usually the Hamilton Anxiety Scale (HAM-A), State-Trait Anxiety Inventory (STAI), or clinical global impression symptom scores. Where NNTs are given, these represent the number of people requiring treatment within a given time period (usually 6–12 weeks) for one additional person to achieve a certain improvement in symptom score. The method for obtaining NNTs was not standardised across studies. Some used a reduction by, for example, 20 points in the HAM-A as a response, while others defined a response as a reduction, for example, by 50% of the premorbid score. We have not attempted to standardise methods but instead have used the response rates reported in each study to calculate NNTs. Similarly, we have calculated NNHs from original trial data.

METHODS   *Clinical Evidence* update search and appraisal May 2000. Recent changes in diagnostic classification make it hard to compare older studies with more recent ones. In the earlier classification system, DSM-III-R, the diagnosis was made only in the absence of other psychiatric disorder. In current systems (DSM-IV and ICD-10 [International Classification of Diseases, 10th revision]), GAD can be diagnosed in the presence of any comorbid condition. All drug studies were short term, at most 12 weeks.

QUESTION   What are the effects of cognitive therapy?

Two systematic reviews of RCTs have found that cognitive therapy, using a combination of behavioural interventions such as exposure, relaxation, and cognitive restructuring, is more effective than remaining on a waiting list (no treatment), anxiety management training alone, or non-directive therapy. We found no evidence of adverse effects.

Benefits: We found two systematic reviews. The first (search date 1996) included 35 RCTs (n = 4002 [60% women]) of medical treatment, cognitive therapy, or both.[10] Thirteen trials included 22 cognitive behavioural therapies, which involved (alone or in combination) cognitive restructuring, relaxation training, exposure, and systematic desensitisation. Combined results from these trials found significantly better results with active treatment compared with control treatments (effect size 0.70, 95% CI 0.57 to 0.83). Controls included remaining on a waiting list, anxiety management training, relaxation training, and non-directive psychotherapy. One year follow up of an RCT found cognitive therapy was associated with better outcomes than analytic psychotherapy and anxiety management training.[10,11] The second systematic review (search date 1998, 8 RCTs, n = 404) found that more participants given individual cognitive therapy maintained recovery after 6 months than those given other treatments (participants maintaining recovery at 6 months: individual cognitive therapy 41%, non-directive therapy 19%, group cognitive therapy 18%, group behaviour therapy 12%, individual behaviour therapy 18%, and analytical psychotherapy 0%; P values not reported).[12]

Harms: We found no evidence of adverse effects.

Comment: None.

QUESTION What are the effects of applied relaxation? New

QUESTION What are the effects of applied relaxation? New

We found no study of applied relaxation (see glossary, p 509) versus placebo treatment. One systematic review of RCTs comparing applied relaxation with cognitive therapy found no significant difference in the proportion of people with clinically important improvement of their anxiety scores over 6 months. The available evidence does not establish or exclude the possibility of clinically important differences in the effects of applied relaxation and cognitive therapy.

Benefits: **Versus placebo:** We found no systematic review or RCT. **Versus other psychological treatments:** We found one systematic review (search date 1998, 6 RCTs, n = 404) of psychological therapy in GAD. The six RCTs all used the State-Trait Anxiety Inventory (STAI). There was significant variation in the type of cognitive therapy (group or individual) and in the comparison therapies (applied relaxation, analytical psychotherapy, behaviour therapy, and non-directive therapy). Only one of the six RCTs included a placebo group, and that RCT did not examine applied relaxation. Two RCTs included individual applied relaxation (n = 38) and four included individual cognitive behavioural therapy (n = 87). The systematic review analysed the raw data from individual studies to calculate the proportion of people who experienced a clinically significant change after treatment and maintained that improvement until 6 months after treatment. Applied relaxation was more likely than individual cognitive behavioural therapy to improve the anxiety inventory after 6 months (52% with applied relaxation v 41%).[12] No statistical tests of significance were performed by the systematic review, but even if the figures presented are taken at face value (see comment below) then the difference between the effects of individual applied relaxation and individual cognitive behavioural therapy may have arisen by chance (recovery maintained to 6 months: 20/38 = 52% with applied relaxation, 41/87 = 41% with cognitive therapy; RR 1.27, 95% CI 0.82 to 1.70).

Harms: No evidence of harms was noted.

Comment: The STAI covers only a restricted range of symptoms, and it may not satisfactorily reflect treatment outcomes in GAD. It is very difficult to interpret the results of the systematic review because the comparison involves arms from different RCTs. This could remove the benefits of randomisation because the groups being compared may have different characteristics. The figures presented in the systematic review produce estimates of relative effectiveness with wide confidence intervals: a clinically important difference has not been established or excluded.

QUESTION What are the effects of drug treatments?

OPTION BENZODIAZEPINES

One systematic review of RCTs has found that, compared with placebo, benzodiazepines are an effective and rapid treatment for GAD. They increase the risk of dependence, sedation, industrial accidents, and road traffic accidents. If used in late pregnancy or while breast feeding, they can cause adverse effects in neonates. One RCT found no significant difference between sustained release alprazolam and bromazepam. One RCT found no evidence of a difference in effectiveness between benzodiazepines and buspirone. One systematic review of RCTs, which looked at long term treatment, found no good evidence that any short term benefit of benzodiazepines was sustained.

Benefits: **Versus placebo:** We found one systematic review (search date January 1996), which identified 24 placebo controlled trials of drug treatments, principally benzodiazepines (in 19 trials), buspirone (in nine trials), antidepressants (ritanserin and imipramine, in three trials), all in people with GAD.[10] Pooled analysis across all studies gave an effect size of 0.60 (95% CI 0.50 to 0.70), whereas for benzodiazepines the mean effect size was 0.70 (no 95% CIs given). The review found no significant differences in effect sizes between different benzodiazepines, although there was insufficient power to rule out a clinically important difference. One of the larger included trials (n = 230) found that the number of people reporting global improvement after 8 weeks (completer analysis, overall dropout rate 35%, no significant difference in withdrawal rates between groups) was greater with diazepam than with placebo (diazepam 67%, placebo 39%, P < 0.026). **Versus each other:** One subsequent RCT (n = 121) compared sustained release alprazolam with bromazepam and found no significant difference in effects (HAM-A scores).[13] **Versus buspirone:** See buspirone option, p 506. **Long term treatment:** We found one systematic review of eight RCTs (any benzodiazepine medication, greater than 2 months duration, people with GAD). The methods of these RCTs included limiting factors that prevent firm conclusions being made.[14]

Harms: **Sedation and dependence:** Benzodiazepines have been found to cause impairment in attention, concentration, and short term memory. One RCT found a high rate of drowsiness (71% with diazepam v 13% with placebo; P = 0.001) and dizziness (29% v 11%; P = 0.001).[10] Sedation can interfere with concomitant psychotherapy. Rebound anxiety on withdrawal has been reported in 15–30% of participants.[15] There is a high risk of substance abuse and dependence with benzodiazepines. **Memory:** Thirty one people with agoraphobia/panic disorder from a placebo controlled trial of 8 weeks' alprazolam were followed up at 3.5 years. Five were still taking benzodiazepines and had significant impairment in memory tasks.[16] There was no difference in memory performance between those who had been in the placebo group and those who had been given alprazolam but were no longer taking the drug. **Road traffic accidents:** We found one systematic review (search date 1997) examining the relation between benzodiazepines and road traffic accidents.[17] In the case control studies identified, the odds ratio for death or emergency medical treatment in those who had taken benzodiazepines compared with those who had not taken them ranged from 1.45 to 2.4. The odds ratio increased with higher doses and more recent intake. In the police and emergency ward studies, benzodiazepine use was a factor in 1–65% of accidents (usually 5–10%). In two studies in which participants had blood alcohol concentrations under the legal limit, benzodiazepines were found in 43% and 65%. For drivers over 65 years, the risk of being involved in reported road traffic accidents was higher if they had taken longer acting and larger quantities of benzodiazepines. These studies are retrospective case control studies and are therefore subject to confounding factors. **Pregnancy and breast feeding:** One systematic review (search date 1997) identified 23 studies looking at the link between cleft lip and palate and use of benzodiazepines in the first trimester of pregnancy.[18] The review found no association. However, use of benzodiazepines in late pregnancy has been found to be associated with neonatal hypotonia and withdrawal syndrome.[19] Benzodiazepines are secreted in breast milk, and there have been reports of sedation and hypothermia in infants.[19] **Other:** A reanalysis of eight RCTs of benzodiazepines compared with placebo or buspirone found a consistent improvement with benzodiazepines. However, recent use of benzodiazepines limited the effectiveness of buspirone.[20]

Comment: All the benzodiazepine studies were short term (at most 12 weeks). There was usually a significant improvement at 6 weeks, but response rates were given at the end of the trials.

| OPTION | BUSPIRONE |

RCTs have found that, compared with placebo, buspirone increases the proportion of people with GAD who improve clinically in the short term. Limited evidence from RCTs found no significant differences in the benefits of buspirone, benzodiazepines or antidepressants. Buspirone had slower onset than benzodiazepines but had fewer adverse effects.

Benefits: **Versus placebo:** We found one systematic review (search date January 1996), which identified nine studies of buspirone but did not report on its effects as distinct from pharmacotherapy in general.[11] One of the included studies was itself a non-systematic meta-analysis of eight placebo controlled trials of buspirone in 520 people with GAD (see comment below). It found that, compared with placebo, buspirone was associated with a greater response rate, defined as the proportion of people much or very much improved as rated by their physician (54% v 28%, P ≤ 0.001). A subsequent double blind placebo controlled trial in 162 people with GAD found similar results (buspirone 55% v placebo 35%, P < 0.05).[21] A reanalysis of pooled data from eight RCTs (n = 735) found a differential response to buspirone depending on whether the participant had been exposed to benzodiazepines (no previous exposure to benzodiazepine: response rate 62% [buspirone] v 31% [placebo]; recent benzodiazepine use: response rate 41% [buspirone] v 21% [placebo]). The latter result was not significant.[20] **Versus benzodiazepines:** The systematic review did not directly compare buspirone with benzodiazepines. One large RCT (n = 230) included in the review found no significant difference between buspirone and benzodiazepines.[10] A recent reanalysis of eight RCTs found no significant difference in the effects of buspirone compared with benzodiazepines.[20] **Versus antidepressants:** See antidepressants, p 507.

Harms: **Sedation and dependence:** The systematic review found that, compared with benzodiazepines, buspirone had a slower onset of action but fewer adverse effects.[10] The subsequent RCT found that, compared with placebo, buspirone caused significantly more nausea (34% v 13%), dizziness (64% v 12%), and somnolence (19% v 7%). We found no reports of dependency on buspirone. **Pregnancy and breast feeding:** We found no evidence.

Comment: All trials in the meta-analysis mentioned above were sponsored by pharmaceutical companies and had been included in new drug applications for buspirone as an antidepressant. Other search criteria were not given. Trial methods were similar.[10]

| OPTION | ANTIDEPRESSANTS |

RCTs have found that imipramine, trazodone, venlafaxine, and paroxetine are effective treatments for GAD. Individual RCTs found that they were more effective than benzodiazepines, with no evidence of a difference in effectiveness compared with buspirone. There is a significant risk of sedation, confusion, and falls with these drugs.

Benefits: **Versus placebo:** We found one systematic review (search date January 1996, 3 placebo controlled RCTs) of antidepressants which found treatment to be significantly associated with a greater response than placebo (pooled effect size 0.57).[10] The review pooled results for trazodone, imipramine, and ritanserin, so limiting the conclusions that may be drawn for trazodone and imipramine alone.[10] In another placebo controlled RCT (n = 230) the NNT for moderate or pronounced improvement after 8 weeks of treatment with imipramine was 3 (completer analysis calculated from data by author) and with trazodone the NNT was 4 (95% CI 3 to 4, calculated from data by author).[22] **Versus benzodiazepines:** We found one RCT comparing paroxetine, imipramine, and 2'-chlordesmethyldiazepam for 8 weeks in 81 people with GAD.[23] Paroxetine and imipramine were significantly more effective than 2'-chlordesmethyldiazepam in improving anxiety scores (mean HAM-A after 8 weeks 11.1 for paroxetine, 10.8 for imipramine, 12.9 for 2'- chlordesmethyldiazepam; P = 0.05). **Versus buspirone:** We found no systematic review. We found one RCT (n = 365) comparing venlafaxine 75 mg and 150 mg/day with buspirone 30 mg/day over 8 weeks, with a small placebo arm. There was no significant difference between the two treatments (venlafaxine 75 mg, NNT 8, 95% CI 6 to 9; venlafaxine 150 mg, NNT 7, 95% CI 6 to 9; buspirone 30 mg, NNT 11, 95% CI 10 to 12).[24] **Sedating tricyclic antidepressants:** We found no systematic review or RCTs evaluating sedating tricyclics in people with GAD.

Harms: Sedation, confusion, dry mouth, and constipation have been reported with both imipramine and trazodone.[22] **Overdose:** In a series of 239 coroner directed necropsies from 1970 to 1989, tricyclic antidepressants were considered to be a causal factor in 12% of deaths and hypnosedatives (primarily benzodiazepines and excluding barbiturates) in 8%.[25] **Accidental poisoning:** From 1958 to 1977 a total of 598 deaths in British children under the age of 10 years from 1958 to 1977 were registered as accidental poisoning. After 1970, tricyclic antidepressants were the most common cause of accidental poisoning in this age group.[26] A study estimated that there was one death for every 44 children admitted to hospital after ingestion of tricyclic antidepressants.[27] **Hyponatraemia:** A case series reported 736 incidents of hyponatraemia in people taking selective serotonin reuptake inhibitors (SSRIs); 83% of episodes were in hospital inpatients aged over 65 years.[28] It is not possible to establish causation from this type of data. **Nausea:** Nausea has been reported in people taking paroxetine.[23] **Falls:** A retrospective cohort study of 2428 elderly residents of nursing homes found an increased risk of falls in new users of antidepressants (adjusted RR for tricyclic antidepressants: 2.0, 95 % CI 1.8 to 2.2, n = 665; for SSRIs: 1.8, 95% CI 1.6 to 2.0, n = 612; and for trazodone: 1.2, 95% CI 1.0 to 1.4, n = 304).[29] The increased rate of falls persisted through the first 180 days of treatment and beyond. A case control study of 8239 people aged 66 years or older treated in hospital for hip fracture found an increased risk of hip fracture in those taking antidepressants.[30] The adjusted odds ratio for hip fracture compared with those not taking antidepressants was 2.4 (95% CI 2.0 to 2.7) for SSRIs, 2.2 (95% CI 1.8 to 2.8) for secondary amine tricyclic antidepressants such as nortriptyline, and 1.5 (95% CI 1.3 to 1.7) for tertiary amine tricyclic antidepressants such as amitriptyline. This study could not control for confounding factors; people taking antidepressants may be at increased risk of hip fracture for other reasons. **In pregnancy:** We found no reports of harmful effects in pregnancy. One case controlled study found no evidence that imipramine or fluoxetine increased the rate of malformations in pregnancy.[31]

Comment: None.

OPTION   ANTIPSYCHOTIC DRUGS

One RCT found that 4 weeks treatment with trifluoperazine lowered anxiety more than placebo but caused more adverse effects.

Benefits: We found no systematic review. We found one RCT (n = 415) comparing 4 weeks of treatment with trifluoperazine 2–6 mg/day with placebo in people with GAD.[32] The trial reported an average reduction of 14 points on the total anxiety rating scale (HAM-A), with no reduction on placebo (P < 0.001).

Harms: Short term treatment with antipsychotic drugs increased the risk of sedation, acute dystonias, akathisia, and parkinsonism. In the longer term, the rate of tardive dyskinesia may be increased, especially if treatment is interrupted.[33]

Comment: None.

OPTION   β BLOCKERS

β Blockers have not been adequately evaluated in people with GAD.

Benefits: We found no systematic review or good RCTs of β blockers in people with GAD.

Harms: We found no good evidence in people with GAD.

Comment: None.

GLOSSARY

Applied relaxation A technique involving imagination of relaxing situations to induce muscular and mental relaxation.

Substantive changes since last issue

Definition One non-systematic review has found that anxiety disorders compromise quality of life.[1]

Incidence and prevalence One non-systematic review found that men have half the incidence of GAD as women.[5] One non-systematic review found a decrease in the prevalence of anxiety disorders associated with increasing age.[6]

Aetiology/risk factors One non-systematic review of psychological sequelae to civilian trauma found rates of GAD were increased significantly.[9]

Cognitive behaviour One systematic review found that individual cognitive therapy was superior to other methods.[12]

Long term benzodiazepines One systematic review found no good evidence for an effective long term treatment.[15]

Harms from benzodiazepines A reanalysis of eight RCTs found recent benzodiazepine use was associated with an increase in nervousness and dizziness.[20]

Buspirone versus placebo A reanalysis of data from 8 RCTs found that previous exposure to benzodiazepines reduced the response to buspirone.[20]

Buspirone versus benzodiazepines A reanalysis of data from 8 RCTs found no difference in the effects of buspirone compared with benzodiazepine.[20]

REFERENCES

1. Mendlowicz MV, Stein MB. Quality of life in individuals with anxiety disorders. *Am J Psychiatry* 2000;157:669–682.
2. Judd LL, Kessler RC, Paulus MP, et al. Comorbidity as a fundamental feature of generalised anxiety disorders: results from the national comorbidity study (NCS). *Acta Psychiatr Scand* 1998;98(suppl 393):6–11.
3. Andrews G, Peters L, Guzman AM, Bird K. A comparison of two structured diagnostic interviews: CIDI and SCAN. *Aust N Z J Psychiatry* 1995;29:124–132.
4. Jessker RC, McGonagle KA, Zhao S, et al. Lifetime and 12-month prevalence of DSM-III-R psychiatric disorders in the United States: results from the national comorbidity survey. *Arch Gen Psychiatry* 1992;51:8–19.
5. Pigott T. Gendere differences in the epidemiology and treatment of anxiety disorders. *J Clin Psychiatry* 1999;60(suppl 18):15–18.
6. Jorm AF. Does old age reduce the risk of anxiety and depression? A review of epidemiological studies across the adult life span. *Psych Med* 2000;30:11–22.
7. Brantley PJ, Mehan DJ, Ames SC, Jones GN. Minor stressors and generalised anxiety disorders among low income patients attending primary care clinics. *J Nerv Ment Dis* 1999;187:435–440.
8. Hoehn-Saric R. Psychic and somatic anxiety: worries, somatic symptoms, and physiological changes. *Acta Psychiatr Scand* 1998;98(suppl 393):32–38.
9. Brown ES, Fulton MK, Wilkeson A, Petty F. The psychiatric sequelae of civilian trauma. *Comp Psychiatry* 2000;41:19–23.
10. Gould RA, Otto MW, Pollack MH, Yap L. Cognitive behavioural and pharmacological treatment of generalised anxiety disorder: a preliminary meta-analysis. *Behav Res Ther* 1997;28:285–305. Search date January 1996; primary sources Psyclit 1974 to 1996; Medline 1966 to January

1996; examination of reference lists; and unpublished articles presented at national conferences.
11. Durham RC, Fisher PL, Trevling LR, Hau CM, Richard K, Stewart JB. One year follow-up of cognitive therapy, analytic psychotherapy and anxiety management training for generalised anxiety disorder: symptom change, medication usage and attitudes to treatment. *Behav Cogn Psychother* 1999;27:19–35.
12. Fisher PL, Durham RC. Recovery rates in generalized anxiety disorder following psychological therapy: an analysis of clinically significant change in the STAI-T across outcome studies since 1990. *Psychol Med* 1999;29:1425–1434. Search date: December 1998; primary sources Medline 1987 to December 1998; Psychlit 1987 to December 1998; and Cochrane Controlled Trials Register 1987 to December 1998.
13. Figueira ML. Alprazolam SR in the treatment of generalised anxiety: a multicentre controlled study with bromazepam. *Hum Psychother* 1999;14: 171–177.
14. Mahe V, Balogh A. Long-term pharmacological treatment of generalized anxiety disorder. *Int Clin Psychopharmacol* 2000;15:99–105.
15. Tyrer P. Current problems with the benzodiazepines. In: Wheatly D, ed. *The anxiolytic jungle: where next?* Chichester: J Wiley and Sons, 1990;23–60.
16. Kilic C, Curran HV, Noshirvani H, Marks IM, Basoglu MB. Long-term effects of alprazolam on memory: a 3.5 year follow-up of agoraphobia/panic patients. *Psychol Med* 1999;29:225–231.
17. Thomas RE. Benzodiazepine use and motor vehicle accidents. Systematic review of reported association. *Can Fam Physician* 1998;44:799–808. Search date 1997; primary sources Medline 1980 to 1997.
18. Dolovich LR, Addis A, Regis Vaillancourt JD, et al.

Benzodiazepine use in pregnancy and major malformations of oral cleft: meta-analysis of cohort and case-control studies. *BMJ* 1998;317: 839–843. Search date December 1998; primary sources Medline 1966 to 1997; Embase 1980 to 1997; Reprotox, references of included studies and review articles.

19. Bernstein JG. *Handbook of drug therapy in psychiatry*, 3rd ed. St Louis, Missouri: Mosby Year Book, 1995:401.

20. DeMartinis N, Rynn M, Rickels K, Mandos L. Prior benzodiazepine use and buspirone response in the treatment of generalized anxiety disorder. *J Clin Psychiatry* 2000;61:91–94.

21. Sramek JJ, Transman M, Suri A, et al. Efficacy of buspirone in generalized anxiety disorder with coexisting mild depressive symptoms. *J Clin Psychiatry* 1996;57:287–291.

22. Rickels K, Downing R, Schweizer E, Hassman H. Antidepressants for the treatment of generalised anxiety disorder: a placebo-controlled comparison of imipramine, trazodone and diazepam. *Arch Gen Psychiatry* 1993;50:884–895.

23. Rocca P, Fonzo V, Scotta M, Zanalda E, Ravizza L. Paroxetine efficacy in the treatment of generalized anxiety disorder. *Acta Psychiatr Scand* 1997;95: 444–450.

24. Davidson JR, DuPont RL, Hedges D, Haskins JT. Efficacy, safety and tolerability of venlafaxine extended release and busperone in outpatients with generalised anxiety disorder. *J Clin Psychiatry* 1999;60:528–535.

25. Dukes PD, Robinson GM, Thomson KJ, Robinson BJ. Wellington coroner autopsy cases 1970–89: acute deaths due to drugs, alcohol and poisons. *N Z Med J* 1992;105:25–27. (Published erratum appears in *N Z Med J* 1992;105:135.)

26. Fraser NC. Accidental poisoning deaths in British children 1958–77. *BMJ* 1980;280:1595–1598.

27. Pearn J, Nixon J, Ansford A, Corcoran A. Accidental poisoning in childhood: five year urban population study with 15 year analysis of fatality. *BMJ* 1984;288:44–46.

28. Lui BA, Mitmann N, Knowles SR, Shear NH. Hyponatremia and the syndrome of inappropriate secretion of antidiuretic hormone associated with the use of selective serotonin reuptake inhibitors: a review of spontaneous reports. *Can Med Assoc J* 1995;155:519–527.

29. Thapa PB, Gideon P, Cost TW, Milam AB, Ray WA. Antidepressants and the risk of falls among nursing home residents. *N Engl J Med* 1998;339: 875–882.

30. Liu B, Anderson G, Mittmann N, To T, Axcell T, Shear N. Use of selective serotonin-reuptake inhibitors of tricyclic antidepressants and risk of hip fractures in elderly people. *Lancet* 1998;351: 1303–1307.

31. Kulin NA, Pastuszak A, Koren G. Are the new SSRIs safe for pregnant women? *Can Fam Physician* 1998;44;2081–2083.

32. Mendels J, Krajewski TF, Huffer V, et al. Effective short-term treatment of generalized anxiety with trifluoroperazine. *J Clin Psychiatry* 1986;47:170–174.

33. Van Harten PN, Hoek HW, Matroos GE, Koeter M, Kahn RS. Intermittent neuroleptic treatment and risk of tardive dyskinesi: Curacao extrapyradimal syndromes study III. *Am J Psychiatry* 1998;155: 565–567.

Christopher Gale
Psychiatrist
Department of Psychiatry, University of Auckland
Auckland
New Zealand

Mark Oakley-Browne
Associate Professor
University of Auckland
Auckland
New Zealand

Competing interests: None declared.

Phillipa Hay and Josue Bacaltchuk

INTERVENTIONS

Key Messages

Psychotherapy

- Two systematic reviews and a subsequent large RCT have found that cognitive behavioural therapy (CBT) reduces specific symptoms of bulimia nervosa and also improves non-specific symptoms, such as depression. One RCT found that the beneficial effects of CBT are maintained for at least 5 years.

- One systematic review of RCTs found that other psychotherapies improve the symptoms of bulimia nervosa.

- Two well designed RCTs found that the onset of the effects of interpersonal psychotherapy is slower than CBT.

Antidepressants

- Two systematic reviews of RCTs have found that antidepressants reduce bulimic symptoms in the short term, but we found insufficient evidence about their role in maintenance treatment.

- We found insufficient evidence about the effects of different classes of antidepressants.

- One systematic review of RCTs comparing antidepressants with psychotherapy found no significant difference in abstinence from binge eating.

Combinations of antidepressants and psychotherapy

- One systematic review of RCTs found that combinations of treatments are more effective than either individual psychotherapy or antidepressants alone. People taking antidepressants, either alone or in combination with psychotherapy, were more likely than people receiving psychotherapy alone to withdraw from treatment.

Bulimia nervosa

DEFINITION Bulimia nervosa is an intense preoccupation with body weight and shape, with regular episodes of uncontrolled overeating of large amounts of food (binge eating associated with use of extreme methods to counteract the feared effects of overeating). If a person also meets the diagnostic criteria for anorexia nervosa, then the diagnosis of anorexia nervosa takes precedence.[1] Bulimia nervosa can be difficult to identify because of extreme secrecy about binge eating and purgative behaviour. Weight may be normal but there is often a history of anorexia nervosa or restrictive dieting. Some people alternate between anorexia nervosa and bulimia nervosa.

INCIDENCE/ PREVALENCE In community based studies, the prevalence of bulimia nervosa is between 0.5% and 1.0%, with an even social class distribution.[2–4] About 90% of people diagnosed with bulimia nervosa are women. The numbers presenting with bulimia nervosa in industrialised countries increased during the decade that followed its recognition in the late 1970s and "a cohort effect" is reported in community surveys[2,5,6] implying an increase in incidence. The prevalence of eating disorders such as bulimia nervosa is lower in non-industrialised populations,[7] and varies across ethnic groups. African-American women have a lower risk of restrictive dieting than white American women, but have a similar risk of recurrent binge eating.[8]

AETIOLOGY/ RISK FACTORS Young women from the developed world who restrict their dietary intake are at highest risk of developing bulimia nervosa and other eating disorders. One community based case control study compared 102 people with bulimia nervosa with 204 healthy controls and found higher rates of the following in people with the eating disorder: obesity, mood disorder, sexual and physical abuse, parental obesity, substance misuse, low self esteem, perfectionism, disturbed family dynamics, parental weight/shape concern, and early menarche.[9] Compared to a control group of 102 women with other psychiatric disorders, women with bulimia nervosa had higher rates of parental problems and obesity.

PROGNOSIS A 10 year follow up study (50 people with bulimia nervosa from a former trial of mianserin treatment) found that 52% had fully recovered, and only 9% continued to experience symptoms of bulimia nervosa.[10] A larger study (222 people from a trial of antidepressants and structured intensive group psychotherapy) found that after a mean follow up of 11.5 years, 11% still met criteria for bulimia nervosa, while 70% were in full or partial remission.[11] Short term studies found similar results: about 50% of people made a full recovery, 30% made a partial recovery, and 20% continued to be symptomatic.[12] There are few consistent predictors of longer term outcome. Good prognosis has been associated with shorter illness duration, a younger age of onset, higher social class, and a family history of alcoholism.[10] Poor prognosis has been associated with a history of substance misuse,[11] premorbid and paternal obesity,[13] and, in some studies, personality disorder.[14–17]

AIMS To reduce symptoms of bulimia nervosa; to improve general psychiatric symptoms; to improve social functioning and quality of life.

OUTCOMES Frequency of binge eating, abstinence from binge eating, frequency of behaviours to reduce weight and counter the effects of binge eating, severity of extreme weight and shape preoccupation, severity of general psychiatric symptoms, severity of depression, improvement in social and adaptive functioning, remission rates, relapse rates, and withdrawal rates.

METHODS *Clinical Evidence* search and appraisal March 2000, and hand-search of reference lists of identified reviews. One RCT in press (since published) was identified through direct contact with an author.[18] One systematic review was not included as it included uncontrolled studies.[19]

QUESTION **What are the effects of treatments for bulimia nervosa in adults?**

OPTION COGNITIVE BEHAVIOURAL THERAPY

Two systematic reviews and one further large RCT have found that cognitive behavioural therapy (CBT) versus remaining on a waiting list reduces specific symptoms of bulimia nervosa, and improves non-specific symptoms, such as depression. Two RCTs found that CBT reduced binge eating in the short term more than interpersonal psychotherapy, but there was no significant difference in the long term.

Benefits: We found three systematic reviews of RCTs of psychotherapy[20–22] and two subsequent RCTs.[18,23] The third systematic review is in German and may be included in a future issue of *Clinical Evidence*.[22] The first systematic review (search date 1999, 20 RCTs) included RCTs of other binge eating disorders, although most studies were of people with bulimia nervosa (18 people with bulimia nervosa characterised by purging behaviour).[20] The second review (search date 1998, 26 RCTs) used a broad definition of CBT, including exposure and response prevention, and included non-randomised trials.[21] **Versus waiting list controls:** The first review (individual analyses included a maximum of 10 RCTs and 396 people) found that CBT compared to remaining on a waiting list increased the proportion of people abstaining from binge eating at the end of the trial (RR 0.64, 95% CI 0.53 to 0.78, 7 RCTs) (see table 1, p 519).[20] CBT compared with remaining on the waiting list was associated with lower depression scores (4 RCTs, 159 people). Weight at the end of treatment was similar with CBT and remaining on the waiting list (3 RCTs). There was insufficient evidence about other outcomes such as social functioning. The second systematic review (9 RCTs of specific CBT, 173 people) found that abstinence from binge eating at the end of treatment ranged from 33% to 92% (mean 55%).[21] Pooled effect sizes (weighted for sample size) ranged from 1.22 to 1.35 for reduction in binge eating frequency, purging frequency, depression, and disturbed eating attitudes. Tests for heterogeneity were not significant. In one study the benefits of CBT were maintained for up to 5 years.[13] **Versus other psychotherapies:** The first review found that more people abstained from binge eating after CBT than after other psychotherapies, but the difference was not significant (6 RCTs; RR 0.79, 95% CI 0.54 to 1.17).[20] CBT in a full or less intensive form was not significantly superior to CBT in a pure self help form (RR 0.94, 95% CI 0.76 to

1.17, 3 trials). CBT was associated with significantly lower depression scores at end of treatment compared with other psychotherapies (SMD −0.52, 95% CI −0.76 to −0.27, 8 RCTs, 273 people). CBT plus exposure therapy was not more effective than CBT alone (RR abstinence from binge eating 0.87, 95% CI 0.65 to 1.16, 4 RCTs). Depression scores were lower at the end of treatment in groups treated with CBT plus exposure therapy than in groups treated with CBT alone (SMD 0.54, 95% CI 0.17 to 0.91, 3 RCTs, 122 people). The first subsequent RCT compared classic CBT for bulimia nervosa with interpersonal psychotherapy in 220 people with bulimia nervosa that involved purging.[18] The trial found that CBT improved abstinence from binge eating at the end of treatment (intention to treat analysis: 29% with CBT v 6% with interpersonal psychotherapy). The differences were not significant at 4, 8, and 12 months' follow up. The benefit of CBT was established fully at the end of treatment and was maintained for up to 1 year. The benefits of interpersonal psychotherapy continued to improve in the year after treatment. The second subsequent RCT compared four sessions of motivational enhancement therapy versus CBT in 125 people with bulimia nervosa. The trial found no significant differences between the treatments.[23] **Versus antidepressants:** See antidepressants option, p 515.

Harms: The RCTs did not report details of the adverse effects.[18,20,21,23] One systematic review found no significant difference in completion rates between interventions,[20] suggesting no major difference in acceptability. However, neither review could exclude infrequent serious adverse effects. An observational study found that group psychotherapy offered very soon after presentation was sometimes perceived as threatening.[10]

Comment: The first review defined CBT as psychotherapy that uses specified techniques and models,[20] but it did not define the number of sessions or specialist expertise.[24] Effect sizes for CBT were large, but over 50% of people were still binge eating at the end of treatment.[20,21] Research is needed to evaluate the specific as well as non-specific effects of CBT and other psychotherapies, to identify individual characteristics that may predict response, and to explore the long term effects of treatment. Rates of abstinence from binge eating were higher in all experimental groups, but the differences reached significance only when compared with those remaining on a waiting list. It is difficult to interpret the clinical importance of the statistically significant changes in depression scores. It is also difficult to interpret directly the clinical importance of the benefits reported as effect sizes, where the individual RCTs used different outcomes. Further limitations are that the quality of trials was variable (e.g. 57% were not blinded and only one was truly double blinded).[20] Sample sizes were often small. None of the studies measured harms rigorously.

Two systematic reviews and one additional RCT have found that non-CBT psychotherapy increases abstinence from binge eating compared with waiting list controls.

Benefits: **Versus waiting list controls:** We found two systematic reviews of psychotherapy,[20,21] and one additional RCT.[25] The first review also included data from studies of other binge eating syndromes, and found that non-CBT psychotherapies (e.g. hypnobehavioural therapy and interpersonal psychotherapy) were associated with significantly greater abstinence rates compared with waiting list controls (RR 0.67, 95% CI 0.56 to 0.81, 3 RCTs, 131 people) and a greater reduction in bulimia nervosa symptom severity measures (SMD −1.2, 95% CI −1.52 to −0.87, 4 RCTs, 177 people). The additional small RCT (17 people with bulimia nervosa) compared structured, behaviour orientated group treatment with a waiting list. The trial found psychotherapy reduced binge eating frequency, depression, and other indices of eating disorder symptom severity.[25]

Harms: The RCTs did not report details of individual adverse events (see harms of cognitive behavioural therapy, p 514). Non-CBT psychotherapies include a large number of options, and it remains to be elucidated which therapies are most effective.

Comment: The quality of trials was variable, few were blinded, sample sizes were small, and none of the studies measured harms rigorously (see comment under cognitive behavioural therapy, p 514).

Two systematic reviews of RCTs have found short term reduction of bulimic symptoms and a small reduction of depressive symptoms. We found insufficient evidence about the persistence of these effects or about the effects of different classes of antidepressants. One systematic review of RCTs comparing antidepressants versus psychotherapy found no significant difference in abstinence from binge eating.

Benefits: We found two systematic reviews,[21,26] two additional RCTs,[27,28] and one subsequent RCT.[29] Versus placebo: Both reviews found that antidepressants reduced bulimic symptoms. The first review (search date 1998, 9 RCTs) found that antidepressants versus placebo significantly reduced binge eating (5 RCTs, 163 people; at the end of the trials 16% not binge eating with antidepressants; effect size weighted for sample size 0.66, 95% CI 0.52 to 0.81).[21] Antidepressants versus placebo improved purging (6 RCTs; effect size 0.39, 95% CI 0.24 to 0.54), depression (effect size 0.73, 95% CI 0.58 to 0.88), and improved scales of eating attitudes. The second review (search date 1997, 8 placebo controlled RCTs) found more frequent remission of bulimic episodes with antidepressants (19% v 8% with placebo; pooled RR 0.88, 95% CI 0.83 to 0.94; NNT 9, 95% CI 6 to 16). The review found no significant difference in effect between different classes of antidepressants, but there were too few trials to exclude a clinically important difference (see table 2, p 519). Fluoxetine was the only selective serotonin reuptake inhibitor (SSRI) included in the review, and only one trial reported remission rates.[26] Two additional RCTs (not in either of the above reviews) found a high relapse rate (30–45%) over 4–6 months.[27,28] Improvement was maintained after withdrawal of treatment that had been continued for 6 months.[30] The subsequent double blind RCT compared fluvoxamine versus placebo.[29] Relapse rates during a 15 week maintenance period after successful psychotherapy treatment were significantly higher applying an intention to treat analysis for placebo, but withdrawal rates were very high (19/33 people randomised to fluvoxamine). Fluvoxamine was associated with fewer relapses of general psychiatric symptoms and depression, but differences were not significant (P < 0.1).[31] **Versus CBT:** See benefits of cognitive behavioural therapy, p 513. **Versus psychotherapy:** We found one systematic review (5 RCTs) of antidepressants versus psychotherapy (all CBT trials) that found no significant difference in remission rates (39% with psychotherapies, 20% with antidepressants; effect size 1.28; P = 0.07), bulimic symptom severity (3 RCTs), or depression symptom severity at the end of the trial (3 RCTs).[25,32] **Antidepressants plus psychotherapy:** See benefits of combination treatment, p 517.

Harms: One systematic review found higher withdrawal rates with antidepressants than with psychotherapy (40% v 18%, 4 trials, 189 people, RR = 2.18, 95% CI 1.09 to 4.35).[33] The second systematic review found significantly higher withdrawal rates in people with bulimia taking antidepressants than with placebo (12 RCTs, 10.5% v 5.1%).[26] The review found no significant difference in withdrawal rates due to adverse effects among and within classes of antidepressants. In pooled analysis, withdrawal due to any cause was more likely with tricyclic antidepressants than with placebo (6 RCTs, 29% v 14.4%, P = 0.01), but more likely with placebo than SSRIs (3 RCTs, 37% v 40%, P = 0.04). We found two RCTs that examined specific adverse effects. One found significant increases in reclining and standing blood pulse rate, lying systolic and diastolic blood pressure, and greater orthostatic effects on blood pressure with desipramine than with placebo.[33] The cardiovascular changes were well tolerated, and few people withdrew because of these effects. Meta-analysis of two double blind RCTs of fluoxetine versus placebo found no significant difference in the incidence of suicidal acts or ideation in people treated with fluoxetine versus placebo.[34] However, the overall incidence of events was low (suicide attempts: 1.2%, none fatal; emergent suicidal ideation: 3.1%).

Comment: We found no consistent predictors of response to treatment. Antidepressants included in the trials were imipramine, amitriptyline, desipramine, phenylzine, isocaboxazid, brofaramine, fluoxetine, mianserin, and buprorion. We found no good evidence on the effects of newer antidepressants, such as venlafaxine and moclobemide. Both reviews commented on the lack of follow up.[21,26]

OPTION	COMBINATION TREATMENT

One systematic review of RCTs has found that combination treatment (antidepressants plus psychotherapy) reduces binge frequency and increases rates of remission from binge eating more than either

intervention alone. Reporting of other outcome measures was poor. Antidepressants alone or in combination with psychotherapy were associated with higher withdrawal rates.

Benefits: We found one systematic review (search date 1997) comparing combination treatment (antidepressants plus psychotherapy) versus either treatment alone.[35] One meta-analysis compared antidepressants versus a combination of psychotherapy plus antidepressants.[35] Combined treatment was associated with significantly greater improvement in binge frequency and depressive symptoms (3 trials, effect size 0.47, P = 0.04), but there was no significant difference in rates of short term remission compared with antidepressants alone (4 RCTs, 141 people, 42% v 23%, RR 1.38, P = 0.06). A second meta-analysis compared psychotherapy alone versus a combination of psychotherapy plus antidepressants.[35] Combination treatment was associated with significantly higher rates of short term remission (6 RCTs, 257 people, 49% v 36%, RR 1.21, P = 0.03) and greater improvement in depressive symptoms, but no significant difference in frequency of binge eating compared with psychotherapy alone.

Harms: Withdrawal rates were lower after psychotherapy plus antidepressants than with antidepressants alone (4 trials, 196 people, 34% v 41%, RR 1.19, 95% CI 0.69 to 2.05).[35] Withdrawal rates were significantly higher with psychotherapy plus antidepressants than with psychotherapy alone (6 trials, 295 people, 30% v 16%, RR 0.57, P = 0.01).[35]

Comment: None.

GLOSSARY

Bulimia nervosa The American Psychiatric Association DSM-IV[1] criteria include recurrent episodes of binge eating; recurrent inappropriate compensatory behaviour to prevent weight gain; frequency of binge eating and inappropriate compensatory behaviour both, on average, at least twice a week for 3 months; self evaluation unduly influenced by body shape and weight; and disturbance occurring not exclusively during episodes of anorexia nervosa.

Types of bulimia nervosa, modified from DSM-IV[1]: purging: using self induced vomiting, laxatives, diuretics, or enemas. Non-purging: fasting, exercise, but not vomiting or other abuse as purging type.

Binge eating Modified from DSM-IV.[1] Eating, in a discrete period (e.g. hours), a large amount of food, and a sense of lack of control during the episode.

REFERENCES

1. American Psychiatric Association. *Diagnostic and statistical manual of mental disorders* 4th ed. Washington DC: American Psychiatric Press, 1994.

2. Bushnell JA, Wells JE, Hornblow AR, Oakley-Brown MA, Joyce P. Prevalence of three bulimic syndromes in the general population. *Psychol Med* 1990;20:671–680.

3. Garfinkel PE, Lin B, Goering P, et al. Bulimia nervosa in a Canadian community sample: Prevalence, co-morbidity, early experiences and psychosocial functioning. *Am J Psychiatry* 1995; 152:1052–1058.

4. Gard MCE, Freeman CP. The dismantling of a myth: A review of eating disorders and socioeconomic status. *Int J Eat Disord* 1996;20: 1–12.

5. Hall A, Hay PJ. Eating disorder patient referrals

from a population region 1977–1986. *Psychol Med* 1991;21:697–701.

6. Kendler KS, Maclean C, Neale M, et al. The genetic epidemiology of bulimia nervosa *Am J Psychiatry* 1991;148:1627–1637.

7. Choudry IY, Mumford DB. A pilot study of eating disorders in Mirpur (Pakistan) using an Urdu version of the Eating Attitude Test. *Int J Eat Disord* 1992;11:243–251.

8. Striegel-Moore RH, Wifley DE, Caldwell MB, Needham ML, Brownell KD. Weight-related attitudes and behaviors of women who diet to lose weight: A comparison for black dieters and white dieters. *Obes Res* 1996;4:109–116.

9. Fairburn CG, Welch SL, Doll HA, Davies BA, O'Connor ME. Risk factors for bulimia nervosa: A community-based case-control study. *Arch Gen Psychiatry* 1997;54:509–517.

10. Collings S, King M. Ten year follow-up of 50 patients with bulimia nervosa. *Br J Psychiatry* 1994;164:80–87.

11. Keel PK, Mitchell JE, Miller KB, Davis TL, Crow SJ. Long-term outcome of bulimia nervosa. *Arch Gen Psychiatry* 1999;56:63–69.

12. Keel PK, Mitchell JE. Outcome in bulimia nervosa. *Am J Psychiatry* 1997;154:313–321.

13. Fairburn CG, Norman PA, Welch SL, et al. A prospective study of outcome in bulimia nervosa and the long-term effects of three psychological treatments. *Arch Gen Psychiatry* 1995;52:304–312.

14. Coker S, Vize C, Wade T, Cooper PJ. Patients with bulimia nervosa who fail to engage in cognitive behaviour therapy. *Int J Eat Disord* 1993;13:35–40.

15. Fahy TA, Russell GFM. Outcome and prognostic variables in bulimia. *Int J Eat Disord* 1993;14:135–146.

16. Rossiter EM, Agras WS, Telch CF, Schneider JA. Cluster B personality disorder characteristics predict outcome in the treatment of bulimia nervosa. *Int J Eat Disord* 1993;13:349–358.

17. Johnson C, Tobin DL, Dennis A. Differences in treatment outcome between borderline and nonborderline bulimics at 1-year follow-up. *Int J Eat Disord* 1990;9:617–627.

18. Agras WS, Walsh BT, Fairburn CG, Wilson GT, Kraemer HC. A multicenter comparison of cognitive-behavioral therapy and interpersonal psychotherapy. *Arch Gen Psychiatry* 2000;54:459–465.

19. Lewandowski LM, Gebing TA, Anthony JL, O'Brien WH. Meta-analysis of cognitive behavioural treatment studies for bulimia. *Clin Psychol Rev* 1997;17:703–718. Search date 1995; primary sources Psyinfo and hand searches of references lists.

20. Hay, PJ, Bacaltchuk J. Psychotherapy for bulimia nervosa and binging. In: The Cochrane Library, Issue 4, 1999. Oxford: Update software. Search dates 1999. Handsearch of *Int J Eat Disord* since its first issue; Medline 1966 to 1998; an Extramed, Embase, Psychlit, Current Contents, Lilacs, Scisearch up to 1998; the Cochrane Collaboration Controlled Trials Register 1997 Internet version; and the Cochrane Collaboration Depression and Anxiety Trials Register up to February 1999; handsearch of all citation lists in identified studies and reviews and personal contact.

21. Whittal ML, Agras WS, Gould RA. Bulimia nervosa: A meta-analysis of psychosocial and pharmacological treatments. *Behavr Ther* 1999;30:117–135. Search dates "to present": presumed 1998 (date of submission); Psyclit 1974–1998; Medline 1966–1998; handsearch of *Int J Eat Disord* 1990–1998; handsearch other relevant (not specified) journals and identified studies. This was reviewed in Waller G. *Evidenced Based Medicine* (September/October 1999).

22. Jacobi C, Dahme B, Rustenbach S. Vergleich kontrollierter Psycho- und Pharmakaotherapiestudien bei Bulimia und Anorexia nervosa. *Psychother Psychosom Med Psychol* 1997;47:346–364. Search dates from 1994; Psych Abstracts, Medline, Psychindex, Psychinfo.

23. Treasure JL, Katzman M, Schmidt U, et al. Engagement and outcome in the treatment of bulimia nervosa: first phase of a sequential design comparing motivation enhancement therapy and cognitive behavioural therapy. *Behav Res Ther* 1999;37:405–418.

24. Wilson GT, Fairburn CG. Treatments for eating disorders. In Nathan PE, Gorman JM, eds. *A Guide to Treatments that Work.* New York: Oxford University Press, 1998:501–530.

25. Laessle RG, Waadt S, Pirke KM. A structured behaviourally orientated group treatment for bulimia nervosa. *Psychother Psychosom* 1987;48:141–145.

26. Bacaltchuk J, Hay P, Mari JJ. Antidepressants versus placebo for the treatment of bulimia nervosa: A systematic review. *Aust N Z J Psychiatry* 2000;34:310–317. Search dates 1997; handsearch of *Int J Eat Disord* since its first issue; Medline 1966–1998; an Extramed, Embase, Psychlit, Current Contents, Lilacs, Scisearch up to 1997; the Cochrane Collaboration Controlled Trials Register 1997 Internet version; and the Cochrane Collaboration Depression and Anxiety Register; handsearch of all citation lists in identified studies and reviews and personal contact.

27. Walsh BT, Hadigan CM, Devlin MJ, Gladis M, Roose SP. Long-term outcome of antidepressant treatment for bulimia nervosa. *Am J Psychiatry* 1991;148:1206–1212.

28. Pyle RL, Mitchell JE, Eckert ED, et al. Maintenance treatment and 6-month outcome for bulimic patients who respond to initial treatment. *Am J Psychiatry* 1990;147:871–875.

29. Fichter MM, Kr ger R, Rief W, Holland R, Döhne J. Fluvoxamine in prevention of relapse in bulimia nervosa: effects on eating specific psychopathology. *J Clin Psychopharmacol* 1996;16:9–18.

30. Agras WS, Rossiter EM, Arnow B, et al. One-year follow-up of psychosocial and pharmacologic treatments for bulimia nervosa *J Clin Psychiatry* 1994;55:179–183.

31. Fichter MM, Leibl C, Kr ger R, Rief W. Effects of fluvoxamine on depression, anxiety, and other areas of general psychopathology in bulimia nervosa. *Pharmacopsychiatry* 1997;30:85–92.

32. Bacaltchuk J, Trefiglio RP, de Oliveira IR, Lima MS, Mari JJ. Antidepressants versus psychotherapy for bulimia nervosa: a systematic review. *J Clin Pharm Ther* 1999;24:23–31. Search dates 1997; handsearch of *Int J Eat Disord* since its first issue; Medline 1966–1998; an Extramed, Embase, Psychlit, Current Contents, Lilacs, Scisearch up to 1997; Cochrane Collaboration Controlled Trials Register 1997 Internet version; Cochrane Collaboration Depression and Anxiety Trials Register; handsearch of all citation lists in identified studies and reviews and personal contact.

33. Agras WS, Rossiter EM, Arnow B, et al. Pharmacologic and cognitive-behavioral treatment for bulimia nervosa: A controlled comparison. *Am J Psychiatry* 1992;149:82–87. Cited in reference 28.

34. Wheadon DE, Rampey AH, Thompson VL, et al. Lack of association between fluoxetine and suicidality in bulimia nervosa. *J Clin Psychiatry* 1992;53:235–241.

35. Bacaltchuk J, Trefiglio RP, Oliveira IR, et al. Combination of antidepressants and psychotherapy for bulimia nervosa: a systematic review. *Acta Psychiatr Scand* 2000;101:256–264. Search dates 1997; handsearch of *Int J Eat Disord* since its first issue; Medline 1966–1998; an Extramed, Embase, Psychlit, Current Contents, Lilacs, Scisearch up to 1997; Cochrane Collaboration Controlled Trials Register 1997 Internet version; Cochrane Collaboration Depression and Anxiety Trials Register; handsearch of all citation lists in identified studies and reviews and personal contact.

Phillipa Hay
Psychiatrist
University of Adelaide
Adelaide
Australia

Josue Bacaltchuk
Psychiatrist
Federal University of Sao Paulo
Sao Paulo
Brazil

Competing interests: PH has received support to attend conferences and meetings from Pfizer PTY LTD, Solvay Pharmaceuticals, and Bristol-Myers Squibb Pharmaceuticals. JB has received fees from Janssen-Cilag Farmaceutica, Brazil.

| TABLE 1 | Comparison of remission rates between cognitive behaviour therapy (CBT) or other active psychotherapy and comparison group (see text, p 513).[20] |

Comparison	Number of RCTs	N	Absolute remission rates	RR (95% CI)
CBT v waiting list	7	300	42% v 6%	0.64 (0.53 to 0.78)
CBT v other psychotherapy	7	474*	40% v 21%	0.80 (0.61 to 1.04)
CBT v pure self help CBT	3	183	45% v 37%	0.92 (0.48 to 1.77)
Other psychotherapy v waiting list	3	131	36% v 3%	0.67 (0.56 to 0.81)

*Updated to include new trial;[18] CBT, cognitive behavioural therapy.
‡Comparisons (RR) were for numbers who did not show remission; N, number of participants.

| TABLE 2 | Comparison of remission rates between active drug and placebo by class of antidepressant (see text, p 515).[26] |

Class: Drug(s)	Number of RCTs	N	RR	95% CI
TCA: desipramine, imipramine	3	132	0.86	0.7 to 1.07
SSRI: fluoxetine	1	398	0.92	0.84 to 1.01
	2	98	0.81	0.68 to 0.96
Other: bupropion, trazodone	2	87	0.86	0.76 to 0.97

MAOI, monoamine oxidase inhibitor; N, number of participants; SSRI, selective serotonin reuptake inhibitor; TCA, tricyclic antidepressant

Depressive disorders

Updated and expanded this issue

John Geddes, Rob Butler and James Warner

INTERVENTIONS

Key Messages

- Systematic reviews of RCTs have found that antidepressant drugs are effective in acute treatment of all grades of depressive disorders in all common treatment settings and in people with or without coexistent physical illness. We found no evidence of a clinically significant difference in the benefits of different antidepressant drugs, although drugs vary in adverse effects.

- One systematic review of RCTs has found that cognitive therapy is effective and may be more effective than drug treatment for mild to moderate depression.

- One systematic review of mixed quality RCTs has found that St John's Wort is an effective treatment for mild to moderate depression.

- One large RCT has found that interpersonal therapy is effective treatment for mild to moderate depression. Less robust RCTs have found that problem solving therapy is also effective. Specific psychological treatments, such as cognitive and interpersonal therapy have been shown to be as effective as drugs.

- We found limited evidence suggesting that other treatments, including exercise, bibliotherapy, befriending, and non-directive counselling, may be effective.

- We found no reliable evidence to suggest that one type of treatment (drug or non-drug) is superior to another. Limited evidence suggests that combining drug and psychological treatments may be effective in severe but not mild to moderate depression.

- Of the interventions examined in this issue, prescription antidepressant drugs are the only treatment for which there is good evidence of effectiveness in severe and psychotic depressive disorders. We found no RCTs comparing drug and non-drug treatments in severe depressive disorder.

- RCTs have found that continuing antidepressant drug treatment for 4–6 months after recovery reduces risk of relapse.

- We found no evidence of a difference between treatments in terms of long term benefits.

DEFINITION   Depressive disorders are characterised by persistent low mood, loss of interest and enjoyment, and reduced energy. They often impair function. **Older adults:** Older adults are generally defined as people aged 65 years or more. The presentation of depression in older adults may be atypical; low mood may be masked and anxiety or memory impairment may be the principal presenting symptoms. Dementia should be considered in the differential diagnosis of depression in older adults.[1]

INCIDENCE/   **Younger adults:** Depressive disorders are common, with a preva-
PREVALENCE lence of major depression between 5–10% of people seen in primary care settings.[2] Two to three times as many people may have depressive symptoms but do not meet criteria for major depression. Women are affected twice as often as men. Depressive disorders are the fourth most important cause of disability worldwide and are expected to become the second most important cause by 2020.[3,4] **Older adults:** 10–15% of older people have significant depressive symptomatology, although major depression is relatively rare in older adults.[5]

AETIOLOGY/   The causes are uncertain but include both childhood events and
RISK FACTORS current psychosocial adversity.

PROGNOSIS   About half of people suffering a first episode of major depressive disorder experience further symptoms in the next 10 years.[6] Different levels of severity[7,8] indicate different prognosis and treatment. **Mild to moderate depression** is characterised by depressive symptoms and some functional impairment. Many people recover in the short term but about half experience recurrent symptoms. **Severe depression** is characterised by additional agitation or psychomotor retardation with marked somatic symptoms. In this review, treatments are considered to have been evaluated in severe depression if the RCTs included inpatients. **Psychotic depression** is characterised by additional hallucinations, delusions, or both. **Older adults:** The prognosis may be especially poor in elderly people with a chronic or relapsing course.[9]

Mental health

AIMS   To improve mood, social and occupational functioning, and quality of life; to reduce morbidity and mortality; to prevent recurrence of depressive disorder; and to minimise adverse effects of treatment. Depression should not be regarded as a natural concomitant of older age.

OUTCOMES   Depressive symptoms rated by the depressed person and clinician, social functioning, occupational functioning, quality of life, admission to hospital, rates of self harm, relapse of depressive symptoms, rates of adverse events. Trials often use continuous scales to measure depressive symptoms (such as the Hamilton Depression Rating Scale and the Beck Depression Inventory). Clinician reports and self reported global outcome measures are also used. Changes in continuous measures can be dealt with in two ways. They can be dichotomised in an arbitrary but clinically helpful manner (e.g. taking a reduction in depressive symptoms of more than 50% as an end point), which allows results to be expressed as relative risks and numbers needed to treat. Alternatively, they can be treated as continuous variables, as is done for systematic analysis. In this case, the pooled estimate of effect (the effect size) expresses the degree of overlap between the range of scores in the control and experimental groups. The effect size can be used to estimate the proportion of people in the control group who had a poorer outcome than the average person in the experimental group. **Older adults:** The Hamilton Depression Rating Scale is not ideal for older people because it includes a number of somatic items that may be positive in older people who are not depressed. It has been the most widely used scale, although specific scales for elderly people (such as the Geriatric Depression Scale) avoid somatic items.

METHODS   A validated search for systematic reviews and RCTs was conducted between May and September 1998 from the Cochrane Database of Systematic Reviews and the Database of Abstract of Reviews of Effectiveness, *Best Evidence* and *Evidence-Based Mental Health*, Medline, PsychLit, and Embase. Studies were included by using epidemiological criteria and relevance to the clinical question. A *Clinical Evidence* update search and appraisal was conducted in May 2000 including a search for data on depression in older adults. To date, few studies have concentrated on older adults as a separate subgroup. Most published evidence for the efficacy of antidepressants includes all ages over 16 or is limited to people aged under 65.

QUESTION   What are the effects of treatments?

OPTION   PRESCRIPTION ANTIDEPRESSANT DRUGS

Updated this issue

Younger adults: Systematic reviews of RCTs have found that antidepressant drugs are effective in acute treatment of all grades of depressive disorders. They have also found no clinically significant difference in effectiveness between different kinds of antidepressant drug. However, the drugs differ in their adverse event profiles. On average, people seem to tolerate selective serotonin reuptake inhibitors

(SSRIs) a little more than older drugs, but this difference is too small to be grounds for a policy of always choosing an SSRI as first line treatment. We found no strong evidence that fluoxetine is associated with increased risk of suicide. Abrupt withdrawal of SSRIs is associated with symptoms, including dizziness and rhinitis in some patients, and this is more likely and probably more severe with drugs with a short half life, such as paroxetine. Older adults: One systematic review has found that heterocyclic antidepressants and SSRIs are effective in older people with mild to moderate depression. However, overall treatment effects were modest. Limitations of this review include the variety of populations studied and the short duration of many studies. Future, high quality RCTs are unlikely for ethical reasons.

Benefits:

In younger adults: Versus placebo: We found two systematic reviews.[10,11] The first review (published in 1996, search date not given, 49 RCTs in people with depressive disorder) included five trials of people admitted to hospital (probably more severely ill); 40 RCTs in a setting outside hospital; one in both settings; and three trials that did not specify the setting. Each RCT compared two antidepressant drugs and included a placebo control group. The review found a mean effect size of 0.50 for antidepressant drugs versus placebo, which means that 69% of those taking placebo did worse than the average person taking antidepressants. Drugs were more effective in those with depressive disorders diagnosed according to standard criteria (mainly *Diagnostic and Statistical Manual of Mental Disorders*, 3rd edition, revised [DSM-III-R]). The second systematic review (updated in 1998, 15 RCTs, 1871 people) compared antidepressant versus placebo in people with dysthymia (chronic mild depressive disorders).[11] Response to treatment was about twice as likely in the antidepressant group (RR versus placebo 1.9, 95% CI 1.6 to 2.3; NNT 4, 95% CI 3 to 5). **Tricyclic antidepressants (TCAs) versus SSRIs:** We found three systematic reviews comparing SSRIs with TCAs.[12-14] These found no significant difference in effectiveness overall. SSRIs seem to be slightly more acceptable overall as measured by the number of people who withdrew from clinical trials (RR 0.88, 95% CI 0.83 to 0.93; NNT 26).[12] The third systematic review (search date 1998, 28 RCTs, 5940 people) compared the efficacy in primary care of newer antidepressants versus placebo and versus older antidepressants.[14] The average response rate was 63% for newer agents, 35% for placebo, and 60% for TCAs (RR for SSRIs compared with placebo 1.6, 95% CI 1.2 to 2.1). One small RCT (152 people) compared adherence on dothiepin with fluoxetine over 12 weeks and found no significant difference between the drugs. However, the study was probably underpowered.[15] **Monoamine oxidase inhibitors (MAOIs) versus TCAs:** We found one systematic review (search date not given, 55 RCTs comparing MAOIs versus TCAs in several subgroups of people with depression).[16] It found that MAOIs were less effective in people with severe depressive disorders but may be more effective in atypical depressive disorders (depressive disorders with reversed biological features—for example, increased sleep, increased appetite, mood reactivity, and rejection sensitivity). **Older adults:** We identified one systematic review (search date 1998, 40 RCTs of pharmacological and psychological treatments of depression in people older than 55 years), in an outpatient or community setting. Of the trials, 26 were of pharmacological treatments and 21 of these were placebo controlled. People were recruited mainly from outpatient clinics. There was significant heterogeneity in the study results (P = 0.03). Nine heterocyclic drug studies had a mean difference in Hamilton Depression Rating scores after treatment of −5.78 (95% CI −8.31 to −3.25). Significant benefits were also found for fluoxetine, trazodone, and phenelzine. Of the 17 drug versus drug comparisons (mainly involving heterocyclic drugs), none showed significant benefit above the others.[17] **In people with depression plus a physical illness versus placebo:** One systematic review (search date 1998, 18 RCTs, n = 838) found that antidepressants were more effective than placebo in people with depression and a physical illness (NNT 4, 95% CI 3 to 7). People allocated to antidepressants were more likely to withdraw from the study than those on placebo (NNH 10, 95% CI 5 to 43).[18]

Harms: **Common adverse events:** One systematic review of RCTs (search date 1996) compared TCAs versus SSRIs in people with all severities of depression (see table 1, p 534).[19] There may also be differences between SSRIs. One large cohort study of people receiving four different SSRIs (fluvoxamine [n = 10 983], fluoxetine [n = 12 692], sertraline [n = 12 734], and paroxetine [n = 13 741]) in British primary care found that reports of common adverse events (nausea/vomiting, malaise/lassitude, dizziness, and headache/migraine) varied between SSRIs (fluvoxamine 78 per 1000 participant months; fluoxetine 23 per 1000 participant months; RR versus fluvoxamine 0.29, 95% CI 0.27 to 0.32; paroxetine 28 per 1000 participant months, RR 0.35, 95% CI 0.33 to 0.37; sertraline 21 per 1000 participant months, RR 0.26, 95% CI 0.25 to 0.28).[20] Only 52% of people responded to the questionnaire, although this response rate was similar for all four drugs. A study of spontaneous reports to the UK Committee on Safety of Medicines found no difference in safety profiles between the same four SSRIs.[21] **Suicide:** One systematic review (which included trials completed by December 1989) pooled data from 17 double blind RCTs in people with depressive disorder comparing fluoxetine (n = 1765) versus a TCA (n = 731) or placebo (n = 569).[22] There was no significant difference in the rate of suicidal acts between the groups (fluoxetine 0.3%, placebo 0.2%, TCAs 0.4%), whereas development of suicidal ideation was less frequent in the fluoxetine group (1.2% fluoxetine v 2.6% placebo, P = 0.042, and v 3.6% TCAs, P = 0.001). One historical cohort study followed 172 598 people who had at least one prescription for one of 10 antidepressants during the study period in general practice in the UK. The risk of suicide was higher in people who received fluoxetine (19 per 10 000 person years, 95% CI 9 to 34) than those receiving dothiepin (RR of suicide v dothiepin 2.1, 95% CI 1.1 to 4.1).[23] In a nested case controlled subanalysis in people with no history of suicidal behaviour or previous antidepressant prescription, the risk remained the same, although the confidence interval broadened to make the result indeterminate (RR 2.1, 95% CI 0.6 to 7.9). Although the apparent association may be due to residual confounding, there remains uncertainty about the possible association between fluoxetine and suicide. However, any absolute increase in risk is unlikely to be large. **Withdrawal effects:** We found one RCT comparing abrupt discontinuation of fluoxetine (n = 96) versus continued treatment (n = 299) in people who had been taking the drug for 12 weeks. Abrupt discontinuation was associated with increased dizziness (7% v 1%), dysmenorrhoea (3% v 0%), rhinitis (10% v 3%), and somnolence (4% v 0%). However, there was a high drop out rate in this study because of return of symptoms of depression (39%), so these may be underestimates of the true rate of withdrawal symptoms.[24] The rate of spontaneous reports of suspected withdrawal reactions per million defined daily doses to the World Health Organization Collaborating Centre for International Drug Monitoring between 1987 and 1995 was higher for paroxetine than for sertraline and fluoxetine.[25] The most common withdrawal effects were dizziness, nausea, paraesthesia, headache, and vertigo. **Older adults:** We found no specific evidence on adverse effects in older adults. **During pregnancy:** One systematic review of the risks of fetal harm of antidepressants in pregnancy found four small prospective studies published since 1993.[26] No evidence of increased risk was found, although the chances of adverse effects with a low incidence cannot be excluded. Decreased birth weights of infants exposed to fluoxetine in the third trimester were identified in one study and direct drug effects and withdrawal syndromes were identified in some neonates.

Comment: A systematic review is under way to examine the efficacy of antidepressants in older people, including data on adverse effects.[17] Metabolic and physical changes with age mean that older people may be more prone to adverse effects such as falls. As older people take more medications, they are at more risk of drug interactions. Suicide is a risk in elderly people.

OPTION   CARE PATHWAYS

Updated this issue

We found limited evidence that effectiveness of drug treatment may be improved by collaborative working between primary care clinicians and psychiatrists, or by intensive patient education.

Benefits: We found no systematic review. We found four RCTs.[27–30] The first in 217 people with mild to moderate depressive disorders in primary care in the USA found that, compared with standard treatment, outcomes were improved by collaborative working between primary care physician and psychiatrist, and by intensive patient education. Clinical outcomes were improved only in the subgroup of people with major depressive disorder (n = 91; AR of clinical response of > 50% reduction on symptom checklist: 74% v 44% with standard treatment; NNT 4, 95% CI 3 to 10).[27] The second (613 people) in a Health Maintenance Organization (HMO) in Seattle compared usual care, feedback (in which doctors received a detailed report on each person at 8 and 16 weeks following randomisation), or feedback plus care management (in which the care manager assessed people with depression by telephone at 8 and 16 weeks, doctors received a detailed report, and care managers facilitated the follow up). The care management group were more likely than those treated with usual care to have a clinically significant reduction in depressive symptoms 6 months after randomisation (estimated event rates 40% of the control group v 56% of the care management group OR 2.22, 95% CI 1.31 to 3.75; NNT 7).[28] The third RCT (1356 people) in 46 primary care clinics in US HMOs compared a multifaceted quality improvement programme with usual care (including mailed practice guidelines). People in the intervention group improved on continuous rating scales. Among people initially employed, 89.7% of the intervention group worked at 12 months compared with 84.7% of the control group (P = 0.05). For people initially not working, there was no difference in employment rates between intervention and control groups at 12 months (17% v 18%).[29] The fourth, a cluster randomised RCT in UK primary care, compared the effects of a clinical practice guideline and practice based education with usual care and found that the intervention did not improve either detection or outcome of depression.[30]

Harms: None reported.

Comment: None.

OPTION ST JOHN'S WORT (*HYPERICUM PERFORATUM*)

One systematic review of RCTs has found that St John's Wort (*Hypericum perforatum*) is more effective than placebo in mild to moderate depressive disorders and as effective as prescription antidepressant drugs. However, these findings have yet to be repeated in fully representative groups of people using standardised preparations.

Benefits: We found one systematic review (updated in 1998, 27 RCTs, 2291 people with mild to moderate depression).[31] Of these trials, 17 were placebo controlled (1168 participants). Ten trials (1123 participants) compared hypericum (8 trials used single preparations, 2 used combinations of hypericum and valeriana) versus other antidepressant or sedative drugs. Hypericum preparations were associated with significant clinical improvement compared with placebo (RR 2.47, 95% CI 1.69 to 3.61) but not compared with standard antidepressants (single preparations RR 1.01, 95% CI 0.87 to 1.16, combinations RR 1.52, 95% CI 0.78 to 2.94).

Harms: We found two systematic reviews (one cited above[31] and one other, search date 1997[32]). The review cited above found that adverse events were poorly reported in the trials. They were reported by 26% of people on hypericum compared with 45% of people on standard antidepressants (RR 0.57, 95% CI 0.47 to 0.69) and 15% on combinations of hypericum and valeriana compared with 27% on amitriptyline or desipramine (RR 0.49, 95% CI 0.23 to 1.04).[31] The second systematic review included RCTs and observational post-marketing surveillance studies of hypericum.[32] The commonest adverse effects of hypericum in the included trials were gastrointestinal symptoms, dizziness/confusion, tiredness/sedation, and dry mouth, although all occurred less frequently than on conventional drugs. Findings from observational studies were consistent with these findings. Photosensitivity is theoretically possible; however only two cases have been reported. Allergic skin reactions seem uncommon.

Comment: The evidence cited above must be interpreted cautiously for the following reasons: (1) it is unclear how closely participants in these trials match people in clinical practice; and (2) the preparations and doses of hypericum and types and doses of standard antidepressants varied. More studies are needed on clearly defined, clinically representative people using standardised preparations. Interactions with other drugs are possible and should be considered.

| OPTION | ELECTROCONVULSIVE THERAPY |

One systematic review of RCTs has found that electroconvulsive therapy (ECT) is effective in the acute treatment of depressive illness.

Benefits: We found two systematic reviews. The first (search date not given) included six RCTs and a total of 205 people with depressive disorder that compared ECT versus simulated ECT (in which people received everything but electric stimulation).[33] People treated with real ECT were more likely to respond to treatment (pooled OR 3.7, 95% CI 2.1 to 6.5; NNT 3, 95% CI 2 to 5, calculated from data in the article). The more recent systematic review (search date 1998) included 11 additional RCTs published between 1987 and 1998, but it did not undertake quantitative analysis.[34]

Harms: We found no adequate systematic review of possible adverse cognitive effects of ECT. However, people often complain of memory impairment after ECT. One of the main difficulties in studying this is that depressive disorders also lead to cognitive impairments that usually improve during the course of treatment. For this reason most of the many small studies in this area find an average improvement in people treated with ECT. This does not rule out the possibility of more subtle, subjective memory impairment secondary to ECT. Adverse memory effects would probably vary according to the dose and electrode used.

Comment: The first review cited above[26] did not include several recent RCTs comparing real versus simulated ECT.[35–39] However, the results of these trials are consistent with the review's findings. A further systematic review is in progress.[40] As ECT may be unacceptable to some people and because it is a short term treatment, there is a consensus that it should normally be reserved for people who cannot tolerate or have not responded to drug treatment, although it may be useful when a rapid response is required.

| OPTION | SPECIFIC PSYCHOLOGICAL TREATMENTS |

Younger adults: One systematic review of RCTs has found that cognitive therapy (see glossary, p 531) is effective, and may be more effective than drug treatment in people with mild to moderate depression. Weaker evidence from RCTs suggests that interpersonal psychotherapy, problem solving therapy and brief, non-directive counselling (see glossary, p 531) may be as effective as drug treatment in mild to moderate depression. We found limited evidence on the relative efficacy of drug and non-drug treatment in severe depression. Older adults: One systematic review of RCTs has found that rational psychological treatments (such as cognitive therapy or cognitive behaviour therapy) are effective for older people with mild to moderate depression. However, people receiving these treatments

improved no more than controls who received similar but non-specific attention. This review was based on a small number of studies, the populations varied (although most were community samples), and many of the studies were short term.

Benefits: **Younger adults:** The evidence comparing psychological treatments versus drug or no treatment is summarised in table 2, p 535.[41–43]
Older adults: We identified one systematic review of 40 controlled trials of pharmacological and psychological treatments in people over the age of 55 in an outpatient or community setting.[44] The review found four comparisons in older adults of psychological treatments (such as psychotherapy) versus untreated controls. None of the trials found a significant difference between treatment and no treatment, measured on the Hamilton Depression Rating Scale. The review also identified six comparisons of different psychological treatments. None found significant differences in effectiveness. Five of six comparisons of "rational" treatments (such as cognitive therapy or cognitive behaviour therapy) versus no treatment in older adults found significant benefit with treatment. Combined, the rational treatments performed significantly better than no treatment, with a mean difference in the Hamilton Depression Rating score of −7.25 (95% CI, −10.1 to −4.4). However, neither of the two rational treatments performed significantly better than non-specific attention.

Harms: See table 2, p 535.

Comment: Large RCTs are needed in more representative people in a range of clinical settings, including primary care. Because of varying exclusion criteria, the generaliseability of the studies is questionable (see table 2, p 535). Other factors to be considered when psychological treatments are compared with drug treatment include whether serum concentrations of drugs reach therapeutic concentrations, whether changes in medication are allowed (reflecting standard clinical practice), and whether studies reflect the natural course of depressive disorders.

OPTION   **SPECIFIC PSYCHOLOGICAL TREATMENTS PLUS DRUG TREATMENT**

Updated this issue

We found evidence from RCTs suggesting that, in severe depression, the addition of drug treatment to interpersonal or cognitive therapy is more effective than either psychological therapy alone. No such effect was observed in mild to moderate depression.

Benefits: We found no systematic review. A non-systematic meta-analysis of six RCTs (595 people) found no advantage in combining drug and specific psychological treatments in mild to moderate depressive disorders, but that in more severe depressive disorders, combining drug and interpersonal therapy or cognitive therapy was more effective than interpersonal therapy or cognitive therapy alone.[45] One recent RCT compared nefazodone or cognitive behavioural–analysis psychotherapy alone with combination treatment in 681 adults with chronic depressive disorder.[46] At 12 weeks, the combined treatment improved the rate of clinical response (at least

50% reduction on the Hamilton Depression Rating Scale and a score of 15 or less, combined therapy v both single interventions, NNT 5, 95% CI 3 to 6).

Harms: We found no evidence of adverse effects.

Comment: A systematic review is needed to address this question.

OPTION   EXERCISE

Updated this issue

RCTs have found that exercise, alone or combined with other treatments, improves mild to moderate depression.

Benefits: We found one systematic review (published in 1990, search date not given), which examined exercise in depressive disorders. However, it was difficult to interpret because it included non-randomised studies and did not clearly describe participants.[47] One small RCT (156 people) compared aerobic exercise, sertraline hydrochloride (an SSRI), and combined treatment for 16 weeks. It found that all groups improved on continuous rating scales, but there was no significant difference in overall improvement between treatments.[48]

Harms: None reported.

Comment: None.

OPTION   BIBLIOTHERAPY

We found limited evidence from a systematic review of RCTs that bibliotherapy (see glossary, p 531) may reduce mild depressive symptoms.

Benefits: We found one systematic review (published in 1997). It identified six small short term RCTs of bibliotherapy in 273 participants recruited by advertisement through the media and probably only mildly ill.[49] The mean effect size of bibliotherapy was 0.82 (95% CI 0.50 to 1.15). This means that 79% of control people had a worse outcome than the average member of the group receiving bibliotherapy.

Harms: None reported.

Comment: Further studies are needed in clinically representative groups.

OPTION   BEFRIENDING   New

Limited evidence from one small RCT found that befriending reduced symptoms of depression.

Benefits: We found one small RCT (86 people) of befriending (see glossary, p 531) of women with chronic depression in London. Initial identification was by postal screening of women registered with but not attending primary care.[50] It found that the befriended group were more likely to experience remission of symptoms at 13 months (65% with befriending v 39% with control; P < 0.05; NNT 4, 95% CI 2 to 18).

Harms: None recorded.

Comment: Less than half of the women screened were interested in befriending as a treatment option.

QUESTION What are the effects of continuation and maintenance treatment with antidepressant drugs?

Updated this issue

RCTs have found that continuation treatment (see glossary, p 531) with antidepressant drugs for 4–6 months after recovery reduces risk of relapse.

Benefits: **Continuation treatment:** We found one systematic review (published in 1991, 6 RCTs, 312 people).[51] Continuation of antidepressant medication for 4–6 months after acute treatment reduced the relapse rate by nearly half (RR 0.6, 95% CI 0.4 to 0.7). Several more recent RCTs confirm this reduction in risk of early relapse with continuing antidepressant treatment for 6–12 months after acute treatment. **Maintenance treatment:** We found no adequate systematic review, but several RCTs have found that maintenance treatment reduced the relapse rate compared with placebo in recurrent depressive disorder. However, they all have problems with their methods (e.g. high withdrawal rates[52]), and will be considered for the next issue of *Clinical Evidence*. **Older adults:** We found one RCT that compared dothiepin versus placebo in 69 older people who had recovered sufficiently and consented to enter a 2 year trial of continuation treatment.[53] Dothiepin reduced the risk of relapse by 55% (RR 0.45, 95% CI 0.22 to 0.96).

Harms: Adverse effects seem to be similar to those reported in trials of acute treatment.

Comment: A systematic review is in progress.[54]

QUESTION Which treatments are most effective at improving long term outcome?

Updated this issue

We found no evidence of a difference between treatments in terms of long term benefits. We found limited evidence that cognitive therapy may be an alternative to drug maintenance therapy in preventing relapse.

Benefits: We found one systematic review (published in 1998, search date not given), which identified eight small RCTs examining long term (at least 1 year) recovery or relapse rates after treatment had stopped. The trials compared cognitive therapy versus antidepressants in people with mainly mild to moderate depressive disorders.[41] Overall, 30% of people [16]treated with cognitive therapy relapsed compared with 60% of those treated with antidepressants. However, the number of people in these trials was too small for this trend to be significant. We found one small additional RCT (40 people) comparing cognitive therapy with normal clinical management for residual depressive symptoms in people who had responded to antidepressants. It also found that at 2 years fewer people relapsed with cognitive therapy than with antidepressants.[55]

Harms: See harms of prescription antidepressant drugs, p 524 and see table 2, p 535.

Comment: The review did not present data on the proportion of people who recovered and remained well in the long term. The largest RCT found that only a fifth of participants remained well over 18 months' follow up, and that there were no significant differences between interpersonal psychotherapy, cognitive therapy, or drug treatment.[43] It is possible that different people respond to different treatments. Further large scale comparative studies are needed of the long term effectiveness of treatments in people with all severities of depressive disorders.

GLOSSARY

Bibliotherapy Consists of advising people to read written material such as *Feeling good: the new mood therapy* by David Burns (New York: New American Library 1980).

Brief, non-directive counselling Aims to help people to express feelings and clarify thoughts and difficulties; therapist suggests alternative understandings and does not give direct advice but tries to encourage people to solve their own problems.

Cognitive therapy Brief (20 sessions over 12–16 weeks) structured treatment aimed at changing the dysfunctional beliefs and negative automatic thoughts that characterise depressive disorders. It requires a high level of training in the therapist.[56]

Continuation treatment Continuation of treatment after successful resolution of a depressive episode to prevent relapse.

Interpersonal psychotherapy Standardised form of brief psychotherapy (usually 12–16 weekly sessions) primarily intended for outpatients with unipolar non-psychotic depressive disorders. It focuses on improving the patient's interpersonal functioning and identifying the problems associated with the onset of the depressive episode.[57]

Maintenance treatment Long term treatment of recurrent depressive disorder to prevent the recurrence of further depressive episodes.

Problem solving Consists of three stages: (1) identifying the main problems for the patient; (2) generating solutions; (3) trying out the solutions. Potentially briefer and simpler than cognitive therapy and may be feasible in primary care.[43]

Befriending Consists of a befriender meeting the patient to talk and socialise for at least 1 hour per week, acting as a friend.

Substantive changes since last issue

TCAs versus SSRIs: Two systematic reviews;[12,13] one new systematic review comparing the efficacy in primary care of newer antidepressants with placebo and older antidepressants;[14] and one new RCT;[15] conclusions unchanged.

People with depression plus a physical illness: One new systematic review found that antidepressants were more effective than placebo.[18]

Pregnancy: One new systematic review of the risks of fetal harm of antidepressants in pregnancy.[26] No evidence of increased risk for intrauterine death or major birth defects was reported. The development of children whose mothers took TCAs or fluoxetine during gestation did not differ from controls. Decreased birth weights of infants exposed to fluoxetine in the third trimester were identified in one study and direct drug effects and withdrawal syndromes were identified in some neonates.

Care pathways: Three new RCTs; conclusions unchanged.[28–30]

Electroconvulsive therapy: Two new RCTs; conclusions unchanged.[38,39]

Specific psychological treatments plus drug treatment: One recent RCT found combination therapy was more effective than nefazodone or cognitive behavioural–analysis psychotherapy alone.[46]

Exercise: One recent RCT; conclusion unchanged.[48]

Improving long term outcome: One new RCT found limited evidence that cognitive therapy may be an alternative to drug maintenance therapy in preventing relapse.[55]

REFERENCES

1. Rosenstein, Leslie D. Differential diagnosis of the major progressive dementias and depression in middle and late adulthood: a summary of the literature of the early 1990s. Neuropsychol Rev 1998;8:109–167.
2. Katon W, Schulberg H. Epidemiology of depression in primary care. Gen Hosp Psychiatry 1992:14:237–247.
3. Murray CJ, Lopez AD. Regional patterns of disability-free life expectancy and disability–adjusted life expectancy: global burden of disease study. Lancet 1997;349:1347–1352.
4. Murray CJ, Lopez AD. Alternative projections of mortality and disability by cause 1990–2020: global burden of disease study. Lancet 1997;349:1498–1504.
5. Beekman ATF, Copeland JRM, Prince MJ. Review of community prevalence of depression in later life. Br J Psychiatry 1999;174:307–11.
6. Judd LL, Akiskal HS, Maser JD, et al. A prospective 12 year study of subsyndromal and syndromal depressive symptoms in unipolar major depressive disorders. Arch Gen Psychiatry 1988;55:694–700.
7. American Psychiatric Association. Diagnostic and statistical manual of mental disorders, 4th ed. Washington, DC: American Psychiatric Association, 1994.
8. World Health Organization. The ICD-10 classification of mental and behavioural disorders. Geneva: World Health Organization, 1992.
9. Cole MG, Bellavance F, Mansour A. Prognosis of depression in elderly community and primary care populations: a systematic review and meta-analysis. Am J Psychiatry 1999;156:1182–1189.
10. Joffe R, Sokolov S, Streiner D. Antidepressant treatment of depression: a meta-analysis. Can J Psychiatry 1996;41:613–616. Search date not given; primary source Medline 1966 to June 1995.
11. Lima MS, Moncrieff J. A comparison of drugs versus placebo for the treatment of dysthymia: a systematic review. In: Cochrane library, Issue 3, 1998. Oxford: Update Software. Search date 1997; primary sources Biological Abstracts 1984 to 1997; Medline 1966 to January 1997; Psychlit 1974 to January 1997; Embase 1980 to January 1997; Lilacs 1982 to January 1997; Cochrane library; personal communication; conference abstracts; unpublished trials from the pharmaceutical industry; and book chapters on the treatment of depression.
12. Geddes JR, Freemantle N, Mason J, Eccles MP, Boynton J SSRIs versus other antidepressants for depressive disorder. In: The Cochrane Library, Issue 3, 2000. Oxford: Update software. Search date 1999; primary source Medline, Embase, Cochrane Group Register of Controlled Trials, hand searches of reference lists of all located studies, and contact with manufacturers.
13. Anderson IM. Selective serotonin reuptake inhibitors versus tricyclic antidepressants: a meta-analysis of efficacy and tolerability. J Affect Disord 2000;58:19–36. Search date 1997; primary sources Medline, and hand searches of reference lists of meta-analyses and reviews.
14. Mulrow CD, Williams JW, Chiqueete E, et al. Efficacy of newer medications for treating depression in primary care patients. Am Med J 2000;108:54–64. Search date 1998; primary source Cochrane Depression Anxiety and Neurosis Group Specialised Register of Clinical Trials, hand searches of trials and 46 pertinent meta-analyses and consultation with experts.
15. Thompson C, Peveler RC, Stephenson D, et al. Compliance with antidepressant medication in the treatment of major depressive disorder in primary care: a randomized comparison of fluoxetine and a tricyclic antidepressant. Am J Psychiatry 2000;157:338–343.
16. Thase ME, Trivedi MH, Rush AJ. MAOIs in the contemporary treatment of depression. Neuropsychopharmacology 1995;12:185–219. Search date not given; primary sources Medline and Psychological Abstracts 1959–July 1992.
17. Wilson K, Mottram P, Sivanthan A. A review of antidepressant drug trials in the treatment of older depressed people (protocol for a Cochrane Review). In: The Cochrane Library. Issue 4, 1998. Oxford: Update software. Search date June 1998; primary sources Cochrane Depression, Neurosis and Anxiety Review Group; hand searched journals, and reference lists. Review not to be published until 2001.
18. Gill D, Hatcher S. Antidepressants for depression in people with physical illness. In: The Cochrane Library, Issue 3, 2000. Oxford: Update software. Search date 1998; primary sources Medline, Cochrane Library Trials Register, Cochrane Depression and Neurosis Group Trials Register, and hand searches of two journals and reference lists.
19. Trindade E, Menon D. Selective serotonin reuptake inhibitors differ from tricyclic antidepressants in adverse events [abstract]. Selective serotonin reuptake inhibitors (SSRIs) for major depression. Part I. Evaluation of the clinical literature. Ottawa: Canadian Coordinating Office for Health Technology Assessment, 1997 August Report 3E. Evidence-Based Mental Health 1998;1:50. Search date 1996; primary sources Medline; Embase; PsycINFO; International Pharmaceutical Abstracts; Pascal; Health Planning and Administration; Mental Health Abstracts; Pharmacoeconomics and Outcomes News; Current Contents databases; scanning bibliographies of retrieved articles; hand searching journals; consulting researchers.
20. Mackay FJ, Dunn NR, Wilton LV, et al. A comparison of fluvoxamine, fluoxetine, sertraline and paroxetine examined by observational cohort studies. Pharmacoepidemiol Drug Safety 1997;6:235–246.
21. Price JS, Waller PC, Wood SM, et al. A comparison of the post marketing safety of four selective serotonin reuptake inhibitors including the investigation of symptoms occurring on withdrawal. Br J Clin Pharmacol 1996;42:757–763.

22. Beasley CM Jr, Dornseif BE, Bosomworth JC, et al. Fluoxetine and suicide: a meta-analysis of controlled trials of treatment for depression. *BMJ* 1991;303:685–692. Search date not given; but included trials that had been completed/analysed by December 1989; primary sources not given in detail but based on clinical report form data from trials and data from the Drug Experience Network Database.

23. Jick SS, Dean AD, Jick H. Antidepressants and suicide. *BMJ* 1995;310:215–218.

24. Zajecka J, Fawcett J, Amsterdam J, et al. Safety of abrupt discontinuation of fluoxetine: a randomised, placebo controlled study. *J Clin Psychopharmacol* 1998;18:193–197.

25. Stahl MM, Lindquist M, Pettersson M, et al. Withdrawal reactions with selective serotonin reuptake inhibitors as reported to the WHO system. *Eur J Clin Pharmacol* 1997;53:163–169.

26. Wisner KL, Gelenberg AJ, Leonard H, et al. Pharmacologic treatment of depression during pregnancy. *JAMA* 1999;282:1264–1269. Search date 1999; primary sources Medline, Healthstar, hand searches of bibliographies of review articles, and discussions with investigators in the field.

27. Katon W, Von Korff M, Lin E, et al. Collaborative management to achieve treatment guidelines: impact on depression in primary care. *JAMA* 1995;273:1026–1031.

28. Simon GE, Vonkorff M, Rutter C, et al. Randomised trial of monitoring, feedback, and management of care by telephone to improve treatment of depression in primary care. *BMJ* 2000;320:550–554.

29. Wells KB, Sherbourne C, Schoenbaum M, et al. Impact of disseminating quality improvement programs for depression in managed primary care: a randomized controlled trial. *JAMA* 2000;283:212–220.

30. Thompson C, Kinmonth AL, Stevens L, et al. Effects of a clinical-practice guideline and practice-based education on detection and outcome of depression in primary care: Hampshire Depression Project randomised controlled trial. *Lancet* 2000;355:185–191.

31. Linde K, Mulrow CD. St John's Wort for depression. In: The Cochrane Library. Issue 4, 1998. Oxford: Update software. Search date 1998; primary sources Medline 1983 to 1997; Embase 1989 to 1997; PsychLit 1987 to 1997; Psychindex 1987 to 1997; specialised databases: Cochrane Complementary Medicine Field, Cochrane Depression and Neurosis CRG, Phytodok; bibliographies of pertinent articles; manufacturers and researchers.

32. Ernst E, Rand JI, Barnes J, et al. Adverse effects profile of the herbal antidepressant St John Wort (*Hypericum perforatum L*) *Eur J Clin Pharmacol* 1998;54:589–594. Search date September 1997; primary sources AMED 1985 to September 1997; Cochrane Library 1997 Issue 2; Embase 1980 to September 1997, Medline 1996 to September 1997; handsearched reference lists; contacted WHO Collaborating Centre for International Drug Monitoring; UK Committee on Safety of Medicines and German Bundesinstitut für Arzneimittel und Medizinproducte plus 12 German manufacturers of hypericum products.

33. Janicak PG, Davis JM, Gibbons RD, et al. Efficacy of ECT: a meta-analysis. *Am J Psychiatry* 1985;142:297–302. Search date not given; primary source Medline.

34. Wijeratne GS, Halliday GS, Lyndon RW. The present status of electroconvulsive therapy: a systematic review. *Med J Austr* 1999;171:250–254. Search date 1998; primary source Medline 1987 to 1998.

35. Johnstone EC, Deakin JF, Lawler P, et al. The Northwick Park electroconvulsive therapy trial. *Lancet* 1980;1:1317–1320.

36. Brandon S, Cowley P, McDonald C, et al. Electroconvulsive therapy: results in depressive illness from the Leicestershire trial. *BMJ* 1984;288:22–25.

37. Gregory S, Shawcross CR, Gill D. The Nottingham ECT study. A double-blind comparison of bilateral, unilateral and simulated ECT in depressive illness. *Br J Psychiatry* 1985;146:520–524.

38. Vaughan McCall W, Reboussin DM, Weiner RD, et al Titrated moderately suprathreshold vs fixed high-dose right unilateral electroconvulsive therapy. *Arch Gen Psychiatry* 2000;57:438–444 .

39. Sackeim HA, Prudic J, Devanand DP, et al. A prospective, randomized, double-blind comparison of bilateral and right unilateral electroconvulsive therapy at different stimulus intensities. *Arch Gen Psychiatry* 2000;57:425–434.

40. Scott AIF, Doris AB. Electroconvulsive therapy for depression (protocol). In: The Cochrane Library. Issue 4, 1998. Oxford: Update software.

41. Gloaguen V, Cottraux J, Cucherat M, et al. A meta-analysis of the effects of cognitive therapy in depressed patients 1998. *J Affect Disord* 1998;49:59–72. Search date not given; primary sources Medline 1966 to December 1996; Embase 1966 to December 1996; references in books and papers; previous reviews and meta-analyses; abstracts from congress presentations; preprints sent by authors.

42. Elkin I, Shea MT, Watkins JT, et al. National Institute of Mental Health treatment of depression collaborative research program: general effectiveness of treatments. *Arch Gen Psychiatry* 1989;46:971–982.

43. Mynors-Wallis LM, Gath DH, Lloyd-Thomas, AR, et al. Randomised controlled trial comparing problem solving treatment with amitriptyline and placebo for major depression in primary care. *BMJ* 1995;310:441–445.

44. Churchill R, Dewey M, Gretton V, et al. Should general practitioners refer patients with major depression to counsellors? A review of current published evidence. *Br J Gen Pract* 1999;49:738–743.

45. Thase ME, Greenhouse JB, Frank E, et al. Treatment of major depression with psychotherapy or psychotherapy—pharmacotherapy combinations. *Arch Gen Psychiatry* 1997;54:1009–1015. Pooled results of six research protocols conducted 1982 to 1992 at the Mental Health Clinical Research Center, University of Pittsburgh School of Medicine.

46. Keller MB, McCullough JP, Klein DN, et al. A comparison of nefazodone, the cognitive behavioral-analysis system of psychotherapy, and their combination for the treatment of chronic depression. *N Engl J Med* 2000;342:1462–1470.

47. North TC, McCullagh P, Tran ZV. Effect of exercise on depression. *Exerc Sport Sci Rev* 1990;18:379–415. Search date not given; primary sources dissertation abstracts online, ERIC, PsychInfo, Medline, books, abstracts from meetings to June 1989.

48. Blumenthal JA, Babyak MA, Moore KA, et al. Effects of exercise training on older patients with major depression. *Arch Intern Med* 1999;159:2349–2356.

49. Cuijpers P. Bibliotherapy in unipolar depression: a meta-analysis. *J Behav Ther Exp Psychiatry* 1997;28:139–147. Search date not given; primary sources Psychlit; Psychinfo; Medline.

50. Harris T, Brown GW, Robinson R. Befriending as an intervention for chronic depression among women in an inner city: Randomised controlled trial. *Br J*

Psychiatry 1999;174:219–224.

51. Loonen AJ, Peer PG, Zwanikken GJ. Continuation and maintenance therapy with antidepressive agents: meta-analysis of research. *Pharm Week Sci* 1991;13:167–175. Search date not given; primary sources references of textbooks and review articles; Medline 1977 to 1988; Embase 1977 to 1988; review of reference lists of primary studies.

52. Keller MB, Kocsis JH, Thase ME, et al. Maintenance phase efficacy of sertraline for chronic depression: a randomized controlled trial. *JAMA* 1998;280:1665–1672.

53. Old age depression interest group. How long should the elderly take antidepressants? A double-blind placebo-controlled study of continuation/prophylaxis therapy with dothiepin. *Br J Psychiatry* 1993;162:175–182.

54. Carney S, Geddes J, Davies D, Furukawa T, Kupfer D, Goodwin G. Duration of treatment with antidepressants in depressive disorder (protocol). In: The Cochrane Library, Issue 3 2000. Oxford: Update software.

55. Fava GA, Rafanelli C, Grandi S, et al. Prevention of recurrent depression with cognitive behavioral therapy: preliminary findings. *Arch Gen Psychiatry* 1998;55:816–820.

56. Haaga DAF, Beck AT. Cognitive therapy. In: Paykel ES, ed. *Handbook of affective disorders*. Edinburgh: Churchill Livingstone, 1992:511–523.

57. Klerman GL, Weissman H. Interpersonal psychotherapy. In: Paykel ES, ed. *Handbook of affective disorders*. Edinburgh: Churchill Livingstone, 1992:501–510.

John Geddes
Senior Clinical Research
Fellow/Honorary Consultant
Psychiatrist
University of Oxford
Oxford
UK

Rob Butler
Lecturer in Old Age Psychiatry

James Warner
Senior Lecturer/Consultant in Old Age
Psychiatry

Imperial College School of Medicine
London
UK

Competing interests: None declared.

| TABLE 1 | Adverse events (% of patients) with selective serotonin reuptake inhibitors (SSRIs) versus tricyclic antidepressants (TCAs) (see text).[20] |

Adverse effects	SSRIs event rates (%)	TCAs event rates (%)
Dry mouth	21	55
Constipation	10	22
Dizziness	13	23
Nausea	22	12
Diarrhoea	13	5
Anxiety	13	7
Agitation	14	8
Insomnia	12	7
Nervousness	15	11
Headache	17	14

TABLE 2 Effects of specific psychological treatments for depressive disorders (see text, p 528).

Intervention	Evidence	Benefits	Harms/disadvantages
Cognitive therapy	One systematic review identified 48 RCTs of psychological therapies (n = 2765 people, mainly outpatients in secondary care therefore probably with mild to moderate depression; people with psychotic or bipolar symptoms were excluded). Twenty RCTs compared cognitive therapy with waiting list or placebo and 17 compared it with drug treatment.[33]	79% of people in the placebo control group were more symptomatic than the average person treated with cognitive therapy (effect size 0.82, 95% CI 0.81 to 0.83).[32] 65% of people treated with cognitive therapy were less symptomatic than the average person treated with antidepressant drugs (effect size −0.38, 95% CI −0.39 to −0.37).[32]	No harms reported. Requires extensive training. Limited availability. RCTs in primary care suggest limited acceptability to some people.
Interpersonal psychotherapy	No systematic reviews. One large RCT, including people with mild to moderate depressive disorders, compared interpersonal psychotherapy versus drug treatment, cognitive therapy, or placebo plus clinical management of 16 weeks' duration.[33]	Recovery rates were: placebo-clinical management (21%); interpersonal psychotherapy (43%, NNT 5, 95% CI 3 to 19), imipramine (42%, NNT 5, 95% CI 3 to 22).[33]	No harms reported. Requires extensive training. Limited availability.
Problem solving therapy	No systematic reviews. Several small RCTs comparing problem solving versus drug treatment in primary care in people with mild depressive disorders.[35]	Problem solving was as effective as drug treatment.	No harms reported. Requires some training. Limited availability.
Non-directive counselling	One systematic review identified five RCTs comparing counselling with routine GP managemenet in UK primary care.[35] The RCTs included people with depressive disorders. There is also a protocol registered with the Cochrane database.[36]	No quantitative results provided in review. No consistent improvement in main outcomes, although studies report higher levels of satisfaction with treatment in counselling.	No harms reported. Requires some training. Limited availability.

Updated this issue

Philip Hazell

INTERVENTIONS

Key Messages

- One systematic review has found evidence of no benefit from tricyclic antidepressants in prepubertal children, and no clear benefit in adolescents. Fluoxetine may be of some benefit in child and adolescent depression, but more research is needed. We found no evidence to support the use of other serotonin reuptake inhibitor drugs. We found equivocal evidence to support the use of the reversible monoamine oxidase inhibitor moclobemide. We found no evidence supporting the use of non-reversible monoamine oxidase inhibitors. Preliminary data do not support the use of the selective noradrenergic reuptake inhibitor venlafaxine, nor the mood stabiliser lithium.

- We found insufficient evidence on the effects of St John's Wort (*Hypericum perforatum*) and electroconvulsive therapy in children and adolescents with depression.

- One systematic review of RCTs has found cognitive behavioural therapy to be superior to non-specific supportive therapies for mild to moderate depression in children and adolescents. Two RCTs of interpersonal therapy also suggested benefit compared with no treatment. We found insufficient evidence to conclude that family therapy, or group treatments other than cognitive behavioural therapy, are effective treatments for depression in children and adolescents.

- We found no systematic reviews or RCTs looking at long term outcomes for psychological or pharmacological treatments.

DEFINITION	See depressive disorders, p 520. Compared with adult depression, depression in children and adolescents may have a more insidious onset, may be characterised more by irritability than sadness, and occurs more often in association with other conditions such as anxiety, conduct disorder, hyperkinesis, and learning problems.[1]
INCIDENCE/ PREVALENCE	Estimates of prevalence of depression among children and adolescents in the community range from 1.7% to 5.9%.[2,3] Prevalence tends to increase with age, with a sharp rise around onset of puberty. Pre-adolescent boys and girls are equally affected by the condition, but depression is seen more frequently among adolescent girls than boys.[4]
AETIOLOGY/ RISK FACTORS	Causes are uncertain, including childhood events and current psychosocial adversity.
PROGNOSIS	See prognosis under depressive disorders, p 520. In children and adolescents, the recurrence rate of depressive episodes first occurring in childhood or adolescence is 70% by 5 years, which is similar to the recurrence rate in adults.[5] Young people experiencing a moderate to severe depressive episode may be more likely than adults to have a manic episode within the next few years.[4] Trials of treatment for child and adolescent depression have found high rates of spontaneous remission (as much as two thirds of people in some inpatient studies).
AIMS	To improve mood, social and occupational functioning, and quality of life; to reduce morbidity and mortality; to prevent recurrence of depressive disorder; and to minimise adverse effects of treatment.
OUTCOMES	See depressive disorders, p 520. In children and adolescents, there are developmentally specific continuous measures such as the Children's Depression Rating Scale and the Children's Depression Inventory. Categorical outcomes are sometimes expressed as patients no longer meeting DSM criteria for depression on a structured psychiatric interview such as the Kiddie-SADS.
METHODS	*Clinical Evidence* update search and appraisal May 2000. Subsequent author search for systematic reviews in The Cochrane Library 2000, Issue 3.

QUESTION What are the effects of treatments?

OPTION PRESCRIPTION ANTIDEPRESSANT DRUGS

One systematic review has found no evidence of benefit from tricyclic antidepressants in prepubertal children, and no clear benefit in adolescents. We have found limited evidence that fluoxetine may be of some benefit for child and adolescent depression. We found no evidence about other serotonin reuptake inhibitor drugs. We found little high quality evidence regarding moclobemide. We found no evidence on the effectiveness of non-reversible monoamine oxidase inhibitors. We have found no evidence that venlafaxine or lithium are beneficial, although the power of the trials was too low to rule out a clinically important difference.

Benefits: **Tricyclic antidepressants:** We found one systematic review (search date 1997, 14 RCTs)[6] and one subsequent RCT.[7] The systematic review found no significant reduction in non-response with the active drug versus placebo (n = 273; OR 0.83, 95% CI 0.48 to 1.42). Analyses for children (2 trials) and adolescents (5 trials) also found no significant benefit of treatment, (children RR of failure to recover 0.9, 95% CI 0.7 to 1.2; adolescents RR of failure to recover 0.9, 95% CI 0.7 to 1.3). However, using the weighted mean difference, trials found a modest but significant difference in adolescents (WMD in depression checklist scores −2.3, 95% CI −3.3 to −1.4) but not in children. Inclusion of the subsequent RCT (meta-analysis personal communication from the author) produced little changes in the estimate of effectiveness but narrowed the 95% confidence intervals.[7] **Pulsed intravenous clomipramine:** We found no systematic review. One small RCT including 16 non-suicidal adolescent outpatients with major depression found that significantly more people responded to intravenous clomipramine 200 mg than to saline.[8] **Monoamine oxidase inhibitors:** We found no systematic review. In one small RCT, 20 adolescents treated with moclobemide showed greater improvement on one clinician rated scale than those treated with placebo, but not on other clinician rated and self report measures.[9] We found no trials of non-reversible monoamine oxidase inhibitors. **Selective serotonin reuptake inhibitors:** We found one systematic review (search date 1998, two RCTs, n = 126).[10] The first RCT in the systematic review (n = 30) found no global benefit. The second RCT (n = 96) found significant benefit on clinician reported global rating and on self reported depressive symptoms, but not on other measures. The systematic review did not pool data from the two RCTs. However, combination of the results for clinician global rating, using a random effects model, found an insignificant pooled odds ratio for non-improvement (0.5, 95% CI 0.22 to 1.12). **Selective noradrenergic reuptake inhibitors:** We found one systematic review (search date 1998, one RCT, n = 33).[10] The one small RCT compared a combination of venlafaxine and psychotherapy with a combination of placebo and psychotherapy. It found no significant difference with regard to improvement. **Lithium:** We found no systematic review. One small placebo controlled RCT compared lithium versus placebo in 30 depressed prepubertal children with a family history of bipolar affective disorder.[11] It found no significant difference of global assessment or of depression scores at follow up.

Harms: See harms of antidepressants under depressive disorders, p 520. One systematic review awaiting publication found that tricyclic antidepressants were more commonly associated with vertigo (OR 8.47, 95% CI 1.40 to 51.0), orthostatic hypotension (OR 4.77, 95% CI 1.11 to 20.5) and dry mouth (OR 5.19, 95% CI 1.15 to 23.5) than placebo (P Hazell et al, personal communication, 2000). It found no significant differences for other adverse effects (tiredness, sleep problems, headache, palpitations, tremor, perspiration, constipation, or problems with micturition). We found single case reports and case series of toxicity and death from tricyclic antidepressants in overdose and therapeutic doses. See harms of antidepressants under depressive disorders, p 520. Of the 17 children randomised to lithium treatment, four were withdrawn because of adverse effects (three had confusion, one had nausea and vomiting).[11]

Comment: Further research is needed to determine long term effects of intravenous clomipramine.

OPTION   ST JOHN'S WORT (*HYPERICUM PERFORATUM*)

We found no evidence about the effects of St John's Wort (*Hypericum perforatum*) in children and adolescents with depression.

Benefits: We found no systematic review and no RCTs in children or adolescents.

Harms: See harms of St John's Wort under depressive disorders, p 520. We found no evidence about adverse effects in children and adolescents.

Comment: None.

OPTION   ELECTROCONVULSIVE THERAPY

We found insufficient evidence about the routine use of electroconvulsive therapy in children and adolescents with depression.

Benefits: We found no systematic reviews or RCTs.

Harms: Despite widespread concern about potentially harmful effects of electroconvulsive therapy, especially on memory loss, we found no evidence about harms in children or adolescents.

Comment: None.

OPTION   SPECIFIC PSYCHOLOGICAL TREATMENTS

One systematic review of RCTs has found cognitive behavioural therapy increases the rate of resolution of the symptoms of depression compared with non-specific supportive therapies for children and adolescents with mild to moderate depression. One RCT of interpersonal therapy found slightly more people recovered than with clinical monitoring alone. A further RCT did not find a significant difference in the recovery rate with interpersonal therapy compared with waiting list control. We found insufficient evidence to conclude that family therapy, or group treatments other than cognitive behavioural therapy, are effective treatments for depression in children and adolescents.

Benefits: **Cognitive behavioural therapy:** See glossary, p 540. We found one systematic review (search date 1997, 6 RCTs, 376 people) of cognitive behavioural therapy compared with "inactive" treatment that ranged from waiting list control to supportive psychotherapy.[12] Cognitive behavioural therapy was associated with increased rate of resolution of symptoms of depression (OR 3.2, 95% CI 1.9 to 5.2; NNT 4, 95% CI 3 to 5) a finding consistent with two non-systematic meta-analytic studies.[13,14] **Interpersonal therapy:** See glossary, p 541. We found no systematic review. We found two RCTs that compared twelve weekly sessions of interpersonal therapy versus clinical monitoring or waiting list control in adolescents with depression. In the first RCT, sessions were augmented by telephone contact. In the first RCT (n = 48) 18 of 24 adolescents receiving treatment interpersonal therapy recovered versus 11 of 24 adolescents receiving clinical monitoring alone (RR 1.64, 95% CI 1.00 to 2.68; ARR 0.29, 95% CI 0.03 to 0.56).[15] In the second RCT (n = 46) 17 of 19 adolescents receiving interpersonal therapy recovered versus 12 of 18 adolescents on the waiting list (RR 1.33, 95% CI 0.94 to 1.93; ARR 0.22, 95% CI –0.03 to +0.49).[16] **Family therapy:** We found no systematic review. One RCT of family therapy versus non-specific supportive therapy did not find a significant difference in remission rates (29% v 34%).[17] **Group administered cognitive behavioural therapy:** We found no systematic review. In one RCT group administered cognitive behavioural therapy for adolescents with depression produced a significantly higher remission rate amongst those receiving treatment (67%) compared with those on a waiting list (48%).[18] **Group therapeutic support versus group social skills training:** We found no systematic review. One RCT in 47 adolescents comparing group therapeutic support versus group social skills training found no significant difference in remission rates (50% v 40%).[19]

Harms: See harms of specific psychological treatments under depressive disorders, p 520. We found no report of harms specifically for children and adolescents.

Comment: See comment of specific psychological treatments under depressive disorders, p 520.

QUESTION   **Which treatments are most effective at improving long term outcome?**

We found no systematic reviews and no RCTs looking at long term outcomes.

Benefits: We found no systematic reviews and no RCTs. We found no trials comparing structured psychotherapy with pharmacotherapy in children and adolescents. We found no trials comparing combined pharmacotherapy and psychotherapy with either treatment alone. We found no trials comparing different psychotherapies.

Harms: See harms of cognitive behavioural therapy, p 539 and harms of prescription antidepressant drugs, p 538.

Comment: See depressive disorders, p 520. We found one prospective cohort study in which adolescents with depression, randomised to cognitive behavioural therapy, systemic behavioural family therapy, or nondirective supportive therapy, were assessed at 3 monthly intervals for the first 12 months and then once again at 24 months. The study found no significant difference between the groups. Of 106 adolescents, 38% experienced sustained recovery, 21% experienced persistent depression, and 41% had a relapsing course.[20]

GLOSSARY

Cognitive behavioural therapy A brief (20 sessions over 12–16 weeks) structured treatment aimed at changing the dysfunctional beliefs and negative automatic thoughts that characterise depressive disorders.[21] Cognitive behavioural therapy requires a high level of training in the therapist, and has been adapted for children and adolescents suffering depression. A course of treatment is characterised by 8–12 weekly sessions in which the therapist and the child collaborate to solve current difficulties. The treatment is structured, and often directed by a manual. Treatment generally includes cognitive elements, such as the challenging of negativistic thoughts, and behavioural elements such as structuring time to engage in pleasurable activity.

Interpersonal therapy A standardised form of brief psychotherapy (usually 12–16 weekly sessions) primarily intended for outpatients with unipolar non-psychotic depressive disorders. It focuses on improving the patient's interpersonal functioning and identifying the problems associated with the onset of the depressive episode.[22] In children and adolescents, interpersonal therapy has been adapted for adolescents to address common adolescent developmental issues, for example separation from parents, exploration of authority in relationship to parents, development of dyadic interpersonal relationships, initial experience with the death of relative or friend, and peer pressure.

Substantive changes since last issue

Tricyclic antidepressants Inclusion of one additional RCT into existing meta-analysis produced little change in estimate of effectiveness but narrowed the 95% confidence intervals.[7]

Selective serotonin reuptake inhibitors One new systematic review; no change in conclusion.[10]

Selective noradrenergic reuptake inhibitors One new systematic review; no change in conclusion.[10]

Tricyclic antidepressants Update on harms from treatment with tricyclic antidepressants from a systematic review in publication (P Hazell et al, personal communication, 2000).

Interpersonal therapy One additional RCT did not find a significant difference in recovery from interpersonal therapy compared with waiting list control.[16]

Long term outcome A 2 year follow up found no difference in long term outcomes between selected psychological treatments in adolescents with depression.[20]

REFERENCES

1. Costello EJ, Angold A, Burns BJ, et al. The Great Smoky Mountains Study of Youth. Goals, design, methods, and the prevalence of DSM-III-R disorders. Arch Gen Psychiatry 1996;53:1129–1136.

2. Costello EJ. Developments in child psychiatric epidemiology. J Am Acad Child Adolesc Psychiatry 1989;28:836–841.

3. Lewinsohn PM, Rohde P, Seely JR. Major depressive disorder in older adolescents: Prevalence, risk factors, and clinical implications. Clin Psychol Rev 1998;18:765–794.

4. Birmaher B, Ryan ND, Williamson DE, Brent DA. Childhood and adolescent depression: A review of the past 10 years, Part I. J Am Acad Child Adolesc Psychiatry 1996;35:1427–1439.

5. Geller B, Fox LW, Fletcher M. Effect of tricyclic antidepressants on switching to mania and on the onset of bipolarity in depressed 6- to 12-year-olds. J Am Acad Child Adolesc Psychiatry 1993; 32:43–50.

6. Hazell P, O'Connell D, Heathcote D, Henry D. Tricyclic drugs for depression in children and adolescents. In: The Cochrane Library 2000 Issue 1. Search date 1997; primary sources: Medline, Excerpta Medica, Cochrane trials database.

7. Bernstein, GA, Borchardt, CM, Perwien, AR, et al. Imipramine plus cognitive-behavioral therapy in the treatment of school refusal. J Am Acad Child Adolesc Psychiatry 2000;39:276–283.

8. Sallee FR, Vrindavanam NS, Deas-Nesmith D, Carson SW, Sethuraman G. Pulse intravenous clomipramine for depressed adolescents: Double-blind, controlled trial. Am J Psychiatry 1997;154: 668–673.

9. Avci A, Diler RS, Kibar M, Sezgin F. Comparison of moclobemide and placebo in young adolescents with major depressive disorder. Ann Med Sci 1999;8:31–40.

10. Williams JW, Mulrow CD, Chiquette E, Noel PH, Aguilar C, Cornell J. A systematic review of newer pharmacotherapies for depression in adults: Evidence report summary. Ann Intern Med 2000; 132:743–756. Search date 1998; primary sources Medline, Embase, Psyclit, Lilacs, Psyindex, Sigle, Cinahl, Biological Abstracts, Cochrane Controled Trials, hand searches, and personal contacts.

11. Geller B, Cooper TB, Zimerman B, et al. Lithium for prepubertal depressed children with family history predictors of future bipolarity: A double-blind, placebo-controlled study. J Affect Disord 1998;51:165–175.

12. Harrington R, Whittaker J, Shoebridge P, Campbell F. Systematic review of efficacy of cognitive behavioural therapies in childhood and adolescent depressive disorder. BMJ 1998;316:1559–1563. Search date 1997; primary sources Medline, Psychlit, Cochrane, and hand searches of reference lists, book chapters, conference proceedings, and relevant journals in the field.

13. Lewinsohn PM, Clarke GN. Psychosocial

treatments for adolescent depression. *Clin Psychol Rev* 1999;19:329–342.

14. Reinecke MA, Ryan NE, DuBois DL. Cognitive-behavioral therapy of depression and depressive symptoms during adolescence: A review and meta-analysis. *J Am Acad Child Adolesc Psychiatry* 1998;37:26–34.

15. Mufson L, Weissman MM, Moreau D, Garfinkel R. Efficacy of interpersonal psychotherapy for depressed adolescents. *Arch Gen Psychiatry* 1999;56:573–579.

16. Rossello J, Bernal G. The efficacy of cognitive-behavioral and interpersonal treatments for depression in Puerto Rican adolescents. *J Consult Clin Psychol* 1999;67:734–745.

17. Brent DA, Holder D, Kolko D, et al. A clinical psychotherapy trial for adolescent depression comparing cognitive, family, and supportive therapy. *Arch Gen Psychiatry* 1997;54:877–885.

18. Clarke GN, Rohde P, Lewinsohn PM, Hops H, Seeley JR. Cognitive-behavioral treatment of adolescent depression: Efficacy of acute group treatment and booster sessions. *J Am Acad Child Adolesc Psychiatry* 1999;38:272–279.

19. Fine S, Forth A, Gilbert M, Haley G. Group therapy for adolescent depressive disorder: a comparison of social skills and therapeutic support. *J Am Acad Child Adolesc Psychiatry* 1991;30:79–85.

20. Birmaher B, Brent DA, Kolko D, et al. Clinical outcome after short-term psychotherapy for adolescents with major depressive disorder. *Arch Gen Psychiatry* 2000;57:29–36.

21. Haaga DAF, Beck AT. Cognitive therapy. In: Paykel ES, ed. *Handbook of affective disorders.* Edinburgh: Churchill Livingstone, 1992;511–523.

22. Klerman GL, Weissman H. Interpersonal psychotherapy. In: Paykel ES, ed. *Handbook of affective disorders.* Edinburgh: Churchill Livingstone, 1992;501–510.

Philip Hazell
Conjoint Professor of Child and
Adolescent Psychiatry/Director, Child and
Youth Mental Health Service
University of Newcastle
New South Wales
Australia

Competing interests: PH has been paid a fee for speaking to general practitioners about the evidence for the treatment of depression in young people by Pfizer, the manufacturer of Sertraline.

Updated this issue

G Mustafa Soomro

Mental health

INTERVENTIONS

Key Messages

- Three systematic reviews of RCTs have found that serotonin reuptake inhibitors improve symptoms. One double blind placebo substitution study found that most participants relapsed within weeks of stopping treatment.

- We found limited evidence from one RCT that sertraline is more effective than clomipramine at reducing symptoms. One systematic review and one RCT found no significant difference between clomipramine and other serotonin reuptake inhibitors. However, clomipramine has more adverse effects than selective serotonin reuptake inhibitors, particularly cholinergic and cardiac effects.

- One systematic review has found that behavioural therapy improves symptoms compared with relaxation. Two follow up studies found that improvement was maintained for up to 2 years.

- We found limited evidence from data pooling within a systematic review, and one RCT which found that cognitive therapy is as effective as behavioural therapy.

- One systematic review found no evidence of a difference between serotonin reuptake inhibitors and behavioural therapy.

- We found limited evidence from RCTs that behavioural therapy plus fluvoxamine is more effective than behavioural therapy alone.

DEFINITION   Obsessive compulsive disorder (OCD) is characterised by obsessions, compulsions, or both, that cause significant personal distress or social dysfunction, and that are not caused by drugs or physical disorder. **Obsessions** are defined as recurrent and persistent ideas, images, or impulses that cause pronounced anxiety and which the person perceives to be self produced. **Compulsions** are intentional repetitive behaviours or mental acts performed in response to obsessions or according to certain rules, and are aimed at reducing distress or preventing certain imagined dreaded events. Obsessions and compulsions are usually recognised as pointless and are resisted by the person. There are minor differences in the criteria for OCD between the third, revised third, and fourth editions of the *Diagnostic and Statistical Manual* (DSM-III, DSM-III-R, and DSM-IV).[1]

INCIDENCE/ PREVALENCE   One national, community based survey of OCD in the UK (1993, n = 10 000) found prevalence to be 1% in men and 1.5% in women.[2] In the USA, the lifetime prevalence of OCD was found to be between 1.9–3.3% in 1984 (n = 18 500).[3] One international study found lifetime prevalence to be 3% in Canada, 3.1% in Puerto Rico, 0.3–0.9% in Taiwan, and 2.2% in New Zealand.[2]

AETIOLOGY/ RISK FACTORS   Aetiology is unknown. Behavioural, cognitive, genetic, and neurobiological factors are implicated.[4–10]

PROGNOSIS   One study that followed 144 people for an average of 47 years found that an episodic (see glossary, p 549) course was more common during the initial years (about 1–9 years), whereas a chronic (see glossary, p 549) course was more common afterwards.[11] Over time, the study found that 39–48% of people showed symptomatic improvement. A 1 year prospective cohort study found 46% of people to have an episodic course and 54% to have a chronic course.[12]

AIMS   To improve symptoms and to reduce impact of illness on social functioning and quality of life.

OUTCOMES   Severity of symptoms, adverse effects of treatment, and social functioning. The most commonly used instruments for measuring symptoms are the Yale–Brown obsessive compulsive scale and the National Institute of Mental Health's global obsessive compulsive scale, both of which are observer rated and well validated.[13–16] Most trials use a 25% decrease in Yale–Brown scale scores from baseline as indicative of clinically significant improvement. Some studies use a 35% reduction.[16]

METHODS   *Clinical Evidence* update search and appraisal May 2000. We reviewed all identified systematic reviews and RCTs.

QUESTION   What are the effects of treatments in adults?

OPTION   SEROTONIN REUPTAKE INHIBITORS

Three systematic reviews and two subsequent RCTs have found good evidence that serotonin reuptake inhibitors (see glossary, p 549) are more effective than placebo in reducing symptoms. Apart from limited evidence from one RCT that sertraline is more effective than

clomipramine, we found no evidence of different efficacy for other serotonin reuptake inhibitors. One systematic review and two subsequent RCTs have found that serotonin reuptake inhibitors are more effective than other kinds of antidepressants. RCTs have found clomipramine to be associated with more adverse effects than selective serotonin reuptake inhibitors. One follow up study found that most people relapsed within a few weeks of stopping drug treatment.

Benefits:
Serotonin reuptake inhibitors versus placebo: We found three systematic reviews and two subsequent RCTs. All found overall benefit of treatment compared with placebo.[17–21] The first review (search date 1994) identified nine RCTs of clomipramine (a non-selective serotonin reuptake inhibitor — see glossary, p 549) in 668 people, with mean treatment duration of 12 weeks. Two RCTs (n = 73) were in children, but the review did not give separate effect sizes.[18] This review found treatment to be more effective than placebo at reducing symptoms (WMD 1.31, 95% CI 1.15 to 1.47). The second review (search date not given) pooled data from eight placebo controlled RCTs of clomipramine (4 trials included in the first review; total of 1131 people with OCD).[18] It found clomipramine to be more effective than placebo (WMD 1.31, CI not given). The first review found fluoxetine, fluvoxamine and sertraline (selective serotonin reuptake inhibitors) to be more effective than placebo (fluoxetine: 1 RCT, 287 people; WMD 0.57, 95% CI 0.33 to 0.81; fluvoxamine: 3 RCTs, 395 people; WMD 0.57, 95% CI 0.37 to 0.77; sertraline: 3 RCTs, 270 people; WMD 0.52, 95% CI 0.27 to 0.77).[17] One subsequent double blind RCT compared fluoxetine 20 mg a day (n = 87) versus 40 mg a day (n = 89) versus 60 mg a day (n = 90) versus placebo (n = 84).[21] It found that people on all doses of fluoxetine improved significantly more than people on placebo (improvement on Yale–Brown scale, fluoxetine 20 mg 19.5%, 40 mg 22.1%, 60 mg 26.6%, placebo 3.3%, CI not given, all P v placebo ≤ 0.001). It also found a significant dose related response (P < 0.001). A second subsequent double blind RCT (164 people) found that sertraline was significantly more effective than placebo in reducing symptoms (P < 0.01, mean reduction on Yale–Brown scale 9 points with sertraline and 4 points with placebo, CI not given). The third review (search date 1997, 3 RCTs of 338 people) found paroxetine (a selective serotonin reuptake inhibitor) to be more effective than placebo over 12 weeks (WMD 0.48, 95% CI 0.24 to 0.72.[19,20] **Serotonin reuptake inhibitors versus each other:** The first review (85 people, three RCTs) found no significant difference in the improvement of obsessive compulsive symptoms between clomipramine and selective serotonin reuptake inhibitors (fluoxetine or fluvoxamine; WMD −0.04, 95% CI −0.43 to +0.35).[17] One subsequent double blind RCT of clomipramine (n = 82) versus sertraline (n = 86) found sertraline to be more effective (associated with a 8% greater mean reduction in obsessive compulsive symptoms; P = 0.036).[22] A second subsequent double blind RCT compared clomipramine (n = 65) with fluvoxamine (n = 68).[23] It found no significant difference in mean improvement in symptoms (improvement on Yale–Brown scale clomipramine 50.2% versus fluvoxamine 45.6%, CI and P not given). **Serotonin reuptake inhibitors versus other antidepressants:** The first systematic review identified seven RCTs comparing clomipramine

with non-serotonin reuptake inhibitor antidepressants (147 people with OCD; 2 trials [n = 67] in children/adolescents without separate results).[17] This review found clomipramine to be more likely to reduce symptoms (WMD 0.65, 95% CI 0.36 to 0.92). One subsequent RCT of fluoxetine (n = 17) versus phenelzine (n = 19) versus placebo (n = 18) found the largest effect from fluoxetine (WMD not given, mean reduction in symptoms was 15% fluoxetine, 9% phenelzine, and 1% placebo).[24] A second subsequent double blind RCT compared sertraline (n = 79) with desipramine (n = 85) in people with concurrent OCD and major depressive disorder.[25] It found sertraline to be more effective at reducing obsessive compulsive and depressive symptoms. The response rate for improvement in obsessive compulsive symptoms (≥40% improvement on Y-BOCS) was 48% with sertraline compared with 31% with desipramine (CI not given, P = 0.01). There was no significant difference in response rate for depressive symptoms (≥50% improvement on Hamilton rating scale for depression) but the remission rate (defined as a score ≤ 7 on Hamilton rating scale for depression) was significantly better with sertraline (49% v 35%, CI not given, P = 0.04). **Serotonin reuptake inhibitors versus behavioural therapy:** We found weak evidence from the third systematic review, which included mixed method studies (number of studies and people not given).[19] This review found no significant difference between effect sizes of serotonin reuptake inhibitors and behavioural therapy (see glossary, p 549) when compared with placebo, but did not make direct comparisons.[19]

Harms: Sixteen RCTs in the second review found a greater incidence of adverse effects with serotonin reuptake inhibitors than placebo (RRI 54% for clomipramine, 11% for fluoxetine, 19% for fluvoxamine, and 27% for sertraline).[18] The third systematic review of controlled and uncontrolled studies found the withdrawal rate due to adverse effects to be 11% for clomipramine, 10% for fluoxetine, 13% for fluvoxamine, 9% for sertraline, and 11% for paroxetine.[19] Anticholinergic adverse effects (dry mouth, blurred vision, constipation, and urinary retention), cardiac adverse effects, drowsiness, dizziness, and convulsions (convulsions usually at doses > 250 mg/day) have been reported to be most common with clomipramine,[26–28] whereas selective serotonin reuptake inhibitors are associated with fewer adverse effects but more nausea, diarrhoea, anxiety, agitation, insomnia, and headache.[26,27] Both clomipramine and selective serotonin reuptake inhibitors were associated with weight change and sexual dysfunction.[26,28] The subsequent RCT comparing sertraline (n = 79) with desipramine (n = 85) found more people discontinued because of adverse effects with desipramine (26% v 10%, P = 0.009).[25] The subsequent RCT comparing clomipramine (n = 65) with fluvoxamine (n = 68) found a higher rate of discontinuation because of adverse effects associated with clomipramine (13.8% v 7.4%, significance not assessed).[23] One non-systematic review identified three prospective cohort studies and five surveys which found fluoxetine during pregnancy did not significantly increase the risk of spontaneous abortion of major malformation (figures not provided).[29] It included one prospective cohort study (n = 174) and three surveys which suggested similar outcomes from other selective serotonin reuptake inhibitors (sertraline, paroxetine, or fluvoxamine). One prospective cohort study (n = 55) found preschool age children exposed to fluoxetine *in utero* showed no significant differences from children not exposed in global IQ, language, or behaviour. It included no long term harms for the other selective serotonin reuptake inhibitors.

Comment: The first systematic review also identified two small RCTs, which found no difference in the effects of placebo and non-serotonin reuptake inhibitors (imipramine and nortriptyline).[17] One small, observer blinded RCT of fluvoxamine (n = 10) versus paroxetine (n = 9) versus citalopram (n = 11) found no significant differences in the effects of these drugs, but the study was too small to exclude a clinically significant effect.[30] **Duration and discontinuation of treatment:** Most RCTs assessed efficacy over 10–12 weeks.[28,31] One prospective, 1 year study found that further significant improvement occurred in the 40 week open label extension, with some continuing adverse effects.[32] One placebo substitution study of clomipramine found that 89% (16/18) of people relapsed within 7 weeks of placebo treatment.[33] **Effects on people without depression:** The first systematic review found that serotonin reuptake inhibitors reduced symptoms in people without depression (5 RCTs including 594 people; WMD 1.37, 95% CI 1.19 to 1.55).[17] **Factors predicting outcome:** Four RCTs found that people who did not respond to treatment had younger age of onset, longer duration of the condition, higher frequency of symptoms, co-existing personality disorders, and a greater likelihood of previous hospital admission. Predictors of good response were older age of onset, history of remissions, no previous drug treatment, more severe OCD, and either high or low score on the Hamilton Depression Rating Scale.[34–37] Two cohort studies of people with OCD found that poor response to serotonin reuptake inhibitors was predicted by concomitant schizotypal personality disorder (see glossary, p 549), by tic disorder (see glossary, p 549) and also by severe OCD with cleaning rituals (OR 4.9, 95% CI 1.1 to 21.2).[38,39] The non-systematic review of effects in pregnancy may have been systematic but did not make explicit how articles were selected.[29]

OPTION   **BEHAVIOURAL THERAPY AND COGNITIVE THERAPY**

One systematic review found behavioural therapy is associated with greater symptom reduction than relaxation. The review found limited evidence of no significant difference in symptom reduction between cognitive therapy (see glossary, p 549) and behavioural therapy. We found limited evidence that behavioural therapy plus fluvoxamine is more effective than behavioural therapy alone. One RCT found no significant difference between cognitive therapy alone and cognitive therapy plus fluvoxamine. Two follow up studies found that after behavioural therapy, significant improvement was maintained for up to 2 years, but that some people required additional behavioural therapy.

Benefits: **Behavioural therapy versus relaxation:** We found one systematic review (search date not given), which pooled results from two RCTs (121 people with OCD, further characteristics not specified). It found evidence that behavioural therapy reduced symptoms more than relaxation (WMD 1.18, P < 0.01, CI not given; 88% of people in the relaxation group did worse than the average improvement on behavioural therapy).[18] **Behavioural therapy versus cognitive therapy:** The same systematic review pooled results from four RCTs (92 people with OCD, further characteristics not specified). It found no significant difference in reduction of symptoms between behavioural therapy and cognitive therapy (WMD –0.19, CI not available).[18] **Combination treatment:** We found weak evidence from one systematic review (search date 1997). It pooled data from mixed method studies (number of studies and people not given) and compared three different regimens with placebo: behavioural therapy plus serotonin reuptake inhibitors; behavioural therapy alone; and serotonin reuptake inhibitors alone. The review found similar reductions in symptoms, but did not make direct comparisons between treatments.[19] One RCT in 99 people in an outpatient setting compared behavioural therapy, cognitive therapy, behavioural therapy plus fluvoxamine, and cognitive therapy plus fluvoxamine.[40] It found no significant differences in outcomes on the Yale–Brown scale (mean reduction in symptoms 32% with behavioural therapy, 47% with cognitive therapy, 49% with behavioural therapy plus fluvoxamine, 43% with cognitive therapy plus fluvoxamine; 16 people per arm would allow detection of a 25% change in the Yale–Brown scale). One double blind RCT (49 people in a teaching hospital setting) found significantly greater improvement in symptoms with behavioural therapy plus fluvoxamine than with behavioural therapy plus pill placebo (88% v 60% achieved a ≥ 35% reduction on the Yale–Brown scale; RR 0.3, 95% CI 0.1 to 0.96; NNT 3).[41] **Maintenance of improvement:** One prospective follow up of 20 people with OCD (specific diagnostic criteria not given) from a 6 month RCT of behavioural therapy found that 79% maintained improvement in obsessive compulsive symptoms at 2 year follow up.[42] One prospective non-inception cohort study of behavioural therapy in 21 people with OCD (specific diagnostic criteria not given) found that after the initial 2 weeks of treatment, 68–79% maintained complete or much improvement in symptoms at 3 months' follow up.[43] In both studies, however, some people required additional behavioural therapy during the follow up period.

Harms: We found no evidence from RCTs or cohort studies of adverse effects from behavioural or cognitive therapy. Case reports have described unbearable and unacceptable anxiety in some people receiving behavioural therapy.

Comment: **Factors predicting outcome:** We found two RCTs of behavioural therapy (duration 2.5 months and 32 weeks; total 96 people) and two retrospective cohort studies (duration 1 year and 11 weeks; total 346 people).[44–47] These found poorer outcome to be predicted by initial severity, depression, longer duration, poorer motivation, and dissatisfaction with the therapeutic relationship. Good outcome was predicted by early adherence to 'exposure homework' (that is, tasks to be carried out outside regular therapy sessions involving contact with anxiety provoking situations), employment, living with one's family, no previous treatment, having fear of contamination, overt ritualistic behaviour, and absence of depression.[44–46] Good outcome for women was predicted by having a co-therapist (someone usually related to the person, who is enlisted to help with treatment outside regular therapy sessions; OR 19.5, 95% CI 2.7 to 139.3).[47] Two systematic reviews of drug, and behavioural, cognitive, and combination treatments for OCD are being prepared.

GLOSSARY

Behavioural therapy Consists of exposure to the anxiety provoking stimuli and prevention of ritual performance.

Chronic Continuous course without periods of remission since first onset.

Cognitive therapy Aims to correct distorted thoughts (such as exaggerated sense of harm and personal responsibility) by Socratic questioning, logical reasoning, and hypothesis testing.

Episodic Episodic course with periods of remission since first onset.

Non-selective serotonin reuptake inhibitor Clomipramine (also classed as a tricyclic antidepressant).

Schizotypal personality disorder Characterised by discomfort in close relationships, cognitive and perceptual distortions, and eccentric behaviour.

Selective serotonin reuptake inhibitors Fluoxetine, fluvoxamine, sertraline, paroxetine, citalopram.

Tic disorder Characterised by motor tics, vocal tics, or both.

Substantive changes since last issue

Serotonin reuptake inhibitors One new RCT found significant improvement in obsessive compulsive symptoms with a range of doses of fluoxetine versus placebo.[21]

Serotonin reuptake inhibitors One new RCT found no significant difference in improvement in obsessive compulsive symptoms with fluvoxamine versus clomipramine. More people withdrew because of adverse events with clomipramine.[23]

Serotonin reuptake inhibitors One RCT found sertraline to be more effective at reducing obsessive compulsive symptoms compared with desipramine. More people withdrew because of adverse events with desipramine.[25]

Serotonin reuptake inhibitors One non-systematic review found limited evidence from cohort studies and surveys that fluoxetine in pregnancy does not increase risk for spontaneous abortion or major malformation. One cohort study and surveys suggest the same for other selective serotonin reuptake inhibitors. One long term cohort of fluoxetine found no evidence of an effect on IQ, language, or behaviour in preschool children exposed *in utero*.[29]

REFERENCES

1. American Psychiatric Association. *Diagnostic and statistical manual of mental disorders*, 4th ed. Washington, DC: American Psychiatric Association, 1994.
2. Bebbington PE. Epidemiology of obsessive–compulsive disorder. *Br J Psychiatry* 1998; 35(suppl):2–6.
3. Karno M, Golding JM, Sorenson SB, Burnam MA. The epidemiology of obsessive–compulsive disorder in five US communities. *Arch Gen Psychiatry* 1988;45:1094–1099.
4. Baer L, Minichiello WE. Behavior therapy for obsessive–compulsive disorder. In: Jenike MA, Baer L, Minichiello WE, eds. *Obsessive–compulsive disorders*. St Louis: Mosby, 1998.
5. Steketee GS, Frost RO, Rheaume J, Wilhelm S. Cognitive theory and treatment of obsessive–compulsive disorder. In: Jenike MA, Baer L, Minichiello WE, eds. *Obsessive–compulsive disorders*. St Louis: Mosby, 1998.
6. Alsobrook JP, Pauls DL. The genetics of obsessive–compulsive disorder. In: Jenike MA, Baer L,

Minichiello WE, eds. *Obsessive–compulsive disorders*. St Louis: Mosby, 1998.
7. Rauch SL, Whalen PJ, Dougherty D, Jenike MA. Neurobiologic models of obsessive compulsive disorder. In: Jenike MA, Baer L, Minichiello WE, eds. *Obsessive–compulsive disorders*. St Louis: Mosby, 1998.
8. Delgado PL, Moreno FA. Different roles for serotonin in anti-obsessional drug action and the pathophysiology of obsessive–compulsive disorder. *Br J Psychiatry* 1998;35(suppl):21–25.
9. Saxena S, Brody AL, Schwartz JM, Baxter LR. Neuroimaging and frontal–subcortical circuitry in obsessive–compulsive disorder. *Br J Psychiatry* 1998;35(suppl):26–37.
10. Rauch SL, Baxter Jr. LR. Neuroimaging in obsessive–compulsive disorder and related disorders. In: Jenike MA, Baer L, Minichiello WE, eds. *Obsessive–compulsive disorders*. St Louis: Mosby, 1998.
11. Skoog G, Skoog I. A 40-year follow-up of patients with obsessive–compulsive disorder. *Arch Gen*

Psychiatry 1999;56:121–127.

12. Ravizza L, Maina G, Bogetto F. Episodic and chronic obsessive–compulsive disorder. *Depress Anxiety* 1997;6:154–158.

13. Goodman WK, Price LH, Rasmussen SA, et al. The Yale–Brown obsessive compulsive scale. I. Development, use, and reliability. *Arch Gen Psychiatry* 1989;46:1006–1011.

14. Insel TR, Murphy DL, Cohen RM, Alterman I, Kilts C, Linnoila M. Obsessive–compulsive disorder. A double-blind trial of clomipramine and clorgyline. *Arch Gen Psychiatry* 1983;40:605–612.

15. Goodman WK, Price LH, Rasmussen SA, et al. The Yale–Brown obsessive compulsive scale. II. Validity. *Arch Gen Psychiatry* 1989;46:1012–1016.

16. Goodman WK, Price LH. Rating scales for obsessive–compulsive disorder. In: Jenike MA, Baer L, Minichiello WE, eds. *Obsessive–compulsive disorders*. St Louis: Mosby, 1998.

17. Piccinelli M, Pini S, Bellantuono C, Wilkinson G. Efficacy of drug treatment in obsessive–compulsive disorder. A meta-analytic review. *Br J Psychiatry* 1995;166:424–443. Search dates 1975 to May 1994; primary sources Medline and Excerpta Medica-Psychiatry.

18. Abramowitz JS. Effectiveness of psychological and pharmacological treatments for obsessive–compulsive disorder: a quantitative review. *J Consult Clin Psychol* 1997;65:44–52. Search date not given; primary sources Medline and PsycLIT.

19. Kobak KA, Greist JH, Jefferson JW, Katzelnick DJ, Henk HJ. Behavioral versus pharmacological treatments of obsessive compulsive disorder: a meta-analysis. *Psychopharmacology (Berl)* 1998; 136:205–216. Search date May 1997; primary sources Medline, PsycINFO, Dissertations, and Abstracts International databases.

20. Kronig MH, Apter J, Asnis G, et al. Placebo controlled multicentre study of sertraline treatment for obsessive–compulsive disorder. *J Clin Psychopharmacol* 1999;19:172–176.

21. Tollefson GD, Rampey AH, Potvin JH, et al. A multicenter investigation of fixed-dose fluoxetine in the treatment of obsessive–compulsive disorder. *Arch Gen Psychiatry* 1994;51:559–567.

22. Bisserbe JC, Lane RM, Flament MF. A double blind comparison of sertraline and clomipramine in outpatients with obsessive–compulsive disorder. *Eur Psychiatry* 1997;12:82–93.

23. Mundo E, Maina G, Uslenghi C. Multicentre, double-blind, comparison of fluvoxamine and clomipramine in the treatment of obsessive–compulsive disorder. *Int Clin Psychopharmacol* 2000;15:69–76.

24. Jenike MA, Baer L, Minichiello WE, Rauch SL, Buttolph ML. Placebo-controlled trial of fluoxetine and phenelzine for obsessive– compulsive disorder. *Am J Psychiatry* 1997;154:1261–1264.

25. Hoehn-Saric R, Ninan P, Black DW, et al. Multcenter double-blind comparison of sertraline and desipramine for concurrent obsessive–compulsive and major depressive disorders. *Arch Gen Psychiatry* 2000;57:76–82.

26. British National Formulary. London: British Medical Association and Royal Pharmaceutical Society of Great Britain, 1999.

27. Trindade E, Menon D. Selective serotonin reuptake inhibitors differ from tricyclics antidepressants in adverse events (Abstract). Selective serotonin reuptake inhibitors for major depression. Part 1. Evaluation of clinical literature. Ottawa: Canadian Coordinating Office for Health Technology Assessment, August 1997 Report 3E. *Evid Based Ment Health* 1998;1:50.

28. Jenike MA. Drug treatment of obsessive–compulsive disorders. In: Jenike MA, Baer L, Minichiello WE, eds. *Obsessive–compulsive disorders*. St Louis: Mosby, 1998:469–532.

29. Goldstein DJ, Sundell K. A review of safety of selective serotonin reuptake inhibitors during pregnancy. *Hum Psychopharmacol Clin Exp* 1999; 14:319–324.

30. Mundo E, Bianchi L, Bellodi L. Efficacy of fluvoxamine, paroxetine, and citalopram in the treatment of obsessive–compulsive disorder: a single-blind study. *J Clin Psychopharmacol* 1997; 17:267–271.

31. Rauch SL, Jenike MA. Pharmacological treatment of obsessive compulsive disorder. In: Nathan PE, Gorman JM, eds. *Treatments that work*. New York: Oxford University Press, 1998:359–376.

32. Rasmussen S, Hackett E, DuBoff E, et al. A 2-year study of sertraline in the treatment of obsessive–compulsive disorder. *Int Clin Psychopharmacol* 1997;12:309–316.

33. Pato MT, Zohar-Kadouch R, Zohar J, Murphy DL. Return of symptoms after discontinuation of clomipramine in patients with obsessive–compulsive disorder. *Am J Psychiatry* 1988;145: 1521–1525.

34. Ravizza L, Barzega G, Bellino S, Bogetto F, Maina G. Predictors of drug treatment response in obsessive–compulsive disorder. *J Clin Psychiatry* 1995;56:368–373.

35. Cavedini P, Erzegovesi S, Ronchi P, Bellodi L. Predictive value of obsessive–compulsive personality disorder in antiobsessional pharmacological treatment. *Eur Neuropsychopharmacol* 1997;7:45–49.

36. Ackerman DL, Greenland S, Bystritsky A. Clinical characteristics of response to fluoxetine treatment of obsessive–compulsive disorder. *J Clin Psychopharmacol* 1998;18:185–192.

37. Ackerman DL, Greenland S, Bystritsky A, Morgenstern H, Katz RJ. Predictors of treatment response in obsessive–compulsive disorder: multivariate analyses from a multicenter trial of clomipramine. *J Clin Psychopharmacol* 1994;14: 247–254.

38. Mundo E, Erzegovesi S, Bellodi L. Follow up of obsessive–compulsive patients treated with proserotonergic agents (letter). *J Clin Psychopharmacol* 1995;15:288–289.

39. Alarcon RD, Libb JW, Spitler D. A predictive study of obsessive–compulsive disorder response to clomipramine. *J Clin Psychopharmacol* 1993;13: 210–213.

40. van Balkom AJ, de Haan E, van Oppen P, Spinhoven P, Hoogduin KA, van Dyck R. Cognitive and behavioral therapies alone versus in combination with fluvoxamine in the treatment of obsessive compulsive disorder. *J Nerv Ment Dis* 1998;186:492–499.

41. Hohagen F, Winkelmann G, Rasche-Ruchle H, et al. Combination of behaviour therapy with fluvoxamine in comparison with behaviour therapy and placebo. Results of a multicentre study. *Br J Psychiatry* 1998;35(suppl):71–78.

42. Marks IM, Hodgson R, Rachman S. Treatment of chronic obsessive–compulsive neurosis by in-vivo exposure. A two year follow-up and issues in treatment. *Br J Psychiatry* 1975;127:349–364.

43. Foa EB, Goldstein A. Continuous exposure and complete response prevention in obsessive–compulsive neurosis. *Behav Ther* 1978;9:821–829.

44. Keijsers GP, Hoogduin CA, Schaap CP. Predictors of treatment outcome in the behavioural treatment of obsessive–compulsive disorder. *Br J Psychiatry* 1994;165:781–786.

45. De Araujo LA, Ito LM, Marks IM. Early compliance and other factors predicting outcome of exposure

for obsessive–compulsive disorder. *Br J Psychiatry* 1996;169:747–752.

46. Buchanan AW, Meng KS, Marks IM. What predicts improvement and compliance during the behavioral treatment of obsessive compulsive disorder? *Anxiety* 1996;2:22–27.

47. Castle DJ, Deale A, Marks IM, Cutts F, Chadhoury Y, Stewart A. Obsessive–compulsive disorder: prediction of outcome from behavioural psychotherapy. *Acta Psychiatr Scand* 1994;89: 393–398.

G Mustafa Soomro
Honorary Research Fellow
Section of Community Psychiatry
St George's Hospital Medical School
London
UK

Competing interests: None declared.

Post-traumatic stress disorder

Updated this issue

Jonathan Bisson

INTERVENTIONS

Key Messages

Prevention

- One systematic review of RCTs found no evidence that debriefing prevents post-traumatic stress disorder (PTSD), and one RCT found that it was associated with an increased risk of PTSD at 1 year.

- We found conflicting evidence on the effects of multiple episode intervention. One small RCT found no evidence of benefit from multiple episode psychological intervention. Two small RCTs found that five sessions of either cognitive behavioural therapy or prolonged exposure are superior to supportive counselling for preventing PTSD in people with acute stress after a traumatic event.

Treatment

- Evidence from mainly small RCTs suggests benefit from psychological treatments compared with supportive counselling, relaxation therapy, or no treatment.

- One systematic review of mainly small RCTs has found that antidepressants reduce symptoms more than placebo. The only anxiolytic drug evaluated, alprazolam, was the least effective drug treatment. We found insufficient evidence on the effects of antipsychotic drugs or carbamazepine.

DEFINITION	Post-traumatic stress disorder (PTSD) occurs after a major traumatic event. Symptoms include upsetting thoughts and nightmares about the traumatic event, avoidance behaviour, numbing of general responsiveness, increased irritability, and hypervigilance.[1]
INCIDENCE/ PREVALENCE	One large cross sectional study in the USA found that one in 10 women and one in 20 men experience PTSD at some stage in their lives.[2]
AETIOLOGY/ RISK FACTORS	Risk factors include major trauma such as rape, a history of psychiatric disorders, acute distress and depression after the trauma, lack of social support, and personality factors (such as neuroticism).[3]
PROGNOSIS	One large cross sectional study in the USA found that over a third of sufferers continued to satisfy the criteria for a diagnosis of PTSD 6 years after diagnosis.[2] Cross sectional studies provide weak evidence about prognosis.
AIMS	To reduce initial distress after a traumatic event; to prevent PTSD and other psychiatric disorders; to reduce levels of distress in the long term; and to improve function and quality of life.
OUTCOMES	Presence or absence of PTSD and severity of symptoms. Scoring systems include impact of event scale and clinician administered PTSD scale.
METHODS	*Clinical Evidence* update search and appraisal May 2000.

QUESTION **What are the effects of preventive psychological interventions?**

One systematic review of RCTs found no evidence that single episode interventions prevent PTSD, and one of these RCTs found an increased risk of PTSD at 1 year. We found conflicting evidence on the effects of multiple episode intervention from three RCTs. One found no significant evidence of benefit, the other two found that five episodes of cognitive behavioural therapy (see glossary, p 556) were superior to supportive counselling (see glossary, p 556).

Benefits: **Single episode intervention ("debriefing"):** We found one systematic review (search date 1997), which identified six RCTs comparing early single episode interventions ("debriefing") with no intervention in 462 people.[4] The trials used psychological debriefing or similar techniques (see glossary, p 556). The review found that more people treated with debriefing still had PTSD at 3–5 months but the difference was not significant (OR 1.5, 95% CI 0.7 to 3.1). One of the trials followed people for 1 year after debriefing and found that debriefing versus no treatment was associated with increased rates of PTSD (OR 2.9, 95% CI 1.1 to 7.5). **Multiple episode intervention:** We found no systematic review. We found three RCTs. The first RCT (151 people) compared 3–6 sessions of educational and cognitive behavioural techniques with no psychological intervention.[5] Intervention began at least 1 month after a road traffic accident. There were no significant differences in outcomes between groups. The second RCT (24 people) compared five sessions of cognitive behavioural therapy (see glossary, p 556) with five sessions of supportive counselling (see glossary, p 556) in people with acute stress disorder within 2 weeks of a road accident or industrial accident.[6] Cognitive behavioural therapy was associated with a large reduction in the number of people who met PTSD diagnostic criteria immediately after treatment (8% v 83% with supportive counselling, P < 0.001) and at 6 months (17% v 67% with supportive counselling, P < 0.05).[7] The third RCT (66 survivors of road accidents or non-sexual assault with acute stress disorder) evaluated five 90 minute sessions of prolonged exposure versus supportive counselling versus prolonged exposure plus anxiety management. Immediately after completion of treatment, significantly lower rates of PTSD were found in the prolonged exposure group (14%) and in the prolonged exposure plus anxiety management group (20%) compared with the supportive counselling group (56%). The differences were still significant at 6 month follow up (15% v 23% v 67%).[8]

Harms: Two trials of single episode intervention found an increased risk of subsequent psychological problems in people receiving the intervention however initial traumatic exposure had been higher in these people.[4]

Comment: The systematic review found that the overall quality of the studies was poor.[4] Problems included lack of blinding, failure to state loss to follow up, and lack of intention to treat analysis despite high withdrawal rates. We found one further RCT of cognitive behavioural therapy in French bus drivers who had been attacked.[9] The trial suggested that early intervention with cognitive behavioural therapy reduces anxiety levels at 6 month follow up. The trial will be fully evaluated for the next edition of *Clinical Evidence*.

QUESTION What are the effects of psychological treatments?

Mainly small RCTs found evidence of benefit from psychological treatments compared with supportive counselling, relaxation therapy (see glossary, p 556), or no treatment.

Benefits: We found one systematic review of psychological treatments for PTSD (search date not given, published in 1998, 17 RCTs, 690 people).[7] They compared a range of specific psychological treatments versus supportive treatment or no intervention. All trials found that psychological treatment was associated with a greater improvement in immediate outcome (using a composite score of PTSD symptoms, anxiety, and depression) compared with supportive counselling or no treatment (overall effect size immediately after treatment 0.54, 95% CI not stated). The difference was still evident at 1 year (overall effect size from 12 studies with long term follow up 0.53, CI not stated). **Cognitive behavioural treatments:** We found one systematic review (search date not given) and two subsequent RCTs.[7,10,11] The review identified 14 RCTs of cognitive behavioural treatments in people with PTSD. Although many were of poor quality, all described a positive effect compared with no treatment. One RCT (n = 45) identified in the review, evaluated three types of cognitive therapy and found that all were better than no treatment at 3 months (effect sizes compared with no treatment: stress inoculation 1.1, 95% CI 0.66 to 1.5; supportive counselling

0.55, 95% CI 0.17 to 0.94; prolonged exposure therapy 1.67, 95% CI 1.2 to 2.1).[12] One subsequent RCT (n = 87) compared exposure or cognitive therapy or both with relaxation therapy.[10] The trial found that all cognitive behavioural treatments reduced symptoms of PTSD more than relaxation therapy, immediately and at 3 months (at 3 months n = 53; no intention to treat analysis performed).[13] The second subsequent RCT (54 people) found that 39% continued to suffer from PTSD one year after 16 one hour sessions of imaginal exposure therapy or cognitive therapy. There was no difference in the prevalence of PTSD between the two treatment groups.[11] **Eye movement desensitisation and reprocessing (EMDR):** We found no systematic review. We found seven small RCTs (257 people in total) evaluating at least three sessions of EMDR (see glossary, p 556). Three found that EMDR was associated with reduced symptoms compared with no treatment.[10,14,15] One found that EMDR was associated with a greater reduction in symptoms compared with relaxation therapy and another found that EMDR reduced symptoms compared with active listening therapy.[15,16] One RCT (n = 36) found a non-significant treatment advantage with EMDR compared with a form of exposure therapy.[14] One RCT found evidence that EMDR was less effective than cognitive behavioural therapy.[17] Three trials compared standard EMDR with EMDR without eye movements.[18-20] Two found that both interventions were associated with a reduction in symptoms (no significant difference between reductions), and one found that standard EMDR was more effective.[18-20] **Affect management:** We found one RCT comparing psychotherapy plus drug treatment with or without affect management (see glossary, p 556) in 48 women. The trial found that symptom control was greater with affect management.[21] The drop-out rate was high (31%) and the analysis was not by intention to treat. **Other psychological treatments:** We found one RCT (112 people), which found no significant difference between psychodynamic psychotherapy (see glossary, p 556), exposure therapy, and hypnotherapy (see glossary, p 556). However, all were slightly better than remaining on the waiting list (no treatment control). The trial did not quantify results.[22] **Inpatient treatment programme:** We found no RCTs. **Drama therapy:** See glossary, p 556. We found no RCTs.

Harms: The studies gave no information on harms. Overall, cognitive behavioural therapy seems well tolerated. However, there have been case reports in some individuals of imaginal flooding (a form of cognitive behavioural therapy) worsening symptoms, leading to calls for caution when assessing people for treatment.[23]

Comment: Most RCTs were of poor quality. We found no theoretical basis for the use of EMDR in people with PTSD.

QUESTION What are the effects of drug treatments?

One systematic review of mainly small RCTs has found that antidepressants versus placebo reduce symptoms more than placebo. One small RCT of alprazolam versus placebo found a small effect. We found insufficient evidence on the effects of antipsychotic drugs or carbamazepine.

Benefits: **Antidepressants and anxiolytics:** We found one systematic review of antidepressants and anxiolytics for PTSD and one subsequent RCT.[24] The review (search date July 1996) identified six placebo controlled trials in 242 people.[25] The effect size for PTSD from all trials and all drugs versus placebo was 0.41 (CI not available). Effect sizes for individual drugs (CI not available) were fluoxetine 0.77 (n = 64, 1 trial), phenelzine 0.39 (n = 63, two trials), tricyclic antidepressants 0.32 (n = 149, 3 trials), and alprazolam 0.25 (n = 16, 1 trial). The review also found that drug treatment reduced depression and anxiety. The subsequent RCT (187 people attending outpatients with PTSD from a variety of traumatic events) compared sertraline, a selective serotonin reuptake inhibitor, with placebo. Sertraline increased the response rate (53% with sertraline v 32% with placebo; P = 0.008), although the actual reduction in traumatic stress symptoms was not very large.[24] **Antipsychotic drugs:** We found no RCTs. **Carbamazepine:** We found no RCTs.

Harms: The trials gave no information on harms. Known adverse effects include the need for dietary restriction and possible hypertensive crisis with monoamine oxidase inhibitors, anticholinergic effects with tricyclic antidepressants, nausea and headache with SSRIs, and dependency with benzodiazepines.

Comment: Small trial sizes and different populations make it difficult to compare results. Other treatments or combinations of drug and psychological treatment await evaluation. It is difficult to interpret effect sizes in terms of clinical importance rather than statistical significance. Some categorise effect sizes of less than 0.5 as small; between 0.5 and 0.8 as medium; and greater than 0.8 as large.

GLOSSARY

Affect management Entails managing mood.

Cognitive behavioural therapy Covers a variety of techniques. *Imaginal exposure* entails exposure to a detailed account or image of what happened. *Real life exposure* involves confronting real life situations that have become associated with the trauma, and cause fear and distress. *Cognitive therapy* entails challenging distorted thoughts about the trauma, the self, and the world. *Stress inoculation* entails instruction in coping skills and some cognitive techniques such as restructuring.

Drama therapy Entails using drama as a form of expression and communication.

Eye movement desensitisation (EMDR) and reprocessing Entails asking the person to focus on the traumatic event, a negative cognition associated with it, and the associated emotions.[26] The person is then asked to follow the therapist's finger as it moves from side to side. We found no theoretical basis for this intervention.

Hypnotherapy Entails hypnosis to allow people to work through the traumatic event.

Jacobson's relaxation therapy A form of muscle relaxation that avoids any exposure to the traumatic event.

Psychodynamic psychotherapy Entails analysis of defence mechanisms, interpretations, and pre-trauma experiences.

Psychological debriefing A technique that entails detailed consideration of the traumatic event and the normalisation of psychological reactions.

Supportive counselling A non-directive intervention dealing with current issues rather than the trauma itself.

Substantive changes since last issue

Preventive psychological interventions One new RCT found that five sessions of prolonged exposure or prolonged exposure with anxiety management resulted in lower rates of PTSD than supportive counselling;[8] conclusion unchanged.

Psychological treatments One new RCT found no difference in effect after 16 one hour sessions of imaginal exposure therapy or cognitive therapy; conclusion unchanged.[11]

Drug treatment One new RCT found sertraline more effective than placebo in reducing traumatic stress symptoms; conclusion unchanged.[24]

REFERENCES

1. American Psychiatric Association. *Diagnostic and statistical manual of mental disorders*. 4th ed. Washington: APA, 1994.
2. Kessler RC, Sonnega A, Bromet E, et al. Posttraumatic stress disorder in the national comorbidity survey. *Arch Gen Psychiatry* 1995;52: 1048–1060.
3. O'Brien S. *Traumatic events and mental health*. Cambridge: Cambridge University Press, 1998.
4. Wessely S, Rose S, Bisson J. A systematic review of brief psychological interventions ('debriefing') for the treatment of immediate trauma related symptoms and the prevention of posttraumatic stress disorder. In: The Cochrane Library, issue 4, 1999. Oxford: Update Software. Search date 1996, primary sources Medline, Embase, Psychlit, Pilots, Biosis, Pascal, *Occup Health Saf*, CDSR and the Trials register of the Cochrane Depression, Anxiety and Neurosis Group; hand search of *J Trauma Stress*, and contact with experts.
5. Brom D, Kleber RJ, Hofman MC. Victims of traffic accidents: incidence and prevention of post-traumatic stress disorder. *J Clin Psychol* 1993;49: 131–140.
6. Bryant RA, Harvey AG, Basten C, Dang ST, Sackville T, Basten C. Treatment of acute stress disorder: a comparison of cognitive behavioural therapy and supportive counselling. *J Consult Clin Psychol* 1998;66:862–866.
7. Sherman JJ. Effects of psychotherapeutic treatments for PTSD: a meta-analysis of controlled clinical trials. *J Trauma Stress* 1998;11:413–436. Search date not given; primary sources Psychlit, ERIC, Medline, Cinahl, Dissertation Abstracts, Pilots Traumatic Stress Database.
8. Bryant RA, Sackville T, Dang ST, Moulds M, Guthrie R. Treating acute stress disorder: an evaluation of cognitive behavior therapy and supportive counselling techniques. *Am J Psychiatry* 1999;156:1780–1786.
9. Andre C, Lelord F, Legeron P, Reigner A, and Delattre A. Controlled study of outcomes after 6 months to early intervention of bus driver victims of aggression [in French]. *Encephale* 1997;23: 65–71.
10. Rothbaum BO. A controlled study of eye movement desensitization and reprocessing in the treatment of posttraumatic stress disordered sexual assault victims. *Bull Menninger Clin* 1997; 61:317–334.
11. Tarrier N, Sommerfield C, Pilgrim H, Humphreys L. Cognitive therapy or imaginal exposure in the treatment of post-traumatic stress disorder. *Br J Psychiatry* 1999;175:571–575.
12. Foa EB, Rothbaum BO, Riggs DS, et al. Treatment of posttraumatic stress disorder in rape victims: a comparison between cognitive-behavioural procedures and counselling. *J Consult Clin Psychol* 1992;59:715–723.
13. Marks I, Lovell K, Noshirvani H, et al. Treatment of posttraumatic stress disorder by exposure and/or cognitive restructuring: a controlled study. *Arch Gen Psychiatry* 1998;55:317–325.
14. Vaughan K, Armstrong MS, Gold R, et al. A trial of eye movement desensitization compared to image habituation training and applied muscle relaxation in post traumatic stress disorder. *J Behav Ther Exp Psychiatry* 1994;25:283–291.
15. Carlson JG, Chemtob CM, Rusnak K, Hedland NL, Muraoka MY. Eye movement desensitization and reprocessing (EMDR) treatment for combat-related posttraumatic stress disorder. *J Trauma Stress* 1998;11:3–24.
16. Scheck MM, Schaeffer JA, Gillette C. Brief psychological intervention with traumatized young women: The efficacy of eye movement desensitization and reprocessing. *J Trauma Stress* 1998;11:25–44.
17. Devilly GJ, Spence SH. The relative efficacy and treatment distress of EMDR and a cognitive-behavior treatment protocol in the amelioration of posttraumatic stress disorder. *J Anxiety Disord* 1999;13:131–157.
18. Renfrey G, Spates CR. Eye movement desensitization: a partial dismantling study. *J Behav Ther Exp Psychiatry* 1994;24:251–259.
19. Pitman RK, Orr SP, Altman B, Longpre RE, Poire RE, Macklin ML. Emotional processing during eye movement densensitisation and reprocessing therapy of Vietnam veterans with chronic posttraumatic stress disorder. *Compr Psychiatry* 1996;37:419–429.
20. Wilson SA, Becker LA, Tinker RH. Eye movement desensitization and reprocessing (EMDR) treatment for psychologically traumatized individuals. *J Consult Clin Psychol* 1995;63:928–937.
21. Zlotnick C, Shea T, Rosen K, et al. An affect-management group for women with posttraumatic stress disorder and histories of childhood sexual abuse. *J Trauma Stress* 1997;10:425–436.
22. Brom D, Kleber RJ, Defares PB. Brief psychotherapy of posttraumatic stress disorders. *J Consult Clin Psychol* 1989;57:607–612.
23. Pitman RK, Altman B, Greenwald E, et al. Psychiatric complications during flooding therapy for posttraumatic stress disorder. *J Clin Psychiatry* 1991;52:17–20.
24. Brady K, Pearlstein T, Asnis GM, et al. Efficacy and safety of sertraline treatment of posttraumatic stress disorder: a randomized controlled trial. *JAMA* 2000;283:1837–1844.
25. Penava SJ, Otto MW, Pollack MH, et al. Current status of pharmacotherapy for PTSD: an effect size analysis of controlled studies. *Depress Anxiety* 1997;4:240–242. Search date July 1994; primary sources Psychlit, Medline.
26. Shapiro, F. Eye movement desensitisation: a new treatment for post-traumatic stress disorder. *J Behav Ther Exp Psychiatry* 1989;20:211–217.

Jonathan Bisson

Consultant Liaison Psychiatrist, Cardiff and the Vale NHS Trust, Cardiff, UK

Competing interests: None declared.

Updated and expanded this issue

Stephen M Lewrie and Andrew McIntosh

INTERVENTIONS

Key Messages

- Most evidence is from systematic reviews of small brief RCTs that report different outcomes. There is a need for larger trials, over longer periods, with well designed end points including standardised, validated symptom scales.
- Systematic reviews of RCTs have found:
  - Chlorpromazine improves clinical outcomes, but adverse effects make it unacceptable to many people.
  - There is limited evidence of benefit from depot haloperidol decanoate compared with placebo.
  - The newer antipsychotic drugs olanzapine, quetiapine, risperidone, ziprasidone, and zotepine are as effective as standard antipsychotics and have different profiles of adverse effects.

- Relapse rates are significantly reduced by continuing antipsychotic medication for at least 6 months after an acute episode and by family interventions. Weaker evidence suggests that social skills training and cognitive behavioural therapy may also reduce relapse rates.
- No intervention has been consistently found to reduce negative symptoms.

■ RCTs have found:
  - Limited evidence that compliance therapy, family therapy, and behavioural therapy may improve adherence with antipsychotic medication.

DEFINITION Schizophrenia is characterised by the "positive symptoms" of auditory hallucinations, delusions, and thought disorder, and the "negative symptoms" of demotivation, self neglect, and reduced emotion.[1]

INCIDENCE/ PREVALENCE Onset of symptoms typically occurs in early adult life (average age 25 years) and is earlier in men than women. Prevalence worldwide is 2–4/1000. One in 100 people will develop schizophrenia in their lifetime.[2,3]

AETIOLOGY/ RISK FACTORS Risk factors include a family history (although no major genes have been identified); obstetric complications; developmental difficulties; central nervous system infections in childhood; cannabis use; and acute life events.[2] The precise contributions of these factors and ways in which they may interact are unclear.

PROGNOSIS About three quarters of people suffer recurrent relapse and continued disability, although outcomes were worse in the pretreatment era.[4] Outcome may be worse in people with insidious onset and delayed initial treatment, social isolation, or a strong family history; in people living in industrialised countries; in men; and in people who misuse drugs.[3] Drug treatment is generally successful in treating positive symptoms, but up to a third of people derive little benefit and negative symptoms are notoriously difficult to treat. About half of people with schizophrenia do not adhere to treatment in the short term. The figure is even higher in the longer term.[5]

AIMS To relieve symptoms and to improve quality of life, with minimal adverse effects of treatment.

OUTCOMES Severity of positive and negative symptoms; global clinical improvement; global clinical impression (a composite measure of symptoms and everyday functioning); rate of relapse; adherence to treatment; adverse effects of treatment.

METHODS *Clinical Evidence* update search and appraisal April 2000. We also searched The Cochrane Library, Issue 2, 2000. Most of the trials we found were small, short term, with many different outcome measures.[6] There were a large number of high quality recent systematic reviews. Therefore, if possible we focused primarily on systematic reviews at the expense of subsequent RCTs and included only the outcomes we thought were the most clinically relevant (because different treatments are associated with different benefits and harms, we used estimates of global effectiveness if they were available). We searched for placebo controlled studies for standard antipsychotic medication, and comparative studies for newer antipsychotics.

Schizophrenia

QUESTION What are the effects of drug treatments?

OPTION CHLORPROMAZINE

One systematic review of RCTs has found that chlorpromazine produces global improvement in the short and medium term.

Benefits: **Versus placebo:** We found one systematic review (updated 1999, 45 RCTs, 3116, mean dose of 511 mg/day, range 25–2000 mg/day.[7] Chlorpromazine was more effective than placebo in terms of psychiatrist rated global improvement by at least 50% (RR 1.3, 95% CI 1.1 to 1.4; NNT 7, 95% CI 5 to 10) and global severity (RR 1.5, 95% CI 1.1 to 2.0; NNT 5, 95% CI 4 to 8) in the short and medium term (up to 6 months).

Harms: The systematic review found that adverse effects include sedation (RR 2.4, 95% CI 1.7 to 3.3; NNH 6, 95% CI 4 to 8), acute dystonias (RR 3.1, 95% CI 1.3 to 7.6; NNH 24, 95% CI 14 to 77), parkinsonism (RR 2.6, 95% CI 1.2 to 5.4; NNH 10, 95% CI 8 to 16), weight gain (RR 4.4, 95% CI 2.1 to 9; NNH 3, 95% CI 2 to 5), skin photosensitivity (RR 5.2, 95% CI 3 to 10; NNH 7, 95% CI 6 to 10), dizziness caused by hypotension (RR 1.9, 95% CI 1.3 to 2.6; NNH 12, 95% CI 8 to 20), and dry mouth (RR 4, 95% CI 1.6 to 10; NNH 19, 95% CI 12 to 37).[7] Chlorpromazine was also associated with a non-significantly higher rate of seizures (RR 2.4, 95% CI 0.4 to 16) and blood dyscrasias (RR 2.0, 95% CI 0.7 to 6). We found no long term data on the risk of tardive dyskinesia or the rare but potentially fatal neuroleptic malignant syndrome. Despite the frequent adverse effects, people receiving active treatment were more likely to stay in trials than those receiving placebo in both the short and the medium term.

Comment: The review did not categorise symptoms as positive or negative as this information was rarely available from included trials. Relative risks and numbers needed to treat were based on 6 months' data.

OPTION DEPOT HALOPERIDOL DECANOATE

One systematic review has found limited evidence from one RCT that depot haloperidol decanoate is more effective than placebo.

Benefits: **Versus placebo:** We found one systematic review, updated in 1998, which identified two RCTs.[8] One RCT (22 people) comparing intramuscular depot haloperidol decanoate (mean dose 150 mg monthly) with placebo found that haloperidol decanoate was more likely to result in a "reduced need for medication" at four months (RR 2.6, 95% CI 1.1 to 5.6; NNT with 4 months' treatment 2, 95% CI 1 to 2).

Harms: Compared with placebo, fewer people receiving haloperidol left the trial early (RR 0.2, 95% CI 0.1 to 0.4; NNT 2, 95% CI 1 to 3).[8]

Comment: How "reduced need for medication" was measured was not described. Depot injection is believed to ensure adherence, but we found no evidence to support this belief.

OPTION DEPOT PIPOTHIAZINE PALMITATE

One systematic review has found limited evidence from two RCTs that there is no significant difference between depot pipothiazine palmitate and standard antipsychotic drugs.

Benefits: **Versus standard oral antipsychotic drugs:** We found one systematic review, updated in 1999, which identified two RCTs, both conducted in the 1970s, comparing intramuscular pipothiazine palmitate with normal treatment ("standard" oral antipsychotic drugs, chosen by physicians).[9] Neither found a significant difference between active treatment and control groups (first trial, 124 people: WMD in composite rating of psychotic symptoms at 18 months −3.1, 95% CI −7.3 to +1.2; second trial, 48 people: no quantified results available).

Harms: One trial (mean dose 90 mg per month) found that the number of people needing to take anticholinergic drugs for unspecified reasons was not significantly different for those taking the depot and for those on standard drugs (RR 0.9, 95% CI 0.7 to 1.1).[9] Meta-analysis combining the first and the second trial (mean dose 113 mg per month for 6 months) found no overall difference in the numbers of people leaving the trial early (25% in both groups, RR 1.0, 95% CI 0.5 to 1.9).

Comment: Several other depot preparations are commercially available in different countries, but we found even less evidence for their efficacy versus placebo or standard antipsychotic drugs.

OPTION LOXAPINE New

One systematic review of 22 small, brief RCTs comparing loxapine and standard antipsychotic drugs found no significant difference in their benefits or harms.

Benefits: **Versus standard antipsychotic drugs:** We found one systematic review (updated in 1999, 22 RCTs, 1073 people), which compared loxapine (dose range 25 to 250 mg daily) with standard antipsychotic drugs, usually chlorpromazine.[10] It found no significant differences in global improvement (9 RCTs, 411 people; RR not improved 0.9, 95% CI 0.7 to 1.2).

Harms: The systematic review found no significant difference in adverse effects.[11]

Comment: All trials were conducted in the USA or India and none lasted longer than 12 weeks.

OPTION   MOLINDONE   New

One systematic review of RCTs found no significant difference between molindone and standard antipsychotic drugs in benefits or harms, but the RCTs were short and of poor quality.

Benefits: **Versus standard antipsychotic drugs:** We found one systematic review of molindone versus standard antipsychotic drugs (updated 2000, 13 RCTs, 469 people).[10] It found no significant differences in global efficacy between molindone and standard antipsychotic drugs (4 RCTs, 150 people; RR no improvement 1.1, 95% CI 0.7 to 1.8).

Harms: No significant differences were found between molindone and standard antipsychotic drugs in terms of total numbers of adverse events. One trial found that the rate of confusion was higher in people taking molindone (RR 3.2, 95% CI 1.4 to 7.3). There were no significant differences in the rates of movement disorders between molindone and standard antipsychotic drugs. Weight loss was more frequent in those taking molindone (2 RCTs, 60 people; RR 2.8, 95% CI 1.1 to 7.0). Molindone was associated with less frequent weight gain than standard antipsychotic drugs (2 RCTs, 60 people; RR 0.4, 95% CI 0.1 to 1.0).

Comment: The RCTs in the review had methodological problems (in four trials it was unclear whether randomisation had been performed, 7/13 trials included people whose diagnosis was not operationally defined) and were brief (all lasted under 13 weeks). We found no reliable evidence comparing molindone with either placebo or new antipsychotic drugs.

OPTION   PIMOZIDE   New

One systematic review of RCTs comparing pimozide with standard antipsychotic drugs found no significant difference in benefits or harms.

Benefits: **Versus standard antipsychotic drugs:** We found one systematic review (updated in 1999, 34 RCTs, 1278 people).[12] It identified trials including 1155 people comparing pimozide (mean dose 7.5 mg daily, range 1 to 75 mg daily) with a variety of standard antipsychotic drugs.[12] It found no significant differences in clinical global impression rates (3 RCTs, 206 people; RR 0.9, 95% CI 0.8 to 1.1).

Harms: Pimozide caused less sedation than standard antipsychotic drugs (RR 0.4, 95% CI 0.2 to 0.7; NNT 6, 95% CI 4 to 16), but was more likely to cause tremor (RR 1.6, 95% CI 1.1 to 2.3; NNH 6, 95% CI 3 to 44).

Comment: Sudden death has been reported in a number of people taking pimozide at doses over 20 mg daily, but we found no evidence that pimozide is more likely to cause sudden death than other antipsychotic drugs. The manufacturer recommends periodic ECG monitoring in all people taking more than 16 mg daily of pimozide and avoidance of other drugs known to prolong the QT interval on an electrocardiogram or cause electrolyte disturbances (other antipsychotics, antihistamines, antidepressants, and diuretics).

| OPTION | POLYUNSATURATED FATTY ACIDS | New |

One systematic review found limited evidence from one small, brief RCT that polyunsaturated fatty acids compared with placebo reduced the subsequent use of antipsychotic medication.

Benefits: **Versus placebo:** We found one systematic review (updated 2000, 4 RCTs). It identified one relevant RCT (30 people) of fatty acid supplementation versus placebo.[13] The need at 12 weeks for subsequent antipsychotic medication was less in those receiving fish oil compared with those receiving placebo (RR 0.6, 95% CI 0.4 to 0.9). The review also found a slight difference in average symptom severity scores favouring fish oil (26 people; WMD −12.5, 95% CI −21.9 to −3.0).

Harms: The RCT did not find significant adverse events.

Comment: The single relevant RCT cited in the systematic review is an unpublished conference proceeding. Other RCTs considered only augmentation of antipsychotic treatment, which may be covered in a later issue of *Clinical Evidence.*

| OPTION | OLANZAPINE |

Two systematic reviews of RCTs have found that olanzapine may be as effective as standard antipsychotic drugs and has fewer adverse effects. We found no evidence that olanzapine is more effective than other new antipsychotic drugs.

Benefits: We found three systematic reviews.[14–16] **Versus standard antipsychotic drugs:** The first review (updated 1999, 15 RCTs, 3282 people) compared olanzapine with standard antipsychotic drugs, usually haloperidol.[14] It found olanzapine 2.5–25 mg daily compared with **standard antipsychotic drugs** did not significantly reduce psychotic symptoms over 6–8 weeks (2778 people; RR of no important response defined as a 40% reduction on any scale: 0.9, 95% CI 0.76 to 1.06). The second review (search date 1998, 4 RCTs, 2914 people) found that olanzapine was associated with slightly greater treatment success than haloperidol on a composite measure of positive and negative symptoms.[15] We found one potentially relevant subsequent RCT comparing olanzapine with haloperidol.[17] It will be appraised for the next issue of *Clinical Evidence.* **Versus other new antipsychotic drugs:** The first review included one trial (84 people) comparing olanzapine with risperidone.[15] It found no evidence of a difference in effectiveness (RR no important clinical response by eight weeks 0.93, 95% CI 0.85 to 1.01). A third systematic review (180 people, 1 trial) comparing olanzapine with clozapine found no significant difference in effectiveness (RR no important clinical response 0.7, 95% CI 0.5 to 1.1).[16]

Harms: **Versus standard antipsychotic drugs:** Olanzapine compared with standard antipsychotic drugs did not significantly reduce the number of people who withdrew from the trials at 6–8 weeks (36% v 49%; RR 0.9, 95% CI 0.7 to 1.1) or at one year (83% v 90%; OR 0.9, 95% CI 0.86 to 1.02).[14] Olanzapine compared with standard antipsychotic drugs caused fewer extrapyramidal adverse effects (in heterogeneous data prone to bias), less nausea (2347 people; RR 0.7, 95% CI 0.6 to 0.9; NNT 25, 95% CI 14 to 85), vomiting (1996 people; RR 0.6, 95% CI 0.4 to 0.8; NNT 20, 95% CI 12 to 46), or drowsiness (2347 people; RR 0.8, 95% CI 0.7 to 0.9) than standard antipsychotic drugs.[14] Olanzapine was associated with a greater increase in appetite (1996 people; RR 1.7, 95% CI 1.4 to 2.0; NNH 10, 95% CI 7 to 15) and weight gain (heterogeneous data) than standard antipsychotic drugs.[14] **Versus other new antipsychotic drugs:** One RCT included in the first review (84 people) found that olanzapine compared with risperidone was associated with fewer extrapyramidal adverse effects (NNT 8), less parkinsonism (NNT 11) and less need for anticholinergic medication (NNT 8); but olanzapine caused more dry mouth (NNH 9) and greater weight gain (NNH 11).[14] RCTs (180 people) found olanzapine compared with clozapine was associated with less nausea (RR 0.1, 95% CI 0.01 to 0.8) and no significant change in the number of people complaining of movement disorders (RR 0.4, 95% CI 0.1 to 1.4).[16]

Comment: The results of the reviews are dominated by one large multicentre RCT reported by drug company employees. Benefits seem to be maximal at a dose of 15 mg daily, and higher doses may be associated with more harms. The results depended on the precise statistical test used. Those presented above are conservative estimates, which seem reasonable given the presence of heterogeneity and other possible biases. Some less conservative statistical methods indicate superior effectiveness for olanzapine compared with standard antipsychotic drugs.

OPTION   QUETIAPINE

Two systematic reviews of RCTs and one subsequent RCT comparing quetiapine with standard antipsychotic drugs have found no significant differences in benefits, but significant reduction of some harms.

Benefits: **Versus standard antipsychotic drugs:** We found two systematic reviews, and one subsequent RCT.[15,18,19] The first review (search date 1998, 6 RCTs, 1414 people) identified two RCTs (809 people) comparing quetiapine with haloperidol and found no evidence of a difference in effectiveness on a composite measure of positive and negative symptoms.[15] The second (updated 1999, 7 RCTs, 2025 people), identified four trials comparing quetiapine (50–800 mg daily) with standard antipsychotic drugs, usually haloperidol.[18] No significant differences in global improvement were reported (310 people; RR no important improvement in mental state 1.1, 95% CI 0.8 to 1.5). The subsequent RCT (448 people) comparing quetiapine with haloperidol found no significant difference in improvement of global impression.[19]

Harms: The review found quetiapine caused less dystonia than standard antipsychotics (558 people; 1% v 5%; RR 0.2, 95% CI 0.1 to 0.9;

NNT 29, 95% CI 13 to 111) but no significant difference in the incidence of dry mouth (649 people; RR 2.5, 95% CI 0.7 to 9) or sleepiness (959 people; RR 1.4, 95% CI 0.8 to 2.5).[18,22] The subsequent RCT found no significant difference in overall adverse effects.[18] It did find significantly less extrapyramidal effects with quetiapine (62% v 14%).[19]

Comment: The evidence comes from a small number of short term trials that had substantial withdrawal rates and did not conduct intention to treat analyses. The Cochrane review has been substantially amended subsequent to our search date; the amendments will be included in the next issue of *Clinical Evidence*.[20]

OPTION   RISPERIDONE

Two systematic reviews of RCTs comparing risperidone with standard antipsychotic drugs (mainly haloperidol) have found limited evidence that risperidone may be more effective than standard antipsychotic drugs and good evidence that at lower doses it has fewer adverse effects.

Benefits: **Versus standard antipsychotic drugs:** We found two systematic reviews, and one additional RCT.[15,21,22] Both systematic reviews found that risperidone was more effective than haloperidol. The first review (updated 1997, 14 RCTs, 3401 people) found that, at 12 weeks, risperidone (mean daily dose range 6.1–12 mg) was more effective than standard antipsychotic drugs, usually haloperidol.[21] Outcome was "clinical improvement," variably defined but usually a 20% reduction in general symptoms (2171 people; 11 RCTs, RR no improvement 0.8, 95% CI 0.7 to 0.9; NNT 10, 95% CI 7 to 16). No benefit was observed for the outcome of global clinical impression. The second review (search date 1998, 9 RCTs, 2215 people) found that risperidone was associated with slightly greater success than haloperidol on a composite measure of positive and negative symptoms.[15] The additional RCT (99 people) comparing a range of doses of risperidone with haloperidol found no overall significant difference in global outcome.[22] **Versus other new antipsychotic drugs:** See olanzapine, p 574. One systematic review found no significant difference between risperidone and clozapine for outcomes such as "improvement in mental state" but only 135 people were involved in the three RCTs.

Harms: The systematic review found that risperidone compared with standard antipsychotic drugs caused no significant change in the number of people who withdrew from treatment (2166 people; RR 0.8, 95% CI 0.6 to 1.1). People taking risperidone developed fewer extrapyramidal effects (2279 people; RR 0.6, 95% CI 0.5 to 0.7; NNT 5, 95% CI 5 to 10), required less antiparkinsonian medication (2436 people; RR 0.6, 95% CI 0.5 to 0.7; NNT 7, 95% CI 5 to 10), and were less likely to develop daytime somnolence (2098 people; RR 0.9, 95% CI 0.7 to 0.99; NNT 22, 95% CI 11 to 500). Risperidone was associated with greater weight gain (1652 people; RR 1.4, 95% CI 1.1 to 1.7; NNH 13, 95% CI 8 to 36).[21] The additional RCT found no overall significant difference in the rate of adverse effects between risperidone and haloperidol.[22]

Comment: The reported benefits in the first review over standard antipsychotic drugs were marginal and it found evidence of publication bias.[21]

Sensitivity analyses found that benefits in clinical improvement and continuing treatment of risperidone compared with standard antipsychotic drugs were no longer significant if studies using more than 10 mg haloperidol daily were excluded.[21] This loss of significance could be because of loss of power when studies were excluded. Exclusion of the higher dosage studies did not remove the difference in rate of extrapyramidal adverse effects.[21]

OPTION   ZIPRASIDONE   New

One systematic review of RCTs comparing ziprasidone with standard antipsychotic drugs found no significant difference in mental state improvement but did find a different profile of adverse effects.

Benefits: We found one systematic review (updated 1999, 7 RCTs, 824 people) **Versus standard antipsychotics:** It identified four RCTs of ziprasidone versus standard antipsychotic drugs.[23] It found no significant differences in mental state improvement in different trials (301 people; RR no important improvement in mental state 0.9, 95% CI 0.7 to 1.0).

Harms: **Versus standard antipsychotics:** The review found no clear difference in total adverse events between ziprasidone and haloperidol.[23] Ziprasidone was less likely to cause akathisia in the short term (438 people; RR 0.3, 95% CI 0.2 to 0.6; NNT 8, 95% CI 5 to 18) or in the long term (301 people; RR 0.3, 95% CI 0.1 to 0.7, NNT 9, 95% CI 5 to 21), and less likely to cause acute dystonia (438 people; RR 0.4, 95% CI 0.2 to 0.9, NNT 16, 95% CI 9 to 166). Ziprasidone was more likely to produce nausea and vomiting in both the short (306 people; RR 3.6, 95% CI 1.8 to 7; NNT 5, 95% CI 4 to 8) and in the long term (301 people; RR 2.1, 95% CI 1 to 4, NNT 9, 95% CI 5 to 33). Intramuscular ziprasidone was significantly more likely to be associated with injection site pain than haloperidol (306 people; RR 5.3, 95% CI 1.3 to 22; NNT 12, 95% CI 7 to 27).

Comment: The duration of RCTs was less than 6 weeks. Most reported a withdrawal rate of over 20% and no RCT clearly described adequate precautions for the blinding of treatment allocation. We found no evidence comparing ziprasidone with other new antipsychotic drugs.

OPTION   ZOTEPINE   New

One systematic review of small, brief RCTs that compared zotepine with standard antipsychotic drugs found weak evidence that zotepine reduced a standard symptom severity score and had fewer adverse effects. This finding was not robust as removal of a single RCT alters the conclusion. We found no evidence comparing zotepine with other new antipsychotic drugs.

Benefits: **Versus standard antipsychotic drugs:** We found one systematic review (updated 1999, 10 RCTs, 537 people). The systematic review included eight RCTs comparing zotepine (75–450 mg daily) with a variety of standard antipsychotic drugs.[24] Zotepine was more likely than standard antipsychotic drugs to bring about "clinically important improvement" as defined by a pre-stated cut off point on the Brief Psychiatric Rating Scale (356 people; 4 RCTs, RR 1.25, 95% CI 1.1 to 1.4; NNT 7, 95% CI 4 to 22).

Harms: The review found zotepine caused less akathisia (396 people; RR 0.7, 95% CI 0.6 to 0.9; NNT 8, 95% CI 5 to 34), dystonia (70 people; RR 0.5, 95% CI 0.2 to 0.9; NNT 4, 95% CI 2 to 56), and rigidity (164 people; RR 0.6, 95% CI 0.4 to 0.9; NNT 7, 95% CI 4 to 360) than standard antipsychotic drugs.[24]

Comment: All but one trial were of 12 weeks or less duration and all were conducted in Europe. Only one RCT favoured zotepine over standard antipsychotic drugs and removal of this RCT from the analysis changed the result from a significant to a non-significant effect. Two RCTs found abnormal ECG results in people taking zotepine, but few additional details were given. We found too few trials to compare zotepine reliably with other new antipsychotics.

OPTION   CLOZAPINE

One systematic review of RCTs has found that clozapine is more effective than standard antipsychotic drugs. It is, however, associated with potentially fatal blood dyscrasias. A second systematic review of RCTs found no strong evidence about the effectiveness or safety of clozapine compared with new antipsychotic drugs.

Benefits: **Versus standard antipsychotics:** We found one systematic review (updated in 1998, 31 RCTs, 2530 people; 73% men).[25] Compared with standard antipsychotics such as chlorpromazine and haloperidol, clozapine was associated with greater clinical improvement both in the short term (4–10 weeks, 14 RCTs, 1131 people; RR no important improvement 0.7, 95% CI 0.7 to 0.8; NNT 6, 95% CI 5 to 7) and the long term (heterogeneous data). **Versus new antipsychotics:** We found one systematic review (updated 2000, 8 RCTs) that compared clozapine with the new antipsychotics, including olanzapine and risperidone.[26] It found no significant difference in efficacy, but the number of people studied was too small to rule out a clinically important difference.

Harms: **Versus standard antipsychotics:** Clozapine was more likely to cause hypersalivation (1419 people; RR 3.0, 95% CI 1.8 to 4.7; NNH 3), temperature increases (1147 people; RR 1.8, 95% CI 1.2 to 2.7; NNH 11), and sedation (1527 people; RR 1.2, 95% CI 1.1 to 1.4; NNH 10), but less likely to cause dry mouth (799 people; RR 0.4, 95% CI 0.3 to 0.6; NNT 6) and extrapyramidal adverse effects (1235 people; RR 0.7, 95% CI 0.5 to 0.9; NNT 6).[26] The review found blood problems occurred more frequently with clozapine than with standard antipsychotics (1293 people; AR 3.6% v 1.9%; ARI 1.7, 95% CI 0.9 to 3.2).[25] In a large observational case series leucopenia was reported in 3% of 99 502 people over 5 years. However, it found monitoring white cell (neutrophil) counts was associated with a lower than expected rate of cases of agranulocytosis (382 v 995, AR 0.38% v 1%) and deaths (12 v 149).[27] Dyscrasias were more common in younger people in a single RCT included in the first systematic review (21 people; RR 5.4, 95% CI 10 to 162; NNH 2.5).[25,28] Despite the requirement for regular

blood tests, fewer people withdrew from treatment with clozapine in the long term (1513 people; RR 0.8, 95% CI 0.6 to 0.9; NNH 3).[25]
Versus new antipsychotics: Compared with new antipsychotic drugs (mainly risperidone), clozapine was less likely to cause extrapyramidal adverse effects (305 people; RR 0.3, 95% CI 0.1 to 0.6; NNT 6, 95% CI 4 to 9). Clozapine may also be less likely to cause dry mouth and more likely to cause fatigue, nausea, dizziness, hypersalivation and hypersomnia, but these findings were from one or at most two trials.[26] The second review found no difference in rates of blood dyscrasias between clozapine and the new antipsychoytics, but the number of people studied was too small (558) to rule out a clinically important difference.[26] It found that compared with new antipsychotics, people on clozapine tended to be more satisfied with their treatment, but also to withdraw from trials more easily.[26]

Comment: Some of the benefits of clozapine were more apparent in the long term, depending on which drug was used for comparison in the trials.

QUESTION   Which interventions reduce relapse rates?

OPTION   CONTINUED TREATMENT WITH ANTIPSYCHOTIC DRUGS

One systematic review of follow up studies has found that continuing antipsychotic medication for at least 6 months after an acute episode significantly reduces relapse rates, and that some benefit of continuing treatment is apparent for up to 2 years. We found no evidence of a difference in relapse rates between standard antipsychotic drugs, but a systematic review of RCTs has found that relapse rates are lower with clozapine.

Benefits: **Versus no treatment or placebo:** We found two systematic reviews.[6,29] Both found evidence that continued treatment was beneficial for prevention of relapse. One review (search date not given, 66 studies, 4365 people taking antipsychotic drugs, mean dose 630 mg chlorpromazine equivalents a day, mean follow up of 6.3 months) included 29 controlled trials with a mean follow up of 9.7 months.[29] It found significantly lower relapse in 1224 people maintained on treatment compared with 1224 withdrawn from treatment (16.2% v 51.5%; ARR 35%, 95% CI 33% to 38%; NNT 3, 95% CI 2.6 to 3.1). Over time, the relapse rate in people maintained on antipsychotic treatment approached that in those withdrawn from treatment, but was still lower in those on treatment at 2 years (ARR 22%; NNT 5). The other review (updated in 1997) found that relapse rates over 6–24 months were significantly lower on chlorpromazine than placebo (3 heterogeneous RCTs; RR 0.7, 95% CI 0.5 to 0.9; NNT 3, 95% CI 2.5 to 4).[6] **Choice of drug:** We found eight systematic reviews which found that the choice of drug or preparation did not seem to affect relapse rates. The first (search date 1995) identified six RCTs comparing oral with depot fluphenazine (see table 1, p 577).[30] A second (updated in 1998) identified seven RCTs comparing haloperidol decanoate with other depot antipsychotics.[8] A third (updated in 1999) identified eight RCTs comparing flupenthixol decanoate with other depot antipsychotics.[31] A fourth (updated in 1999) identified seven RCTs comparing pipothiazine palmitate with other depots and two RCTs comparing pipothiazine palmitate with oral antipsychotics.[9] A fifth (updated in 1999) identified one RCT comparing fluspirilene decanoate with oral chlorpromazine and three studies comparing fluspirilene decanoate with other depot preparations.[32] A sixth (updated in 1999) found one RCT comparing perphenazine enanthate with clopenthixol decanoate.[33] The reviews comparing pimozide and olanzapine versus typical antipsychotic drugs also found no significant difference in relapse rates.[12–14] The number of people studied was too small to rule out clinically important differences. One systematic review comparing clozapine with standard antipsychotic drugs (search date 1998) found that relapse rates up to 12 weeks were significantly lower with clozapine (19 RCTs; RR 0.6, 95% CI 0.5 to 0.8; NNT 20).[25] Another systematic review found that significantly fewer people taking depot zuclopenthixol decanoate relapsed over 12 weeks to 1 year compared with people taking other depot preparations (3 RCTs, 296 people; RR 0.7, 95% CI 0.6 to 1.0; NNT 9, 95% CI 5 to 53).[34]

Harms: Mild transient nausea, malaise, sweating, vomiting, insomnia, and dyskinesia were reported in an unspecified number of people after sudden drug cessation, but were usually acceptable with gradual dose reduction.[35] Annual incidence of tardive dyskinesia was 5%.[34]

Comment: In the systematic review of continued versus withdrawal of treatment, meta-analysis of the 29 controlled trials gave similar results to those obtained when all 66 studies were included (ARR 37%, NNT 3).[34] The review was weakened because all RCT results were used rather than weighted comparisons, no length of time was given since the last acute episode, and no distinction was made between people experiencing a first episode and those with chronic illness.[34] Some clinicians use depot antipsychotic medication in selected people to ensure adherence with medication. We found no evidence from RCTs to support this practice.

OPTION   FAMILY INTERVENTIONS

One systematic review of RCTs has found that family intervention significantly reduces relapse rates compared with usual care.

Benefits: We found one systematic review (updated 1999, 13 RCTs) and one additional RCT comparing family interventions with usual care.[36,37] Family interventions consisted mainly of education about the illness and training in problem solving over at least six weekly sessions. Three of the trials included substantial proportions of people experiencing their first episode. Family interventions significantly reduced relapse rates at 12 and 24 months. At 12 months, the risk of relapse was reduced (6 RCTs, 516 people; RR 0.7, 95% CI 0.5 to 1.0), such that seven families would have to be treated to avoid one additional relapse (and likely hospitalisation) in the family member with schizophrenia (NNT 7, 95% CI 4 to 14).[38] We found one potentially relevant additional RCT of family interventions compared with psychoeducation.[39] It will be assessed for the next issue of *Clinical Evidence*.

Harms: No harms were reported, although illness education could possibly have adverse consequences on morale and outlook.[38]

Comment: These results are likely to overestimate treatment effect because of the difficulty of blinding people and investigators and the likelihood of publication bias.[36] The trend over time is for results to tend to the null. The mechanism for the effects of family intervention remains unclear. It is thought to work by reducing "expressed emotion" (hostility and criticism) in relatives of people with schizophrenia, but may act through improved adherence to medication. The time consuming nature of this intervention, which must normally take place at evenings or weekends, can limit its availability. It cannot be applied to people who have little contact with home based carers.

OPTION   SOCIAL SKILLS TRAINING

Limited evidence from RCTs suggests that social skills training may reduce relapse rates.

Benefits: We found one non-systematic review and meta-analysis of 27 RCTs (search date not given) comparing social skills training with usual care.[40] The trials were mainly in men admitted to hospital, not all of whom had schizophrenia, using different techniques that generally included instruction in social interaction. Four studies provided quantitative information, of which three defined relapse as rehospitalisation. Social skills training significantly reduced relapse rates (WMD 0.47). However, sensitivity analysis indicated that five null results (in studies not identified by a search) would render the difference non-significant. One systematic review (search date 1988) identified 73 RCTs in people with a variety of psychiatric disorders and found similar results, but suggested that motivation was an important predictor of benefit from treatment.[41]

Harms: None reported.

Comment: Many of the trials simultaneously compared the effects of other interventions (medication, education), so the effects of individual interventions are difficult to assess. Overall, it remains uncertain whether people at different stages of illness and function require different approaches. Selected people may benefit even from interventions of short duration.

OPTION   COGNITIVE BEHAVIOURAL THERAPY

Limited evidence from RCTs suggests that cognitive behavioural therapy may reduce relapse rates.

Benefits: We found one systematic review (search date 1998, 4 small RCTs) comparing cognitive behavioural therapy plus standard care with standard care alone.[42] All trials incorporated the challenging of key beliefs, problem solving, and enhancement of coping. Relapse rates were significantly reduced in the short, medium, and long term. In the long term (up to 18 months), cognitive behavioural therapy plus standard care reduced the risk of relapse (3 RCTs, 183 people; RR 0.7, 95% CI 0.5 to 0.9; NNT 6, 95% CI 3 to 30).

Harms: None reported.

Mental health

Comment: None of the three trials contributing long term results were blinded, and each concentrated on different clinical issues — symptoms, adherence to treatment, or general rehabilitation. The fourth trial blinded outcome raters and included an additional supportive psychotherapy control group. It found non-significantly lower relapse rates with cognitive behavioural therapy (1 RCT, 59 people; RR 0.6, 95% CI 0.2 to 2.1).

QUESTION   **Which interventions are effective in people resistant to standard treatment?**

One systematic review of RCTs has found clozapine to benefit people who are resistant to standard treatment.

Benefits: **Clozapine:** We found one systematic review (updated 1998, 6 RCTs) comparing clozapine with standard antipsychotic drugs in people who were resistant to standard treatment.[25] Clozapine achieved improvement both in the short term (6–12 weeks: 370 people; 4 RCTs, RR for no improvement compared with standard antipsychotic drugs 0.7, 95% CI 0.6 to 0.8; NNT 5) and in the longer term (12–24 months: 648, 2 RCTs, RR 0.8, 95% CI 0.6 to 1.0). There was no difference in relapse rates in the short term. **Other interventions:** We found no good evidence on the effects of other interventions in people resistant to standard treatment.

Harms: See harms of clozapine, p 567.

Comment: Trials are under way to clarify the mode of action of cognitive behavioural therapy and establish its effects in people who are resistant to standard treatments.

QUESTION   **Which interventions improve adherence to antipsychotic medication?**

OPTION   COMPLIANCE THERAPY   New

We found limited evidence from three RCTs that compliance therapy (see glossary, p 574) may increase adherence with antipsychotic medication.

Benefits: We found no systematic review. We found one RCT of compliance therapy versus supportive counselling, that included 47 people with acute psychoses, although the majority fulfilled criteria for schizophrenia or had been admitted with the first episode of a psychotic illness.[38,43] People treated with compliance therapy were significantly more likely to attain at least passive acceptance of antipsychotic medication compared with people who received non-specific counselling, both immediately after the intervention (OR 6.3, 95% CI 1.6 to 24.6) and at six months follow up (OR 5.2, 95% CI 1.5 to 18.3). At 18 months (for an extended sample of 74 people) a significant improvement on a seven point scale of medication adherence was found for people treated with compliance therapy (mean difference 1.4, 95% CI 0.9 to 1.6).

Harms: None reported.

Comment: Other studies have examined the potential benefits of compliance therapy but either did not employ a standardised measure of adherence or adherence was not rated in a blind fashion. The RCT above requires independent replication. About one third of each group did not complete the trials and missing data are estimated from the mean scores in each group. Calculation of NNTs was not possible due to missing data.

OPTION   FAMILY THERAPY   New

Limited evidence from three RCTs suggests that family therapy is an effective intervention for improving adherence with antipsychotic medication.

Benefits: We found no systematic review. We found three RCTs of family therapy in schizophrenia that directly assessed its impact on adherence to antipsychotic medication.[39,44,45] The first trial, conducted in the UK, compared family therapy with individual supportive therapy in 32 people recently discharged from hospital who all had at least one parent who exhibited high "expressed emotion".[39] People were followed up for six months. Those receiving family therapy were significantly more likely to take at least half of their prescribed antipsychotic dose than those receiving supportive therapy (ARI 0.54, NNT 2, 95% CI 2 to 5) as judged by tablet counts, reports from people with schizophrenia, their family, and blood levels. The second and third RCTs were conducted in China and used comparison with standard care only. The two trials may have included some or all of the same people. The first of these (63 people) measured adherence as "compliance with medication for at least 75% of the non-hospitalised follow up period".[44] The trial found no advantage of family therapy over standard care using the numbers of people in each group compliant with 50% of their medication dose, or when using the months of medication as an outcome measure. The third RCT was in 78 men with schizophrenia admitted to hospital for the first time.[45] Adherence was measured according to a criterion of "people taking at least 33% of the dose prescribed at the time of the index discharge for at least six days per week". The trial found an increase in medicated adherence with family therapy compared with standard care (ARI 0.23; NNT 5, 95% CI 3 to 34).

Harms: None reported.

Comment: The first trial was conducted in the UK and found that family therapy also improved attendance at clinic appointments. Both of the Chinese studies refer to the unique family structure in China. How adherence to medication was judged is unclear, but appears to have been rated blind to treatment allocation.

OPTION   PSYCHOEDUCATIONAL THERAPY   New

Two RCTs have found that psychoeducational therapy has no significant effect on adherence to antipsychotic medication.

Benefits: We found no systematic review. **Versus usual treatment:** We found one RCT (36 men) comparing psychoeducation versus behavioural therapy versus usual treatment.[46] It found no significant difference between psychoeducation and usual treatment (quantified results not presented). **Versus behavioural therapy:** We found three RCTs.[46–48] One RCT compared behavioural therapy with psychoeducation (36 men) and with usual treatment.[46] The behavioural training method comprised being told the importance of complying with antipsychotic medication and instructions on how to take medication. Each participant was given a self-monitoring spiral calendar, which featured a dated slip of paper for each dose of antipsychotic. Adherence was estimated by pill counts. After three months fewer people had high pill adherence after psychoeducation compared with behaviour therapy (3/11 v 8/11 had pill adherence scores of 80% measured by pill counts). The second RCT (39 people) compared a behavioural intervention given individually, a behavioural intervention involving the person with schizophrenia and their family, and a psychoeducational intervention.[47] The behavioural intervention consisted of specific written guidelines, and oral instructions, given to people to use a pill box consisting of 28 compartments for every medication occasion during a week. The behavioural intervention, when given to the individual and their family, also consisted of instructions for the family member to compliment the person with schizophrenia for taking their prescribed medication. The primary outcome measure was pill count at two months. Medication adherence was more likely with behavioural interventions than with psychoeducation (over 90% adherence at 2 months, 25/26 with behavioural methods versus 6/13 with psychoeducation; ARR 0.5, RR 2.1, NNT 2 95% CI 2 to 5). We found one subsequent RCT which may be relevant.[48] It will be appraised for the next issue of *Clinical Evidence*.

Harms: None reported.

Comment: The first trial found low correlation between the different measures of compliance. The second trial also included some people with non-psychotic chronic psychiatric disorders and some people who were not taking antipsychotic medication. Both trials involved small numbers of people.

| OPTION | BEHAVIOURAL THERAPY | New |

One RCT found that behavioural interventions improved adherence to antipsychotic medication compared with usual treatment. One RCT found that behavioural interventions improved adherence compared with psychoeducational therapy.

Benefits: We found no systematic review. **Versus usual treatment:** We found one RCT (36 men).[46] The behavioural training method comprised being told the importance of complying with antipsychotic medication and instructions on how to take medication. Each participant was given a self-monitoring spiral calendar, which featured a dated slip of paper for each dose of antipsychotic. Adherence was estimated by pill counts. After 3 months fewer people had high pill adherence after usual treatment compared with behaviour therapy (figures not presented). **Versus psychoeducational therapy:** see above.

Schizophrenia

Harms: None reported.

Comment: See above.

GLOSSARY

Compliance therapy A treatment based on cognitive behaviour therapy and motivational interviewing techniques with a view to improving concordance to medication.

Substantive changes since last issue

Chlorpromazine Updated systematic review[7] includes three additional RCTs (total 45 RCTs); no change in conclusion.

Clozapine Updated systematic review[26] includes four additional RCTs (total 8 RCTs); no change in conclusion.

Continued treatment with antipsychotic drugs Three additional systematic reviews (total 8 systematic reviews); no change in conclusion.[9–33]

Additional RCTs have subsequently been identified and may be included in future issues of *Clinical Evidence*.

REFERENCES

1. Andreasen NC. Symptoms, signs and diagnosis of schizophrenia. *Lancet* 1995;346:477–481.
2. Cannon M, Jones P. Neuroepidemiology: schizophrenia. *J Neurol Neurosurg Psychiatry* 1996;61:604–613.
3. Jablensky A, Sartorius N, Ernberg G, et al. Schizophrenia: manifestations, incidence and course in different cultures. A World Health Organisation ten-country study. *Psychol Med* 1992;monograph supplement 20:1–97.
4. Hegarty JD, Baldessarini RJ, Tohen M, Waternaux C, Oepen G. One hundred years of schizophrenia: a meta-analysis of the outcome literature. *Am J Psychiatry* 1994;151:1409–1416.
5. Johnstone EC. Schizophrenia: problems in clinical practice. *Lancet* 1993; 341:536–538.
6. Thornley B, Adams C. Content and quality of 2000 controlled trials in schizophrenia over 50 years. *BMJ* 1998;317:1181–1184.
7. Thornley B, Adams CE, Awad G. Chlorpromazine versus placebo for those with schizophrenia. In: The Cochrane Library, Issue 2, 2000. Oxford: Update Software. Search date 1999; primary sources Biological Abstracts; Embase; Medline; Psyclit; SciSearch; Cochrane Library; Cochrane Schizophrenia Groups register; and hand searches of reference lists; and personal contact with pharmaceutical companies and authors of trials.
8. Quraishi S, David A. Depot haloperidol decanoate for schizophrenia. In: The Cochrane Library, Issue 2, 2000. Oxford: Update Software. Search date 1998; primary sources Biological Abstracts; Embase; Medline; Psyclit; SciSearch; Cochrane Library; reference lists; authors of studies; pharmaceutical companies.
9. Quraishi S, David A. Depot pipothiazine palmitate and undeclynate for schizophrenia. In: The Cochrane Library, Issue 2, 2000. Oxford: Update Software. Search strategy 1998; primary sources Biological Abstracts; Cochrane Library; Cochrane Schizophrenia Group's Register; Embase; Medline; and Psyclit; and hand searches of reference lists; and personal communication with pharmaceutical companies.
10. Bagnall A-M, Fenton M, Lewis R, Leitner ML, Kleijnen J. Molindone for schizophrenia and severe mental illness. In: The Cochrane Library, Issue 2, 2000. Oxford: Update Software. Search date 1999; primary sources; Biological Abstracts; The Cochrane Library Central, The Cochrane Schizophrenia Group's Register, Cinahl; Embase; Psyclit; and pharmaceutical databases and hand searches of reference lists and personal contact with authors of trials.
11. Fenton M, Murphy B, Wood J, Bagnell A-M, Schou P, Leitner M. Loxapine for schizophrenia. In: The Cochrane Library, Issue 2, 2000. Oxford: Update Software. Search date 1999; primary sources Biological Abstracts; The Cochrane Library; The Cochrane Schizophrenia Group's Register; Embase; Lilacs; Psyndex; and PsycLIT; and hand searches of reference lists.
12. Sultana A, McMonagle T. Pimozide for schizophrenia or related psychoses. In: The Cochrane Library, Issue 2, 2000. Oxford: Update Software. Search date 1999; Biological Abstracts; The Cochrane Schizophrenia Group's Register; Embase; Janssen-Cilag UK's register of studies; Medline; and hand searches of reference lists and personal contact with pharmaceutical companies.
13. Joy CB, Mumby-Croft R, Joy LA. Polyunsaturated fatty acid (fish or evening primrose oil) for schizophrenia. In: The Cochrane Library, Issue 2, 2000. Oxford: Update Software. Search date 2000; primary sources Biological Abstracts; Cinahl; The Cochrane Library; The Cochrane Schizophrenia Group's Register; Embase; and Psyclit; and hand searches of reference lists; and personal contact with the authors.
14. Duggan L, Fenton M, Dardennes RM, El-Dosoky A, Indran S. Olanzapine for schizophrenia. In: The Cochrane Library, Issue 2, 2000. Oxford: Update Software. Search date June 1998; primary sources Biological Abstracts; Embase; Medline; Psyclit; Cochrane Library; and hand searches of reference lists and conference abstracts; personal communication with authors of trials and pharmaceutical companies.
15. Leucht S, Pitschel-Walx G, Abraham D, Kissling W. Efficacy and extrapyramidal side-effects of the new antipsychotics olanzapine, quetiapine, ripseridone and sertindole compared to conventional antipsychotics and placebo. A meta-analysis of randomised controlled trials. *Schizophr Res* 1999; 35:51–68. Search date 1999; primary sources Medline; Current Contents; and hand searches of reference lists; and personal communication with pharmaceutical companies.
16. Tuunainen A, Gilbody SM. Newer atypical antipsychotic medication versus clozapine for

schizophrenia. In: The Cochrane Library, Issue 2, 2000. Oxford: Update Software. Search date May 1998; primary sources Biological Abstracts; Cochrane Schizophrenia Group's register; Cochrane Library; Embase; Lilacs; Medline; Psyclit; and hand searches of reference lists; and personal contact with authors of trials and pharmaceutical companies.

17. Revicki D, Genduso L, Hamilton S, Ganoczy D, and Beasley C. Olanzapine versus haloperidol in the treatment of schizophrenia and other psychotic disorders: quality of life and clinical outcomes of a randomized clinical trial. *Qual Life Res* 1999;8: 417–426.

18. Srisurapanont M, Disayavanish C, Taimkaew K. Quetiapine for schizophrenia. In: The Cochrane Library, Issue 2, 2000. Oxford: Update Software. Search date 1998; primary sources Biological Abstracts; Embase; Medline; Psyclit; Cochrane Library; Cinahl; Sigle; Sociofile; hand searches of journals; personal communication with authors of studies and pharmaceutical companies.

19. Copolov DL, Link CGG, Kowalcyk B. A multicentre, double-blind, randomized comparison of quetiapine (ICI 204,636, "Seroquel") and haloperidol in schizophrenia. *Psychol Med* 2000; 30:95–105.

20. Barbui C. Quetiapine for schizophrenia. (Commentary). *Evid Based Mental Health* 1999;2: 52.

21. Kennedy E, Song F, Hunter R, Clarke Q, Gilbody S. Risperidone versus typical antipsychotic medication for schizophrenia. In: The Cochrane Library, Issue 2, 2000. Oxford: Update Software. Search date 1997; primary sources Biological Abstracts; The Cochrane Trials Register; Embase; Medline; and Psyclit; and hand searches of reference lists; and hand searches of reference lists; and personal communication with pharmaceutical companies.

22. Lopez Ibor JJ, Ayuso JL, Gutierrez M, et al. Risperidone in the treatment of chronic schizophrenia: multicenter study comparative to haloperidol. *Actas Luso Esp Neurol Psiquiatr Cienc Afines* 1996;24:165–172.

23. Bagnall A-M, Lewis RA, Leitner ML, Kleijnen J. Ziprasidone for schizophrenia and severe mental illness. In: The Cochrane Library, Issue 2, 2000. Oxford: Update Software. Search date 1999; primary sources Biological Abstracts; The Cochrane Library; The Cochrane Schizophrenia Group's Register; Embase; Lilacs; Psyndex; and Psyclit; pharmaceutical databases; and hand searches of reference lists; and personal contact with authors of trials.

24. Fenton M, Morris F, De Silva P, et al. Zotepine for schizophrenia. In: The Cochrane Library, Issue 2, 2000. Oxford: Update Software. Search date 1999; primary sources Biological Abstracts; The Cochrane Library; The Cochrane Schizophrenia Group's Register; Embase; Dialog Corporation Datastar service; Medline; and Psyclit; and hand searches of reference lists; and personal contact with authors of trials and pharmaceutical companies.

25. Wahlbeck K, Cheine M, Essali MA. Clozapine versus typical neuroleptic medication for schizophrenia. In: The Cochrane Library, Issue 2, 2000. Oxford: Update Software. Search date 1999; primary sources Biological Abstracts; Cochrane Schizophrenia Group's register; Cochrane Library; Embase; Lilacs; Medline; Psyclit; SciSearch — Science Citation Index; and hand searches of reference lists; and personal communication with pharmaceutical companies.

26. Tuunainen A, Gilbody SM. Newer atypical antipsychotic medication versus clozapine for schizophrenia. In: The Cochrane Library, Issue 2, 2000. Oxford: Update Software. Search date 1998; primary sources Biological Abstracts; Cochrane Schizophrenia Group's register; Cochrane Library; Embase; Lilacs; Medline; Psyclit; and hand searches of reference lists; and personal communicatio with authors of trials and pharmaceutical companies.

27. Honigfeld G, Arellano F, Sethi J, Bianchini A, Schein J. Reducing clozapine-related morbidity and mortality: five years experience of the Clozaril national registry. *J Clin Psychiatry* 1998;59(suppl 3):3–7.

28. Kumra S, Frazier JA, Jacobsen LK, et al. Childhood-onset schizophrenia. A double-blind clozapine-haloperidol comparison. *Arch Gen Psychiatry* 1996;53:1090–1097.

29. Gilbert PL, Harris MJ, McAdams LA, Jeste DV. Neuroleptic withdrawal in schizophrenic people: a review of the literature. *Arch Gen Psychiatry* 1995; 52:173–188. Search date not given; primary source Medline.

30. Adams CE, Eisenbruch M. Depot fluphenazine versus oral fluphenazine for those with schizophrenia. In: The Cochrane Library, Issue 2, 2000. Oxford: Update Software. Search date May 1995; primary sources Biological Abstracts; Cochrane Library; Cochrane Schizophrenia Group's register; Embase; Medline; Psyclit; Science Citation Index; hand searches of reference lists and personal communication with pharmaceutical companies.

31. Quraishi S, David A. Depot flupenthixol decanoate for schizophrenia or similar psychotic disorders. In: The Cochrane Library, Issue 2, 2000. Oxford: Update Software. Search date 1998; primary sources Biological Abstracts; Cochrane Library; Cochrane Schizophrenia Group's register; Embase; Medline; Psyclit; SciSearch; references, personal communication with authors of trials and pharmaceutical companies.

32. Quraishi S, David A. Depot fluspirilene for schizophrenia. In: The Cochrane Library, Issue 2, 2000. Oxford: Update Software. Search date 1998; primary sources Biological Abstracts; Cochrane Library; The Cochrane Schizophrenia Group's Register; Embase; Medline; and Psyclit; and hand searches of reference lists.

33. Quraishi S, David A. Depot perphenazine decanoate and enanthate for schizophrenia. In: The Cochrane Library, Issue 2, 2000. Oxford: Update Software. Search date 1998; primary sources Biological Abstracts; The Cochrane Library; The Cochrane Schizophrenia Group's Register; Embase; Medline; and Psyclit; and hand searches of reference lists; and personal communication with the pharmaceutical companies.

34. Coutinho E, Fenton M, Quraishi S. Zuclopenthixol decanoate for schizophrenia and other serious mental illnesses. In: The Cochrane Library, Issue 2, 2000. Oxford: Update software. Search date April 1998; primary sources Biological Abstracts 1982 to 1998, CINAHL 1982 to 1998), The Cochrane Library Issue 2, 2000, The Cochrane Schizophrenia Group's Register April 1998, Embase 1980 to 1998, Medline 1966 to 1998, Psyclit 1974 to 1998. References of all eligible studies were searched for further trials. The manufacturer of zuclopenthixol was contacted.

35. Jeste D, Gilbert P, McAdams L, Harris M. Considering neuroleptic maintenance and taper on a continuum: need for an individual rather than dogmatic approach. *Arch Gen Psychiatry* 1995; 52:209–212.

36. Pharaoh FM, Mari JJ, Streiner D. Family intervention for schizophrenia. In: The Cochrane

Library, Issue 2, 2000. Oxford: Update Software. Search date 1998; primary sources Medline; Embase; Cochrane Library; Cochrane Schizophrenia Group's Register of Trials; reference lists of articles.

37. McFarlane WR, Lukens E, Link B, et al. Multiple-family groups and psychoeducation in the treatment of schizophrenia. Arch Gen Psychiatry 1995;52:679–687.

38. Kemp R, Kirov G, Everitt B, Hayward P, David A. Randomised controlled trial of compliance therapy. 18-month follow-up. Br J Psychiatry 1998;172:413–419.

39. Strang JS, Falloon IRH, Moss HB, Razani J, Boyd JL. Drug treatment and family intervention during the aftercare treatment of schizophrenics. Psychopharmacology Bull 1981;17:87–88.

40. Benton MK, Schroeder HE. Social skills training with schizophrenics: a meta-analytic evaluation. J Consult Clin Psychol 1990;58:741–747. Search date not given.

41. Corrigan PW. Social skills training in adult psychiatric populations: a meta-analysis. J Behav Ther Exp Psychiatry 1991;22:203–210. Search date 1988; primary sources Psychological Abstracts.

42. Jones C, Cormac I, Mota J, Campbell C. Cognitive behavioural therapy for schizophrenia. In: The Cochrane Library, Issue 2, 2000. Oxford: Update Software. Search date July 1998; primary sources Biological abstracts; Cochrane Schizophrenia Group's Register of Trials; Cinahl; Cochrane Library; Medline; Embase; Psyclit; Sigle; Sociofile; reference lists of articles; and personal communication with authors of trials.

43. Kemp R, Hayward P, Applewhaite G, Everitt B, David A. Compliance therapy in psychotic people: randomised controlled trial. BMJ 1996;312:345–349.

44. Xiong W, Phillips MR, Hu X, et al. Family-based intervention for schizophrenic people in China. A randomised controlled trial. Br J Psychiatry 1994;165:239–247.

45. Zhang M, Wang M, Li J, Phillips MR. Randomised-control trial of family intervention for 78 first-episode male schizophrenic people. An 18-month study in Suzhou, Jiangsu. Br J Psychiatry 1994;165:96–102.

46. Boczkowski JA, Zeichner A, DeSanto N. Neuroleptic compliance among chronic schizophrenic outpeople: an intervention outcome report. J Consult Clin Psychol 1985;53:666–671.

47. Azrin NH, Teichner G. Evaluation of an instructional program for improving medication compliance for chronically mentally ill outpatients. Behaviour Res Ther 1998;36:849–861.

48. Liberman RP, Wallace CJ, Blackwell G, Kopelowicz A, Vaccaro JV. et al. Mintz skills training versus psychological occupational therapy for persons with persistent schizophrenia. Am J Psychiatry 1998;155;8:1087–1091.

Stephen M Lawrie
Senior Clinical Research Fellow and
Honorary Consultant Psychiatrist
University of Edinburgh
Edinburgh
UK

Andrew McIntosh
Lecturer in Psychiatry
Department of Psychiatry
University of Edinburgh
Edinburgh
UK

Competing interests: Stephen Lawrie has been paid for speaking about critical appraisal, has had travel expenses for a conference reimbursed by Janssen the manufacturers of Risperidone, and has been paid for speaking about critical appraisal and chairing a symposium by Eli Lilly, the manufacturer of olanzapine.

TABLE 1 Continued treatment with antipsychotic drugs: choice of drugs (see text, p 568).

Review	Search Date	Number of RCTs	Comparisons	Main Conclusion
30	1995	6	Oral v depot fluphenazine	No significant difference
8	1998	7	Haloperidol decanoate v other depots	No significant difference
31	1998	8	Flupenthixol decanoate v other depots	No significant difference
9	1998	7	Pipothiazine palmitate v other depots	No significant difference
9	1998	2	Pipothiazine palmitate v oral antipsychotics	No significant difference
32	1998	1	Fluspirilene decanoate v oral chlorpromazine	No significant difference
32	1998	3	Fluspirilene decanoate v other depots	No significant difference
33	1998	1	Perphenazine enanthate v clopenthixol decanoate	No significant difference
12	1999	11	Pimozide v standard antipsychotics	No significant difference
14	1998	1	Olanzapine v standard antipsychotics	No significant difference
34	1998	3	Zuclopenthixol decanoate v other depots	People taking zuclopenthixol had lower relapse rates over 12 weeks to 1 year
25	1999	19	Clozapine v standard antipsychotics	Relapse rates up to 12 weeks were lower with clozapine

Chronic fatigue syndrome

Updated this issue

Steven Reid, Trudie Chalder, Anthony Cleare, Matthew Hotopf and Simon Wessely

INTERVENTIONS

Key Messages

- Limited data from four RCTs provide insufficient evidence to support the use of antidepressants in people with chronic fatigue syndrome (CFS).

- Limited data from three RCTs provide insufficient evidence to support the use of corticosteroids in people with CFS. Any benefit from low dose glucocorticoid treatment seems to be short lived, and higher doses are associated with adverse effects.

- One small RCT found limited benefit from oral nicotinamide adenine dinucleotide (NADH).

- Two RCTs found that a graded exercise programme produced substantial improvements in measures of fatigue and physical functioning in people with CFS.

- We found no evidence that prolonged rest is an effective treatment for CFS. We found indirect evidence suggesting that prolonged rest may be harmful.

- Limited data from three small RCTs provide no clear evidence of benefit from magnesium injections or oral evening primrose oil in people with CFS.

- Four small RCTs of Immunoglobulin G (IgG) in people with CFS found only limited benefit and adverse effects. RCTs of other forms of immunotherapy found no evidence of an advantage over placebo.

- A systematic review has found that cognitive behavioural therapy administered by highly skilled therapists in specialist centres is effective in people with CFS, with a number needed to treat of 2. This finding may be of limited relevance to less specialised settings.

DEFINITION	Chronic fatigue syndrome (CFS) is characterised by severe, disabling fatigue and other symptoms, including musculoskeletal pain, sleep disturbance, impaired concentration and headaches. Two widely used definitions of CFS (see table 1, p 586) from the US Centers for Disease Control and Prevention [1] and Oxford, UK[2] were developed as operational criteria for research. There are two important differences between these definitions. The UK criteria insist upon the presence of mental fatigue, whereas the US criteria include a requirement for several physical symptoms, reflecting the belief that CFS has an underlying immunological or infective pathology.
INCIDENCE/ PREVALENCE	Community and primary care based studies have reported the prevalence of CFS to be 0.2–2.6%, depending on the criteria used.[3,4] Systematic population surveys have found similar rates of CFS in people of different socioeconomic status, and in all ethnic groups.[4,5] Women are at higher risk than men (RR 1.3 to 1.7 depending on diagnostic criteria used).[6]
AETIOLOGY/ RISK FACTORS	The cause of CFS is poorly understood.
PROGNOSIS	Studies have focused on people attending specialist clinics. A systematic review of studies of prognosis (search date 1996) found that children with CFS had a notably better outcome than adults; 54–94% of children showed definite improvement (after up to 6 years' follow up) whereas 20–50% of adults showed some improvement in the medium term and only 6% returned to premorbid levels of functioning.[7] Despite the considerable burden of morbidity associated with CFS, we found no evidence of increased mortality. The systematic review found that outcome was influenced by the presence of psychiatric disorders and beliefs about causation and treatment.[7]
AIMS	To reduce levels of fatigue and associated symptoms; to increase levels of activity; to improve quality of life.
OUTCOMES	Severity of symptoms and their effects on physical function and quality of life. These outcomes are measured in several different ways: the medical outcomes survey short form general health survey (SF-36),[8] a rating scale measuring limitation of physical functioning caused by ill health; the Karnofsky scale,[9] a modified questionnaire originally developed for the rating of quality of life in people undergoing chemotherapy for malignancy; the Beck Depression Inventory;[10] the sickness impact profile,[11] a measure of the influence of symptoms on social and physical functioning; and self reported severity of symptoms and levels of activity.
METHODS	*Clinical Evidence* update search and appraisal May 2000.

QUESTION What are the effects of treatments?

OPTION ANTIDEPRESSANTS

Limited data from four RCTs provide insufficient evidence to support the use of antidepressants in people with CFS.

Benefits:
We found no systematic reviews. We found three RCTs. One compared fluoxetine versus placebo in 96 people.[12] It found no significant benefit in terms of the Beck Depression Inventory and the sickness impact profile. Another RCT allocated 136 people to four groups: exercise plus fluoxetine; exercise plus placebo; appointments to review activity diary with physiotherapist plus fluoxetine; and appointments to review activity diary with physiotherapist plus placebo. It found no significant difference in outcome (level of fatigue), although there was a trend indicating some benefit and there were modest improvements in measures of depression.[13] A third RCT compared the monoamine oxidase inhibitor phenelzine versus placebo in 24 people with CFS, using a modified Karnofsky scale and other outcome measures.[14*] This also found a non-significant trend towards improvement. We found one RCT comparing sertraline versus clomipramine in people with CFS. There was no placebo group, making it difficult to draw useful conclusions.[15]

Harms:
Up to 15% of participants withdrew from active treatment because of adverse drug effects.[12–15]

Comment:
To date, clinical trials have taken place in specialist clinics, which may actively select for people whose condition is more resistant to treatment. The first trial[12] used shorter treatment and studied people with a long duration of illness than the second trial.[13]

OPTION CORTICOSTEROIDS

Limited data from three RCTs provide insufficient evidence about the effects of corticosteroids in people with CFS. Any benefit from low dose glucocorticoids seems to be short lived, and higher doses are associated with adverse effects.

Benefits:
We found no systematic review. **Versus placebo:** We found three placebo controlled RCTs in people with CFS. One, a crossover RCT of fludrocortisone in 20 people, measured outcomes as change in symptom severity, on a visual analogue scale, and functional status (using the SF-36).[16] It found no significant difference between active treatment and placebo. The other two trials evaluated hydrocortisone. One compared hydrocortisone 25–35 mg daily versus placebo in 65 people and found a greater improvement in a self rated scale of "wellness" in the active treatment group. Other self rating scales did not show significant benefit.[17] The other trial used a lower dose of hydrocortisone (5 or 10 mg daily) in 32 people and found short term improvement in fatigue. Nine people (28%) taking hydrocortisone improved, as measured by a self report fatigue scale, compared with three (9%) taking placebo. The benefit rapidly attenuated when treatment was stopped.[18]

Harms: The trial using the higher doses of hydrocortisone found that 12 people (40%) on active treatment experienced adrenal suppression.[17] Minor adverse effects were reported in up to 10% of people in the other trials.[16,18]

Comment: The RCT of fludrocortisone may have had too few participants to detect a difference. The trials used different reasons for their choice of active treatment. The use of fludrocortisone, a mineralocorticoid, was based on the hypothesis that CFS is associated with neurally mediated hypotension.[19] The use of hydrocortisone in the other trials was based on evidence of underactivity of the hypothalamic-pituitary-adrenocortical axis in some people with CFS.[20]

OPTION   ORAL NADH

One small RCT found limited benefit from oral NADH.

Benefits: We found no systematic review. We found one randomised cross-over trial comparing NADH 10 mg per day) versus placebo for 4 weeks.[21] Of the 33 people with CFS who completed the trial, 26 were included in the analysis. Using a symptom rating scale, 8/26 attained a 10% improvement on active treatment compared with 2/26 on placebo.

Harms: Minor adverse effects (loss of appetite, dyspepsia, flatulence) were reported on active treatment but did not lead to cessation of treatment.

Comment: The rationale for this treatment is that NADH facilitates generation of adenosine triphosphate, which it is suggested may be depleted in CFS.[21] The authors are planning a larger trial.

OPTION   EXERCISE

Two RCTs found that a graded exercise programme substantially improved measures of fatigue and physical functioning in people with CFS.

Benefits: We found no systematic review. We found two RCTs. The first compared aerobic exercise versus flexibility training (control intervention) in 66 people.[22] The programmes involved individual weekly sessions over 12 weeks. The exercise group built up their level of activity to 30 minutes of exercise a day, with a maximum energy expenditure of 60% of maximum oxygen consumption (VO_2max). Using the self rated clinical global impression scales as an outcome measure, 55% of the aerobic exercise group reported feeling much better or very much better compared with 27% of the flexibility training group ($P = 0.05$). Significantly better outcomes were also reported as measured by physical fatigue and levels of physical functioning on SF-36. The flexibility training group crossed over to aerobic exercise at the end of the trial, and significant improvements from baseline were found. The second trial randomised 136 people with CFS to one of four groups: exercise plus fluoxetine; exercise plus placebo; appointments plus fluoxetine; and appointments plus placebo.[13] The exercise group undertook graded aerobic exercise for 20 minutes three times a week up to an energy expenditure of 75% of VO_2max. Exercise was associated with significant improvements in fatigue and functional work capacity. This trial was complicated by a high withdrawal rate, particularly in the exercise groups (37% v 22% in the appointment groups), but the differences remained significant after intention to treat analysis.

Harms: Neither trial reported data on adverse effects, and we found no evidence that exercise is harmful in people with CFS.

Comment: Experience suggests that symptoms of CFS may be exacerbated by over ambitious or over hasty attempts at exercise.

OPTION   **PROLONGED REST**

We found no evidence that prolonged rest is an effective treatment for CFS. We found considerable indirect evidence suggesting that prolonged rest may be harmful.

Benefits: We found no systematic reviews or RCTs of prolonged rest in people with CFS.

Harms: We found no direct evidence of harmful effects of rest in people with CFS. We found observational evidence suggesting that prolonged inactivity may perpetuate or worsen fatigue and its associated symptoms in both healthy volunteers[23] and in people recovering from viral illness.[24]

Comment: None.

OPTION   **DIETARY SUPPLEMENTS**

One small RCT found limited evidence of benefit from magnesium injections. Two small RCTs of oral evening primrose oil found mixed results.

Benefits: We found no systematic review. **Magnesium:** We found one RCT (n = 32) comparing intramuscular injections of magnesium versus placebo in people with CFS over a 6 week period.[25] This trial found significant benefits with magnesium: 12/15 people on active treatment compared with 3/17 on placebo. **Evening primrose oil:** We found two RCTs comparing evening primrose oil versus placebo in people with a diagnosis of postviral fatigue syndrome or CFS. One RCT (n = 63) compared evening primrose oil (4 g orally per day) versus placebo in people with a diagnosis of postviral fatigue syndrome.[26] At 3 months, 85% of the people on active treatment had improved compared with 17% on placebo, a significant benefit. The other RCT (n = 50) found no significant difference between evening primrose oil (4 g orally per day) and placebo, in people with CFS, at 3 months (using the Oxford, UK diagnostic criteria).[27]

Harms: These trials reported no adverse effects.

Comment: Subsequent studies have failed to find a deficiency of magnesium in people with CFS.[28–30] The difference in outcome for the studies of evening primrose oil may be partly explained by participant selection; the second study used currently accepted diagnostic criteria.[27] Also, whereas the first study used liquid paraffin as a placebo,[26] the second study used sunflower oil, which is better tolerated and less likely to affect the placebo response adversely.[27]

| OPTION | IMMUNOTHERAPY |

Four small RCTs of Immunoglobulin G (IgG) in people with CFS found only limited benefit and considerable adverse effects. RCTs of other forms of immunotherapy have found no evidence of a benefit over placebo.

Benefits: We found no systematic review. **IgG:** We found four RCTs comparing IgG versus placebo. In the first, 30 people were given either intravenous IgG 1 g/kg or albumin (placebo) every 30 days.[31] After 6 months no differences were found in measures of fatigue or physical and social functioning. A similar study randomised 49 people to three infusions of either intravenous IgG (2 g/kg) or placebo (a maltose solution).[32] Treatment was given monthly. Nearly half (10/23) of the immunoglobulin recipients improved in terms of a physician rated assessment of symptoms and disability, compared with 3/26 placebo recipients. A subsequent attempt by the same group to replicate the results was unsuccessful.[33] A further trial compared IgG 1 g/kg versus placebo in 71 adolescents aged 11–18 years.[34] Three infusions were given 1 month apart. There was a significant difference between the active treatment and control groups in mean functional outcome determined by taking the mean of clinician ratings from four areas of the participants' activities. Both groups showed significant improvements from baseline, however, continuing to the 6 month assessment after treatment. **Other immunotherapies:** We found one RCT comparing α interferon versus placebo (n = 30).[35] In this study, treatment benefit was found only on subgroup analysis. Other RCTs found no significant advantage over controls from dialysable leucocyte extract (in a factorial design with cognitive behavioural therapy)[36] or terfenadine.[37]

Harms: Considerable adverse effects (gastrointestinal complaints, headaches, arthralgia, and worsening fatigue) were reported with IgG in up to 82% of trial participants.[31] Adverse effects were also notable with α interferon, and two of 13 participants on active treatment developed neutropenia.[35]

Comment: The first two studies differed in that the second used twice the dose of IgG, did not require that participants fulfil the operational criteria for CFS, and made no assessments of them during the study, waiting until 3 months after completion.[32] Terfenadine, particularly in increased blood concentrations, is associated with rare hazardous cardiac arrhythmias. Terfenadine has been withdrawn from sale in the US and UK.[38]

| OPTION | COGNITIVE BEHAVIOURAL THERAPY |

A systematic review has found that cognitive behavioural therapy administered by highly skilled therapists in specialist centres is effective in people with CFS, with a number needed to treat of 2. This finding may be of limited relevance to less specialised settings.

Benefits: We found one systematic review (updated August 1998, 13 RCTs) of cognitive behavioural therapy in people with CFS.[39] Three trials met the reviewers' inclusion criteria (all participants fulfilled diagnostic criteria for CFS, use of adequate randomisation, and use of controls).[30,36,40] The earliest trial (n = 90) used the Australian diagnostic criteria and evaluated cognitive behavioural therapy and immunotherapy using a factorial design.[36] The comparison group received standard medical care. Cognitive behavioural therapy was given every 2 weeks for six sessions lasting 30–60 minutes each. Treatment involved encouraging participants to exercise at home and feel less helpless. There was no significant difference in outcomes between cognitive behavioural therapy and standard care, using the Karnofsky scale and symptom report on a visual analogue scale. The second trial (n = 60) used the Oxford, UK diagnostic criteria and compared cognitive behavioural therapy versus normal general practice care in people attending a secondary care centre.[41] The active treatment consisted of a cognitive behavioural assessment, followed by 16 weekly sessions of behavioural experiments, problem solving activity, and re-evaluation of thoughts and beliefs inhibiting return to normal functioning. At 12 months, using the Karnofsky scale, 73% of those receiving cognitive behavioural therapy were improved compared with 27% receiving standard care. The relative benefit increase was 175% (95% CI 54% to 432%), with three people needing to be treated with cognitive behavioural therapy for one additional person to achieve normal functioning (NNT 3, 95% CI 2 to 5). The third trial (n = 60) was in people attending a different secondary care centre.[40] Cognitive behavioural therapy was given in 13 weekly sessions. The control group received relaxation therapy. Outcome was assessed using the medical outcomes survey short form. A good outcome was found in 63% of those treated with cognitive behavioural therapy compared with 17% receiving relaxation therapy. The relative benefit increase was 270% (95% CI 137% to 531%, NNT 3, 95% CI 1 to 7). In both the second and third trials, improvement continued over 6–12 months' follow up.[30,40]

Harms: No harmful effects were reported.

Comment: The negative results of the Australian trial[36] may have been because the therapy was less intense and no attempts at cognitive reappraisal were offered, and because routine care was itself reasonably effective. The conflict between the differing illness models for the two active treatments being evaluated, cognitive behavioural therapy and immunotherapy, may also have had an impact on effectiveness. The Australian diagnostic criteria are no longer widely used. The other two trials [40,41] took place in centres with highly skilled cognitive behavioural therapists. The applicability of their positive results to settings outside specialist centres remains uncertain. A large Dutch RCT (G Bleijenberg, personal communication, 1999) and a UK RCT based in primary care (L Ridsdale et al, personal communication, 1999) are due to report soon.

REFERENCES

1. Fukuda K, Straus S, Hickie I, et al. The chronic fatigue syndrome: a comprehensive approach to its definition and study. *Ann Intern Med* 1994; 121:953–959.
2. Sharpe M, Archard LC, Banatvala JE. A report - chronic fatigue syndrome: guidelines for research. *J R Soc Med* 1991;84:118–121.
3. Wessely S, Chalder T, Hirsch S, et al. The prevalence and morbidity of chronic fatigue and chronic fatigue syndrome: a prospective primary care study. *Am J Public Health* 1997;87:1449–1455.
4. Steele L, Dobbins JG, Fukuda K, et al. The epidemiology of chronic fatigue in San Francisco. *Am J Med* 1998;105(suppl 3A):83–90.
5. Lawrie SM, Pelosi AJ. Chronic fatigue syndrome in the community: prevalence and associations. *Br J Psychiatry* 1995;166:793–797.

6. Wessely S. The epidemiology of chronic fatigue syndrome. *Epidemiol Rev* 1995;17:139–151.

7. Joyce J, Hotopf M, Wessely S. The prognosis of chronic fatigue and chronic fatigue syndrome: a systematic review. *QJM* 1997;90:223–133. Search date March 1996; primary sources Medline; Embase; Current Contents; Psyclit.

8. Stewart AD, Hays RD, Ware JE. The MOS short-form general health survey. *Med Care* 1988;26: 724–732.

9. Karnofsky DA, Burchenal JH. MacLeod CM, eds. *The clinical evaluation of chemotherapeutic agents in cancer.* New York Academy of Medicine. New York: Columbia University Press, 1949:191–206.

10. Beck AT, Ward CH, Mendelson M, Mock JE, Erbaugh JK. An inventory for measuring depression. *Arch Gen Psychiatry* 1961;4:561–571.

11. Bergner M, Bobbit RA, Carter WB, et al. The sickness impact profile: development and final revision of a health status measure. *Med Care* 1981;19:787–805.

12. Vercoulen J, Swanink C, Zitman F. Randomised, double-blind, placebo-controlled study of fluoxetine in chronic fatigue syndrome. *Lancet* 1996;347:858–861.

13. Wearden AJ, Morriss RK, Mullis R, et al. Randomised, double-blind, placebo controlled treatment trial of fluoxetine and a graded exercise programme for chronic fatigue syndrome. *Br J Psychiatry* 1998;172:485–490.

14. Natelson BH, Cheu J, Pareja J, et al. Randomised, double blind, controlled placebo-phase in trial of low dose phenelzine in the chronic fatigue syndrome. *Psychopharmacology* 1996;124:226–230.

15. Behan PO, Hannifah H. 5-HT reuptake inhibitors in CFS. *J Immunol Immunopharmacol.* 1995;15:66–69.

16. Peterson PK, Pheley A, Schroeppel J, et al. A preliminary placebo-controlled crossover trial of fludrocortisone for chronic fatigue syndrome. *Arch Intern Med* 1998;158:908–914.

17. McKenzie R, O'Fallon A, Dale J, et al. Low-dose hydrocortisone for treatment of chronic fatigue syndrome. *JAMA* 1998;280:1061–1066.

18. Cleare AJ, Heap E, Malhi G, et al. Low-dose hydrocortisone in chronic fatigue syndrome: a randomised crossover trial. *Lancet* 1999;353: 455–458.

19. Bou-Holaigah I, Rowe P, Kan J, et al. The relationship between neurally mediated hypotension and the chronic fatigue syndrome. *JAMA* 1995;274:961–967.

20. Demitrack M, Dale J, Straus S, et al. Evidence for impaired activation of the hypothalamic-pituitary-adrenal axis in patients with chronic fatigue syndrome. *J Clin Endocrinol Metab* 1991;73: 1224–1234.

21. Forsyth LM, Preuss HG, MacDowell AL, et al. Therapeutic effects of oral NADH on the symptoms of patients with chronic fatigue syndrome. *Ann Allergy Asthma Immunol* 1999;82:185–191.

22. Fulcher KY, White PD. A randomised controlled trial of graded exercise therapy in patients with the chronic fatigue syndrome. *BMJ* 1997;314:1647–1652.

23. Sandler H, Vernikos J. *Inactivity: physiological effects.* London: Academic Press, 1986.

24. Dalrymple W. Infectious mononucleosis: 2. relation of bed rest and activity to prognosis. *Postgrad Med* 1961;35:345–349.

25. Cox IM, Campbell MJ, Dowson D. Red blood cell magnesium and chronic fatigue syndrome. *Lancet* 1991;337:757–760.

26. Behan PO, Behan WMH, Horrobin D. Effect of high doses of essential fatty acids on the postviral fatigue syndrome. *Acta Neurol Scand* 1990;82: 209–216.

27. Warren G, McKendrick M, Peet M. The role of essential fatty acids in chronic fatigue syndrome. *Acta Neurol Scand* 1999;99:112–116.

28. Clague JE, Edwards RHT, Jackson MJ. Intravenous magnesium loading in chronic fatigue syndrome. *Lancet* 1992;340:124–125.

29. Hinds G, Bell NP, McMaster D, et al. Normal red cell magnesium concentrations and magnesium loading tests in patients with chronic fatigue syndrome. *Ann Clin Biochem* 1994;31:459–461.

30. Swanink CM, Vercoulen JH, Bleijenberg G, et al. Chronic fatigue syndrome: a clinical and laboratory study with a well matched control group. *J Intern Med* 1995;237:499–506.

31. Peterson PK, Shepard J, Macres M, et al. A controlled trial of intravenous immunoglobulin G in chronic fatigue syndrome. *Am J Med* 1990;89: 554–560.

32. Lloyd A, Hickie I, Wakefield D, et al. A double-blind, placebo-controlled trial of intravenous immunoglobulin therapy in patients with chronic fatigue syndrome. *Am J Med* 1990;89:561–568.

33. Vollmer-Conna U, Hickie I, Hadzi-Pavlovic D, et al. Intravenous immunoglobulin is ineffective in the treatment of patients with chronic fatigue syndrome. *Am J Med* 1997;103:38–43.

34. Rowe KS. Double-blind randomized controlled trial to assess the efficacy of intravenous gammaglobulin for the management of chronic fatigue syndrome in adolescents. *J Psychiatr Res* 1997;31:133–47.

35. See DM, Tilles JG. Alpha interferon treatment of patients with chronic fatigue syndrome. *Immunol Invest.* 1996;25:153–164.

36. Lloyd A, Hickie I, Boughton R, et al. Immunologic and psychological therapy for patients with chronic fatigue syndrome. *Am J Med* 1993;94:197–203.

37. Steinberg P, McNutt BE, Marshall P, et al. Double-blind placebo-controlled study of efficacy of oral terfenadine in the treatment of chronic fatigue syndrome. *J Allergy Clin Immunol* 1996;97:119–126.

38. British National Formulary 2000;40. London: British Medical Association and Royal Pharmaceutical Society of Great Britain.

39. Price JR, Couper, J. Cognitive behaviour therapy for CFS. In: The Cochrane Library, Issue 4, 1998. Oxford: Update Software. Search date May 1998; primary sources Medline; Embase; Biological Abstracts; SIGLE (System for Information on Grey Literature in Europe); Index to Theses of Great Britain and Ireland; Index to Scientific and Technical Proceedings; Science Citation Index; Trials Register of the Depression; Anxiety and Neurosis Group plus citation lists and personal contacts.

40. Deale A, Chalder T, Marks I, et al. Cognitive behaviour therapy for chronic fatigue syndrome: a randomized controlled trial. *Am J Psychiatry* 1997; 154:408–414.

41. Sharpe M, Hawton K, Simkin S, et al. Cognitive behaviour therapy for chronic fatigue syndrome: a randomized controlled trial. *BMJ* 1996;312:22–26.

Chronic fatigue syndrome

Steven Reid
Clinical Research Fellow

Trudie Chalder
Senior Lecturer

Anthony Cleare
Senior Lecturer

Matthew Hotopf
Senior Lecturer

Simon Wessely
Professor of Epidemiological and
Liaison Psychiatry

Guys, Kings and St Thomas's School
of Medicine and Institute of Psychiatry
London
UK

Competing interests: None declared.

TABLE 1	Diagnostic criteria for chronic fatigue syndrome (see text, p 579).

CDC 1994[1]

Clinically evaluated, medically unexplained fatigue of at least 6 months' duration that is:

- of new onset
- not a result of ongoing exertion
- not substantially alleviated by rest
- a substantial reduction in previous levels of activity

The occurrence of four or more of the following symptoms:

- subjective memory impairment
- tender lymph nodes
- muscle pain
- joint pain
- headache
- unrefreshing sleep
- postexertional malaise (> 24 hours)

Oxford, UK[2]

Severe, disabling fatigue of at least 6 months' duration that:

- affects both physical and mental functioning
- was present for more than 50% of the time

Other symptoms, particularly myalgia, sleep, and mood disturbance, may be present

Exclusion criteria

- active, unresolved, or suspected disease likely to cause fatigue
- psychotic, melancholic, or bipolar depression (but not uncomplicated major depression)
- psychotic disorders
- dementia

- anorexia or bulimia nervosa
- alcohol or other substance misuse
- severe obesity
- same as US CDC, apart from substance misuse and obesity

New topic

Olivier Bruyere and Jean-Yves Reginster

QUESTIONS

INTERVENTIONS

PREVENTION

Likely to be beneficial

Unknown effectiveness

To be covered in future issues of *Clinical Evidence*

Fracture prevention in men and premenopausal women
Prevention of pathological fractures
Effects of dietary intervention
Effects of exercise
Use of hip protectors, helmets, joint and limb pads
Environmental manipulation
Non-hormonal drug treatment

Key Messages

Prevention

- Two RCTs have found that hormone replacement therapy (HRT) reduces the risk of vertebral fracture by 40–60% compared with placebo. Similar reductions have been found in observational studies.

- For hip fracture, two RCTs and several observational studies presented conflicting results.

DEFINITION	A fracture is a break or disruption of bone or cartilage. Symptoms may include immobility, pain, tenderness, numbness, bruising, joint deformity, joint swelling, and limb shortening.
INCIDENCE/ PREVALENCE	The lifetime risk of fracture in white women is 20% for the spine, 15% for the wrist, and 18% for the hip.
AETIOLOGY/ RISK FACTORS	Fractures usually arise from trauma. Risk factors include those associated with an increased tendency to fall (such as ataxia, drug and alcohol intake, loose carpets), age, osteoporosis, bony metastases, and other disorders of bone.
PROGNOSIS	Fractures may result in pain, short or long term disability, haemorrhage, shock, and death. Vertebral fractures are associated with pain, physical impairment, changes in body shape, loss of physical function, and lower quality of life. Around 20% of women die in the year after a hip fracture, representing an increase in mortality of 12–20% compared with women of similar age and no hip fracture. Half of elderly women who had been independent become partly dependent after hip fracture. One third become totally dependent.
AIMS	To prevent fractures with minimal adverse effects from treatment.
OUTCOMES	Incidence of hip, wrist, and vertebral fractures.
METHODS	We identified RCTs and systematic reviews using Medline (1970 to 1999) and Embase (1980 to 1999). We also hand searched journals of bone diseases and carried out manual searches using the bibliographies of review articles published after 1985. We considered all studies assessing the effects of HRT on fracture rates.

QUESTION What are the effects of treatment to prevent fractures in postmenopausal women?

OPTION HORMONE REPLACEMENT THERAPY

Two RCTs found fewer vertebral fractures after HRT than after placebo. For non-vertebral fractures, two RCTs and several observational studies found conflicting results. Reduced risk of hip fracture seems significant only in women who started HRT within 5 years of menopause and who have used it continuously.

Benefits: **Vertebral fractures:** We found no systematic review of RCTs. We found two RCTs. One RCT in 75 postmenopausal women (47–75 years of age with one or more vertebral fractures) evaluated transdermal HRT (17β oestradiol and oral medroxyprogesterone acetate).[1] After 12 months it found fewer vertebral fractures with HRT than with placebo (8 fractures in 7 women with HRT v 20 fractures in 12 women with placebo; RR 0.39; 95 % CI 0.16 to 0.95). The second RCT (100 postmenopausal women) found that, over a median of 9 years, oestrogen reduced total spine score, an indirect measurement of vertebral fracture rate (P < 0.01) but had no effect on the number of women with a vertebral crush fracture (1/57 with oestrogen, 5/42 with placebo; RR 0.15, 95% CI 0.02 to 1.15).[2] **Non-vertebral fractures:** We found two RCTs and several observational studies. One RCT (2763 postmenopausal women, age less than 80 years) compared HRT versus placebo for an average of 4.1 years in the secondary prevention of coronary artery disease; prevention of fracture was a secondary end point.[3] It found that oestrogen had no effect on the number of women with a hip fracture (0.9% with HRT, 0.8% with placebo; RR 1.09, 95% CI 0.48 to 2.46) or on the number with any fracture (9% with HRT, 10% with placebo; RR 0.94, 95% CI 0.75 to 1.18). The other RCT randomised 464 postmenopausal women to one of four groups: HRT alone (oestradiol and cyproterone), vitamin D alone, HRT plus vitamin D, or placebo.[4] At a mean of 4.3 years follow up, 32 women had 39 non-vertebral fractures (HRT 4, vitamin D 10, HRT plus vitamin D 8, placebo 17). Women on HRT alone had fewer fractures but this did not quite reach significance on intention to treat analysis (RR 0.41, 95% CI 0.16 to 1.05). However, comparison of the two HRT groups versus the two groups not receiving HRT did find a reduction in the number of non-vertebral fractures (RR 0.44, 95% CI 0.21 to 0.93).

Harms: See hormone replacement therapy in secondary prevention of ischaemic cardiac events, p 83. In the second RCT of non-vertebral fractures, 96 women withdrew from the trial, 72 of whom were in groups receiving HRT. The most common reasons cited for withdrawal were menstrual disorders (n = 19) and headache (n = 14).[4]

Comment: In addition to these RCTs, we found many observational studies with conflicting results.[5–11] One non-systematic review[7] of 11 observational studies found a reduced risk of hip fracture in women taking oestrogen compared with non-users (RR 0.75; 95% CI 0.68 to 0.84). Other observational studies found no differences.[12,13] We found no observational studies that detected an increased risk of fracture with HRT. Several observational studies found that only 8%–20% of women continued HRT for at least 3 years.[14,15]

REFERENCES

1. Lufkin E, Wahner H, O'Fallon W, et al. Treatment of postmenopausal osteoporosis with transdermal estrogen. *Ann Intern Med* 1992;117:1–9.

2. Lindsay R. Prevention of spinal osteoporosis in oophorectomised women. *Lancet* 1980;1:1152–1154.

3. Hulley S, Grady D, Bush T, et al. Randomized trial of estrogen plus progestin for secondary prevention of coronary heart disease in postmenopausal women. *JAMA* 1998;31:45–54.

4. Komulainen M, Kröger H, Tuppurainen M, et al. HRT and vitamin D in prevention of non-vertebral fractures in postmenopausal women; a 5 year randomized trial. *Maturitas* 1998;31:45–54.

5. Ettinger B, Genant H, Cann C. Long-term estrogen replacement therapy prevents bone loss and fractures. *Ann Intern Med* 1985;102:319–324.

6. Maxim P, Ettinger B, Spitalny M. Fracture protection provided by long-term estrogen treatment. *Osteoporos Int* 1995;5:23–29.

7. Grady D, Rubin S, Petitti D, et al. Hormone therapy to prevent disease and prolong life in postmenopausal women. *Ann Intern Med* 1992;117:1016–1037.

8. Cauley J, Seeley D, Ensrud K, et al. Estrogen replacement therapy and fractures in older women. *Ann Intern Med* 1995;122:9–16.

9. Kanis J, Johnell O, Gullberg B, et al. Evidence for efficacy of drugs affecting bone metabolism in preventing hip fracture. *BMJ* 1992;305:1124–1128.

10. Michaëlsson K, Varon J, Farahmand B, et al. on behalf of the Swedish Hip Fracture Study Group. Hormone replacement therapy and risk of hip fracture: population based case-control study. *BMJ* 1998;316:1858–1863.

11. Michaëlsson K, Baron J, Johnell O, et al. for the Swedish Hip Fracture Study Group. Variation in the efficacy of hormone replacement therapy in the prevention of hip fracture. *Osteoporos Int* 1998;8: 540–546.

12. Nguyen T, Jones G, Sambrook N, et al. Effects of estrogen exposure and reproductive factors on bone mineral density and osteoporotic fractures. *J Clin Endocrin Metab* 1995;80:2709–2714.

13. Kiel D, Baron J, Anderson J, et al. Smoking eliminates the protective effect of oral estrogens on the risk for hip fracture among women. *Ann Intern Med* 1992;116:716–721.

14. Ettinger B, Li D, Lein R. Continuation of postmenopausal hormone replacement therapy: comparison of cyclic versus continuous combined schedules. *Menopause* 1996;3:185–189.

15. Groeneveld F, Bareman F, Barentsen R, et al. Duration of hormonal replacement therapy in general practice: a follow up study. *Maturitas* 1998;29:125–131.

Olivier Bruyere
Research Fellow
WHO Collaborating Center for Public
Health Aspects of Osteoarticular
Diseases
Liege
Belgium

Jean-Yves Reginster
Professor of Epidemiology and
Public Health
Bone and Cartilage Metabolism Unit
University of Liege
Liege
Belgium

Competing interests: OB, none declared. J-Y R has carried out consultancy and research work for the following companies: Merck Sharp and Dohme Ltd, Procter and Gamble Pharmaceuticals, Novartis, Hologic, Negma, Rotta Research, IBSA, Eli Lilly and Co Ltd, Wyeth, and AHP.

INTERVENTIONS

Beneficial
Osteotomy 594

Likely to be beneficial
Absorbable pin fixation (similar
  to standard bone fixation) . .595
Early weightbearing 596
Crepe postoperative bandage .596

Trade off between benefits and harms
Keller's arthroplasty 593
Chevron osteotomy 594

Unknown effectiveness
Orthoses to treat hallux valgus in
  adults 592
Chevron osteotomy with additional
  tenotomy 594

Continuous passive motion . . .595

Unlikely to be beneficial
Orthoses to prevent hallux valgus in
  high risk adults 592
Night splints 593

Likely to be ineffective or harmful
Antipronatory orthoses in
  children. 592

To be covered in future issues of Clinical Evidence
Mitchell's osteotomy
Individual adaptation of standard
  surgical procedures

See glossary, p 597

Key Messages

- We found no strong evidence about optimal treatment for hallux valgus.
- Few conservative treatments have been evaluated by RCT and those that have show no clear benefit compared with placebo.
- One systematic review of RCTs has found that Keller's arthroplasty and the chevron osteotomy have poor radiographic outcomes when compared with other types of operation for hallux valgus.
- One RCT found no evidence of a difference between absorbable pin bone fixation and standard methods.
- Three RCTs found that new postoperative regimens (the use of crepe bandages, continuous passive motion and allowing early weightbearing) are of similar effectiveness as older techniques (plaster slipper casts, routine physiotherapy and delayed weightbearing).

DEFINITION   **Hallux valgus** is a deformity of the great toe characterised by a lateral deviation (abduction) and valgus rotation with adduction and varus rotation of the first metatarsal.[1] Radiological criteria for hallux valgus vary, but a commonly accepted criterion is a metatarsal joint angle >14.5°.[2] **Bunion** is the lay term used to describe a prominent and often inflamed metatarsal head and overlying bursa. Symptoms include pain, limitation in walking, and problems with wearing normal shoes.

INCIDENCE/   The prevalence of hallux valgus varies in different populations. In a
PREVALENCE   recent study of 6000 British school children aged 9 to 10 years, 2.5% had clinical evidence of hallux valgus, and 2% met both clinical and radiological criteria for hallux valgus. An earlier[2] study found hallux valgus in 48% of adults. Different prevalences may be due to different methods of measurement, varying age groups, or different diagnostic criteria (e.g. metatarsal joint angle > 10° or > 15°).[3]

AETIOLOGY/   Nearly all population studies have found that hallux valgus is more
RISK FACTORS common in women. Footwear may contribute to the deformity, but studies comparing people who wear shoes with those who do not have been contradictory. Hypermobility of the first ray (see glossary, p 597) and excessive foot pronation are associated with hallux valgus.[4]

PROGNOSIS   We found no studies that looked at progression of hallux valgus. Progression of deformity and symptoms is rapid in some people, others remain asymptomatic. One study found that hallux valgus is often unilateral initially, but usually progresses to bilateral deformity.[2]

AIMS   To reduce symptoms and deformity with minimum adverse effects.

OUTCOMES   Hallux abductus angle (the angle, usually measured from radiographs, between the shaft of the metatarsal and the hallux). The first intermetatarsal angle (the angle measured radiographically between the first and second metatarsal shafts). Range of motion of the first metatarsophalangeal joint (the total range of both dorsiflexion and plantarflexion). Incidence of complications such as infection; reoperation; non-union; avascular necrosis; pain; general satisfaction and satisfaction with appearance; requirement for specialist or extra-width footwear; proportion of people with mobility problems; time to healing; development of transfer lesions; and adverse effects of treatment.

METHODS   *Clinical Evidence* search and appraisal March 2000. An earlier search (October 1998) was also made using a strategy developed by the Cochrane Musculoskeletal Injuries Group. We also hand-searched podiatry journals up to March 2000.

QUESTION   **What are the effects of conservative treatments?**

OPTION   ORTHOSES

Two RCTs have evaluated the use of antipronatory orthoses (see glossary, p 597) in the treatment and prevention of hallux valgus. In children, deterioration of the deformity has been shown to occur regardless of

orthotic intervention. In adult males with rheumatoid arthritis, orthoses have been shown to reduce the chance of developing hallux valgus.

Benefits: We found no systematic reviews. We found two RCTs. **In Children:** One RCT screened 6000 British school children aged 9–10 years. Based on clinical examination, 150 were selected for x-ray examination. Children (n = 122, 13% boys) with metatarsophalangeal joint angles >14.5° were randomised either to antipronatory orthoses for 3 years, or to no treatment.[2] For children with bilateral deformity (n = 46), the hallux abductus angle increased for both treatment groups but the difference was not significant. For children with unilateral deformity (n = 47), orthoses were associated with greater deterioration in joint position. **In Adults:** We found no RCTs of orthoses in adults who already had hallux valgus. We found one RCT which compared the use of orthoses with no treatment in preventing the development of hallux valgus in 102 men with rheumatoid arthritis.[5] None of the men had hallux valgus at inclusion. Hallux valgus was less frequent in those treated with orthoses compared with the control group, but the difference was not significant (AR 5/50 [10%] for adults with orthoses v 12/48 [25%] no treatment; RR 0.4, 95% CI 0.2 to 1.1). Orthoses did not improve pain, disability or function.

Harms: The RCT of orthoses in children gave no information on complications.[2] A few men with rheumatoid arthritis experienced mild discomfort with orthoses.[5]

Comment: The use of this type of antipronatory orthoses in children is questionable since earlier studies have found that hallux valgus in children is not related to pronation but is due to positional changes in the first ray (see glossary, p 597).[6] Twenty nine children (mainly from the control group) were lost to follow up. The study in adults with rheumatoid arthritis only included men, although rheumatoid arthritis is more frequent in women. Generalisations from the results may be limited.

OPTION   NIGHT SPLINTS

One RCT has found no significant difference in deformity or pain with night splints compared with no treatment in people with hallux valgus.

Benefits: We found no systematic review. One RCT in 28 people compared the use of night splints no treatment with follow up for 6 months.[6] It found no significant difference between groups in the hallux abductus angle or pain.

Harms: Eleven people (39%) failed to complete the trial; seven were from the treatment group.

Comment: None.

QUESTION   What are the effects of surgical treatments?

OPTION   KELLER'S ARTHROPLASTY

One systematic review of RCTs found little good evidence on the effects of surgical treatments for hallux valgus.

Benefits: We found one systematic review (search date 1998, 3 RCTs).[7] The first RCT (n = 81) compared Keller's arthroplasty (see glossary, p 597) with arthrodesis. There was no significant difference between procedures for any of the outcomes used except limitation in walking, where the Keller's arthroplasty was associated with significantly less reduction in mobility position (AR 11/37 [30%] for arthrodesis v 4/44 [9%] for Keller's arthroplasty; RR 3.3, 95% CI 1.1 to 9.4; NNH 5, 95% CI 3 to 29). The second RCT (n = 29) compared Keller's arthroplasty with distal metatarsal osteotomy. The osteotomy gave better results for many outcomes but these were significant only for intermetatarsal angle, (WMD –5.00°, 95% CI –1.1° to –8.9°), and for range of movement (WMD –13°; 95% CI –5.0° to –21.1°). **Plus joint distraction:** The third RCT compared the use of a Kirschner wire to distract the joint during healing after Keller's arthroplasty. It found no evidence of improvement in the hallux abductus angle and no improvement of intermetatarsal angle, pain, or movement. However, a subjective assessment score for symptoms and activity was significantly better in the non-wire group (P < 0.05). A significant decrease in interphalangeal joint movement was noted when wire distraction was used (P < 0.05).

Harms: No particular complications were described. Reduced toe function has been described after Keller's procedure.[7] The systematic review reported high levels of dissatisfaction (up to 33%) in most trials.[7]

Comment: Most of the people having surgery were under 50 years old and were followed up for no more than 3 years. Longer term outcomes remain unclear. Many of the RCTs reported results for numbers of feet, and did not always report standard deviations of the results. The systematic review analysed the results by numbers of people.

OPTION   CHEVRON OSTEOTOMY

One systematic review of RCTs found limited evidence that chevron osteotomy (see glossary, p 597) was likely to produce poor outcomes compared with comparable operations.

Benefits: We found one systematic review (search date 1998, 4 RCTs).[7] The first RCT (n = 75) compared proximal chevron osteotomy (see glossary, p 597) with proximal crescentic osteotomy (see glossary, p 597). It found no significant difference between the procedures for the hallux abductus angle, intermetatarsal angle, transfer lesions (see glossary, p 597), or number of complications after 22 months in 66 people who were assessed. Chevron osteotomy was associated with significantly faster healing time (P < 0.001) and significantly less postoperative dorsiflexion at the healed site (P = 0.005). The second RCT (n = 68) compared chevron osteotomy with proximal osteotomy (see glossary, p 597). After 2 years it found significantly better hallux abductus angle with the proximal osteostomy (WMD –5.0°, 95% CI –0.5° to –9.5°), and intermetatarsal angle (WMD –3.00°, 95% CI –1.00 to –5.00). It found no difference between the procedures for pain, satisfaction, footwear, or limited walking. The third RCT compared chevron versus Wilson osteotomy (see glossary, p 597). Forty six people were examined after 38 months. Wilson osteotomy significantly improved the hallux abductus angle (WMD −12.4°, 95% CI −17.5° to −7.5°). It found no significant differences in complications, footwear, or limited walking. **Additional adductor tenotomy:** The fourth RCT (n = 84) considered the use of an additional adductor tenotomy in the chevron osteotomy. There were no significant differences in hallux abductus angle, range of motion, complications, pain, satisfaction, footwear, or limited walking.

Harms: Complications were found in most RCTs. Overcorrection (4 v 5) and pin tract infections (1 v 2) were reported in one trial. In the trial of proximal osteotomy versus chevron osteotomy, there was one wound infection and two stress fractures in the chevron group, and eleven complications in the proximal osteotomy group that consisted mostly of development of pain in other areas of the forefoot (metatarsalgia). In the trial of Wilson osteotomy versus chevron osteotomy, complications were found in both groups. Transfer pain and lesions were recurring problems in both groups (18 v 17). Although Wilson osteotomy resulted in a significantly shortened metatarsal (P = 0.02) with metatarsal dorsiflexion in 20% of people, this change in position did not correlate with development of new lesions or pain. In the RCT of additional adductor tenotomy in the chevron osteostomy, about 25% of both groups remained dissatisfied during follow up. This may be related to greater postoperative reduction in the circumference of the ball of the foot; the ball circumference of dissatisfied patients was greater than that of satisfied patients (P > 0.005).[7]

Comment: No trial included long term follow up.

OPTION   DIFFERENT METHODS OF BONE FIXATION

One RCT found that absorbable pin versus a standard fixation method (vicryl bone sutures or K wire) produces no significant difference in clinical or radiological benefits, or in the number of surgical complications.

Benefits: We found no systematic review. One trial (n = 28, 39 feet) compared a standard method of fixation with absorbable pin fixation following Mitchell's osteotomy.[8] The mean follow up was 11 months (2–24 months) and included radiological outcomes: hallux abductus angle, intermetatarsal angle and the ratio of the 1st to 2nd metatarsal length; and clinical outcomes: range of movement, pain, metatarsalgia, walking ability, and cosmetic appearance. No significant differences were found.

Harms: Complications occurred in 14/17 feet (standard fixation method) versus 16/22 feet (absorbable pin fixation). These included recurrence of deformity (3 v 2); problems primarily resulting in pain (5 v 6); and continued swelling (3 v 0).

Comment: The trial used participants as the unit of randomisation and feet as the unit of analysis.

QUESTION   What are the effects of postoperative care?

OPTION   CONTINUOUS PASSIVE MOTION

One systematic review (1 small RCT) found no significant difference between continuous passive motion versus routine rehabilitation on joint

range of motion or return to normal footwear, but was too small to rule out a clinically important effect.

Benefits: We found one systematic review (search date 1998, 1 RCT).[7] For 3 months the RCT (n = 39) compared continuous passive motion plus physiotherapy with physiotherapy alone. It found no significant difference in the range of motion (WMD −6.7°, 95% CI −13.6° to +0.3°) or in the number of people who returned to normal footwear.

Harms: No complications were found in the trial.

Comment: None.

OPTION   **EARLY WEIGHTBEARING**

One systematic review found that early weightbearing after surgery was not detrimental to non-union at the site of arthrodesis.

Benefits: We found one systematic review (search date 1998, 1 RCT).[7] The RCT (n = 56) compared early with late weightbearing. One group (29 people) began to bear weight in a cast for 2 to 4 weeks after the operation while 27 people did not bear weight until 4 weeks postoperatively. The only outcome assessed was non-union at the site of arthrodesis (see harms below).

Harms: The only complication considered was non-union at the site of arthrodesis. This occurred in one person allowed early weightbearing and in two from the late weightbearing group. The RCT found no significant difference in the number of new complications.[7]

Comment: None.

OPTION   **SLIPPER CAST**

One RCT comparing crepe bandage with plaster cast slippers following a Wilson osteotomy found no significant difference in any outcome, but was too small to rule out a clinically important significant effect.

Benefits: We found no systematic review. We found one trial (54 feet) that compared the use of plaster slipper cast (27 feet) with crepe bandage (27 feet) following a Wilson osteotomy.[9] Cast and dressings were changed 12 days after surgery and then kept on for a further 4 weeks. There was no significant difference between the groups for hallux valgus angle, pain, overall assessment, joint range of movement, or return to normal activities.

Harms: One failed union occurred in the crepe group versus none in the plaster group. Two people in the plaster group had a superficial wound infection.[9]

Comment: The RCT was small and could not exclude a small but clinically important difference between the groups.

GLOSSARY

Antipronatory orthoses Insoles designed to reduce the amount of in-roll or flattening of the foot during gait.

Chevron osteotomy A v-shaped wedge of bone is removed from the distal end of the metatarsal shaft allowing the metatarsal head to be realigned on the shaft.

First ray The first metatarsal and medial cuneiform function as a single unit called the first ray.

Keller's arthroplasty A procedure involving removal of the medial side of the metatarsal head and straight resection of the base of the proximal phalanx.

Proximal chevron osteotomy Removal of a v-shaped wedge of bone from the base of the metatarsal shaft followed by displacement and fixation of the distal portion of bone.

Proximal crescentic osteotomy A curved cut is made across the base of the metatarsal shaft. The distal portion of bone is slid across the proximal end of bone and fixed in a corrected position.

Proximal osteotomy A similar procedure to the proximal chevron osteotomy.

Transfer lesions Areas of corns or callus that develop when the weightbearing forces are transferred from one area of the foot to another.

Wilson osteotomy A double oblique cut is made in the distal portion of the metatarsal shaft and the metatarsal head is slid into a corrected position.

REFERENCES

1. Dykyj D. Pathological anatomy of hallux abducto valgus. *Clin Podiatr Med Surg* 1989;6:1–15.
2. Kilmartin TE, Barrington RL, Wallace WA. A controlled prospective trial of a foot orthosis for juvenile hallux valgus. *J Bone Joint Surg (Br)* 1994;76:210–214.
3. Morris JB, Brash LF, Hird MD. Chiropodial survey of Geriatric and Psychiatric hospital in-patients – Angus District. *Chiropodist* 1980;128–139.
4. LaPorta G, Melillo T, Olinsky D. X-ray evaluation of hallux abducto valgus deformity. *J Am Podiatr Med Assoc* 1974;64:544–566.
5. Budiman-Mak E, Conrad KJ, Roach KE, et al. Can orthoses prevent hallux valgus deformity in rheumatoid arthritis? A randomised clinical trial. *J Clin Rheumatol* 1995;1:313–321.
6. Juriansz AM. Conservative treatment of hallux valgus: a randomised controlled trial of a hallux valgus night splint. MSc Thesis 1996: Faculty of Science, Kings College, London University.
7. Ferrari J, Higgins JPT, William RL. Interventions for treating hallux valgus (abductovalgus) and bunions. In: The Cochrane Library, Issue 4, 1999. Oxford: Update Software. Search date 1998; primary sources Medline, Embase, Cinahl, Amed, Cochrane Controlled Trials Register, Cochrane Musculoskeletal Injuries Trials Register, bibliographies of identified trials, and hand searching of podiatry journals.
8. Prior TD, Grace DL, MacLean JB, et al. Correction of hallux abductovalgus by Mitchell's osteotomy: comparing standard fixation methods with absorbable polydioxanone pins. *Foot* 1997;7:121–125.
9. Meek RMD, Anderson EG. Plaster slipper versus crepe bandage after Wilson's osteotomy for hallux valgus. *Foot* 1999;9:138–141.

Jill Ferrari
Department of Podiatry
University College London
London
UK

Competing interests: None declared.

Hip fracture

New topic

William Gillespie

Musculoskeletal disorders

INTERVENTIONS

Key Messages

Surgical treatment

- One systematic review of RCTs has found that regional anaesthesia compared with general anaesthesia may reduce short term mortality and deep venous thrombosis after hip fracture surgery.

- Limited evidence from a systematic review of randomised and observational studies suggests that arthroplasty for displaced intracapsular fractures of the hip has no significant effect on mortality or morbidity compared with internal fixation.

- A systematic review of RCTs has found that leg deformity is more common after conservative treatment of extracapsular hip fractures. From limited data we found no evidence of a difference between conservative and operative management in terms of medical complications, mortality, or long term pain.

- We found insufficient evidence from RCTs to determine whether replacement arthroplasty has any advantage over the sliding hip screw for extracapsular hip fractures.

- One systematic review of RCTs has found that sliding hip screws are associated with significantly fewer complications than fixed nail plates in the treatment of extracapsular hip fractures.

- One systematic review found that compared with cephalocondylic intramedullary devices, extramedullary fixation of hip fractures using sliding hip screw devices is associated with similar benefits and significantly fewer operative complications.

- One systematic review found that condylocephalic nails are less effective than extramedullary fixation for extracapsular hip fractures.

Preoperative medical treatment

- We found no evidence that routine preoperative traction causes any significant benefit or harm.

- A systematic review has found that nerve blocks for pain control reduce total analgesic intake.

- Systematic reviews of RCTs have found that multidose perioperative and single dose preoperative antibiotic prophylaxis is effective in reducing nosocomial infection following hip surgery.

- A systematic review of RCTs has found that prophylaxis with unfractionated heparin or low molecular weight heparin after hip fracture significantly reduces the incidence of deep venous thrombosis identified by imaging. We found insufficient evidence to confirm the effect on clinical outcomes (pulmonary thromboembolism or postphlebitic leg).

- A systematic review has found that aspirin is likely to be effective in reducing the risk of deep venous thrombosis and pulmonary embolism in patients undergoing hip fracture surgery when administered as preoperative prophylaxis.

- We found no RCT of thromboembolism stockings versus no stockings for hip fracture in elderly people. One systematic review of RCTs has found that graduated elastic compression versus no compression in elective total hip replacement reduces the risk of deep venous thrombosis by a third.

- A systematic review has found that cyclical compression devices (foot or calf pumps) reduce deep venous thrombosis in people with hip fracture. Problems with skin abrasion and compliance have been reported.

Hip fracture

- One systematic review found that high specification foam mattresses and pressure relieving mattresses on operating tables prevent pressure sores.
- One systematic review of poor quality RCTs found weak evidence that nutritional supplementation (oral protein and energy feeds) reduce unfavourable outcomes after hip fracture surgery.

Rehabilitation programmes

- RCTs comparing geriatric orthopaedic rehabilitation units (GORU) versus conventional care found inconclusive results. Limited evidence from observational studies suggest that GORU may reduce the frequency of readmission to hospital, improve the rate of return to previous residence, and provide improved function in mobility and activities of daily living.
- A systematic review of RCTs and observational studies has found limited evidence that geriatric hip fracture programmes (GHFP) versus control programmes may return more elderly people who have suffered hip fracture to their previous residence, and restore mobility and competence in activities of daily living. GHFP may reduce length of hospital stay and the incidence of hospital complications. We found no evidence of reduced mortality or readmission to hospital.
- One systematic review found that early supported discharge programmes (ESD) increase the number of people returning to their previous residence after hip fracture and reduce the length of hospital stay, but increase the number of people readmitted to hospital.

DEFINITION	Hip fracture is a fracture of the femur above a point 5 cm below the distal part of the lesser trochanter.[1] **Intracapsular fractures** occur proximal to the point at which the hip joint capsule attaches to the femur, and can be subdivided into displaced and undisplaced fractures. Undisplaced fractures include impacted or adduction fractures. Displaced intracapsular fractures may be associated with disruption of the blood supply to the head of the femur. Numerous subdivisions and classification methods exist for these fractures. In the most distal part of the proximal femoral segment (below the lesser trochanter), the term "subtrochanteric" is used. **Extracapsular fractures** occur distal to the hip joint capsule.
INCIDENCE/ PREVALENCE	Hip fractures may occur at any age but are most common in elderly people. In industrialised societies, the lifetime risk of hip fracture is about 18% in women and 6% in men.[2] A recent study reported that prevalence increases from about three per 100 women aged 65–74 to 12.6 per 100 women aged 85 years and above.[3] The age stratified incidence has also increased in some societies during the past 25 years; not only are people living longer, but the incidence of fracture in each age group may have increased.[4]
AETIOLOGY/ RISK FACTORS	Hip fractures are usually sustained through a fall from standing height or less. The pattern of incidence is consistent with two main risk factors: increased risk of falling, and loss of skeletal strength from osteoporosis. Both are associated with ageing.
PROGNOSIS	One in five people die in the first year after a hip fracture,[5] and one in four elderly people require a higher level of long term care after a fracture.[5,6] Those who do return to live in the community after a hip fracture have greater difficulty with activities of daily living than age and sex matched controls.[3]

AIMS	To improve survival and quality of life; to minimise complications and disability associated with hip fracture.
METHODS	We searched for any systematic reviews and randomised or quasi-randomised trials that evaluated a treatment or strategy relating to the prevention, management, or rehabilitation of proximal femoral fracture. This included any type of surgical or non-surgical intervention applied in the treatment of hip fracture, as well as any type of prophylactic treatment or dietary supplementation hypothesised to reduce the occurrence of complications of surgery or bed rest (e.g. antibiotic prophylaxis, prophylaxis against venous thromboembolism, dietary supplements, rehabilitation after acute treatment of hip fracture. We searched the following databases: Current Contents to March 2000, Medline to end February 2000, Embase to August 1999, CINAHL to December 1999, Cochrane Library to 2000 Issue 1, and *Best Evidence* to March 2000. We also scanned the bibliographies of included studies for additional references, and contacted known trialists for up to date information.

QUESTION **What are the effects of specific surgical interventions in the treatment of hip fracture?**

OPTION **GENERAL VERSUS REGIONAL ANAESTHESIA FOR HIP FRACTURE SURGERY**

One systematic review of RCTs has found that regional anaesthesia may reduce short term mortality after hip fracture surgery compared with general anaesthesia, and may be associated with a lower rate of deep venous thrombosis.

Benefits:	We found one systematic review (search date 1998, 15 RCTs, 2162 participants).[7] Regional anaesthesia was associated with lower mortality at 1 month, (49/766 with regional anaesthesia *v* 76/812 with general anaesthesia; RR 0.68, 95% CI 0.49 to 0.97; ARR 0.03; NNT 33). Too few people were seen at 1 year's follow up to confirm any long term benefit. Regional anaesthesia was associated with a reduced risk of deep venous thrombosis (39/129 *v* 61/130 with general anaesthesia; RR 0.64, 95% CI 0.48 to 0.86; ARR 0.169; NNT 6).
Harms:	Regional anaesthesia was associated with a marginally longer operation time (WMD 4.8 minutes, 95% CI 1.1 minutes to 8.6 minutes).
Comment:	Although the pooled data indicated a significant reduction in risk of deep venous thrombosis, the three trials contributing data for this outcome had methodological limitations (probable selection and performance biases). Therefore, this association may be insecure.

OPTION **INTERNAL FIXATION VERSUS JOINT ARTHROPLASTY FOR INTRACAPSULAR HIP FRACTURES**

A systematic review of randomised and observational studies has found limited evidence that arthroplasty for displaced intracapsular fractures of the hip has no significant difference in mortality or morbidity compared with internal fixation.

Hip fracture

Benefits: **Arthroplasty versus internal fixation:** We found one systematic review comparing internal fixation versus arthroplasty in people aged over 65 with a displaced intracapsular fracture (search date 1997, 1 RCT, 105 non-randomised studies).[8] Overall, the review found no significant differences between the two options in terms of mortality, mobility, deep vein thrombosis, or pulmonary embolism. No health related quality of life data were available. Deep infection was slightly but significantly more common after arthroplasty than after internal fixation (no data provided). **Unipolar versus bipolar hemiarthroplasty:** We found no systematic review. We found two RCTs.[9,10] One RCT (250 people aged over 80, followed for 2 years) found that significantly more unipolar participants returned to preinjury status (numbers not given; OR 1.94, 95% CI 1.03 to 3.67).[9] The other RCT (48 people, mean age 77 years) found that at 6 months, performance in a 6 m walk was better after bipolar hemiarthroplasty (unipolar 1.93 feet/second, range 1.16–3.30 v bipolar 2.67 feet/second, range 0.77–4.86).[10]

Harms: The need for reoperation was higher after internal fixation by 12–15 months (3 studies, arthroplasty 36/285 v fixation 75/170; RR 2.9, 95% CI 1.7 to 5.3) and by 24 months (2 studies, arthroplasty 26/144 v fixation 61/194; RR 2.6, 95% CI 1.4 to 4.6).[8]

Comment: The review included only one RCT. Protocols have been published for systematic reviews dealing with the management of displaced intracapsular fractures.

OPTION **CONSERVATIVE VERSUS OPERATIVE TREATMENT FOR EXTRACAPSULAR HIP FRACTURES**

A systematic review of RCTs has found that leg deformity is more common after conservative treatment of extracapsular hip fractures. From limited data we found no evidence of a difference between conservative and operative management in terms of medical complications, mortality, or long term pain.

Benefits: We found one systematic review (search date 1997, 4 RCTs).[11] Only one RCT (106 people) used a fixation device with the dynamic features used in contemporary practice (sliding nail plate). Operative treatment was associated with shorter hospital stay, but no data were provided.

Harms: Conservative treatment was associated with leg shortening (conservative 29/39 v operative fixation 11/37; RR 2.5, 95% CI 1.47 to 4.24) and varus deformity (conservative 19/39 v operative fixation 3/35; RR 5.7, 95% CI 1.8 to 17.6).

Comment: Operative treatment was introduced in the 1950s with the expectation of improved functional outcome and reduced incidence of complications of immobilisation and prolonged bed rest. Although we found only limited evidence from RCTs about short term benefits of operation, the additional benefits of early mobilisation and early supported discharge (see option, p 611) can be realised only after surgery.

OPTION ARTHROPLASTY VERSUS INTERNAL FIXATION FOR EXTRACAPSULAR FRACTURES

We found insufficient evidence from RCTs to determine whether replacement arthroplasty has any advantage over the sliding hip screw for extracapsular hip fractures.

Benefits: We found one systematic review (search date 1996, 1 RCT, 90 people).[12] Participants with unstable extracapsular hip fractures were randomised to arthroplasty or a sliding hip screw. From the limited data available, there were no significant differences between the two methods of treatment for operating time, local wound complications, mortality at 12 months (RR 0.99, 95% CI 0.47 to 2.10; AR 23.4% for arthroplasty v 23.4% for sliding hip screw), or mobility at discharge (RR 0.80, 95% CI 0.45 to 1.42; AR 40% v 50%) of previously independent patients.

Harms: More participants required blood transfusion in the arthroplasty group (arthroplasty 34/143 v fixation 27/47; RR 1.38, 95% CI 1.03 to 1.84).

Comment: The RCT had methodological limitation (the method of randomisation was not specified, there was no blinding, analysis was not by intention to treat, and the outcome measures were not defined clearly).[12]

OPTION FIXED VERSUS DYNAMIC (SLIDING) EXTRAMEDULLARY FIXATION FOR EXTRACAPSULAR HIP FRACTURE

One systematic review of RCTs has found that sliding hip screws are associated with significantly fewer complications than fixed nail plates in the treatment of extracapsular hip fractures.

Benefits: We found one systematic review (search date 1998).[13] Three RCTs compared a fixed nail plate (Jewett or McLaughlin) versus the sliding hip screw. There were no significant differences in mortality or reported pain at follow up.

Harms: The use of fixed nail plates was associated with increased risk of fixation failure (2 trials, 38/62 v 12/83 with sliding hip screw; RR 4.27, 95% CI 2.44 to 7.45). Postoperative mobility was non-significantly poorer in participants whose fractures were fixed with fixed nail plates (1 trial, 15/36 v 11/42 with sliding hip screw; RR 1.59, 95% CI 0.84 to 3.01).

Comment: None.

OPTION CEPHALOCONDYLIC NAILS VERSUS EXTRAMEDULLARY FIXATION FOR EXTRACAPSULAR HIP FRACTURE

One systematic review found that compared with cephalocondylic intramedullary devices, extramedullary fixation of hip fractures using sliding hip screw devices is associated with similar benefits and significantly fewer operative complications.

Benefits: We found one systematic review (search date 1998)[14] and one subsequent RCT.[15] **Intramedullary (Gamma nail) fixation versus**

extramedullary (sliding hip screw) fixation: The review identified 14 RCTs (1977 people, follow up 3–12 months). The pooled data showed no evidence of difference between cephalocondylic nails and sliding hip screws in terms of mortality, incidence of wound infection, medical complications of surgery, need for blood transfusion, or functional outcomes at follow up. Radiological screening time, a measure of radiation exposure, was shorter in the Gamma nail group (Gamma 172 people, sliding hip screw 172 people; WMD –22.6 seconds, 95% CI –25.7 seconds to –19.5 seconds). **Intramedullary hip screw versus sliding hip screw:** The review identified two trials (231 people). Results for postoperative complications, mortality, and functional outcomes were similar in the two groups. The subsequent RCT (110 people) compared intramedullary hip screw with a sliding hip screw and found no difference between groups in fracture healing or functional outcomes.

Harms: The Gamma nail was associated with an increased risk of fracture of the femur during the operative procedure (RR 3.75, 95% CI 1.69 to 8.31) or later (RR 6.26, 95% CI 2.55 to 15.4) and an increased reoperation rate (RR 1.99, 95% CI 1.27 to 3.11). In the comparisons of intramedullary hip screw and sliding hip screw, more fracture fixation complications, including all of the intraoperative and later femur fractures, occurred in the intramedullary hip screw group, but the difference was not significant.

Comment: We found no evidence that the theoretical mechanical advantages of intramedullary cephalocondylic devices for operative fixation of extracapsular hip fractures have so far been confirmed. The designs tested have been associated with higher risk of fracture fixation complications than alternative devices. The data refer to extracapsular hip fractures in the trochanteric region; their relevance to the subtrochanteric fracture subgroup is not known.

| OPTION | CONDYLOCEPHALIC NAILS OR EXTRAMEDULLARY FIXATION FOR EXTRACAPSULAR HIP FRACTURE |

One systematic review found that condylocephalic nails are less effective than extramedullary fixation for extracapsular hip fractures.

Benefits: We found one systematic review (search date 1997, 11 RCTs, 1667 people).[16] The advantages of condylocephalic nails were a reduced deep wound sepsis rate (condylocephalic 5/554 v extramedullary 23/549; RR 0.26, 95% CI 0.11 to 0.62), shorter length of surgery (326 people; WMD –22.8 minutes, 95% CI –27.7 minutes to –17.8 minutes), and lower operative blood loss (326 people; WMD –208 ml, 95% CI –262 to –154 ml).

Harms: Use of condylocephalic nails was associated with several adverse outcomes: higher risk of reoperation for fixation failure (8 trials, condylocephalic 118/564 v extramedullary 31/566; RR 3.72, 95% CI 2.54 to 5.44), greater incidence of leg shortening (7 trials, condylocephalic 44/401 v extramedullary 19/442; RR 2.71, 95% CI 1.65 to 4.59), and higher incidence of external rotation deformity (5 trials, condylocephalic 86/345 v extramedullary 28/396; RR 3.73, 95% CI 2.47 to 5.64).

Comment: None.

QUESTION What are the effects of perisurgical medical interventions on surgical outcome and prevention of complications?

OPTION TEMPORARY TRACTION BEFORE SURGERY FOR HIP FRACTURE

We found no evidence that routine preoperative traction to the injured limb is associated with any significant benefit or harm.

Benefits: We found one systematic review[6] (search date 1998, 4 RCTs, 515 people with recent hip fracture). Traction had no effect on the number of people requiring analgesia in the 24 hours following admission (1 RCT, traction 54/101 v control 71/151; RR 1.14, 95% CI 0.89 to 1.46) or the difficulty of fracture reduction at time of surgery (1 RCT, traction 5/45 v control 7/64; RR 1.02, 95% CI 0.34 to 3.00). In the one trial that compared skeletal with skin traction, there was a small but significant reduction in the mean number of analgesic doses used by those treated with skeletal traction (1 RCT, skin traction 40 people, mean 2.50, SD 1.6 v skeletal traction 38 people, mean 1.7, SD 1.4; WMD 0.80, 95% CI 0.13 to 1.46).

Harms: Two of the trials compared skeletal traction with skin traction. Although no important difference was identified between these two methods, initial skeletal traction was more painful and most costly.

Comment: Routine preoperative traction to the injured limb of hip fracture patients in hospital should be reconsidered.

OPTION NERVE BLOCKS FOR PAIN CONTROL BEFORE AND AFTER HIP FRACTURE

One systematic review found that nerve blocks for pain control reduce total analgesic intake.

Benefits: We found one systematic review (search date 1998, 6 RCT/CCTs, 229 people with recent hip fracture).[17] One small trial studied the impact of a nerve block at hospital admission, and the remaining five examined perioperative blocks. Use of nerve blocks was associated with a reduced use of other forms of pain management. Evidence for other clinical benefit was limited. Nerve blocks reduced the use of parenteral or oral analgesia to control pain from the fracture/operation or during surgery. Reduced analgesic use was found with lateral cutaneous block (2 trials, block 19/26 v control 25/25; RR 0.73, 95% CI 0.58 to 0.92) and with triple block (1 trial, block 13/25 v control 22/24; RR 0.57, 95% CI 0.38 to 0.84). It is not clear whether this reduction in analgesia was associated with clinical benefit, although the small trial of femoral nerve block on admission reduced incidence of respiratory infection (block 2/25 v control 11/25; RR 0.18, 95% CI 0.04 to 0.74).

Harms: None reported.

Comment: The trials had few participants, used different types of nerve blocks, and had varying times of insertion. It is unclear whether nerve blocks confer any benefit compared with other methods of analgesia in hip fracture. The possible reduction of respiratory infection is worthy of further study.

OPTION   PERIOPERATIVE ANTIBIOTICS

Systematic reviews of RCTs have found that multidose perioperative and single dose preoperative antibiotic prophylaxis is effective in reducing nosocomial infection following hip surgery.

Benefits: **Multiple dose perioperative regimens:** We found one systematic review (search date 1998, 11 RCTs, 1896 people with recent hip fracture) of multiple dose regimens versus placebo or no prophylaxis.[18] The review found significant reduction in the incidence of deep wound infection (antibiotic 12/961 v control 40/935; RR 0.36, 95% CI 0.21 to 0.65; ARR 2.9% 95% CI 1.3% to 4.4%), superficial wound infection (antibiotic 22/705 v control 38/661; RR 0.48, 95% CI 0.28 to 0.81), and urinary tract infection (antibiotic 31/259 v control 44/241; RR 0.66, 95% CI 0.43 to 1.00). The review found no significant reduction in the incidence of respiratory infection (antibiotic 14/259 v control 16/241; RR 0.81, 95% CI 0.41 to 1.63). **Single dose preoperative regimens:** We found one systematic review[18] (search date 1998, 6 RCTs, 3276 people with recent hip fracture, including 2195 people from one multicentre trial). Compared with placebo or no treatment, single dose prophylaxis significantly reduced deep wound infection (antibiotic 20/1628 v control 49/1648; RR 0.41, 95% CI 0.25 to 0.69; ARR 1.8%, 95% CI 0.8% to 2.8%), superficial wound infection (antibiotic 56/1628 v control 84/1648; RR 0.68, 95% CI 0.49 to 0.95), urinary tract infection (antibiotic 127/1376 v control 206/1375; RR 0.63, 95% CI 0.53 to 0.76), and respiratory infection (antibiotic 41/1376 v control 91/1375; RR 0.47, 95% CI 0.33 to 0.66).

Harms: Adverse effects (allergy, rashes, gastrointestinal complaints) were rarely reported but were more common in people given multiple dose perioperative antibiotics (antibiotic 24/520 v control 12/362; RR1.83, 95% CI 0.96 to 3.50).[18]

Comment: Many different antimicrobials were studied (all active against *Staphylococcus aureus*). The absolute risk reduction with single dose regimens was not significantly less than with multiple dose regimens.

OPTION   UNFRACTIONATED HEPARIN VERSUS LOW MOLECULAR WEIGHT HEPARIN

A systematic review of RCTs has found that prophylaxis with unfractionated heparin or low molecular weight heparin (LMWH) after hip fracture significantly reduces the incidence of deep venous thrombosis identified by imaging. We found insufficient evidence to confirm the effect on clinical outcomes (pulmonary thromboembolism or postphlebitic leg).

Benefits: We found one systematic review (search date 1996, 22 RCTs in elderly people undergoing surgery for hip fracture).[19] Overall, trial quality was poor. **Heparin versus placebo or no treatment:** Ten trials evaluated unfractionated heparin and four trials evaluated LMWH. The trials found fewer lower limb deep vein thromboses (identified by imaging) with unfractionated heparin (103/407 with heparin v 166/409 with control; RR 0.59, 95% CI 0.49 to 0.72; ARR 0.169; NNT 6) and with LMWH (18/104 with heparin v 37/110 with control; RR 0.55, 95% CI 0.34 to 0.88; ARR 0.147; NNT 7). **Unfractionated heparin versus LMWH:** Five trials compared unfractionated heparin versus LMWH. LMWH significantly reduced deep venous thrombosis identified by imaging (47/252 v 64/227 with unfractionated heparin; RR 0.67, 95% CI 0.48 to 0.94; ARR 0.09, 95% CI 0.02 to 0.16; NNT 11).

Harms: There was a non-significant increase in overall mortality after hip fracture in the group receiving heparin (heparin 46/420 v control 35/423 [8%]; RR 1.31, 95% CI 0.88 to 1.97).[19] One systematic review (search date not stated) summarised the risk of bleeding or transfusion in all RCTs of prophylactic subcutaneous unfractionated heparin in general, orthopaedic, and urological surgery.[20] Overall, excessive bleeding or need for transfusion was significantly increased with heparin (heparin 419/7027 v control 244/6504; OR 1.66). Another systematic review (search date 1991) included comparisons of unfractionated heparin and LMWH in general and orthopaedic surgery and found insufficient evidence from published RCTs to confirm a difference in the rate of bleeding complications.[21]

Comment: We found no trials that reported the incidence of postphlebitic leg or wound complications.

OPTION   **ANTIPLATELET AGENTS**

One systematic review has found that aspirin is likely to be effective in reducing the risk of deep venous thrombosis and pulmonary embolism in patients undergoing hip fracture surgery when administered as preoperative prophylaxis.

Benefits: We found one systematic review (10 trials reported before March 1990, 898 people) that compared prophylaxis versus an antiplatelet agent versus placebo or no prophylaxis after fracture.[22] Most people in the review had a hip fracture. For this group of people, the reduction in deep venous thrombosis incidence was not significant (antiplatelet 163/454 v control 186/444; odds reduction 31%), but for pulmonary embolism it was significant (antiplatelet 14/504 v control 34/494, odds reduction 60%).

Harms: The systematic review[22] summarised the bleeding complications reported across all surgical procedures. Fatal bleeds were extremely rare (antiplatelet group 2/4441 v controls 0/4450). The need for transfusion was significantly more frequent in the antiplatelet group (28/2798 v controls 15/3808), as were other bleeding related complications (reoperation, haematoma, or infection because of a bleed), (antiplatelet agents 177/2269 v controls 129/2306).

Comment: A large RCT was published after the search was performed for this review.[23] This trial included 13 356 people having surgery for hip fracture and found that aspirin versus placebo started preoperatively and continued for 35 days reduces the risk of deep venous thrombosis by about a third. Full analysis will be included in the next issue of *Clinical Evidence*, and on the website http://www.clinicalevidence.org).

OPTION GRADUATED ELASTIC COMPRESSION (THROMBOEMBOLISM STOCKINGS)

We found no randomised trial evaluating thromboembolism stockings for hip fracture in elderly people. One systematic review of RCTs has found that graduated elastic compression in elective total hip replacement reduces the risk of deep venous thrombosis by a third compared with placebo.

Benefits: We found one overview with pooling of data from four trials evaluating the use of graduated elastic compression.[24] Graduated elastic compression significantly reduced deep venous thrombosis in people undergoing elective total hip replacement (stockings 32/125 v control 61/111; RR 0.43, 95%CI 0.30 to 0.61; ARR 0.29; NNT 4).

Harms: The overview found that manufacturers of stockings advise against their use in patients with an ankle : brachial pressure of less than 0.7. Patients with peripheral arterial disease and diabetics with neuropathy were stated to be particularly at risk of worsening ischaemia, but we found no evidence in RCTs to quantify this risk.

Comment: It is unclear whether extrapolation from hip replacement studies is appropriate for hip fracture patients.

OPTION CYCLICAL COMPRESSION OF THE FOOT OR CALF

The systematic review found that cyclical compression devices (foot or calf pumps) reduce deep venous thrombosis in people with hip fracture. Problems with skin abrasion and compliance have been reported.

Benefits: We found one systematic review (4 trials, 442 people) comparing mechanical pumping devices versus no intervention.[19] Cyclical compression devices reduced the risk of deep venous thrombosis (compression 12/202 v control 42/212; RR 0.30, 95% CI 0.17 to 0.53). We found no adequate evidence about any effect on the incidence of pulmonary embolism and overall mortality.

Harms: Problems with skin abrasion and compliance were reported in all four trials of cyclical compression devices.

Comment: None.

OPTION BEDS, MATTRESSES, AND CUSHIONS FOR PREVENTING PRESSURE SORES

One systematic review found that high specification foam mattresses and pressure relieving mattresses on operating tables prevent pressure sores.

Benefits: We found one systematic review (updated 1999, search date not stated).[25] High specification foam mattresses compared with "standard hospital" foam mattresses significantly reduced pressure sores (4 trials, high specification 52/678 v standard 57/172; RR

0.29, 95% CI 0.19 to 0.43). Pressure relieving mattresses for high risk patients in the operating theatre reduced postoperative pressure sores. Three RCTs evaluated different methods of pressure relief on the operating table. A viscoelastic polymer (gel) pad compared with a standard table reduced postoperative pressure sores (gel 22/205 v control 43/211; RR 0.53, 95% CI 0.33 to 0.85; ARR 0.096; NNT 11). Two RCTs compared an alternating system (applied both during surgery and postoperatively) with a gel pad used during surgery plus standard mattress postoperatively. Use of alternating pressure throughout significantly reduced pressure sores (alternation 3/188 v control 14/180; RR 0.21, 95% CI 0.06 to 0.7; ARR 6.2%; NNT 16)

Harms: None identified.

Comment: None.

| OPTION | NUTRITIONAL SUPPLEMENTATION AFTER HIP FRACTURE |

One systematic review has found that nutritional supplementation (oral protein and energy feeds) reduces unfavourable outcomes after surgery for hip fracture.

Benefits: We found one systematic review (updated October 1999, 15 RCTs, 943 people).[26] Oral multinutrient feeds (providing non-protein energy, protein, some vitamins and minerals), evaluated by six trials, reduced the overall incidence of death or complications by the end of the study (14/66 v 26/73; RR 0.52, 95% CI 0.32 to 0.84), but did not find an effect on mortality (12/91 v 14/97; RR 0.85, 95% CI 0.42 to 1.70). Three RCTs comparing nasogastric multinutrient feeding versus control found no evidence for an effect on mortality (RR 0.99, 95% CI 0.50 to 1.97), but the studies were heterogeneous and included people with differing characteristics. Two RCTs found that protein in an oral feed did not reduce mortality significantly (RR 0.94, 95% CI 0.35 to 2.52) but may have reduced days spent in rehabilitation wards. Two RCTs, one testing intravenous thiamine (vitamin B1) and other water soluble vitamins, the other testing 1-α-hydroxycholecalciferol, found no evidence of benefit for either vitamin supplement.

Harms: We found little evidence about harms. Nasogastric feeds were sometimes tolerated poorly. Complications, described in only one trial, included bloating and anorexia. We found no reports of feed induced diarrhoea or aspiration pneumonia.

Comment: The quality of trials reported in the review was poor. Defects included inadequate size, method problems (inadequate allocation concealment, assessor blinding and intention to treat analysis), and limited outcome assessment.

| QUESTION | What are the effects of rehabilitation programmes and treatment protocols after hip fracture? |

| OPTION | INPATIENT REHABILITATION IN A GERIATRIC ORTHOPAEDIC REHABILITATION UNIT |

Overall, the evidence from RCTs for effectiveness of geriatric orthopaedic rehabilitation units (GORU) is inconclusive. Limited evidence from

observational studies suggest that GORU may reduce the frequency of readmission to an acute facility, improve the rate of return to previous residence, and provide improved function in mobility and activities of daily living.

Benefits: We found one systematic review (search date 1998, 41 comparative studies, including 14 RCTs) that included seven studies (4 RCTs, 3 cohort studies) of GORU.[27] **Length of hospital stay:** Significant heterogeneity was present between results of RCTs.[27] The pooled results from RCTs (GORU 333 people *v* control 375; WMD 1.6 days, 95% CI −28.0 days to +31 days) were similar to those found in a cohort study. There was no evidence of a significant difference in total hospital stay between programmes with access to a GORU and those without. **Readmission to acute care facility:** The systematic review found a significant reduction in rate of readmission for acute care (GORU 36/182 *v* control 57/196; RR 0.68, 95% CI 0.47 to 0.97). **Return to previous residence after discharge:** There was a marginally significant improvement in the return to previous residence in the GORU group (4 RCTs, GORU 254/343 *v* control 255/380; RR 1.11, 95% CI 1.01 to 1.22). **Death:** The review found no reduction in death by follow up with rehabilitation in a GORU (GORU 79/383 *v* control 90/433; RR 0.98, 95% CI 0.75 to 1.28). **Hospital morbidity:** Two cohort studies found no significant difference in postoperative complications as a whole (1 study, GORU 102 events from 521 admissions *v* control 95 events from 202 admissions). **Mobility and activities of daily living:** One cohort study found that the proportion of participants independently mobile at 6 months was significantly higher with the orthopaedic unit (GORU 221/336 *v* control 104/127; RR 1.25, 95% CI 1.11 to 1.39). Rehabilitation in the GORU reduced loss of daily living ability score at 12 months (22/44 had loss of ability with GORU *v* 28/36 with control; RR 0.64, 95% CI 0.46 to 0.91). **Health related quality of life (HRQL):** The systematic review included one RCT (108 people) and one cohort study (723 people) that compared HRQL scores for GORU versus control. They both found no significant difference.

Harms: Broken pressure sores were more common in GORU (1 study, GORU 17/142 *v* control 8/193, RR 2.89, 95% CI 1.28 to 6.50).

Comment: None.

OPTION	GERIATRIC HIP FRACTURE PROGRAMME WITHIN AN ACUTE ORTHOPAEDIC UNIT

The systematic review of randomised and observational studies found limited evidence that geriatric hip fracture programmes (GHFP) versus control programmes may return more elderly people who have suffered hip fracture to their previous residence, and restore mobility and competence in activities of daily living. GHFP may be effective in reducing length of hospital stay and the incidence of hospital complications. We found no evidence of difference in readmission to an acute facility or mortality.

Benefits: We found one systematic review (41 comparative studies, including 14 RCTs) that compared five studies of GHFP versus control.[27]

Length of hospital stay: The introduction of GHFP was associated with a reduction in length of hospital stay in four of the five included studies. The crude average reduction from the published data was 9 days. **Readmission for acute care:** One RCT found no significant effect on readmission rate by 4 months. (GHFP 16/127 v control 11/125; RR 1.43, 95% CI 0.69 to 2.96). **Return to previous residence after discharge:** GHFP reduced the risk of failing to return home (2 RCTs, GHFP 121/139 v control 100/131; RR 0.88, 95% CI 078 to 0.99). **Mortality:** Two RCTs found no significant reduction in mortality with a GHFP (GHFP 27/165 v control 30/158; RR 0.87, 95% CI 0.54 to 1.39). **Morbidity:** The number of participants sustaining one or more complications in hospital was lower in the GHFP group (GHFP 162/431 v control 39/60; RR 0.58, 95% CI 0.46 to 0.72). **Mobility and activities of daily living:** One RCT found that GHFP was associated with a non-significant reduction in number failing to walk independently by discharge (1 RCT, GHFP 63/127 v control 51/125; RR 0.70, 95% CI 0.43 to 1,15). Another RCT found that performance of a 20 m walk was quicker (1 RCT, GHFP mean 45 seconds v control 59 seconds, no SD provided). A third RCT found that the modified Barthel Index was higher in GHFP participants (1 RCT, GHFP mean 92.8, 95% CI 90 to 95.6 v control 85.6, 95% CI 81.3 to 89.8). **Health related quality of life:** The systematic review found no studies of this outcome.

Harms: We found no evidence of harms.

Comment: None.

| OPTION | EARLY SUPPORTED DISCHARGE PROGRAMMES |

One systematic review found that early supported discharge programmes (ESD) after hip fracture increased the number of people returning to their previous residence and reduced length of hospital stay, but increased the frequency of readmission to hospital.

Benefits: We found one systematic review (41 comparative studies, including 14 RCTs), which included six studies of ESD.[27] **Lengths of hospital stay:** The introduction of ESD was associated with a reduction in length of both acute hospital stay and total number of days in hospital. The crude average reduction (no standard deviations provided) was 6.9 days in acute hospital stay and 2 days in total duration of care. **Return to previous residence after discharge:** ESD was associated with a significantly increased rate of return to previous residence (3 cohort studies, ESD 203/247 v control 129/197; RR 1.25, 95% CI 1.11 to 1.41). **Mortality:** There was no evidence of benefit or disadvantage from introduction of ESD (1 RCT, ESD 12/160 v control 6/81; RR 1.01, 95% CI 0.39 to 2.60). **Morbidity:** One cohort study found no evidence of a significant difference in incidence of one or more hospital complications between ESD and control participants (ESD 17/63 v control 15/66; RR 1.19, 95% CI 0.65 to 2.17). **Mobility and activities of daily living:** One cohort study found no evidence of difference in Nottingham Health Profile mobility dimension mean score (ESD 48 v control 50, no SD provided). One RCT found no evidence of

Hip fracture

difference in improvement of Barthel Index over 3 months (ESD 160 people, mean change 1.9, SD 3.22 v control 81 people, mean change 1.7, SD 2.68). **HRQL:** Two studies reported HRQL scores. There was no evidence of difference in mean Nottingham Health Profile dimension score (1 cohort study, 110 people). One RCT found no evidence of difference in EUROQOL score at 3 months (mean difference −0.04, 95% CI −0.13 to +0.06).

Harms: ESD was associated with a significant increase in the frequency of readmission to hospital (3 cohort studies; 69/922 with ESD v 17/406 with control; RR 1.91, 95% CI 1.11 to 3.29).

Comment: None.

OPTION SYSTEMATIC MULTICOMPONENT HOME REHABILITATION AFTER HIP FRACTURE

One RCT comparing a systematic home based rehabilitation programme with existing services found no important differences.

Benefits: We found no systematic review, but we found one RCT[28] (304 people who had surgery for hip fracture and returned home within 100 days, follow up 12 months) that compared a systematic home based multicomponent rehabilitation strategy addressing physical impairments and activities of daily living versus "usual care". The trial found no significant difference between groups in recovery to prefracture levels of self care, home management, social activity, balance, or lower extremity strength. The systematic programme was associated with slightly greater upper arm strength, and marginally better gait performance.

Harms: None reported.

Comment: The RCT examined whether systematising home assessment and treatment according to a protocol made a difference compared with "usual care". The failure of this trial to find a difference between the systematic programme and "usual care" may be contextual, indicating that "usual care" was already being delivered competently.

REFERENCES

1. Parker MJ, Pryor GA. Hip fracture management. Oxford: Blackwell Scientific Publications, 1993.
2. Meunier PJ. Prevention of hip fractures. Am J Med 1993;95(suppl):75–78.
3. Hochberg MC, Williamson J, Skinner EA, et al. The prevalence and impact of self-reported hip fracture in elderly community-dwelling women: The Women's Health and Aging Study. Osteoporos Int 1998;8:385–389.
4. Boyce WJ, Vessey MP. Rising incidence of fracture of the proximal femur. Lancet 1985;1:150–151.
5. Schurch M-A, Rizzoli R, Mermillod B, et al. A prospective study on the socio-economic aspects of fracture of the proximal femur. J Bone Miner Res 1996;11:1935–1942
6. Parker MJ, Handoll HHG. Pre-operative traction for fractures of the proximal femur. In: The Cochrane Library, Issue 1, 2000. Oxford: Update software. Search date 1998; primary sources Cochrane Musculoskeletal Injuries Group trials register, Medline and hand searches of reference bibliographies.
7. Parker MJ, Urwin SC, Handoll HHG, Griffiths R.

General versus spinal/epidural anaesthesia for surgery for hip fractures in adults. In: The Cochrane Library, Issue 1, 2000. Oxford: Update software. Search date 1998; primary sources Cochrane Musculoskeletal Injuries Group trials register, Medline, and hand searching of selected orthopaedic and anaesthetic journals, conference proceedings, and reference lists of relevant articles.
8. Lu-Yao GL, Keller RB, Littenberg B, Wenberg JE. Outcomes after displaced fractures of the femoral neck. A meta-analysis of one hundred and six published reports. J Bone Joint Surg Am 1994; 76A:15–25 Search date 1990; primary sources Medline and hand searches of reference lists.
9. Calder SJ, Anderson GH, Jagger C, et al. Unipolar or bipolar prosthesis for displaced intracapsular hip fracture in octagenarians; a randomised prospective study. J Bone Joint Surg Br 1996; 78B:391–394.
10. Cornell CN, Levine D, O'Doherty J, Lyden J. Unipolar versus bipolar arthroplasty for the treatment of femoral neck fractures in the elderly.

Clin Orthop 1998;348;67–71.

11. Parker MJ, Handoll HHG. Conservative versus operative treatment for extracapsular hip fractures. In: The Cochrane Library, Issue 1, 2000. Oxford: Update software. Search date 1997; primary sources Cochrane Musculoskeletal Injuries Group trials register, hand searches of reference bibliographies, and personal contact with trialists.

12. Parker MJ, Handoll HHG. Replacement arthroplasty versus internal fixation for extracapsular hip fractures. In: The Cochrane Library, Issue 1, 2000. Oxford: Update software. Search date 1996; primary sources Cochrane Musculoskeletal Injuries Group trials register, hand searches of reference bibliographies, and personal contact with colleagues.

13. Parker MJ, Handoll HHG, Chinoy MA. Extramedullary fixation implants for extracapsular hip fractures. In: The Cochrane Library, Issue 1, 2000. Oxford: Update software. Search date 1998; primary sources Cochrane Musculoskeletal Injuries Group trials register and hand searches of reference lists of relevant articles.

14. Parker MJ, Handoll HHG. Gamma and other cephalocondylic intramedullary nails versus extramedullary implants for extracapsular hip fractures. In: The Cochrane Library, Issue 1, 2000. Oxford: Update software. Search date 1998; primary sources Cochrane Musculoskeletal Injuries Group trials register, Medline, hand searching of selected orthopaedic journals, conference proceedings, and reference lists of relevant articles, and personal contact with trialists, colleagues, and implant manufacturers.

15. Hoffmann R, Schmidmaier G, Schulz R, Schutz M, Sudkamp NP. Classic nail versus DHS. A prospective randomised study of fixation of trochanteric femur fractures. *Unfallchirurg* 1999; 102:182–190.

16. Parker MJ, Handoll HHG, Bhonsle S, Gillespie WJ. Condylocephalic nails versus extramedullary implants for extracapsular hip fractures. In: The Cochrane Library, Issue 1, 2000. Oxford: Update software. Search date 1997; primary sources Cochrane Musculoskeletal Injuries Group trials register, Medline, and hand searches of reference lists of relevant articles.

17. Parker MJ, Griffiths R, Appadu BN. Nerve blocks (subcostal, lateral cutaneous, femoral, triple, psoas) for hip fractures. In: The Cochrane Library, Issue 1, 2000. Oxford: Update software. Search date 1998; primary sources Cochrane Musculoskeletal Injuries Group trials register, Medline, and hand searches of trial bibliographies.

18. Gillespie WJ, Walenkamp G. Antibiotic prophylaxis for surgery for proximal femoral and other closed long bone fractures. In: The Cochrane Library, Issue 1, 2000. Oxford: Update software. Search date 1998; primary sources Medline, Embase, Current Contents, Dissertation Abstracts, Index to UK theses, and hand searches of bibliographies of identified articles.

19. Handoll HHG, Farrar MJ, McBirnie J, et al. Heparin, low molecular weight heparin and physical methods for preventing deep vein thrombosis and pulmonary embolism following surgery for hip fractures. In: The Cochrane Library, Issue 1, 2000. Oxford: Update software. Search date 1996; primary sources Cochrane Musculoskeletal Injuries Group trials register, Medline, Embase, hand searches of published papers and books, and personal contact with trialists and other workers in the field.

20. Collins R, Scrimgeour A, Yusuf S, Peto R. Reduction in fatal pulmonary embolism and venous thrombosis by perioperative administration of subcutaneous heparin. *N Engl J Med* 1988; 318:1162–1173. Search date not stated; primary sources Medline, hand searches of reference lists, and personal contact with colleagues, investigators, and manufacturers of heparin.

21. Jorgensen LN, Wille-Jorgensen P, Hauch O. Prophylaxis of postoperative thromboembolism with low molecular weight heparins. *Br J Surg* 1993;80:689–704. Search date 1991; primary sources Medline, Current Contents, hand searches of reference lists, and personal contact with authors of trials.

22. Antiplatelet Trialists' Collaboration. Collaborative review of randomized trials of antiplatelet therapy. III: Reduction in venous thrombosis and pulmonary embolism by antiplatelet prophylaxis among surgical and medical patients. *BMJ* 1994;308: 235–246.

23. Anon. Prevention of pulmonary embolism and deep vein thrombosis with low dose aspirin: Pulmonary Embolism Prevention (PEP) trial. Lancet 2000;355:1295–1302.

24. Agu O, Hamilton G, Baker D. Graduated compression stockings in the prevention of venous thromboembolism. *Br J Surg* 1999;86:992–1004.

25. Cullum N, Deeks J, Sheldon TA, Song F, Fletcher AW. Beds, mattresses and cushions for pressure sore prevention and treatment. In: The Cochrane Library, Issue 1, 2000. Oxford: Update software. Search date 1999; primary sources Cochrane Wounds Group specialist trials register, hand searching of wound care journals, and relevant conference proceedings.

26. Avenell A, Handoll HHG. Nutritional supplementation for hip fracture aftercare in the elderly (Cochrane Review). In: The Cochrane Library, Issue 1, 2000. Oxford: Update Software. Search date: January 2000; primary sources: Cochrane Musculoskeletal Injuries Group trials register, The Cochrane Controlled Trials register, Medline, Nutrition Abstracts and Reviews, Healthstar, Embase, Biosis, Cinahl, hand searching of reference lists of selected nutrition journals.

27. Cameron I, Crotty M, Currie C, et al. Geriatric rehabilitation following fractures in older people: a systematic review. *Health Technol Assess* 2000;4. Search date 1988; primary sources: Cochrane Musculoskeletal Injuries Group trials register, The Cochrane Controlled Trials register, Medline, Cinahl, hand searches of reference lists.

28. Tinetti ME, Baker DI, Gottschalk M, et al. Home-based multi-component rehabilitation program for older persons after hip fracture: a randomized trial. *Arch Phys Med Rehab* 1999;80:916–922

William Gillespie
Professor
Dunedin School of Medicine
University of Otago
Dunedin
New Zealand

Competing interests: WG is co-ordinating editor of the Cochrane Musculo-skeletal Injuries Group, and has participated in several of the cited systematic reviews.

Low back pain and sciatica

Updated this issue

Maurits van Tulder and Bart Koes

INTERVENTIONS

Key Messages

Acute low back pain

- Systematic reviews of RCTs have found:
  - That NSAIDs and muscle relaxants relieve pain more than placebo.
  - That advice to stay active speeds up symptomatic recovery and reduces chronic disability.
  - No evidence that bed rest, specific back exercises, or other interventions (traction or acupuncture) are effective.

Chronic low back pain

- Systematic reviews of RCTs have found:
  - That back exercises, back schools, behavioural therapy, and multidisciplinary pain treatment programmes are effective.
  - No evidence that other interventions (such as antidepressants, facet joint injections, and EMG biofeedback) are effective.

DEFINITION   Low back pain is pain, muscle tension, or stiffness localised below the costal margin and above the inferior gluteal folds, with or without leg pain (sciatica).[1] It may be acute or chronic (persisting for 12 weeks or more).[2] Non-specific low back pain is low back pain not attributed to recognisable pathology (such as infection, tumour, osteoporosis, rheumatoid arthritis, fracture, or inflammation).[1] This review excludes low back pain or sciatica with symptoms or signs that suggest a specific underlying condition.

INCIDENCE/   Over 70% of people in developed countries will experience low back
PREVALENCE   pain at some time in their lives.[3] Each year, 15–45% of adults suffer low backache, and one in 20 people present with a new episode. Low back pain is most common between the ages of 35 and 55.[3]

AETIOLOGY/   Symptoms, pathology, and radiological appearances are poorly
RISK FACTORS   correlated. Pain is non-specific in about 85% of people. About 4% with low back pain in primary care have compression fractures, and about 1% have a neoplasm. Ankylosing spondylitis and spinal infections are rarer.[4] The prevalence of prolapsed intervertebral disc is about 1–3%.[3] Risk factors include heavy physical work, frequent bending, twisting, lifting, pulling and pushing, repetitive work, static postures, and vibrations. Psychosocial risk factors include anxiety, depression, job dissatisfaction, and mental stress at work.[3,5]

PROGNOSIS   Acute low back pain is usually self limiting (90% recover within 6 weeks) but 2–7% develop chronic pain. One study found recurrent pain accounted for 75–85% of absenteeism.[6]

AIMS   To relieve pain; to improve function; to learn to cope with pain, with minimal adverse effects from treatment.[2,7]

OUTCOMES   Pain intensity (visual analogue or numerical rating scale); overall improvement (self reported or observed); back pain specific functional status (such as Roland Morris questionnaire, Oswestry questionnaire); impact on employment (days of sick leave, number of people returned to work); functional status (sickness impact profile); medication use; strength, mobility, fitness; intervention specific outcomes (such as coping and pain behaviour for behavioural treatment, strength and flexibility for exercise therapy, depression for antidepressants, and muscle spasm for muscle relaxants and EMG biofeedback).

METHODS We searched Medline (1966 to December 1998), Embase drugs and pharmacology database (1980 to September 1998), and Psyclit (1984 to December 1998), using the search strategy recommended by the Cochrane Back Review Group.[8] *Clinical Evidence* update search and appraisal May 2000. We examined the references in relevant publications and reviewed the titles and abstracts of identified articles to determine their relevance. In doubtful cases we read the article. We excluded abstracts and unpublished studies. We included all relevant systematic reviews and RCTs. Most RCTs of treatments for low back pain were small (< 50 people per intervention group, range 9–169), short term (mostly < 6 months' follow up), and of low overall quality. Problems included lack of power, no description of randomisation procedure, incomplete analysis with failure to describe dropouts, and lack of blinding.[9]

QUESTION **What are the effects of oral drug treatments?**

OPTION **ANALGESICS (PARACETAMOL, OPIOIDS)**

One placebo controlled trial of tramadol found decreased pain and improved function in people with chronic low back pain. Systematic reviews have found no clear difference between analgesics and non-steroidal anti-inflammatory drug (NSAIDs) in people with low back pain. Analgesics were less effective than electroacupuncture (see glossary, p 628) or ultrasound. There is considerable evidence from studies of other acute pain conditions that analgesics provide short term pain relief. One RCT found that analgesics were less effective than NSAIDs in people with chronic low back pain.

Benefits: We found two systematic reviews (search date not given,[2] search date 1995;[9] no placebo controlled RCTs, seven comparative RCTs, no statistical pooling) and one subsequent RCT.[10] **Acute low back pain:** Of six RCTs identified in the reviews (329 people), three compared analgesics versus NSAIDs. Two of these (110 people) found no significant difference in the pain reduction from meptazinol, paracetamol, or diflunisal (an NSAID). The third trial found that mefenamic acid reduced pain more than paracetamol. One small trial (40 people) found that electroacupuncture reduced pain slightly more than paracetamol after 6 weeks. One RCT (73 people) found that ultrasound treatment substantially increased the proportion of people who were pain free after 4 weeks compared with (unspecified) analgesics. **Chronic low back pain:** One small RCT identified in the review (29 people, paracetamol versus diflunisal) found that more people treated with diflunisal rated the treatment as good or excellent. One subsequent RCT (254 people) found that tramadol decreased pain and increased functional status more than placebo.[10]

Harms: The trials found adverse effects (constipation and drowsiness) with analgesics in about 50% of people. One systematic review compar-

ing combinations of paracetamol and weak opioids versus paracetamol alone found that combination therapy increased the risk of
adverse effects (single dose studies OR 1.1, 95% CI 0.8 to 1.5;
multiple dose studies OR 2.5, 95% CI 1.5 to 4.2).[11]

Comment: None.

| OPTION | ANTIDEPRESSANTS |

**We found insufficient evidence on the effects of antidepressants in acute
low back pain. RCTs of antidepressants found conflicting results for relief
of pain and depressive symptoms associated with chronic low back pain.**

Benefits: We found four systematic reviews[2,7,9,12] and five additional RCTs
(no statistical pooling of data).[13–18] **Acute low back pain:** We
found no RCTs. **Chronic low back pain:** Overall, from four systematic reviews that did not pool data, and from additional RCTs, we
identified seven placebo controlled RCTs (328 people) evaluating
an antidepressant (imipramine, trazodone, nortriptyline, doxepin, or
clomipramine) in people with chronic low back pain. Five trials
reported on pain relief; three of these found no evidence that
antidepressants reduced pain more than placebo, and two found
that antidepressants were more effective. Six trials reported on
antidepressant effects; five (one of which was not included in the
systematic reviews[13]) found no evidence of benefit whereas one
reported a significant reduction in depression with antidepressants
compared with placebo.[14,15] We found three head to head RCTs.
One (36 people) compared different antidepressants (doxepin v
desipramine) and found no differences in pain relief or depression.
The second RCT (67 people) also compared antidepressants and
found better pain relief with maprotiline versus paroxetine.[18] The
other (n = 39) compared antidepressants versus paracetamol in
people with mild depression and chronic low back pain and found
that antidepressants reduced pain more.[16]

Harms: Adverse effects of antidepressants included dry mouth, drowsiness,
constipation, urinary retention, orthostatic hypotension, and
mania.[2] One of the RCTs not included in the systematic reviews
found that the prevalence of dry mouth, insomnia, sedation, and
orthostatic symptoms was between 60–80% with tricyclic antidepressants; however, rates were only slightly lower in the placebo
group and none of the differences was significant.[13]

Comment: None.

| OPTION | COLCHICINE |

**We found insufficient evidence on the effects of colchicine in acute or
chronic low back pain.**

Benefits: We found one systematic review, which identified three RCTs
(n = 135).[2] Two of the identified trials did not distinguish between
acute and chronic low back pain. Of these, one (n = 48, intravenous colchicine v intravenous saline) found greater short term pain
relief with colchicine. The other (n = 60, intravenous plus oral
colchicine v placebo) found greater pain relief with colchicine.

Acute low back pain: One identified trial (n = 27) compared oral colchicine with placebo and found no evidence of an effect; however, the trial was too small to rule out a clinically important difference.[2] **Chronic low back pain:** We found no RCTs.

Harms: The trials reported gastrointestinal irritation and skin problems in about 33% of people.[2] Other adverse effects included chemical cellulitis and agranulocytosis.[19]

Comment: None.

OPTION   MUSCLE RELAXANTS/BENZODIAZEPINES

Systematic reviews of RCTs have found that muscle relaxants reduce acute low back pain but have found no evidence to distinguish different muscle relaxants. One small RCT found that muscle relaxants reduced chronic low back pain in the short term.

Benefits: We found two systematic reviews (search date not given,[2] search date 1995;[9] 15 RCTs, no statistical pooling). **Acute low back pain:** Of 14 identified trials (total n = 1160), nine (n = 762) compared a muscle relaxant (tizanidine, cyclobenzaprine, dantrolene, carisoprodol, baclofen, orphenadrine, diazepam) versus placebo. Seven of these found that muscle relaxants reduced pain and muscle tension and increased mobility more than placebo between 1 and 2 weeks; two found no evidence of benefit. Three trials (total n = 236) compared different types of muscle relaxants. Two of these found that overall improvement was equivalent with cyclobenzaprine and with carisoprodol, both being better for overall improvement than diazepam. The trials found that all three treatments provided similar reductions in pain intensity. One RCT found no evidence of difference between methocarbamol and chlormezanone. **Chronic low back pain:** One trial in the reviews (n = 50, tetrazepam versus placebo) found that tetrazepam was associated with greater overall improvement (64% v 29% improved people) and reduced pain more than placebo after 10 days.

Harms: Adverse effects included drowsiness or dizziness in up to 70% of people and a risk of dependency even after 1 week of treatment.[2,9] Adverse effects were more common with muscle relaxants than placebo; 68% of people taking baclofen experienced one or more adverse reactions compared with 30% of those taking placebo. One RCT found more adverse effects (dyspepsia and drowsiness) with chlormezanone (14 of 52 people) than with methocarbamol (six of 55 people).[2,9]

Comment: None.

OPTION   NON-STEROIDAL ANTI-INFLAMMATORY DRUGS (NSAIDS)

RCTs in people with acute low back pain have found that NSAIDs are more effective than placebo for pain relief and overall improvement. They have found no evidence to distinguish different NSAIDs, no evidence that NSAIDs relieve radicular pain, and conflicting evidence for benefit compared with paracetamol, opioids, muscle relaxants, antidepressants, and non-drug treatments. Two RCTs in people with chronic low back pain found that NSAIDs were more effective than paracetamol for overall

improvement and more effective than placebo for pain, and that NSAIDs plus vitamin B were more effective than NSAIDs alone.

Benefits: We found four systematic reviews and 25 additional RCTs (51 RCTs in total, statistical pooling only for NSAIDs versus placebo in acute low back pain).[2,9,20,21] (References for individual RCTs available on www.clinicalevidence.org). **Acute low back pain, NSAIDs versus placebo:** Nine RCTs (n = 1135) found that NSAIDs increased the number of people experiencing global improvement (pooled OR after 1 week 2.0, 95% CI 1.4 to 3.0) and reduced the number needing additional analgesics (pooled OR 0.64, 95% CI 0.45 to 0.91). Four RCTs (n = 313) found no evidence that NSAIDs relieved radicular pain. **Versus paracetamol:** Of three conflicting trials, two (n = 93) found no evidence of significant differences in recovery, and one (n = 60) found greater pain reduction with mefenamic acid than paracetamol. **Versus muscle relaxants and opioid analgesics:** Five out of six RCTs (n = 399 out of 459) found no evidence of significant differences in pain and overall improvement. One RCT (n = 60) found that mefenamic acid reduced pain more than dextropropoxyphene plus paracetamol. **Versus non-drug treatments:** We found three trials (n = 461). One (n = 110) found that NSAIDs improved range of movement more than bed rest and reduced the need for further treatment, although another trial (n = 241) found no evidence of an effect on these outcomes. Both this RCT and one further trial (total n = 354) found no evidence of benefit versus physiotherapy or spinal manipulation in terms of pain and mobility. **Versus each other:** 15 RCTs (n = 1490) found no evidence of significant differences in efficacy. **Versus NSAID plus adjuvant treatment:** Three RCTs (n = 232, NSAIDs v NSAIDs plus muscle relaxants) found no evidence of significant differences in efficacy between NSAID/muscle relaxant combinations versus NSAIDs alone. Two RCTs (n = 123) (one of which was not included in the systematic reviews[22]) comparing NSAIDs with NSAID/vitamin B combinations found no evidence of significant differences in pain, although one of these trials found that combination therapy was associated with a greater return to work within a week (78% of people with combination therapy v 35% with NSAIDs alone). **Chronic low back pain:** One RCT (n = 37) found that naproxen reduced pain more than placebo, but found no evidence that diflunisal was better than placebo for pain. One small RCT (n = 30) found more overall improvement with diflunisal compared with paracetamol. Three trials (n = 262) compared different NSAIDs and found no evidence of a significant difference. One RCT (n = 252, diclofenac versus diclofenac plus vitamins B1, B6, B12) found greater overall improvement for the NSAID/B complex combination.

Harms: Adverse effects (particularly at high doses and in elderly people) may be serious. Effects included gastritis and other gastrointestinal complaints (in 10% of people). Ibuprofen and diclofenac had the lowest gastrointestinal complication rate, mainly because of the low doses used in practice (pooled OR for adverse effects compared with placebo 1.3, 95% CI 0.91 to 1.8).[2,18,23] In two trials, adverse effects were more frequent with NSAID/muscle relaxant combinations.

Comment: None.

QUESTION What are the effects of local injections for acute and chronic non-specific low back pain?

OPTION EPIDURAL STEROID INJECTIONS

In people with acute low back pain, we found no evidence that epidural steroids are effective in the absence of sciatica. In chronic low back pain with sciatica, we found conflicting evidence on the effects of epidural steroids.

Benefits: We found four systematic reviews.[2,9,24,25] **Acute low back pain:** We found two RCTs. One trial (n = 57, epidural steroids v subcutaneous lignocaine injections in people with acute pain and sciatica) found no differences after 1 month, but more people were pain free in the steroid group at 3 months. The second trial (n = 63, epidural steroids v epidural saline, bupivacaine, and dry needling) found no difference in the number of people improved or cured. **Chronic low back pain:** Seven trials were common to all four systematic reviews (n = 216, 3 RCTs of epidural steroids versus epidural saline, 4 RCTs of epidural steroids versus epidural bupivacaine, procaine, midazolam, or lignocaine and morphine). Three of the reviews (no statistical pooling) found insufficient evidence to draw conclusions. The fourth review found that steroids reduced pain in more people than the control interventions in the short term (pooled OR 2.60, 95% CI 1.9 to 3.8).[25]

Harms: Adverse effects were infrequent and included headache, fever, subdural penetration, and more rarely epidural abscess and ventilatory depression.[2,24]

Comment: Trials were small (range 22–73 participants) and included people with a variety of indications (chronic low back pain with and without sciatica, sciatica alone, lumbar radicular pain syndrome, postlaminectomy pain syndrome).

OPTION FACET JOINT INJECTIONS

One systematic review of RCTs has found no evidence that facet joint injections improve pain or function in people with chronic low back pain. We found insufficient evidence in people with acute low back pain.

Benefits: We found one systematic review (search date not stated, published 1994, 5 RCTs, no statistical pooling).[2] Two trials did not distinguish between acute and chronic pain.[2] **Acute low back pain:** We found no RCTs. **Chronic low back pain:** Two trials (n = 206, intra-articular corticosteroid versus intra-articular saline) found no significant differences in pain, disability, and flexibility after 1, 3, and 6 months. One trial (n = 86) compared facet joint injections versus facet nerve block and found no significant difference in pain relief after 2 weeks, 1 month, and 3 months.

Harms: Adverse effects included pain at injection site, infection, haemorrhage, neurological damage, and chemical meningitis.[2]

Comment: None.

OPTION   **TRIGGER POINT AND LIGAMENTOUS INJECTIONS**

One systematic review of RCTs in chronic low back pain has found limited evidence that combined steroid and local anaesthetic injection of trigger points provides greater pain relief after 3 months than injection of local anaesthetic alone. It also found limited evidence that phenol injection of the lumbar interspinal ligament reduces disability compared with saline injection. We found insufficient evidence in acute low back pain.

Benefits: We found one systematic review (search date not given, published 1994, two RCTs, 138 people).[2] **Acute low back pain:** We found no RCTs. **Chronic low back pain:** One trial (n = 57) compared trigger point injection with methylprednisolone or triamcinolone plus lignocaine versus lignocaine alone. It found that combined lignocaine and steroid completely relieved pain in more people than lignocaine alone (60–80% v 20%). The other RCT (n = 81) compared injection of dextrose-glycerine-phenol into the lumbar interspinal ligament versus injection of saline. It found that phenol reduced pain and disability more than saline at 1, 3, and 6 months.

Harms: Potential harms included nerve or other tissue damage, infection, and haemorrhage.[2]

Comment: None.

QUESTION   **What are the effects of non-drug treatments?**

OPTION   **ADVICE TO STAY ACTIVE**

Systematic reviews of RCTs have found that, in people with acute low back pain, advice to stay active speeds symptomatic recovery, reduces chronic disability and results in less time off work compared with bed rest or usual care. We found insufficient evidence in people with chronic low back pain.

Benefits: We found two systematic reviews (search dates not given, no statistical pooling).[2,26] **Acute low back pain:** Two RCTs (n = 228) found faster rates of recovery, less pain, and less disability in people advised to stay active than in people receiving no advice. Five RCTs (n = 1500) found that advice to stay active led to less sick leave and less chronic disability compared with traditional medical treatment (analgesics as required, advice to rest and "let pain be your guide"). **Chronic low back pain:** We found no RCTs.

Harms: Harms were not addressed.

Comment: Limitations in methods preclude meaningful quantification of effect sizes. Advice to stay active was either provided as a single treatment or in combination with other interventions such as back schools, a graded activity programme, or behavioural counselling.

OPTION   **BACK SCHOOLS**

Systematic reviews of RCTs have found conflicting evidence on the effects of back schools in people with acute or chronic low back pain. In occupational settings, back schools have been shown to be more effective than no treatment in people with chronic low back pain.

Benefits: We found one systematic review (16 RCTs, no statistical pooling),[27] and one subsequent RCT.[28] **Acute low back pain:** Two RCTs (n = 242) compared back schools versus McKenzie exercises (see glossary, p 628) and physical therapy. They found no evidence of improvements in pain, recovery rate, and rates of sick leave. One trial (n = 100, ongoing McKenzie exercises v one 45 minute session of back school) found that exercises improved pain and reduced sick leave more than back school up to 5 years. The other trial (n = 145) found that back schools speeded recovery and reduced sick leave in the short term compared with placebo (shortwave diathermy at lowest intensity). **Chronic low back pain:** Of 10 RCTs, five (861 people) compared back schools versus exercises, manipulation, NSAIDs, or physiotherapy. They found that back schools were better at reducing pain and disability up to 6 months, but found no evidence of an effect after 1 year. Of seven trials (529 people) comparing back schools versus no treatment, waiting list control, or detuned shortwave diathermy, four reported positive short term outcomes for the back school treatment, two found no short term differences, and two found no long term differences. Five RCTs (880 people) found that intensive back school programmes in an occupational setting improved pain and disability more than no treatment, but found no evidence that they were better than other treatments (physical therapy, calisthenics group training, usual care).

Harms: We found no evidence.

Comment: The risk of adverse effects is considered to be low.[2]

OPTION　BED REST

Systematic reviews of RCTs have found no evidence that bed rest is better, and found evidence that it may be worse than back exercises, physiotherapy, spinal manipulation, NSAIDs, or no treatment in people with acute low back pain. We found insufficient evidence on the effects of bed rest in people with chronic low back pain.

Benefits: We found five systematic reviews (no statistical pooling).[2,7,9,26,29] **Acute low back pain:** Five RCTs (n = 921) compared bed rest versus other treatments (back exercises, physiotherapy, spinal manipulation, or NSAIDs). They found either no evidence of benefit or that bed rest was worse (using outcomes of pain, recovery rate, time to return to daily activities, and sick leave). Five RCTs (n = 663) found that bed rest was no different or worse than no treatment or placebo. Two RCTs (n = 254) found that 7 days of bed rest was no different from 2–4 of bed rest. **Chronic low back pain:** We found no RCTs.

Harms: Adverse effects of bed rest were joint stiffness, muscle wasting, loss of bone mineral density, pressure sores, and venous thromboembolism. Prolonged bed rest may lead to chronic disability and may impair rehabilitation.[26]

Comment: None.

| OPTION | BEHAVIOURAL THERAPY |

Two RCTs found that behavioural therapy reduced acute low back pain more than traditional care or EMG feedback. In people with chronic back pain, systematic reviews of RCTs have found that behavioural therapy has a moderate effect on pain and a mild effect on disability compared with no treatment. We found conflicting evidence comparing behavioural therapy with other treatments (usual care, back exercises), and found no evidence that one type of behavioural therapy is superior to another.

Benefits: We found five systematic reviews and additional RCTs (no statistical pooling).[2,7,9,30,31] (References for additional RCTs available on www.clinicalevidence.org) **Acute low back pain:** One RCT (n = 107) found that behavioural treatment reduced pain and perceived disability (at 9–12 months) more than traditional care (analgesics and back exercises until pain had subsided). A second RCT (50 people) found better pain relief in people with acute sciatica with risk factor based cognitive behavioural treatment (see glossary, p 628) than with EMG feedback.[32] **Chronic low back pain:** We found 9 RCTs that compared different types of behavioural therapy (cognitive behavioural treatment, operant behavioural treatmentsand respondent behavioural treatment, n = 308). They found no overall differences among the treatments (using functional status, pain, and behavioural outcomes, including anxiety, depression, pain behaviour, and coping). Eleven trials (n = 1223) found that behavioural treatment had a moderate effect on pain intensity and small effects on functional status and behavioural outcomes compared with no treatment, waiting list controls, or placebo. Of two RCTs (n = 202) comparing behavioural treatment versus other treatments, one found that a higher proportion of people returned to work within 12 weeks with operant behavioural treatment compared with traditional care (rest, analgesics, physical therapy). The other RCT found no evidence of differences in pain and depression after 6 and 12 months between operant behavioural treatment and back exercises. Six RCTs (n = 343) evaluated behavioural therapy in combination with other treatments (physiotherapy and back education, multidisciplinary treatment programmes, inpatient pain management programmes, and back exercises). These found that the addition of behavioural therapy had a small positive short term effect on functional status but no significant effect on pain or behavioural outcomes compared with the other treatments alone.

Harms: The trials did not assess harms.

Comment: None.

| OPTION | ELECTROMYOGRAPHIC (EMG) BIOFEEDBACK |

One small RCT found that EMG biofeedback (see glossary, p 628) produced less pain relief than cognitive behavioural treatment in acute low back pain. One systematic review found conflicting evidence in chronic low back pain.

Benefits: We found one systematic review (search date 1995, 5 RCTs, no statistical pooling)[9] and one subsequent RCT.[32] **Acute low back pain:** We found one small RCT (50 people) that found better pain relief in people with acute sciatica with risk factor based cognitive behavioural treatment than EMG biofeedback.[32] **Chronic low back pain:** The review found five small trials (total n = 168).[9] Three (n = 102) found no differences between EMG biofeedback and placebo or waiting list control (outcomes were pain and functional status). Two trials (n = 30) compared biofeedback versus progressive relaxation training and found conflicting effects on pain and functional status; one trial found EMG biofeedback better than relaxation training, and the other found the converse. One trial (n = 30) found no evidence of differences in pain and range of movement between rehabilitation programmes with and without biofeedback.

Harms: The trials did not address harms.

Comment: None.

OPTION   BACK EXERCISES

Systematic reviews of RCTs have found no evidence that specific back exercises (flexion, extension, aerobic, or strengthening exercises) are more effective than other conservative treatments in people with acute low back pain. RCTs have found that back exercises are more effective than other conservative measures in people with chronic low back pain.

Benefits: We found five systematic reviews and additional[2,7,9,33,34] RCTs (no statistical pooling). (References for additional RCTs available on www.clinicalevidence.org) Results for acute and chronic low back pain were not reported separately in three trials. **Acute low back pain:** Of 12 identified trials (n = 1894), eight compared specific back exercises (flexion, extension, aerobic or strengthening programmes, such as McKenzie exercises) versus other conservative treatments (usual care by the general practitioner, continuation of ordinary activities, bed rest, manipulation, NSAIDs, mini back school, or short wave diathermy). Seven of these found either no significant differences or that exercise mildly increased pain intensity and disability. The eighth trial found that exercise therapy improved pain and return to work compared with a mini back school. The four other trials (n = 1234) found no evidence that exercises had significant effects on pain, global improvement, or functional status compared with "inactive" treatment (bed rest, educational booklet, and placebo ultrasound). **Chronic low back pain:** We found four systematic reviews.[7,9,33,34] Three systematic reviews found 23 RCTs (2240 people) and found that overall, exercises improved pain, disability, and physical outcomes (e.g. strength and flexibility) in the short term, but the effects were small.[7,9,33] The fourth systematic review concluded that it is still unclear whether back exercises are more effective than inactive treatment for chronic low back pain.[34] Nine of the RCTs (1020 people) compared exercises versus conservative treatment. Three trials found no evidence that exercises had significant effects on pain, functional status, overall improvement, or return to work compared with conventional physiotherapy. Three trials found that exercises improved pain, functional status, and return to work compared with "usual care" by the general practitioner. The remaining three RCTs found that exercises improved pain and functional status more than back school education and early morning lumbar flexion control. Six trials (n = 587) compared exercises versus inactive treatments (hot packs and rest, semi hot packs and sham traction, waiting list controls, TENS, sham TENS, detuned ultrasound, or detuned shortwave diathermy). Three found better overall improvement or more pain reduction with exercises, whereas three found no evidence of significant differences. Three small trials (153 people) compared extension versus flexion exercises; two found no evidence of a significant difference in pain intensity and one found better global improvement with flexion exercises. One RCT (148 people) found no significant difference between active physiotherapy muscle reconditioning and low impact aerobics.[35]

Harms: Potential harms include increased stress on the spine.[2] Most trials did not assess harms.

Comment: None.

OPTION	LUMBAR SUPPORTS

We found insufficient evidence on the effects of lumbar supports in acute or chronic back pain.

Benefits: We found five systematic reviews and additional RCTs (six RCTs in total, no statistical pooling).[2,7,9,25,28–30,36] Five trials (1200 people) did not differentiate between acute and chronic pain. These compared lumbar supports for 3–6 weeks versus no treatment or versus treatments such as manipulation, physiotherapy, and analgesics.[2,7,37,38] Results for overall improvement, return to work, and functional status were conflicting. **Acute low back pain:** We found no RCTs specifically including people with acute low back pain. **Chronic low back pain:** One RCT (n = 19) evaluated a lumbar corset with or without a synthetic support. It found that the inclusion of a support improved symptom severity and functional disability, but found no evidence that it improved range of movement.

Harms: Adverse effects of prolonged lumbar support include decreased strength of the trunk musculature, a false sense of security, heat, skin irritation, and general discomfort.[2] The trials did not assess these.

Comment: None.

OPTION	MULTIDISCIPLINARY TREATMENT PROGRAMMES

One systematic review of two RCTs found limited evidence that multidisciplinary treatment (see glossary, p 628), which includes a workplace visit, leads to faster recovery from acute low back pain. A systematic review found that multidisciplinary treatment programmes improve pain, functional status, and return to work in people with chronic low back pain.

Benefits: **Acute low back pain:** We found one systematic review (search date 1998, 2 RCTs, 233 people).[39] It found that multidisciplinary treatment which includes a workplace visit leads to faster return to work and less sick leave than usual care. **Chronic low back pain:**

We found one systematic review and two additional RCTs (10 trials, n = 1691).[7,40–42] These found that, in people with severe chronic low back pain, multidisciplinary treatment programmes improved pain, functional status, and return to work moderately more than traditional inpatient rehabilitation (see glossary, p 629) or usual care, up to 1 year.

Harms: The trials gave no information on adverse effects.

Comment: None.

OPTION   **PHYSICAL TREATMENTS (SHORT WAVE DIATHERMY, ULTRASOUND, ICE, HEAT, MASSAGE)**

We found insufficient evidence on the effects of physical treatments in acute and chronic low back pain.

Benefits: We found two systematic reviews, which found no RCTs.[2,43]

Harms: Insufficient information.

Comment: None.

OPTION   **SPINAL MANIPULATION**

We found conflicting evidence on the effects of spinal manipulation in acute and chronic low back pain.

Benefits: We found five systematic reviews of 36 RCTs (no statistical pooling).[2,7,9,44,45] **Acute low back pain:** Of five placebo controlled trials (n = 383), two found slightly more pain relief with manipulation up to 3 weeks and two found no evidence of pain reduction compared with placebo. The remaining trial found slightly faster recovery in the manipulation group. The reviews identified 12 RCTs (n = 899) comparing manipulation versus short wave diathermy, massage, exercises, back school, or drug treatment. Four systematic reviews found that the results of these RCTs were conflicting.[2,7,9,44] The other review (7 RCTs, n = 731, manipulation versus other conservative treatments) found that manipulation increased recovery at 2–3 weeks (NNT 5, 95% CI 4 to 14).[45] **Chronic low back pain:** Four trials (n = 514) compared manipulation versus placebo. Eight trials (n = 545) compared manipulation versus other conservative treatments (such as usual care, short wave diathermy, massage, exercises, back schools, and drug treatment). Of four systematic reviews in chronic low back pain, three found that the results of these RCTs were conflicting.[7,44,45] One systematic review (no statistical pooling) found manipulation slightly more effective than placebo in five trials (n = 543).[9]

Harms: In the studies that used a trained therapist to select and manipulate people, the risk of serious complication was low (estimated risk: vertebrobasilar strokes 1 in 20 000 to 1 in 1 000 000; cauda equina syndrome < 1 in 1 000 000).

Comment: Current guidelines contraindicate manipulation in people with severe or progressive neurological deficit.[2,19]

OPTION TRACTION

Systematic reviews of RCTs have found no evidence that traction is effective in either acute or chronic back pain.

Benefits: We found three systematic reviews[7,9,46] and two additional RCTs.[47–48] Of the 16 RCTs identified, 12 (n = 921) did not distinguish between acute and chronic low back pain. Ten of these trials found no significant differences between traction and placebo traction, exercises, hot packs, massage, interferential therapy or rest. Two found slightly better overall improvement after treatment. **Acute low back pain:** Two RCTs (total n = 225) compared traction versus bed rest plus corset, and traction versus infrared treatment. One study found more overall improvement after 1 and 3 weeks with traction, but the other found no significant difference in overall improvement after 2 weeks. **Chronic low back pain:** Two studies (total n = 176) compared traction versus placebo traction of maximum 25% of body weight. They found no significant differences in global improvement, pain or functional status after 5–9 weeks.[1,49]

Harms: The trials gave no information on harms. Potential adverse effects include debilitation, loss of muscle tone, bone demineralisation, and thrombophlebitis.[2]

Comment: None.

OPTION TRANSCUTANEOUS ELECTRICAL NERVE STIMULATION (TENS)

We found insufficient evidence on the effects of TENS in either acute or chronic low back pain.

Benefits: We found three systematic reviews of five RCTs.[2,9,50] **Acute low back pain:** Of two identified RCTs, one (n = 58) compared rehabilitation programmes with and without TENS and found no difference in pain and functional status. The other (n = 40) found that TENS improved pain and mobility significantly more than paracetamol after 6 weeks of treatment. **Chronic low back pain:** Four identified RCTs (n = 253) compared TENS versus placebo. One trial (n = 42) found better pain relief with TENS after 1 week but not after 3 and 6 months, and one crossover trial (n = 33) found slightly better overall improvement with TENS. The other two trials (n = 178) found no differences in pain, functional status, or mobility. Two of the systematic reviews found that these RCTs conflicted (no statistical pooling performed).[2,9] The other review pooled the data and found that TENS did not significantly reduce the number of people with pain compared with placebo (OR no pain 1.62, 95% CI 0.90 to 2.68).[50]

Harms: The reviews gave no information on adverse effects.[2,9,50]

Comment: None.

OPTION ACUPUNCTURE

We found no RCTs of acupuncture (see glossary, p 628) in people with acute low back pain. Two systematic reviews of RCTs found conflicting evidence of its effects in people with chronic low back pain.

Benefits: We found two systematic reviews (search dates 1996, 12 RCTs in total, of which six RCTs were unsuitable; see comment below),[51,52] and one subsequent RCT.[53] **Acute low back pain:** No RCTs. **Chronic low back pain:** Seven RCTs (380 people) compared acupuncture versus no treatment or waiting list or transcutaneous electrical nerve stimulation or placebo acupuncture in people with chronic low back pain. One systematic review (no statistical pooling) found that the overall quality of the RCTs was low, and found no evidence that acupuncture was more effective than placebo or no treatment.[52] The other review found that acupuncture was better than all other interventions analysed together (OR for overall improvement 2.3, 95% CI 1.3 to 4.1). It found no significant difference between acupuncture and placebo acupuncture (OR 1.4, 95% CI 0.84 to 2.3).[51] The subsequent RCT included 60 elderly people aged 60 or over found that acupuncture versus transcutaneous electrical nerve stimulation significantly reduced pain measured on a visual analogue scale ($P < 0.001$), pain measured on the pain subscale of the Nottingham Health Profile ($P < 0.001$) and the number of analgesic tablets consumed per week ($P < 0.05$).[53]

Harms: Acupuncture has been found to have fewer adverse effects than spinal manipulation.[51] One systematic review (search date 1996) found that serious, rare, adverse effects included infections (HIV, hepatitis, bacterial endocarditis) and trauma (pneumothorax, cardiac tamponade).[54]

Comment: Three of the identified RCTs combined acute and chronic low back pain and two did not specify the duration of symptoms. One RCT included people with back and neck pain.[51,52]

GLOSSARY

Acupuncture Needling of the skin at traditional "meridian" acupuncture points. Modern acupuncturists also use non-meridian points and trigger points (tender sites occurring in the most painful areas). The needles may be stimulated manually or electrically. Placebo acupuncture is needling of traditionally unimportant sites or non-stimulation of the needles once placed.

Cognitive behavioural treatment This aims to identify and modify patients' cognitions regarding their pain and disability using cognitive restructuring techniques (such as imagery and attention diversion) or by modifying maladaptive thoughts, feelings, and beliefs.

Electroacupuncture Non-penetrative electrical stimulation of classical acupuncture points with low amplitude, pulsed electrical current.

Electromyographic (EMG) biofeedback A person receives external feedback of their own electromyogram (using visual or auditory scales), and uses this to learn how to control the electromyogram, and hence the tension within their own muscles. Electromyogram biofeedback for low back pain aims to relax the paraspinal muscles.

McKenzie exercises Extension exercises that use self generated stresses and forces to centralise pain from the legs and buttocks to the lower back. This method emphasises self care.

Multidisciplinary treatment Intensive physical and psychosocial training by a team (e.g. a physician, physiotherapist, psychologist, social worker, and occupational therapist). Training is usually given in groups and does not involve passive physical therapy.

Operant behavioural treatments These include positive reinforcement of healthy behaviours and consequent withdrawal of attention from pain behaviours, time-contingent instead of pain-contingent pain management, and spouse involvement, while undergoing a programme aimed at increasing exercise tolerance towards a preset goal.

Respondent behavioural treatment This aims to modify physiological responses directly (e.g. reducing muscle tension by explaining the relation between tension and pain, and using relaxation techniques).

Traditional inpatient rehabilitation The components of inpatient rehabilitation may vary from country to country, and may include passive physical therapy (massage, ultrasound, electrotherapy, heat, traction), muscle training, relaxation exercises, pool exercises, back school education, and may last for about 3 weeks.

Substantive changes since last issue

Analgesics One new RCT of tramadol versus placebo that found decreased pain and increased function in peoples with acute low back pain.[10] First placebo controlled RCT of analgesics in low back pain.

Antidepressants One new small RCT of maprotiline versus paroxetine in 67 people with chronic low back pain. The result is not consistent with previous systematic reviews in 328 people that found no overall benefit from antidepressants.[18]

NSAIDs One new systematic review; conclusion unaltered.[21]

Back schools One new RCT of back school versus no treatment; conclusion that back schools can be beneficial strengthened.[28]

Behavioural therapy One new systematic review; conclusion unaltered.[31]

Behavioural therapy New RCT that found more benefit with cognitive behavioural therapy than with EMG feedback; conclusion unaltered.[32]

EMG feedback New RCT that found more benefit with cognitive behavioural therapy than with EMG feedback; conclusion changed.[32]

Back exercises Additional systematic review concluding that the effects of back exercises remain unclear.[34]

Back exercises One new RCT that found no difference between active physiotherapy, muscle reconditioning, and low impact aerobics; conclusion unaltered.[35]

Lumbar supports one new systematic review; conclusion unaltered.[38]

Multidisciplinary treatment One systematic review of two RCTs; additional evidence, and conclusion modified.[39]

Traction One additional RCT of traction and massage versus interferential therapy; conclusion unaltered.[48]

Acupuncture One new RCT of acupuncture versus transcutaneous electrical nerve stimulation for chronic back pain in the elderly; conclusion unaltered.[53]

REFERENCES

1. Van der Heijden GJMG, Bouter LM, Terpstra-Lindeman E. De effectiviteit van tractie bij lage rugklachten. De resultaten van een pilotstudy. Ned T Fysiotherapie 1991;101:37–43.

2. Bigos S, Bowyer O, Braen G, et al. Acute low back problems in adults. Clinical Practice Guideline no.14. AHCPR Publication No. 95–0642. Rockville MD: Agency for Health Care Policy and Research, Public Health Service, US, Department of Health and Human Services. December 1994. Search date not given; primary sources The Quebec Task Force on Spinal Disorders Review to 1984; search carried out by National Library of Medicine from 1984; and references from expert panel.

3. Andersson GBJ. The epidemiology of spinal disorders. In: Frymoyer JW, ed. The adult spine: principles and practice. 2nd ed. New York: Raven Press, 1997:93–141.

4. Deyo RA, Rainville J, Kent DL. What can the history and physical examination tell us about low back pain? JAMA 1992;268:760–765.

5. Bongers PM, de Winter CR, Kompier MA, et al. Psychosocial factors at work and musculoskeletal disease. Scand J Work Environ Health 1993;19:297–312.

6. Frymoyer JW. Back pain and sciatica. N Engl J Med 1988;318:291–300.

7. Evans G, Richards S. Low back pain: an evaluation of therapeutic interventions. Bristol: Health Care Evaluation Unit, University of Bristol, 1996. Search date 1995; primary sources Medline; Embase; A-Med; Psyclit; and hand searched references.

8. Van Tulder MW, Assendelft WJJ, Koes BW, et al, and the Editorial Board of the Cochrane Collaboration Back Review Group. Method guidelines for systematic reviews in the Cochrane Collaboration back review group for spinal disorders. Spine 1997;22:2323–2330.

9. Van Tulder MW, Koes BW, Bouter LM. Conservative treatment of acute and chronic nonspecific low back pain: a systematic review of randomized controlled trials of the most common interventions. *Spine* 1997;22:2128–2156. Search date 1995; primary sources Medline; Embase; Psychlit; and hand searched references.

10. Schnitzer TJ, Gray WL, Paster RZ, et al. Efficacy of tramadol in treatment of chronic low back pain. *J Rheumatol* 2000;27:772–778.

11. De Craen AJM, Di Giulio G, Lampe-Schoenmaeckers AJEM, et al. Analgesic efficacy and safety of paracetamol–codeine combinations versus paracetamol alone: a systematic review. *BMJ* 1996;313:321–325. Search date 1995; primary sources Medline; Embase; International Pharmaceutical Abstracts; Biosis; contact with pharmaceutical companies, and hand searched references.

12. Turner JA, Denny MC. Do antidepressant medications relieve chronic low back pain? *J Fam Pract* 1993;37:545–553. Search date 1992; primary sources Medline; Psyclit; hand searches of bibliographies; and inquiries to researchers and drug companies.

13. Atkinson JH, Slater MA, Williams RA, et al. A placebo-controlled randomized clinical trial of nortriptyline for chronic low back pain. *Pain* 1998; 76:287–296.

14. Hameroff SR, Cork RC, Scherer K, et al. Doxepin effects on chronic pain, depression and plasma opioids. *J Clin Psychiatry* 1982;43:22–27.

15. Hameroff SR, Weiss JL, Lerman JC, et al. Doxepin's effects on chronic pain and depression: a controlled study. *J Clin Psychiatry* 1984;45:47–52.

16. Stein D, Peri T, Edelstein E, et al. The efficacy of amitriptyline and acetaminophen in the management of acute low back pain. *Psychosomatics* 1996;37:63–70.

17. Treves R, Montane De La Roque P, Dumond JJ, et al. Prospective study of the analgesic action of clomipramine versus placebo in refractory low back pain and sciatica (68 cases). *Rev Rhum* 1991;58:549–552 (in French).

18. Atkinson JH, Slater MA, Wahlgren DR, et al. Effects of noradrenergic and serotonergic antidepressants on chronic low back pain intensity. *Pain* 1999;83:137–145.

19. Waddell G, Feder G, McIntosh A, et al. Low back pain evidence review. London: Royal College of General Practitioners, 1996. Search date 1996; primary sources Medline; Embase; Science Citation Index; Social Sciences Citation Index; correspondence with experts and researchers, and hand searched references.

20. Koes BW, Scholten RJPM, Mens JMA, et al. Efficacy of non-steroidal anti-inflammatory drugs for low back pain: a systematic review of randomised clinical trials. *Ann Rheum Dis* 1997; 56:214–223. Search date 1994; primary sources Medline 1966 to 1994; Embase 1980 to 1994, and hand searched references.

21. Van Tulder MW, Scholten RJPM, Koes BW, et al. Non-steroidal anti-inflammatory drugs (NSAIDs) for non-specific low back pain. In: The Cochrane Library, Issue 3, 2000. Oxford: Update Software. Search date 1998; primary sources Medline; Embase; Cochrane Controlled Trials Register; and hand searches of reference lists.

22. Bruggemann G, Koehler CO, Koch EM. Results of a double-blind study of diclofenac + vitamin B1, B6, B12 versus diclofenac in patients with acute pain of the lumbar vertebrae: a multicenter study. *Klinische Wochenschrift* 1990;68:116–120.

23. Henry D, Lim LLY, Rodriguez LAG, et al. Variability in risk of gastrointestinal complications with individual non-steroidal anti-inflammatory drugs: results of a collaborative meta-analysis. *BMJ* 1996;312:1563–1566. Search date 1994; primary sources Medline, contact with study authors, and hand searched references.

24. Koes BW, Scholten RJPM, Mens JMA, et al. Efficacy of epidural steroid injections for low back pain and sciatica: a systematic review of randomized clinical trials. Pain 1995;63:279–288. Search date 1993; primary sources Medline 1966 to 1993, and hand searched references.

25. Watts RW, Silagy CA. A meta-analysis on the efficacy of epidural corticosteroids in the treatment of sciatica. *Anaesth Intensive Care* 1995;23:564–569.

26. Waddell G, Feder G, Lewis M. Systematic reviews of bed rest and advice to stay active for acute low back pain. *Br J Gen Pract* 1997;47:647–652. Search date not given; primary sources Medline; contacted recently published authors and pharmaceutical company; and hand searched references.

27. Van Tulder MW, Esmail R, Bombardier C, Koes BW. Back schools for non-specific low back pain. In: The Cochrane Library, Issue 3, 2000. Oxford: Update Software. Search date 1997; primary sources Medline, Embase, and hand searched references.

28. Dalichau S, Scheele K, Perrey RM, et al. Ultraschallgest tzte Haltungs- und Bewegungsanalyse der Lendenwirbelsa le zum Nachweis der Wirksamkeit einer R ckenschule. *Zentralbl Arbeitsmed* 1999;49:148–156.

29. Koes BW, van den Hoogen HMM. Efficacy of bed rest and orthoses of low back pain. A review of randomized clinical trials. *Eur J Phys Med Rehabil* 1994;4:86–93. Search date not given; primary sources Medline 1966 to 1992, and hand searched references.

30. Turner JA. Educational and behavioral interventions for back pain in primary care. *Spine* 1996;21:2851–2859. Search date 1994; primary sources Medline; Psyclit; handsearches; and inquiries to pharmaceutical companies and expert researchers in the field.

31. Van Tulder MW, Ostelo R, Vlaeyen JWS, Linton SJ, Morley SJ, Assendelft WJJ. Behavioural treatment for chronic low back pain. In: The Cochrane Library, Issue 3, 2000. Oxford: Update Software. Search date 1999; primary sources Medline; Psyclit; Cochrane Controlled Trials Register; Embase; and hand searches of reference lists.

32. Hasenbring M, Ulrich HW, Hartmann M, et al. The efficacy of a risk factor-based cognitive behavioral intervention and electromyographic biofeedback in patients with acute sciatic pain: an attempt to prevent chronicity. *Spine* 1999;24:2525–2535.

33. Faas A. Exercises: which ones are worth trying, for which patients and when? *Spine* 1996;21:2874–2879. Search date 1995; primary source Medline.

34. Van Tulder MW, Malmivaara A, Esmail R, Koes BW. Exercise therapy for non-specific low back pain. In: The Cochrane Library, Issue 3, 2000. Oxford: Update Software. Search date 1999; primary sources Medline; Psychlit; Cochrane Controlled Trials Register; Embase; and hand searches of reference lists.

35. Mannion AF, M ntener M, Taimela S, et al. A randomized clinical trial of three active therapies for chronic low back pain. *Spine* 1999;24:2435–2448.

36. Van Tulder MW, Jellema P, van Poppel MNM, et al. Lumbar supports for prevention and treatment of low back pain. In: The Cochrane Library, Issue 3, 2000. Oxford: Update Software. Search date 1999; primary sources Medline; Cinahl; Current

Contents; Cochrane Controlled Trials Register; Embase; Science Citation Index; and hand searches of reference lists.

37. Penrose KW, Chook K, Stump JL. Acute and chronic effects of pneumatic lumbar support on muscular strength, flexibility, and functional impairment index. *Sports Train Med Rehab* 1991; 2:121–129.

38. Pope MH, Phillips RB, Haugh LD, et al. A prospective randomized three week trial of spinal manipulation, transcutaneous muscle stimulation, massage and corset in the treatment of subacute low back pain. *Spine* 1994;19:2571–2577.

39. Karjalainen K, Malmivaara A, van Tulder M, et al. Multidisciplinary biopsychosocial rehabilitation for subacute low back pain among working age adults. In: The Cochrane Library, Issue 3, 2000. Oxford: Update Software. Search date 1998; primary sources Medline; Embase; Psyclit; Cochrane Register of Controlled Clinical Trials; Science Citation Index; and hand searches of reference lists and personal contact with experts.

40. Bendix AF, Bendix T, Ostenfeld S, et al. Active treatment programs for patients with chronic low back pain: a prospective, randomized, observer-blinded study. *Eur Spine J* 1995;4:148–152.

41. Bendix AF, Bendix T, Vaegter K, et al. Multidisciplinary intensive treatment for chronic low back pain: a randomized, prospective study. *Cleve Clin J Med* 1996;63:62–69.

42. Bendix AF, Bendix T, Labriola M, et al. Functional restoration for chronic low back pain: two-year follow-up of two randomized clinical trials. *Spine* 1998;23:717–725.

43. Gam AN, Johannsen F. Ultrasound therapy in musculoskeletal disorders: a meta-analysis. *Pain* 1995;63:85–91. Search date 1992; primary sources Index Medicus, Medline, and hand searched references.

44. Koes BW, Assendelft WJJ, van der Heijden GJMG, et al. Spinal manipulation for low back pain. An updated systematic review of randomized clinical trials. *Spine* 1996;21:2860–2871. Search date 1995; primary sources Medline, and hand searched references.

45. Shekelle PG, Adams AH, Chassin MR, et al. Spinal manipulation for low back pain. *Ann Intern Med* 1992;117:590–598. Search date not given; primary sources Medline and Index Medicus from 1952; contacted experts; and hand searched references.

46. Van der Heijden GJMG, Beurskens AJHM, Koes BW, et al. The efficacy of traction for back and neck pain: a systematic, blinded review of randomized clinical trial methods. *Phys Ther* 1995;75:93–104. Search date 1992; primary sources Medline 1966 to 1992; Embase 1974 to 1992; Index to Chiropractic Literature 1980 to 1992; Physiotherapy Index 1986 to 1992; and hand searched non-indexed journals.

47. Ljunggren E, Weber H, Larssen S. Autotraction versus manual traction in patients with prolapsed lumbar intervertebral discs. *Scand J Rehabil Med* 1984;16:117–124.

48. Werners R, Pynsent PB, Bulstrode CJK. Randomized trial comparing interferential therapy with motorized lumbar traction and massage in the management of low back pain in a primary care setting. *Spine* 1999;24:1579–1584.

49. Beurskens AJ, de Vet HCW, Köke AJ, et al. Efficacy of traction for non-specific low back pain: a randomised clinical trial. *Lancet* 1995;346:1596–1600.

50. Gadsby JG, Flowerdew MW. The effectiveness of transcutaneous electrical nerve stimulation (TENS) and acupuncture-like transcutaneous electrical nerve stimulation (ALTENS) in the treatment of patients with chronic low back pain. In: The Cochrane Library, Issue 3, 2000. Oxford: Update Software. Search date 1999; primary sources Medline; Embase; AMED; CISCOM; contacted investigators; hand searched references, conference proceedings and textbooks.

51. Ernst E, White AR. Acupuncture for back pain. A meta-analysis of randomized controlled trials. *Arch Intern Med* 1998;158:2235–2241. Search date 1996; primary sources Medline 1969 to 1996; Cochrane Controlled Trials Register; CISCOM November 1996; contacted authors and experts; and hand searched references.

52. Van Tulder MW, Cherkin DC, Berman B, et al. Acupuncture low back pain. In: The Cochrane Library, Issue 3, 2000. Oxford: Update Software. Search date 1996; primary sources Medline; Embase; Cochrane Complementary Medicine Field trials register; Cochrane Controlled Trials Register; Science Citation Index; and hand searched references.

53. Grant DJ, Bishop-Miller J, Winchester DM, et al. A randomized comparative trial of acupuncture versus transcutaneous electrical nerve stimulation for chronic back pain in the elderly. *Pain* 1999;82: 9–13.

54. Ernst E, White A. Life-threatening adverse reactions after acupuncture? A systematic review. *Pain* 1997;71:123–126. Search date 1996; primary sources Medline; CISCOM; other specialised databases; contacted experts and hand searched references.

Maurits van Tulder
Institute for Research in Extramural
Medicine
Vrije Universiteit
Amsterdam
The Netherlands

Bart Koes
Department of General Practice
Eramus University
Rotterdam
Netherlands

Competing interests: None declared.

Musculoskeletal disorders

Neck pain

Updated this issue

Allan Binder

Key Messages

- We found little good quality evidence, highlighting the need for prospective studies with standardised validation of diagnosis and good study design.

DEFINITION Neck pain can be divided into uncomplicated pain, whiplash, and pain with radiculopathy. Neck pain often occurs with limitation of movement and poorly defined neurological symptoms affecting the upper limbs. The pain can be severe and intractable, and can occur with radiculopathy or myelopathy.

INCIDENCE/ PREVALENCE About two thirds of people will experience neck pain at some time in their lives.[1,2] Prevalence is highest in middle age. In the UK, about 15% of hospital based physiotherapy, and in Canada 30% of chiropractic referrals are for neck pain.[3,4] In the Netherlands neck pain contributes up to 2% of general practitioner consultations.[5]

AETIOLOGY/ RISK FACTORS Most uncomplicated pain is associated with poor posture, anxiety and depression, neck strain, or occupational or sport injuries. With chronic pain, mechanical and degenerative factors, often referred to as cervical spondylosis, become more evident. Some neck pain results from soft tissue trauma, most typically seen in whiplash syndrome. Rarely disc prolapse and inflammatory, infective, or malignant conditions affect the cervical spine and present with neck pain with or without neurological features.

PROGNOSIS Neck pain usually resolves within days or weeks but can recur or become chronic. In some industries, neck related disorders account for as much time off work as low back pain[6] See low back pain and sciatica, p 614. The percentage of people in whom neck pain becomes chronic depends on the cause but is thought to be around 10%,[1] similar to low back pain. It causes severe disability in 5% of affected people.[2] One systematic review of the clinical course and prognostic factors of non-specific neck pain identified six observational studies and 17 RCTs.[7] In people who had had pain for at least 6 months, a median of 46% (22–79%) improved with treatment. Whiplash injuries were more likely to cause disability; up to 40% of sufferers reported symptoms even after 15 years of follow up.[8] Factors associated with a poorer outcome after whiplash are not well defined.[9]

OUTCOMES Pain, range of movement, function, adverse effects of treatment.

METHODS *Clinical Evidence* update search and appraisal May 2000. We also searched the following databases: Chirolars (now called Mantis) for English language articles from 1966 to November 1999; the Cochrane database;[10] Index Medicus (1966 to 1997); Bioethics-line (1973 to 1997); Cumulative Index to Nursing and Allied Health (Cinahl) (1982 to 1997); and Current Contents (1994 to 1997). Criteria for assessment of RCTs were based on those suggested by Koes, et al.[11]

QUESTION	What are the effects of treatments for people with uncomplicated neck pain without severe neurological deficit?

OPTION	PHYSICAL TREATMENTS

We found insufficient evidence about the effects of most physical treatments—heat or cold, traction, biofeedback, spray and stretch, acupuncture, and laser—in people with uncomplicated neck pain without neurological deficit. Two RCTs found benefit from physiotherapy, and one RCT found limited evidence for benefit from pulsed electromagnetic field therapy.

Benefits:
We found four systematic reviews[10,12-14] and one subsequent RCT.[15] Two of the systematic reviews[10,12] considered all physical modalities and the other two considered traction only[13] or acupuncture only.[14] The first systematic review (search date 1993) identified 13 RCTs (in 760 people with neck pain but without neurological deficit) that evaluated at least one form of physical treatment. It found no significant benefit from any of the following physical treatments: heat or cold, traction, electrotherapy (pulsing electromagnetic field [PEMF] or transcutaneous electrical nerve stimulation), biofeedback, spray and stretch, acupuncture, or laser.[10] The second general systematic review (search date 1995) identified 17 RCTs (1202 people) and found possible benefit for pulsed electromagnetic field therapy and active physiotherapy but not for traction, acupuncture or other physical therapies.[12] One RCT included in both reviews involved 47 people and found that active physiotherapy and exercise significantly reduced pain immediately after treatment compared with passive treatment (P < 0.05).[16] One RCT included in the second systematic review compared true and sham pulsed electromagnetic field therapy (given for at least 1 year) in 81 people with neck pain and radiographic evidence of cervical osteoarthritis and in 86 people with osteoarthritis of the knee.[17] In people with chronic neck pain, the RCT found that after 18 episodes of treatment there were significant reductions in pain (P < 0.04) and pain on passive motion (P = 0.03) but not in difficulty with activities of daily living, tenderness, self assessment of improvement, or physicians' global assessment with active versus sham treatment. It found no significant differences between the effects in people with knee or neck problems and, after the results were pooled, found that more people had improved in at least three of six variables with active compared with sham therapy (57/82 [70%] v 37/82 [45%]; ARI 24%, 95% CI 9% to 36%; RR 1.54, 95% CI 1.21 to 1.80; NNT 4, 95% CI 3 to 11). This benefit was sustained up to 1 month in many more treated than control patients (see comment below). The third systematic review (search date 1992) identified three RCTs in 639 people comparing traction versus a range of alternative treatments, including heat, mobilisation, exercise, no treatment, collar, and analgesics. The RCTs found no consistent pain reduction from traction compared with any of the alternatives.[13] The fourth review (search date 1998) identified 13 RCTs comparing needle or laser acupuncture with a range of control procedures (sham therapies, diazepam, and physiotherapy) but

found no consistent benefit for the acupuncture groups.[14] The subsequent RCT included 103 women with work related neck pain comparing the effect of three exercise regimes (training strength, endurance or coordination) over 10 weeks with a control group. Pain decreased significantly (P < 0.05) on the visual analogue scale in each exercise group when compared with controls, with no advantage for any exercise programme. Comparison of exercisers (82 women) and controls (21 women) showed significantly larger pain reductions among exercisers.[15]

Harms: We found no good data on harms. The incidence of serious adverse events seems to be low for all physical treatments considered.

Comment: The RCT comparing true and sham pulsed electromagnetic field therapy was double blinded and used random numbers to allocate people to groups. By chance, the baseline characteristics of treated and placebo groups were different: the people allocated to active treatment had higher pain scores, more tenderness, and more difficulty with the activities of daily living than the placebo group. The analysis in the RCT was based on changes from the baseline value, and it is not known how much of the observed effect was caused by bias introduced by the baseline differences.

OPTION	MANUAL TREATMENTS: MOBILISATION AND MANIPULATION

Four systematic reviews found evidence to suggest benefit from manipulation and mobilisation that did not require instrumentation or anaesthesia. Rare but serious adverse effects have been reported following manipulation of the cervical spine.

Benefits: We found four systematic reviews (search dates 1990,[11] 1993,[18] 1995,[19] and 1995[12]), which evaluated mobilisation (defined as any manual treatment to improve joint function that does not involve high velocity movement, anaesthesia, or instrumentation) and manipulation (the use of short or long lever high velocity thrusts directed at one or more of the cervical spine joints that does not involve anaesthesia or instrumentation). **Mobilisation:** One RCT (included in all four systematic reviews) in 30 people with acute pain found no significant pain reduction with mobilisation compared with analgesics, collar, or transcutaneous nerve stimulation.[20] However, the trial was too small to rule out a beneficial effect. Two other RCTs included people with chronic neck pain and found modest benefit from mobilisation in the short term. The first of these compared mobilisation plus analgesia versus less active physiotherapy plus analgesia in 63 people.[21] It found significant pain reduction with mobilisation in the first month but not thereafter; 83% of the mobilisation group improved compared with 60% of the physiotherapy group (P < 0.05, 95% CIs not available). The second RCT compared manual treatment (mobilisation, manipulation, or both) versus physical treatment (heat, electrotherapy, ultrasound, shortwave diathermy), placebo (detuned shortwave diathermy or ultrasound), or usual medical care (analgesics, advice, home exercise, and bed rest) in 256 people with chronic neck and back pain, 64 having chronic neck pain alone.[22] The study found significant benefit from manual treatment, which was sustained for 12 months. However, it was not possible to compare directly the effects of the two manual treatments, and more people received manipulation. **Manipulation:** We found one meta-analysis within one of the systematic reviews of three RCTs in 155 people with chronic pain.[19] The RCTs compared manipulation versus diazepam,[23] anti-inflammatory drugs,[24] or usual medical care.[22] The review found no significant difference; there was greater improvement with manipulation compared with the other treatments (a benefit of 12.6 mm on a 100 mm visual analogue scale), but the confidence interval spanned zero (95% CI −0.15 to +25.5).[19] **Mobilisation versus manipulation:** We found one RCT comparing a single mobilisation treatment versus a single manipulation treatment in 100 people with mainly chronic neck pain.[25] It found no significant difference between groups (immediate improvement in pain found in 69% of people with mobilisation v 85% with manipulation, RR of improvement in pain with manipulation compared with mobilisation 1.23, P = 0.05, but corrected to P = 0.16 after adjusting for pretreatment differences between the groups). People in the manipulation group had improved range of movement, but the result was not significant. We found one RCT published after the systematic reviews, which included 119 people with chronic neck pain treated with mobilisation physiotherapy, manipulation, or intensive training.[26] It found reduced pain in all three groups compared with baseline. Pain was measured on a 30 point scale and the median score dropped from 12 to 6 with intensive training or mobilisation and from 13 to 6 with manipulation. There was no significant difference between groups at the end of treatment (P = 0.44) or at 12 months. The lack of a placebo control group makes the impact of treatment hard to determine in this study.

Harms: **Mobilisation:** We found occasional reports of increased pain, but no serious adverse effects or deaths. **Manipulation:** Rare but serious adverse effects have been reported, including death and serious disability caused by vertebrobasilar and other strokes, dissection of the vertebral arteries, disc herniation, and other serious neurological complications. The estimated risk from case reports of cerebrovascular accident is 1 to 3 per million manipulations[27] and of all serious adverse effects is 5 to 10 per 10 million manipulations.[19] A non-systematic review of reported cases of injury attributable to manipulation of the cervical spine identified 116 articles published between 1925 and 1997 with 177 cases of injury. The most frequently reported injuries involved arterial dissection or spasm, lesions of the brain stem and Wallenberg's syndrome (see glossary, p 639); death occurred in 32 (18%) of the cases. However, the method of data collection and analysis makes it impossible to assess the frequency of complications with this treatment.[28]

Comment: None.

QUESTION   **What are the effects of treatments for acute whiplash injury?**

One systematic review of RCTs found that, in people with acute whiplash injury, electrotherapy was more effective than placebo, early mobilisation

physiotherapy was more effective than immobilisation, and return to normal activity was more effective than rest.

Benefits: We found one systematic review of treatment of whiplash injury (search date 1993), which highlighted the paucity of evidence on all treatment modalities.[9] **Physical treatments:** One RCT included in the review compared PEMF versus placebo PEMF in 40 people with acute whiplash.[29] All participants received analgesia and collar. People in the active PEMF group had significantly better pain relief after 4 weeks (P < 0.05) but not after 3 months. **Early mobilisation versus immobilisation or less active treatment:** Two RCTs included in the review compared early mobilisation physiotherapy versus immobilisation, analgesics, rest, and education in 165 people.[30,31] Those in the mobilisation group had significantly better pain relief and improved range of movement at 4 and 8 weeks (P < 0.01). **Early resumption of normal activity versus immobilisation and rest:** We found one recent single blinded RCT of 201 people presenting to an emergency department with acute whiplash, which compared an "act as usual" group (advice plus anti-inflammatory drugs) versus an immobilisation group (also given 14 days' sick leave).[32] The "act as usual" group did better for subjective symptoms, including pain during daily activities, neck stiffness, memory, concentration, and headache at 6 months, but with no benefit in terms of objective variables such as neck range and length of sick leave. At 6 months, 11% of the "act as usual" group still had severe symptoms compared with 15% of the immobilisation group. The difference, however, was not significant (RRR 0.25, 95% CI −0.42 to +0.92). The systematic review found no evidence of benefit from immobilisation, rest, traction, or other physical treatments in acute whiplash.[9]

Harms: Adverse effects are not well documented, but early mobilisation physiotherapy is not always well tolerated.[33]

Comment: The management of acute whiplash injury remains controversial, and needs further investigation.

QUESTION **What are the effects of treatment for chronic whiplash injury?**

We found little good quality information on the management of chronic whiplash injury, although one RCT found limited evidence that percutaneous radiofrequency neurotomy may be beneficial for zygapophyseal joint pain.

Benefits: We found one systematic review of treatment of whiplash injury (search date 1993), which highlighted the paucity of evidence on all treatment modalities.[9] It identified one RCT in 24 people with chronic whiplash (9 men; mean age 43 years) in whom the source of pain was confirmed by placebo controlled diagnostic blocks to be the zygapophyseal (excluding C2/3) joints.[34] Percutaneous radiofrequency neurotomy was compared with a similar placebo procedure. The median time taken for more than half of the pain to return was 263 days in the active group compared with 8 days in the control group (P = 0.04). At 27 weeks more people were free of pain in the active group then in the control group (AR 58% with active treatment v 8% with placebo; ARR 50%, 95% CI 3% to 85%; NTT 2, 95% CI 1 to 29).

Harms: Adverse effects are not well documented.

Comment: Few studies have considered treatment for chronic whiplash, and many people with whiplash are included in general studies of chronic mechanical neck pain.

QUESTION What are the effects of treatments for neck pain with radiculopathy?

OPTION CONSERVATIVE TREATMENT VERSUS SURGERY

We found insufficient evidence comparing the effects of conservative treatment and surgery in people with neck pain and radiculopathy.

Benefits: We found no systematic review. One non-blinded RCT in 81 people with severe radicular symptoms for at least 3 months (number with disc prolapse not stated) compared surgery versus physiotherapy or immobilisation in a collar.[35] Participants were reviewed at 12 months. Although the surgery group had more rapid pain reduction (P < 0.01), there was no difference between the groups at 1 year follow up. Between 3 and 12 months, people who did not improve were given additional treatments: one patient in the physiotherapy group and five in the collar group underwent surgery; eight people in the surgery group underwent a second operation; and 12 people in the surgery group and 11 in the collar group received physiotherapy.

Harms: The study gave no information on adverse effects.

Comment: Conservative treatment needs further assessment, particularly in people considered to be poor risk candidates for surgery.

OPTION PERIRADICULAR AND/OR CERVICAL EPIDURAL STEROID INJECTION

We found insufficient evidence on the effects of epidural steroid injection in people with neck pain and radiculopathy.

Benefits: We found no systematic review or RCTs comparing epidural injection versus placebo, conservative treatment, or surgery. One prospective study lacked a control group.[36]

Harms: Case reports have documented occasional complications, such as infection or bleeding after cervical epidural injection. The incidence of adverse events after different cervical injection techniques is unknown.

Comment: None.

GLOSSARY

Wallenberg's syndrome (lateral medullary syndrome) An infarction of the dorsolateral aspect of the medulla. Manifestations may include loss of pain and temperature sensation in the same side of the face and opposite side of the body.

Substantive changes since last issue

Physical treatments One new RCT indicating that exercise significantly reduces neck pain compared with no exercise.[15]
Mobilisation/manipulation One new non-systematic review of injuries attributable to manipulation of cervical spine.[28]

REFERENCES

1. M kel M, Heliövaara M, Sievers K, Impivaara O, Knekt P, Aromaa A. Prevalence, determinants, and consequences of chronic neck pain in Finland. *Am J Epidemiol* 1991;134:1356–1367.
2. Cote P, Cassidy D, Carroll L. The Saskatchewan health and back pain survey: the prevalence of neck pain and related disability in Saskatchewan adults. *Spine* 1998;23:1689–1698.
3. Hackett GI, Hudson MF, Wylie JB, et al. Evaluation of the efficacy and acceptability to patients of a physiotherapist working in a health centre. *BMJ* 1987;294:24–26.
4. Waalen D, White P, Waalen J. Demographic and clinical characteristics of chiropractic patients: a 5-year study of patients treated at the Canadian Memorial Chiropractic College. *J Can Chiropract Assoc* 1994;38:75–82.
5. Lamberts H, Brouwer H, Groen AJM, Huisman H. Het transitiemodel in de huisartspraktijk. *Huisart Wet* 1987;30:105–113.
6. Kvarnstrom S. Occurrence of musculoskeletal disorders in a manufacturing industry with special attention to occupational shoulder disorders. *Scand J Rehabil Med* 1983(suppl 8):1–114.
7. Borghouts JA, Koes BW, Bouter LM. The clinical course and prognostic factors of non-specific neck pain: a systematic review. *Pain* 1998;77:1–13. Search date 1996; primary sources Medline, Embase.
8. Squires B, Gargan MF, Bannister GC. Soft-tissue injuries of the cervical spine: 15 year follow-up. *J Bone Joint Surg Br* 1996;78:955–957.
9. Spitzer WO, Skovron ML, Salmi LR, et al. Scientific monograph of the Quebec Task Force on whiplash-associated disorders: redefining "whiplash" and its management. *Spine* 1995;20(suppl 8):1–73. Search date 1993; primary sources Medline, TRIS, NTIS, plus personal contacts and Task Force reference lists.
10. Gross AR, Aker PD, Goldsmith CH, Peloso P. Physical medicine modalities for mechanical neck disorders. In: The Cochrane Library, Issue 2, 1999. Oxford: Update Software. Search date, 1985–1993; primary sources Medline, Embase, Chirolars, Index to Chiropractic Literature, Cinahl, Science Citation Index
11. Koes BW, Assendelft WJ, Van Der Heijden GJ, Bouter LM, Knipschild PG. Spinal manipulation and mobilisation for back and neck pain: a blinded review. *BMJ* 1991;303:1298–1303. (Comment in *BMJ* 1992;304:184; discussion 185, and *BMJ* 1992;304:184–185.) Search date 1990; primary sources Medline.
12. Kjellman GV, Skargren EI, Oberg BE. A critical analysis of randomised clinical trials on neck pain and treatment efficacy. A review of the literature. *Scand J Rehabil Med* 1999;31:139–152. Search date 1995; primary sources Medline, Cinahl and hand searches of reference lists.)
13. Van der Heijden GJ, Beurskens AJ, Koes BW,

Assendelft WJ, de Vet HC, Bouter LM. The efficacy of traction for back and neck pain: a systematic, blinded review of randomized clinical trial methods. *Phys Ther* 1995;75:93–104. Search date 1992; primary sources Medline, Embase, Index to Chiropractic Literature, Physiotherapy Index.
14. White AR, Ernst E. A systematic review of randomized controlled trials of acupuncture for neck pain. *Rheumatology* 1999;38:143–147. Search date 1998; primary sources Medline, Embase, Cochrane Library, and CISCOM (a database specialising in complementary medicine).
15. Waling K, Sundelin G, Ahlgren C, Jarvholm B. Perceived pain before and after three exercise programs–a controlled clinical trial of women with work-related trapezius myalgia. *Pain* 2000;85: 201–207.
16. Levoska S, Kein nen-Kiukaanniemi S. Active or passive physiotherapy for occupational cervicobrachial disorders? A comparison of two treatment methods with a 1-year follow-up. *Arch Phys Med Rehabil* 1993;74:425–430.
17. Trock DH, Bollet AJ, Markoll R. The effect of pulsed electromagnetic fields in the treatment of osteoarthritis of the knee and cervical spine. Report of randomized double-blind placebo controlled trials. *J Rheumatol* 1994;21:1903–1911.
18. Aker PD, Gross AR, Goldsmith CH, Peloso P. Conservative management of mechanical neck pain: systematic overview and meta-analysis. *BMJ* 1996;313:1291–1296. Search date 1985–1993; primary sources Medlars, Embase, Cinahl, Chirolars.
19. Hurwitz EL, Aker PD, Adams AH, Meeker WC, Shekelle PG. Manipulation and mobilization of the cervical spine: a systematic review of the literature. *Spine* 1996;21:1746–1760. Search dates 1966–1995; primary sources Medline, Embase, Chirolars, Cinahl.
20. Nordemar R, Thörner C. Treatment of acute cervical pain: a comparative group study. *Pain* 1981;10:93–101.
21. Brodin H. Cervical pain and mobilization. *Manipulative Med* 1985;2:18–22.
22. Koes BW, Bouter LM, van Mameren H, et al. Randomised clinical trial of manipulative therapy and physiotherapy for persistent back and neck complaints: results of one year follow up. *BMJ* 1992;304:601–605.
23. Sloop PR, Smith DS, Goldenberg E, Dore C. Manipulation for chronic neck pain: a double-blind controlled study. *Spine* 1982;7:532–535.
24. Howe DH, Newcombe RG, Wade MT. Manipulation of the cervical spine: a pilot study. *J R Coll Gen Pract* 1983;33:574–579.
25. Cassidy JD, Lopes AA, Yong-Hing K. The immediate effect of manipulation versus

mobilization on pain and range of motion in the cervical spine: a randomised controlled trial. *J Manipulative Physiol Ther* 1992;15:570–575.

26. Jordan A, Bendix T, Nielsen H, Hansen F R, Host D, Winkel A. Intensive training, physiotherapy, or manipulation for patients with chronic neck pain. A prospective, single-blinded, randomized clinical trial. *Spine* 1998;23:311–319.

27. Dabbs V, Lauretti W J. A risk assessment of cervical manipulation vs NSAIDS for the treatment of neck pain. *J Manipulative Physiol Ther* 1995; 18:530–536.

28. Di Fabio RP. Manipulation of the cervical spine: risks and benefits. *Phys Ther* 1999;79:50–65.

29. Foley-Nolan D, Moore K, Codd M, Barry C, O'Connor P, Coughlun RJ. Low energy high frequency pulsed electromagnetic therapy for acute whiplash injuries. A double blind randomised controlled study. *Scand J Rehabil Med* 1992;24: 51–59.

30. Mealy K, Brennan H, Fenelon GC. Early mobilization of acute whiplash injuries. *BMJ* 1986; 292:656–657.

31. McKinney LA, Dornan JO, Ryan M. The role of physiotherapy in the management of acute neck sprains following road-traffic accidents. *Arch Emerg Med* 1989;6:27–33.

32. Borchgrevink GE, Kaasa A, McDonagh D, Stiles TC, Haraldseth O, Lereim I. Acute treatment of whiplash neck sprain injuries: a randomised trial of treatment during the first 14 days after a car accident. *Spine* 1998;23:25–31.

33. Pennie BH, Agambar LJ. Whiplash injuries: a trial of early management. *J Bone Joint Surg Br* 1990; 72:277–279.

34. Lord SM, Barnsley L, Wallis BJ, McDonald GJ, Bogduk N. Percutaneous radio-frequency neurotomy for chronic cervical zygapophyseal-joint pain. *N Engl J Med*. 1996;335:1721–1726.

35. Persson LC, Carlsson CA, Carlsson JY. Long-lasting cervical radicular pain managed with surgery, physiotherapy, or a cervical collar: a prospective randomised study. *Spine* 1997;22:751–758.

36. Bush K, Hillier S. Outcome of cervical radiculopathy treated with periradicular/epidural corticosteroid injections: a prospective study with independent clinical review. *Eur Spine J* 1996;5: 319–325.

Allan Binder
Consultant Rheumatologist
Lister Hospital
Stevenage
UK

Competing interests: None declared.

Last updated Issue 3

Peter Gøtzsche

Musculoskeletal disorders

INTERVENTIONS

Key Messages

Differences between NSAIDs

- Systematic reviews of RCTs have found no important differences in effect
  between different NSAIDs or doses but have found differences in toxicity
  related to increased doses and possibly to the nature of the NSAID itself.

- In acute musculoskeletal syndromes, we found no large double blind trial that
  compared an NSAID with paracetamol.

Preventing gastrointestinal adverse effects

- One large RCT has found that misoprostol slightly reduces the incidence of
  clinically significant gastrointestinal complications of oral NSAIDs.

- One large RCT has found that omeprazole 20 mg and 40 mg daily and
  misoprostol 800 µg daily produce similar reductions of endoscopically diagnosed ulceration. RCTs have found that misoprostol causes more adverse
  effects than placebo, omeprazole, and ranitidine (mostly diarrhoea and
  abdominal pain).

- RCTs have found H_2 blockers to be inferior to omeprazole and misoprostol at
  preventing adverse effects of NSAIDs.

Topical NSAIDs

- One systematic review of RCTs has found that topical NSAIDs are effective compared with placebo in acute pain conditions (NNT 5 to obtain good pain relief) and chronic pain conditions (NNT 3).
- We found no high quality trials of topical NSAIDs versus oral forms of the same drug, or against paracetamol.

DEFINITION	NSAIDs have anti-inflammatory, analgesic, and antipyretic effects, and inhibit platelet aggregation. The drugs have no documented effect on the disease process itself.
INCIDENCE/ PREVALENCE	NSAIDs are widely used. Almost 10% of people in the Netherlands used a non-aspirin NSAID in 1987, and the overall use was 11 defined daily doses defined daily doses (see glossary, p 647) per 1000 persons a day.[1] In Australia in 1994, overall use was 35 defined daily doses per 1000 persons a day, with 36% of the people receiving NSAIDs for osteoarthritis, 42% for sprain and strain or low back pain, and 4% for rheumatoid arthritis; 35% were aged over 60 years.[2]
AIMS	To reduce symptoms in rheumatic disorders; to avoid severe gastrointestinal adverse effects.
OUTCOMES	**Primary outcomes:** pain intensity; person's preference for one drug over another; global efficacy; clinically significant gastrointestinal complications. **Secondary outcomes:** number of tender joints; perforation; gastrointestinal haemorrhage; dyspepsia; and ulcer detected by routine endoscopy.
METHODS	We searched Medline and the Cochrane Library in November 1999 for systematic reviews and RCTs. More than 100 systematic reviews and thousands of RCTs have compared various NSAIDs. Many trials are unpublished, or published in sources that are not indexed in publicly available databases. The quality of the trials is variable and bias is common, both in the design and analysis of the trials, to such an extent that a systematic review identified false significant findings favouring new drugs over control drugs in 6% of trials.[3] We have therefore focused on systematic reviews that have not been sponsored or authored by industry, and have included large trials only when they provided clinically important information that was not already covered in the systematic reviews.

QUESTION **Are there any important differences between available NSAIDs?**

Systematic reviews have found no important differences in effect between different NSAIDs or doses, but found differences in toxicity related to increased doses, and to the nature of the NSAID itself. In acute musculoskeletal syndromes, we found no large double blind trials that compared an NSAID with paracetamol. We found no evidence that NSAIDs are more effective than simple analgesics.

Benefits: **Rheumatoid arthritis:** We found two systematic reviews[4,5] and one subsequent RCT.[6] One systematic review (published in 1989, search date 1985) of 37 crossover trials compared indomethacin with 10 newer NSAIDs. It included 1416 people treated for a median of 2 weeks with each drug.[4] Only 5% more people (95% CI 0% to 10%) preferred the newer NSAID to indomethacin. Four of the trials included a placebo period and one trial compared four drugs. Another systematic review (search date 1988) of 88 trials comparing two NSAIDs, and 27 trials comparing an NSAID with placebo, in a total of 6440 people, found no differences in the number of tender joints among 17 different NSAIDs.[5] One subsequent RCT in 1149 people that compared three doses of the COX-2 inhibitor celecoxib versus naproxen 1 g found a similar beneficial effect with fewer endoscopically detected ulcers (5% *v* 26%; ARR 21%, 95% CI 13% to 29%). Only one of the ulcers was clinically significant and only 7/692 people taking celecoxib and 5/225 people taking naproxen withdrew because of gastrointestinal adverse effects.[6] **Osteoarthritis:** Two systematic reviews (search date 1994, search date 1996) found no clear differences between various NSAIDs used to treat osteoarthritis of the hip (39 trials)[7] or the knee (16 trials).[8] One systematic review (search date 1990) of tenoxicam versus three other NSAIDs for osteoarthritis found superiority of tenoxicam over piroxicam both for global efficacy (10 trials, 834 people; OR 1.46, 95% CI 1.08 to 2.03), and for global tolerability (7 trials, 974 people; OR 1.46, 95% CI 1.01 to 2.15).[9] This result is at variance with a large RCT of 1328 people with osteoarthritis or rheumatoid arthritis, which found no significant differences in global efficacy or tolerability between the two drugs. Improvement was noted for 55% of people on tenoxicam versus 53% of people on piroxicam (95% CI for the difference −5% to +9%) (see NSAIDs under osteoarthritis, p 649).[10] One review of eight RCTs (5435 people) of rofecoxib versus other NSAIDs found a cumulative incidence of clinically significant gastrointestinal adverse events of 1.3% versus 1.8% (CI not available; P = 0.46).[11] Fewer people taking rofecoxib withdrew because of gastrointestinal adverse effects (3.5% *v* 4.8%, ARR 1.3%, 95% CI 0.1% to 2.8%; RR 0.73, 95% CI 0.55 to 0.97; NNT with rofecoxib versus other NSAIDs to avoid one additional withdrawal because of gastrointestinal adverse effects 78, 95% CI 46 to 790). **Acute musculoskeletal syndromes:** The RCTs were generally of poor quality,[12] and we found few systematic reviews. One review of 17 NSAID trials for shoulder pain was inconclusive (see NSAIDs under osteoarthritis, p 649).[13] Another systematic review (search date 1993) of 84 studies included 32 025 people with soft tissue injuries of the ankle; the authors were unable to pool data to perform a statistical analysis of the different forms of treatment.[12] We found no good evidence that NSAIDs are more effective than paracetamol in acute musculoskeletal syndromes. **Dose response relation:** One systematic review of 19 trials (search date 1989) in which participants were randomised to more than one dose of nine different NSAIDs found a dose response relation that saturated at high doses.[14] This and another systematic review (search date 1992) found that the recommended dosages were close to providing a ceiling effect.[14,15] The review of the 115 trials mentioned above found no differences between various doses of drugs;[5] 10 of 21 studies of ibuprofen had used a daily dosage of 1200 mg or less.[5]

Harms: **Versus placebo:** One systematic review of 100 trials (12 853 people) found an increased risk of gross haemorrhage (ARI for

NSAID v placebo 0.7%, 95% CI −0.1% to +1.5%) and for proven ulcer (ARI for NSAID v placebo 0.05%, 95% CI −0.01% to +0.11%). The effect was not significant but mean treatment duration was only 2 months.[16] For 40 aspirin trials (22 234 people, mean treatment duration 1 year) the review found an increased risk of gross haemorrhage (ARI 0.6%, 95% CI 0.2% to 1.0%) and for proven ulcer (ARI 0.6%, 95% CI 0% to 1.2%).[16] The number needed to harm was in the range 100–1000. One systematic review of 38 placebo controlled trials found that NSAIDs raised mean blood pressure by 5.0 mm Hg (95% CI 1.2 mm Hg to 8.7 mm Hg).[17]

Versus other NSAIDs: One meta-analysis of 11 case control studies and one cohort study found that ibuprofen was significantly less toxic than other NSAIDs. The 11 comparator drugs were associated with a 1.6–9.2 fold increase in risk of serious upper gastrointestinal complications.[18] COX-2 inhibitors are associated with less gastrointestinal toxicity than older NSAIDs, but the clinical significance is not clear (see above).[6,11] **Dose response relation:** Three systematic reviews found no ceiling effect for adverse effects; the incidence of adverse effects increased in an approximately linear fashion with dose.[15,18,19]

Comment: Important differences in adverse effects seem to exist between different NSAIDs. In contrast, the beneficial effects of NSAIDs seem similar. The only meta-analysis that found one drug to be more effective than another was funded by the manufacturer;[9] the studies it included were small and the result was not replicated in a large RCT. People's preferences for particular drugs have not been replicated and could therefore be due to chance or to natural fluctuations in disease activity.[20,21] The evidence suggests that if the NSAID is unsatisfactory, switching to another NSAID will not solve the problem.[10] Likewise, doubling the dose of an NSAID leads to only a small increase in effect, which may not be clinically relevant. In acute musculoskeletal problems it is doubtful whether NSAIDs have any clinically relevant anti-inflammatory effect; we found no large double blind RCT comparing an NSAID with paracetamol. Paracetamol has been studied in osteoarthritis where it had much the same effect as ibuprofen or naproxen (see simple analgesics v NSAIDs under osteoarthritis, p 649) We are aware of reviews of COX-2 inhibitors published subsequent to the *Clinical Evidence* search. They will be appraised for Issue five of *Clinical Evidence*.

| QUESTION | What are the effects of co-treatments to reduce the risk of gastrointestinal adverse effects of NSAIDs? |

One large RCT found that misoprostol slightly reduced the incidence of clinically significant gastrointestinal complications of oral NSAIDs. One large RCT found that omeprazole 20 mg and 40 mg daily and misoprostol 800 µg daily had similar effects in reducing endoscopically diagnosed adverse effects. However, misoprostol caused more adverse effects (mostly diarrhoea and abdominal pain). RCTs found H$_2$ blockers to be inferior to omeprazole and misoprostol. The absolute risk of serious upper gastrointestinal complications is approximately doubled for people over 75 years of age, and for those with a history of peptic ulcer, bleeding, or cardiovascular disease.

Benefits: We found one systematic review and four large subsequent RCTs. **Misoprostol versus placebo:** The systematic review (24 RCTs, search date 1994) included 5005 people who all received NSAIDs.[22] In trials lasting more than 4 weeks, misoprostol compared with placebo reduced the development of gastric ulcer detected by routine endoscopy (ARR 8%, 95% CI 1% to 18%). H_2 blockers had no effect on gastric ulcer (ARR 1%, 95% CI −2% to +3%) but reduced the risk of duodenal ulcer (ARR 2%, 95% CI 0% to 5%). Misoprostol also reduced duodenal ulcer risk with long term use (ARR 3%, 95% CI 0% to 6%) but not with short term use (ARR 2%, 95% CI −2% to +6%). In a 6 month RCT published after the systematic review, 8843 people with rheumatoid arthritis (mean age 68 years, all treated with NSAIDs) were randomised to misoprostol 800 µg daily or placebo.[23] Serious upper gastrointestinal complications (such as perforation, gastric outlet obstruction, or bleeding detected by clinical symptoms or investigation) were reduced by misoprostol compared with placebo (AR 0.6% in misoprostol group, 1.0% in placebo group; ARR 0.4%, 95% CI 0% to 0.7%; NNT 263). The risk of serious upper gastrointestinal complications was approximately doubled for people above 75 years of age, and for those with a history of peptic ulcer, bleeding, or cardiovascular disease. People with all four risk factors had an absolute risk of 9% for a major complication in 6 months, corresponding to a number needed to treat with misoprostol rather than placebo of 28 people. **Misoprostol versus omeprazole:** In another RCT of 935 people treated with NSAIDs who had ulcers or more than 10 erosions at endoscopy, treatment success was defined as fewer than five erosions at each site, no ulcers, and not more than mild dyspepsia.[24] At 8 weeks, treatment was successful in 76% of individuals given omeprazole 20 mg daily, 75% given omeprazole 40 mg daily, and 71% given misoprostol 800 µg daily. People (n = 732) in whom treatment was successful were re-randomised to maintenance treatment for 6 months. More people remained in remission with omeprazole 20 mg (61%) than with misoprostol 400 µg (48%), and with either drug than with placebo (27%; ARR for omeprazole v placebo 34%, 95% CI 25% to 43%; NNT 3; ARR for misoprostol v placebo 21%, 95% CI 12% to 30%; NNT 5). **H_2 blockers:** In a similarly designed trial in 541 people, treatment was successful in 80%, 79%, and 63% of people given omeprazole 20 mg, omeprazole 40 mg, or ranitidine 300 mg daily, respectively.[25] The estimated proportions in remission after 6 months were 72% with omeprazole 20 mg and 59% with ranitidine 300 mg (ARR for omeprazole v ranitidine 13%, 95% CI 4% to 22%; NNT 8). In an 8 week study, 538 people with NSAID related upper gastrointestinal pain without endoscopic evidence of ulcers were randomised to either misoprostol 800 µg or ranitidine 300 mg daily.[26] One third were excluded from analysis because of problems with adherence and missing endoscopic examinations. Gastric ulcers at least 3 mm in diameter were found in 1% of people taking misoprostol and in 6% of people taking ranitidine (ARR for misoprostol v ranitidine 5%, 95% CI 2% to 9%; NNT 20). Duodenal ulcer rate was 1% with both drugs.

Harms: In one of the large trials, more people receiving misoprostol than placebo withdrew from the study because of adverse events, primarily diarrhoea and abdominal pain (27% v 20%).[23] There were 17 versus 21 deaths. One death was a direct result of gastrointestinal toxicity. In another trial, adverse events were noted in 48%, 46%, and 59% of people receiving omeprazole 20 mg, omeprazole 40 mg, and misoprostol; treatment discontinuations (all causes) occurred in 10%, 11%, and 17%.[22] Few adverse events were reported in the trial comparing omeprazole with rantidine; treatment discontinuations (all causes) occurred in 10%, 10%, and 14% of people taking omeprazole 20 mg, omeprazole 40 mg, and rantidine.[25] In the trial comparing misoprostol with ranitidine, adverse events (mostly gastrointestinal) occurred in 77% of people taking misoprostol and 66% taking ranitidine, with withdrawal rates of 13% and 7%, respectively (ARR for ranitidine v misoprostol 6%, 95% CI 1% to 11%; NNT 17).[26]

Comment: The clinical relevance of these findings is doubtful. The only trial that used clinically relevant outcomes found little difference between active drug and placebo, except for people at high risk.[23] The rate of ulcers was more than 10 times higher in the studies where the investigators looked for them with regular endoscopy, than in earlier trials of NSAIDs.[18] These ulcers were sometimes defined as endoscopic lesions with a size of only 3 mm, or as any lesion of an unequivocal depth, or no definition was provided at all.[22]

QUESTION What are the effects of topical NSAIDs?

One systematic review of RCTs has found that topical NSAIDs are effective compared with placebo in acute pain conditions (NNT 5 to obtain good pain relief) and chronic pain conditions (NNT 3). We found no high quality trials of topical versus oral formulations of the same drug, and found no direct comparisons of topical NSAIDs versus paracetamol. It is therefore uncertain whether topical treatment is advantageous over these alternatives.

Benefits: **Versus placebo:** We found one systematic review (86 RCTs, search date 1996) in 10 160 people,[27] that primarily compared a topical NSAID with placebo. The review was partly sponsored by two manufacturers. Many trials of acute pain conditions (soft tissue trauma, strains, and sprains) were small; in 37 trials, the average number of actively treated people was 32, and the effect declined significantly with sample size. In seven trials with more than 80 people per group, the number of people that would need to be treated for one extra good outcome was five (RR 1.6, 95% CI 1.3 to 1.9, NNT 5, 95% CI 4 to 6). In 12 trials in chronic pain conditions (osteoarthritis, tendinitis) the number of people that would need to be treated for one extra good outcome was three (RR 2.0, 95% CI 1.5 to 2.7, NNT 3, 95% CI 3 to 4). In one additional trial, which was not included in this review, copper salicylate gel or placebo was applied to the forearm of 116 people with osteoarthritis of the hip or knee.[28] It found no significant difference in effect (22% v 21% participants reported good effect). **Versus oral NSAIDs:** Five trials in the systematic review compared topical versus oral NSAIDs, but they all had inadequate design and power.[27] **Versus paracetamol:** We found no RCTs.

Harms: In the systematic review, local adverse effects occurred in 3% of people in both groups and systemic adverse events in 1%.[27] In the trial of copper salicylate gel, more people receiving treatment reported adverse reactions, most commonly skin reactions (83% v 52%), and more people withdrew from the trial because of these reactions (17% v 2%).[28]

Comment: Sample size bias hampers the interpretation of the available trials. We found no high quality trials comparing topical versus systemic administration of the same NSAID, and no trials comparing a topical NSAID with paracetamol.

GLOSSARY

Defined daily dose The assumed average daily dose for the main indication of a specified drug. The defined daily dose per 1000 population per day is an estimate of the proportion of that population receiving treatment with that drug.

REFERENCES

1. Leufkens HG, Ameling CB, Hekster YA, Bakker A. Utilization patterns of non-steroidal anti-inflammatory drugs in an open Dutch population. *Pharm Weekbl Sci* 1990;12:97–103.
2. McManus P, Primrose JG, Henry DA, et al. Pattern of non-steroidal anti-inflammatory drug use in Australia 1990–1994. A report from the drug utilization sub-committee of the pharmaceutical benefits advisory committee. *Med J Aust* 1996; 164:589–592.
3. Gøtzsche PC. Methodology and overt and hidden bias in reports of 196 double-blind trials of nonsteroidal anti-inflammatory drugs in rheumatoid arthritis (published erratum appears in *Control Clin Trials* 1989;10:356). *Control Clin Trials* 1989;10:31–56. Search date May 1985; primary source Medline.
4. Gøtzsche PC. Patients' preference in indomethacin trials: an overview. *Lancet* 1989;i:88–91. Search date 1985; primary sources Medline, and personal contact with companies that marketed proprietary products, and hand searching of reference lists of collected articles.
5. Gøtzsche PC. Meta-analysis of NSAIDs: contribution of drugs, doses, trial designs, and meta-analytic techniques. *Scand J Rheumatol* 1993;22:255–260. Search dates May 1985 and September 1988; primary source Medline.
6. Simon LS, Weaver AL, Graham DY, et al. Anti-inflammatory and upper gastrointestinal effects of celecoxib in rheumatoid arthritis. *JAMA* 1999;282: 1921–1928.
7. Towheed T, Shea B, Wells G, Hochberg M. Analgesia and non-aspirin, non-steroidal anti-inflammatory drugs in osteoarthritis of the hip. In: The Cochrane Library, Issue 4, 1999. Oxford: Update Software. Search date 1994; primary sources Cochrane Controlled Trials Register; Medline 1966 to August 1994; and hand searched references.
8. Watson MC, Brookes ST, Kirwan JR, Faulkner A. Osteoarthritis: the comparative efficacy of non-aspirin non-steroidal anti-inflammatory drugs for the management of osteoarthritis of the knee. In: The Cochrane Library, Issue 4, 1999. Oxford: Update Software. Search date November 1996; primary sources Medline 1966 to 1995; and Embase 1980 to 1995.
9. Riedemann PJ, Bersinic S, Cuddy J, Torrance GW, Tugwell PX. A study to determine the efficacy and safety of tenoxicam versus piroxicam, diclofenac and indomethacin in patients with osteoarthritis: a meta-analysis. *J Rheumatol* 1993;20:2095–2103. Search date up to 1990; primary source Medline.
10. Simpson J, Golding DN, Freeman AM, et al. A large multicentre, parallel group, double-blind study comparing tenoxicam and piroxicam in the treatment of osteoarthritis and rheumatoid arthritis. *Br J Clin Pract* 1989;43:328–333.
11. Langman MJ, Jensen DM, Watson DG, et al. Adverse upper gastrointestinal effects of rofecoxib compared with NSAIDs. *JAMA* 1999;282:1929–1933.
12. Ogilvie Harris DJ, Gilbart M. Treatment modalities for soft tissue injuries of the ankle: a critical review. *Clin J Sport Med* 1995;5:175–186. Search date up to 1993; primary sources Medline and Embase.
13. Green S, Buchbinder R, Glazier R, Forbes A. Interventions for shoulder pain. In: The Cochrane Library, Issue 4, 1999. Oxford: Update Software. Search date up to May 1998; primary sources Cochrane Musculoskeletal Group trials register; Cochrane Controlled Trials Register; Medline; Embase; Cinahl; and Science Citation Index.
14. Gøtzsche PC. Review of dose-response studies of NSAIDs in rheumatoid arthritis. *Dan Med Bull* 1989;36:395–399.
15. Eisenberg E, Berkey CS, Carr DB, Mosteller F, Chalmers TC. Efficacy and safety of nonsteroidal antiinflammatory drugs for cancer pain: a meta-analysis. *J Clin Oncol* 1994;12:2756–2765. Search date up to 1992; primary source Medline.
16. Chalmers TC, Berrier J, Hewitt P, et al. Meta-analysis of randomized controlled trials as a method of estimating rare complications of non-steroidal anti-inflammatory drug therapy. *Aliment Pharmacol Ther* 1988;2(suppl 1):9–26. Search date not available; primary source Medline.
17. Johnson AG, Nguyen TV, Day RO. Do nonsteroidal anti-inflammatory drugs affect blood pressure? A meta-analysis. *Ann Intern Med* 1994;121:289–300.
18. Henry D, Lim LL, Garcia Rodriguez LA, et al. Variability in risk of gastrointestinal complications with individual non-steroidal anti-inflammatory drugs: results of a collaborative meta-analysis. *BMJ* 1996;312:1563–1566. Search date up to 1994; primary source Medline.
19. Cappelleri JC, Lau J, Kupelnick B, Chalmers TC. Efficacy and safety of different aspirin dosages on vascular diseases in high-risk patients. A meta-regression analysis. *Online J Curr Clin Trials* 1995; Doc No 174:(6442 words; 55 paragraphs). Search date up to 1992; primary sources Medline; Current Contents.
20. Huskisson EC, Woolf DL, Balme HW, Scott J, Franklin S. Four new anti-inflammatory drugs:

responses and variations. *BMJ* 1976;i:1048–1049.

21. Cooperating Clinics Committee of the American Rheumatism Association. A seven-day variability study of 499 patients with peripheral rheumatoid arthritis. *Arthritis Rheum* 1965;8:302–334.

22. Koch M, Dezi A, Ferrario F, Capurso I. Prevention of nonsteroidal anti-inflammatory drug-induced gastrointestinal mucosal injury. A meta-analysis of randomized controlled clinical trials. *Arch Intern Med* 1996;156:2321–2332. Search date up to 1994; primary source Medline.

23. Silverstein FE, Graham DY, Senior JR, et al. Misoprostol reduces serious gastrointestinal complications in patients with rheumatoid arthritis receiving nonsteroidal anti-inflammatory drugs. A randomized, double-blind, placebo-controlled trial. *Ann Intern Med* 1995;123:241–249.

24. Hawkey CJ, Karrasch JA, Szczepanski L, et al. Omeprazole compared with misoprostol for ulcers associated with nonsteroidal antiinflammatory drugs. Omeprazole versus misoprostol for NSAID-induced ulcer management (OMNIUM) study group. *N Engl J Med* 1998;338:727–734.

25. Yeomans ND, Tulassay Z, Juhasz L, et al. A comparison of omeprazole with ranitidine for ulcers associated with nonsteroidal antiinflammatory drugs. Acid suppression trial: ranitidine versus omeprazole for NSAID associated ulcer treatment (ASTRONAUT) study group. *N Engl J Med* 1998;338:719–726.

26. Raskin JB, White RH, Jaszewski R, Korsten MA, Schubert TT, Fort JG. Misoprostol and ranitidine in the prevention of NSAID-induced ulcers: a prospective, double-blind, multicenter study. *Am J Gastroenterol* 1996;91:223–227.

27. Moore RA, Tramer MR, Carroll D, Wiffen PJ, McQuay HJ. Quantitative systematic review of topically applied non-steroidal anti-inflammatory drugs. *BMJ* 1998;316:333–338. Search date 1996; primary sources Medline 1966 to September 1996; Embase 1981 to September 1996; Oxford Pain Relief Database 1950 to 1994; and contacted pharmaceutical companies and hand searched references.

28. Shackel NA, Day RO, Kellett B, Brooks PM. Copper-salicylate gel for pain relief in osteoarthritis: a randomised controlled trial. *Med J Aust* 1997;167:134–136.

Peter Gøtzsche
Director
The Nordic Cochrane Centre
Copenhagen
Denmark

Competing interests: None declared.

Updated this issue

Paul Dieppe, Jiri Chard, Alex Faulkner and Stefan Lohmander

INTERVENTIONS

Key Messages

Non surgical treatments

- Systematic reviews of RCTs have found that non-steroidal anti-inflammatory drugs (NSAIDs) and simple analgesics such as paracetamol (acetaminophen) reduce the pain of osteoarthritis. We found no good evidence that non-steroidal anti-inflammatory drugs (NSAIDs) are superior to simple analgesics such as paracetamol (acetaminophen), or that any one of the many NSAIDs is more effective than the others in relieving the pain of osteoarthritis.

- One systematic review of RCTs has found that topical agents relieve pain in people with osteoarthritis and have fewer adverse effects than systemic treatments. However, we found no evidence that prescribed agents are superior to cheaper non-prescription alternatives or to other local treatments such as heat or cold packs.

- Systematic reviews and subsequent RCTs have found that both exercise and education may help reduce the burden of pain and disability in people with hip or knee osteoarthritis.

- Systematic reviews of RCTs have found no clear evidence of benefit from intra-articular injection of various drugs over placebo injection in people with osteoarthritis of the knee.

Surgical treatments

- Systematic reviews have found that hip and knee replacements are effective in relieving pain and improving function in a wide range of people.

- We found limited evidence suggesting that hip replacement is less effective in younger people.

- We found conflicting evidence from observational studies about the effects of old age and obesity on the balance of benefits and harms from knee surgery.

DEFINITION Osteoarthritis is a heterogeneous condition for which the prevalence, risk factors, clinical manifestations, and prognosis vary according to the joints affected. It most commonly affects hands, knees, hips, and spinal apophyseal joints. It is usually defined by pathological or radiological criteria rather than clinical features, and is characterised by focal areas of damage to the cartilage surfaces of synovial joints, associated with remodelling of the underlying bone and mild synovitis. When severe, there is characteristic joint space narrowing and osteophyte formation, with visible subchondral bone changes on radiography.

INCIDENCE/ PREVALENCE Osteoarthritis is common and an important cause of pain and disability in older adults.[1,2] Radiographic features are practically universal in at least some joints in people aged over 60 years, but significant clinical disease probably affects 10–20% of people. Knee disease is about twice as prevalent as hip disease in people aged over 60 (about 10% v 5%).[3,4]

AETIOLOGY/ RISK FACTORS The main initiating factors are abnormalities in joint shape or injury.

PROGNOSIS The natural history of osteoarthritis is poorly understood. Only a minority of people with clinical disease of the hip or knee joint progress to surgery.

AIMS	To reduce pain, stiffness, and disability; to limit the risk of progressive joint damage; to improve quality of life, with minimal adverse effects.
OUTCOMES	Frequency and severity of joint pain (particularly activity related pain and night pain); stiffness; functional impairment and disability; quality of life; perioperative complications (infection, bleeding, venous thromboembolism and death); prosthesis survival and the need for revision surgery. A global knee rating scale that includes measures of pain, function and range of movement. A modified Knee Society score: this instrument combines three different domains (pain, function and joint status) into a single score (patient function [walking ability, stair climbing etc] accounts for about 50% of the total, with pain and joint status [stability, deformity etc] each accounting for about 25%).[5] The Western Ontario and McMaster osteoarthritis index (WOMAC) is a validated instrument for assessing lower limb (hip and knee) osteoarthritis and is sensitive to change. It is a self-assessment questionnaire and includes questions on pain, stiffness and physical function (such as walking ability). WOMAC is disease specific, but not intervention specific; it can be used to assess any intervention in osteoarthritis.[6–9]
METHODS	*Clinical Evidence* update search and appraisal April 2000.

QUESTION What are the effects of exercise and physical therapy?

Evidence from systematic reviews and subsequent RCTs suggests that exercise and physical therapy reduces pain and disability in people with hip or knee osteoarthritis.

Benefits: We found three systematic reviews and three subsequent RCTs of exercise in people with osteoarthritis of the knee or hip. The first review (search date 1997, 11 RCTs) concluded that exercise regimens were beneficial but that more evidence was needed. (see table 2, p 663) [10] The second systematic review (search date 1993) of non-medicinal and non-invasive treatments for hip and knee osteoarthritis concluded that, of seven modalities reviewed, exercise had the strongest evidence of benefit.[11] The third systematic review (search date 1994) of aerobic exercises for osteoarthritis of the knee found only three admissible RCTs.[12] The review concluded that, despite a favourable impression, the evidence currently available was inadequate. We found three subsequent RCTs. The first examined the effects of a structured exercise programme on self reported disability. Participants (439 people aged over 60 years with osteoarthritis of the knee) were randomised to one of three programmes: an aerobic exercise programme; a resistance exercise programme; or a health education programme. The two exercise groups experienced significant but modest reductions in disability and pain compared with the education group.[13] The second RCT examined physical therapy and exercise versus placebo (83 people with osteoarthritis of the knee). After 8 weeks follow up, significant improvements were seen in WOMAC score for the treatment group over the control group (P < 0.001).[14] The third RCT (n = 98) compared an isokinetic exercise regime versus generic information lectures given by health professionals over 12 weeks. There was no significant difference in leg strength, pain, or function between the groups. Both groups improved from base-line.[15]

Harms: We found no evidence of harm.

Comment: We found few well designed RCTs, and the participants in many trials were not representative of those in the general population.

QUESTION **What are the effects of education and behavioural change?**

Evidence from one systematic review and three RCTs suggests that education reduces pain and disability in people with hip or knee osteoarthritis.

Benefits: We found one systematic review and three subsequent RCTs. The systematic review (search date 1993) included 10 controlled trials of education over 2–48 weeks. One trial, which found benefit from a combination of exercise and education, was excluded from the main analysis (see comment). Effect sizes associated with educa-tion were non-significant for pain (0.16, 95% CI −0.69 to +1.02) and disability (0.0, 95% CI −0.61 to +0.61).[16] We found three subsequent RCTs. The first (n = 211 people with osteoarthritis of the knee) compared self care education (see glossary, p 659) versus attention only education (see glossary, p 659) over 1 year. The self care education group derived greater benefit for both pain and disability.[17] The second RCT (n = 252) assessed methods to improve adherence to treatment plans. The trial compared a tar-geted education programme versus an information pack, both delivered via computer over 8 weeks, and found no significant difference in quality of life, pain, or disability between groups. The targeted education programme was associated with significant improvement in stiffness compared with controls (effect size −0.63, 95% CI −0.81 to −0.45 v −0.39, 95% CI −0.53 to −0.25).[18] The third RCT (n = 98) compared an isokinetic exercise regime versus generic information lectures given by health professionals over 12 weeks. There was no significant difference in leg strength, pain, or function between the groups; both improved from baseline.[15]

Harms: We found no evidence of harm.

Comment: We found few well designed RCTs, and the participants in many trials were not representative of those in the general population. Individual patient education studies in the systematic review also included biofeedback, exercises, and social support.[16] One trial that found a very large improvement for pain and disability was excluded from the analysis because its results were so different from the others. It also included exercise in the intervention. The remaining nine trials showed no evidence of heterogeneity of effects.

QUESTION **What are the effects of physical aids?**

We found limited evidence on the effectiveness of these interventions. Physical aids refer to shoe wedges/insole, walking aids, joint braces, and

taping of the joint. These interventions either support or modify the weight distribution/loading through the joint.

Benefits: We found no systematic reviews. We found two RCTs on the use of physical aids. One RCT (n = 119) compared two forms of valgus knee bracing (neoprene sleeve and unloader-brace) against a control group. Results showed that both the knee brace groups did significantly better than the control group in disease specific quality of life (P = 0.001) and function (P < 0.001). No significant difference was found between WOMAC scores for the two braces (P = 0.062).[19] The second small RCT (n = 14) found that taping of the knee was associated with a 25% reduction in pain compared with a control group.[20]

Harms: We found no evidence of adverse effects from using physical aids.

Comment: In addition to the two RCTs identified, we found several observational studies, which all found positive effects from using physical aids.

QUESTION **What are the effects of oral drug treatments?**

OPTION ANALGESICS

Three systematic reviews found that simple analgesics such a paracetamol (acetaminophen) are effective for controlling short term pain associated with osteoarthritis.

Benefits: We found one systematic review evaluating analgesics in osteoarthritis of the hip (search date 1994, 3 RCTs[21]) and one systematic review (search date 1994[22]) in osteoarthritis of the knee. The reviews found limited evidence that, compared to placebo, simple analgesics were effective in controlling pain associated with osteoarthritis. A small RCT (included in the review,[22] 44 people with osteoarthritis of the knee) found that paracetamol (acetaminophen) was superior to placebo for short term pain relief (improvement in pain at rest in 73% knees with paracetamol v 5% of knees with control) and global responses of the people treated (improved global response 18/22 [82%] with paracetamol v 1/22 [5%] with control; ARI 77%, 95% CI 27% to 93%; RR 18, 95% CI 6.9 to 22; NNT 1, 95% CI 1 to 4).[23]

Harms: Liver damage results from overdose, or at lower doses in people with existing liver damage.[24]

Comment: None.

OPTION NON-STEROIDAL ANTI-INFLAMMATORY DRUGS

Three systematic reviews of RCTs have found that NSAIDs are effective for short term pain relief in osteoarthritis (see NSAIDs, p 641).

Benefits: We identified three systematic reviews evaluating analgesic and anti-inflammatory treatment in osteoarthritis of the hip (search date 1994, 14 RCTs[21]) and knee (search dates 1996, 16 RCTs,[25] and search date 1994, 45 RCTs[22]). The reviews found that NSAIDs were effective at relieving short term pain. We identified hundreds of RCTs comparing NSAIDs with other NSAIDs or placebo for treatment of osteoarthritis. Most of these trials showed benefit from using NSAIDs for the treatment of osteoarthritis. **Oral versus topical NSAIDs:** See topical agents, p 655.

Harms: Indomethacin (and possibly other NSAIDs) may accelerate joint damage in osteoarthritis, and there is a risk of gastrointestinal or renal damage in older people with osteoarthritis, particularly those with intercurrent disease.[26] Case control data from several thousand people suggest that the relative risk of gastrointestinal haemorrhage when taking any NSAID is around 4–5, the risk increasing with certain drugs and with increased doses.[27,28] A meta-analysis (search date 1994) ranked the risk from different drugs and found it to be dose dependent (see table 1, p 662).[29] We found insufficient data on GI effects of COX-2 inhibitors versus traditional NSAIDs to calculate the comparative risk for more recently introduced NSAIDs (see COX-2 option under NSAIDs, p 641).

Comment: Despite the many studies of NSAID use in osteoarthritis, the evidence we found on efficacy remains poor and difficult to generalise. Most RCTs suffer from weak methods, including: short duration; exclusion of older people, those with intercurrent disease or those at risk of gastrointestinal and other drug complications; variable outcome measures; comparison of one drug versus another rather than versus placebo; and funding bias.[30,31] In the absence of clear evidence of the superiority of one type of treatment or product, other considerations, such as safety (particularly the risk of gastrointestinal bleeding with NSAIDs) and cost should determine the choice of drug (see NSAIDs, p 641).

OPTION   **ANALGESICS VERSUS NON-STEROIDAL ANTI-INFLAMMATORY DRUGS**

Two systematic reviews found that simple analgesics and NSAIDs produce short term pain relief in osteoarthritis. However, we found no good evidence that NSAIDs are superior to simple analgesics such as paracetamol (acetaminophen) (see NSAIDs, p 641).

Benefits: We found two systematic reviews (14 RCTs in one review of which 1 is a comparison of NSAIDs versus other analgesics[21]; 48 RCTs in the other review[22] of which two[32,33] compared NSAIDs and analgesics). The systematic reviews found no evidence for the superiority of NSAIDs over simple analgesics. One RCT (n = 178 people with knee osteoarthritis) compared naproxen versus paracetamol (acetaminophen) over 2 years. The trial found no significant difference in effects.[32] Another RCT (n = 184 people with osteoarthritis) compared two doses of ibuprofen versus paracetamol. The trial concluded that there were no differences in the three groups.[33] Twenty crossover trials of one person each ("n of 1" trials) compared paracetamol (acetaminophen) versus diclofenac and concluded that although some people's pain was adequately controlled by paracetamol (acetaminophen) alone, others responded better to an NSAID.[34]

Harms: See above.

Comment: None.

QUESTION What are the effects of topical agents?

We found limited evidence that topical agents provide some pain relief for people with osteoarthritis and that they are less toxic than systemic drug treatments. We found no evidence comparing different topical agents or comparing topical agents with other local treatments such as heat or cold packs.

Benefits: **Topical NSAIDs versus placebo:** See NSAIDs, p 641. We found one recent systematic review (search date 1996, 86 trials) comparing topically applied agents containing NSAIDs versus placebo.[35] It found that these agents were beneficial (RR for relief of chronic musculoskeletal pain due to osteoarthritis and tendinitis 2.0, 95% CI 1.5 to 2.7). One subsequent RCT (n = 119 people with osteoarthritis) found the topical NSAID (diclofenac-hyaluronan gel) to be more effective in relieving pain than placebo gel (P = 0.057).[36] One further RCT (n = 70 people with mild knee osteoarthritis) showed a significant improvement (measured by WOMAC) in the treatment group receiving diclofenac gel compared to the control group receiving vehicle gel (P = 0.05).[37] **Topical NSAIDs versus oral NSAIDs:** One good quality RCT (included in the review) in 235 people with mild osteoarthritis of the knee compared topical piroxicam gel versus oral ibuprofen 1200 mg daily and found no significant difference in pain relief between the two groups (good or excellent relief in 60% v 64%).[38] **Capsaicin:** One non-systematic meta-analysis of three RCTs of topically applied capsaicin found that capsaicin cream reduced pain compared with placebo (OR 4.4, 95% CI 2.8 to 6.9).[39] One RCT (n = 70 people with osteoarthritis) compared 0.025% capsaicin cream versus non-medicated cream. Active treatment resulted in significantly greater pain reduction than placebo (no quantified estimates of benefit available).[40] **Versus other local treatments:** We found no systematic review or RCTs that compared agents containing NSAIDs or capsaicin with simple rubefacients (see glossary, p 659), or local applications such as hot packs.

Harms: The main adverse effect of topical treatment is local skin irritation; systemic adverse effects were no more common than with placebo.[35] We found no reports of gastric or renal problems.

Comment: The evidence is poor, most studies being short term, including a mixture of patient groups, and comparing different agents with no placebo control.

QUESTION What are the effects of intra-articular injection of the knee?

Systematic reviews found no clear evidence of benefit from intra-articular injection of various drugs over placebo injection in people with osteoarthritis of the knee.

Benefits: **Glucocorticoids:** We found one systematic review (published in 1997, 10 RCTs)[41] and one subsequent RCT.[42] The systematic review found that intra-articular injection of glucocorticoids into the knee (one trial used four injections, the rest used single injections) provided little additional pain relief compared with placebo. Pain reduction lasted from 1 week to 1 month.[41] The subsequent RCT evaluated a single injection with 24 weeks' follow up.[42] The trial found a short term benefit (1–4 weeks) of the steroid injection compared with placebo for both pain and for a functional index.[41] **Hyaluronan:** We found one systematic reviews[41] and four subsequent RCTs.[43–46] The review identified 10 trials of hyaluronan in the knee joint.[41] Treatment consisted of several injections of high molecular weight hyaluronan complexes over several weeks. The review found slightly greater benefit than placebo at 1–6 months after treatment. A subsequent non-systematic review (published in 1995) identified 13 trials of hyaluronan injections and included many of the RCTs reported in the first review.[47] It confirmed the conclusions of the systematic review. Three of the four subsequent RCTs of hyaluronan injections versus placebo found no significant difference at 2–5 months' follow up, but both active and placebo groups improved compared with baseline.[43–45] One of the trials (n = 240) included a subgroup analysis of people aged over 60 years with moderate to severe symptoms; these benefited more with active treatment than placebo.[43] The fourth subsequent RCT (n = 100) found significant benefit on the Lequense index with hyaluronan versus placebo, both at 5 weeks (P = 0.030) and 4 months (P = 0.0431).[46] **Other intra-articular treatments:** Several other intra-articular treatments exist, but we found only limited evidence on their effects. Treatments include radioactive isotopes, glycosaminoglycan polysulfuric acid, orgotein, and morphine.[4,48,49]

Harms: We found no reports of serious adverse effects. Localised discomfort after injection is common. A theoretical risk of infection exists, but we found no evidence on this.

Comment: There seems to be little benefit from intra-articular injection over and above a placebo effect. Placebo injection seems to have a substantial beneficial effect. Whether simple aspiration of the knee would be as beneficial as injection remains to be established.

QUESTION What are the effects of joint replacement surgery?

OPTION TOTAL HIP REPLACEMENT

One systematic review and observational studies have found that hip replacement is effective for at least 10 years. Many uncontrolled, observational studies suggest that even better results can be obtained over longer time periods.

Benefits: We found one systematic review (search date 1995, 17 RCTs, 61 observational studies of hip replacements).[50] Mean ages of people in the trials ranged from 43–71 years. The review found that at least 70% of people without prosthetic failure were rated "good/excellent" for pain and function at 10 year follow up (see comment).

Harms: **Death:** We found one recent systematic review (search date 1995). It pooled data on 130 000 people who had undergone hip replacement and had not received thromboprophylaxis, and found that the rate of fatal pulmonary embolism was 0.1–0.2%, and the overall death rate was 0.3–0.4%.[51] One retrospective cohort study

(11 607 hip replacements) found death rates to be higher in the first 3 months after surgery than in the subsequent 9 months.[52] **Revision and infection:** Two good observational studies found that the risk of a revision operation was about 1% per annum, ranging from 0.2–2.0%.[50,53] Most studies found that revisions were not required until at least 10 years after implantation. One large study, using data from a patient register in Sweden, found that the proportion of revised hip replacements that were caused by deep infection fell to less than 0.5% between 1978 and 1990. It also found that aseptic loosening accounted for about 80% of all requirements for replacement or revision surgery after the immediate postoperative period.[54] Observational studies found that the initial results of revision surgery were only slightly worse than primary surgery. However, the prostheses deteriorated more quickly.[55–57]

Comment: A second systematic review (search date 1995) identified 11 RCTs and 180 observational studies comparing different prostheses.[58] It found wide variations in outcome with primary evidence too weak to make valid comparisons. We also found a weak narrative review of 20 mainly small uncontrolled studies evaluating self assessed quality of life (at least two out of: physical, social, emotional, economic, and overall satisfaction).[59] It found that improvement in non-physical measures occurred most often within 3 months. Benefit was sustained for up to 5 years after surgery. We found no longer term data. Most studies did not distinguish between hip replacement for osteoarthritis, and hip replacement for other reasons, which may confound data for osteoarthritis. Outcome of hip replacement for osteoarthritis differs significantly from that for other conditions (e.g. hip fracture in the very elderly and frail, or replacement for rheumatoid arthritis).

OPTION	TOTAL KNEE REPLACEMENT

Two systematic reviews of RCTs have found that knee joint replacement is effective. Most studies concentrated on prosthesis survival rather than clinical outcomes.

Benefits: **Tricompartmental prostheses:** We found one systematic review (search date 1992), which identified 154 studies (4 RCTs, 130 cohort studies, 20 others) of 37 different tricompartmental prostheses in 9879 people (63% with osteoarthritis, mean follow up 4.1 years). Good or excellent outcomes (improved function 5 years after surgery; pain relief after 5 years; mortality rate at 30 days and at 1 year; thromboembolism by 30 days after surgery; no failure of knee prosthesis) were reported in 89% of people.[60] **Uni- or bicompartmental prostheses:** We found one systematic review (search date 1992), which identified no RCTs. It identified 46 cohort studies of unicompartmental prostheses in 2391 people, and 18 cohort studies of bicompartmental prostheses in 884 people.[61] The review found that both procedures were effective (based on a global knee rating scale that includes measures of pain, function and range of movement) with better outcomes from unicompartmental operations, particularly since 1987.[61] **Quality of life:** Two observational studies published since the reviews found improvement in quality of life after all forms of total knee replacement. The first found that function, as measured by WOMAC, improved from 58.2 before surgery to 18.4 at time of survey.[62] The second, a cross sectional community survey, found that 361/487 people (74%) had moderate to severe pain (assessed using a modified Knee Society score) before surgery, compared with 100/487 (21%) 1 or more years after surgery.[63]

Harms: **Death:** In one 6 year cohort of 338 736 US Medicare patients, the death rate within 30 days of hospital admission for total knee replacement was 2147 (0.63%).[60] The same study reported a mean mortality of 1.5% per annum (no comparative data available).[60] **Thrombosis:** We found one RCT[64] and one prospective cohort study,[58] which reported rates of venous thrombosis: about 24% of people who had a total knee replacement developed a deep vein thrombosis.[65] **Revision and infection:** This is the main long term risk. The first review, mentioned above, found a revision rate of 3.8% during 4.1 years of follow up after tricompartmental replacements.[60] The second review found a revision rate of 9.2% over 4.6 years for unicompartmental prostheses and 7.2% over 3.6 years for bicompartmental prostheses.[61] Data from large patient register based studies in Sweden found that the cumulative 10 year risk for revision surgery due to infection was decreasing, and was now less than 1%. The majority of implant revision surgery was due to aseptic loosening. For unicompartmental osteoarthritis, unicompartmental knee replacement is an effective alternative to total knee replacement.[66,67] **Postoperative pain:** This was rarely recorded, but seemed to be absent or mild in most people. **Wound infection:** We found no good evidence on the frequency of wound infections. One large retrospective cohort study found lower complication rates in centres with a higher volume of procedures.[68]

Comment: We found hundreds of observational studies that reported the time to prosthesis failure or revision surgery, but less evidence on patient related outcomes. The evidence suggests that benefits and harms of knee replacement now appear to be comparable to that of hip replacement.

QUESTION   **Which people are most likely to benefit from hip replacement?**

Observational studies have found younger age (under 45 years), old age (over 75 years), and obesity to be associated with worse outcomes from hip replacement, in terms of self assessed satisfaction and failure rates.

Benefits: We found no RCTs. One systematic review (published in 1998) identified 40 observational studies (number of people not stated) relating individual characteristics to outcome after hip replacement.[69] It found that the following factors predicted better outcomes in terms of pain relief and function: age 45–75 years; weight less than 70 kg; good social support; higher educational level; and less preoperative morbidity. **Obesity:** One prospective cohort study (n = 176) found no difference in the quality of life after a primary hip replacement between the non-obese and moderately obese either at 1 or 3 years but the study reported no data in people with body mass index 40 kg/m^2.[70] **Age:** We found a few large observational studies. They found conflicting evidence, which suggested that older people had good self reported outcomes in terms of pain and function, but spent longer in hospital, needed more rehabilitation, and experienced more perioperative complications.[59,71–76]

Harms: **Revision and infection:** One Swedish cohort study found that younger people and those doing heavy physical work were at greater risk of revision.[54] Another study found lower rates of long term survival of the implant in obese people.[56]

Comment: Consensus groups have reported from Sweden, USA, Canada, and New Zealand.[77–80] Constant pain, particularly night or rest pain, with or without substantial functional impairment, are the generally agreed criteria for joint replacement (see table 3, p 663). In practice, most surgeons prefer to have radiographic evidence of joint damage as well.

QUESTION   **Which people are most likely to benefit from knee replacement?**

We found limited and conflicting evidence from observational studies.

Benefits: **Obesity:** We found limited and conflicting evidence from observational studies on the effects of obesity on outcome of knee replacement.[81–84] **Age:** We found limited evidence from observational studies suggesting that knee replacement is effective in elderly people.[13]

Harms: None found.

Comment: None.

GLOSSARY

Self care education Individualised arthritis self care instruction based on patients needs assessment.
Attention only education Information about arthritis but no guidance on self treatment.
Rubefacient An agent that produces mild irritation and redness of the skin.

Substantive changes since last issue

Major restructuring since last issue in order to provide a more logical layout.

REFERENCES

1. Petersson IF. Occurrence of osteoarthritis of the peripheral joints in European populations. *Ann Rheum Dis* 1996;55:659–661.
2. Felson DT. Epidemiology of hip and knee osteoarthritis. *Epidemiol Rev* 1988;10:1–28.
3. Gaffney KL. Intra-articular triamcinolone hexacetonide in knee osteoarthritis: factors influencing the clinical response. *Ann Rheum Dis* 1995;54:379–381.
4. Pavelka JKS. Glycosaminoglycan polysulfuric acid (GAGPS) in osteoarthritis of the knee. *Osteoarthritis Cartilage* 1995;3:15–23.
5. Insall JN, Dorr LD, Scott RD, Scott WN. Rationale of the Knee Society clinical rating system. *Clin Orthopaed Rel Res* 1988;248:13–14.
6. Bellamy N, Buchanan WW, Goldsmith CH, et al. Validation study of WOMAC: a health status instrument for measuring clinically important, patient relevant outcomes following total hip or knee arthroplasty in osteoarthritis. *J Rheumatol* 1988;1:95–108.
7. Bellamy N, Buchanan WW, Goldsmith CH, et al. Validation study of WOMAC: A health status instrument for measuring clinically important patient relevant outcomes to antirheumatic drug therapy in patients with osteoarthritis of the hip or knee. *J Rheumatol* 1988;15:1833–1840.
8. Dougados M, Devogelaer JP, Annefeldt M, et al. Recommendations for the registration of drugs used in the treatment of osteoarthritis. *Ann Rheum Dis* 1996;55:552–557.
9. Altman R, Brandt K, Hochberg M, et al. Design and conduct of clinical trials in patients with osteoarthritis: recommendations from a task force of the Osteoarthritis Research Society. *Osteoarthritis Cartilage* 1996;4:217–243.
10. Van Baar ME, Assendelft WJJ, Dekker J, et al. Effectiveness of exercise therapy in patients with osteoarthritis of the hip or knee: a systematic

review of randomized clinical trials. *Arthritis Rheum* 1999;42:1361–1369. Search date September 1997; primary sources Medline, Embase, Cinahl, Cochrane Controlled Trials Register.

11. Puett DW, Griffin MR. Published trials of non-medicinal and non-invasive therapies for hip and knee osteoarthritis. *Ann Intern Med* 1994;121: 133–140. Search date 1993; primary source: Medline.

12. La Mantia K, Marks R. The efficacy of aerobic exercises for treating osteoarthritis of the knee. *NZ J Physiother* 1995;23:23–30. Search date 1994; primary sources Medline, Cinahl, hand searched references, personal contacts.

13. Ettinger WH Jr, Burns R, Messier SP, et al. A randomized trial comparing aerobic exercise and resistance exercise with a health education program in older adults with knee osteoarthritis. The fitness arthritis and seniors trial (FAST). *JAMA* 1997;277:25–31.

14. Deyle GD, Henderson NE, Matekel RL, et al. Effectiveness of manual physical therapy and exercise in osteoarthritis of the knee: A randomized, controlled trial. *Ann Intern Med* 2000;132:173–181.

15. Maurer BT, Stern AG, Kinossian B, et al. Osteoarthritis of the knee: Isokinetic quadriceps exercise versus and educational intervention. *Arch Phys Med Rehab* 1999;80:1293–1299.

16. Superio-Cabuslay E, Ward MM, Lorig KR. Patient education interventions in osteoarthritis and rheumatoid arthritis: a meta-analytic comparison with non-steroidal anti-inflammatory drug treatment. *Arthritis Care Res* 1996;9:292–301. Search date 1993; primary sources Medline and hand searched references.

17. Mazzuca SA, Brandt KD, Katz BP, et al. Effects of self-care education on the health status of inner-city patients with osteoarthritis of the knee. *Arthritis Rheum* 1997;40:1466–1474.

18. Edworthy SM, Devins GM. Improving medication adherence through patient education distinguishing between appropriate and inappropriate utilization. Patient Education Study Group. *J Rheumatol* 1999;26:793–1801.

19. Kirkley A, Websterbogaert S, Litchfield R, et al. The effect of bracing on varus gonarthrosis. *J Bone Joint Surg* 1999;81a:539–548.

20. Cushnaghan J, McCarthy C, Dieppe P. Taping the patella medially - a new treatment for osteoarthritis of the knee-joint. *BMJ* 1994;308: 753–755.

21. Towheed T, Shea B, Wells G, Hochberg M. Osteoarthritis: a systematic review of randomized controlled trials of analgesia and anti-inflammatory therapy in osteoarthritis of the hip. In The Cochrane Library, Issue 4, 1999. Search date 1994; primary sources Medline; Cochrane Library; and Controlled Clinical Trials Register.

22. Towheed TE, Hochberg MC. A systematic review of randomized controlled trials of pharmacological therapy in osteoarthritis of the knee, with an emphasis on trial methodology. *Semin Arthritis Rheum* 1997;26:755–770. Search date August 1994, primary sources Medline, and hand searched references.

23. Amadio P, Cummings DM. Evaluation of acetaminophen in the management of osteoarthritis of the knee. *Curr Ther Res Clin Exp* 1983;34:59–66.

24. Hawton K, Ware C, Mistry H, et al. Why patients choose paracetamol for self poisoning and their knowledge of its dangers. *BMJ* 1995;310:164.

25. Watson MC, Brookes ST, Kirwan JR, Faulkner A. Osteoarthritis: the comparative efficacy of non-aspirin non-steroidal anti-inflammatory drugs for the management of osteoarthritis of the knee. In The Cochrane Library, Issue 4, 1999. Search dates and primary sources Medline January 1980 to December 1995; BIDS 1996; Embase 1995.

26. Huskisson EC, Berry H, Gishen P, et al. Effects of anti-inflammatory drugs on the progression of osteoarthritis of the knee. *J Rheumatol* 1995;22: 1941–1946.

27. Langman MJ. Non-steroidal anti-inflammatory drugs and peptic ulcer. Hepatogastroenterology 1992;39(suppl 1):37–39.

28. Garcia Rodriguez LA, Williams R, Derby LE, et al. Acute liver injury associated with non-steroidal anti-inflammatory drugs and the role of risk factors. *Arch Intern Med* 1994;154:311–316.

29. Henry D, Lim LL, Garcia Rodriguez LA, et al. Variability in risk of gastrointestinal complications with individual non-steroidal anti-inflammatory drugs: results of a collaborative meta-analysis. *BMJ* 1996;312:1563–1566.

30. Brandt KD. Nonsurgical management of osteoarthritis, with an emphasis on nonpharmacologic measures. *Arch Fam Med* 1995;4:1057–1064.

31. Wollheim FA. Current pharmacological treatment of osteoarthritis. *Drugs* 1996;52(suppl 3):27–38.

32. Williams HJ, Ward JR, Egger MJ, et al. Comparison of naproxen and acetaminophen in a 2-year study of treatment of osteoarthritis of the knee. *Arthritis Rheum* 1993;36:1196–1206.

33. Bradley JD, Brandt KD, Katz BP, et al. Comparison of an anti-inflammatory dose of ibuprofen, an analgesic dose of ibuprofen, and acetaminophen in the treatment of patients with osteoarthritis of the knee. *N Engl J Med* 1991;325:87–91.

34. March L, Irwig L, Schwarz J, et al. N of 1 trials comparing non-steroidal anti-inflammatory drug with paracetamol in osteoarthritis. *BMJ* 1993; 309:1041–1046.

35. Moore RA, Tramer MR, Carroll D, et al. Quantitative systematic review of topically applied non-steroidal anti-inflammatory drugs. *BMJ* 1998; 316:333–338. Search date September 1996; primary sources Embase, Medline, Oxford Pain Relief Database, hand searched references, librarians and medical directors of 12 pharmaceutical companies asked for reports of their products.

36. Roth SH. A controlled clinical investigation of 3% diclofenac/2.5% sodium hyaluronate topical gel in the treatment of uncontrolled pain in chronic oral NSAID users with osteoarthritis. *Int J Tissue React* 1995;17:129–132.

37. Grace D, Rogers J, Skeith K, et al. Topical diclofenac versus placebo: A double blind, randomized clinical trial in patients with osteoarthritis of the knee. *J Rheumatol* 1999;26: 2659–2663.

38. Dickson DJ. A double-blind evaluation of topical piroxicam gel with oral ibuprofen in osteoarthritis of the knee. *Curr Ther Res Clin Exp* 1991;49: 199–207.

39. Zhang WY, Po ALW. The effectiveness of topically applied capsaicin: a meta-analysis. *Eur J Clin Pharmacol* 1994;46:517–522. Search date 1994; primary sources BIDS 1980 to 1994; Medline 1980 to 1994, and hand searches of relevant published references.

40. Deal CL, Schnitzer TJ, Lipstein E, et al. Treatment of arthritis with topical capsaicin: a double-blind trial. *Clin Ther* 1991;13:383–395.

41. Kirwan JRR. Intra-articular therapy in osteoarthritis. *Baillieres Clin Rheumatol* 1997;11: 769–794. Search date not stated. RCTs cited from 1958 to 1996; primary sources Medline, Embase.

42. Ravaud P, Moulinier L, Giraudeau B, et al. Effects

of joint lavage and steroid injection in patients with osteoarthritis of the knee: results of a multicenter, randomized, controlled trial. *Arthritis Rheum* 1999;42:475–82.

43. Lohmander LSD. Intra-articular hyaluronan injections in the treatment of osteoarthritis of the knee: a randomised, double blind, placebo controlled multicentre trial. *Ann Rheum Dis* 1996; 55:424–431.

44. Corrado EM, Peluso GF, Gigliotti S. The effects of intra-articular administration of hyaluronic acid on osteoarthritis of the knee: a clinical study with immunological and biochemical evaluations. *Eur J Rheumatol Inflamm* 1995;15:47–56.

45. Formiguera SSE. Intra-articular hyaluronic acid in the treatment osteoarthritis of the knee: a short term study. *Eur J Rheumatol Inflamm* 1995;15: 33–38.

46. Huskisson EC, Donnelly S. Hyaluronic acid in the treatment of osteoarthritis of the knee. *Rheumatology* 1999;38:602–607.

47. Maheu E. Hyaluronan in knee osteoarthritis: a review of the clinical trials with Hyalgan. *Eur J Rheumatol Inflamm* 1995;15:17–24.

48. McIlwain HSJ. Intra-articular orgotein in osteoarthritis of the knee: a placebo-controlled efficacy, safety, and dosage comparison. *Am J Med* 1989;87:295–300.

49. Likar RS. Intraarticular morphine analgesia in chronic pain patients with osteoarthritis. *Anesth Analg* 1997;84:1313–1317.

50. Faulkner A, Kennedy LG, Baxter K, et al. Effectiveness of hip prostheses in primary total hip replacement: a critical review of evidence and an economic model. *Health Technol Assess* 1998;2: 1–33. Search date 1995; primary sources Embase, Medline, in-house database on epidemiology and service provision for total hip replacement; additional search on Embase 1990–1996.

51. Murray DW, Britton AR, Bulstrode CJ. Thromboprophylaxis and death after total hip replacement. *J Bone Joint Surg Br* 1996;78:863–870. Search date 1995; primary source Medline.

52. Seagroatt V, Soon Tan H, Goldacre M, et al. Elective total hip replacement: incidence, emergency readmission rate, and postoperative mortality. *BMJ* 1991;303:1431–1435.

53. Chang RW, Pellissier JM, Hazen GB. A cost-effectiveness analysis of total hip arthroplasty for osteoarthritis of the hip. *JAMA* 1996;275:858–865.

54. Malchau H, Herberts P, Ahnfelt L. Prognosis of total hip replacement in Sweden. Follow up of 92 675 operations performed 1978–1990. *Acta Orthop Scand* 1993;64:497–506.

55. Robinson AH, Palmer CR, Villar RN. Is revision as good as primary hip replacement? A comparison of quality of life. *J Bone Joint Surg Br* 1999;81: 42–45.

56. Espehaug B, Havelin LI, Engesaeter LB, et al. Patient-related risk-factors for early revision of total hip replacements. A population register-based case-control study of 674 revised hips. *Acta Orthop Scand* 1997;68:207–215.

57. Johnsson R, Franzen H, Nilsson LT. Combined survivorship and multivariate analyses of revisions in 799 hip prostheses. A 10- to 20-year review of mechanical loosening *J Bone Joint Surg Br* 1994; 76:439–443.

58. Fitzpatrick R, Shortall E, Sculpher M, et al. Primary total hip replacement surgery: a systematic review of outcomes and modelling of cost-effectiveness associated with different prostheses. *Health Technol Assess* 1998;2:1–64. Search date 1995; primary sources Medline, and hand searched references.

59. Towheed TE, Hochberg MC. Health-related quality of life after total hip replacement. *Semin Arthritis Rheum* 1996;26:483–491.

60. Callahan CM, Drake BG, Heck DA, et al. Patient outcomes following tricompartmental total knee replacement; a meta-analysis. *JAMA* 1994;271: 1349–1357. Search date 1992; primary sources Medlars and hand searched references.

61. Callahan CM, Drake BG, Heck DA, et al. Patient outcomes following unicompartmental or bicompartmental knee arthroplasty: a meta-analysis. *J Arthroplasty* 1995;10:141–150. Search date 1992; primary sources Medlars and hand searched references.

62. Kiebzak GM, Vain PA, Gregory AM, et al. SF-36 general health status survey to determine patient satisfaction at short-term follow up after total hip and knee arthroplasty. *J South Orthop Assoc* 1997;6:169–172.

63. Hawker G, Wright J, Coyte P, et al. Health related quality of life after knee replacement. *J Bone Joint Surg* 1998;80(A):163–173.

64. Kim YH. The incidence of deep vein thrombosis after cementless and cemented knee replacement. *J Bone Joint Surg* 1990;72:779–783.

65. Fauno P, Suomalained O, Rehnberg V, et al. Prophylaxis for the prevention of venous thromboembolism after total knee arthroplasty. *J Bone Joint Surg* 1994;76(A):1814–1818.

66. Knutson K, Lewold S, Robertsson O, Lidgren L. The Swedish knee arthroplasty register. A nation-wide study of 30 003 knees *Acta Orthop Scand* 1994;65:375–386.

67. Robertsson O, Borgquist L, Knutson K, et al. Use of unicompartmental instead of tricompartmental prostheses for unicompartmental arthrosis of the knee is a cost-effective alternative. 15,437 primary tricompartmental prostheses were compared with 10 624 primary medical or lateral unicompartmental prostheses. *Acta Orthop Scand* 1999;70:170–175.

68. Norton EC, Garfinkel SA, McQuay LJ, et al. The effect of hospital volume on the in-hospital complication rate in knee replacement patients. *Health Serv Res* 1998;33:1191–1210.

69. Young NL, Cheah D, Waddell JP, et al. Patient characteristics that affect the outcome of total hip arthroplasty: a review. *Can J Surg* 1998;41:188–195. Search date not stated; primary sources Medline, and hand search of references.

70. Chan CL, Villar RN. Obesity and quality of life after primary hip arthroplasty. *J Bone Joint Surg Br* 1996;78:78–81.

71. Espehaug B, Havelin LI, Engesaeter LB, et al. Patient satisfaction and function after primary and revision total hip replacement. *Clin Orthop* 1998; 351:135–148.

72. Garellick G, Malchau H, Herberts P, et al. Life expectancy and cost utility after total hip replacement. *Clin Orthop* 1998;346:141–151.

73. Brander VA, Malhotra S, Jet J, et al. Outcome of hip and knee arthroplasty in persons aged 80 years and older. *Clin Orthop* 1997;345:67–78.

74. Levy RN, Levy CM, Snyder J, et al. Outcome and long-term results following total hip replacement in elderly patients. *Clin Orthop* 1995;316:25–30.

75. Boettcher WG. Total hip arthroplasties in the elderly – morbidity, mortality, and cost-effectiveness. *Clin Orthop* 1992;274:30–34.

76. Donnell ST, Neyret P, Dejour H, et al. The effect of age on the quality of life after knee replacement. *Knee* 1998;5:125–112.

77. Swedish web site: http://www.sos.se/sosmenye.htm (in Swedish).

78. National Institutes of Health. Total hip replacement. NIH consensus development panel

on total hip replacement. *JAMA* 1995;273:1950–1956.

79. Naylor CD, Williams JI. Primary hip and knee replacement surgery: Ontario criteria for case selection and surgical priority. *Qual Health Care* 1996;5:20–30.

80. Hardorn DC, Holmes AC. The New Zealand priority criteria project. *BMJ* 1997;314:131–134.

81. Braeken AM, Lochaas-Gerlach JA, et al. Determinants of 6–12 month postoperative functional status and pain after elective total hip

replacement. *Int J Qual Health Care* 1997;9:413–418.

82. De Leeuw JM, Villar RN. Obesity and quality of life after primary total knee replacement. *Knee* 1998;5:119–23.

83. Lubitz R, Dittus R, Robinson R, et al. Effects of severe obesity on health status 2 years after knee replacement. *J Gen Intern Med* 1996;11:145.

84. Winiarsky R, Barth P, Lotke P. Total knee arthroplasty in morbidly obese patients. *J Bone J Surg* 1998;80A;1770–1774.

Paul Dieppe
Director

Jiri Chard
Research Associate

MRC Health Services Research Collaboration, University of Bristol
Bristol
UK

Alex Faulkner
Research Fellow
University of Wales
Cardiff
UK

Stefan Lohmander
Professor
Department of Orthopaedics
Lund University
Lund
Sweden
Competing interests: None declared.

TABLE 1   **Estimated relative risk of gastrointestinal adverse effects with the use of individual NSAIDs (pooled data from 12 studies) (see text, p 654).[29]**

Drug	Pooled RR	95% CI for pooled RR
Ibuprofen (low dose)*	1.0	–
Fenoprofen	1.6	1.0 to 2.5
Aspirin	1.6	1.3 to 2.0
Diclofenac	1.8	1.4 to 2.3
Sulindac	2.1	1.6 to 2.7
Diflunisal	2.2	1.2 to 4.1
Naproxen	2.2	1.7 to 2.9
Indomethacin	2.4	1.9 to 3.1
Tometin	3.0	1.8 to 4.9
Piroxicam	3.8	2.7 to 5.2
Ketoprofen	4.2	2.7 to 6.4
Azapropazone	9.2	4.0 to 21.0

*Comparative data used low dose ibuprofen as the reference control for calculating the relative risk of other drugs.

TABLE 2	Effect sizes (95% CI) of exercise in osteoarthritis of the knee and hip: results of the best three RCTs identified in a systematic review (see text, p 651).[10]

RCT	Pain	Observed disability
1	0.31 (0.28 to 0.34)	0.31 (0.28 to 0.34)
2	0.47 (0.44 to 0.50)	0.89 (0.85 to 0.93)
3	0.58 (0.54 to 0.62)	0.28 (0.24 to 0.32)

TABLE 3	Summary of New Zealand priority criteria for joint replacement (see text, p 659).[80]

Severity is scored out of a possible 100 on the basis of:

Pain: severity 0–20; duration 0–20

Function: walking difficulty 0–10, other 0–10

Joint damage: pain on passive movement 0–10, other/X ray 0–10

Other: other joints 0–10, work, care giving, independence 0–10

Plantar heel pain (including plantar fasciitis)

New topic

Fay Crawford

Key Messages

- RCTs have found that symptoms resolve spontaneously in most people allocated to placebo.

- One systematic review found limited evidence of short term improvement in pain for steroid injections plus lignocaine versus local anaesthetic alone. This small clinical effect was not found in the group receiving lignocaine plus local anaesthetic plus nerve block, and no evidence of medium to long term benefit was found.

- Observational studies have found a high rate of plantar fascia rupture and other complications associated with steroid injections, which may lead to chronic disability in some people.

- We found conflicting evidence on the effect of steroid plus local anaesthetic injections versus pads. One RCT found limited evidence of effectiveness for short term improvement in pain for steroid plus lignocaine injections versus pads. A second RCT using a different type of pad and different outcomes found no significant difference. Neither RCT found medium to long term benefit from steroid plus lignocaine injections.

Musculoskeletal conditions

- We found no evidence from systematic reviews or RCTs of medium to long term benefit for steroid injections with or without local anaesthetics versus placebo or other treatments.
- We found conflicting evidence about the benefit of orthoses versus heel pads. Trials involved different regimens.
- One systematic review of one weak RCT found limited evidence of a benefit with extra corporeal shock wave therapy (ESWT) versus placebo.
- We found no RCTs of surgery.
- One systematic review found no significant benefit from laser, ultrasound, or night splints versus placebo or no treatment.

DEFINITION Plantar heel pain is soreness or tenderness of the heel. It often radiates from the central part of the heel pad or the medial tubercle of the calcaneum but may extend along the plantar fascia into the medial longitudinal arch of the foot. Severity may range from an irritation at the origin of the plantar fascia, noticeable on rising after rest, to an incapacitating pain. This review excludes clinically evident underlying disorders, foe example, infection, calcaneal fracture, and calcaneal nerve entrapment, which can be distinguished by their characteristic history and signs. (A calcaneal fracture may present after trauma, whereas calcaneal nerve entrapment gives rise to shooting pains and feelings of "pins and needles" on the medial aspect of the heel.)

INCIDENCE/ The incidence and prevalence of plantar heel pain is uncertain.
PREVALENCE Plantar heel pain primarily affects those in mid to late life.[1]

AETIOLOGY/ Unknown.
RISK FACTORS

PROGNOSIS One systematic review (search date 1998) found that almost all the included trials reported an improvement in discomfort regardless of the intervention received (including placebo).[1] A telephone survey of 100 people treated conservatively (average follow up 47 months) found that 82 people had resolution of symptoms, 15 had continued symptoms but no limitations of activity or work), and three had continued symptoms that limited activity or changed work status.[2] Thirty one people said that they would have seriously considered surgical treatment at the time medical attention was sought. The three people still with limitation had bilateral symptoms but no other clear risk factors.

AIMS To reduce pain and immobility, with minimal adverse effects.

OUTCOMES Pain reduction (using visual analogue scales); walking distance.

METHODS *Clinical Evidence* search and appraisal February 2000. Searches of Medline and BIDs were performed in 1996 and updated in 2000 to identify systematic reviews and RCTs. The reference list of trials was searched. Schools of podiatry were contacted for unpublished studies.

Plantar heel pain (including plantar fasciitis)

QUESTION What are the effects of treatments for plantar heel pain?

OPTION STEROID INJECTIONS

One systematic review of one small RCT found no significant reduction in pain with steroid injection versus placebo. One systematic review of one small RCT found no significant difference in pain relief with steroid injection versus heel pads (see glossary, p 672).

Benefits: We found one systematic review (search date 1998).[1] **Versus placebo or no treatment:** The review found one small RCT of steroid (hydrocortisone acetate 25 mg) versus saline injection in 19 people with recalcitrant heel pain but not arthritis.[1] It found no significant difference in pain relief (RR 0.52, 95% CI 0.15 to 1.79). **Versus orthoses:** The review found no RCTs. **Versus pads:** The review found one small RCT (n = 17) of steroid (20 mg triamcinolone 2%) versus a prefabricated silicone type heel pad. Although more people improved after treatment with the heel pad (66% v 33% at 12 weeks) the difference was not significant at 1, 2, or 12 weeks. **Versus pain medication alone:** The review found no RCTs.

Harms: Steroid injections can be painful. In one study of 106 people, all heels were injected through the medial aspect of the heel pad. Half of the participants were given a tibial nerve block to reduce discomfort during the injection, but there was no significant difference in pain at time of injection between those who received the nerve block and those who did not. Local steroid injection may lead to infection, subcutaneous fat atrophy, skin pigmentation changes, fascial rupture, infection, peripheral nerve injury, or muscle damage.[3] Observational studies have reported rupture of the plantar fascia in people receiving steroid injections.[4,5] One study reported a 10% incidence of rupture out of 122 injected heels,[4] and a second study reported ruptures in 33% of 37 people given injections.[5] The original heel pain may be relieved after rupture, but arch and midfoot strain, lateral plantar nerve dysfunction, stress fracture, deformity, and swelling may result from plantar fascia rupture, and may persist.

Comment: All trials were small. Heterogeneity of interventions prevented data pooling. The evidence from observational studies makes it difficult to define the clinical importance of rupture of the plantar fascia, and may incorporate confounding factors.

OPTION STEROID INJECTIONS PLUS LOCAL ANAESTHESIA

One systematic review and a subsequent RCT found no evidence of a significant long term benefit from steroid plus local anaesthetic injections versus alternative treatments, and only limited evidence of a short term benefit.

Benefits: We found one systematic review (search date 1998), which included RCTs of injected steroid plus local anaesthetic versus various other treatments.[1] **Versus placebo or no treatment:** The review found no RCTs. **Versus heel pads:** See glossary, p 672. The review[1] found one RCT, and we found one subsequent RCT.[6] The first RCT included people with pain on the plantar aspect of the heel but excluded people on anti-inflammatory medication, people who had a steroid injection in the last 6 months, people with rheumatoid arthritis, and people with pain that radiated along the plantar fascia more distally. It compared three arms, a heel pad alone versus an injection alone (triamcinolone hexacteonide + 2% lignocaine) versus injection plus pad. Analysis was not by intention to treat, and four people (5%) were lost to follow up. After 1 month, the greatest improvement in pain was in people who received the injection alone (n = 22) with the least improvement in people who had the pad alone (n = 26) (100 mm VAS scale, injection alone v pad alone WMD −45 mm, 95% CI −59 to −31). At 24 weeks, there was greater pain reduction with the injection alone versus the pad alone, but the difference was not significant (85% v 75%). The subsequent RCT included 103 people with plantar heel tenderness, a history of pain upon rising in the morning (first step pain), and no history of trauma in the previous 3 months.[6] Analysis was not intention to treat and 18 people were lost to follow up. It compared three arms: NSAIDs plus three steroid plus local anaesthetic injections into the heel (anti-inflammatory, n = 35) versus heel pads plus paracetamol (acetaminophen) as required (accommodative, n = 33) versus a heel pad prior to fitting of custom made orthoses (see glossary, p 672) (mechanical, n = 35). The anti-inflammatory regimen consisted of 2 x 300 mg capsules of etodolac and 0.5 ml dexamethasone sodium phosphate 4 mg/ml plus 0.55 bupivacaine hydrochloride without epinephrine. If there was no response then 0.2 ml of dexamethasone acetate 16 mg/ml injection was added cumulatively to the second (2 weeks) and third (4 weeks) injections. The RCT found slightly greater pain relief among people treated by the anti-inflammatory regimen compared with the accommodative regimen at 3 months but the difference was not significant (10 cm VAS, WMD −1.2 cm, 95% CI −2.8 to +0.4). **Versus heel pad and orthoses:** The review found no RCTs. We found no RCTs versus orthoses alone. We found one subsequent RCT comparing an anti-inflammatory regimen versus mechanical regimen.[6] At 3 months, people treated with a heel pad and orthoses had improved more, but the difference was not significant (WMD −1, 95% CI −2.5 to +0.5). **Versus local anaesthetic alone:** The review found no RCTs. We found one subsequent RCT (n = 106).[7] It compared a single injection of 1 ml 25 mg/ml prednisolone acetate plus 1 ml 2% lignocaine hydrochloride versus 2 ml 2% lignocaine hydrochloride alone. It found a small benefit with the combined injection at 1 month, the clinical relevance of which is considered small (10 cm

VAS, WMD −0.8, 95% CI −1.5 to −0.2) but no significant difference in pain thereafter (3 months, WMD 0.1, 95% CI −1.2 to +1.3 and 6 months, 0.5, 95% CI −0.8 to +1.7). **Versus steroid alone:** The review found no RCTs. **Versus steroid plus local anaesthetic plus pad:** The review[1] found one RCT in 76 people, which found significantly worse results at 1 month after treatment with the heel pad plus injection versus steroid injection plus local anaesthetic (100 mm VAS, WMD −16 mm, 95% CI −31 to −1). However, at 24 weeks, people treated with pad plus injection versus injection alone had less pain, but this did not reach statistical significance (94% v 85%). **Steroid plus local anaesthetic plus pad versus pad alone:** The review[1] found one RCT in 76 people. It found a significantly better response with injection plus pad versus pad alone at 4 weeks and 12 weeks, but not at 24 weeks (100 mm VAS; at 4 weeks figures not available; at 24 weeks WMD −10.7 mm, 95% CI −25.5 to +4.1, 94% v 75% pain reduction).

Harms: No trials reported on harms.

Comment: All trials were small. Heterogeneity of interventions prevented data pooling. A recent survey of UK rheumatologists found that corticosteroid injections are the most common treatment of heel pain and are used by 98% of UK rheumatologists (F Crawford, personal communication, 2000), confirming the results of similar surveys.[3] We found no placebo controlled RCTs of steroid injections plus local anaesthesia, and no evidence of medium to long term efficacy in RCTs comparing this treatment with other options. We found evidence from two observational studies of high rates of moderate harms from this treatment (see harms of steroid injections). This is also consistent with evidence about harms of steroid injections in other areas.[3] These harms are particularly relevant because the evidence of benefit is poor, and spontaneous resolution of symptoms is common. The RCTs have many flaws (lack of intention to treat analysis, high drop-out rates, and lack of placebo control). The weaknesses of the available evidence make the use of steroid injections in heel pain difficult to categorise.

OPTION   **CUSTOM MADE ORTHOSES**

A systematic review found no evidence about the benefit of orthoses versus placebo or no treatment for heel pain. A few RCTs found limited evidence about the benefit of orthoses versus other treatments for heel pain.

Benefits: We found one systematic review (search date 1998).[1] **Versus placebo or no treatment:** The review found no RCTs. **Orthoses plus heel pad versus steroid plus pain medication:** The review[1] found no RCTs. We found one subsequent RCT, which found no significant difference in pain improvement.[6] **Orthoses plus heel pad versus heel pads plus pain medication:** The review found one RCT of a heel pad applied for 4 weeks prior to fitting of custom made orthoses heel pad (n = 28) versus a viscoelastic heel pad plus paracetamol (acetaminophen) as required (n = 26). It found significantly better pain reduction with pad plus orthoses (10 cm VAS; WMD −2.2 mm 95% CI −3.8 to −0.5). **Orthoses plus**

stretching versus heel pad plus stretching: The review found no RCTs. We found one subsequent RCT (n = 236, 5 groups) in people with maximal tenderness over the medial calcaneal tuberosity for which they had received no previous treatment.[8] People with systemic disease, sciatica, or local nerve entrapment were excluded. The RCT compared customised orthoses plus stretching exercises versus prefabricated shoe inserts made from three different materials (silicone, felt, and rubber) plus stretching exercises (achilles and plantar fascial stretching for 10 minutes twice daily). It found significantly less pain at 8 weeks in people who were assigned to prefabricated inserts (results combined) versus orthoses (P = 0.007). **Orthoses plus stretching versus stretching alone:** The review found no RCTs. We found one subsequent RCT of custom made orthoses plus stretching exercises versus stretching exercises alone. It found no significant difference in pain improvement at 8 weeks (100 mm VAS; WMD −3.2 mm 95% CI −17.4 to +11.0).

Harms: No trials reported on harms.

Comment: Subgroup analysis in the RCT comparing orthoses versus heel pads found that, among people who stood for more than 8 hours daily, a greater reduction in pain was achieved with stretching alone than with customised insoles.[8] It found no significant difference in people who stood for less than 8 hours a day. This hypothesis requires testing as the primary outcome in an RCT. Only half the participants in this subgroup analysis responded to the pain questionnaire.

OPTION	HEEL PADS AND HEEL CUPS

One systematic review found no evidence about heel pads and heel cups (see glossary, p 672) versus placebo or no treatment for heel pain. A few small RCTs of heel pads and heel cups versus other treatments for heel pain provided no strong evidence.

Benefits: We found one systematic review (search date 1998)[1], which included RCTs of heel pads and heel cups versus various treatments. **Versus placebo or no treatment:** The review found no RCTs.[1] **Versus steroid:** The review found one small RCT, which found no significant difference in pain improvement (see benefits of steroids versus heel pads, p 672 and benefits of steroids plus pain mediation versus heel pads, p 667). **Versus steroid plus pain medication:** The review found one RCT, which found better short term outcomes with steroid plus lignocaine injections.[1] One subsequent RCT found no significant difference in pain improvement between steroid injection plus NSAIDs versus pads plus paracetamol (see benefits under steroids plus local anaesthesia, p 667).[6] **Versus customised orthoses:** The review found one RCT[1] and we found one subsequent RCT.[6] They found conflicting evidence on improvement in pain (see benefits under customised orthoses, p 668). **Heel pad plus steroid plus local anaesthetic versus steroid plus local anaesthetic:** The review found one RCT.[1] It found a short term benefit with the steroid plus local anaesthetic injection alone (see benefits under steroids plus local anaesthesia, p 667).

Harms: None of the trials reported harms.

Comment: Heel cups and heel pads can be made from several different materials, but rubber, viscoelastic, and silicone can be bought as prefabricated shoe inserts. Podiatrists or orthotists sometimes use felt and foam to construct heel pads.

OPTION   LOCAL ANAESTHETIC INJECTION

One systematic review found no evidence about the benefit of local anaesthesia versus placebo or no treatment for heel pain. A few small RCTs found limited evidence about the benefit of local anaesthesia versus other treatments.

Benefits: We found one systematic review (search date 1998).[1] **Local anaesthetic versus placebo or no treatment:** The review found no RCTs.[1] **Local anaesthetic versus steroids plus local anaesthetic:** The review found one RCT (see benefits of steroids plus local anaesthesia, p 667), which found a short term benefit with combined treatment.[1] **Local anaesthetic plus steroid versus orthoses:** The review found one RCT of NSAIDs plus up to three steroid injections versus orthoses (see benefits under customised orthoses, p 668 or heel pads, p 669).[1] It found no advantage with NSAIDs. **Local anaesthetic plus steroid versus local anaesthetic plus steroid plus pad:** The review identified one RCT, which found a better result at 1 month without the pad (see benefits under steroids plus local anaesthesia, p 667).[1] **Local anaesthetic plus steroid plus pad versus pad alone:** The review found one RCT, which found a better result at 1 month with lignocaine plus pads versus pads alone (see benefits under steroids plus local anaesthesia, p 667).[1]

Harms: None of the trials reported on harms.

Comment: Adrenaline is not recommended in local anaesthetics for procedures involving the appendages because of the risk of ischaemic necrosis.[9]

OPTION   EXTRA CORPOREAL SHOCK WAVE THERAPY

One systematic review of one poor quality RCT found limited evidence of a benefit with ESWT versus sham ESWT (see glossary, p 672). One subsequent RCT found a small, non significant reduction of pain with ESWT versus sham ESWT. Two RCTs found limited evidence of a greater improvement with high dose versus low dose ESWT.

Benefits: **Versus placebo:** We found one systematic review (search date 1998)[1] and one subsequent RCT of extracorporeal shock wave therapy (ESWT).[10] The review found one single blind RCT in 36 people with recalcitrant heel pain, which compared 1000 impulses (0.06 mJ/mm^2) versus placebo (sham ESWT) three times at weekly intervals. It found that pain on manual pressure and pain free walking ability were significantly improved at 6 weeks (P < 0.005). Six people withdrew from the trial and analysis was not intention to treat. The small subsequent RCT in people with recalcitrant heel pain found no significant difference between ESWT at 1500 pulses at 3 Hz versus sham treatment (n = 37, 100 mm VAS; WMD −15 mm, 95% CI −45 to +15).[10] **Different doses:** The review identified one non-blinded RCT [1] and one additional RCT.[12] The RCT in the review (n = 119) compared 1000 impulses of 0.08 mJ/mm^2 versus 10 impulses of 0.08 mJ in people with recalcitrant heel pain. All treatments were given three times at weekly intervals. It found greater improvements in pressure pain between weeks 0–12 with the higher dose (100 mm VAS, WMD −47 mm, −54 to −40). The additional RCT (n = 50) compared 3 x 500 impulses of ESWT versus 3 x 100 impulses (both at intensity 0.08 mJ/mm^2) in people with recalcitrant heel pain.[12] It found no significant difference in pain on pressure at 6 weeks (10 cm VAS: WMD −0.4, 95% CI −2.0 to +1.2) or at 12 weeks (WMD −1.4, 95% CI −3.0 to 0.2). There was also no significant difference in walking pain at 6 weeks (WMD −0.8, 95% CI −2.4 to +0.7) or at 12 weeks (WMD −0.9, 95% CI −2.5 to +0.7). Self reported walking pain at 12 months suggested a marginal long term benefit from higher doses of ESWT (10 cm VAS: WMD −2.0 cm, 95% CI −3.7 to −0.2).

Harms: ESWT without local anaesthetic can be painful.

Comment: All trial participants had recalcitrant heel pain. Availability of ESWT is limited. RCTs and reviews are mainly from German speaking countries. Pain associated with ESWT and differences in procedures mean the single blinding in the first placebo controlled RCT was probably not maintained.[1]

OPTION   **SURGERY**

One systematic review found no RCTs of surgery for heel pain.

Benefits: We found one systematic review (search date 1998).[1] It identified no RCTs of surgery for heel pain.

Harms: We found no evidence.

Comment: One systematic review (search date 1998) identified many observational studies of surgery for chronically painful heels.[1] One of the largest observational studies (n = 76) compared postoperative complication rates after endoscopic fasciotomy versus traditional plantar fasciotomy.[11] It found that serious complications were more common in people treated with endoscopic fasciotomy (35% *v* 17%).

OPTION   **LASERS**

One systematic review of one small RCT found no evidence of benefit with lasers versus placebo.

Benefits: One systematic review (search date 1998) identified one small RCT of laser therapy versus placebo (treatment with a disabled laser) in 32 people with pain of at least 1 months' duration, tenderness to pressure at the origin of the plantar fascia, on the mid-anterior inferior border of the calcaneus and sharp shooting, and/or localised inferior foot pain made worse with activity or on rising in the morning.[1] It found no evidence of a significant effect.

Harms: The RCT[1] reported that 96% of people had no adverse effects and the rest (4%) reported a mild sensation during or after treatment.

Comment: None.

OPTION   ULTRASOUND

One systematic review of one small RCT found no evidence of a significant effect.

Benefits: One systematic review (search date 1998) included one small RCT in 19 people (7 with bilateral heel pain) of eight treatments of true ultrasound versus the same number of applications of placebo (sham ultrasound).[1] Inclusion criteria were pain radiating from the medial tubercle of the calcaneum in response to both pressure and weight bearing first thing in the morning. The trial found no significant effect (WMD 0.1, 95% CI −1.8 to +2.1).

Harms: The trial did not look for harms.

Comment: None.

OPTION   NIGHT SPLINTS

One RCT found no evidence of an effect from wearing night splints.

Benefits: One systematic review found no good quality trials. We found one additional RCT in 116 people with recalcitrant heel pain (people with bilateral presentations of heel pain were excluded).[13] All participants received ankle dorsiflexion exercises and piroxicam 20 mg daily for 30 days, with (n = 54) or without (n = 59) a night splint which dorsiflexed the ankle joint by 5°. The night splint was worn for 3 months. The trial found no evidence of an effect on pain (RR 1.0, 95% CI 0.8 to 1.3).

Harms: The trial did not look for harms.

Comment: The trial excluded people with bilateral disease because of potential inconvenience and poor compliance from wearing two night splints simultaneously.

GLOSSARY

Custom made orthoses Made from polyurethene or similar material to a negative cast of a person's foot.

Heel pads Prefabricated viscoelastic heel pads made of malleable material.

Heel cups Prefabricated rubber heel cups (firmer than viscoelastic heel pads) that extend up the sides of the heel and enclose the fibro fatty heel pad.

Extra corporeal shock wave therapy (ESWT) Shock waves are pulsed acoustic waves that dissipate mechanical energy at the interface of two substances with different acoustic impedance.

REFERENCES

1. Atkins D, Crawford F, Edwards J, et al. A systematic review of treatments for the painful heel. *Rheumatology* 1999;38:968–973. Search date 1998; BIDS database, and hand searches of *The Chiropodist*, *The Journal of British Podiatric Medicine*, and *The Foot* and personal contact with experts.

2. Wolgin M, Cook C, Graham C, et al. Conservative treatment of plantar heel pain: long term follow up. *Foot Ankle Int* 1994;15:97–102.

3. Fadale PD, Wiggins MD. Corticosteroid Injections: their use and abuse. *J Am Acad Orthop Surg* 1994;2:133–140.

4. Acevedo JI, Beskin JL. Complications of plantar fascial rupture associated with steroid injection. *Foot Ankle Int* 1998;19:91–97.

5. Sellman JR. Plantar fascial rupture associated with corticosteroid injection. *Foot Ankle Int* 1994;15: 376–381.

6. Lynch DM, Goforth WP, Martin JE, et al. Conservative treatment of plantar fasciitis. A prospective study. *J Am Podiatr Assoc* 1998;88: 377–380.

7. Crawford F, Atkins D, Young P, et al. Steroid injection for heel pain: evidence of short term effectiveness. A randomised controlled trial. *Rheumatology* 1999;38:974–977.

8. Pfeffer G, Bacchetti P, Deland J, et al. Comparison of custom and prefabricated orthoses in the initial treatment of proximal plantar fasciitis. *Foot Ankle Int* 1999;20:214–221.

9. McCauley WA, Gerace RV, Scilley C. Treatment of accidental digital injection of epinephrine. *Ann Emerg Med* 1991;6:665–668.

10. Speed CA, Nichols DW, Burnett SP, et al Extracorporeal shock wave therapy (ESWT) in plantar fasciitis. A pilot double blind randomised placebo controlled study [abstract]. *Rheumatology* 2000;39 (suppl 123).

11. Krischeck O, Rompe JD, Herbsthrofer B, et al. Symptomatic low-energy shockwave therapy in heel pain and ragiologically detected plantar heel spur [in German]. *Z Orthop* 1998;136:169–174.

12. Kinley S, Frascone S, Calderone D, et al. Endoscopic plantar fasciotomy versus traditional heel spur surgery: a prospective study. *J Foot Ankle Surg* 1993;32:595–603.

13. Probe RA, Baca M, Adams R, et al. Night splint treatment for plantar fasciitis. *Clin Orthop* 1999; 368:191–195.

Fay Crawford
MRC Fellow
University of York
York
UK

Competing interests: None declared.

Updated this issue

Maria Suarez-Almazor and Wednesday Foster

Key Messages

- Systematic reviews of RCTs have found that early intervention with a disease modifying antirheumatic drug (DMARD) improves outcome at one year.

- Most DMARDs have been shown to be more effective than placebo in reducing disease activity and joint inflammation, but the effect of prolonged treatment with DMARDs (for more than a year) has not been adequately evaluated in RCTs.

- Systematic reviews of RCTs have found no evidence of a difference in effectiveness between most DMARDs, although auranofin seems to be the least effective.

- One systematic review and five subsequent RCTs found that some combinations of two or more DMARDs might be beneficial. The long term effects of these combined therapies have not been established.

- Systematic reviews of RCTs have found that low dose oral steroids relieve symptoms and may slow radiological progression. However, long term use carries the risk of serious adverse effects.

- Five RCTs have found that tumour necrosis factor antagonists reduce disease activity and joint inflammation. Short term toxicity was low, but the long term risk is unknown. Optimal dosages and duration of treatment have not been clearly established.

DEFINITION Rheumatoid arthritis is a chronic inflammatory disorder. It is characterised by a chronic polyarthritis affecting primarily the peripheral joints and related periarticular tissues. It usually starts as an insidious symmetric polyarthritis, often with non-specific systemic symptoms. Diagnostic criteria include arthritis lasting longer than 6 weeks, positive rheumatoid factor, and radiological damage.[1]

INCIDENCE/ PREVALENCE Prevalence ranges from 0.5 to 1.5% of the population in industrialised countries.[2,3] Rheumatoid arthritis occurs more frequently in women than men (ratio 2.5 to 1).[2,3] The annual incidence in women was recently estimated at 36/100 000 and in men 14/100 000.[3]

AETIOLOGY/ RISK FACTORS The evidence suggests that the cause is multifactorial in people with genetic susceptibility.[4]

PROGNOSIS The course of rheumatoid arthritis is variable and unpredictable. Some people experience flares and remissions and others a progressive course. Over the years, structural damage may occur, often leading to articular deformities and functional impairment. About half of people will be disabled or unable to work within 10 years.[5] Rheumatoid arthritis shortens life expectancy.[6]

AIMS To relieve symptoms and to prevent or limit disease activity, joint inflammation, joint damage, and disability, with minimum adverse effects.

OUTCOMES Number of swollen or tender joints; pain score; acute phase reactants such as erythrocyte sedimentation rate (ESR); functional status; patient and physician global assessments; radiological progression; and rates of withdrawal from treatment. Many of the RCTs in rheumatoid arthritis use, as some of their primary outcomes, proxy measures such as acute phase reactants and radiological progression. These measures are normally not clinically relevant to people with rheumatoid arthritis. In subsequent editions *Clinical Evidence* will address the issue of including more quality of life measures and measures of function. The American College of Rheumatology (ACR) has established criteria for improvement to be used in clinical trials. ACR20 criteria specify a 20% reduction in swollen and tender joints and 20% improvement in at least three of the following: pain, function, patient and physician global assessments and acute phase reactants. ACR50 and ACR70 use a 50% or 70% improvement in the same parameters. Trials of many new treatments, such as biological agents use these aggregate indices as primary end points.[7] Radiological progression is assessed in many RCTs by reference to standard films. The Larsen score, for instance, provides six grades of severity ranging from normal

(Larsen Grade 0) to mutilating abnormality (Larsen Grade V). However, the question of what constitutes a clinically important change remains unresolved.

METHODS *Clinical Evidence* update search and appraisal May 2000.

QUESTION What are the effects of disease modifying antirheumatic drugs?

OPTION METHOTREXATE

One systematic review of short term RCTs has found that methotrexate is more effective than placebo in reducing joint inflammation and radiological progression, and improving functional status in people with rheumatoid arthritis. Four systematic reviews of RCTs have found no consistent differences between methotrexate and other disease modifying antirheumatic drugs (DMARDs), but observational studies have found that people are more likely to continue therapy with methotrexate than with other DMARDs.

Benefits: **Versus placebo:** We found one systematic review (search date 1997), which identified five placebo controlled RCTs of low dose methotrexate (usually < 20 mg per week) for 12–18 weeks in 161 people.[8] It found a significant improvement in the number of swollen and tender joints, pain score, physician and patient global assessment, and functional status. There was no significant difference in ESR. **Versus other DMARDs:** We found four systematic reviews of comparative RCTs (search dates 1989,[9] 1990,[10] 1988,[11] not specified).[12] These reported no consistent differences between methotrexate and other DMARDs. One systematic review of observational studies comparing the effect of methotrexate versus other DMARDs on radiological progression found a significant benefit from methotrexate only when compared with azathioprine (P = 0.049).[13] No significant difference was observed between methotrexate and parenteral gold (results not quantified). In RCTs, methotrexate was as effective as leflunomide (and better than placebo) in reducing radiological progression (see benefits of leflunomide, p 682).[14]

Harms: In the systematic review of placebo controlled trials, 22% of patients on methotrexate withdrew because of adverse effects (mainly liver enzyme abnormalities) compared with 7% taking placebo (AR for liver abnormalities 11% on methotrexate, 2.6% on placebo; ARI 9%, 95% CI 1.5% to 26%; RRI 347%, 95% CI 60% to 998%; NNH 11, 95% CI 4 to 65).[8] Other common adverse effects were mucocutaneous, gastrointestinal, or haematological. Pulmonary toxicity, hepatic fibrosis, and infections occur occasionally, even at the low dosages usually used in rheumatoid arthritis. Another systematic review found that concurrent administration of folic acid decreased the risk of gastrointestinal and mucocutaneous adverse effects (AR 51% with folic acid, 83% without folic acid; ARR 33%, 95% CI 14% to 51%; NNT 3, 95% CI 2 to 7) with no adverse impact on the efficacy of methotrexate.[15] Although some studies reported an increased risk of tumours, results have not been consistent.

Comment: Observational studies (3 prospective, 1 retrospective) have found that people with rheumatoid arthritis are more likely to continue methotrexate than any other DMARD.[16–19]

| OPTION | ANTIMALARIALS |

One systematic review of RCTs has found that hydroxychloroquine is more effective than placebo in reducing disease activity and joint inflammation in people with rheumatoid arthritis. Older, poorer quality RCTs also found benefit from chloroquine compared with placebo. Two trials provided no evidence of a beneficial effect on functional status and radiological progression. Systematic reviews of RCTs found no evidence of a difference in effectiveness between antimalarials and other DMARDs.

Benefits: **Versus placebo:** We found one systematic review (search date 1997, 4 placebo controlled RCTs of hydroxychloroquine given for 6–12 months, 371 people).[20] The review reported a significant improvement in the number of swollen and tender joints, pain score, physician and patient global assessment, and ESR. One trial measured functional status, and another evaluated radiological progression. No significant differences were observed for these outcomes. **Versus other DMARDs:** We found four systematic reviews of RCTs (search dates 1989,[9] 1990,[10] 1988,[11] not specified.[12] They found no significant differences between antimalarials and other DMARDs. Individual trials failed to show consistent advantage for any one drug, although some reported better results with penicillamine and sulfasalazine than with antimalarials. **Hydroxychloroquine versus chloroquine:** We found no RCTs adequately comparing chloroquine versus hydroxychloroquine; one older trial included both drugs but did not report a direct comparison.

Harms: Antimalarials at currently recommended dosages seem to have limited toxicity. The systematic review, search date 1997, of 4 placebo controlled trials found no difference between groups in the number of withdrawals because of adverse effects.[20] **Ocular toxicity:** No participants discontinued treatment because of ocular adverse effects, and mild toxicity was reported in only one person.[20] One long term retrospective observational study (97 people) found that 6 of 31 people receiving chloroquine alone and 0 of 66 receiving hydroxychloroquine alone developed retinopathy.[21] The optimal frequency for eye examinations has not been reliably established; expert opinion ranges from every 6 months to 2 years. **Non-ocular adverse effects:** The most common are gastrointestinal disturbances, occurring in around 25% of people. Skin reactions and renal abnormalities occasionally occur. Mild neurological abnormalities include non-specific symptoms such as vertigo and blurred vision. Cardiomyopathy and severe neurological disease are extremely rare.

Comment: Older trials of chloroquine compared with placebo (not included in the systematic review because of weak methods) found a beneficial effect. Observational studies (two prospective, one retrospective) found that people with rheumatoid arthritis were more likely to continue on other DMARDs than on antimalarials.[16–18] Most people discontinued treatment because of lack of efficacy. Typical figures for median duration of courses were around 20 months for hydroxychloroquine, 25 months for parenteral gold, and 60 months for methotrexate.[17] One recent RCT found that dose loading for 6 weeks at a higher dose than that usually recommended when initiating treatment with hydroxychloroquine increased the clinical response.[22]

OPTION SULFASALAZINE

One systematic review of RCTs has found that sulfasalazine is more effective than placebo in reducing disease activity and joint inflammation. We found inadequate evidence on its effects on radiological progression and functional status. Six systematic reviews have found no consistent evidence of a difference between sulfasalazine and other DMARDs.

Benefits:
Versus placebo: We found two systematic reviews. The first review (search date 1997, 6 RCTs, 252 people) of sulfasalazine given for 6 months found improvement in the number of tender and swollen joints, pain score, and ESR.[23] Only some trials included global assessments and evaluation of radiological progression, with inconclusive results. None evaluated functional status. The second review (search date 1998, 8 RCTs, 903 people) of sulfasalazine compared with placebo found treatment better than control in all outcome measures used (decrease in number of swollen joints; 51% in the sulfasalazine group v 26% in the placebo group, P < 0.0001).[24] **Versus other DMARDs:** We found six systematic reviews of sulfasalazine compared with other DMARDs. They found no significant differences between sulfasalazine and other DMARDs.[9–12,24] One RCT (60 people) comparing sulfasalazine versus hydroxychloroquine found that sulfasalazine was significantly better in controlling radiological damage, although progression occurred with both drugs (median erosion scores at week 48; hydroxychloroquine 16, sulphasalazine 5, P < 0.02). However, hydroxychloroquine was given at a lower dose than is usually recommended.[25] In one RCT sulfasalazine was as effective as leflunomide and better than placebo in reducing radiological progression.[26]

Harms:
Common adverse effects included gastrointestinal discomfort, rash, and liver enzyme abnormalities.[23] More serious haematological or hepatic toxicity was uncommon. Reversible leucopenia or agranulocytosis was occasionally observed. Treatment was discontinued for adverse effects less often than with other DMARDs, with the exception of antimalarials.

Comment:
Observational studies have reported lower long term efficacy of sulfasalazine compared with other DMARDs such as methotrexate or parenteral gold, with most people who withdrew from treatment doing so because of lack of efficacy.[19]

OPTION PARENTERAL GOLD

Systematic reviews of RCTs have found that parenteral gold is more effective than placebo in reducing disease activity and joint inflammation in people with rheumatoid arthritis, and that parenteral gold slows

radiological progression. We found no evidence on its effect on long term functional status. Systematic reviews provide no evidence of a difference between parenteral gold and other DMARDs.

Benefits: **Versus placebo:** We found one systematic review (search date 1997, 4 placebo controlled RCTs of parenteral gold given for 6 months, 309 people).[27] The review found significant improvement in the number of swollen joints, patient and physician global assessments, and ESR. Functional status was not evaluated. One overview of nine RCTs and one observational study that included radiological assessment found that parenteral gold decreased the rate of radiological progression.[28] **Versus other DMARDs:** We found four systematic reviews of RCTs.[9–12] These reported no consistent differences between parenteral gold and other DMARDs. Parenteral gold was found in some trials to be more effective but also more toxic than its oral counterpart, auranofin. A few trials comparing parenteral gold versus methotrexate found no difference in short term efficacy.

Harms: In the systematic review of four placebo controlled trials (search date 1997) about 30% of people receiving gold discontinued treatment because of adverse effects, including dermatitis, stomatitis, proteinuria, and haematological changes, compared with 15% taking placebo.[27] Life threatening reactions such as aplastic anaemia or nephrotic syndrome are rare.

Comment: Use of parenteral gold is limited mainly by toxicity.

OPTION **AURANOFIN (ORAL GOLD)**

We found limited evidence from systematic reviews of RCTs suggesting that auranofin (oral gold) reduces disease activity and joint inflammation. We found no evidence of its effect on radiological progression or long term functional status. We found limited evidence from direct comparisons suggesting that auranofin is less effective than other DMARDs.

Benefits: **Versus placebo:** We found two systematic reviews (search dates 1989 and 1990), which identified several RCTs. These found that auranofin was superior to placebo.[9,10] **Versus other DMARDs:** Clinical trials comparing auranofin versus other DMARDs such as antimalarials found no consistent differences. However, one systematic review of RCTs (published in 1992) concluded that auranofin was significantly less effective than other DMARDs.[10] Data pooling found auranofin to be less effective than parenteral gold in controlling disease activity.[29] One RCT (200 people) compared auranofin with sulfasalazine over 5 years. The trial found that participants were more than twice as likely to continue with sulfasalazine than auranofin (% participants continuing treatment over 5 years; sulfasalazine 31%, auranofin 15%).[30]

Harms: The major adverse effects of auranofin were diarrhoea and gastrointestinal discomfort.[9,10] Serious adverse effects, such as those associated with parenteral gold, were rare with auranofin (number of participants developing serious organ specific toxicity was < 0.5%; blood 0.2%, renal 0.1%, lung 0.1%, and hepatic 0.4%).[31]

Comment: None.

OPTION	MINOCYCLINE

We found limited evidence from three RCTs suggesting that minocycline is more effective than placebo in controlling disease activity in people with rheumatoid arthritis. We found no evidence of its effect on radiological progression or functional status. It has not been directly compared with other DMARDs.

Benefits:
Versus placebo: We found no systematic review. Three placebo controlled RCTs found that minocycline was superior to placebo in controlling disease activity.[32–34] Different outcomes were reported in the trials: a typical result was that minocycline compared with placebo at least halved the proportion of people who did not improve (AR 3/23 [13%] with minocycline, 11/20 [55%] with placebo; ARR 42%, 95% CI 15% to 52%; RRR 76%, 95% CI 27% to 94%; NNT 2, 95% CI 2 to 7).[34] **Versus other DMARDs:** We found no RCTs.

Harms:
Adverse reactions included nausea (AR at 26 weeks 50% with minocycline, 13% with placebo), dyspepsia, and dizziness (AR 40% with minocycline, 15% with placebo).[32] No serious adverse effects were observed.

Comment:
The magnitude of the beneficial effects of minocycline seems moderate, similar to that observed with antimalarials or sulfasalazine. However, we found no direct comparisons with other DMARDs.

OPTION	PENICILLAMINE

One systematic review of RCTs has found that penicillamine is effective compared with placebo in reducing disease activity and joint inflammation. We found no evidence of its effect on radiological progression or long term functional status. Systematic reviews of RCTs have found no evidence of a difference compared with other DMARDs. Common and potentially serious adverse effects limit its usefulness.

Benefits:
Versus placebo: We found one systematic review (published 1999, 6 placebo controlled RCTs of penicillamine, 683 people).[35] The review found significant improvement in the number of swollen joints and ESR. Only some of the studies evaluated global assessment and functional status, with inconclusive results. **Versus other DMARDs:** We found two systematic reviews of RCTs.[9,10] The second review (search date 1990, 79 RCTs, 6518 people, 22 treatment arms using penicillamine, 583 people completing the trial), an update of the first, found no consistent differences between penicillamine and other drugs, although some trials found it to be superior to antimalarials.[10]

Harms:
Adverse effects were common and sometimes serious. Reactions included mucocutaneous reactions, altered taste, gastrointestinal reactions, proteinuria, haematological effects, myositis, and autoimmune induced disease.

Comment:
The use of penicillamine is limited by the frequency of serious adverse effects. Observational studies found that most people discontinued the drug within the first 2 years of treatment.[16–19]

| **OPTION** | AZATHIOPRINE |

One systematic review of three small RCTs has found that azathioprine is more effective than placebo in reducing disease activity. We found no evidence of its effect on radiological progression or long term functional status. We found no evidence that it is superior to other DMARDs. Toxicity limits its usefulness.

Benefits: **Versus placebo:** We found one systematic review (published in 1999, 3 placebo controlled RCTs of azathioprine, 81 people).[36] The review found a significant benefit in the tender joint score from azathioprine compared with placebo. However, not all trials reported all outcomes, and benefits were observed in only one trial. **Versus other DMARDs:** One RCT found azathioprine to be less effective than methotrexate. No other consistent differences between azathioprine and other DMARDs have been reported.

Harms: Nausea and abnormal liver enzymes were commonly reported adverse effects. Serious haematological adverse reactions included leucopenia, thrombocytopenia, and anaemia. Azathioprine is an immunosuppressive drug and its use has been associated with increased risk of infection and tumours.

Comment: Because of its toxicity profile, azathioprine tends to be reserved for people who have not responded to other DMARDs.

| **OPTION** | CYCLOPHOSPHAMIDE |

One systematic review of three small RCTs has found that cyclophosphamide is more effective than placebo in reducing disease activity and joint inflammation in people with rheumatoid arthritis. It may also reduce the rate of radiological progression, but the evidence we found was limited. We found no evidence of its effect on long term functional status. We found no evidence that it is more effective than other DMARDs. Severe toxicity limits its usefulness.

Benefits: **Versus placebo:** We found one systematic review (search date 1997, 3 placebo controlled RCTs of cyclophosphamide given for 6 months).[37] Pooled data from 70 people found significant reduction in number of tender and swollen joints. One trial reported radiological progression, which appeared to be delayed in the cyclophosphamide group. **Versus other DMARDs:** Only a few RCTs compared cyclophosphamide versus other DMARDs.[9,10] These provide no good evidence of a difference.

Harms: Adverse effects included nausea or vomiting (58%), alopecia (26%), dysuria (26%) and amenorrhoea.[37] Severe reactions included leucopenia, thrombocytopenia, and anaemia. People on cyclophosphamide were at increased risk of infections such as herpes zoster. Prolonged use has been associated with increased risk of cancer.

Comment: Because of its cytotoxic effects, cyclophosphamide is usually reserved for people who have not responded to other DMARDs. Another related drug, chlorambucil, has also been used in people with severe rheumatoid arthritis that is unresponsive to other DMARDs.

| OPTION | CYCLOSPORIN |

One systematic review of three RCTs have found that, compared with methotrexate, cyclosporin reduces disease activity and joint inflammation, improves functional status, and may decrease the rate of radiological progression. Severe toxicity limits its usefulness.

Benefits: **Versus placebo:** We found one systematic review (search date 1997, 3 RCTs of cyclosporin given for a minimum of 4 months, 318 people).[38] The review found significant improvement in the number of tender and swollen joints and in functional status. Radiological progression was also reduced. **Versus other DMARDs:** Only a few trials compared cyclosporin with other DMARDs such as methotrexate, antimalarials, and gold, with no clear evidence of a difference.[39]

Harms: **Renal toxicity:** People given cyclosporin may develop nephropathy, which can be irreversible, and hypertension. **Other adverse reactions:** These included nausea and dyspepsia, hypertrichosis, gingival hyperplasia, and hepatotoxicity. Cyclosporin has been associated with increased risk of infections and tumours.

Comment: Cyclosporin is usually reserved for people with severe disease or those who do not respond to other less toxic DMARDs.

| OPTION | LEFLUNOMIDE |

One RCT found that in people with rheumatoid arthritis, leflunomide compared with placebo reduced disease activity and joint inflammation, improved functional status and health related quality of life, and decreased radiological progression.

Benefits: **Versus placebo:** We found no systematic review but found three RCTs.[14,26,40] The first RCT (402 people with active rheumatoid disease) compared leflunomide (two dosages) to placebo.[40] Leflunomide was significantly more effective than placebo in reducing the number of swollen joints (leflunomide 25 mg or 10 mg –20, placebo –13, $P < 0.05$). The second RCT (358 people) compared leflunomide versus placebo or sulfasalazine.[26] The trial found a significant reduction in the number of swollen joints with leflunomide (44%) versus placebo (21%) ($P < 0.0001$). The third RCT (482 people) compared leflunomide with methotrexate or placebo over 12 months.[14] Twenty per cent improvement (ACR20 criteria) was achieved by 52%, 46%, and 26% respectively in the leflunomide, methotrexate, and placebo groups. ACR50 response criteria were achieved by 34%, 23%, and 8% respectively ($P \leq 0.001$). Radiological progression was also reduced in people receiving leflunomide compared to placebo. Significant improvements in the quality of life of the treated people were also reported.[41] **Versus other DMARDs:** We found no evidence of significant differences between leflunomide and sulfasalazine or methotrexate in controlling disease activity or radiological progression.[14,26]

Harms: In one of the trials, adverse effects included diarrhoea (17% with leflunomide v 5% with placebo) nausea (10% v 7%), rash (10% v 4%), alopecia (8% v 2%), and liver enzyme abnormalities (2% v

0%).[26] Adverse reactions were observed more frequently in the study comparing leflunomide with methotrexate but the rate of serious adverse events was similar for all three groups (methotrexate, leflunomide, and placebo).[14] We found no evidence on long term adverse effects.

Comment: Leflunomide is a new drug, which seems to be as effective as other DMARDs in the short term. Studies of longer duration are required to adequately evaluate the efficacy of leflunomide against that of other drugs.

QUESTION   Which DMARD is the treatment of choice?

We found no good evidence to suggest that one DMARD is more effective than another for initial treatment of rheumatoid arthritis, although auranofin seems to be the least effective. Penicillamine, azathioprine, cyclophosphamide, and cyclosporin are considered too toxic for first line treatment.

Benefits: We found two systematic reviews evaluating placebo controlled RCTs of various different DMARDs. The first review (search date 1988, 33 RCTs, 3409 people) found the efficacy of most drugs to be modest, with overall risk of discontinuing treatment greater for active drug than for placebo.[11] The second review (search date not given, published 1998) found no significant differences between most DMARDs compared with placebo; only methotrexate seemed slightly better for some outcomes such as joint inflammation.[12] We found two systematic reviews comparing the efficacy and toxicity of various DMARDs (search dates 1989[9], 1990[10]; 66 trials with 117 treatment groups). When results were pooled, auranofin was significantly less effective than other drugs, although more effective than placebo. The differences between methotrexate, penicillamine, parenteral gold, and sulfasalazine were not significant. One recent RCT (541 people) compared hydroxychloroquine, parenteral gold, penicillamine, and auranofin over 5 years.[42] No major differences were observed between these drugs. In observational studies, more participants are likely to continue with methotrexate compared to other DMARDs.[16–19]

Harms: Two systematic reviews found that parenteral gold had the highest withdrawal rate because of toxicity, whereas auranofin had the lowest withdrawal rate.[9,10] These three drugs had a lower toxicity profile than others, although methotrexate had more adverse effects than antimalarials or sulfasalazine.

Comment: The method of analysis used in the two systematic reviews of comparative RCTs removed the benefit of randomisation, and the summary results cannot truly be considered as summary measures of RCTs.[9,10] The approach recommended by the Cochrane Collaboration is to conduct various meta-analyses, one for each specific group of comparisons, and to evaluate the effects of each drug within each group. The various interventions can then be compared by examining the magnitude of the effect sizes. Observational studies found that the DMARDs most frequently prescribed as initial treatment were methotrexate, sulfasalazine, and antimalarials.[16–19]

QUESTION What are the effects of combining DMARDs?

One systematic review of RCTs has found that combining certain DMARDs is more effective than using individual drugs alone. However, the evidence remains conflicting, and the balance between benefits and harms varies between combinations.

Benefits:
We found one systematic review[41] and five subsequent RCTs.[43–48] The review (published in 1998, 20 RCTs, 1956 people) concluded that many combinations of DMARDs may be useful. Nine of the RCTs (1240 people) compared methotrexate plus another DMARD versus methotrexate or the other DMARD alone. A wide range of other DMARDs were included. The review found that methotrexate combined with most other DMARDs was more beneficial than treatment with a single drug.[41] Five subsequent RCTs have found that combinations of different agents (antimalarials, sulfasalazine, methotrexate, cyclosporin, and steroids) have a greater beneficial effect than monotherapy.[44–48] Some RCTs included in the systematic review have not found significant differences between combinations of different agents and monotherapy.[43]

Harms:
Toxicity of combination treatments depends on the drugs used. Potential synergistic interactions should also be considered. Combination treatments may be worse than using a single drug because of interactions between drugs.

Comment:
An additional meta-analysis (search date 1992) pooled data from RCTs that compared single versus combination drug treatment.[49] However, the analysis did not provide adequate data on specific combinations. We found no evidence that any one or more DMARD combination therapy is more effective than of the other combination therapies.

QUESTION When should DMARDs be introduced?

We found limited evidence from RCTs suggesting that people with active rheumatoid arthritis should start treatment with DMARDs early in the course of their disease.

Benefits:
We found no systematic review but found four RCTs. One RCT (238 people with recently diagnosed rheumatoid arthritis) compared early treatment with DMARDs (within 1 year of symptom onset) versus delayed treatment.[50] People who received early treatment had significantly better outcomes at 12 months, including improved measures of disability, pain, joint inflammation, and ESR. No differences were observed in radiological progression between the early and delayed groups. A second RCT compared early treatment of auranofin versus early treatment with placebo for 2 years followed by open treatment with DMARDs for a further 3 years. Five year follow up found better outcomes with the active drug. However, this analysis included only 75 of the original 137 people.[51] A third prospective 3 year follow up of 119 people with early disease who participated in a placebo controlled trial of hydroxychloroquine found that a 9 month delay in instituting DMARD treatment had a significant detrimental effect on pain intensity and patient global

well being.[52] A fourth RCT in 38 people with early disease (< 1 year) compared minocycline versus placebo.[53] All participants were given DMARDs at the end of the 3 month study. After 4 years of follow up, eight people who originally received minocycline were in remission compared with one in the placebo group (P = 0.02). The need for DMARDs at 4 years was also reduced in the minocycline group.

Harms: We found no evidence comparing the harms of early versus delayed DMARDs.

Comment: About 10% of people with rheumatoid arthritis experience a short illness that resolves and remains largely quiescent. Early treatment may expose them to adverse effects unnecessarily.

QUESTION   For how long should DMARDs be given?

We found no good evidence about optimum duration of treatment with DMARDs. Few trials have followed people for more than a year, and most people discontinue treatment with an individual drug within a few years because of toxicity or lack of effectiveness.

Benefits: We found one review of 122 studies of DMARDs (including 57 single or double blinded RCTs, 35 open label RCTs, and 19 observational studies) in 16 071 people. The review found that 90% of participants had been followed for 1 year or less.[54] Short term clinical trials in people with rheumatoid arthritis found beneficial effects for most DMARDs, but in the longer term, effectiveness of these drugs seemed to decline. Observational studies have found that after a few years, most people discontinued the prescribed DMARD, either because of toxicity or lack of effectiveness. We found limited evidence suggesting that discontinuing DMARDs, even for people in remission, may result in disease exacerbation or flare. These effects may vary according to the DMARD being discontinued. One RCT comparing gold and methotrexate found that people discontinuing methotrexate because of adverse effects were more likely to relapse than people discontinuing gold (joint counts as % of baseline; gold 30%, methotrexate 70%, P < 0.05).[55] One additional RCT (51 people, 24 weeks follow up) suggests that, for people with early disease and in remission, maintenance on low dose methotrexate (7.5 mg), could be given every second week rather than weekly.[56]

Harms: Serious adverse effects were common, limiting long term usefulness of DMARDs.

Comment: Trials of longer duration may not be feasible because many people will eventually receive a different or additional DMARD, contaminating the original groups.

QUESTION   What are the effects of low dose oral corticosteroids?

Three systematic reviews of RCTs have found benefit from both short and longer term treatment (more than 3 months) with low dose oral corticosteroids. Short term treatment reduces disease activity and joint inflammation. Longer term treatment may reduce radiological progression while treatment continues. However, long term use is associated with considerable adverse effects.

Benefits: **Versus placebo or non-steroidal anti-inflammatory drugs (NSAIDs):** We found two systematic reviews. One review (search date 1997, 10 RCTs, 402 people) compared short term treatment with low dose prednisolone (15 mg/day for several weeks) versus placebo or NSAIDs.[57] The review found that, in the short term, prednisolone had a greater effect than placebo or NSAIDs in controlling disease activity. Prednisolone compared to placebo improved pain, grip strength, and joint tenderness (WMD for the number of tender joints −12, 95% CI −18 to −6). The second review (search date 1998, 7 RCTs, 508 people) evaluated longer term treatment with corticosteroids (for at least 3 months). The review found that moderate term treatment with prednisolone was superior to placebo (WMD for tender joints −0.37, 95% CI −0.59 to −0.14; swollen joints −0.41, 95% CI −0.67 to −0.16; pain −0.43, 95% CI −0.74 to −0.12; and functional status −0.57, 95% CI −0.92 to −0.22). The review also found that prednisolone was comparable to aspirin or chloroquine.[58] One RCT (128 people), included in the review, evaluated radiological damage. The trial found a significant decrease in the rate of progression in people treated with prednisolone 7.5 mg daily compared with placebo over 2 years.[59] One follow up study of people in this trial found that joint destruction resumed after discontinuing prednisolone.[60] **Versus chloroquine:** One systematic review found no significant difference between oral prednisolone and chloroquine in improving disease activity.[58]

Harms: Serious long term adverse effects of corticosteroids include hypertension, diabetes, osteoporosis, infections, gastrointestinal ulcers, obesity, and hirsutism. Observational studies of people with rheumatoid arthritis have suggested that mortality may be increased by long term treatment with steroids.[61] However, many of these studies included people receiving dosages over 7.5 mg, which were higher than those currently recommended. One systematic review found that bone loss was limited when lower dosages were prescribed.[62]

Comment: The decision to give oral corticosteroids should balance the potential for increased comorbidity, which is affected by individual risk factors, and the potential improvement in disease activity.

QUESTION What are the effects of biological agents?

OPTION TUMOUR NECROSIS FACTOR ANTAGONISTS   New

Five RCTs have found that tumour necrosis factor (TNF) antagonists (etanercept and infliximab) reduce disease activity and joint inflammation. Short term toxicity is low, but long term safety is unknown. Optimal dosages and duration of treatment have not been clearly established.

Benefits: **Etanercept:** We found no systematic review. We found two 6 month placebo controlled RCTs. One RCT (234 people who had failed to respond to other DMARDs) compared two doses of etanercept (25 mg and 10 mg) versus placebo.[63] More people improved by at least 20% (ACR20 criteria) with etanercept 25 mg than with the lower dose or with placebo (59% v 51% v 11%: placebo v

10 mg, P < 0.001; placebo v 25 mg, P < 0.001; 10 mg v 25 mg, P = 0.2). Improvement by at least 50% (ACR50 criteria) was found in 40% of people with high dose etanercept, 24% with low dose etanercept, and 5% with placebo (placebo v 10 mg, P < 0.001; placebo v 25 mg, P < 0.001; 10 mg v 25 mg, P = 0.032). The trial also found that etanercept improved functional status (disability index; 25 mg v placebo, P < 0.05) and quality of life (general health status; 25 mg v placebo, P < 0.05). The other trial (89 people with inadequate response to methotrexate) compared etanercept (25 mg) versus placebo.[64] People were allowed to continue methotrexate. More people achieved ACR20 criteria with etanercept (71%) than with placebo (27%) (P < 0.001). **Infliximab:** We found three placebo controlled RCTs. The first RCT (73 people) compared infliximab 1 mg/kg, infliximab 10 mg/kg versus placebo over 4 weeks.[65] More people experienced at least 20% improvement in the 10 mg group (79%) than in the 1 mg group (44%) or in the placebo group (8%) (placebo v 1 mg/kg, P = 0.0083; placebo v 10 mg/kg P < 0.0001). A second RCT (1010 people) compared 1, 3, or 10 mg/kg of infliximab with or without methotrexate versus placebo (ACR 20 improvement; 60% in people taking 3 or 10 mg/kg infliximab v 15% in people taking placebo).[66] A third large multicentre RCT (428 people with active disease not responsive to methotrexate) compared five groups over 7 months: placebo versus infliximab at 3 mg or 10 mg/kg, administered every 4 or 8 weeks.[67] All continued to receive methotrexate. ACR20 criteria were reached by 50–58% receiving infliximab/methotrexate and 20% with the methotrexate/placebo group. ACR50 was attained by 26–31% of the people receiving infliximab and 5% in the placebo group (P < 0.001).

Harms: **Etanercept:** The most common adverse effect was mild injection site reaction: 42–49% in the treated group versus 7–13% in the placebo group. Other adverse effects included upper respiratory symptoms or infections, headache, and diarrhoea. Auto-antibodies to double stranded DNA developed in 5–9% of the treated group. Less than 1% of people developed malignancies or infections within the 6 months of the trials. We found no long term studies. **Infliximab:** In the RCTs common adverse reactions were upper respiratory infections, headache, diarrhoea, and abdominal pain. Reactions during or immediately after the injection (headache, nausea, and urticaria) were also observed in the placebo groups, but were more frequent with infliximab. Antibodies to double stranded DNA were found in about 16% of people taking infliximab. The rates of serious adverse effects in treated and placebo groups were not significantly different, but there was insufficient power to detect clinically important differences.

Comment: Etanercept and infliximab, were administered by injection (twice weekly subcutaneous for etanercept and intravenously every 4 or 8 weeks for infliximab). The effects on disease activity occurred within weeks, unlike other DMARDs which may take several months to act. The optimal dosage and duration of treatment are unclear. We found insufficient evidence to estimate the rates and severity of adverse reactions.

Substantive changes since last issue

Sulfasalazine New systematic review comparing sulfasalazine versus hydrochloroquine found no significant difference in withdrawal rates to lack of efficacy; no change in conclusion.[24]

Auranofin One RCT comparing auranofin with sulfasalazine found that participants were twice as likely to continue therapy with sulfasalazine.[30]

Combination therapy Two additional RCTs show benefit of DMARD combination therapy compared with monotherapy, no change in conclusion.[47,48]

Duration of treatment One additional RCT suggests that, for people with early disease and in remission, the monthly methotrexate dosage could be halved.[56]

REFERENCES

1. Arnett FC, Edworthy SM, Bloch DA, et al. The American Rheumatism Association 1987 revised criteria for the classification of rheumatoid arthritis. *Arthritis Rheum* 1987;31:315–324.
2. Lawrence RC, Helmick CG, Arnett FC, et al. Estimates of the prevalence of arthritis and selected musculoskeletal disorders in the United States. *Arthritis Rheum* 1998;41:778–781.
3. Symmons DP, Barrett EM, Bankhead CR, Scott DG, Silman AJ. The incidence of rheumatoid arthritis in the United Kingdom: results from the Norfolk Arthritis Register. *Br J Rheumatol* 1994; 33:735–739.
4. Winchester R, Dwyer E, Rose S. The genetic basis of rheumatoid arthritis: the shared epitope hypothesis. *Rheum Dis Clin North Am* 1992;18: 761–783.
5. Yelin E, Henke C, Epstein W. The work dynamics of the person with rheumatoid arthritis. *Arthritis Rheum* 1987;30:507–512.
6. Mutru O, Laakso M, Isom ki H, Koota K. Ten year mortality and causes of death in patients with rheumatoid arthritis. *BMJ* 1985;290:1811–1813.
7. Felson DT, Anderson JJ, Boers M, et al. American College of Rheumatology preliminary definition of improvement in rheumatoid arthritis. *Arthritis Rheum* 1995;38:727–735.
8. Suarez-Almazor ME, Belseck E, Shea B, Wells G, Tugwell P. Methotrexate for rheumatoid arthritis. In: The Cochrane Library, Issue 1, 2000. Oxford: Update Software. Search date 1997; primary sources Medline; Embase; Cochrane Controlled Trials Register; and hand search of reference lists.
9. Felson DT, Anderson JJ, Meenan RF. The comparative efficacy and toxicity of second-line drugs in rheumatoid arthritis: results of two meta-analyses. *Arthritis Rheum* 1990;33:1449–1461. Search date 1989; primary sources Medline 1966 to August 1989; hand search of two key journals and reference lists.
10. Felson DT, Anderson JJ, Meenan RF. Use of short-term efficacy/toxicity trade-offs to select second-line drugs in rheumatoid arthritis: a meta-analysis of published clinical trials. *Arthritis Rheum* 1992; 35:1117–1125. Search date 1990; primary sources Medline 1966 to December 1990; hand search of two key journals and reference lists.
11. Gotzsche PC, Podenphant J, Olesen M, Halberg P. Meta-analysis of second-line antirheumatic drugs: sample size bias and uncertain benefit. *J Clin Epidemiol* 1992;45:587–594. Search date 1988; primary source Medline September 1966 to 1988; hand searching of reference lists and drug companies contacted for unpublished trials.
12. Suarez-Almazor ME, Belseck E, Wells G, Shea B, Tugwell P. Meta-analyses of placebo controlled trials of disease-modifying antirheumatic drugs (DMARD) for the treatment of rheumatoid arthritis (RA). *Arthritis Rheum* 1998;41:S153. Search date

not specified; primary sources Medline and Embase.
13. Alarcon GS, Lopez-Mendez A, Walter J, et al. Radiographic evidence of disease progression in methotrexate treated and nonmethotrexate disease modifying antirheumatic drug treated rheumatoid arthritis patients: a meta-analysis. *J Rheumatol* 1992;19:1868–1873. Search date 1991; primary sources Medline 1970 to May 1991. Handsearch of bibliographies and meetings abstract of the American College of Rheumatology 1988–1991.
14. Strand V, Cohen S, Schiff M, et al. Treatment of active rheumatoid arthritis with leflunomide compared with placebo or methotrexate. *Arch Intern Med* 1999;159:2542–2550.
15. Ortiz Z, Shea B, Suarez-Almazor ME, Moher D, Wells GA, Tugwell P. The efficacy of folic acid and folinic acid in reducing methotrexate gastrointestinal toxicity in rheumatoid arthritis: a meta-analysis of randomised controlled clinical trials. *J Rheumatol* 1998;25;36–43. Search date 1996; primary sources Medline 1966 to December 1996; hand search bibliographic references; Current Contents June 1996 to December 1996; and abstracts selected rheumatology meetings and journals.
16. Wolfe F, Hawley DJ, Cathey MA. Termination of slow acting anti-rheumatic therapy in rheumatoid arthritis: a 14 year prospective evaluation of 1017 starts. *J Rheumatol* 1990;17:994–1002.
17. Pincus T, Marcum SB, Callahan LF. Long-term drug therapy for rheumatoid arthritis in seven rheumatology private practices: II. second line drugs and prednisone. *J Rheumatol* 1992;19: 1885–1894.
18. Fries JF, Williams CA, Ramey D, Bloch DA. The relative toxicity of disease-modifying antirheumatic drugs. *Arthritis Rheum* 1993;36:297–306.
19. Suarez-Almazor ME, Soskolne CL, Saunders LD, Russell AS. Use of second-line drugs in the treatment of rheumatoid arthritis in Edmonton, Alberta: patterns of prescription and long-term effectiveness. *J Rheumatol* 1995;22:836–843.
20. Suarez-Almazor ME, Belseck E, Shea B, Homik J, Wells G, Tugwell P. Antimalarials for rheumatoid arthritis. In: The Cochrane Library, Issue 1, 2000. Oxford: Update Software. Search date 1997; primary sources Medline; Embase; Cochrane Controlled Trials Register; and hand search of reference lists.
21. Finbloom DS, Silver K, Newsome DA, Gunke R. Comparison of hydroxychloroquine and chloroquine use and the development of retinal toxicity. *J Rheumatol* 1985;12:692–694.
22. Furst DE, Lindsley H, Baethge B, et al. Dose-loading with hydroxychloroquine improves the rate of response in early, active rheumatoid arthritis: A randomized, double-blind six-week trial with

eighteen-week extension. *Arthritis Rheum* 1999; 42:357–365.

23. Suarez-Almazor ME, Belseck E, Shea B, Wells G, Tugwell P. Sulfasalazine for rheumatoid arthritis. In: The Cochrane Library; Issue 1, 2000. Oxford: Update Software. Search date 1997; primary sources Medline; Embase; Cochrane Controlled Trials Register; and hand search of reference lists.

24. Weinblatt ME, Reda D, Henderson W, et al. Sulfasalazine treatment for rheumatoid arthritis: a metaanalysis of 15 randomized trials. *J Rheumatol* 1999;26:2123–2130. Search date 1998; primary sources Medline 1966 to 1998, Excerpta Medica 1974 to 1998; and Derwent Drug File 1964 to 1998.

25. Van der Heijde DM, van Riel PL, Nuver-Zwart IH, Gribnau FW, van de Putte LB. Effects of hydroxychloroquine and sulphasalazine on progression of joint damage in rheumatoid arthritis. *Lancet* 1989;1:1036–1038.

26. Smolen JS, Kalden JR, Scott, DL, et al. Efficacy and safety of leflunomide compared with placebo and sulphasalazine in active rheumatoid arthritis: A double-blind, randomised, multicentre. Trial. *Lancet* 1999;353:259–266.

27. Clark P, Tugwell P, Bennet K, et al. Injectable gold for rheumatoid arthritis In: The Cochrane Library, Issue 1, 2000. Oxford: Update Software. Search date 1997; primary sources Medline and hand search of reference lists and bibliographies in selected textbooks.

28. Rau R. Does parenteral gold retard radiological progression in rheumatoid arthritis? *Z Rheumatol* 1996;55:307–318.

29. Berkey CS, Anderson JJ, Hoaglin DC. Multiple outcome meta-analysis of clinical trials. *Stat Med* 1996;15:537–557.

30. McEntegart A, Porter D, Capell HA, Thomson EA. Sulfasalazine has a better efficacy/toxicity profile than auranofin — evidence from a 5 year prospective randomized trial. *J Rheumatol* 1996; 23:1887–1890.

31. Singh G, Fieis JF, Williams CA, et al. Toxicity profiles of disease modifying antirheumatic drugs in rheumatoid arthritis. *J Rheumatol* 1991;18: 188–194.

32. Kloppenburg M, Breedveld FC, Terwiel JP, Mallee C, Dijkmans BA. Minocycline in active rheumatoid arthritis: a double-blind, placebo-controlled trial. *Arthritis Rheum* 1994;37:629–636.

33. Tilley BC, Alarcon GS, Heyse SP, et al. Minocycline in rheumatoid arthritis: a 48-week, double-blind, placebo-controlled trial. MIRA trial group. *Ann Intern Med* 1995;122:81–89.

34. O'Dell JR, Haire CE, Palmer W, et al. Treatment of early rheumatoid arthritis with minocycline or placebo: results of a randomized, double-blind, placebo-controlled trial. *Arthritis Rheum* 1997;40: 842–848.

35. Suarez-Almazor ME, Spooner C, Belseck E. Penicillamine for rheumatoid arthritis. In: The Cochrane Library, Issue 1, 2000. Oxford: Update Software. Search date 1998; primary sources Cochrane Musculoskeletal Group's Trials Register; Cochrane Controlled Trials Register; Medline; Embase; and hand searching of reference lists of trials retrieved.

36. Suarez-Almazor ME, Spooner C, Bekseck E. Azathioprine for rheumatoid arthritis. In: The Cochrane Library, Issue 1, 2000. Oxford: Update Software. Search date 1998; primary sources Cochrane Musculoskeletal Group's Trials Register; Cochrane Controlled Trials Register; Medline; Embase; and hand searching of reference lists of trials retrieved.

37. Suarez-Almazor ME, Belseck E, Shea B, Wells G, Tugwell P. Cyclophosphamide for rheumatoid arthritis. In: The Cochrane Library, Issue 1, 2000. Oxford: Update Software. Search date 1997; primary sources Medline; Embase; and hand search of reference lists.

38. Wells G, Haguenauer D, Shea B, Suarez-Almazor ME, Welch VA, Tugwell P. Cyclosporin for rheumatoid arthritis. In: The Cochrane Library, Issue 1, 2000. Oxford: Update Software. Search date 1997; primary sources Medline; hand search of reference lists; consultation with experts.

39. Drosos A.A, Voulgari PV, Papadopoulos IA, Politi EN, and Georgiou PE. Cyclosporin A in the treatment of early rheumatoid arthritis. A prospective, randomized 24-month study. *Clin Exp Rheumatol* 1998;16:695–701.

40. Mladenovic V, Domljan Z, Rozman B, et al. Safety and effectiveness of leflunomide in the treatment of patients with active rheumatoid arthritis. *Arthritis Rheum* 1995;38:1595–1603.

41. Strand V, Tugwell P, Bombardier C, et al. Function and health-related quality of life: results from a randomized controlled trial of leflunomide versus methotrexate or placebo in patients with active rheumatoid arthritis. *Arthritis Rheum* 1999;42: 1870–1878.

42. Jessop JD, O'Sullivan MM, Lewis PA, et al. A long-term five-year randomized controlled trial of hydroxychloroquine, sodium aurothiomalate, auranofin and penicillamine in the treatment of patients with rheumatoid arthritis. *Br J Rheumatol* 1998;37:992–1002.

43. Verhoeven AC, Boers M, Tugwell P. Combination therapy in rheumatoid arthritis: updated systematic review. *Br J Rheumatol* 1998;37:612–619. Search date 1997; primary source Medline, and hand searches of article bibliographies.

44. Van den Borne BE, Landewe RB, Goei HS, et al. Combination therapy in recent onset rheumatoid arthritis: a randomized double blind trial of the addition of low dose cyclosporin to patients treated with low dose chloroquine. *J Rheumatol* 1998;25:1493–1498.

45. Boers M, Verhoeven AC, Markusse HM, et al. Randomised comparison of combined step-down prednisolone, methotrexate and sulphasalazine with sulphasalazine alone in early rheumatoid arthritis. *Lancet* 1997;350:309–318.

46. Mottonen T, Hannonen P, Leirisalo-Repo M, et al. Comparison of combination therapy with single-drug therapy in early rheumatoid arthritis: a randomised trial. FIN-RACo trial group. *Lancet* 1999;353:1568–1573.

47. Calguneri M, Pay S, Caliskaner Z, et al. Combination therapy versus monotherapy for the treatment of patients with rheumatoid arthritis. *Clin Exp Rheumatol* 1999;17:699–704.

48. O'Dell JR, Haire CE, Erikson N, et al. Treatment of rheumatoid arthritis with methotrexate alone, sulfasalazine and hydroxychloroquine, or a combination of all three medications. *N Engl J Med* 1996; 334:1287–1291.

49. Felson DT, Anderson JJ, Meenan RF. The efficacy and toxicity of combination therapy in rheumatoid arthritis: a meta-analysis. *Arthritis Rheum* 1994; 37:1487–1491. Search date 1992; primary sources: Medline; hand searches of five international rheumatology journals; abstracts of rheumatology society meetings.

50. Van Der Heide A, Jacobs JWG, Bijlsma JWJ, et al. The effectiveness of early treatment with 'second-line' antirheumatic drugs: a randomized, controlled trial. *Ann Intern Med* 1996;124:699–707.

51. Egsmose C, Lund B, Borg G, et al. Patients with rheumatoid arthritis benefit from early second line therapy: 5 year follow up of a prospective double

blind placebo controlled study. *J Rheumatol* 1995; 22:2208–2213.

52. Tsakonas E, Fitzgerald AA, Fitzcharles MA, et al. Consequences of delayed therapy with second line agents in rheumatoid arthritis: a 3 year follow up on the hydroxychloroquine in early rheumatoid arthritis (HERA) study. *J Rheumatol* 2000;27: 623–629.

53. O'Dell JR, Paulsen G, Haire CE, et al. Treatment of early seropositive rheumatoid arthritis with minocycline: four-year follow up of a double blind, placebo-controlled trial. *Arthritis Rheum* 1999;42: 1691–1695.

54. Hawley DJ, Wolfe F. Are the results of controlled clinical trials and observational studies of second line therapy in rheumatoid arthritis valid and generalizeable as measures of rheumatoid arthritis outcomes? An analysis of 122 studies. *J Rheumatol* 1991;18:1008–1014.

55. Sander O, Herborn G, Bock E, Rau R. Prospective six year follow up of patients withdrawn from a randomised study comparing parenteral gold salt and methotrexate. *Ann Rheum Dis* 1999;58:281–287.

56. Luis M, Pacheco-Tena C, Cazarin-Barrientos J, et al. Comparison of two schedules for administering oral low-dose methotrexate (weekly versus every-other-week) in patients with rheumatoid arthritis in remission: a twenty-four week, single blind, randomized study. *Arthritis Rheum* 1999;42: 2160–2165.

57. Gotzsche PC, Johansen HK. Meta-analysis of short term low dose prednisolone versus placebo and non-steroidal anti-inflammatory drugs in rheumatoid arthritis. *BMJ* 1998;316:811–818. Search date 1997; primary sources Medline 1966 to Sept 1997; Cochrane Controlled Trials Register searched up to September 1997; and hand search of reference lists.

58. Criswell LA, Saag KG, Sems KM, et al. Moderate-term low dose corticosteroids for rheumatoid arthritis. In: The Cochrane Library, Issue 1, 2000. Oxford: Update Software. Search date 1998; primary sources Medline; and hand search of selected journals.

59. Kirwan JR. Arthritis and Rheumatism Council low dose glucocorticoid study group: the effect of glucocorticoids on joint destruction in rheumatoid arthritis. *N Engl J Med* 1995;333:142–146.

60. Hickling P, Jacoby RK, Kirwan JR, et al. Joint destruction after glucocorticoids are withdrawn in early rheumatoid arthritis. *Br J Rheumatol* 1998; 37:930–936.

61. Wolfe F, Mitchell DM, Sibley JT, et al. The mortality of rheumatoid arthritis. *Arthritis Rheum* 1994;37: 481–494.

62. Verhoeven AC, Boers M. Limited bone loss due to corticosteroids: a systematic review of prospective studies in rheumatoid arthritis and other diseases. *J Rheumatol* 1997;24:1495–1503. Search date 1995; primary source Medline.

63. Moreland LW, Schiff MH, Baumgartner SW, et al. Etanercept therapy in rheumatoid arthritis. A randomized, controlled trial. *Ann Intern Med* 1999;130:478–486.

64. Weinblatt ME, Kremer JM, Bankhurst AD, et al. A trial of etanercept, a recombinant tumor necrosis factor receptor:Fc fusion protein, in patients with rheumatoid arthritis receiving methotrexate. *N Engl J Med* 1999;340:253–259.

65. Elliott MJ, Maini RN, Feldmann M, et al. Randomised double-blind comparison of chimeric monoclonal antibody to tumour necrosis factor alpha (cA2) versus placebo in rheumatoid arthritis. *Lancet* 1994;344:1105–1110.

66. Maini RN, Breedveld FC, Kalden JR, et al. Therapeutic efficacy of multiple intravenous infusions of anti-tumor necrosis factor alpha monoclonal antibody combined with low-dose weekly methotrexate in rheumatoid arthritis. *Arthritis Rheum* 1998;41:1552–1563.

67. Maini RN, St Clair EW, Breedweld F, et al. Infliximab (chimeric anti-tumour necrosis factor alpha monoclonal antibody) versus placebo in rheumatoid arthritis patients receiving concomitant methotrexate: a randomized phase III trial. ATTRACT study group. *Lancet* 1999;354: 1932–1939.

Maria Suarez-Almazor
Associate Professor of Medicine
Baylor College of Medicine
Houston, Texas
USA

Wednesday Foster
Research Health Science Specialist
Veterans Affairs Medical Center and
Baylor College of Medicine
Houston, Texas
USA

Competing interests: The author has been reimbursed by Sanofi-Winthrop, manufacturer of hydroxychloroquine, for attending conferences and as a consultant, and has received research funds from Connetics, manufacturer of auranofin.

Cathy Speed and Brian Hazelman

INTERVENTIONS

Key Messages

- Systematic reviews have emphasised a lack of uniformity of studies, poor methods, and pronounced heterogeneity of study populations and outcome measures.

- Shoulder pain is not a diagnosis. Well designed, double blind RCTs of specific interventions in specific shoulder disorders are needed.

- We found insufficient evidence on the effects of most interventions in people with non-specific shoulder pain.

- One systematic review of two small RCTs and one additional small RCT found that subacromial corticosteroid injections improved range of movement but found no evidence of an effect on pain compared with placebo.

- One small RCT found that, in people with frozen shoulder, distending the glenohumeral joint, in addition to intra-articular corticosteroid injection, may increase range of movement and reduce severity of symptoms.

- We found no evidence that ultrasound for shoulder pain improved pain or quality of life compared with sham treatment.

- One small RCT found limited evidence that extracorporeal shock wave therapy may improve function in calcifying tendinitis.

- Four small RCTs found conflicting evidence on effects of laser treatment in people with shoulder pain.

- One small RCT found limited evidence that intra-articular guanethidine reduced pain more than placebo 8 weeks after treatment.

- One small RCT found limited evidence that high intensity transcutaneous nerve stimulation (TNS) during distension arthrography reduced pain of the procedure compared with low intensity treatment or placebo in people with frozen shoulder.

- We found no evidence on most surgical interventions in shoulder pain. We found limited evidence from one small RCT that forced manipulation and intra-articular corticosteroid injection reduced the number of people with disability due to frozen shoulder at 3 months' follow up compared with intra-articular corticosteroid injection alone.

DEFINITION Shoulder pain arises in or around the shoulder from the gleno-humeral, acromioclavicular, sternoclavicular, "subacromial", and scapulothoracic articulations and surrounding soft tissues. Regardless of the disorder, pain is the reason for most consultations. In adhesive capsulitis (frozen shoulder), pain is associated with pronounced restriction of movement. For most shoulder disorders, diagnosis is based on clinical features, with imaging studies playing a role in some. Non-articular shoulder disorders are the most common, involving rotator cuff, subacromial bursa, joint capsule, glenoid labrum, or ligaments within the shoulder complex.

INCIDENCE/ PREVALENCE Each year in primary care in the UK, about 1% of adults aged over 45 years present with a new episode of shoulder pain.[1] Prevalence is uncertain, with estimates from 4–20%.[2–6] One survey reported a 1 month prevalence of shoulder pain of 34% in a general community sample of 392 people.[7] The age distribution of specific shoulder disorders in the community is unknown. A second community survey (644 elderly people aged over 70) reported a point prevalence of 21%.[8] It was more common in women than men (25% v 17%). Seventy per cent of cases involved the rotator cuff. One survey of 134 people in a community based rheumatology clinic found that 65% of cases were rotator cuff lesions; 11% were caused by localised tenderness in the pericapsular musculature; 10% acromioclavicular joint pain; 3% glenohumeral joint arthritis; and 5% were referred pain from the neck.[9] One survey found that in adults the annual incidence of frozen shoulder was about 2%, with those aged 40–70 years most commonly affected.[10]

AETIOLOGY/ RISK FACTORS Rotator cuff disorders are associated with excessive overloading, instability of the glenohumeral and acromioclavicular joints, muscle imbalance, adverse anatomical features, such as a narrow coracoacromial arch and a hooked acromion, cuff degeneration with ageing, ischaemia, and musculoskeletal diseases that result in attrition of the cuff.[11–14] Risk factors for frozen shoulder include female sex, age, shoulder trauma, and surgery.[10,15] It is associated with diabetes, cardiorespiratory disorders, cerebrovascular events, thyroid disease, and hemiplegia.[10,16] Arthritis of the glenohumeral joint can occur in numerous forms, including primary and secondary osteoarthritis, rheumatoid arthritis, and crystal arthritides.[11]

PROGNOSIS One community survey in an elderly community found that most people with shoulder pain were still affected 3 years after the initial survey.[17] One prospective cohort study of 122 people in primary care found that a quarter of people with shoulder pain reported previous episodes and 49% reported full recovery at 18 months' follow up.[18]

AIMS   To reduce pain and to improve range of movement and function, with minimal adverse effects.

OUTCOMES   Pain scores (overall score, on activity, at night, at rest, during the day, analgesia count); range of movement measures; assessment of overall severity (self assessed or by blinded assessor); functional score; global improvement scores (self assessed or by blinded assessor); tenderness; strength; stiffness; and adverse effects of treatment. The shoulder pain and disability index (SPADI) is a validated, shoulder related pain and disability questionnaire.[19–24] Other validated patient rated disability scores have been developed.[20]

METHODS   *Clinical Evidence* update search and appraisal May 2000.

QUESTION   What are the effects of treatments?

OPTION   SIMPLE ANALGESICS (PARACETAMOL OR OPIATES)

We found no evidence about the effect of analgesics specifically for shoulder disorders.

Benefits: We found no systematic reviews or RCTs of analgesics in shoulder pain.

Harms: We found no evidence.

Comment: None.

OPTION   ORAL NON-STEROIDAL ANTI-INFLAMMATORY DRUGS (NSAIDS)

Two systematic reviews found weak evidence for short term benefits with non-steroidal anti-inflammatory drugs (NSAIDs) in shoulder pain (see acute musculoskeletal syndromes under NSAIDs topic, p 641).

Benefits: **NSAIDs versus placebo:** We found two systematic reviews of NSAIDs in shoulder pain.[25,26] One of the reviews (search date 1995, 4 RCTs, 151 people) compared oral NSAIDs versus placebo in shoulder pain lasting more than 72 hours.[25] Data pooling from two small RCTs (90 people with rotator cuff tendinitis) found no significant effect at 4 weeks for pain measured using a visual analogue scale (WMD 3%, 95% CI –19% to +25%, positive values represent deterioration) and no significant effect on abduction (WMD +26, 95% CI –9 to +61, positive values represent improvement).[27,28] The third RCT found a small improvement in pain and no change in abduction; the final RCT did not allow assessment of pain or abduction. The other systematic review (search date 1993) identified three RCTs, including two trials pooled in the first review.[26] The third RCT (69 people) compared oral NSAIDs versus placebo for 14 days in acute shoulder pain of < 96 hours' duration. NSAIDs were associated with a higher rate of effective pain relief as judged by the investigator (86% of people v 56% with placebo; ARR 30%, 95% CI 10% to 50%).[29]

Harms: One systematic review of NSAIDs in shoulder pain (search date 1993, 5 RCTs, 14 comparative studies) found adverse events reported in 10 studies that involved NSAIDs in shoulder pain. The review noted a wide range in the incidence of adverse events across studies (8–76%). Adverse events were generally mild to moderate. Withdrawal due to adverse events was less than 10% in most studies. However, three trials reported that withdrawal, due to adverse events, was up to 20%. Adverse events were mostly gastrointestinal, skin rash, headache, or dizziness.[26] The review found no evidence that agents differed with respect to the incidence or nature of adverse effects. One RCT (not included in either review, 224 adults with musculoskeletal sprains or tendinitis) compared two NSAIDs and found adverse events in 12–18%, causing 5–7% of people to withdraw.[30] We found no systematic review of the adverse effects of cyclo-oxygenase type II selective agents (see cyclo-oxygenase under NSAIDs topic, p 641).

Comment: The quality of research on the effects of NSAIDs in shoulder disorders is limited by the lack of standardised approaches to research in this field: diverse disorders are considered under the universal term shoulder pain, different types of NSAIDs are used, and outcome measures and follow up periods vary.

OPTION TOPICAL NSAIDS

We found insufficient evidence about the effects of topical NSAIDs specifically in shoulder pain (see topical NSAIDS under NSAIDs topic, p 641).

Benefits: We found no systematic review or RCTs of topical NSAIDs specifically in shoulder disorders.

Harms: We found no systematic review or RCTs of the harms of topical NSAIDs specifically in shoulder disorders.

Comment: None.

OPTION INTRA-ARTICULAR NSAIDS

We found insufficient evidence on the effects of intra-articular injection of NSAIDs in people with shoulder pain.

Benefits: We found no systematic review. One RCT (80 people with acute or subacute rotator cuff tendinitis) found that local injection of NSAIDs was more effective than placebo for pain control, and found no significant difference in active abduction.[3] At 4 weeks, active treatment was associated with greater improvement than placebo in mean pain at rest (visual analogue scale, range not stated, from 4.7 [95% CI 3.8 to 5.6] to 1.7 [95% CI 0.95 to 2.5] v from 4.8 [95% CI 4.1 to 5.6] to 3.2 [95% CI 2.3 to 4.1]; WMD and 95% CI not available), greater improvement in mean pain during active movement (from 7.4 [95% CI 6.9 to 7.8] to 2.4 [95% CI 1.5 to 3.2] v from 7.0 [95% CI 6.5 to 7.5] to 5.0 [95% CI 4.1 to 5.9]), greater improvement in mean active abduction (from 111° [95% CI 98° to 124°] to 142° [95% CI 130° to 153°] v from 116° [95% CI 105° to 128°] to 129° [95% CI 116° to 142°]). Participants were offered further injections at weekly intervals if the assessor felt this was indicated. There were no differences in the total number of injections per group.

Harms: The trial reported episodes of a vagal reaction (2/80 people) and one episode of nausea in the treatment group, and single separate episodes of nausea, hotness, gastric pain, and flu-like symptoms in the placebo group after injection (time interval not stated). There were no withdrawals from the study as a result.[31]

Comment: Eight people did not complete the study (3 in the treatment group, 5 on placebo) and follow up was limited to 4 weeks after the initial injection. The clinical importance of the benefits found in the trial is uncertain.

OPTION	SUBACROMIAL CORTICOSTEROID INJECTIONS

One systematic review found limited evidence of improved range of abduction but no evidence of an effect on pain. One additional RCT found no evidence of an effect on pain or abduction.

Benefits: **Versus placebo:** We found one systematic review (search date 1995), which identified two placebo controlled RCTs of corticosteroid injections for shoulder pain with 4 weeks' follow up.[25] One RCT (50 people with rotator cuff tendinitis) was of subacromial bursa injection (triamcinolone 40 mg) and the other (40 people with rotator cuff tendinitis) was of subacromial and intra-articular injection (2 ml of 0.5% lignocaine plus 1 ml of triamcinolone).[27,28] The review found that abduction improved at 4 weeks (WMD 35°, 95% CI 14° to 55°) but there was no evidence of an effect on pain (WMD 7%, 95% CI −33% to +47%). We found one additional RCT (55 people with rotator cuff tendinitis), which compared subacromial methylprednisolone plus lignocaine versus lignocaine alone. It found no evidence of a significant effect on pain or abduction at 12 weeks (median pain improved by 8 with active treatment v 8 with placebo, visual analogue scale 0–30). Range of abduction did not change from baseline with either active treatment or placebo.[32]

Harms: One RCT in which 20 people with rotator cuff tendinitis received subacromial corticosteroid injections reported no adverse effects apart from mild postinjection discomfort.[27] In another study in which 25 people with rotator cuff tendinitis received subacromial corticosteroid injection and placebo tablets, one person developed mild gastrointestinal upset, one developed pityriasis rosea 2 days after the injection, and one experienced increased frequency of urination. This compared with adverse effects in 3/25 people in the placebo group (subacromial lignocaine and placebo tablets). One person had mild gastrointestinal upset, one had diarrhoea, and one had a vasovagal reaction after the injection.

Comment: Range of movement is not a satisfactory surrogate measure of function.

Shoulder pain

OPTION   INTRA-ARTICULAR CORTICOSTEROID INJECTIONS

Two systematic reviews found no evidence of an effect. We found limited evidence from one small RCT in people with frozen shoulder that distending the glenohumeral joint, in addition to intra-articular steroid injection, may increase range of movement and reduce severity of symptoms.

Benefits: **Versus placebo:** We found two systematic reviews (search dates 1995[25] and 1993[26]), which identified the same two RCTs.[33,34] Both the first RCT (24 people with shoulder pain, 4 week follow up) and the second RCT (30 people with adhesive capsulitis, 24 week follow up) found no benefit in either pain or range of movement. In the first trial, mean pain scores, assessed on a 100 mm visual analogue scale, improved from 39 mm at baseline to 27 mm at week 4 with active treatment, compared with 52 mm at baseline and 22 mm at week 4 with placebo; mean range of shoulder abduction was 86° at baseline and 101° at week 4 with active treatment, compared with 92° and 121° with placebo (no CI available).[33] The second trial assessed pain using a six point rating system, on which 0 was no pain and 5 was extreme pain. Mean pain improved from 3.9 at baseline to 3.2 at 24 weeks with active treatment (n = 15), compared with 4.1 at baseline to 3.0 at 24 weeks with placebo (n = 15).[34] Mean total degrees of shoulder movement improved from 303° at baseline to 351° at 24 weeks with active treatment compared with 300° at baseline to 347° at 24 weeks with placebo (no CI available). **Different doses:** One RCT compared low dose versus higher dose triamcinolone injections in people with adhesive capsulitis (10 mg, 32 people; 40 mg, 25 people). It found the higher dose more effective for relieving pain, movement restriction, and functional impairment.[35] Pain scores improved over 6 weeks (100 mm visual analogue scale) by 31 mm (low dose) compared with 49 mm (high dose); movement restriction improved by 0.7 compared with 1.1; and patient rated functional impairment was reduced by 0.7 compared with 1.3 (four point ordinal scale; no CI available). The trial found no significant difference in sleep disturbance between treatment and control groups (four point ordinal scale, both improved from baseline).[36] **Combined intra-articular and subacromial corticosteroid injections versus placebo:** Two systematic reviews of interventions in shoulder pain[25,26] identified two RCTs (42 people with adhesive capsulitis and 101 people with shoulder pain) of combined intra-articular and subacromial corticosteroid.[35,37] Data could not be pooled because of diversity in study designs. Both found no significant benefit from injections at 6 weeks' follow up (figures not available). **Hydrodistension with corticosteroid versus corticosteroid alone:** We found no systematic review. We found one small RCT in people with frozen shoulder comparing intra-articular corticosteroid alone (8 people) or in combination with hydrodistension (12 people) given weekly for 6 weeks or until symptoms resolved.[38] Hydrodistension involved injection of 19 ml of 0.5% lignocaine. Distension of the glenohumeral joint was confirmed by ultrasound. At 12 weeks, distension of the joint was associated with a significant increase in the number of people with a range of external rotation in the affected shoulder of at least 75%

of that in the opposite shoulder (10/12 with distension, 1/8 with steroid alone; RR for improvement 3.33, 95% CI 1.4 to 3.9; NNT 2, 95% CI 1 to 10). There were also significant improvements in physicians' impression of severity of symptoms (number with light or no symptoms 12/12 with distension v 3/8 with steroid alone; NNT 2, 95% CI 2 to 9) and in the use of analgesics. No significant improvement was found in visual analogue scores of function or pain at rest.

Harms: Intra-articular injections were associated with infection in up to 1 in 14 000–50 000 injections.[39,40] An acute self limited synovitis was reported in up to 2%. Prevalence of tendon rupture, including rupture of the bicipital tendon and rotator cuff, has been reported at less than 1% after local injection.[39] Prevalence of subcutaneous fat necrosis or skin atrophy was estimated at less than 1%. There are reports of corticosteroid arthropathy and osteonecrosis, which are rare (< 0.8%) and seem to affect mostly weight bearing joints.[27] One RCT of corticosteroid injection versus physiotherapy in painful stiff shoulders reported facial flushing in 9/52 (17%) people treated with corticosteroid injections versus 1/56 (2%) treated with physiotherapy, and new menstrual irregularities in 6/52 (12%) people treated with local corticosteroid injections versus none after physiotherapy.[41] Two of the 12 people treated with intra-articular corticosteroid and hydrodistension complained of unacceptable pain after the injection.[38]

Comment: The systematic reviews of interventions in shoulder pain emphasise the lack of adequately designed studies on the subject. One case control study found that clinical outcome correlated with accuracy of injection.[42] Another case control study found that only 10% of intra-articular injections were placed correctly even with experienced operators.[43] Confirmation of injection accuracy can be obtained through fluoroscopy or ultrasound. We found no evidence on the accuracy of placement of subacromial injections. The RCT of hydrodistension included only 20 people with frozen shoulder, but it used specific inclusion criteria (only 26 people with frozen shoulder were recruited out of 120 referred). They were recruited from a hospital rheumatology clinic and may not be representative of people with frozen shoulder in the community. Twenty two people were randomised, but one dropped out of each group. The reported results were not analysed on an intention to treat basis, but they remain significant even when reanalysed in that way. There was no placebo group, and it is not clear whether any effect of distension was dependent on the intra-articular steroid injection.[38] We found no other RCTs of hydrodistension. The possibility of publication and other biases cannot be assessed until the results have been replicated in other studies.

OPTION   ORAL CORTICOSTEROIDS

Two small RCTs found no evidence of an effect from oral corticosteroids.

Benefits: **Versus placebo:** We found no systematic review. One placebo controlled RCT of oral corticosteroids (32 people with frozen shoulder) found no evidence of an effect.[44] Active treatment was associated with a mean pain improvement from 1.4 at baseline to 0.5 at 18 weeks, compared with 1.4 to 0.6 with placebo (four point rating scale, 0 is no pain and 3 is severe), and an improvement in mean range of abduction from 75° at baseline to 154° at 18 weeks, compared with 82° to 153° with placebo (no CI available). Another RCT (40 people with frozen shoulder) of 4 weeks' oral corticosteroid treatment versus no treatment found no benefit at 8 months' follow up in pain and range of motion (no figures available).[45]

Harms: The adverse effect of corticosteroids are well documented (see rheumatoid arthritis, p 674, and asthma, p 828). One RCT (40 people with adhesive capsulitis) reported mild indigestion in two people in the oral corticosteroid group that settled on reducing the dose from 10 mg.[45] No other adverse events were reported. The other RCT did not report adverse events.[44]

Comment: None.

OPTION PHYSIOTHERAPY (MANUAL THERAPY AND EXERCISES)

One small RCT found no evidence of an effect for manual therapy and exercises in shoulder pain.

Benefits: We found two systematic reviews (search dates 1995 and 1993), which identified one small RCT (19 people) of manual therapy and exercises in frozen shoulder.[25,26,35] The RCT compared a particular type of physiotherapy (Maitland mobilisations, 11) versus no treatment. It found no significant difference in shoulder pain between the groups at 3 months (no figures available).

Harms: One RCT of corticosteroid injection versus physiotherapy in people with painful stiff shoulders found adverse events in 56% of the 57 people treated with physiotherapy. These effects lasted longer than two days in 13%.[41] Fever during treatment was found in 1% and local skin irritation in 2%; 4% reported tingling, radiation of pain down the arm, or slight swelling after treatment.

Comment: The quality of research on the effects of physiotherapy in shoulder disorders is limited by the lack of standardised approaches to research in this field: diverse disorders are considered under the universal term shoulder pain, widely diverse forms of physiotherapy are evaluated, and outcome measures and follow up periods vary.

OPTION ULTRASOUND

One systematic review and two subsequent RCTs found no evidence of an effect for ultrasound.

Benefits: We found one systematic review and two subsequent RCTs. The systematic review (search date July 1997, 5 RCTs, 136 people) compared ultrasound versus placebo treatment for shoulder disorders.[46] Follow up was 4–6 weeks. Clinical heterogeneity and insufficient data on outcome measures precluded pooling of results, but none of the individual trials found evidence of a clinically important effect of ultrasound versus placebo. The subsequent RCT involved 180 people with shoulder disorders who had failed to respond to six sessions of exercise therapy.[47] It compared pulsed ultrasound versus dummy ultrasound and bipolar interferential electrotherapy versus dummy electrotherapy in a blinded two by two factorial design. It also included an additional control group that received no active or dummy treatments. Thirty nine people received only pulsed ultrasound and 68 received no active treatment (either no treatment or two dummy treatments). After 6 weeks, ultrasound was not significantly associated with improvement on a seven point Likert scale (improvement occurred in 7/35 [20%] with no treatment, 19/73 [26%] with active ultrasound, 14/72 [19%] with dummy ultrasound; ARR for failure to improve with ultrasound v control treatments 6%, 95% CI –5% to +22%). Follow up at 12 months found no significant effect of ultrasound versus control treatments on proportion reporting substantial improvement in functional status, pain, or range of movement. One additional double blind RCT (63 people, 70 shoulders) found no evidence that ultrasound for shoulder pain improved pain or quality of life scores at 9 months compared with sham treatment. Shoulders, not individuals, were randomised to pulsed ultrasound (frequency 0.89 MHz; intensity 2.5 W/cm^2; pulsed mode 1 : 4) or an indistinguishable sham treatment over the area of calcification. The first 15 treatments were given daily (5 times per week) and the remainder 3 times weekly for 3 weeks. The treating therapist was blinded. Sixty one shoulders completed the study. At 6 weeks, greater decreases were noted in the treatment group in pain (mean change in 15 point pain score: 6.4, 95% CI 5.1 to 7.7 [ultrasound] v 1.6, 95% CI 0.01 to 3.1 [sham]; P < 0.001) in quality of life (mean change in 10 cm quality of life visual analogue scale: 2.6, 95% CI 1.7 to 3.6 [ultrasound] v 0.4, 95% CI 0.6 to 1.4 [sham]; P = 0.002) and in function (mean change in total Constant score—a functional shoulder score 17.8, 95% CI 12.0 to 23.8 [ultrasound] v 3.7, 95% CI –3.3 to +10.7 [sham]; P = 0.002). At 9 months there were no significant differences between the treatment and sham groups for any of the three outcomes of pain (5.7, 95% CI 4.0 to 7.3 [ultrasound] v 4.0, 95% CI 1.8 to 6.2 [sham]; P = 0.23), quality of life (2.4, 95% CI 1.2 to 3.5 [ultrasound] v 1.9, 95% CI 0.8 to 2.9; P = 0.52) or function (mean change in total Constant score: 15.7, 95% CI 8.5 to 22.9 [ultrasound] v 12.4, 95% CI 4.8 to 19.9 [sham]; P = 0.52). Nine people (nine shoulders) did not complete the treatment; three in the ultrasound group and six in the sham group, two in the latter due to pain.[48]

Harms: We found no systematic review and no RCTs specifically addressing adverse effects. The trials described above gave no information on adverse events.

Comment: In most studies, with the exception of the most recent RCT,[48] there was considerable heterogeneity of the groups, interventions, and follow up duration among the RCTs. It is not clear that ultrasound machines were always adequately calibrated before use.

OPTION   **LASER TREATMENT**

We found conflicting evidence from four small RCTs.

Benefits: We found no systematic review. We found four placebo controlled RCTs. One RCT (35 people) found no significant effect of laser treatment at 8 weeks. With active treatment, pain score on a 10 cm visual analogue scale improved by 3.6 cm compared with 1.2 cm with placebo (P = 0.34), and range of movement improved by 36° compared with 29° with placebo (P = 0.23).[49] The second trial (91 people) found that more people recovered at 1 month follow up with laser treatment than with placebo (42/47 v 18/44; mean difference 48%, 95% CI 31% to 65%).[50] The third RCT (20 people with rotator cuff tendinitis) of low level laser treatment versus placebo found less pain at 2 weeks with treatment (mean score difference of 2.5% (95% CI 2% to 3%).[51] The fourth RCT (24 people with supraspinatus tendinitis) of low level laser treatment versus placebo found no significant difference in shoulder pain at 12 weeks' follow up (no figures available).[52]

Harms: We found no evidence on harms.

Comment: As with other interventions, the quality of research on the effects of laser treatment in shoulder disorders is limited by the lack of standardised approaches to research in this field.

OPTION   ELECTROTHERAPY

We found no evidence of a significant effect.

Benefits: We found no systematic review. **Pulsed electromagnetic field treatment versus placebo:** One RCT (29 people with rotator cuff tendinitis) of pulsed electromagnetic field treatment (5–9 hours daily for 4 weeks) versus placebo found no difference in the number recovered at 4 weeks (figures not available).[53] **Bipolar interferential electrotherapy versus ultrasound:** One RCT (see ultrasound, p 698) involved 180 people with shoulder disorders who had failed to respond to six sessions of exercise therapy.[48] It compared pulsed ultrasound versus dummy ultrasound and bipolar interferential electrotherapy versus dummy electrotherapy in a blinded two by two factorial design. At 6 weeks, there was no difference between the groups with respect to the percentage reporting large improvements (20% without electrotherapy or ultrasound, 23% and 22% with active and dummy electrotherapy, 26% and 19% with active and dummy ultrasound).

Harms: We found no evidence on harms.

Comment: As with other interventions, the quality of research on the effects of pulsed electromagnetic field treatment in shoulder disorders is limited by the lack of standardised approaches to research in this field.

OPTION   ICE

We found insufficient evidence on the effects of ice.

Benefits: We found no systematic review or RCTs.

Harms: We found no evidence.

Comment: None.

OPTION INTRA-ARTICULAR GUANETHIDINE

One small RCT of intra-articular guanethidine found significant pain benefit 8 weeks after treatment, but no evidence of an effect on range of abduction.

Benefits: We found no systematic review. One RCT (18 people with resistant shoulder pain) found that intra-articular sympathetic block with guanethidine improved pain over time more than placebo, reaching significance at 8 weeks (P < 0.05; mean reduction in pain 10 cm on a vertical visual analogue scale: 9% *v* 7 % at week 1, 15% *v* 6% at week 4, 36% *v* 16% at week 8).[54] No significant change in range of movement was found. Mean range of abduction was 53° at baseline and 52° at 8 weeks with active treatment compared with 57° and 56° with placebo (no CI available).

Harms: Not reported.

Comment: This single study involved a heterogeneous population, including people with osteoarthritis, frozen shoulder, and rotator cuff tendinitis. The effects of treatment in individual disorders remain uncertain.

OPTION TRANSDERMAL GLYCERYL TRINITRATE

We found insufficient evidence that transdermal glyceryl trinitrate is superior to placebo for pain relief in people with supraspinatus tendinitis.

Benefits: We found no systematic review. One RCT (20 people with supraspinatus tendinitis) of local transdermal glyceryl trinitrate versus placebo found significant decreases in pain scores at 24 hours.[55] Mean pain intensities with active treatment (measured on a 0 to 10 analogue scale) were 7.1 at baseline compared with 4.5 at 24 hours (P < 0.001) and 2.0 at 48 hours (P < 0.001). The trial reported no changes in the placebo group (data not given). Relief was maintained at 15 days follow up (values not reported). Mean duration of pain was also significantly reduced with active treatment (figures not available). Mean mobility (assessor rated four point scale) significantly improved with active treatment (2.0 at baseline *v* 0.1 at 5 days; P < 0.0001) but not with placebo (1.2 at baseline *v* 1.2 at 15 days).

Harms: Headaches were reported in 20% of the treatment group 24 hours after the treatment was started (no comparative figures available).[55]

Comment: The significance figures quoted are not direct comparisons. Significance figures for treatment versus placebo are not stated.

OPTION TRANSCUTANEOUS NERVE STIMULATION

One RCT of transcutaneous nerve stimulation (TNS) during distension arthrography found improved pain relief with high intensity TNS compared with low intensity treatment or placebo.

Benefits: We found no systematic review. One RCT of TNS (60 people with frozen shoulder) compared high intensity TNS versus low intensity treatment or placebo.[56] Pain of the procedure (distension arthrography) was measured using a 0 to 100 mm visual analogue scale. No baseline measures were taken. Mean pain scores after the procedure were 19 (high intensity), 23.5 (low intensity), and 37.5 (placebo); (no CI available). Difference from the control groups was significant (P < 0.001 for high intensity and P < 0.05 for low intensity TNS). No further data were available.

Harms: We found no adverse events reported in RCTs.

Comment: None.

OPTION PHONOPHORESIS

One small RCT found no evidence of an effect of phonophoresis (see glossary, p 703).

Benefits: We found no systematic review. One RCT (24 people: 13 with rotator cuff tendinitis, 1 with tendinitis of the biceps, 1 triceps, and 9 with a knee tendinitis) compared phonophoresis using a coupling medium of dexamethasone, lignocaine, and aqueous gel (5 sessions of treatment lasting 5–10 days) versus placebo.[57] It found no significant difference for perceived pain (measured on 10 cm visual perception scale from 0 no pain to 10 extreme pain). Between sessions 1 and 5, active treatment was associated with a reduction in pain from 2.4 (95% CI 1.5 to 3.3) to 1.3 (95% CI 0.7 to 1.9), compared with placebo (2.6, 95% CI 1.4 to 3.8, to 1.5, 95% CI 0.77 to 2.3). No significant effect was found in punctate tenderness (degree of force [ounces] before pain elicited). With active treatment, this rose from 7.0 (95% CI 5.8 to 8.3) at session 1 to 7.2 (95% CI 6.0 to 8.4) at session 5, compared with 6.9 (95% CI 5.4 to 8.3) to 8.8 (95% CI 7.8 to 9.7) with placebo.

Harms: Adverse effects were not reported.

Comment: None.

OPTION EXTRACORPOREAL SHOCK WAVE THERAPY

Limited evidence from one RCT suggests that extracorporeal shock wave therapy (ESWT) may improve function in calcifying tendinitis.

Benefits: We found no systematic review. We found one RCT with two parts.[58] The first compared three different ESWT regimens (low energy treatment in a single session, a single high energy session, and two high energy sessions 1 week apart) versus placebo in 80 people with calcifying tendinitis. It found that more people experienced subjective improvement of pain after high energy treatment than after less intense treatment (0/20 with placebo, 6/21 with low energy treatment, 12/20 with one high energy session, 14/20 with two high energy sessions; NNT 2 for high energy treatment compared with placebo, 95% CI 1 to 21 for single session and 1 to 14 for two session treatment). A combined measure of pain and function in activities of daily living (the Constant score) showed significant improvement for both high energy groups versus the placebo group (P < 0.0001). The second part compared one versus two high energy sessions in 115 people with calcifying tendinitis (91 followed for 6 months). More people experienced relief of pain with two sessions than with a single session, but the result was not significant (19/42 [45%] with one session v 26/49 [53%] with two sessions; RR of continued pain 0.85, 95% CI 0.50 to 1.23). The difference in Constant scores after 6 months was also not significant.

Harms: High intensity ESWT may be painful during treatment. Small haematomas were reported in the RCT, but the incidence was not stated and they may have been related to subcutaneous infiltration of local anaesthetic before treatment.[58]

Comment: The mechanism of action of ESWT remains unclear. There was radiological disappearance or disintegration of calcium deposits in a significantly greater proportion of people who received high energy treatment than control treatment: 77% of those receiving two sessions of treatment had radiological disappearance or disintegration of calcium deposits after 6 months, compared with 47% who had one session (P = 0.05).

OPTION   SURGERY

We found no evidence on most surgical interventions in shoulder pain. One small RCT found that forced manipulation was more effective in the short term management of frozen shoulder (3 months) than intra-articular injection of corticosteroid, although we found no placebo controlled trials.

Benefits: We found one RCT (30 people with frozen shoulder, 15 in each group).[59] It compared forced manipulation and intra-articular hydrocortisone injection versus intra-articular hydrocortisone injection alone. Manipulation and injection versus injection alone increased the number of people who completely recovered (no disability) at 3 months (7/15 v 2/15; ARI 33%, 95% CI 1% to 65%.[59]

Harms: Adverse effects were not reported.

Comment: There is a need for RCTs of specific surgical interventions in people with specific shoulder disorders.

GLOSSARY

Phonophoresis This is the application of topical medication followed by ultrasound to the same area, the theory being that the ultrasound energy drives the medication through the skin.

Substantive changes since last issue

Ultrasound One additional RCT found no evidence that ultrasound for shoulder pain improved pain or quality of life scores at 9 months compared with sham treatment.[48]

REFERENCES

1. Royal College of General Practitioners; Office of Populations, Censuses and Surveys. Third National Morbidity Survey in General Practice, 1980–1981; Department of Health and Social Security, series MB5 No 1. London; HMSO.

2. Bergunnud H, Lindgarde F, Nilsson B, Petersson CJ. Shoulder pain in middle age. *Clin Orthop* 1988;231:234–238.

3. McCormack RR, Inman RD, Wells A, Bernsten C, Imbus HR. Prevalence of tendinitis and related disorders of the upper extremity in a manufacturing workforce. *J Rheumatol* 1990;17:958–964.

4. Allander E. Prevalence, incidence and remission rates of some common rheumatic diseases or syndromes. *Scand J Rheumatol* 1974;3:145–153.

5. Badley EM, Tennant A. Changing profile of joint disorders with age: findings from a postal survey of the population of Calderdale, West Yorkshire, UK. *Ann Rheum Dis* 1992;51:366–371.

6. Andersson HI, Ejlertsson G, Leden I, Rosenberg C. Chronic pain in a geographically defined general population: studies of differences in age, gender, social class and pain localisation. *Clin J Pain* 1993;9:174–182.

7. Pope DP, Croft PR, Pritchard CM, Macfarlane GJ, Silman AJ. The frequency of restricted range of movement in individuals with self-reported shoulder pain: results from a population-based survey. *Br J Rheumatol* 1996;35:1137–1141.

8. Chard M, Hazleman R, Hazleman BL, King RH, Reiss BB. Shoulder disorders in the elderly: a community survey. *Arthritis Rheum* 1991;34:766–769.

9. Vecchio-P, Kavanagh R, Hazleman BL, King RH. Shoulder pain in a community-based rheumatology clinic. *Br J Rheumatol* 1995;34:440–442.

10. Lundberg B. The frozen shoulder. *Acta Orthop Scand* 1969(suppl 119).

11. Riordan J, Dieppe PA. Arthritis of the glenohumeral joint. In: *The shoulder joint. Baillieres Clin Rheumatol* 1989;3:607–626.

12. Bonutti PM, Hawkins RJ. Rotator cuff disorders. *Baillieres Clin Rheumatol* 1989;3:535–550.

13. Jobe FW, Kvitne RS. Shoulder pain in the overhand or throwing athlete: the relationship of anterior instability and rotator cuff impingement. *Orthop Rev* 1989;18:963–975.

14. Soslowsky LJ, An CH, Johnston SP, Carpenter JE. Geometric and mechanical properties of the coracoacromial ligament and their relationship to rotator cuff disease. *Clin Orthop* 1994;304:10–17.

15. Nash P, Hazleman BL. Frozen shoulder. *Baillieres Clin Rheumatol* 1989;3:551–566.

16. Wohlgethan JR. Frozen shoulder in hyperthyroidism. *Arthritis Rheum* 1987;30:936–939.

17. Vecchio PC, Kavanagh RT, Hazleman BL, King RH. Community survey of shoulder disorders in the elderly to assess the natural history and effects of treatment. *Ann Rheumatol Dis* 1995;54:152–154.

18. Croft P, Pope D, Silman A. The clinical course of shoulder pain: prospective cohort study in primary care. *BMJ* 1996;313:601–602.

19. Roach KE, Budiman-Mak E, Songsiridej N, Lertratanakul Y. Development of a shoulder pain and disability index. *Arthritis Care Res* 1991;4:143–149.

20. Croft P, Pope D, Zonca M, O'Neill T, Silman A. Measurement of shoulder related disability: results of a validation study. *Ann Rheum Dis* 1994;53:525–528.

21. Beaton DE, Richards RR. Measuring function of the shoulder. A cross-sectional comparison of five questionnaires. *J Bone Joint Surg Am* 1996;78;882–890.

22. Gerber C. Integrated scoring systems for the functional assessment of the shoulder. In: Matsen III FA, Fu EH, Hawkins RJ, eds. *The shoulder: a balance of mobility and stability*. Rosemont, Illinois: The American Academy of Orthopaedic Surgeons, 1993:531–550.

23. Richards RR, An KN, Bigliani LU, et al. A standardbased method for the assessment of shoulder function. *J Shoulder Elbow Surg* 1994;3:347–352.

24. L'Insalata JC, Warren RF, Cohen SF, et al. A self-administered questionnaire for assessment of symptoms and function of the shoulder. *J Bone Joint Surg* 1997;79:738–748.

25. Green S, Buchbinder R, Glazier R, Forbes A. Systematic review of randomised controlled trials of interventions for painful shoulder: selection criteria, outcome assessment and efficacy. *BMJ* 1998;316:354–360. Search date 1995; primary sources Medline, Embase, Cinahl, hand searched references, and conference proceedings.

26. Van der Windt DAWM, Van der Heijden GJMG, Scholten RJPM, Koes BW, Bouter, LM. The efficacy of non-steroidal anti-inflammatory drugs (NSAIDs) for shoulder complaints. A systematic review. *J Clin Epidemiol* 1995;48:691–704. Search date 1993; primary sources Medline and hand searched references.

27. Adejabo AO, Nash P, Hazleman BL. A prospective blind dummy placebo controlled study comparing triamcinolone hexacetonide injection with oral diclofenac 50 mg tds in patients with rotator cuff tendinitis. *J Rheumatol* 1990;17:1207–1210.

28. Petri M, Dobrow R, Neiman R, Whiting-O'Keefe Q, Seaman WE. Randomised double blind, placebo controlled study of the treatment of the painful shoulder. *Arthritis Rheum* 1987;30:1040–1045.

29. Mena HR, Lomen PL, Turner LF, et al. Treatment of acute shoulder syndrome with flurbiprofen. *Am J Med* 1986;80:141–144.

30. Auvinet B, Crielaard JM, Manteuffel GE, Muller P. A double-blind comparison of piroxicam fast-dissolving dosage form and diclofenac enteric-coated tablets in the treatment of patients with acute musculoskeletal disorders. *Curr Ther Res Clin Exp* 1995;56:1142–1153.

31. Itzkowitch D, Ginsberg F, Leon M, Bernard V, Appelboom T. Peri-articular injection of tenoxicam for painful shoulders: a double-blind, placebo controlled trial. *Clin Rheumatol* 1996;15:604–609.

32. Vecchio PC, Hazleman BL, King RH. A double-blind trial comparing subacromial methylprednisolone and lignocaine in acute rotator cuff tendinitis. *Br J Rheumatol* 1993;32:743–745.

33. Berry H, Fernandes L, Bloom B, Clarke R, Hamilton E. Clinical study comparing acupuncture, physiotherapy, injection and oral anti-inflammatory therapy in the shoulder. *Curr Med Res Opin* 1980;7:121–126.

34. Rizk T, Pinals R, Talaiver A. Corticosteroid injections in adhesive capsulitis: investigation of their value and site. *Arch Phys Med* 1991;72:20–22.

35. Bulgen D, Binder A, Hazleman B, Dutton J, Roberts S. Frozen shoulder: prospective clinical study with an evaluation of three treatment regimes. *Ann Rheum Dis* 1984;43:353–360.

36. de Jong BA, Dahmen R, Hogeweg JA, Marti RK. Intra-articular triamcinolone acetonide injection in patients with capsulitis of the shoulder: a comparative study of two dose regimens. *Clin Rehabil* 1998;12:211–215.

37. Richardson AT. The painful shoulder. *Proc R Soc Med* 1975;68:11–16.

38. Gam AN, Schydlowsky P, Rossel I, Remvig L, Jensen EM. Treatment of "frozen shoulder" with distension and glucocorticoid compared with glucocorticoid alone. *Scand J Rheumatol* 1998;27:425–430.

39. Gray RG, Gottlieb NL. Intra-articular corticosteroids. An updated assessment. *Clin Orth* 1983;177:235–263.

40. Hollander JL. The use of intra-articular hydrocortisone, its analogues, and its higher esters in arthritis. *Md Med J* 1970;61:511.

41. van der Windt DA, Koes BW, Deville W, Boeke AJP, de Jong BA, Bouter LM. Effectiveness of corticosteroid injections versus physiotherapy for treatment of painful stiff shoulder in primary care: randomised trial. *BMJ* 1998;317:1292–1296.

42. Eustace JA, Brophy DP, Gibney RP, Bresnihan B, FitzGerald O. Comparison of the accuracy of steroid placement with clinical outcome in patients with shoulder symptoms. *Ann Rheum Dis* 1997;56:59–63.

43. Jones A, Regan M, Ledingham J, Patrick M, Manhire A, Doherty M. Importance of placement of intra-articular steroid injections. *BMJ* 1993; 307:1329–1330.

44. Blockey N, Wright J. Oral cortisone therapy in periarthritis of the shoulder. *BMJ* 1954;i:1455–1457.

45. Binder A, Hazleman BL, Parr G, Roberts S. A controlled study of oral prednisolone in frozen shoulder. *Br J Rheum* 1986;25:288–292.

46. van der Windt DAWM, van der Heijden GJMG, van der Berg SGM, ter Riet G, de Winter AF, Bouter LM. Ultrasound therapy for musculoskeletal disorders: a systematic review. *Pain* 1999;81: 257–271. Search date July 1997; primary sources, Medline, Embase, Cochrane Database of Randomised Clinical Trials.

47. van der Heijden GJMG, Leffers P, Wolters PJMC, et al. No effect of bipolar interferential electrotherapy and pulsed ultrasound for soft tissue shoulder disorders: a randomised controlled trial. *Ann Rheum Dis* 1999;58:530–540.

48. Ebenbichler GR, Erdogmus CB, Resch KL, et al. Ultrasound therapy for calcific tendinitis of the shoulder. *N Engl J Med* 1999;340:1533–1588.

49. Vecchio P, Cave C, King V, et al. A double blind study of the effectiveness of low level laser treatment of rotator cuff tendinitis. *Br J Rheumatol* 1993;32:740–742.

50. Gudmundssen J, Vikne J. Laser treatment for epicondylitis humeri and rotator cuff syndrome. *Nord Tidskr Idrettsmed* 1987;2:6–15.

51. England S, Farrell A, Coppock J, Struthers G, Bacon P. Low laser therapy of shoulder tendonitis. *Scand J Rheumatol* 1989;18:427–443.

52. Saunders L. The efficacy of low level laser therapy in supraspinatus tendinitis. *Clin Rehabil* 1995;9: 126–134.

53. Binder A, Parr G, Hazleman B. Pulsed electromagnetic field therapy of persistent rotator cuff tendonitis. *Lancet* 1984;1:695–698.

54. Gado I, Emery P. Intra-articular guanethidine injection for resistant shoulder pain: a preliminary double blind study of a novel approach. *Ann Rheum Dis* 1996;55:199–201.

55. Berrazueta JR, Losada A, Poveda J, et al. Successful treatment of shoulder pain syndrome due to supraspinatus tendinitis with transdermal nitroglycerin. A double blind study. *Pain* 1996;66: 63–67.

56. Nash TP, Williams JD, Machin D. TENS: does the type of stimulus really matter? *Pain Clinic* 1990;3: 161–168.

57. Penderghest CE, Kimura IF, Gulick DT. Double-blind clinical efficacy study of pulsed phonophoresis on perceived pain associated with symptomatic tendinitis. *J Sport Rehab* 1998;7:9–19.

58. Loew M, Daecke W, Kusnierczak D, Rahmanzadeh M, Ewerbeck V. Shock-wave therapy is effective for chronic calcifying tendinitis of the shoulder. *J Bone Joint Surg Br* 1999;81:863–867.

59. Thomas D, Williams R, Smith D. The frozen shoulder. A review of manipulative treatment. *Rheumatol Rehab* 1980;19:173–179.

Cathy Speed
Rheumatologist/Director of Sports and
Exercise Medicine Unit

Brian Hazelman
Senior Consultant

Addenbrooke's Hospital
Cambridge
UK

Competing interests: None declared.

Bell's palsy

Updated this issue

Rodrigo Salinas

QUESTIONS
Effects of medical treatments in adults and children. 707

INTERVENTIONS

Unknown effectiveness

Steroids 707
Antiviral treatment. 708

To be covered in future issues of
Clinical Evidence
Surgery

See glossary, p 708

Key Messages

- One systematic review of RCTs and one subsequent RCT found no good evidence that steroids provide long term benefit compared with placebo.
- One RCT has found limited evidence that prednisone is more effective than aciclovir in improving recovery of facial motor function.
- One RCT has found limited evidence that aciclovir is more effective than placebo in people receiving prednisone.

DEFINITION   Bell's palsy is an acute, unilateral paresis or paralysis of the face in a pattern consistent with peripheral nerve dysfunction, without detectable causes.[1] Additional symptoms may include pain in or behind the ear, numbness in the affected side of the face, hyperacusis, and disturbed taste on the ipsilateral anterior part of the tongue.[2–5]

INCIDENCE/   The incidence is around 23 per 100 000 people per year, or about
PREVALENCE   1 in 60–70 people in a lifetime.[6] Bell's palsy affects men and women more or less equally, with a peak incidence between the ages of 10 and 40 years. It occurs with equal frequency on the right and left sides of the face.[7]

AETIOLOGY/   The cause is unclear. Viral infection, vascular ischaemia, autoim-
RISK FACTORS mune inflammatory disorders, and heredity have been proposed as the underlying causes.[2,8,9] A viral cause has gained popularity since the isolation of the herpes simplex virus-1 genome from facial nerve endoneurial fluid in people with Bell's palsy.[10]

PROGNOSIS   More than two thirds of people with Bell's palsy achieve full spontaneous recovery. The largest series of people with Bell's palsy who received no specific treatment (n = 1011) found the first signs of improvement within 3 weeks of onset in 85% of people.[11] For the other 15%, some improvement occurred 3–6 months later. The same series found that 71% of people recovered normal function of the face, 13% had insignificant sequelae, and the remaining 16% had permanently diminished function, with contracture and synkinesis (see glossary, p 708). These figures are roughly similar to those of other series of people receiving no specific treatment for Bell's palsy.[7,8,12]

AIMS   To maximise recovery of facial function and to reduce the risk of complications, with minimum adverse effects.

OUTCOMES   Grade of recovery of motor function of the face; presence of sequelae (motor synkinesis, autonomic dysfunction, and hemifacial spasm); time to full recovery.

METHODS   *Clinical Evidence* update search and appraisal May 2000. All identified trials were reviewed. Trials used different scoring systems for reporting outcomes.

QUESTION	What are the effects of treatments in adults and children?

OPTION	CORTICOSTEROIDS

A systematic review of RCTs found no significant difference between steroids and placebo either in the proportion of people achieving good recovery of facial motor function, or in the proportion left with permanent complications. One poor quality RCT found that steroids decreased the frequency of motor synkinesis (see glossary, p 708) and autonomic dysfunction.

Benefits: **Versus placebo or no specific treatment:** We found one systematic review (search date 1995, 4 RCTs, n = 390, 180 people given steroids v 210 controls).[13] Two of the trials were of good quality, and we found one subsequent RCT of sufficient quality.[14] The review found that steroids significantly improved the recovery of facial motor function. However, this conclusion was affected by the inclusion of an RCT in which 29% of participants were lost to follow up.[15] If this trial was excluded, the result was no longer significant. Pooled results of the two high quality RCTs (n = 75, both double blind) and one subsequent trial of sufficient quality (n = 42, not blind) found recovery of facial motor function in 46/59 people taking steroids and 46/58 controls (RR 0.97, 95% CI 0.71 to 1.34). They found no significant difference in the time to recovery. **Versus aciclovir:** See antiviral treatment below.

Harms: No serious adverse effects were reported in these trials.

Comment: None.

OPTION	ANTIVIRAL TREATMENT

One RCT found that aciclovir in combination with prednisone was better than placebo in improving recovery of facial motor function.

Benefits: We found no systematic review. **Versus placebo:** We found two RCTs.[16,17] The first enrolled 119 participants, of which 20 people (16%) were lost to follow up, 53 people received aciclovir (400 mg 5 times daily for 10 days), and 46 people received placebo. All participants received prednisone. The proportion of people with good recovery of facial motor function was significantly higher in those receiving the aciclovir and prednisone combination (good recovery AR 49/53 [93%] with aciclovir plus prednisone v 35/46 [76%] with prednisone alone; RR 1.22, 95% CI 1.02 to 1.45; ARR 16%; NNT 6, 95% CI 3 to 50). There was no significant difference in the incidence of sequelae (AR 7/53 [13%] receiving aciclovir and prednisone v 13/46 [28%] with prednisone alone; RR 0.47, 95% CI 0.20 to 1.07).[16] The second trial enrolled 30 people, of whom 14 received prednisone and aciclovir (200 mg 5 times daily for 10 days) and 16 received prednisone alone. All achieved good recovery of facial motor function.[17] **Versus prednisone:** We found one RCT.[18] The trial was not blinded or placebo controlled, and the randomisation technique was not stated. Of the 113 people enrolled, 12 (11%) were lost to follow up, 54 (48%) received aciclovir, and 47 (41%) received prednisone. Prednisone was associated with a significantly higher rate of good facial motor recovery (AR 44/47 [94%] good recovery with prednisone v 42/54 [78%] with aciclovir; RR 1.2, 95% CI 1.03 to 1.41; NNT 6 95% CI 3 to 56).

Harms: No serious adverse effects were reported in these trials.

Comment: The final trial comparing aciclovir versus prednisone was of poor quality and should be interpreted cautiously.[18]

GLOSSARY

Synkinesis Involuntary movement accompanying a voluntary movement.

Substantive changes since last issue

Corticosteroids One additional RCT identified and included; no change in conclusions.[14]

REFERENCES

1. Niparko JK, Mattox DE. Bell's palsy and herpes zoster oticus. In: Johnson RT, Griffin JW, eds. *Current therapy in neurologic disease*. St. Louis: Mosby, 1993:355–361.
2. Burgess LPA, Capt MC, Yim DWS, Lepore ML. Bell's Palsy: the steroid controversy revisited. *Laryngoscope* 1984;94:1472–1476.
3. Knox GW. Treatment controversy in Bell's Palsy. *Arch Otolaryngol Head Neck Surg* 1998;124:821–824.
4. May M, Klein SR, Taylor FH. Idiopathic (Bell's) facial palsy: natural history defies steroid or surgical treatment. *Laryngoscope* 1985;95:406–409.
5. Rowland LP. Treatment of Bell's Palsy. *N Engl J Med* 1972;287:1298–1299.
6. Victor M, Martin J. Disorders of the cranial nerves. In: Isselbacher KJ, et al, eds. *Harrison's principles of internal medicine* 13th ed. New York: McGraw-Hill, 1994:2347–2352.
7. Prescott CAJ. Idiopathic facial nerve palsy. *J Laryngol Otol* 1988;102:403–407.
8. Adour KK. Diagnosis and management of facial paralysis. *N Engl J Med* 1982;307:348–351.
9. Lorber B. Are all diseases infectious? *Ann Intern Med* 1996;125:844–851.
10. Murakami S, Mizobuchi M, Nakashiro Y, et al. Bell Palsy and herpes simplex virus: identification of viral DNA in endoneurial fluid and muscle. *Ann Intern Med* 1996;124:27–30.
11. Peitersen E. The natural history of Bell's palsy. *Am J Otol* 1982;4:107–111.
12. Brown JS. Bell's Palsy: a 5 year review of 174 consecutive cases: an attempted double blind study. *Laryngoscope* 1982;92:1369–1373.
13. Williamson IG, Whelan TR. The clinical problem of Bell's Palsy: is treatment with steroids effective? *Br J Gen Pract* 1996;46:743–747. Search date 1995; primary sources Medline, BIDS, science citation index, and communication with manufacturers and specialists.
14. Ünüvar E, Oduz F, Sidal M, Kilic A. Corticosteroid treatment of childhood Bell's palsy. *Pediatr Neurol* 1999; 21:814–816.
15. Austin JR, Peskind SP, Austin S, Rice DH. Idiopathic facial nerve paralysis: a randomized double blind controlled study of placebo versus prednisone. *Laryngoscope* 1993;103:1326–1333.
16. Adour KK, Ruboyianes JM, Von Doersten PG, et al. Bell's palsy treatment with acyclovir and prednisone alone: a double blind, randomized, controlled trial. *Ann Otol Rhinol Laryngol* 1996; 105:371–378.
17. Ramos-Macias A, De Miguel Martinez I, Martin Sanchez AM, Gomez Gonzalez JI, Martin Galan A. Incorporación del aciclovir en el tratamiento de la parálisis periférica. Un estudio de 45 casos. *Acta Otorrinolaringol Esp* 1992;43:117–120.
18. De Diego JI, Prim MP, De Sarriá MJ, Madero R, Gavilán J. Idiopathic facial paralysis; a randomized, prospective, and controlled study using single-dose prednisone versus acyclovir three times daily. *Laryngoscope* 1998;108:573–575.

Rodrigo Salinas
Ministry of Health
Chile

Competing interests: None declared.

Chronic tension-type headache

New topic

Anish Bahra and Peter Goadsby

INTERVENTIONS

Key Messages

- We found only limited evidence about the treatment of chronic tension-type headache (CTTH).

- Systematic reviews of limited evidence from small, brief RCTs have found that amitriptyline may improve CTTH. It is difficult to interpret older studies that were carried out without standard patient inclusion criteria (International Headache Society criteria).

- We found insufficient evidence about other tricyclic antidepressants and serotonin reuptake inhibitors.

- We found insufficient evidence about any benefits of benzodiazepines to outweigh the harms associated with their regular use.

- A systematic review of observational studies has suggested that regular analgesic medication may lead to a daily headache and reduce the effectiveness of prophylactic medication.

- Small, earlier, mainly poor quality RCTs have found modest improvement with relaxation and electromyographic (EMG) biofeedback therapy in a selective group of patients.

- We found insufficient evidence about the use of cognitive behavioural therapy for CTTH.

DEFINITION	The 1988 International Headache Society criteria for CTTH are headaches on 15 or more days per month (180 days per year) for at least 6 months; pain that is bilateral, pressing or tightening in quality, of mild or moderate intensity, that does not prohibit activities, and that is not aggravated by routine physical activity; presence of no more than one additional clinical feature (nausea, photophobia, or phonophobia); and no vomiting.[1] CTTH is distinguished from the other causes of chronic daily headache (e.g. migraine, analgesic related headache).[2] In contrast to CTTH, episodic tension-type headache can last for 30 minutes to 7 days and occurs for fewer than 180 days per year. Terms based on assumed mechanisms (muscle contraction headache, tension headache) are not operationally defined, and old studies that used these terms may have included people with many different types of headache.
INCIDENCE/ PREVALENCE	The prevalence of chronic daily headache from a survey of the general population in the USA was 4.1%. Half of sufferers met the criteria for CTTH.[3] In a survey of 2500 undergraduate students in the USA, the prevalence of CTTH was 2%.[4] The prevalence of CTTH was 2.5% in a Danish population based survey of 975 individuals.[5]
AETIOLOGY/ RISK FACTORS	Tension-type headache is more prevalent in women.[6] Symptoms begin before the age of 10 years in 15% of people with CTTH. The prevalence declines with age.[7] There is a family history of some form of headache in 40% of people with tension-type headache.[8]
PROGNOSIS	The prevalence of CTTH declines with age.[7]
AIMS	To reduce frequency, severity, and duration of headache, with minimal adverse effects from treatment.
OUTCOMES	Headache frequency, intensity and duration.
METHODS	We searched the Cochrane Library, Medline, and EMBASE from 1966 to August 2000, and performed a hand search of the references in recent books on headache. We reviewed all systematic reviews and RCTs. Unless stated otherwise, we selected studies that used a definition of headache consistent with current International Headache Society criteria,[1] and which excluded patients with concomitant analgesic or other drug misuse. One systematic review of chronic daily headache (a term that includes, but is not limited to, CTTH) was not included.[9]

QUESTION	What are the effects of treatments for chronic tension-type headache?

OPTION	PHARMACOLOGICAL TREATMENTS

Small, short duration RCTs have found benefit from amitriptyline compared with placebo for the treatment of CTTH. We found insufficient evidence on the effects of other types of tricyclic antidepressants, serotonin reuptake inhibitors, or benzodiazepines.

Benefits:	**Tricyclic antidepressants versus placebo:** We found one systematic review[10] (search date 1994, 2 RCTs), a non-systematic review (published in 1997, 4 further RCTs),[11] and two additional RCTs.[12,13] Six of the eight RCTs looked at amitriptyline specifically.

All six had methodological flaws (see additional table on clinicalevidence.org web site).[13–18] Treatment duration ranged from 4 to 32 weeks. Doses of amitriptyline ranged from 10 mg to 150 mg daily. Outcomes used in the trials varied considerably. The two RCTs of highest quality[12,19] found significant improvement in headache duration and frequency with amitriptyline (see table 1, p 716). The other four RCTs showed variable results. All RCTs had methodological problems. **Serotonin reuptake inhibitors versus tricyclic antidepressants or placebo:** We found one RCT, which found no significant benefit from citalopram versus placebo in headache duration, frequency; or severity.[12] It also found amitriptyline improved headache duration, frequency, and severity more than citalopram (see table 1, p 716). **Regular analgesics:** We found no RCTs (see comment below). **Benzodiazepines:** We found no systematic reviews and two RCTs.[20,21] One small RCT (16 people) found that diazepam versus placebo produced modest improvement over 12 weeks.[20] The dose of diazepam was not stated, and International Headache Society criteria were not used. The other RCT (crossover design) compared alprazolam 250 µg three times daily versus placebo over 16 weeks.[21] The trial also found a modest short term improvement.

Harms: **Tricyclic antidepressants:** One RCT found increased rates of dry mouth (54% with amitriptyline 75 mg daily v 17% with placebo, $P < 0.05$), drowsiness (62% v 27%, $P < 0.05$), and weight gain (16% v 0%, NS).[19] Similar results have been found for amitriptyline[12] and other tricyclic antidepressants.[15,22] **Serotonin reuptake inhibitors:** Four of eight people taking fluvoxamine in a cohort study had transient nausea, two complained of anorexia, and three complained of irritability.[22] **Regular analgesics:** We found no RCTs but found one systematic review of 29 observational studies (2612 people).[23] Maintained frequent analgesic use (2–3 times per week) in people with episodic headache was associated with chronic headache and reduced effectiveness of prophylactic treatment. Many, but not all, people improved following withdrawal of the acute relief medication. **Benzodiazepines:** Harms of benzodiazepines found in studies for other indications include increased risk of motor vehicle accidents, falls and fractures, fatal poisonings, depression, dependency, decline in functional status, cognitive decline, confusion, bizarre behaviour, and amnesia.[24]

Comment: Most RCTs were small, short term, and used different outcome measures. Not all studies excluded people taking regular analgesics. The quality of the studies often did not conform to current International Headache Society guidelines. Observational studies are also difficult to interpret. One cohort study found significant benefit from fluvoxamine, but the people recruited were not randomised, and those responding to placebo were excluded before the trial.[22] The available evidence supports the view that prophylactic treatment with amitriptyline is likely to be superior to the habitual use of short term analgesics. It is not clear whether benzodiazepines alone might contribute to the development of a daily headache, but the modest benefit found in the two small RCTs is unlikely to outweigh the risk of dependence with prolonged use.

| OPTION | RELAXATION THERAPY AND ELECTROMYOGRAPHIC BIOFEEDBACK THERAPY |

Small, mainly poor quality RCTs have found modest improvement with relaxation and electromyographic (EMG) biofeedback therapy (see glossary, p 714). People most likely to benefit seem to be younger individuals, women, and those who volunteer for treatment.

Benefits: We found two systematic reviews (published in 1986[25] and 1994[10]) and one subsequent RCT.[4] **Adults:** The first systematic review evaluated 37 small, short term, prospective studies of relaxation and EMG biofeedback therapy in people with CTTH.[25] The review found results from 66 treatment groups. Only a third reported criteria used for diagnosing "tension headache". Three treatments were used: EMG biofeedback training (26 treatment groups), relaxation training (15 groups), and combined EMG biofeedback and relaxation training (9 groups). Two control conditions were used: non-contingent biofeedback (see glossary, p 714) training (6 groups), and headache monitoring (see glossary, p 714) (10 groups). Pooling the results from many studies found that improvement in headache frequency, intensity, and duration varied between the interventions (46% with EMG biofeedback, 45% with relaxation, 57% with both EMG biofeedback and relaxation, 15% with non-contingent biofeedback and −4% with headache monitoring or other control treatments). However, the apparent difference in effectiveness of the different interventions was explained best by differences in the people recruited to the studies rather than by differences in the effectiveness of the interventions or study designs. Outcomes were better in groups with mean age below 35 years, a greater proportion of women, small size, lower withdrawal rates, and when people were asked to enter the study rather than being referred. Half the studies reported follow up data; greater improvement was reported at follow up than immediately after treatment for at least 3–6 months. The second review included 29 EMG biofeedback treatment groups, 38 treated with relaxation therapy (see glossary, p 714), 11 with both, 17 control groups (no treatment), and 28 sham treatment or placebo groups from many small studies. The review found that EMG biofeedback and relaxation therapy alone or in combination were better than no treatment, sham treatments, or placebo. Retrospective analysis found greater improvements in younger people with short duration of headache but no greater improvement with gender, method of recruitment, quality of the study, sample size, diagnostic criteria, or withdrawal rate. The review selected studies that used specified diagnostic criteria, but did not differentiate between episodic tension-type headache or CTTH. Treatment outcome measures were variable. Concomitant analgesic use was not considered. Smaller benefits of treatment were reported in the most recent studies. The subsequent RCT compared six sessions of relaxation plus EMG biofeedback therapy versus three sessions of assessment only in 44 paid undergraduate college students (mean age 19 years, 86% women in both groups, all with International Headache Society defined CTTH).[4] Of the 30 people in the treatment group, 52% had at least a 50% reduction in headache activity (based on headache intensity and indirectly on frequency) compared with

15% of the controls. EMG biofeedback versus control treatment significantly increased the number of headache free days ($P < 0.05$) and non-significantly reduced analgesic consumption ($P = 0.065$).

Harms: We found no reported adverse effects of EMG biofeedback or relaxation therapy.

Comment: Relaxation and biofeedback require additional trained staff and are time consuming. The finding of smaller benefits in recently published studies may reflect publication bias (earlier studies with negative results failing to be published) or possibly because recent studies are less prone to systematic bias.

OPTION COGNITIVE BEHAVIOURAL THERAPY

One systematic review found limited evidence from three small RCTs that cognitive therapy versus no treatment is effective for the treatment of CTTH.

Benefits: **Versus placebo:** We found one systematic review (published in 1994, 3 small RCTs), which found greater improvement with cognitive therapy compared with no treatment, sham treatment, or placebo groups.[10] **Versus another treatment:** Nine additional comparative studies of relaxation and/or EMG biofeedback therapy compared with either cognitive therapy alone (2 studies) or in combination with relaxation or EMG biofeedback therapy (7 studies) found inconclusive results.

Harms: We found no reported adverse effects of cognitive behavioural therapy.

Comment: The studies were small and had as few as five people in a group. The evidence is too limited to define the role of cognitive therapy in CTTH.

GLOSSARY

Electromyographic (EMG) biofeedback Feedback of the amplified EMG signal from forehead and neck muscles through earphones or a loudspeaker to enable people to reduce the amount of muscle contraction.
Non-contingent biofeedback Sounds uncorrelated with muscle activity are played to the person.
Relaxation therapy Includes Jacobson's progressive relaxation exercises, meditation, passive relaxation, and autogenic training.[25]
Headache monitoring People in a study who make daily recordings of headache symptoms without additional therapeutic intervention.

REFERENCES

1. Headache Classification Committee of the International Headache Society. Classification and diagnostic criteria for headache disorders, cranial neuralgias and facial pain. *Cephalalgia* 1988;8:1–96.
2. Silberstein SD, Lipton RB, Sliwinski M. Classification of daily and near-daily headaches: field trial of revised IHS criteria. *Neurology* 1996;47:871–875.
3. Schwartz BS, Stewart WF, Simon D, Lipton RB. Epidemiology of tension-type headache. *JAMA* 1998;279:381–383.
4. Rokicki LA, Holroyd KA, France CR, et al. Change mechanisms associated with combined relaxation/EMG biofeedback training and chronic tension-type headache. *Appl Psychophysiol Biofeedback* 1997;22:21–187.
5. Rasmussen BK, Jensen R, Olesen J. A population-based analysis of the diagnostic criteria of the International Headache Society. *Cephalalgia* 1991;11:129–134.
6. Friedman AP, von Storch TJC, Merritt HH. Migraine and tension headaches: a clinical study of two thousand cases. *Neurology* 1954;4:773–788.

7. Lance JW, Curran DA, Anthony M. Investigations into the mechanism and treatment of chronic headache. Med J Aust 1965;2:909–914.

8. Russell MB, Ostergaard S, Bendtsen L, Olesen J. Familial occurrence of chronic tension-type headache. Cephalalgia 1999;19:207–210.

9. Redillas C, Solomon S. Prophylactic treatment of chronic daily headache. Headache 2000;40:83–102. Search date not given; primary sources Medline 1988 to search date for open studies; Medline 1966 to date for double-blind studies.

10. Bogaards MC, Moniek M, ter Kuile M. Treatment of recurrent tension-type headache: A meta-analytic review. Clin J Pain 1994;10:174–190. Search date 1994; primary sources Compact Cambridge, Psyclit and reference lists of relevant articles.

11. Schoenen J, Wang W. Tension-type headache. In: Goadsby PJ, Silberstein SD, eds. Headache. 1st ed. Newton: Butterworth-Heinemann, 1997:177–200.

12. Bendtsen L, Jensen R, Olesen J. A non-selective (amitriptyline), but not a selective (citalopram), serotonin reuptake inhibitor is effective in the prophylactic treatment of chronic tension-type headache. J Neurol Neurosurg Psychiatry 1996; 61:285–290.

13. Holroyd KA, O'Donnell FJ, Lipchik GL, Cordingley GE, Carlson B. Management of chronic tension-type headache with (tricyclic) antidepressant medication, stress-management therapy and their combination: a randomized controlled trial [abstract]. Cephalalgia 2000;20 (in press).

14. Diamond S, Baltes BJ. Chronic tension headache treated with amitriptyline: A double-blind study. Headache 1971;11:110–116.

15. Fogelholm R, Murros K. Maprotiline in chronic tension headache: a double-blind cross-over study. Headache 1985;25:273–275.

16. Langemark M, Loldrup D, Bech P, Oleson J. Clompramine and mianserin in the treatment of chronic tension headache. A double-blind, controlled study. Headache 1990;30:118–21.

17. Pfaffenrath V, Essen D, Islet H, et al. Amitriptyline versus amitriptyline-N-oxide versus placebo in the treatment of chronic tension-type headache : A multi-centre randomised parallel-group double-blind study. Cephalalgia 1991;11(suppl).

18. Lance JW. Mechanism and Management of Headache. London: Butterworth, 1973.

19. Gobel H, Hamouz V, Hansen C, et al. Chronic tension-type headache: amitriptyline reduces clinical headache-duration and experimental pain sensitivity but does not alter pericranial muscle activity readings. Pain 1994;59:241–249.

20. Paiva T, Nunes JS, Moreira A, et al. Effects of frontalis EMG biofeedback and diazepam in the treatment of tension headache. Headache 1982; 22:216–220.

21. Shukla R, Nag D, Ahuja RC. Alprazolam in chronic tension-type headache. J Assoc Physician India 1996;44:641–644.

22. Manna V, Bolino F, Di Cicco L. Chronic tension-type headache, mood depression and serotonin: therapeutic effects of fluvoxamine and mianserine. Headache 1994;34:44–49.

23. Diener H-C, Tfelt-Hansen P. Headache associated with chronic use of substances. In: Oleson J, Tfelt-Hansen P, Welch KMA, eds. The Headaches. New York: Raven, 1993:721–727.

24. Holbrook AM, Crowther R, Lotter A, et al. The diagnosis and management of insomnia in clinical practice: a practical evidence-based approach. CMAJ 2000;162:216–220.

25. Holroyd KA, Penzien DB. Client variables and the behavioural treatment of recurrent tension headache: A meta-analytic review. J Behav Med 1986;9:515. Search date not stated; primary sources Eric, Medlars, Psycinfo, Psycalert, and hand searches of key journals, book reviews and conference proceedings.

Anish Bahra
Research Fellow
Institute of Neurology
London
UK

Peter Goadsby
Professor of Clinical Neurology
Institute of Neurology
London
UK

Competing interests: None declared.

TABLE 1 RCTs of tricyclic antidepressants versus placebo for the treatment of chronic tension-type headache, including a comparative study with serotonin reuptake inhibitor (see text, p 712).

RCT	Treatment	Number of people	CTTH definition	Analgesic overuse excluded?	Total duration and type of study	Outcome	Effect of drug compared with placebo
19	Amitriptyline 75 mg placebo	2429	*IHS[1]	Yes	6 weeks Parallel group	Mean daily headache duration	At 6 weeks, pain reduced by 3.2 hours per day with amitriptyline v 0.28 hours per day with placebo (P < 0.01)
12	Amitriptyline 75 mg citalopram 20 mg placebo	34	*IHS[1]	Yes	32 weeks total Cross-over	Headache duration and intensity, analgesic intake	Reduced analgesic intake (P = 0.01), and headache duration and frequency (P = 0.002) with amitriptyline; no significant difference in headache intensity. No significant difference in headache duration, frequency, and severity with citalopram.

CTTH, chronic tension-type headache; *IHS, International Headache Society criteria.

Updated this issue

Anthony Marson

INTERVENTIONS

Beneficial

Antiepileptic monotherapy in
  partial epilepsy* 719
Antiepileptic monotherapy in
  generalised epilepsy* 720
Addition of second line drugs for
  drug resistant partial
  epilepsy 721

**Trade off between benefits and
  harms**

Antiepileptic drugs after a single
  seizure 718

**To be covered in future issues of
  *Clinical Evidence***

Treatment of infantile spasms
Treatment of drug resistant
  generalised epilepsy
Temporal lobe surgery and vagus
  nerve stimulation for drug
  resistant epilepsy

* We found no placebo controlled
  RCTs. However, widespread
  consensus holds that these
  drugs are effective.

Key Messages

- RCTs have found that treatment of single seizures reduces the risk of further seizures by about half. However, we found no evidence that treatment alters long term prognosis. Long term antiepileptic drug treatment is potentially harmful.

- We found no placebo controlled trials of the main antiepileptic drugs (carbamazepine, lamotrigine, phenobarbitone, phenytoin, primidone, valproate) in people with newly diagnosed partial or generalised epilepsy. We found no good evidence on which to base a choice between drugs in terms of efficacy. RCTs have found that phenobarbitone and primidone are less well tolerated than other drugs.

- One systematic review of RCTs has found that the addition of second line drugs significantly reduces the seizure frequency in people with partial epilepsy who have not responded to usual treatment. Each additional drug increases the frequency of adverse effects, the need for withdrawal of additional treatment, or both. We found no good evidence from RCTs on which to base a choice between drugs.

- One systematic review of observational studies and one RCT have found that antiepileptic drug withdrawal for people in remission is associated with a higher risk of seizure recurrence than continued treatment. Clinical predictors of relapse after drug withdrawal include age, seizure type, number of antiepileptic drugs being taken, whether seizures have occurred since antiepileptic drugs were started, and the period of remission before drug withdrawal.

DEFINITION   Epilepsy is a group of disorders rather than a single disease. Seizures can be partial (categorised as simple partial, complex partial, and secondary generalised tonic clonic seizures) or generalised (categorised as generalised tonic clonic, absence, myoclonic, tonic, and atonic seizures).[1]

INCIDENCE/   Epilepsy is common, with an estimated prevalence in the developed
PREVALENCE world of 5–10/1000 and an annual incidence of 50/100 000.[2] About 3% of people will be given a diagnosis of epilepsy at some time in their lives.[3]

AETIOLOGY/   Epilepsy can also be classified by cause.[1] Idiopathic generalised
RISK FACTORS epilepsies (such as juvenile myoclonic epilepsy or childhood absence epilepsy) are largely genetic. Symptomatic epilepsies result from a known cerebral abnormality — for example, temporal lobe epilepsy may result from a congenital defect, mesial temporal sclerosis, or a tumour. Cryptogenic epilepsies are those that cannot be classified as idiopathic or symptomatic and in which no causative factor has been identified, but is suspected.

PROGNOSIS   For most people with epilepsy the prognosis is good. About 70% go into remission, defined as being seizure free for 5 years on or off treatment. This leaves 20–30% who develop chronic epilepsy, often treated with multiple antiepileptic drugs.[4] About 60% of untreated people suffer no further seizures in the 2 years after their first seizure.[5]

AIMS   To reduce the risk of subsequent seizures and to improve the prognosis of the seizure disorder; in people in remission, to withdraw antiepileptic drugs without causing seizure recurrence; and to minimise adverse effects of treatment.

OUTCOMES   For treatment after a single seizure: time to subsequent seizures; time to achieve remission; proportion achieving remission. For treatment of newly diagnosed epilepsy: retention on allocated treatment or time to withdrawal of allocated treatment; time to remission; time to first seizure after treatment. For treatment of drug resistant epilepsy: percentage reduction in seizure frequency; proportion of responders (response defined as ≥ 50% in reduction in seizure frequency). For drug withdrawal: time to seizure recurrence.

METHODS   *Clinical Evidence* update search and appraisal May 2000. Three reviews to be published in the next issue of the Cochrane Library will be discussed in the next issue of *Clinical Evidence*.

QUESTION   Should single seizures be treated?

RCTs have found that treatment with antiepileptic drugs reduces the risk of further seizures by about half. However, we found no evidence that treatment alters long term prognosis. Long term antiepileptic drug treatment is potentially harmful.

Benefits: We found no systematic review examining the effects of treatment (see comment below). We found three RCTs, the largest of which compared immediate with no treatment in 419 people (42% women, 28% aged 16 years or under, 65% aged 16–65 years, 6%

aged 60 years or over).[6,7] Participants were randomised within 7 days of their first tonic clonic seizure and were followed for a minimum of 3 years. At 2 years, there were half as many second seizures in the treatment group compared with the control group (HR 0.36, 95% CI 0.24 to 0.53). However, there was no significant difference in the proportion of people achieving a 2 year remission (AR 60% v 68%; RR 0.82, 95% CI 0.64 to 1.03; RR adjusted for time of starting treatment 0.96, 95% CI 0.77 to 1.22).

Harms: The largest RCT gave no information on adverse effects.[6,7] However, these are well known and include idiosyncratic reactions, teratogenesis, and cognitive effects.

Comment: One systematic review of prospective observational studies (search date not given) concluded that, at 2 years from their first seizure, 40% (95% CI 37% to 43%) of people will have had further seizures.[5] The largest RCT was too small to rule out the possibility that treating a first seizure alters the long term prognosis of epilepsy.[6,7]

QUESTION What are the effects of monotherapy in newly diagnosed partial epilepsy?

We found no placebo controlled RCTs of the main antiepileptic drugs (carbamazepine, lamotrigine, phenobarbitone, phenytoin, primidone, valproate) used as monotherapy in people with partial epilepsy. Trials comparing one drug with another have found that phenobarbitone and primidone are less well tolerated than other drugs. With respect to efficacy, we found no evidence on which to base a choice between drugs in partial epilepsy.

Benefits: We found no systematic review. **Versus placebo:** We found no RCTs. **Versus each other:** We found more than 20 RCTs, although many were small and methodologically weak. The two largest RCTs are summarised here. The first randomised 622 people (mean age 41 years, 87% men) to either carbamazepine, phenobarbitone, phenytoin, or primidone.[8] At 36 months, people allocated to primidone did significantly worse for the outcome "retention on allocated treatment" (P < 0.001). When the subgroup of people with predominantly simple and/or complex partial seizures was considered, those allocated to phenobarbitone and primidone did significantly worse for this outcome (P < 0.02). At 3 years, 39% of participants had remained seizure free, and no overall difference was found between groups. For people with predominantly tonic clonic seizures, the proportion remaining seizure free was similar in all treatment groups (43–48%), and no significant differences were found (no P values were quoted). For people with predominantly complex partial seizures, those taking carbamazepine fared significantly better than those taking phenobarbitone or primidone (proportions remaining seizure free 43%, 16%, 15%; P < 0.03). The second RCT randomised 480 people (mean age 47 years, 93% male) to either valproate or carbamazepine.[9] At 12 months, no significant difference was found for the outcome "retention on allocated treatment", with 70–80% of people continuing to take allocated treatment (no P value quoted). People with predominantly complex partial seizures taking carbamazepine did significantly better for the outcome "time to first seizure" ($P < 0.02$). However, the proportion of people remaining seizure free at 12 months did not differ (no P value quoted).

Harms: See above.

Comment: Placebo controlled trials of these drugs would now be considered unethical. People recruited into the two largest comparative trials were predominantly male veterans and were therefore more likely to have epilepsy as a consequence of brain trauma, which may result in a more resistant form of partial epilepsy.

QUESTION   **What are the effects of monotherapy in newly diagnosed generalised epilepsy (generalised tonic clonic seizures with or without other generalised seizure types)?**

We found no placebo controlled trials of the main antiepileptic drugs (carbamazepine, lamotrigine, phenobarbitone, phenytoin, valproate) used as monotherapy in people with generalised epilepsy. Trials comparing one drug with another have failed to find consistent differences between drugs.

Benefits: We found no systematic review. **Versus placebo:** We found no RCTs. **Versus each other:** We found four RCTs of monotherapy, two in adults, and two in children, comparing carbamazepine with valproate.[10–13] One, in 200 adults, found that at 3 years, retention on allocated treatment was more likely with valproate than carbamazepine (RR of a change in treatment 0.34, 95% CI 0.16 to 0.72).[11] Another trial, in 160 children aged 5–16 years, found no difference in retention on allocated treatment (no measure of significance quoted).[13] Both trials found that about 80% of participants achieved remission at 3 years, with no significant difference between groups.[11,13] The other two studies did not present results separately for partial and generalised epilepsy. However, on regression analysis they found no interaction between epilepsy type and drug, for either retention on allocated treatment or time to first seizure.[10,12]

Harms: The overall prevalence of adverse events was similar on the two drugs.[11,13] Rashes occurred more often in people on carbamazepine than on sodium valproate (11.2% v 1.7%, $P < 0.05$)[11] (6.3% v 3.4%, NS),[13] and more people on sodium valproate reported weight gain (12.1% v 1.1%, $P < 0.05$);[11] (10.2% v 3.9%, NS),[13] usually after at least 3 months of treatment. Other adverse events with carbamazepine were dizziness (6.7% v 2.9%, NS);[11] (6.3% v 0.8%, $P < 0.05$),[13] headaches (6.1% v 3.4%), ataxia (2.2% v 0%), somnolence (19.7% v 9.3%, $P < 0.05$), fatigue (10.2% v 5.1%, NS), diplopia (3.9% v 0%, NS), and insomnia (3.9% v 0%, NS).[11,13] Other drug related adverse events with sodium valproate were tremor (5.2% v 1.7%, NS), alopecia (2.9% v 0.6%, NS, 4.2% v 1.6%, NS), and appetite increase (2.3% v 0%, NS; 9.3% v 0%, $P < 0.01$).[11,13] Treatment was withdrawn because of adverse events in 9.3% of people on valproate compared with 17.7% on carbamazepine (18 v 15 people).[11,13]

Comment: None.

QUESTION Does the addition of second line drugs benefit people with drug resistant partial epilepsy?

Four systematic reviews have found that the addition of second line drugs significantly reduces the seizure frequency in people with partial epilepsy who have not responded to usual treatment. Each additional drug increases the frequency of adverse effects, the need for withdrawal of additional treatment, or both. We found no good evidence from RCTs on which to base a choice between these drugs.

Benefits: We found four systematic reviews (search dates 1995, 1998, 1999, and 1999). For gabapentin the systematic reviews identified four RCTs (n = 750 people with drug resistant partial epilepsy), for lamotrigine 10 RCTs (n = 1044), for tiagabine three RCTs (n = 769), for topiramate six RCTs (n = 743), for vigabatrin four RCTs (n = 495), and for zonisamide three RCTs (n = 499).[14–17] These reviews found that the addition of each drug to usual treatment significantly reduced seizure frequency compared with placebo (see table 1, p 723).

Harms: Adverse effects were more frequent with additional treatment compared with placebo (see table 1, p 723).[15,16] Lamotrigine is associated with a rash, which may be avoided by slower titration of the drug. Vigabatrin is associated with concentric visual field abnormalities in about 40% of people, which is probably irreversible.[18]

Comment: Few RCTs have compared these drugs directly with each other. Consensus about the irreversibility of the visual field abnormalities with vigabatrin have meant that few neurologists recommend this drug.

QUESTION Which people are at risk of relapse on withdrawal of drug treatment?

Observational studies have found that nearly a third of people will relapse within 2 years if antiepileptic drugs are withdrawn. Clinical predictors of relapse after drug withdrawal include age, seizure type, number of antiepileptic drugs being taken, whether seizures have occurred since antiepileptic drugs were started, and the period of remission before drug withdrawal.

Benefits: One systematic review of observational studies (search date not specified) found that, at 2 years, 29% (95% CI 24% to 34%) of people in remission from all types of epilepsy would relapse if antiepileptic drugs were withdrawn.[19] We found no systematic review of RCTs. The largest single RCT compared continued antiepileptic treatment with slow antiepileptic drug withdrawal in 1013 people who had been seizure free for at least 2 years.[20,21] At 2 years, 78% of people who continued treatment remained seizure free, compared with 59% in the withdrawal group. Risk reductions with 95% confidence intervals for the main factors predicting recurrence of seizures are given in table 2 (see table 2, p 724).

Harms: Sixteen people died during the trial, 10 in the continued treatment group, and six in the withdrawal group.[20,21] Only two deaths were attributed to epilepsy, and both of these occurred in people randomised to continued treatment.

Comment: There were no significant differences in psychosocial outcomes between groups. People with a seizure recurrence were less likely to be in paid employment at 2 years.[20,21]

REFERENCES

1. Commission on classification and terminology of the international league against epilepsy. Proposal for revised classification of epilepsies and epileptic syndromes. *Epilepsia* 1989;30:389–399.
2. Hauser AW, Annegers JF, Kurland LT. Incidence of epilepsy and unprovoked seizures in Rochester, Minnesota 1935–84. *Epilepsia* 1993;34:453–468.
3. Hauser WA, Kurland LT. The epidemiology of epilepsy in Rochester, Minnesota, 1935 through 1967. *Epilepsia* 1975;16:1–66.
4. Cockerell OC, Johnson AL, Sander JW, Hart YM, Shorvon SD. Remission of epilepsy: results from the national general practice study of epilepsy. *Lancet* 1995;346:140–144.
5. Berg AT, Shinnar S. The risk of seizure recurrence following a first unprovoked seizure: a quantitative review. *Neurology* 1991;41:965–972. Search date not given; primary sources Cumulated Index Medicus and bibliographies of relevant papers.
6. First Seizure Trial Group (FIRST Group). Randomized clinical trial on the efficacy of antiepileptic drugs in reducing the risk of relapse after a first unprovoked tonic clonic seizure. *Neurology* 1993;43:478–483.
7. Musicco M, Beghi E, Solari A, Viani F, for the FIRST group. Treatment of first tonic clonic seizure does not improve the prognosis of epilepsy. *Neurology* 1997;49:991–998.
8. Mattson RH, Cramer JA, Collins JF, et al. Comparison of carbamazepine, phenobarbital, phenytoin, and primidone in partial and secondarily generalized tonic-clonic seizures. *N Engl J Med* 1985;313:145–151.
9. Mattson R, Cramer J, Collins J. A comparison of valproate with carbamazepine for the treatment of complex partial seizures and secondarily generalized tonic clonic seizures in adults: Department of Veterans Affairs epilepsy cooperative study No. 264 group. *N Engl J Med* 1992;327:765–771.
10. Heller AJ, Chesterman P, Crawford P, Chadwick D, Johnson AL, Reynolds EH. Phenobarbitone, phenytoin, or sodium valproate for newly diagnosed epilepsy: a randomized comparative monotherapy trial. *J Neurol Neurosurg Psychiatry* 1995;8:44–50.
11. Richens A, Davidson DL, Cartlidge NE, Easter DJ. A multicentre comparative trial of sodium valproate and carbamazepine in adult onset epilepsy: adult EPITEG collaborative group. *J Neurol Neurosurg Psychiatry* 1994;57:682–687.
12. de Silva M, MacArdle B, McGowan M, et al. Randomised comparative monotherapy trial of phenobarbitone, phenytoin, carbamazepine, or sodium valproate for newly diagnosed childhood epilepsy. *Lancet* 1996;347:709–713.
13. Verity CM, Hosking G, Easter DJ. A multicentre comparative trial of sodium valproate and carbamazepine in paediatric epilepsy: the paediatric EPITEG collaborative group. *Dev Med Child Neurol* 1995;37:97–108.
14. Marson AG, Kadir ZA, Hutton JL, Chadwick DW. The new antiepileptic drugs: a systematic review of their efficacy and tolerability. *Epilepsia* 1997;38:859–880. Search date 1995; primary sources Medline 1966 to December 1995; hand search of key journals, and contacting pharmaceutical companies.
15. Marson AG, Kadir ZA, Hutton JL, Chadwick DW. Gabapentin for drug-resistant partial epilepsy. In: The Cochrane Library, Issue 2, 2000. Oxford: Update Software. Search date 1999; primary sources Cochrane Controlled Trials Register, Cochrane Epilepsy Group Trials Register, and personal contact with Johnson and Johnson, manufacturer of topiramate, and experts in the field.
16. Jette NJ, Marson AG, Kadir ZA, Hutton JL. Topiramate in drug-resistant partial epilepsy. In: The Cochrane Library, Issue 2, 2000. Oxford: Update Software. Search date 1998; primary sources Cochrane Epilepsy Group Trial Register, Cochrane Controlled Trials Register, and personal contact with Parke Davis, manufacturer of gabapentin, and experts in the field.
17. Chadwick DW, Marson AG. Zonisamide for drug-resistant partial epilepsy. In: The Cochrane Library, Issue 2, 2000. Oxford: Update Software. Search date 1999; primary sources Cochrane Controlled Trials Register, Cochrane Epilepsy Group Trials Register, and personal contact with Dainippon and Elan Pharma, manufacturers of zonisamide, and experts in the field.
18. Kalviainen R, Nousiainen I, Mantyjarvi M, et al. Vigabatrin, a gabaergic antiepileptic drug, causes concentric visual field defects. *Neurology* 1999;53:922–926.
19. Berg AT, Shinnar S. Relapse following discontinuation of antiepileptic drugs. *Neurology* 1994;44:601–608. Search date not given; primary sources Index Medicus and bibliographies of relevant papers.
20. Medical Research Council Antiepileptic Drug Withdrawal Study Group. Prognostic index for recurrence of seizures after remission of epilepsy. *BMJ* 1993;306:1374–1378.
21. Medical Research Council Antiepileptic Drug Withdrawal Study Group. Randomised study of antiepileptic drug withdrawal in patients in remission. *Lancet* 1991;337:1175–1180.

Anthony Marson
Lecturer in Neurology
University of Liverpool
Liverpool
UK

Competing interests: The author has been paid for speaking at meetings by Johnson and Johnson, manufacturer of topiramate, and by Janssen Cilag, Sanofi, and Glaxo Wellcome for attending conferences.

TABLE 1 Effects of additional drug treatment in people not responding to usual treatment: results of four systematic reviews (see text, p 721).[14]*, [15-17]

Drug added to usual treatment	Daily dose (mg)	Proportion of people responding (≥ 50% reduction in seizure frequency) % (95% CI)	OR of overall rate of treatment withdrawal (95% CI)‡	OR of significant adverse effects (95% CI)	Comment
Gabapentin	Placebo	9.9 (7.2 to 13.5)	1.36	Dizziness 2.25 (1.28 to 3.98)	4 RCTs. Efficacy increased with increasing dose. No plateauing of therapeutic effect, so doses tested may not have been optimal
	600	14.4 (12.0 to 17.3)	(0.75 to 2.49)	Fatigue 2.25 (1.09 to 4.63)	
	900	17.3 (14.6 to 20.3)		Somnolence 2.04 (1.21 to 3.44)	
	1200	20.6 (17.1 to 24.6)			
	1800	28.5 (21.5 to 36.7)			
Lamotrigine†	200–500	OR versus placebo	1.19	Ataxia 2.98 (1.86 to 4.77)	10 RCTs
		2.32 (1.47 to 3.68)	(0.79 to 1.79)	Diplopia 3.39 (2.05 to 5.61)	
				Dizziness 2.38 (1.63 to 3.48)	
				Nausea 1.70 (1.08 to 2.68)	
Tiagabine	Placebo	6.2 (3.9 to 9.7)	1.81	Dizziness 1.88 (1.18 to 2.99)	3 RCTs
	16	9.8 (4.5 to 20.1)	(1.21 to 2.70)	Tremor 3.17 (1.15 to 8.75)	
	30–32	21.6 (17.7 to 26.0)			
	56	29.8 (19.4 to 42.8)			
Topiramate	Placebo	11.6 (8.0 to 16.6)	2.56	Dizziness 1.99 (1.20 to 3.28)	6 RCTs. There was a clear plateauing of therapeutic effect. Doses above 400 mg showed no significant advantage
	200	26.7 (15.8 to 41.3)	(1.64 to 4.00)	Fatigue 2.52 (1.47 to 4.31)	
	400–1000	45.7 (41.3 to 50.1)		Somnolence 2.86 (1.71 to 4.79)	
				Difficulty thinking 3.95 (1.86 to 8.39)	
Vigabatrin	Placebo	13.8 (9.7 to 19.2)	2.58	No adverse effects were significantly more frequent with vigabatrin, however 40% of patients treated with vigabatrin develop concentric visual field abnormalities.[18]	4 RCTs
	1000 or 2000	22.8 (14.5 to 34.0)	(1.26 to 5.27)		
	3000 or 6000	45.9 (39.5 to 52.5)			
Zonisamide	400 mg	OR versus placebo	1.74	Ataxia 3.94 (1.23 to 12.57)	3 RCTs
		2.72 (1.74 to 4.25)	(1.03 to 2.95)	Somnolence 2.11 (1.11 to 3.98)	
				Agitation 2.43 (1.04 to 5.66)	
				Anorexia 2.98 (1.3 to 6.42)	

*Results were generated from regression models rather than from multiple subgroup analyses.
†Lamotrigine has been evaluated in several crossover trials and one parallel group trial. As a result we were unable to investigate the effects of different lamotrigine doses in regression models.
‡OR of overall treatment withdrawal of usual treatment plus active drug versus usual treatment plus placebo.

TABLE 2 Relative risks of seizure recurrence within 2 years of treatment withdrawal, according to prognostic variable (see text, p 721).[20,21]

Prognostic variable	RR (95% CI) of seizure recurrence within 2 years
Age < 16 years	1.75 (1.30 to 2.36)
Tonic clonic seizures	1.56 (1.09 to 2.22)
Myoclonus	1.84 (1.12 to 3.02)
Treatment with more than one antiepileptic drug	1.85 (1.38 to 2.40)
Seizures since antiepileptic drugs were started	1.56 (1.18 to 2.05)
Any electroencephalographic abnormality	1.32 (1.00 to 1.75)

Risk of recurrence also declined as the seizure free period increased, but in a complex manner.

Updated this issue

Helen Ford and Mike Boggild

INTERVENTIONS

Key Messages

Relapse rates and disability

- We found no evidence that any treatment alters long term outcome in multiple sclerosis (MS).

- Large RCTs in people with active relapsing and remitting MS have found that interferon beta-1a/b reduces relapse rates by a third and may delay development of neurological disability.

- One RCT in people with secondary progressive MS found that interferon beta-1b delayed development of disability by 9–12 months.

- One systematic review of RCTs has found that azathioprine has a modest effect on relapse rates.

- Evidence from single RCTs suggests modest benefit from glatiramer acetate, intravenous immunoglobulin (Ig), and methotrexate.

- Limited evidence from small RCTs suggests that pulsed intravenous mitoxantrone improves outcome in people with very active MS, in whom the risk of severe neurological disability may outweigh the risks of cytotoxic treatment.

© *Clinical Evidence* 2000;4:725–736.

- We found insufficient evidence about the effects of plasma exchange on neurological disability.
- We found no evidence about the effects of corticosteroids on long term outcome.

Fatigue

- One short term RCT found that amantadine modestly reduced MS related fatigue. It found no evidence of a benefit from pemoline.
- We found insufficient evidence on the effects of behavioural modification therapy or exercise in people with MS related fatigue.

Spasticity

- Two RCTs have found that tizanidine reduces spasticity in people with MS.
- We found insufficient evidence on the effects of other oral drug treatments or of physical therapy in people with MS related spasticity.
- One small RCT found benefit from intrathecal baclofen in non-ambulant patients with symptomatic spasticity resistant to oral drug treatment.

Multidisciplinary care

- Limited evidence from two RCTs suggests that 3–4 weeks of inpatient rehabilitation results in short term improvements in disability, despite no evidence of an effect on neurological impairment. The duration of this effect is uncertain.
- One small RCT found that prolonged outpatient rehabilitation reduced MS symptom frequency and fatigue.

DEFINITION MS is a chronic inflammatory disease of the central nervous system. Diagnosis requires evidence of lesions that are separated in both time and space and the exclusion of other inflammatory, structural, or hereditary conditions that might give a similar clinical picture. The disease takes three main forms: relapsing and remitting MS, characterised by episodes of neurological dysfunction interspersed with periods of stability; primary progressive MS, where progressive neurological disability occurs from the outset; and secondary progressive MS, where progressive neurological disability occurs later in the course of the disease.

INCIDENCE/ PREVALENCE Prevalence varies with geography and racial group; it is highest in white populations in temperate regions.[1] In Europe and North America, prevalence is 1 in 800 people, with an annual incidence of 2–10 per 100 000, making MS the most common cause of neurological disability in young adults. Age of onset is broad, peaking between 20 and 40 years.[2]

AETIOLOGY/ RISK FACTORS The cause remains unclear, although current evidence suggests that MS is an autoimmune disorder of the central nervous system resulting from an environmental stimulus in genetically susceptible individuals. MS is currently regarded as a single disorder with clinical variants, but there is some evidence that it may comprise several related disorders with distinct immunological, pathological, and genetic features.[1,3]

PROGNOSIS In 90% of people, early disease is relapsing and remitting. Although some people follow a relatively benign course over many years, most develop secondary progressive disease, usually 6–10 years after onset. In 10% of people, initial disease is primary progressive.

Apart from a minority of people with "aggressive" MS, life expectancy is not greatly affected, and the disease course is often of more than 30 years' duration.

AIMS	To prevent or delay disability; to improve function; to alleviate symptoms of spasticity; to prevent complications (contractures, pressure sores); to optimise quality of life.

OUTCOMES Neurological disability, spasticity, fatigue, general health, relapse rate, quality of life. **Neurological disability:** In clinical trials, disability in MS is usually measured using the disease specific expanded disability status scale (EDSS), which ranges from 0 (no disability) to 10 (death from MS) in half point increments.[4] Lower scores (0–4) reflect specific neurological impairments and disability; higher scores reflect reducing levels of mobility (4–7) and upper limb and bulbar function (7–9.5). The scale is non-linear and has been criticised for indicating change poorly, for emphasising neurological examination and mobility, and for failing to reflect other disabilities (such as fatigue and sexual disability). Some timed outcomes include ambulation (time taken to walk a specified short distance), the nine-hole peg test (time taken to place some pegs into holes in a block), and the box and block test (time taken to transfer blocks between boxes). **Sustained disease progression:** This is reported when an increase in disability from either disease progression or incomplete recovery from relapse is sustained for 3 or 6 months. A relapse that resolves within this time period constitutes non-sustained progression. **Spasticity:** A variety of clinical measures are used, the most common being the Ashworth scale, which scores muscle tone on a scale of 0–4 with 0 representing normal tone and 4 severe spasticity. Other measures include examination findings, neurophysiological techniques, and patient/physician ratings. **General health:** Attempts have been made to customise generic health status scales, but these scales have not been widely used.[5]

METHODS *Clinical Evidence* update search and appraisal May 2000. We included only trials focusing on clinical outcomes (disability, relapses, and symptoms) and commonly used drug treatments.

QUESTION	What are the effects of treatments aimed at reducing relapse rates and disability?

OPTION	INTERFERON BETA-1A/B

We found three large RCTs in people with active relapsing and remitting MS have found that interferon beta-1a/b reduces relapse rates by a third and may delay development of neurological disability. Limited evidence from one RCT in people with secondary progressive disease suggests that interferon beta-1b delays development of disability by 9–12 months. The effect of interferon beta on long term outcome and quality of life is unknown.

Benefits: We found no systematic review. **Relapsing and remitting MS:** We found three large placebo controlled RCTs with 2–3 years' follow up in people with active relapsing and remitting MS.[6–8] One RCT (560 people, disability range EDSS 0–5) compared interferon beta-1a

(22 µg and 44 µg given subcutaneously on alternate days) versus placebo.[6] The trial found significant reductions in relapse rate with both doses over 2 years (22 µg ARR 27%, 95% CI 14% to 39%; 44 µg ARR 33%, 95% CI 21% to 44%) and delayed time to sustained progression of disability (1 or more steps in the EDSS, sustained for at least 3 months). The average time to progression with placebo was 11.9 months versus 18.5 months with 22 µg (P < 0.05, RR progression within 6 months 0.68, 95% CI 0.48 to 0.98) and 21.4 months with 44 µg (P 0.05, RR progression within 6 months 0.62, 95% CI 0.43 to 0.91). A second RCT (372 people, EDSS 0–5.5) compared interferon beta-1b 1.6 MIU and 8 MIU given subcutaneously on alternate days versus placebo.[7] The trial found no significant effect of the lower dose compared with placebo. With the higher dose, the exacerbation rate was significantly reduced (RRR 33%, average number of exacerbations per year 0.84 v 1.27) on placebo, and at 2 years more people were relapse free (OR 2.38, 95% CI 1.25 to 4.25). A third RCT (301 people, EDSS 1–3.5) compared interferon beta-1a 6 MIU given intramuscularly every week versus placebo.[8] At 2 years' follow up (172 people), the trial found a significant reduction in the exacerbation rate (RRR 32%, average number of exacerbations per year 0.61 v 0.9 on placebo) and fewer people had sustained progression of disability (21.9% v 34.9% on placebo, OR not reported). **Secondary progressive MS:** We found one large RCT comparing interferon beta-1b (8 MIU on alternate days) versus placebo in 718 people with secondary progressive MS (EDSS 3–6.5).[9] The average length of follow up was 30 months. It found that average time to sustained progression of disability (as measured by EDSS) was longer with active treatment by 9–12 months (OR 0.65, 95% CI 0.52 to 0.83). To prevent one additional person becoming wheelchair bound, 13 people need to be treated over 30 months (NNT 13, 95% CI 8 to 49). The treatment effect was apparent in people of all levels of baseline disability. There were a large number of withdrawals from both groups (27% placebo and 25% interferon), and no data on quality of life were reported.

Harms: The trials did not report any major adverse effects.[6–9] Mild to moderate effects included early flu-like symptoms (50% of people) and, rarely, leucopenia and asymptomatic elevation of transaminases. Injection site reactions occurred with subcutaneous administration in 80% of people.

Comment: None.

OPTION GLATIRAMER ACETATE

One RCT found a modest effect on relapse rate over 2 years, but found no evidence of an effect on disability.

Benefits: We found no systematic review. **Relapsing and remitting MS:** We found one placebo controlled RCT in 251 people (EDSS 0–5.0).[10] At 2 years, the trial found significantly reduced relapse rates with glatiramer acetate 20 mg daily (ARR 29%, P = 0.007). No significant effect on disability was found. **Secondary progressive MS:** We found no good large RCTs.

Harms:	Glatiramer acetate seems to be well tolerated. A self limiting allergic type reaction (flushing, chest tightness, and anxiety) lasting up to 30 minutes was reported by 15% of people on active treatment on at least one occasion (maximum 7 reactions).[10]
Comment:	None.

OPTION   INTRAVENOUS IMMUNOGLOBULIN

We found limited evidence from one RCT in people with relapsing and remitting MS suggesting that monthly intravenous immunoglobulin (Ig) reduced disability compared with placebo.

Benefits:	We found no systematic review. **Relapsing and remitting MS:** We found one RCT comparing intravenous Ig 0.2 g/kg per month versus placebo in 150 people with relapsing and remitting MS.[11] Treatment was for a maximum of 2 years, but average duration was 21 months. The level of disability decreased in the experimental group (change in EDSS −0.23, 95% CI −0.43 to −0.03) compared with no significant change in the placebo group (change in EDSS 0.12, 95% CI −0.13 to +0.37). The trial did not report data on the time to development of sustained progression of disability. **Secondary progressive MS:** We found no good large RCTs.
Harms:	No significant adverse effects were reported.[11] However, higher dosages of intravenous Ig have been associated with aseptic meningitis and several other systemic reactions.[12]
Comment:	None.

OPTION   AZATHIOPRINE

One systematic review of RCTs has found a modest reduction in relapse rates but no evidence of a significant effect on disability over 2–3 years.

Benefits:	We found one systematic review of azathioprine (search date 1989, 7 RCTs, 793 people with both relapsing remitting MS and progressive MS).[13] At 2 years, the trial found that azathioprine reduced the relapse rate compared with placebo or no treatment (OR 2.04, 95% CI 1.42 to 2.93) and just failed to reduce disability significantly (EDSS mean score difference −0.22, 95% CI −0.43 to +0.003).
Harms:	About 10% of people were unable to tolerate therapeutic doses of azathioprine. Well documented adverse effects include hepatotoxicity and bone marrow suppression.[13] There are concerns about long term cancer risk.[14] In one large RCT, 21% of people on azathioprine withdrew after 1 year compared with 12% on placebo.[15]
Comment:	The methods used in MS trials have improved over the past 10 years, making it hard to compare older and more recent studies. Trials in the review included people with different categories of MS and used different definitions of relapse.[13]

OPTION   METHOTREXATE

We found weak evidence from one small RCT suggesting that low dose, weekly methotrexate may delay disease progression marginally in people with secondary progressive disease.

Benefits: We found no systematic review. We found one RCT comparing low dose methotrexate (7.5 mg) versus placebo in 60 people with primary or secondary progressive disease.[16] The trial found that methotrexate reduced the risk of progression (ARR 31%, P = 0.01), defined by a composite outcome measure, including EDSS, ambulation, nine-hole peg test, and box and block test.

Harms: No major toxicity was reported in the RCT, but marrow suppression and hepatotoxicity can occur with low dose methotrexate; regular monitoring is advised.[16]

Comment: The trial's findings mainly reflected changes in upper limb function.[16] Studies of other drugs have not used composite outcome measures, which makes comparisons difficult. Relative risks for treatment failure were not reported.

OPTION   MITOXANTRONE

Limited evidence from small RCTs suggests that pulsed intravenous mitoxantrone reduces disease activity in people with very active MS, in whom the risk of severe neurological disability may outweigh the risks of cytotoxic treatment.

Benefits: We found no systematic review. Several small RCTs have evaluated this cytotoxic antibiotic in people with MS, finding a positive or neutral effect. One non-blinded RCT in 42 people with very active disease compared 6 months of treatment with monthly intravenous mitoxantrone 20 mg plus methylprednisolone 1 g versus methylprednisolone alone.[17] The trial found mitoxantrone plus methylprednisolone significantly reduced disease activity (as assessed by appearance on magnetic resonance imaging) and lower annual clinical relapse rates (0.7 v 3.0, P < 0.01) compared with methylprednisolone alone.

Harms: The major risk is dose related cardiotoxicity, but this is rare at the doses used in trials in people with MS. Leucopenia, nausea, and amenorrhoea are commonly reported.[18]

Comment: A larger blinded RCT has recently been completed and results are awaited.

QUESTION   What are the effects of treatments for acute relapse?

OPTION   CORTICOSTEROIDS

We found evidence from a large RCT in people with acute optic neuritis, and several small RCTs in people with acute MS relapse, that pulsed intravenous methylprednisolone improves recovery at 4 weeks. We found no evidence that steroids affect long term outcome. None of the available studies of steroids include quantitative data on the effects of treatment.

Benefits: We found no systematic review. **Oral steroids versus placebo:** We found one RCT comparing oral methylprednisolone (500 mg daily for 5 days with 10 day taper) versus placebo in 51 people with acute MS relapse.[19] The trial found that oral steroid treatment improved outcome at 3 and 8 weeks, as measured by EDSS, Scripps neurological rating scale (derived from the neurological examination), and visual analogue scores. **Intravenous steroids versus placebo:** Two small RCTs (45 people) compared intravenous methylprednisolone (500 mg for 5 days or 15 mg/kg per day) versus placebo for acute relapses.[20,21] In both trials, methylprednisolone improved the chance of recovery (no OR or RR given). One large RCT in 457 people with acute optic neuritis compared intravenous methylprednisolone (151 people, 1 g daily for 3 days followed by an oral steroid taper 11 days) versus oral prednisolone (156 people, 1 mg/kg per day for 14 days) versus placebo (150 people). Compared with placebo, intravenous methylprednisolone significantly improved the visual fields at 4 weeks (P = 0.0001) but not at 6 months. **Oral versus intravenous steroids:** We found two small RCTs comparing intravenous versus oral methylprednisolone.[23,24] These trials found no significant differences between the effects of each treatment on functional or disability scores, as measured by the EDSS. The first RCT (35 people with acute relapse) compared identical doses of methylprednisolone (500 mg/day for 5 days).[23] At 4 weeks' follow up, there was no significant difference in disability scores between the groups. The second RCT (n = 80) compared high dose intravenous methylprednisolone (1 g for 3 days) versus intermediate dose oral methylprednisolone.[24] The trial found no significant difference between treatments in terms of EDSS at predetermined time points after relapse.

Harms: In the trial in people with acute optic neuritis, oral steroids were associated with an increased risk of recurrence of optic neuritis at 2 years (RR of a "new episode" of optic neuritis in either eye with oral steroids versus placebo 1.79, 95% CI 1.08 to 2.95).[22] This effect was no longer evident at 3 years. Occasional serious complications of intravenous methylprednisolone include acute psychosis, avascular necrosis of the femoral head, and sudden death caused by cardiac arrhythmia. A retrospective analysis of 350 treatment courses in people with MS found one episode of psychotic depression and one case of severe duodenitis, but no cardiac events or avascular necrosis.[25]

Comment: In one RCT, minor adverse effects from steroid treatment were common and may have compromised blinding.[19]

| OPTION | PLASMA EXCHANGE | New |

We found insufficient evidence on the effectiveness of plasma exchange in people with acute demyelinating episodes who had previously failed to respond to intravenous steroids.

Benefits: We found no systematic review. We found one randomised, double blinded crossover trial of plasma exchange versus a sham control in people with acute relapses of MS (n = 12) or other demyelinating disease (n = 10) who had previously failed to respond to intravenous steroids.[26] The trial found moderate or greater improvement in neurological disability in people receiving plasma exchange compared with sham treatment (8/19 [42%] v 1/17 [6%]; ARI 36%, 95% CI 1% to 81%; RR 7.2, 95% CI 1.2 to 15; NNT 3, 95% CI 1 to 68).

Harms: The trial reported no major complications.[26]

Comment: At the time of randomisation, all patients had failed to respond to standard doses of intravenous corticosteroids, and were within 3 months of onset of the acute deficit. This is a small study in a difficult area and further data are needed.

QUESTION What are the effects of treatments for fatigue in multiple sclerosis?

OPTION DRUG TREATMENT: AMANTADINE AND PEMOLINE

One short term RCT found that amantadine modestly reduced MS related fatigue. This trial, and a small crossover RCT, found no evidence of benefit from pemoline.

Benefits: We found no systematic review but found two RCTs.[27,28] One RCT (119 people) compared amantadine and pemoline versus placebo.[27] Amantadine significantly reduced fatigue, measured by the MS specific fatigue scale ($P = 0.04$), but there was no significant difference in the effects of pemoline and placebo. After a 2 week washout period, the proportions of people who reported feeling better on than off the study medication were 79% (15/19) with amantadine, 32% (7/22) with pemoline, and 52% with placebo. Neither amantadine nor pemoline affected the secondary outcome measures of sleep or depression. A crossover RCT in 46 people found no significant benefit of pemoline over placebo.[28]

Harms: Two people taking amantadine withdrew from the trial because of rash or anxiety. Other reported adverse effects of amantadine included sleep disturbance (2 people) and palpitations (1 person).[27]

Comment: None.

OPTION BEHAVIOURAL MODIFICATION THERAPY

We found insufficient evidence on the effects of behavioural modification therapy in people with MS related fatigue.

Benefits: We found no systematic review and no RCTs.

Harms: None reported.

Comment: None.

OPTION EXERCISE

We found insufficient evidence on the effects of exercise in people with MS related fatigue.

Benefits: We found no systematic review. We found one RCT (46 people, EDSS 0–6.0), which compared 15 weeks of aerobic training versus no exercise.[29] Using a scale that measures mental and physical fatigue, there was a significant reduction in fatigue at 10 weeks but not after completion of the exercise programme. A different scale that measured only physical fatigue remained unchanged in both groups of people. The trial found improvements in emotional behaviour and quality of life.

Harms: None reported.

Comment: People with moderate disability or severe fatigue may have difficulty adhering to an aerobic exercise programme.

QUESTION **What are the effects of treatments for spasticity?**

OPTION **PHYSICAL THERAPY**

One small RCT of inpatient physiotherapy found no evidence of benefit in terms of mobility or activities of daily living.

Benefits: We found no systematic review. One non-blinded RCT compared early versus delayed physiotherapy (9 weeks of inpatient treatment) in 45 people with progressive MS.[30] The trial found no evidence of an effect of treatment on measures of mobility (timed walk, Rivermead mobility index) or activities of daily living. Treated people reported reduced mobility related stress (P < 0.001).

Harms: None reported.

Comment: The study lacked the power to detect a small effect of treatment on mobility.

OPTION **ORAL DRUG TREATMENT**

Two RCTs have found that tizanidine reduces spasticity in people with MS, but with no evidence of a beneficial effect on mobility. We found insufficient evidence to assess other oral drug treatments.

Benefits: **Versus placebo:** We found no systematic review. We found two large RCTs comparing tizanidine versus placebo in people with MS related spasticity.[31,32] One RCT (220 people, tizanidine 2–36 mg daily) found no significant difference in Ashworth scores (see Outcomes, p 727) but found that tizanidine reduced self reported clonus and spasm.[31] The other RCT (187 people, tizanidine 24–36 mg daily) found that tizanidine significantly reduced muscle tone (P < 0.05), although the trial found no impact of tizanidine on mobility related activities of daily living.[32] **Versus each other:** We found one systematic review (published 1998, 10 European RCTs, 70 people with both cerebrovascular disease and MS) comparing tizanidine versus baclofen (7 RCTs) or diazepam (3 RCTs). The review found no difference between the three drugs in their effects on muscle tone.[33] The trials were too small to rule out clinically important differences.

Harms: Comparative studies of baclofen and tizanidine found similar levels of adverse effects (including muscle weakness, sedation, and dry mouth), but tizanidine may be less likely than baclofen to cause muscle weakness.[33]

Comment: Increased muscle tone is not always detrimental or disabling; mild or moderate spasticity may aid standing or transfers.

OPTION INTRATHECAL BACLOFEN

Limited evidence from one small RCT suggests benefit in non-ambulant people with symptomatic spasticity resistant to oral drug treatment.

Benefits:
We found no systematic review. We found one small RCT comparing intrathecal baclofen versus intrathecal saline in 20 (19 non-ambulant) people with spasticity resistant to oral baclofen.[34] Participants suffered from MS or spinal cord injury. Baclofen significantly reduced spasticity and spasm frequency. Average Ashworth scores (see Outcomes, p 727) fell from 4.0 to 1.2 (P < 0.0001), with scores for all participants improving from baseline.

Harms:
Potential problems include pump failure, infection, and, rarely, baclofen overdose.

Comment:
We found no evidence on the role of intrathecal baclofen in ambulant patients.

QUESTION What are the effects of a multidisciplinary approach to patient management?

OPTION INPATIENT REHABILITATION

Two RCTs found that 3–4 weeks of inpatient rehabilitation resulted in short term improvements in disability, despite no evidence of an effect on levels of neurological impairment. The duration of this effect is uncertain.

Benefits:
We found no systematic review but found two RCTs.[35,36] The first trial compared a short period of inpatient rehabilitation (average 25 days) versus remaining on the waiting list (non-treatment control group) in 66 people with progressive MS who were selected as "good candidates" for rehabilitation.[35] Rehabilitation significantly improved disability, assessed by the functional independence measure and the London handicap scale, despite unchanged levels of neurological impairment (EDSS). Follow up of these people found that benefit persisted for up to 9 months. The second RCT compared 3 weeks of inpatient rehabilitation versus exercises at home in 50 (ambulant) people. The trial found improvements in disability, as measured by the functional independence measure (P < 0.004), which persisted at 9 but not at 15 weeks' follow up.[36]

Harms:
None reported.

Comment:
Many centres lack appropriate rehabilitation facilities.

OPTION OUTPATIENT REHABILITATION

One small RCT found that prolonged outpatient rehabilitation reduced MS symptom frequency and fatigue.

Benefits:
We found no systematic review. We found one RCT comparing outpatient rehabilitation (5 hours per week for 1 year) versus remaining on the waiting list (non-treatment control group) in 46 people with progressive MS. Rehabilitation reduced the frequency

of fatigue (effect size –0.27) and MS symptoms (effect size –0.32), despite no evidence of a change in neurological impairment in either group.[37]

Harms: None reported.

Comment: Future trials need to record effects on disability and quality of life as well as impairment.

REFERENCES

1. Compston A. Genetic epidemiology of multiple sclerosis. *J Neurol Neurosurg Psychiatry* 1997;62: 553–561.
2. Weinshenker BG, Bass B, Rice GPA, et al. The natural history of multiple sclerosis: a geographically based study. 1. Clinical course and disability. *Brain* 1989;112:133–146.
3. Lucchinetti CF, Bruck W, Rodriguez M, Lassmann H. Distinct patterns of multiple sclerosis pathology indicates heterogeneity in pathogenesis. *Brain Pathol* 1996;6:259–274.
4. Kurtzke JF. Rating neurological impairment in multiple sclerosis: an expanded disability status scale (EDSS). *Neurology* 1983;33:1444–1452.
5. Vickrey BG, Hays RD, Genovese BJ, Myers LW, Ellison GW. Comparison of a generic to disease-targeted health-related quality-of-life measures for multiple sclerosis. *J Clin Epidemiol* 1997;50:557–569.
6. PRISMS Study Group. Randomised double-blind placebo-controlled study of interferon beta-1a in relapsing/remitting multiple sclerosis. *Lancet* 1998;352:1498–1504.
7. The IFNB Multiple Sclerosis Study Group. Interferon beta-1b is effective in relapsing-remitting multiple sclerosis. Clinical results of a multicenter, randomised, double-blind, placebo-controlled trial. *Neurology* 1993;43:655–661.
8. Jacobs LD, Cookfair DL, Rudick RA, et al. Intramuscular interferon beta-1a for disease progression in relapsing multiple sclerosis. *Ann Neurol* 1996;39:285–294.
9. European Study Group on Interferon Beta-1b in Secondary Progressive MS. Placebo-controlled multicentre randomised trial of interferon beta-1b in treatment of secondary progressive multiple sclerosis. *Lancet* 1998;352:1491–1497.
10. Johnson KP, Brooks BR, Cohen JA, et al. Copolymer-1 reduces relapse rate and improves disability in relapsing-remitting multiple sclerosis: results of a phase III multicenter, double-blind, placebo-controlled trial. *Neurology* 1995;45:1268–1276.
11. Fazekas F, Deisenhammer F, Strasser-Fuchs S, Naylor G, Mamoli M, for the Austrian Immunoglobulin in Multiple Sclerosis Study Group. Randomised placebo-controlled trial of monthly intravenous immunoglobulin therapy in relapsing-remitting multiple sclerosis. *Lancet* 1997;349:589–593.
12. Stangel M, Hartung HP, Marx P, Gold R. Side-effects of high-dose intravenous immunoglobulins. *Clin Neuropharmacol* 1997;20:385–393.
13. Yudkin PL, Ellison GW, Ghezzi A, et al. Overview of azathioprine treatment in multiple sclerosis. *Lancet* 1991;338:1051–1055. Search date 1989; primary sources Medline 1966 to 1989; and hand searched references.
14. Confavreux C, Saddier P, Grimaud J, et al. Risk of cancer from azathioprine therapy in multiple sclerosis: a case-control study. *Neurology* 1996; 46:1607–1612.
15. British and Dutch Multiple Sclerosis Azathioprine Trial Group. Double masked trial of azathioprine in

16. Goodkin DE, Rudick RA, VanderBrug Medendorp S, et al. Low-dose (7.5 mg) oral methotrexate reduces the rate of progression in chronic progressive multiple sclerosis. *Ann Neurol* 1995; 37:30–40.
17. Edan G, Miller D, Clanet M, et al. Therapeutic effect of mitoxantrone combined with methylprednisolone in multiple sclerosis: a randomised multicentre study of active disease using MRI and clinical criteria. *J Neurol Neurosurg Psychiatry* 1997;62:112–118.
18. MacDonald M, Posner LE, Dukart G, et al. A review of the acute and chronic toxicity of mitoxantrone. *Future Trends Chemother* 1985;6: 443–450.
19. Sellebjerg F, Frederiksen JL, Nielsen PM, Olesen J. Double-blind, randomised, placebo-controlled study of oral, high-dose methylprednisolone in attacks of MS. *Neurology* 1998;51:529–534.
20. Milligan NM, Newcombe R, Compston DAS. A double-blind controlled trial of high dose methylprednisolone in patients with multiple sclerosis: 1. Clinical effects. *J Neurol Neurosurg Psychiatry* 1987;50:511–516.
21. Durelli L, Cocito D, Riccio A, et al. High-dose intravenous methylprednisolone in the treatment of multiple sclerosis. *Neurology* 1986;36:238–243.
22. Beck RW, Cleary PA, Anderson MM, et al. A randomised controlled trial of corticosteroids in the treatment of acute optic neuritis. *N Engl J Med* 1992;326:581–588.
23. Alam SM, Kyriakides T, Lawden M, Newman PK. Methylprednisolone in multiple sclerosis: a comparison of oral with intravenous therapy at equivalent high dose. *J Neurol Neurosurg Psychiatry* 1993;56:1219–1220.
24. Barnes D, Hughes RAC, Morris RW, et al. Randomised trial of oral and intravenous methylprednisolone in acute relapses of multiple sclerosis. *Lancet* 1997;349:902–906.
25. Lyons PR, Newman PK, Saunders M. Methylprednisolone therapy in multiple sclerosis; a profile of adverse events. *J Neurol Neurosurg Psychiatry* 1988;51:285–287.
26. Weinshenker BG, O'Brien PC, Petterson TM, et al. A randomised trial of plasma exchange in acute central nervous system inflammatory demyelinating disease. *Neurology* 1999;46:878–886.
27. Fuller KJ, Dawson K, Wiles CM. Physiotherapy in chronic multiple sclerosis: a controlled trial. *Clin Rehabil* 1996;10:195–204.
28. Krupp LB, Coyle PK, Doscher C, et al. Fatigue therapy in multiple sclerosis: results of a double-blind, randomised parallel trial of amantadine, pemoline and placebo. *Neurology* 1995;45: 1956–1961.
29. Weinshenker BG, Penman M, Bass B. A double-blind, randomised, crossover trial of pemoline in fatigue associated with multiple sclerosis. *Neurology* 1992;42:1468–1471.
30. Petajan JH, Gappmaier E, White AT, et al. Impact

multiple sclerosis. *Lancet* 1988;2:179–183.

of aerobic training on fitness and quality of life in multiple sclerosis. *Ann Neurol* 1996;39:432–441.

31. Smith C, Birnbaum G, Carter JL, Greenstein J, Lublin FD. Tizanidine treatment of spasticity caused by multiple sclerosis: results of a double-blind, placebo-controlled trial. US tizanidine study group. *Neurology* 1994;44(suppl):34–42.

32. UK Tizanidine Trial Group. A double-blind, placebo-controlled trial of tizanidine in the treatment of spasticity caused by multiple sclerosis. *Neurology* 1994;44:S70–S78.

33. Groves L, Shellenberger MK, Davis CS. Tizanidine treatment of spasticity: a meta-analysis of controlled, double-blind, comparative studies with baclofen and diazepam. *Adv Ther* 1998;15:241–251. Search date not given; primary sources records of Sandoz (now Novartis).

34. Penn RD, Savoy SM, Corcos D, et al. Intrathecal baclofen for severe spinal spasticity. *N Engl J Med* 1989;320:1517–1521.

35. Freeman JA, Langdon DW, Hobart JC, Thompson AJ. The impact of inpatient rehabilitation on progressive multiple sclerosis. *Ann Neurol* 1997; 42:236–244.

36. Solari A, Fillipini G, Gasco P, et al. Physical rehabilitation has a positive effect on disability in multiple sclerosis patients. *Neurology* 1999;52: 57–62.

37. Di Fabio RP, Soderberg J, Choi T, Hanson CR, Schapiro RT. Extended outpatient rehabilitation: its influence on symptom frequency, fatigue and functional status for persons with progressive multiple sclerosis. *Arch Phys Med Rehabil* 1998; 79:141–146.

Helen Ford
Consultant Neurologist
St James's Hospital
Leeds
UK

Mike Boggild
Consultant Neurologist
The Walton Centre for Neurology and Neurosurgery
Liverpool
UK

Competing interests: HF has been paid by Schering and Biogen for speaking at meetings, and by Serono Pharmaceuticals and Biogen for attending conferences; MB has received financial support for attending scientific meetings from Biogen, Serono Pharmaceuticals, and Teva Pharmaceuticals, and has organised educational sessions for Serono.

Updated this issue

A Moore and Carl Clarke

INTERVENTIONS

Beneficial

Dopamine agonists instead of levodopa in younger people with early disease 740

Trade off between benefits and harms

Levodopa combined with a dopa decarboxylase inhibitor in initial treatment 740

Dopamine agonists in later disease. 741

Unknown effectiveness

Selegiline 739

Pallidotomy. 742

Unlikely to be beneficial

Modified release levodopa (compared with immediate release levodopa) 740

To be covered in future issues of *Clinical Evidence*

Non-medical interventions

Catechol-O-methyltransferase inhibitors

Other types of surgery

See glossary, p 743

Key Messages

- We found no good evidence that any drug delays the progression of Parkinson's disease.

- Five RCTs found that selegiline delays the need for levadopa, one of which found increased mortality in people with early Parkinson's disease.

- Two RCTs found no evidence of a difference in long term motor complications with controlled release or immediate release levodopa monotherapy in people with early Parkinson's disease.

- One systematic review and three RCTs have found that dopamine agonists are less likely to cause long term motor complications than levodopa. The strategy of starting younger people on dopamine agonists and deferring the use of levodopa needs further evaluation.

- Two systematic reviews and two additional RCTs have found that, when used in later stage disease, adjuvant dopamine agonists reduce "off" time (see glossary, p 743), improve motor impairments and activities of daily living, and reduce levodopa dose, but increase dopaminergic adverse events and dyskinesia. Newer dopamine agonists await evaluation.

- We found limited evidence suggesting that pallidotomy (see glossary, p 743) may be effective for the control of tremor, rigidity, and dyskinesias, although serious complications of surgery are considerable.

DEFINITION Idiopathic Parkinson's disease is an age related neurodegenerative disorder and the most common cause of the parkinsonian syndrome: a combination of asymmetric bradykinesia, hypokinesia, and rigidity, sometimes combined with rest tremor and postural changes. Clinical diagnostic criteria have a sensitivity of 80% and specificity of 30% compared with the gold standard of diagnosis at autopsy.[1] The primary pathology is progressive loss of dopaminergic cells from the substantia nigra in the brainstem. Treatment aims to replace or compensate for the lost dopamine. A good response to treatment supports, but does not confirm, the diagnosis. Several other catecholaminergic neurotransmitter systems are also deranged in Parkinson's disease.

INCIDENCE/ PREVALENCE Parkinson's disease occurs worldwide with equal incidence in both sexes. In 5–10% of people who develop Parkinson's disease it manifests itself before the age of 40 years ("young onset"), with a mean age of onset of about 65 years. Overall age adjusted prevalence is 1% worldwide and 1.6% in Europe, rising from 0.6% at age 60–64 years to 3.5% at age 85–89 years.[2,3] First-degree relatives of affected people may have twice the risk of developing Parkinson's disease (17% chance of developing the condition in their lifetime) compared with people in the general population.[4–6]

AETIOLOGY/ RISK FACTORS The cause is unknown. Parkinson's disease may represent different conditions with a final common pathway. People may be affected differently by a combination of genetic and environmental factors (viruses, toxins, 1-methyl-4-phenyl-1,2,3,6-tetrahydropyridine [MPTP], well water, vitamin E, and smoking).[7–10] Purely genetic varieties probably comprise a small minority of people with Parkinson's disease.[11,12]

PROGNOSIS Parkinson's disease is currently incurable. Disability is progressive and associated with increased mortality (RR death compared with the general population ranges from 1.6 to 3).[13] Treatment may reduce symptoms and slow progression but rarely achieves complete control. The question of whether treatment reduces mortality remains controversial.[14] Levodopa seemed to reduce mortality in the UK for 5 years after its introduction, before a "catch up" effect was noted and overall mortality rose towards previous levels. This suggested a limited prolongation of life.[15] An Australian cohort study followed 130 treated people for 10 years. The standardised mortality ratio was 1.58 (P < 0.001). At 10 years, 25% had been admitted to a nursing home and only four were still employed. The mean duration of disease until death was 9.1 years.[16] In a similar Italian cohort study[17] over 8 years, the relative risk of death for affected people versus healthy controls was 2.3 (95% CI 1.60 to 3.39). Age at initial census date was the main predictor of outcome: for age under 75 years, RR death was 1.80 (95% CI 1.04 to 3.11); for age over 75 years, RR was 5.61 (95% CI 2.13 to 14.8).

AIMS To improve symptoms and quality of life; to slow disease progression; to limit short and long term adverse effects of treatment, such as motor fluctuations (see glossary, p 743).

OUTCOMES Disease severity, severity of drug induced symptoms or signs, rate of progression of symptoms, need for levodopa or other treatment, adverse effects of treatment, withdrawals from treatment, and quality of life measures. There are no universal scales, but commonly used scales are the Hoehn and Yahr scale, Webster scale, the Unified Parkinson's Disease Rating Scale (UPDRS), the Core Assessment Programme for Intracerebral Transplantation (CAPIT),[18,19] the Parkinson's Disease Quality of Life questionnaire (PDQL),[20] and the UK Parkinson's Disease Quality of Life questionnaire 39 (PDQ-39).[21]

METHODS *Clinical Evidence* update search and appraisal May 2000. We included all RCTs that met *Clinical Evidence* criteria. Unless stated otherwise, we have used the term "levodopa" to refer to a combination of levodopa and a peripheral decarboxylase inhibitor.

QUESTION **What are the effects of drug treatments in people with early Parkinson's disease?**

OPTION SELEGILINE

Five large RCTs have found that selegiline delays the need for levodopa, but one of these trials found increased mortality in people with early Parkinson's disease.

Benefits: We found no systematic review. We found five large placebo controlled RCTs in people with early Parkinson's disease. The first (n = 800) found that selegiline delayed the need for levodopa for 9 months (HR 0.50 for requiring levodopa in each time period, 95% CI 0.41 to 0.62, P < 0.001).[22] The second trial (n = 101), in people newly diagnosed with Parkinson's disease, found that after 12 months of treatment and 2 months of washout there was a significantly smaller deterioration in total UPDRS score with selegiline compared with placebo.[23] The third trial (n = 782) found no evidence of a clinically important difference after 4 years of selegiline.[24] The fourth trial (n = 116) found that significantly fewer people randomised to selegiline required a 50% or greater increase in their levodopa dose after 5 years (50% on selegiline v 74% on placebo, P = 0.027).[25] A recent fifth trial (n = 163) found significantly better motor function in those treated with selegiline for 5 years.[26] The absence of any deterioration on selegiline withdrawal argues against any symptomatic effect after 5 years of treatment. Other studies of early selegiline treatment were either too small or too brief to reach a conclusion.[27]

Harms: One large RCT and one non-systematic review (see comment below) found no evidence of a difference in mortality between selegiline and placebo.[27,28] Another RCT found (at interim analysis after 5.6 years of follow up) higher mortality in those treated with selegiline (HR 1.57, 95% CI 1.07 to 2.31); the selegiline arm of the trial was terminated early.[24] Updated analysis (including blinded assessment of cause-specific mortality) found that the increase in mortality did not quite reach significance (HR 1.30, 95% CI 0.99 to 1.72), perhaps because the study was stopped when, by chance, mortality was high.[29,30] One retrospective observational study in 12 621 people who had taken an antiparkinsonian drug (excluding those also taking antipsychotic drugs) found increased mortality in people prescribed selegiline, but the confidence interval included zero (ARI 11%, 95% CI 0% to 23%).[31]

Comment: The review[27] claimed to be systematic but omitted at least one relevant study. A systematic review is under way and a large RCT is planned.

OPTION   MODIFIED RELEASE LEVODOPA

Two RCTs found no evidence that modified release levodopa reduced motor complications or improved disease control at 5 years versus immediate release levodopa in people with early Parkinson's disease.

Benefits: We found no systematic review. Two long term RCTs compared modified versus immediate release levodopa preparations (co-beneldopa and co-careldopa) in 134 and 618 people with early Parkinson's disease.[32,33] At 5 years, the trials found no significant differences in the incidence of dyskinesia (see glossary, p 743) (41% with modified release *v* 34% with immediate release co-beneldopa), motor fluctuations (see glossary, p 743) (59% *v* 57%), motor impairment, or activities of daily living.

Harms: The co-careldopa trial found that nausea was more common with the immediate release preparation.[33]

Comment: In both trials, levodopa was combined with a peripheral decarboxylase inhibitor.[32,33]

OPTION   DOPAMINE AGONIST VERSUS LEVODOPA IN EARLY DISEASE

Widespread experience suggests that dyskinesias and fluctuations in motor response are related to long term levodopa treatment and are irreversible. One systematic review and three long term RCTs (one unblinded) found that dopamine agonists reduce the incidence of dyskinesias and may delay their onset.

Benefits: We found two systematic reviews published in abstract form only (full reviews awaited). The first review (published in 1999) identified six RCTs comparing bromocriptine with levodopa, and found that bromocriptine delayed motor complications and dyskinesias.[34] The second review (published in 1999) identified eight RCTs comparing bromocriptine plus levodopa versus levodopa alone, and found a trend towards reduced dyskinesia with combination treatment but no difference in duration of "off" time.[35] Neither review recorded effects on disability or motor impairment. We found three additional long term RCTs. One compared ropinirole plus rescue levodopa if needed versus levodopa alone (n = 268) and found that at 5 years dyskinesias were more common with levodopa alone (OR 3.8, 95% CI 2.1 to 6.9).[36] It found no difference in disability at 5 years (UPDRS activities of daily living scale) and a small increase in motor impairments with ropinirole. The second RCT compared cabergoline plus rescue levodopa versus levodopa alone (n = 419) and found that motor complications occurred in 22% of people in the cabergoline group and 34% in the levodopa group.[37] Activities of daily living scores were worse with cabergoline. The third RCT was small (n = 90) and unblinded. It compared lisuride plus levodopa if needed versus levodopa alone, and found fewer motor complications after lisuride treatment.[38]

Harms: Adverse events were similar in all treatment groups, except that motor complications were less frequent with lisuride and cabergoline than with levodopa.[37,38]

Comment: We found no direct comparisons of individual dopamine agonists. A large, UK based RCT is planned to examine quality of life with agonist monotherapy in people likely to develop motor complications. A multicentre North American study is also planned to investigate the effect of levodopa on dopaminergic cell death.[39]

QUESTION   **What are the effects of adding a dopamine agonist in people with a fluctuating response to levodopa?**

Systematic reviews and RCTs have found that certain dopamine agonists reduce "off" time (see glossary, p 743), improve motor impairment and activities of daily living, and reduce requirement for levodopa, but increase dopaminergic adverse effects (see glossary, p 743) and dyskinesia.

Benefits: **Versus placebo:** We found four systematic reviews of placebo controlled RCTs. The first (search date January 1998) identified seven trials comparing adjuvant bromocriptine versus placebo in a total of 396 people with later Parkinson's disease.[40] Heterogeneity in trial design and outcomes made it impossible to draw conclusions. The second review (search date November 1998) identified no trials comparing lisuride versus placebo.[41] The third review (search date January 1999) identified one RCT comparing pergolide versus placebo in a total of 376 people.[42] It found that pergolide reduced daily "off" time (mean difference 1.6 hours, P < 0.001), reduced daily levodopa dose (mean 184 mg, P < 0.001), and improved activities of daily living scores. The fourth review (search date March 1999) identified four trials comparing pramipexole versus placebo in a total of 669 people.[43] Pramipexole reduced daily "off" time (WMD 1.8 hours, 95% CI 1.2 hours to 2.3 hours), reduced levodopa dose (WMD 115 mg, 95% CI 87 mg to 143 mg), and improved activities of daily living scores. We found two additional RCTs. One (n = 149) found that, compared with placebo, ropinirole reduced "off" time (proportion of participants achieving a 20% reduction in "off" time 35% v 13%, P = 0.003) and levodopa dose.[44] The other trial (n = 188) found that cabergoline increased "on" time (see glossary, p 743), and improved motor impairment (proportion of participants who improved at 6 months: 16% v 6%, P = 0.031) and activities of daily living scores (19% v 4%, P = 0.032).[45] **Versus each other:** One systematic review (search date January 1999) identified three short RCTs, which found that pergolide slightly improved motor impairment compared with bromocriptine; this small advantage may not be clinically important.[46] One systematic review (search date November 1998) found insufficient evidence to compare lisuride with bromocriptine.[41]

Harms: **Versus placebo:** The systematic reviews found increased rates of dopaminergic adverse events and dyskinesia with pramipexole (OR

2.1, 95% CI 1.5 to 2.9) and pergolide (OR 4.6, 95% CI 3.1 to 7.0) compared with placebo.[42,43] Rates of withdrawal from treatment were lower for pramipexole compared with placebo (OR 0.64, 95% CI 0.44 to 0.93) but not for pergolide (OR 0.88, 95% CI 0.5 to 1.51).[42,43] One RCT found that ropinirole was associated with increased dyskinesia compared with placebo (34% v 7%, P = 0.006), although other adverse events were reported equally in both groups.[44] One RCT found that, compared with placebo, cabergoline was significantly more likely to cause autonomic (25% v 11%, P = 0.02) and cardiovascular (7% v 0%, P = 0.05) adverse events.[45] **Versus each other:** One systematic review (search date 1998) found no difference in adverse events between pergolide and bromocriptine.[46]

Comment: Systematic reviews of ropinirole and cabergoline versus placebo are under way. The published RCTs comparing ropinirole and cabergoline versus bromocriptine were small. Larger phase III studies are currently in press. Cochrane systematic reviews will assess all of these studies. We found no direct comparisons of these drugs in people with later Parkinson's disease.

QUESTION   **What are the effects of surgery in people with later Parkinson's disease?**

OPTION   **PALLIDOTOMY**

Two systematic reviews including two RCTs provide limited evidence that pallidotomy (see glossary, p 743) reduces contralateral tremor, rigidity, and dyskinesia, but with significant risk of morbidity and mortality. Bilateral surgery is associated with a variety of axial problems including mutism.

Benefits: **Versus medical treatment:** We found two systematic reviews,[47,48] which between them included evidence from two short term RCTs[49,50] (64 people) and 15 uncontrolled trials (551 people), mainly evaluating unilateral posteroventral pallidotomy in people with advanced Parkinson's disease. One RCT, published only as an abstract, compared medical treatment versus pallidotomy with 6 months' follow up.[49] Pallidotomy achieved greater improvements in tremor, bradykinesia, rigidity, gait, postural stability, and "off" time. It found no evidence that pallidotomy reduced the need for medical treatment. The other RCT, in 37 patients with advanced Parkinson's disease, compared unilateral pallidotomy with best medical treatment over 6 months' follow up.[50] Pallidotomy was associated with improved "off" phase median motor score (UPDRS part 3) from 47 to 32.5, compared with a deterioration from 52.5 to 56.6 in those receiving medical treatment only (P < 0.001); improved contralateral dyskinesia, which decreased in duration by 50% compared with no change on medical treatment; improved duration of independence, which increased by 2.2 hours/day compared with a decrease of 0.4 hours/day with medical treatment (difference 2.6 hours/day, 95% CI 0.0 to 5.3, P < 0.05); and improved quality of life (PDQL) (P < 0.004). Unilateral pallidotomy had no cognitive or behavioural effects, except that left-sided pallidotomy reduced verbal fluency.[51] One recent non-systematic review and consensus statement (evaluating one RCT[52] plus 13 uncontrolled studies) suggested that gait, balance disorders, and hypophonia were less responsive to surgery.[53] **Versus stimulation of the posteroventral pallidum:** One small RCT (n = 13) over 3 months found no significant difference between lesioning and deep brain stimulation (see glossary, p 743) but was probably too small to exclude a clinically important difference.[54] **Versus stimulation of the subthalamic nucleus:** We found no RCTs.

Harms: The incidence of permanent adverse effects of pallidotomy was 4–46%, with a risk of a serious complication (including death) of 3–10%.[47] Complication rates decline with experience.[53] Bilateral procedures may worsen axial symptoms, including dysarthria, dysphonia, and gait disturbances.

Comment: The studies cited in the reviews followed different protocols.[47] Transplants or implants of dopaminergic tissue remain experimental. Most reports of stereotactic lesioning (see glossary, p 743) or stimulation are uncontrolled. A North American controlled trial of pallidotomy versus delayed pallidotomy is currently under way.[52]

GLOSSARY

Deep brain stimulation Prolonged focal electrical brain stimulation through a stereotactically implanted wire.

Dopaminergic adverse effects Include dyskinesia, hallucinations, and psychosis.

Dyskinesia Normal or involuntary writhing or jerky movements distinct from tremor.

"On" time Periods when treatment is working.

"Off" time Periods when treatment is not working.

Pallidotomy Making a permanent surgical lesion, usually thermally or electrically, in the globus pallidum.

Motor fluctuations Fluctuations in motor symptoms, such as bradykinesia, rigidity, and tremor during a day. Response fluctuations are fluctuations in a person's overall response to treatment during a day.

Stereotactic lesioning Placing a lesion using stereotactic techniques; a kind of three-dimensional triangulation.

Axial effects Changes affecting axial body sections such as head and trunk, rather than the limbs.

Substantive changes since last issue

Selegiline One new RCT found;[26] no change in overall conclusions.

Pallidotomy New systematic review found;[48] no change in overall conclusions.

REFERENCES

1. Hughes AJ, Daniel SE, Blankson S, Lees AJ. A clinico-pathologic study of 100 cases of Parkinson's disease. *Arch Neurol* 1993;50:140–148.
2. Zhang Z, Roman G. Worldwide occurrence of Parkinson's disease: an updated review. *Neuroepidemiology* 1993;12:195–208.
3. De Rijk MC, Tzourio C, Breteler MMB, et al. Prevalence of parkinsonism and Parkinson's disease in Europe: the EUROPARKINSON collaborative study. *J Neurol Neurosurg Psychiatry* 1997;62:10–15.
4. Marder K, Tang M, Mejia H, et al. Risk of Parkinson's disease among first degree relatives: a community based study. *Neurology* 1996;47:155–160.
5. Jarman P, Wood N. Parkinson's disease genetics comes of age. *BMJ* 1999;318:1641–1642.
6. Lazzarini A, Myers R, Zimmerman T, et al. A clinical genetic study of Parkinson's disease: evidence for dominant transmission. *Neurology* 1994;44:499–506.
7. Ben-Shlomo Y. How far are we in understanding the cause of Parkinson's disease? *J Neurol Neurosurg Psychiatry* 1996;61:4–16.
8. De Rijk M, Breteler M, den Breeilnen J, et al. Dietary antioxidants and Parkinson's disease: the Rotterdam study. *Arch Neurol* 1997;54:762–765.
9. Hellenbrand W, Seidler A, Robra B, et al. Smoking

and Parkinson's disease: a case-control study in Germany. *Int J Epidemiol* 1997;26:328–339.

10. Tzourio C, Rocca W, Breteler M, et al. Smoking and Parkinson's disease: an age-dependent risk effect? *Neurology* 1997;49:1267–1272.

11. Gasser T, M ller-Myhsok B, Wszolek Z, et al. A susceptibility locus for Parkinson's disease maps to chromosome 2p13. *Nat Genet* 1998;18:262–265.

12. Tanner C, Ottman R, Goldman S, et al. Parkinson's disease in twins. An etiologic study. *JAMA* 1999; 281:341–346.

13. Parkinson Study Group. Mortality in DATATOP: a multicenter trial in early Parkinson's disease. *Ann Neurol* 1998;43:318–325.

14. Rajput A, Uitti J, Offord K. Timely levodopa (LD) administration prolongs survival in Parkinson's disease. *Parkinsonism Related Disord* 1997;3: 159–165.

15. Clarke CE. Does levodopa therapy delay death in Parkinson's disease? A review of the evidence. *Mov Disord* 1995;10:250–256.

16. Hely MA, Morris JGL, Traficante R, et al. The Sydney multicentre study of Parkinson's disease: progression and mortality at 10 years. *J Neurol Neurosurg Psychiatry* 1999;67:300–307.

17. Morgante L, Salemi G, Meneghini F, et al. Parkinson disease survival. A population-based study. *Arch Neurol* 2000;57:507–512.

18. Fahn S, Elton L, for the UPDRS Development Committee. Unified Parkinson's disease rating scale. In: Fahn S, Marsden C, Calne D, et al, eds. *Recent developments in Parkinson's disease*, Vol. 2. Florham Park, NJ, USA: Macmillan Healthcare Information, 1987:153–163.

19. Langston JW, Widner H, Goetz CG, et al. Core Assessment Program for Intracerebral Transplantations (CAPIT). *Mov Disord* 1992;7:2–13.

20. De Boer A, Wijker W, Speelman J, de Haes JCJM. Quality of life in people with Parkinson's disease: development of a questionnaire. *J Neurol Neurosurg Psychiatry* 1996;61:70–74.

21. Peto V, Jenkinson C, Fitzpatrick R, Greenhall R. The development and validation of a short measure of functioning and well being for individuals with Parkinson's disease. *Qual Life Res* 1995;4:241–248.

22. The Parkinson's Disease Study Group. Effects of tocopherol and deprenyl on the progression of disability in early Parkinson's disease. *N Engl J Med* 1993;328:176–183.

23. Olanow CW, Hauser RA, Gauger L, et al. The effect of deprenyl and levodopa on the progression of Parkinson's disease. *Ann Neurol* 1995;38:771–777.

24. Lees AJ, for the Parkinson's Disease Research Group of the United Kingdom. Comparison of therapeutic effects and mortality data of levodopa and levodopa combined with selegiline in patients with early, mild Parkinson's disease. *BMJ* 1995; 311:1602–1607.

25. Przuntek H, Conrad B, Dichgans J, et al. SELEDO: a 5-year long-term trial on the effect of selegiline in early Parkinsonian patients treated with levodopa. *Eur J Neurol* 1999;6(2):141–150.

26. Larson JP, Boas J, Erdal JE, et al. Does selegiline modify the progression of early Parkinson's disease? Results from a five-year study. *Eur J Neurol* 1999;6:539–547.

27. Olanow CW, Mylla V, Sotaniemi K, et al. Effect of selegiline on mortality in patients with Parkinson's disease. *Neurology* 1998;51:825–830.

28. Penny J, for the Parkinson Study Group. Impact of deprenyl and tocopherol treatment for Parkinson's disease in DATATOP patients requiring levodopa. *Ann Neurol* 1996;39:37–45.

29. Ben-Shlomo Y, Churchyard A, Head J, et al. Investigation by Parkinson's Disease Research Group of United Kingdom into excess mortality seen with combined levodopa and selegiline treatment in patients with early, mild Parkinson's disease: further results of randomised trial and confidential inquiry. *BMJ* 1998;316:1191–1196.

30. Counsell C. Effect of adding selegiline to levodopa in early, mild Parkinson's disease. *BMJ* 1998;17: 1586.

31. Thorogood M, Armstrong B, Nichols T, et al. Mortality in people taking selegiline: observational study. *BMJ* 1998;317:252–254.

32. Dupont E, Andersen A, Boas J, et al. Sustained-release Madopar HBS compared with standard Madopar in the long-term treatment of de novo Parkinsonian patients. *Acta Neurol Scand* 1996; 93:14–20.

33. Block G, Liss C, Reines S, Irr J, Nibbelink D, for the CR First Study Group. Comparison of immediate release and controlled release carbidopa/levodopa in Parkinson's disease. *Eur Neurol* 1997;37:23–47.

34. Ramaker C, van Hilten J. Bromocriptine versus levodopa in early Parkinson's disease. *Parkinson Related Disord* 1999;5(suppl):83. Search dates and primary sources not available.

35. Ramaker C, van Hilten J. Bromocriptine/levodopa versus levodopa in early Parkinson's disease. Parkinso Related Disord 1999;5(suppl):82. Search dates and primary sources not available.

36. Rascol O, Brooks D, Korczyn A, et al. Ropinirole reduces the risk of dyskinesia compared to L-dopa when used in early Parkinson's disease. *Parkinson Related Disord* 1999;5(suppl):83.

37. Rinne U. A 5-year double-blind study with cabergoline versus levodopa in the treatment of early Parkinson's disease. *Parkinson Related Disord* 1999;5(suppl):84.

38. Rinne U. Lisuride, a dopamine agonist in the treatment of early Parkinson's disease. *Neurology* 1989;39:336–339.

39. Fahn S. Parkinson's disease, the effect of levodopa and the ELLDOPA trial. *Arch Neurol* 1999;56:529–535.

40. Van Hilten J, Beek W, Finken M. Bromocriptine for levodopa-induced motor complications in Parkinson's disease. In: The Cochrane Library, Issue 4, 1999. Oxford: Update software. Search date January 1998; primary sources Cochrane Controlled Trials Register, Medline 1974–1998, Scisearch, pharmaceutical companies, experts for unpublished studies, and hand searched references.

41. Clarke C, Speller J. Lisuride for levodopa-induced complications in Parkinson's disease. In: The Cochrane Library, Issue 4, 1999. Oxford: Update software. Search date November 1998; primary sources Medline, Embase, Cochrane Controlled Trials Register, pharmaceutical companies, and hand searched references.

42. Clarke C, Speller J. Pergolide for levodopa-induced complications in Parkinson's disease. In: The Cochrane Library, Issue 4, 1999. Oxford: Update software. Search date January 1999; primary sources Medline, Embase, Cochrane Controlled Trials Register, pharmaceutical companies, and hand searched references.

43. Clarke C, Speller J. Pramipexole for levodopa-induced motor complications in Parkinson's disease. *Parkinsonism and Related Disorders* 1999;5(suppl):71. Search date March 1999; primary sources Medline, Embase, Cochrane Controlled Trials Register, pharmaceutical companies, and hand searched references.

44. Lieberman A, Olanow C, Sethi K, et al. A multicentre trial of ropinirole as adjunct treatment

for Parkinson's disease. *Neurology* 1998;51: 1057–1062.

45. Hutton JT, Koller WC, Ahlskog JE, et al. Multicenter, placebo-controlled trial of cabergoline taken once daily in the treatment of Parkinson's disease. *Neurology* 1996;46:1062–1065.

46. Clarke C, Speller J. Pergolide versus bromocriptine for levodopa-induced motor complications in Parkinson's disease. In: The Cochrane Library, Issue 4, 1999. Oxford: Update software. Search date 1998; primary sources Medline 1966– December 1997, Embase, Cochrane Controlled Trials Register (Issue 4, 1997), pharmaceuticals companies, and hand searched references.

47. Gregory R. Posteroventral pallidotomy for advanced Parkinson's disease: a systematic review. *Neurology Reviews International* 1999; 3(1):8–12.

48. Development and Evaluation Committee. Report 105. *Pallidotomy, thalotomy and deep brain stimulation for severe Parkinson's disease.* Southampton: Wessex Institute for Health Research and Development, 1999. Search date September 1999; primary sources Cochrane Library 1999; Health Technology Assessment database July 1999; Medline 1966 to June 1999; Science Citation Index January 1999 to September 1999; BIOSIS September 1999; Embase 1980 to May 1999; Index to Scientific and Technical Proceedings August 1999 September 1999; Inspec January 1999 to September 1999; Best Evidence 1999.

49. Vitek J, Bakay R, Freeman A, et al. Randomised clinical trial of pallidotomy for Parkinson's disease. *Neurology* 1998; 50(4[suppl 4]):A80.

50. De Bie R, de Haan R, Nijssen P, et al. Unilateral pallidotomy in Parkinson's disease: a randomised, single-blind, multicentre trial. *Lancet* 1999;354: 1665–1669.

51. Schmand B, de Bie R, Koning-Haanstra M, et al. Unilateral pallidotomy in PD. A controlled study of cognitive and behavioural effects. *Neurology* 2000;54:1058–64.

52. Vitek J, Bakay R, Freeman A, et al. Randomised clinical trial of pallidotomy versus medical therapy for Parkinson's disease (abstract). *Mov Disord* 1998;13(suppl 2):266.

53. Bronstein JM, DeSalles A, DeLong MR. Sterotactic pallidotomy in the treatment of Parkinson's disease. *Arch Neurol* 1999;56:1064–1069.

54. Merello M, Nouzeilles MI, Kuzis G, et al. Unilateral radiofrequency lesion versus electrostimulation of posteroventral pallidum: a prospective randomized comparison. *Mov Disord* 1999;14:50–56.

A Moore
Senior Lecturer in Neurology
University of Liverpool
Liverpool
UK

Carl Clarke
Reader in Clinical Neurology
University of Birmingham
Birmingham
UK

Competing interests: AM and CC have been paid by various manufacturers of the drugs dealt with above for speaking at meetings and attending conferences.

Aphthous ulcers: recurrent

Updated this issue

Stephen Porter and Crispian Scully

INTERVENTIONS

Likely to be beneficial
Chlorhexidine (but no effect on
  recurrence rates).........748

Unknown effectiveness
Topical corticosteroids.......747

Unlikely to be beneficial
Hexidine................748

To be covered in future issues of
  Clinical Evidence
Other drug treatments
Low intensity ultrasound
Novel toothpastes
Barrier techniques
Laser

Key Messages

- Nine small RCTs found no consistent effect of topical corticosteroids on the incidence of new ulcers, compared with control preparations. They found weak evidence that topical corticosteroids may reduce duration of ulcers and hasten pain relief without causing notable local or systemic adverse effects.

- RCTs have found that chlorhexidine gluconate mouth rinses may reduce the duration and severity of each episode of ulceration, but do not effect the incidence of recurrent ulceration.

- Single RCTs provide no evidence of benefit from hexidine mouthwash or from a proprietary antiseptic mouthwash compared with control mouthwashes.

DEFINITION	Recurrent aphthous ulcers are superficial and rounded, with painful mouth ulcers usually occurring in recurrent bouts at intervals of a few days to a few months.[1]
INCIDENCE/ PREVALENCE	The point prevalence of recurrent aphthous ulcers in Swedish adults has been reported as 2%.[1] Prevalence may be 5–10% of some groups of children. Up to 66% of young adults give a history consistent with recurrent aphthous ulceration.[1]
AETIOLOGY/ RISK FACTORS	The causes of aphthous ulcers remain unknown. Associations with haematinic deficiency, infections, gluten sensitive enteropathy, food sensitivities, and psychological stress have rarely been confirmed. Similar ulcers are seen in Behçet's syndrome.
PROGNOSIS	About 80% of people with recurrent aphthous ulcers develop a few ulcers smaller than 1 cm in diameter that heal within 5–14 days without scarring (the pattern known as minor aphthous ulceration). The episodes recur typically after an interval of 1–4 months. One in 10 sufferers has a more severe form (major aphthous ulceration) with lesions larger than 1 cm that may recur after a shorter interval and can cause scarring. Likewise perhaps one in 10 people with such recurrent ulceration may have multiple minute ulcers (herpetiform ulceration).
AIMS	To reduce pain, frequency, and duration of ulceration, with minimal adverse effects.
OUTCOMES	Number of new ulcers appearing within a specified period, usually 4–8 weeks; ulcer day index (the sum of the number of ulcers each day over a period, usually 4–8 weeks, which indicates the severity of the episode and reflects the mean prevalence and duration of ulcers); symptom score based on subjective pain severity recorded in categories on a questionnaire (e.g. from 0 to 3, ranging from no pain to severe pain) or on a 10 cm visual analogue scale; mean duration of individual ulcers (difficult to determine because of uncertainty in detecting the point of complete resolution); number of ulcer free days during a specified period; preference of people for one treatment over another. Diameter of lesions is a proxy measure of these clinical outcomes.
METHODS	*Clinical Evidence* update search and appraisal May 2000.

QUESTION	What are the effects of treatments for recurrent aphthous ulcers?

OPTION	TOPICAL CORTICOSTEROIDS

Nine small RCTs found no consistent effect of topical corticosteroids on the incidence of new ulcers compared with control preparations. They found weak evidence that topical corticosteroids may reduce duration of ulcers and hasten pain relief without causing notable local or systemic adverse effects.

Benefits: We found no systematic review but found nine RCTs of corticosteroids versus placebo that reported relevant clinical outcomes in the management of recurrent aphthous ulcers.[2–9] Overall, one trial found larger effect sizes than the others.[2] **Incidence of new**

ulcers: Five randomised crossover trials (102 people) found inconsistent effects on the incidence of new ulcers (see table 1, p 751). **Ulcer duration:** Six RCTs reported data on ulcer duration, but the data were not presented in comparable forms.[3,4,6–9] Four trials reported the mean duration of ulcers, and no consistent effect was seen (see table 1, p 751). One RCT found that more people using topical steroid had a mean ulcer duration below 6 days (25/33 [76%] with topical steroid v 14/30 [47%] with control preparations; ARI 29%, 95% CI 5% to 43%; RRI 45%, 95% CI 19% to 91%; NNT 3, 95% CI 2 to 20).[6] One crossover trial found that 13 out of 15 people had shorter mean duration with topical steroid than with the control preparation.[8] **Ulcer days index:** Four trials found that topical steroids reduced the number of ulcer days compared with control; the reduction was significant in two of the trials (see table 1, p 751).[2,4,5,7] **Symptom scores:** Four trials reported symptom scores with topical steroids versus control, but all four presented their results in different ways.[6–9] One found that more people using steroids had symptom relief compared with those using a control preparation (29/33 v 18/30; ARI 27%, 95% CI 5% to 43%; RRI 46%, 95% CI 19% to 91%; NNT 4, 95% CI 2 to 20).[6] One crossover trial found that symptom scores were lower with topical steroids than the control preparation (2.77 v 3.54), but the results were not significantly different.[7] Another crossover trial found that 11 out of 15 people had lower pain scores while using topical steroid than while using the control preparation.[8] One further crossover trial found that the pain score fell with time whether using topical steroids or control applications, but that the rate of fall was significantly faster when using topical steroids.[9] **User preference:** Two crossover trials found that more users preferred topical steroids than control preparations (20/26 in one study[4] and 10/17 in the other[6]).

Harms:
The nine trials reported no serious adverse effects. Long term use of corticosteroid mouth rinses was occasionally associated with oral candidiasis (rate not specified). Limited studies of adrenal function found no evidence that 0.05% fluocinonide in adhesive paste and betamethasone-17-valerate mouth rinse caused adrenal suppression.[8,10] One RCT reported adrenal suppression in one man using betamethasone disodium phosphate.[5]

Comment:
The trials differed in many ways: selection of people, type of topical corticosteroid and formulation used, control preparation used (although this was usually a base without topical steroid), duration of treatment, reported outcomes, and design (double or single blind, parallel group or crossover, use of washout period or not). Withdrawal rates were high. Most people in the trials had more severe ulceration than the average person with recurrent aphthous ulceration.

OPTION   CHLORHEXIDINE AND SIMILAR AGENTS

RCTs have found that chlorhexidine gluconate mouth rinses may reduce the duration and severity of each episode of ulceration, but did not effect the incidence of recurrent ulceration. Single RCTs found no significant benefit from hexidine mouthwash or a proprietary antiseptic mouthwash compared with control mouthwashes.

Benefits: We found no systematic review but found five RCTs of chlorhexidine gluconate or similar preparations versus assumed inactive control preparations in 203 people with recurrent aphthous ulceration.[11-15] Four of the RCTs used a crossover design with randomised sequence comparing a control preparation versus 1% chlorhexidine gel,[11] 0.2% chlorhexidine gel,[12] 0.2% chlorhexidine mouthwash,[13] or 0.1% hexetidine mouthwash.[14] One trial was a parallel group RCT of a proprietary antiseptic rinse versus a hydroalcoholic control.[15] **Incidence of ulceration:** All trials reported the number of ulcers as either the total number of ulcers or the number of new ulcers with each treatment (see table 1, p 751). Only one of the five trials found significantly fewer ulcers with active treatment.[13] Three trials noted that the number of ulcers fell during the course of the study, irrespective of the treatment received.[13-15] The crossover trial that found a significant difference in numbers of ulcers did not overtly account for this effect: data were available from only 12 out of 26 people who were recruited, and it is not clear if there was a balanced sequencing of active and placebo treatments among these people. **Duration of ulceration:** The mean duration of individual ulcers was reported in four of the RCTs (see table 1, p 751). The mean duration of individual ulcers was reduced by active treatment in all four trials, but the difference was significant in only one trial and the mean difference was less than 1 day in the others. **Ulcer days index:** Three RCTs reported the ulcer days index. Both studies of chlorhexidine versus control found significant reduction in the ulcer day index. One trial found that chlorhexidine significantly increased the number of ulcer free days compared with an inert preparation, from a mean of 17.5 to 22.9 over 6 weeks — an extra 5.4 ulcer free days per 6 weeks of treatment.[13] Another RCT found that hexidine had no significant effect.[14] **Severity of pain:** All five RCTs reported severity scores (see table 1, p 751). Two trials found that chlorhexidine significantly reduced the mean severity of pain compared with an inert preparation.[11] One RCT of a proprietary antiseptic mouthwash versus the alcohol containing control preparation found no difference between the treatment groups, but found a large improvement in clinical outcomes in both groups compared with baseline levels.[15] The evidence relating to other antibacterial agents such as triclosan will be reviewed in future issues of *Clinical Evidence*.

Harms: The RCTs reported few adverse events. Chlorhexidine had a bitter taste and was associated with brown staining of teeth and tongue, and with nausea.[12]

Comment: Four of the RCTs used a crossover design. A consistent observation was that outcomes improved during the course of the trials irrespective of the treatment received. One of the studies did not make clear if the effect of sequencing had been allowed for.[12] The withdrawal rates in the crossover trials were high. The parallel group trial had fewer withdrawals; 106 people with recurrent aphthous ulceration were recruited and 96 completed the study. Analysis was not by intention to treat and the method of randomisation was not specified.[15] People recruited to the trials might not be typical of the average person with recurrent aphthous ulceration.

Oral health

REFERENCES

1. Porter SR, Scully C, Pedersen A. Recurrent aphthous stomatitis. *Crit Rev Oral Biol Med* 1998; 9:306–321.
2. Cooke BED, Armitage P. Recurrent Mikulicz's aphthae treatment with topical hydrocortisone hemisuccinate sodium. *BMJ* 1960;1:764–766.
3. Walter T, McFall JR. Effect of flurandrenolone on oral aphthae. *J Periodontol* 1968;39:364–365.
4. Browne RM, Fox EC, Anderson RJ. Topical triamcinolone acetonide in recurrent aphthous stomatitis. *Lancet* 1968;1:565–567.
5. MacPhee IT, Sircus W, Farmer ED, Harkness RA, Cowley GC. Use of steroids in treatment of aphthous ulceration. *BMJ* 1968;2:147–149.
6. Merchant HW, Gangarosa LP, Glassman AB, Sobel RE. Betamethasone-17-benzoate in the treatment of recurrent aphthous ulcers. *Oral Surg Oral Med Oral Pathol* 1978;45:870–875.
7. Pimlott SJ, Walker DM. A controlled clinical trial efficacy of topically applied fluocinonide in the treatment of recurrent aphthous ulceration. *Br Dent J* 1983;154:174–177.
8. Thompson AC, Nolan A, Lamey P-J. Minor aphthous oral ulceration: a double-blind cross-over study of beclomethasone diproprionate aerosol spray. *Scot Med J* 1989;34:531–532.
9. Miles DA, Bricker SL, Razmus TF, Potter RH. Triamcinolone acetonide versus chlorhexidine for treatment of recurrent stomatitis. *Oral Surg Oral Med Oral Pathol* 1993;75:397–402.
10. Lehner T, Lyne C. Adrenal function during topical oral corticosteroid treatment. *BMJ* 1969;4:138–141.
11. Addy M, Carpenter R, Roberts WR. Management of recurrent aphthous ulceration – a trial of chlorhexidine gluconate gel. *Br Dent J* 1976;141:118–120.
12. Addy M. Hibitane in the treatment of recurrent aphthous ulceration. *J Clin Periodontol* 1977;4:108–116.
13. Hunter L, Addy M. Chlorhexidine gluconate mouthwash in the management of minor aphthous stomatitis. *Br Dent J* 1987;162:106–110.
14. Chadwick B, Addy M, Walker DM. Hexetidine mouthrinse in the management of minor aphthous ulceration and as an adjunct to oral hygiene. *Br Dent J* 1991;171:83.
15. Meiller TF, Kutcher MJ, Overholser CD, Niehaus C, DePaola LG, Siegel MA. Effect of an antimicrobial mouthrinse on recurrent aphthous ulcerations. *Oral Surg Oral Med Oral Pathol* 1991;72:425–429.

Stephen Porter
Professor of Oral Medicine

Crispian Scully
Professor

Eastman Dental Institute for Oral Health
Care Sciences
University College London
London
UK

Competing interests: None declared.

TABLE 1 Effects of treatments on different outcomes: results of RCTs (see text, p 748).

Intervention	Study	Number	Treatment duration (weeks)	Outcomes Treatment	Outcomes Control	Effect (%)* (significance)
Incidence new ulcers (ulcers per week): topical corticosteroids versus inert preparations	2	17	8	0.51	1.15	−55% (P < 0.05)
	4	26	8	0.84	0.94	−11% (NS)
	5 pilot	8	4	2.07	1.85	+12% (NS)
	5 main	31†	4	0.73	0.82	−11% (NS)
	5	20	6	1.27	1.92	+6% (NS)
Mean ulcer duration (days): topical corticosteroids versus inert preparations	3	50	Until complete healing	6	6	0% (NS)
	4	26	8	8.07	8.94	−10% (NS)
	7	20	6	4.93	7.83	−37% (P < 0.001)
	9	19	12	5.93	5.92	0% (NS)
Ulcer days index: topical corticosteroids versus inert preparations	2	17	8	26.3	65.9	−60% (P < 0.01)
	4	26	8	58.3	71.3	−18% (NS)
	5 main	25	4	24.0	30.7	−22% (NS)
	7	20	6	48.3	70.6	−32% (P < 0.05)

TABLE 1 continued

Intervention	Study	Number	Treatment duration (weeks)	Outcomes		Effect (%)* (significance)
				Treatment	Control	
Number of ulcers (ulcers/person/week): antiseptic versus presumed inert preparations	11	20	5	1.04	1.40	NS
	12	12	5	0.6	1.02	P < 0.05
	13	38	6	1.26	1.38	NS
	14	37	6	1.48	1.39	NS
	15	96	26	0.09	0.13	NS
Mean duration of ulcers (days): topical antibacterial versus inert preparation	11	20	5	4.8	7.8	P < 0.01
	13	38	6	5.02	5.78	NS
	14	37	6	6.64	6.80	NS
	15	96	26	Median fall in ulcer duration from start of trial 2.42 days	Median fall in ulcer duration from start of trial 1.58 days	NS
Ulcer days index: topical antibacterial versus inert preparations	12	12	5	9.5	17	P < 0.05
	13	38	6	42.8	52.3	P < 0.05
	14	37	6	79.7	65.7	NS

†Each participant received one treatment for 4 weeks, a blank month, then another treatment with another drug. The trial compared an inert base, two local steroids and two other preparations. The figures given here are those during treatment with local steroids, and with the inert base.
*Defined as difference between outcome measures for control and treatment, expressed as a fraction of the control; NS, not significant.

Burning mouth syndrome

Updated this issue

John Buchanan and Joanna Zakrzewska

QUESTIONS
Effects of treatments. 755

INTERVENTIONS

Beneficial
Cognitive behavioural therapy. .755

Unknown effectiveness
Hormone replacement therapy in
    postmenopausal women. . . .755
Vitamin B replacement or
    supplementation 755

Antidepressants 756
Benzydamine hypochloride. . . .756
Subsequent issues
Atypical facial pain

Key Messages

- We found insufficient evidence about the effects of any treatment for people with burning mouth syndrome.
- One small RCT found that cognitive behavioural therapy reduced symptom intensity.

© *Clinical Evidence* 2000;4:753–757.

DEFINITION Burning mouth syndrome is a psychogenic or idiopathic burning discomfort or pain affecting people with clinically normal oral mucosa in whom a medical or dental cause has been excluded.[1–3] Terms previously used to describe what is now called burning mouth syndrome include glossodynia, glossopyrosis, stomatodynia, stomatopyrosis, sore tongue, and oral dysaesthesia.[4] A survey of 669 men and 758 women randomly selected from 48 500 people aged between 20 and 69 years found that people with burning mouth also have subjective dryness (66%), take some form of medication (64%), report other systemic illnesses (57%), and have altered taste (11%).[5] Many studies of people with symptoms of burning mouth do not distinguish those with burning mouth syndrome (i.e. idiopathic disease) from those with other conditions (such as vitamin B deficiency), making results unreliable.

INCIDENCE/ PREVALENCE Incidence and prevalence vary according to diagnostic criteria.[4] A recent population based study found a prevalence of 3.7% (men 1.6%, mean age 59 years; women 5.5%, mean age 57 years). The prevalence was highest in women aged 60–69 years (12%).[5] Reported prevalence in general populations varies from 15%[6] to 0.7%[7] and mostly relates to the symptom of burning mouth rather than to burning mouth syndrome as defined above. Most studies suggest that burning mouth syndrome mainly affects women,[6,8,9] particularly after the menopause, when its prevalence may increase to 18–33%.[10]

AETIOLOGY/ RISK FACTORS The cause is unknown, and we found no good aetiological studies. Hormonal disturbances associated with the menopause[8–10] and psychogenic factors (including anxiety, depression, stress, life events, personality disorders, and phobia of cancer) are possible causal factors.[11–13] Local and systemic factors (such as infections, allergies, ill fitting dentures,[12] hypersensitivity reactions,[14] and hormone and vitamin deficiencies[15–17]) may cause the symptom of burning mouth and should be excluded before diagnosing burning mouth syndrome.

PROGNOSIS We found no prospective cohort studies or other reliable evidence describing the natural history of burning mouth syndrome.[18] We found anecdotal reports of at least partial spontaneous remission in about half of people with burning mouth syndrome within 6–7 years.[12]

AIMS To alleviate symptoms, with minimal adverse effects.

OUTCOMES Self reported relief of symptoms (burning mouth, altered taste, xerostomia); incidence and severity of anxiety and depression; quality of life using a validated ordinal scale.

METHODS *Clinical Evidence* update search and appraisal May 2000, using the terms burning mouth, burning mouth syndrome, dysaesthesia or dysesthesia, stomatodynia or glossopyrosis, sore tongue, glossodynia or glossalgia.

OPTION   COGNITIVE BEHAVIOURAL THERAPY

One small RCT found that cognitive behavioural therapy relieved symptoms.

Benefits:	We found no systematic review. We found one small, attention controlled RCT in 30 people with resistant burning mouth syndrome.[19] This trial found that 12–15 sessions of cognitive behavioural therapy for 1 hour per week significantly reduced intensity of symptoms from baseline, as measured on a visual analogue scale, compared with no effect in the control group. The difference remained at 6 month follow up (mean pretreatment score 5.0 v 4.3 on placebo; mean score 6 months after treatment 1.4 v 4.7 on placebo, 4 versus 0 people symptom free).
Harms:	The trial gave no information on adverse effects.[19]
Comment:	The trial was small and individual characteristics of the two groups were not described, so the groups may not have been comparable. The visual analogue scale for assessing oral burning was not validated.[19]

OPTION   HORMONE REPLACEMENT THERAPY IN POSTMENOPAUSAL WOMEN

We found insufficient evidence on the effects of hormone replacement therapy in postmenopausal women with burning mouth syndrome.

Benefits:	We found no systematic review and no RCTs of sufficient quality.
Harms:	Adverse effects of hormone replacement therapy are well documented (see oestrogen under menopausal symptoms, p 1091).
Comment:	We found three non-randomised intervention studies with no clear diagnostic criteria or outcome measures.[20–22]

OPTION   VITAMIN B REPLACEMENT OR SUPPLEMENTATION

We found no reliable evidence about the effects of vitamin B supplementation in people with burning mouth with or without vitamin B deficiency.

Benefits:	We found no systematic reviews or RCTs, either in people with burning mouth syndrome, or in people with vitamin B deficiency and symptoms of burning mouth (see comment below).
Harms:	We found no reliable evidence.
Comment:	People with vitamin B group deficiencies and symptoms of burning mouth should no longer be classified as having burning mouth syndrome (see definition, p 754). One case control study in 70 people found that people with symptoms of burning mouth were more likely to have vitamin B deficiency (28/70 v 6/80).[16] One study of 16 people with vitamin deficiencies given vitamins or placebo found no improvement.[17]

| OPTION | ANTIDEPRESSANTS |

We found insufficient evidence on the effects of antidepressants in people with burning mouth syndrome.

Benefits: We found no systematic review. **Clomipramine and mianserin:** We found one short term RCT comparing clomipramine versus mianserin versus placebo for 6 weeks in 253 people with chronic idiopathic pain syndrome, including 77 people with burning mouth syndrome.[23] After 6 weeks, there was no significant improvement in any group. **Trazodone:** One double blind RCT compared trazodone (200 mg/day) versus placebo in 37 women with burning mouth syndrome.[24] After 8 weeks there was no significant difference in pain or related symptoms between groups: mean pain on a visual analogue scale decreased in both the trazodone group (from 59.2 to 45.3 at 8 weeks) and the placebo group (from 46.6 to 34.3).

Harms: The first RCT did not report on adverse effects.[23] Adverse effects caused 7/18 people taking trazodone to withdraw from the trial compared with 2/19 taking placebo. Adverse effects reported with trazodone were dizziness (11 people) and drowsiness (9 people).[24] Adverse effects of clomipramine, mianserin, and other antidepressants are well documented.

Comment: The trial of clomipramine and mianserin versus placebo was too small to exclude an effect of treatment, did not use adequate diagnostic criteria, was of short duration, and had limited follow up.[23] It therefore does not provide sufficient evidence to determine the role of antidepressants in treating burning mouth syndrome. Although the trial of trazodone versus placebo was well conducted and used several pertinent outcome measures, including psychological ones, it was too small and short term to detect clinically important effects.[24] The widespread use of antidepressants in burning mouth syndrome may be due to their effects on neuropathic pain[25] and the association of burning mouth syndrome with generalised anxiety disorder, depression, and adverse life events.[26]

| OPTION | BENZYDAMINE HYPOCHLORIDE | New |

New

We found insufficient evidence on the effects of benzydamine hypochloride in burning mouth syndrome.

Benefits: We found no systematic review. We found one small RCT, which compared benzydamine hypochloride (15 ml of 0.15%, for 1 minute 3 times daily for 4 weeks) versus placebo versus no treatment in 30 people with burning mouth syndrome.[27] The trial found no significant difference among groups for symptoms (using visual analogue scale 0 to 8, where 0 = no symptoms and 8 = severe burning sensation), but the power of the trial was too low to rule out a clinical difference.

Harms: No adverse effects were reported.

Comment: Inclusion criteria were well defined. The trial was incompletely blinded, because the third group received no treatment.

REFERENCES

1. Fox H. Burning tongue glossodynia. *N Y State J Med* 1935;35:881–884.
2. Zakrzewska JM. The burning mouth syndrome remains an enigma. *Pain* 1995;62:253–257.
3. van der Waal I. *The burning mouth syndrome.* 1st ed. Copenhagen: Munksgaard, 1990.
4. Merksey H, Bogduk N, eds. *Classification of chronic pain.* 2nd ed. Seattle: International Association for the Study of Pain Press, 1994.
5. Bergdahl M, Bergdahl J. Burning mouth syndrome: prevalence and associated factors. *J Oral Pathol Med* 1999 Sep;28:350–354.
6. Tammiala-Salonen T, Hiidenkarii T, Parvinen T. Burning mouth in a Finnish adult population. *Community Dent Oral Epidemiol* 1993;21:67–71.
7. Lipton JA, Ship JA, Larach-Robinson D. Estimated prevalence and distribution of reported orofacial pain in the United States. *J Am Dent Assoc* 1993; 124:115–121.
8. Basker RM, Sturdee DW, Davenport JC. Patients with burning mouths. A clinical investigation of causative factors, including the climacteric and diabetes. *Br Dent J* 1978;145:9–16.
9. Grushka M. Clinical features of burning mouth syndrome. *Oral Surg Oral Med Oral Pathol Oral Radiol Endod* 1987;63:30–36.
10. Wardrop RW, Hailes J, Burger H, Reade PC. Oral discomfort at the menopause. *Oral Surg Oral Med Oral Pathol Oral Radiol Endod* 1989;67:535–540.
11. Rojo L, Silvestre FJ, Bagan JV, De Vicente T. Psychiatric morbidity in burning mouth syndrome. Psychiatric interview versus depression and anxiety scales. *Oral Surg Oral Med Oral Pathol Oral Radiol Endod* 1993;75:308–311.
12. Grushka M, Sessle BJ. Burning mouth syndrome. *Dent Clin North Am* 1991;35:171–184.
13. Lamey PJ, Lamb AB. The usefulness of the HAD scale in assessing anxiety in patients with burning mouth syndrome. *Oral Surg Oral Med Oral Pathol* 1989;67:390–392.
14. Bergdahl J, Anneroth G, Anneroth I. Clinical study of patients with burning mouth. *Scad J Dent Res* 1994; 102:299–305.
15. Maragou P, Ivanyi L. Serum zinc levels in patients with burning mouth syndrome. *Oral Surg Oral Med Oral Pathol* 1991;71:447–450.
16. Lamey PJ, Allam BF. Vitamin status of patients with burning mouth syndrome and the response to replacement therapy. *Br Dent J* 1986;168:81–84.
17. Hugoson A, Thorstensson B. Vitamin B status and response to replacement therapy in patients with burning mouth syndrome. *Acta Odontol Scand* 1991;49:367–375.
18. Zakrzewska JM, Hamlyn PJ. Facial pain. In: Crombie IK, Croft PR, Linton SJ, Le Resche L, Von Korff M. *Epidemiology of pain.* Seattle: International Association for the Study of Pain Press, 1999:177–202.
19. Bergdahl J, Anneroth G, Perris H. Cognitive therapy in the treatment of patients with burning mouth syndrome: a controlled study. *J Oral Pathol Med* 1995;24:213–215.
20. Pisanty S, Rafaely B, Polshuk WZ. The effects of steroid hormones on buccal mucosa of menopausal women. *Oral Surg Oral Med Oral Pathol Oral Radiol Endod* 1975;40:346–353.
21. Ferguson MM, Boyle P, Hart D McK, Lindsay R. Oral complaints related to climacteric symptoms in oophorectomized women. *J R Soc Med* 1981;74: 492–497.
22. Forabosco A, Crisculo M, Coukos G, et al. Efficacy of hormone replacement therapy in postmenopausal women with oral discomfort. *Oral Surg Oral Med Oral Pathol Oral Radiol Endod* 1992;73:570–574.
23. Loldrup D, Langemark M, Hansen HJ, Olesen J, Bech P. Clomipramine and mianserin in chronic idiopathic pain syndrome. A placebo controlled study. *Psychopharmacology* 1989;99:1–7.
24. Tammiala-Salonen T, Forssell H. Trazodone in burning mouth pain: placebo-controlled, double-blind study. *J Orofac Pain* 1999;13:83–88.
25. McQuay HJ, Tramer M, Nye BA, Carroll D, Wiffen PJ, Moore RA. A systematic review of antidepressants in neuropathic pain. *Pain* 1996; 68:217–227.
26. Bogetto F, Maina G, Ferro G, Carbone M, Gandolfo S. Psychiatric comorbidity in patients with burning mouth syndrome. *Psychosom Med* 1998;60:378–385.
27. Sardella A, Uglietti D, Demarosi F, Lodi G, Bez C, Carrassi A. Benzydamine hypochloride oral rinses in management of burning mouth syndrome. A clinical trial. *Oral Surg Oral Med Oral Pathol Oral Radiol Endod* 1999;88:683–686.

John Buchanan
Clinical Lecturer in Oral Medicine

Joanna Zakrzewska
Senior Lecturer/Honorary Consultant in Oral Medicine

St Bartholomew's and The Royal London
School of Medicine and Dentistry
London
UK

Competing interests: None declared.

Impacted wisdom teeth

Updated this issue

Stephen Worrall

QUESTIONS

INTERVENTIONS

Likely to be ineffective or harmful

Key Messages

- We found limited evidence suggesting that harms of removing asymptomatic impacted wisdom teeth outweigh the benefits.

DEFINITION	Wisdom teeth are third molars that develop in almost all adults by about the age of 20. In some people, the teeth become partially or completely impacted below the gumline because of lack of space, obstruction, or abnormal position. Impacted wisdom teeth may be diagnosed because of pain and swelling, or incidentally by routine dental radiography.
INCIDENCE/ PREVALENCE	Third molar impaction is common. Over 72% of Swedish people aged 20–30 have at least one impacted lower third molar.[1] The surgical removal of impacted third molars (symptomatic and asymptomatic) is the most common procedure performed by oral and maxillofacial surgeons. It is performed on about 4/1000 people per year in England and Wales, making it one of the top ten inpatient and day case procedures.[2–4] Up to 90% of people on oral and maxillofacial surgery hospital waiting lists in the UK are awaiting removal of wisdom teeth.[3]
AETIOLOGY/ RISK FACTORS	Impacted wisdom teeth are partly a result of improved oral hygiene and changes in diet. Less gum disease and dental caries, and less wear and tear on teeth because of more refined diet, have increased the likelihood of retaining teeth into adult life, leaving less room for wisdom teeth.
PROGNOSIS	Impacted wisdom teeth can cause pain, swelling, and infection, as well as destroying adjacent teeth and bone. The removal of diseased and symptomatic wisdom teeth alleviates pain and improves oral health and function. We found no good data on what happens without treatment in people with asymptomatic impacted wisdom teeth.
AIMS	To reduce morbidity associated with impacted wisdom teeth with minimal adverse effects of treatments.
OUTCOMES	Pain; rates of infection; oral health and function.
METHODS	*Clinical Evidence* update search and appraisal May 2000.

QUESTION **Effects of prophylactic removal of impacted wisdom teeth**

We found no RCTs on the effects of prophylactic removal of asymptomatic impacted wisdom teeth. Non-randomised studies provide no evidence of benefit. Removal of lower wisdom teeth causes permanent numbness of the lower lip or tongue in about one in 200 people.

Benefits:
We found one systematic review (published in 1997), which identified 12 published reviews concerning the surgical removal of third molars.[5] No RCTs were found. There was no good evidence of benefit from the removal of impacted third molars that were free from disease. Two formal decision analyses also concluded that non-intervention was the optimal treatment for disease free, asymptomatic third molars.[6,7]

Harms:
Pain and swelling are almost universal after removing impacted wisdom teeth.[8,9] Removing lower wisdom teeth carries the risk of damage to the inferior alveolar nerve (injured in 1.3–7.8% of people,[10,11] permanently injured in 0.5–1%[12]), and to the lingual nerve (permanently injured in up to 0.8% of people[13]). The risks

appear to be greater with greater depth of impaction. The risks are the same whether the wisdom tooth is symptomatic or asymptomatic.

Comment: All studies identified in the review were of poor quality. It is likely to require an RCT with 10 years follow up to reliably answer the question. Anecdotal accounts and evidence from developing countries suggest that the answer would not be in favour of surgery.[5] Surgical morbidity following third molar removal increases with age. Where there are compelling reasons to remove them, it is prudent to do so in early adulthood.[14] Surgical morbidity is operator and technique sensitive.[15] A recently reported 20 year follow up including more than 2000 procedures reported no cases of permanent sensory lingual nerve disturbance.[15,16]

REFERENCES

1. Hugoson A, Kugelberg CF. The prevalence of third molars in a Swedish population. An epidemiological study. *Community Dent Health* 1988;5:121–138.
2. Mercier P, Precious D. Risks and benefits of removal of impacted third molars. *Int J Oral Maxillofac Surg* 1992;21:17–27.
3. Shepherd JP, Brickley M. Surgical removal of third molars. *BMJ* 1994;309:620–621.
4. Worrall SF, Riden K, Corrigan AM. UK National Third Molar project: the initial report. *Br J Oral Maxillofac Surg* 1998;36:14–18.
5. Song F, Landes DP, Glenny A-M, et al. Prophylactic removal of impacted third molars: an assessment of published reviews. *Br Dent J* 1997;182:339–346.
6. Tulloch JFC, Antczak AA, Wilkes JW. The application of decision analysis to evaluate the need for extraction of asymptomatic third molars. *J Oral Maxillofac Surg* 1987;45:855–863.
7. Brickley M, Kay E, Shepherd JP, et al. Decision analysis for lower third molar surgery. *Med Decis Making* 1995;15:143–151.
8. Bramley P. Sense about wisdoms? *J R Soc Med* 1981;74:867–868.
9. Capuzzi P, Montebugnoli L, Vaccaro MA. Extraction of impacted third molars. *Oral Surg Oral* 1994;77:341–343.
10. Schultze-Mosgau S, Reich RH. Assessment of inferior alveolar and lingual nerve disturbances after dentoalveolar surgery, and recovery of sensitivity. *Int J Oral Maxillofac Surg* 1993;22:214–217.
11. Rood JP. Permanent damage to inferior alveolar nerves during the removal of impacted mandibular third molars: comparison of two methods of bone removal. *Br Dent J* 1992;172:108–110.
12. Blackburn CW, Bramley PA. Lingual nerve damage associated with removal of lower third molars. *Br Dent J* 1989;167:103–107.
13. Robinson PP, Smith KG. Lingual nerve damage during lower third molar removal: a comparison of two surgical methods. *Br Dent J* 1996;180:456–461.
14. Bruce RA, Frederickson GC, Small GS. Age of patients and morbidity with mandibular third molar surgery. *J Am Dent Assoc* 1980;101:240–245.
15. Sisk AL, Hammer WB, Shelton DW, et al. Complications following removal of impacted third molars: the role of the experience of the surgeon. *J Oral Maxillofac Surg* 1986;44:855–859.
16. Moss CE , Wake MJC. Lingual access for third molar surgery: a 20-year retrospective audit. *Br J Oral Maxillofac Surg* 1999;37:255–258.

Stephen Worrall
Consultant Surgeon
St Luke's Hospital
Bedford
UK

Competing interests: None declared.

Updated this issue

Caroline Pankhurst

INTERVENTIONS

PREVENTION
Beneficial
Antifungal prophylaxis in advanced
HIV disease 769

Likely to be beneficial
Antifungal prophylaxis in
immunocompromised infants
and children 766

Unknown effectiveness
Chlorhexidine oral rinse in
neutropenic adults undergoing
treatment for cancer 765
Preventive interventions in
people with diabetes 767
Continuous prophylaxis versus
intermittent treatment in people
with HIV infection and acute
episodes of oropharyngeal
candidiasis (in terms of
preventing antifungal
resistance) 771

TREATMENT
Beneficial
Antifungal prophylaxis in
neutropenic adults undergoing
treatment for cancer 764
Antifungal treatment in
immunocompetent and
immunocompromised infants
and children 766
Oral suspension of systemic azoles
in people with HIV infection .770

Likely to be beneficial
Denture hygiene and removing
dentures while sleeping for
denture stomatitis 768
Oral polyenes for denture
stomatitis 768

Unknown effectiveness
Fluconazole versus amphotericin B
in adults undergoing
treatment for cancer 765
Treatments in people with
diabetes mellitus 767
Miconazole dental lacquer for
denture stomatitis 768

**To be covered in future issues of
*Clinical Evidence***
Treatment of systemic candidiasis
Prevention in people with dentures
Prevention and treatment in
neonates

In people receiving chemotherapy or radiotherapy

- One systematic review of RCTs has found that antifungal drugs prevent oropharyngeal candidiasis in neutropenic adults with cancer. RCTs have found that fluconazole is more effective than topical oral polyenes. Two RCTs found conflicting evidence of the preventive value of chlorhexidine versus placebo.
- Limited evidence from one small RCT suggests that fluconazole is more effective than amphotericin B lozenges for treatment of oropharyngeal candidiasis in people undergoing treatment for cancer.
- Two systematic reviews have found that antifungal drugs prevent oropharyngeal candidiasis in people with neutropenia and in people with cancer.

In infants and children

- One RCT has found that fluconazole is more effective than oral polyenes in prevention of oropharyngeal candidiasis in immunocompromised infants and children.
- Two RCTs have found that, in immunocompetent infants, miconazole gel is superior to nystatin suspension in the speed and effectiveness of treating oropharyngeal candidiasis. One RCT has found that fluconazole is more effective than oral polyenes in the treatment of oropharyngeal candidiasis in immunocompromised infants and children.

In people with diabetes mellitus

- We found no systematic reviews or RCTs on the prevention or treatment of oropharyngeal candidiasis in people with diabetes.

In people with denture stomatitis

- One small RCT found weak evidence that oral polyenes (nystatin, amphotericin B) were more effective than placebo at curing denture stomatitis. One RCT found no good evidence that miconazole dental lacquer benefits denture stomatitis. We found weak observational evidence that denture hygiene and not wearing dentures during sleep may cure denture stomatitis.

In people with HIV infection

- RCTs have found that daily or weekly antifungal prophylaxis with fluconazole or nystatin reduces the incidence of oropharyngeal candidiasis. Most absolute benefit was found in people with AIDS who had low CD4 cell counts ($\leq 200/mm^3$) and a history of recurrent oropharyngeal candidiasis.
- RCTs have found that topical preparations of itraconazole, fluconazole, and clotrimazole effectively treat oropharyngeal candidiasis in people with HIV infection. One RCT found that topical nystatin was inferior to fluconazole.
- RCTs have found daily or weekly antifungal prophylaxis with fluconazole, itraconazole, and nystatin reduce the incidence of oropharyngeal candidiasis.

Reducing risk of antifungal resistance

- One RCT in people with HIV infection and acute episodes of oropharyngeal candidiasis found no significant difference between continuous prophylaxis and intermittent treatment in terms of the emergence of antifungal resistance.

DEFINITION	Oropharyngeal candidiasis is an opportunistic mucosal infection, caused in over 85% of cases by *Candida albicans*. The four main types of oropharyngeal candidiasis are: (1) pseudomembranous (thrush), comprising white discrete plaques on an erythematous background, located on the buccal mucosa, throat, tongue, or gingivae; (2) erythematous, comprising smooth red patches on hard or soft palate, dorsum of tongue, or buccal mucosa; (3) hyperplastic, comprising white firmly adherent patches or plaques, usually bilateral on the buccal mucosa; (4) denture induced stomatitis, presenting as either a smooth or granular erythema confined to the denture bearing area of the hard palate. Symptoms vary, ranging from none to a sore, painful mouth with a burning tongue and altered taste, which can impair speech, nutritional intake, and quality of life.
INCIDENCE/ PREVALENCE	Candida species are commensals in the gastrointestinal tract. Transmission occurs directly between infected people or on fomites. Candida is found in the mouth of 31–60% of healthy people.[1] Denture stomatitis associated with Candida is prevalent in 65% of denture wearers.[1] Oropharyngeal candidiasis affects 15–60% of people with haematological or oncological malignancies during periods of immunosuppression.[2] Oropharyngeal candidiasis occurs in 7–48% of people with HIV infection and in over 90% of those with advanced disease. In severely immunosuppressed people, relapse rates are high (30–50%) and usually occur within 14 days of treatment cessation.[3]
AETIOLOGY/ RISK FACTORS	Risk factors associated with symptomatic oropharyngeal candidiasis include local or systemic immunosuppression, haematological disorders, broad spectrum antibiotic use, inhaled or systemic steroids, xerostomia, diabetes, and wearing dentures, obturators, or orthodontic appliances. The same strain may persist for months or years in the absence of infection. In people with HIV infection there is no direct correlation between the number of organisms and the presence of clinical disease. Symptomatic oropharyngeal candidiasis associated with in vitro resistance to fluconazole occurs in 5% of people with advanced HIV disease.[4] Resistance to azole antifungals is associated with severe immunosuppression (≤ 50 CD4 cell/ mm^3), more episodes treated with antifungal drugs, and longer median duration of systemic azole treatment.[5]
PROGNOSIS	Untreated candidiasis persists for months or years unless associated risk factors are treated or eliminated. In neonates, spontaneous cure of oropharyngeal candidiasis usually occurs after 3–8 weeks.
AIMS	To resolve signs and symptoms of oropharyngeal candidiasis; to prevent or delay relapse in immunocompromised people; and to minimise drug induced resistance, with minimum adverse effects.
OUTCOMES	Resolution of signs and symptoms; rate of recurrence on the basis of scoring of signs and symptoms. Many RCTs report the results of mycological culture but, whenever possible, this review has not used these intermediate outcomes because the relation between the clinical and mycological culture findings is uncertain.

METHODS *Clinical Evidence* update search and appraisal May 2000, supplemented by a literature search of Medline and the author's library, selecting publications in English, from 1975–1999. We included only systematic reviews and RCTs that specified oropharyngeal candidiasis in the protocol design and outcome measurements; those dealing with oesophagitis and invasive, systemic candidal infections were excluded.

QUESTION **What are the effects of interventions to prevent and treat oropharyngeal candidiasis in people receiving chemotherapy or radiotherapy?**

OPTION **ANTIFUNGAL PROPHYLAXIS**

Two systematic reviews of RCTs have found that antifungal drugs prevent oropharyngeal candidiasis in neutropenic adults and cancer patients undergoing treatment. RCTs have found that fluconazole is more effective than topical oral polyenes. Two RCTs found conflicting evidence of the value of chlorhexidine oral rinse.

Benefits: We found two systematic reviews.[6,7] The earlier review (search date 1991, 9 RCTs, n = 710) compared systemic or topical antifungal agents with placebo in the prevention of oropharyngeal candidiasis in people with cancer and neutropenia.[6] Participants were immunosuppressed; they were not selected according to their fungal colonisation status before initiation of treatment. Treatments included amphotericin B, clotrimazole, miconazole, ketoconazole, fluconazole, and itraconazole. The duration of the prophylaxis was not stated in the review. No eligible RCTs of nystatin were identified. Continuing colonisation of the throat after starting treatment was found to be a risk factor for development of oropharyngeal candidiasis (OR 3.66, 95% CI 1.74 to 5.18). Compared with placebo, antifungal drugs reduced the number of episodes of oropharyngeal candidiasis (AR 17/372 [5%] with antifungal v 109/338 [32%] with placebo; ARR 26%, 95% CI 23% to 28%; OR 0.15, 95% CI 0.10 to 0.22; NNT 4). Subgroup analysis for clotrimazole or fluconazole versus placebo was consistent with the global result. The second review (search date 1999, 15 RCTs, n = 1164) compared 3–10 weeks of oral and topical prophylaxis with placebo or no treatment in people of all ages with cancer (excluding people with head and neck cancer) who were receiving chemotherapy. The review found significant reduction of oral candidiasis compared with placebo or no treatment for drugs that were partially absorbed from the gastrointestinal tract (miconazole, clotrimazole: RR 0.13, 95% CI 0.06 to 0.27; NNT3, 95% CI 3 to 5) and for fully absorbed drugs (fluconazole, itraconazole and metoconazole: RR 0.36, 95% CI 0.19 to 0.69) but not for unabsorbed drugs (nystatin, amphotericin B, natamycin, chlorhexidine: RR 0.81, 95% CI 0.58 to 1.12).[7]
Azoles versus polyenes: We found no systematic review but found three RCTs (see table 1, p 774).[7–10] One multicentre RCT compared prophylaxis for 30 days with fluconazole 50 mg daily with the oral polyenes amphotericin B (2 g/day), nystatin (4 x 106 units/day), or both, for the prevention of oropharyngeal candidiasis and invasive fungal infection.[8] It included 536 people with cancer and neutro-

penia associated with chemotherapy, radiotherapy, or bone marrow transplant. Oropharyngeal candidiasis was less likely in people treated with fluconazole. Two smaller RCTs in people with liver transplant compared the prevention of oropharyngeal candidiasis by azoles with prevention by polyenes.[9,10] One was a multicentre trial involving 143 people given prophylaxis for 28 days after liver transplantation. It found that fluconazole compared with nystatin reduced the incidence of oropharyngeal candidiasis, but the result was not significant.[9] The other RCT found no significant difference between nystatin and clotrimazole for prophylaxis during hospital stay after transplantation.[10] However, the two smaller RCTs had insufficient power individually to show a clinically important difference. We found no systematic review, but the results of the three RCTs were consistent with each other and the pooled results suggest that use of azoles instead of polyenes reduces the risk of oropharyngeal candidiasis by at least 40%. **Chlorhexidine oral rinse:** We found two RCTs in people who had received bone marrow transplants.[11,12] One RCT (51 people) compared prophylaxis for 60 days with chlorhexidine oral rinse versus a placebo rinse. All participants received oral nystatin suspension 100 000 units. Compared with placebo, chlorhexidine reduced oropharyngeal candidiasis (2/24 [8%] with chlorhexidine v 15/27 [56%] with control; ARR 47%, 95% CI 24% to 54%; RR 15%, 95% CI 3% to 57%; NNT 2, 95% CI 2 to 4) and mucositis.[11] The other RCT found no significant difference in the development of oropharyngeal candidiasis in 86 adults with leukaemia and bone marrow transplant randomly assigned to rinses containing saline alone, chlorhexidine alone, nystatin alone, or nystatin with chlorhexidine (no statistical analysis available).[12]

Harms: In one RCT with no placebo arm, the rates of adverse reactions over 30 days were 5.6% with fluconazole and 5.2% with oral polyenes.[8] The most common adverse events were abdominal pain, nausea and vomiting, and skin rash. There was no increased hepatoxicity, cyclosporin interaction, or emergence of clinically relevant resistant strains reported in people receiving antifungal prophylaxis after liver transplantation.[9]

Comment: We found no RCTs comparing nystatin against placebo. The trials of chlorhexidine found conflicting results regarding its value in reducing oropharyngeal candidiasis and mucositis,[11,12] but the second RCT had four parallel arms and was not powered to detect a clinically important difference.[12]

OPTION ANTIFUNGAL TREATMENT

Limited evidence from one small RCT suggests that fluconazole is more effective than amphotericin B lozenges for treating oropharyngeal candidiasis in people undergoing treatment for cancer.

Benefits: We found no systematic review. We found one RCT, which compared fluconazole 50 mg tablets daily for 1 week with amphotericin B 10 mg lozenges four times daily for 2 weeks in people with oropharyngeal candidiasis undergoing radiotherapy for head and neck cancer.[13] Clinical cure was more likely with fluconazole (34/37

[92%] *v* 26/36 [72%] with amphotericin; RR of cure 1.27, 95% CI 1.02 to 1.35; NNT with fluconazole rather than amphotericin to cure one additional person 5, 95% CI 4 to 60). For both treatments, cure rate was lower in denture wearers than in non-denture wearers.

Harms: The trial did not give details of adverse effects.

Comment: None.

QUESTION What are the effects of interventions to prevent and treat oropharyngeal candidiasis in infants and children?

OPTION ANTIFUNGAL PREVENTION IN IMMUNOCOMPROMISED INFANTS AND CHILDREN

One RCT found that fluconazole was more effective than oral polyenes in prevention of oropharyngeal candidiasis in immunocompromised infants and children.

Benefits: We found no systematic review. We found one large, unblinded, multicentre RCT (n = 502) comparing fluconazole 3 mg/kg with oral polyenes (nystatin 50 000 units/kg four times daily, oral amphotericin B 25 mg/kg four times daily, or both) for the prevention of fungal infections, including oropharyngeal candidiasis. Participants were immunocompromised infants and children, aged 6 months to 17 years, admitted to hospital and scheduled within the next 48 hours to undergo initial or repeat courses of chemotherapy or radiotherapy for haematological or oncological malignancies.[2] The mean duration of prophylaxis was 28 days. Fluconazole was associated with reduced incidence of oropharyngeal candidiasis (3/236 [1.3%] for fluconazole, 15/249 [6.0%] for oral polyenes; RR 0.21, 95% CI 0.06 to 0.72; NNT with fluconazole instead of oral polyene to prevent one additional episode of oropharyngeal candidiasis 21, 95% CI 18 to 58).[2]

Harms: Eight of 245 children on fluconazole and three of 257 on an oral polyene were withdrawn from the trial because of adverse events.[2]

Comment: None.

OPTION ANTIFUNGAL TREATMENT IN CHILDREN

Two RCTs have found that, in immunocompetent infants, miconazole gel is superior to nystatin suspension in the speed and effectiveness of treating oropharyngeal candidiasis. One RCT has found that fluconazole is more effective than oral polyenes in treatment of oropharyngeal candidiasis occurring in immunocompromised infants and children.

Benefits: We found no systematic review. **Immunocompetent infants and children:** We found no placebo controlled RCTs and no RCTs in children. We found two RCTs in immunocompetent infants, which compared miconazole with nystatin for treatment of oropharyngeal candidiasis.[14,15] In both studies, miconazole resulted in higher rates of clinical cure. In the larger trial (n = 183), quicker clinical cure was obtained with miconazole (at day 5: cure rate 83/98

[85%] for miconazole gel 25 mg 4 times daily v 18/85 [21%] for nystatin suspension 100 000 units 4 times daily; at day 12: 97/98 [99%] for miconazole v 46/85 [54%] for nystatin).[14] The clinical cure rates were not significantly influenced by the presence or absence of nappy rash. **Immunocompromised infants and children:** We found no placebo controlled RCTs. We found one multi-centre RCT (32 centres, 182 immunocompromised infants and children aged 6 months to 17 years), which compared fluconazole suspension 3 mg/kg with nystatin 400 000 units four times daily for 14 days for the treatment of oropharyngeal candidiasis. The participants were a heterogeneous group: 64 were infected with HIV, 92 had a malignancy, and 26 were receiving immunosuppressive treatment.[16] Fluconazole was associated with a higher clinical cure rate than nystatin (78/86 [91%] with fluconazole, 37/73 [51%] with nystatin; RR of cure 1.79, 95% CI 1.59 to 1.89; NNT 2, 95% CI 2 to 3). In subgroup analyses, clinical cure with fluconazole was superior to nystatin for children with HIV infection (28/35 [80%] with fluconazole v 6/29 [21%] for nystatin) and for people with malignancy (49/50 [98%] for fluconazole v 30/42 [71%] for nystatin). Clinical relapse rates after 2 weeks were similar (18% for fluconazole v 24% for nystatin).

Harms: The most common adverse events with both miconazole and nystatin were vomiting or, more rarely, diarrhoea, affecting under 4.5% of immunocompetent infants.[14,15] Two of 94 immunocompromised children were withdrawn from the fluconazole group and none of 88 children from the nystatin group as a result of adverse events.[15]

Comment: **Immunocompetent infants and children:** The trials were conducted as open studies without placebo controls.[14,15] There is potential for observer bias, but the clinical results were corroborated by the mycological findings, which were blinded.[14] The larger RCT was carried out in 26 general practices,[14] so is representative of the context in which most otherwise healthy infants with oropharyngeal candidiasis would be treated, especially regarding compliance and cure rate. **Immunocompromised infants and children:** The RCT showed the benefit of fluconazole for infants and children presenting with a wide range of different haematological malignancies, solid tumours, or HIV infection with no apparent age, sex, or race differences.[16]

QUESTION What are the effects of interventions to prevent and treat oropharyngeal candidiasis in people with diabetes?

OPTION ANTIFUNGAL DRUGS

We found insufficient evidence on prevention or treatment of oropharyngeal candidiasis in people with diabetes.

Benefits: We found no systematic reviews or RCTs.

Harms: Insufficient data.

Comment: None.

Oropharyngeal candidiasis

QUESTION	What are the effects of treatments for oropharyngeal candidiasis in people with dentures?

One small RCT found weak evidence that oral polyenes (nystatin, amphotericin B) were more effective than placebo at curing denture stomatitis. One RCT found no good evidence that miconazole dental lacquer benefits denture stomatitis. We found weak observational evidence that denture hygiene and not wearing dentures during sleep may cure denture stomatitis.

Benefits:
We found no systematic review but several RCTs. **Versus placebo:** Four RCTs compared topical oral antifungals with placebo for the treatment of denture stomatitis.[17–20] One (n = 46) found that topical oral polyenes (nystatin, amphotericin B) were associated with a significant improvement in the clinical cure of denture stomatitis.[19] The second RCT (n = 22) found no significant difference between polyenes and placebo in the clinical appearance of denture stomatitis.[18] The third RCT (n = 49) compared amphotericin B with and without a hydrogen peroxide denture cleanser versus placebo. No combination was better than placebo for clinical cure.[17] The fourth RCT (n = 36) compared miconazole dental lacquer applied to the fit surface of an upper denture as a single application with a placebo lacquer but found no significant difference in the resolution of palatal symptoms by day 14 (symptom resolution in 54% with lacquer v 23% with placebo; RR 2.42, 95% CI 0.89 to 3.8).[20] **Different antifungal treatments:** We found three small RCTs. One RCT compared miconazole dental lacquer with 2% miconazole gel applied to the denture four times a day and found no significant difference in palatal erythema after 14 days of treatment (13/20 [65%] with lacquer v 16/21 [76%] with gel; RR of erythema with lacquer v gel 0.85, 95% CI 0.42 to 1.15).[21] The second RCT in 19 elderly, chronically ill, institutionalised adults compared nystatin denture soaking solution (10 000 units/ml) with tap water as a soaking solution; both groups were given nystatin pastilles (10 000 units/g 3 times daily).[22] It found no additional advantage from the use of nystatin as a soaking agent: all participants in both groups were clinically cured at 7 days.[22] The third RCT (n = 29) compared fluconazole 50 mg daily for 14 days with amphotericin B lozenges plus denture cream for 28 days.[23] At 28 days there was no significant difference in the clinical cure rate (84% for fluconazole v 90% for amphotericin B). Clinical relapse was common in both groups at 12 weeks. We found one large multicentre RCT (305 elderly people from 56 investigational sites; 176 wore dentures). It compared daily administration of fluconazole (50 mg) suspension with amphotericin B (0.5 g) oral suspension three times daily for 2 weeks. It found no significant difference between fluconazole and amphotericin for either clinical or mycological cure. Wearing dentures did not affect the response to antifungal therapy (clinical cure rate 151/176 [86%] of denture wearers v 102/124 [82%] of non-denture wearers).[24]

Harms:
None of the trials exclusively enrolling denture patients was large enough to report accurately on the incidence of adverse effects. In the large RCT of elderly people[24] 6/150 in the fluconazole arm and 0/155 in the amphotericin arm experienced adverse events, includ-

ing diarrhoea, buccal bitterness, aggravation of pre-existing renal dysfunction (one, withdrawn from study), and increased liver transaminases (one, not withdrawn).

Comment: The high clinical cure rate with placebo may be attributable to professional cleaning of the dentures at the start of the study combined with advice on denture hygiene and advice not to wear the dentures while asleep at night. There was poor correlation between clinical cure and mycological cure. The trials comparing different antifungals were not sufficiently powerful to detect clinically important differences.

QUESTION **What are the effects of interventions to prevent and treat oropharyngeal candidiasis in people with HIV infection?**

OPTION CONTINUOUS ANTIFUNGAL PROPHYLAXIS

RCTs have found that daily or weekly antifungal prophylaxis with fluconazole, itraconazole, or nystatin reduces the incidence of oropharyngeal candidiasis in people with HIV infection. Most absolute benefit was found in people with AIDS who had low CD4 cell counts ($\leq 200/mm^3$) and a history of recurrent oropharyngeal candidiasis.

Benefits: We found no systematic review. We found eight RCTs using different prophylaxis protocols with follow up from 3–29 months.[25–32] All trials enrolled people with AIDS, AIDS related complex, or CD4 cell counts ≤ 300 cells/mm^3. **Fluconazole versus placebo:** Five RCTs using daily or weekly regimens found significant reduction in oropharyngeal candidiasis with fluconazole.[25,26,28–30] Three of these trials compared weekly fluconazole with placebo. Clinical relapse during 6 months' prophylaxis was reduced by fluconazole 150 mg weekly (relapse: 4/9 with fluconazole, 5/5 with placebo;[25] 13/31 with fluconazole, 25/26 with placebo;[28] pooled AR 43% with fluconazole, 95% with placebo; RR 0.45, 95% CI 0.09 to 0.89; NNT 2, 95% CI 1 to 9). The third RCT (323 women infected with HIV) compared fluconazole 200 mg weekly versus placebo and found similar results: fluconazole reduced the risk of recurrent oropharyngeal candidiasis over 29 months (RR 0.50, CI 0.33 to 0.74).[26] For people with a history of oropharyngeal candidiasis, the absolute benefit of treatment with weekly fluconazole was higher than in those with no history of infection (ARR 25.6 per 100 person years for those with previous infection v 11.2 per 100 person years for those with no history of infection).[26] In one RCT, the median time to relapse was 168 days with fluconazole versus 37 days with placebo ($P \leq 0.0001$).[28] We found no RCTs comparing weekly with daily regimens. No significant difference was found between 50 mg or 100 mg daily doses (oropharyngeal candidiasis: 2/18 [11%] with 50 mg v 4/19 [21%] with 100 mg; RR 0.53, 95% CI 0.09 to 2.09).[29] **Itraconazole versus placebo:** One placebo controlled RCT found that daily prophylaxis with 200 mg of itraconazole for 24 weeks reduced the number of people who relapsed (5/24 [21%] with itraconazole v 14/20 [70%] with placebo; ARR 49%, 95% CI 19% to 64%; NNT 2, 95% CI 2 to 5) and increased the time interval before relapse occurred (median time to relapse 8.0 with placebo v

> 10.4 weeks with itraconazole, P = 0.001).[32] **Nystatin versus placebo:** One RCT found that, compared with placebo, prophylaxis with nystatin 200 000 unit pastille once daily over 20 weeks delayed the onset of oropharyngeal candidiasis (HR 0.56, no 95% CI given).[27] **Fluconazole versus clotrimazole:** One large RCT (428 people from 29 sites) compared fluconazole 200 mg/day versus clotrimazole 10 mg five times/day over 35 months and found that fluconazole was associated with reduced recurrent oropharyngeal candidiasis (fluconazole 5.7 episodes per 100 person years, clotrimazole 38.1, P ≤ 0.001).[31]

Harms: The most commonly reported adverse events were gastrointestinal symptoms, rash, and headache, but data on adverse effects were incomplete and were not presented in all trials. No participants withdrew due to adverse changes in liver function or haematological variables. Concomitant medication and severe underlying disease may have confounded attribution of adverse events.

Comment: Many of the trials were small and not blinded, and most did not adjust for confounding factors such as antiretroviral treatment and other established risk factors for oropharyngeal candidiasis. No trials used quality of life scores. The optimal dosage schedule and frequency of administration of preventive treatment have not been established.

OPTION	TOPICAL TREATMENT

RCTs have found that topical preparations of itraconazole, fluconazole, and clotrimazole effectively treat oropharyngeal candidiasis in people with HIV infection. One RCT found that topical nystatin was inferior to fluconazole.

Benefits: We found no systematic review. We found four RCTs comparing topical (suspensions or pastilles) with orally absorbed antifungals for treatment of oropharyngeal candidiasis in people with HIV infection. Three RCTs found itraconazole oral solution 100 mg or 200 mg used in a swish and swallow mode was as effective as fluconazole 100 mg once daily for 14 days or clotrimazole 10 mg five times a day. All three trials achieved clinical response rates over 90%.[33–35] The fourth RCT found that complete resolution of signs and symptoms of oropharyngeal candidiasis was more common with fluconazole 100 mg daily than with nystatin liquid for 14 days (fluconazole 60/69 [87%] v 36/69 [52%] for nystatin liquid; ARI 35%, 95% CI 22% to 42%; RR 1.67, 95% CI 1.42 to 1.80; NNT 3, 95% CI 2 to 5).[36]

Harms: No consistent changes in results of haematology tests or blood or urine biochemistry tests were noted in any of the trials. The most frequently reported adverse effects were gastrointestinal symptoms (nausea, diarrhoea, and vomiting). Altered taste, dry mouth, headache, and rashes were also recorded. On the basis of data from the six trials (n = 861), in which adverse events were considered to be drug induced and resulted in withdrawal from the study, adverse events were reported with fluconazole (n = 4), itraconazole (n = 14), clotrimazole (n = 12), and nystatin (n = 1).[27,31,33–36]

Comment: Once daily dosing is associated with good adherence to treatment. Non-adherence because of the inconvenience of taking multiple doses was documented with clotrimazole.

QUESTION Which treatments reduce the risk of acquiring resistance to antifungal drugs?

OPTION CONTINUOUS ANTIFUNGAL PROPHYLAXIS VERSUS INTERMITTENT ANTIFUNGAL TREATMENT

One RCT in people with HIV infection and acute episodes of oropharyngeal candidiasis found no significant difference between continuous antifungal prophylaxis and intermittent antifungal treatment in terms of the emergence of antifungal resistance.

Benefits: We found no systematic review. We found one RCT comparing the effect of different treatment regimens on the development of acquired resistance in people with HIV infection over a mean follow up of 11 months.[37] Antifungal sensitivity testing followed the National Committee for Clinical Laboratory Standards guidelines.[38] Continuous prophylaxis compared with intermittent treatment with fluconazole 200 mg/day reduced median annual relapse rates (0 episodes/year for continuous prophylaxis v 4.1 episodes/year for intermittent treatment, $P \leq 0.001$). Antifungal resistance developed in more people on continuous prophylaxis than on intermittent treatment, but the difference was not significant (9/16 [56%] for continuous v 13/28 [46%] for intermittent, $P = 0.75$).

Harms: No adverse reactions were reported.

Comment: Optimal treatment regimens to reduce the risk of acquiring resistance have not yet been adequately evaluated. In a prospective observational study of protease inhibitor treatment, 93 people with HIV and with a history of recurrent oropharyngeal candidiasis were followed up for 1 year. Oropharyngeal candidiasis was diagnosed in 2/30 [7%] of people given protease inhibitors and 23/63 [37%] given other treatment ($P \leq 0.001$, no 95% CI given).[39] Immuno-modulating antiretroviral treatments (e.g. highly active antiretrovial therapy), by reducing the number of recurrences of oropharyngeal candidiasis, are acting indirectly as antifungal sparing agents, thereby reducing exposure to antifungals and the potential risk of resistance.

Substantive changes since last issue

Antifungal prophylaxis Additional systematic review; no change to conclusions.[7]
Effects of treatment in people with dentures Subgroup analysis of additional RCT. Found no significant difference between fluconazole and amphoteracin oral suspensions. Also reported on adverse effects.[24]
Effects of interventions to prevent and treat oropharyngeal candidiasis in people with HIV infection Additional RCT. Found that daily itraconazole reduced relapse compared with placebo.[32]

REFERENCES

1. Webb BC, Thomas CJ, Willcox MD, et al. Candida-associated denture stomatitis. Aetiology and management: a review. Part 3. Treatment of oral candidosis. Aust Dent J 1998;43:244–249.
2. Ninane JA. Multicentre study of fluconazole versus oral polyenes in the prevention of fungal infection in children with hematological or oncological malignancies. Multicentre study group. Eur J Clin Microbiol Infect Dis 1994;13:330–337.
3. Philips P, Zemcov J, Mahmood W, et al. Itraconazole cyclodextrin solution for fluconazole-refractory oropharyngeal candidiasis in AIDS: correlation of clinical response with in vitro susceptibility. AIDS 1996;10:1369–1376.
4. Rex JH, Rinald MG, Pfaler MA. Resistance of candida species to fluconazole. Antimicrob Agents Chemother 1995;39:1–8.
5. Maenza JR, Keruly JC, Moore RD, et al. Risk factors for fluconazole-resistant candidiasis in human immuno-deficiency virus-infected patients. J Infect Dis 1996;173:219–225.
6. Meunier F, Paesmans M, Autier P. Value of antifungal prophylaxis with antifungal drugs against oropharyngeal candidiasis in cancer patients. Eur J Cancer B Oral Oncol 1994;30: 196–199. Search dates 1975–1991; primary sources English language papers from Medline and authors' library.
7. Clarkson JE, Worthington HV, Eden OB. Prevention of oral mucositis or oral candidiasis for patients with cancer receiving chemotherapy (excluding head and neck cancer). In: The Cochrane Library, Issue 2, 2000. Oxford: Update Software. Search Dates from 1963 to July 1999; primary sources: Medline (from 1966), Embase (from 1989), CINAHL (from 1982), Cancerlit (from 1963), and the Cochrane Controlled Trials Register and the Cochrane Oral Health Group Specialist Register.
8. Philpott-Howard JN, Wade JJ, Mufti GJ, et al. Randomized comparison of oral fluconazole versus oral polyenes for the prevention of fungal infection in patients at risk of neutropenia. Multicentre study group. J Antimicrob Chemother 1993;31: 973–984.
9. Lumbreras C, Cuervas-Mons V, Jara P, et al. Randomized trial of fluconazole versus nystatin for the prophylaxis of candida infection following liver transplantation. J Infect Dis 1996;174:583–588.
10. Ruskin JD, Wood RP, Bailey MR, et al. Comparative trial of oral clotrimazole and nystatin for oropharyngeal candidiasis prophylaxis in orthotopic liver transplant patients. Oral Surg Oral Med Oral Pathol Oral Radiol Endod 1992;74: 567–571.
11. Ferretti GA, Ash RC, Brown AT, Parr MD, Romond EH, Lillich TT. Control of oral mucositis and candidiasis in marrow transplantation: a prospective, double-blind trial of chlorhexidine digluconate oral rinse. Bone Marrow Transplant 1988;3:483–493.
12. Epstein JB, Vickars L, Spinelli J, Reece D. Efficacy of chlorhexidine and nystatin rinses in prevention of oral complications in leukemia and bone marrow transplantation. Oral Surg Oral Med Oral Pathol Oral Radiol Endod 1992;73:682–689.
13. Finlay PM, Richardson MD, Robertson AG. A comparative study of the efficacy of fluconazole and amphotericin B in the treatment of oropharyngeal candidosis in patients undergoing radiotherapy for head and neck tumours. Br J Oral Maxillofac Surg 1996;34:23–25.
14. Hoppe J, Burr R, Ebeling H, et al. Treatment of oropharyngeal candidiasis in immunocompetent infants: a randomized multicenter study of miconazole gel vs. nystatin suspension. Pediatr Infect Dis J 1997;16:288–293.
15. Hoppe JE, Hahn H. Randomized comparison of two nystatin oral gels with miconazole oral gel for treatment of oral thrush in infants. Antimycotics study group. Infection 1996;24:136–139.
16. Flynn PM, Cunningham CK, Kerkering T, et al. Oropharyngeal candidiasis in immunocompromised children: a randomized, multicenter study of orally administered fluconazole suspension versus nystatin. The multicenter fluconazole study group. J Pediatr 1995;127:322–328.
17. Walker DM, Stafford GD, Huggett R, et al. The treatment of denture stomatitis: evaluation of 2 agents. Br Dent J 1981;151:416–419.
18. Nairn RI. Nystatin and amphotericin B in the treatment of denture-related candidiasis. Oral Surg Oral Med Oral Pathol Oral Radiol Endod 1975;40:68–75.
19. Johnson GH, Taylor TD, Heid DW. Clinical evaluation of a nystatin pastille for treatment of denture-related oral candidiasis. J Prosthet Dent 1989;61:699–703.
20. Konsberg R, Axell T. Treatment of candida-infected denture stomatitis with a miconazole lacquer. Oral Surg Oral Med Oral Pathol 1994;78:306–311.
21. Budtz-Jorgensen E, Carlino P. A miconazole lacquer in the treatment of Candida-associated denture stomatitis. Mycoses 1994;37:131–135.
22. Banting DW, Greenhorn PA, McMinn JG. Effectiveness of a topical antifungal regimen for the treatment of oral candidiasis in older, chronically ill, institutionalized, adults. J Can Dent Assoc 1995;61:199–195.
23. Bissell V, Felix DH, Wray D. Comparative trial of fluconazole and amphotericin B in the treatment of denture stomatitis. Oral Surg Oral Med Oral Path Oral Radiol Endod 1993;76:35–39.
24. Taillandier J, Esnault Y, Alemanni M, and the multicentre study group. A comparison of fluconazole oral suspension and amphotericin B oral suspension in older patients with oropharyngeal candidosis. Age Ageing 2000;29: 117–123.
25. Leen CLS, Dunbar EM, Ellis ME, et al. Once-weekly fluconazole to prevent recurrence of oropharyngeal candidiasis in patients with AIDS and AIDS-related complex: a double-blind placebo controlled study. J Infect 1990;21:55–60.
26. Schuman P, Capps L, Peng G, et al. Weekly fluconazole for the prevention of mucosal candidiasis in women with HIV infection. A randomized, double-blind, placebo-controlled trial. Terry Beirn community programs for clinical research on AIDS. Ann Intern Med 1997;126: 689–696.
27. MacPhail LA, Hilton JF, Dodd CL, et al. Prophylaxis with nystatin pastilles for HIV-associated oral candidiasis. J Acquir Immune Defic Syndr 1996; 12:470–476.
28. Marriott DJE, Jones PD, Hoy JF, et al. Fluconazole once a week as secondary prophylaxis against oropharyngeal candidiasis in HIV-infected patients. A double-blind placebo-controlled study. Med J Aust 1993;158:312–316.
29. Just-Nubling G, Gentschew G, Meissner K, et al. Fluconazole prophylaxis of recurrent oral candidiasis in HIV-positive patients. Eur J Clin Microbiol Infect Dis 1991;10:917–921.
30. Stevens DA, Greene SI, Lang OS. Thrush can be prevented in patients with acquired immunodeficiency syndrome and the acquired immunodeficiency syndrome-related complex. Randomized, double-blind, placebo-controlled study of 100 mg oral fluconazole daily. Arch Intern

Med 1991;151:2458–2464.

31. Powderly WG, Finklestein DM, Feinberg J, et al. A randomised trial comparing fluconazole with clotrimazole troches for the prevention of fungal infection in patients with advanced human immunodefiency virus infection. *N Engl J Med* 1995;332:700 705.

32. Smith D, Midgley J, Gazzard B. A randomised, double-blind study of itraconazole versus placebo in the treatment and prevention of oral or oesophageal candidosis in patients with HIV infection. *Int J Clin Pract* 1999;53:349–352.

33. Graybill JR, Vazquez J, Darouiche RO, et al. Randomized trial of itraconazole oral solution for oropharyngeal candidiasis in HIV/AIDS patients. *Am J Med* 1998;104:33–39.

34. Phillips P, De Beule K, Frechette G, et al. A double-blind comparison of itraconazole oral solution and fluconazole capsules for the treatment of oropharyngeal candidiasis in patients with AIDS. *Clin Infect Dis* 1998;26:1368–1373.

35. Murray PA, Koletar SL, Mallegol I, et al. Itraconazole oral solution versus clotrimazole troches for the treatment of oropharyngeal candidiasis in immunocompromised patients. *Clin Ther* 1997;19:471–480.

36. Pons V, Greenspan D, Lozada-Nur F, et al. Oropharyngeal candidiasis in patients with AIDS: randomized comparison of fluconazole versus nystatin oral suspensions. *Clin Infect Dis* 1997; 24:1204–1207.

37. Revankar SG, Kirkpatrick WR, McAtee RK, et al. A randomized trial of continuous or intermittent therapy with fluconazole for oropharyngeal candidiasis in HIV-infected patients: clinical outcomes and development of fluconazole resistance. *Am J Med* 1998;105:7–11.

38. National Committee for Clinical Laboratory Standards. *Reference method for broth dilution antifungal susceptibility testing of yeasts: approved standard*. Wayne, Penn: NCCLS, 1997 (document M27-A).

39. Cauda R, Tacconelli E, Tumbarello M, et al. Role of protease inhibitors in preventing recurrent oral candidiasis in patients with HIV infections: a prospective case control study. *J Acquir Immune Defic Syndr* 1999;21:20–25.

Caroline Pankhurst
Guy's, King's College, and St Thomas's
Dental Institute
London
UK

Competing interests: CP has been reimbursed for a conference registration fee in 1994 by Pfizer, the manufacturer of fluconazole.

TABLE 1 RCTs of azoles versus polyenes in prevention of oropharyngeal candidiasis in people with impaired immunity (see text, p764).

RCT	AR with azole	AR with nystatin	ARR	RR	NNT
Fluconazole v amphotericin and/or nystatin[8]	4/256 (1.6 %)	22/255 (8.6%)	7% (4.2% to 8.1%)	0.18 (0.06 to 0.52)	14 (12 to 24)
Fluconazole v nystatin[9]	7/76 (9%)	14/67 (21%)	12%	0.44 (0.18 to 1.01)	–
Clotrimazole v nystatin[10]	1/17 (6%)	1/17 (6%)	0%	1.00 (0.06 to 8.86)	–
Pooled results	**12/349 (3%)**	**37/339 (11%)**	**7.5% (4.4% to 9.1%)**	**0.32 (0.16 to 0.59)**	**13 (11 to 23)**

New topic

Michael Eddleston and Nick Buckley

INTERVENTIONS

Key Messages

- We found no good evidence on the effectiveness of ipecac, gastric lavage, or activated charcoal in paracetamol poisoning.

- One small RCT found that acetylcysteine reduced mortality in people with established paracetamol induced liver failure. One observational study found that people given early treatment with acetylcysteine were less likely to develop liver damage than untreated historical controls.

- One small RCT found that the risk of hepatotoxicity was lower with methionine than with supportive care.

DEFINITION Paracetamol poisoning occurs as a result of either accidental or intentional overdose with paracetamol (acetaminophen).

INCIDENCE/ PREVALENCE Paracetamol is the commonest drug used for self poisoning in the UK.[1] It is also a common means of self poisoning in Europe, North America, and Australasia. An estimated 41 200 cases of poisoning with products containing paracetamol occurred in 1989–1990 in England and Wales, with a case fatality rate of 0.4% (95% CI 0.38% to 0.46%). Overdoses due to paracetamol alone result in an estimated 150–200 deaths and 15–20 liver transplants each year in England and Wales.

AETIOLOGY/ RISK FACTORS Most cases in the UK are impulsive acts of self harm in young people.[1,2] In one study of 80 people, 42 had obtained the tablets for the specific purpose of taking an overdose, and 33 had obtained them less than 1 hour before the act.[2]

PROGNOSIS People with blood paracetamol concentrations above the standard treatment line (defined in the UK as a line joining 200 mg/l at 4 hours and 30 mg/l at 15 hours on a semilogarithmic plot) have a poor prognosis without treatment (see figure 1, p 780).[3,4] In one study of 57 untreated people with blood concentrations above this line, 33 developed severe liver damage and three died.[3] People with a history of chronic alcohol misuse, use of enzyme inducing drugs, eating disorders, or multiple paracetamol overdoses may be at risk of liver damage with blood concentrations below this line.[5] In the USA, a lower line is used as an indication for treatment, but we found no data relating this line to prognostic outcomes.[6] **Dose effect:** The dose ingested also indicates the risk of hepatotoxicity. People ingesting less than 125 mg/kg had no significant hepatotoxicity with a sharp dose dependent rise for higher doses.[7]

AIMS To prevent liver failure; liver transplantation; or death, with minimal adverse effects.

OUTCOMES Rates of death, liver failure, liver transplantation, or hepatotoxicity (most commonly defined by the objective criterion of an aspartate aminotransferase of > 1000 U/l).

METHODS *Clinical Evidence* search and appraisal February 2000. We searched Medline, Embase, and Cochrane databases, and contacted experts in the field to identify unpublished studies. We evaluated only interventions that are currently in common use (not for example cysteamine, cimetidine, or dimercaprol).

QUESTION What are the effects of treatments for acute paracetamol poisoning?

OPTION IPECAC

We found no evidence of the effectiveness of ipecac in paracetamol poisoning.

Benefits: We found no systematic review and no RCTs that reported clinical end points.

Harms: We found no large study of complications in paracetamol poisoned people receiving ipecac. Specific complications of ipecac may include aspiration, diarrhoea, ileus, arrhythmia during vomiting, dystonia from treatment for vomiting, and haematemesis from vomiting.[8]

Comment: Human simulated overdose studies suggest that ipecac given within 1 hour could reduce paracetamol absorption but no studies have shown a change in clinical outcome.[9] One non-systematic review of ipecac in all forms of poisoning found no evidence that ipecac improved outcome in poisoned people.[9] Administration of ipecac may delay the administration of activated charcoal and oral antidotes.

OPTION   GASTRIC LAVAGE

We found no evidence of the effectiveness of gastric lavage in paracetamol poisoning.

Benefits: We found no systematic review and no RCTs that reported clinical outcomes.

Harms: We found no large study of complications in paracetamol poisoned people receiving gastric lavage. Harms may include aspiration of stomach contents, hypoxia, and oesophageal perforation.[8]

Comment: Studies of simulated overdose in human volunteers suggest that gastric lavage carried out within 1 hour removes a variable number of paracetamol tablets and that the number diminishes with time.[10] One cohort study in 450 consecutive people who took at least 10 g or more of paracetamol, found that those given activated charcoal were significantly less likely to have high risk blood paracetamol concentrations (OR 0.36, 95% CI 0.23 to 0.58).[11] However, the addition of gastric lavage did not further decrease the risk (OR 1.12, 95% CI 0.57 to 2.20). One non-systematic review of gastric lavage in all forms of poisoning found no evidence that gastric lavage improved outcome in poisoned people.[10]

OPTION   ACTIVATED CHARCOAL (SINGLE OR MULTIPLE DOSE)

We found no evidence of the effectiveness of activated charcoal, whether in single or multiple dose regimens, in paracetamol poisoning.

Benefits: We found no systematic review and no RCT that reported clinical outcomes.

Harms: We found no large study of complications in paracetamol poisoned people receiving single doses of activated charcoal. We found no large, high quality RCT comparing activated charcoal with placebo in any form of poisoning that might have allowed calculation of the incidence of complications. Harms may include aspiration pneumonia, vomiting, diarrhoea, constipation, ileus, and interference with regular medications.

Comment: Single dose regimens: Studies of simulated overdose in human volunteers suggest that activated charcoal given within 2 hours decreases paracetamol absorption by a variable amount and that this amount diminishes with time.[12,13] One cohort study in consecutive people who had taken 10 g or more of paracetamol found that those who had been given activated charcoal were significantly less likely to have high risk blood paracetamol concentrations (OR 0.36, 95% CI 0.23 to 0.58).[11] The effect was seen only in those treated within 2 hours and the study was not large enough to assess the effect of numerous potential confounders.[11] One non-systematic review of activated charcoal in all forms of poisoning found no evidence that activated charcoal improved outcome in poisoned people.[12] Multiple dose regimens: We found no studies of simulated overdose that evaluated multiple dose regimens in paracetamol poisoning. The rapid absorption and short half-life of paracetamol suggest a beneficial effect is unlikely.

OPTION   ACETYLCYSTEINE

One small RCT found that acetylcysteine reduced mortality in people with established paracetamol induced liver failure. One observational study found that people given early treatment with acetylcysteine were less likely to develop liver damage than untreated historical controls.

Benefits: We found no systematic review. We found one RCT in 50 people with established paracetamol induced liver failure, which compared intravenous acetylcysteine (150 mg/kg over 15 minutes, 50 mg/kg over 4 hours and then 100 mg/kg over 16 hours, continued until death or recovery) versus a placebo infusion of 5% dextrose.[14] It found that significantly more people survived in the treated group compared with controls (48% v 20%; ARR 28%, 95% CI 3% to 53%).

Harms: The RCT did not specifically assess adverse outcomes and none were noted. Four case series suggested that the incidence of adverse effects from intravenous acetylcysteine is 5–15%.[15–18] These were predominantly rash, urticaria, and occasionally more serious anaphylactoid reactions occurring with the initial "loading" dose. In most or all cases, adverse effects responded to temporary cessation of infusions and symptomatic treatment, and did not recur when treatment was recommenced. Vomiting is common after oral acetylcysteine and occurred in 63% of people in one series despite prior administration of metoclopramide.[18] Oral acetylcysteine can also cause hypersensitivity and anaphylactoid reactions.[19] Two deaths have been reported due to a tenfold miscalculation of the dose, although only half of the loading dose was given in one case.[20]

Comment: In the RCT, allocation was concealed but treatment was not blinded. There were differences between the groups in prognostic variables (prothrombin time, coma grade) and other treatments, but a possible confounding effect could not be adequately assessed because of the small size of the study.[14] One observational study evaluated the use of intravenous acetylcysteine in people presenting early to hospital. It found that people treated within 10 hours of ingestion were less likely to develop liver damage than untreated historical controls (1.6% in treated group v 57.9% controls; ARR 56%, 95% CI 47% to 58%; RRR 97%, 95% CI 81% to 99.6%; NNT

2, 95% CI 2 to 3).[3] As a result, subsequent RCTs were considered unethical. A systematic review of numerous case series found evidence that acetylcysteine is beneficial in paracetamol poisoning.[15] For both oral and intravenous acetylcysteine, the overall rate of hepatotoxicity was worse if treatment was delayed beyond 8 to 10 hours (1% in those treated within 8 hours v 46% in those treated after 16 hours).[3,15] We found no RCTs of different regimens and no evidence of a difference between oral and intravenous routes of administration.[15] The optimal dose, route, and duration of treatment is unknown.

| OPTION | METHIONINE |

One RCT was too small to detect a clinically important effect of methionine on the death rate in people with blood paracetamol concentrations above the UK standard treatment line. The RCT found a lower risk of hepatotoxicity with methionine than supportive care.

Benefits: We found no systematic review. One RCT (n = 40) compared methionine (2.5 g 4 hourly for four doses), cysteamine, and supportive care in people with blood paracetamol concentrations above the UK standard treatment line.[21] There was no significant effect on death (0 deaths in the methionine group compared with one in the supportive care group). Only 27 people had a liver biopsy. Fewer people suffered grade III hepatic necrosis (0/9 v 6/10 after supportive care), or had peak aspartate aminotransferase greater than 1000 U (1/13 [7%] v 8/13 [62%] with supportive care; ARR 54%, 95% CI 16% to 61%; RRR 88%, 95% CI 25% to 99%; NNT 2, 95% CI 2 to 6).

Harms: No serious adverse effects associated with treatment were reported in the RCT, but vomiting after administration of methionine occurred in 8 of 13 people. The incidence of adverse effects in the control group was not reported.

Comment: Interpretation of liver biopsy results from the RCT was difficult as not all people were tested and an intention to treat analysis was not possible. We found one case series in people treated with methionine in early and late paracetamol poisoning, but there was no comparison group.[22]

REFERENCES

1. Gunnell D, Hawton K, Murray V, et al. Use of paracetamol for suicide and non-fatal poisoning in the UK and France: are restrictions on availability justified? J Epidemiol Community Health 1997; 51:175–179.
2. Hawton K, Ware C, Mistry H, et al. Paracetamol self-poisoning. Characteristics, prevention and harm reduction. Br J Psychiatry 1996;168:43–48.
3. Prescott LF, Illingworth RN, Critchley JAJH, Stewart MJ, Adam RD, Proudfoot AT. Intravenous N-acetylcysteine: the treatment of choice for paracetamol poisoning. BMJ 1979;ii:1097–1100.
4. Rumack BH, Matthew H. Acetaminophen poisoning and toxicity. Pediatrics 1975;55:871–876.
5. Vale JA, Proudfoot AT. Paracetamol (acetaminophen) poisoning. Lancet 1995;346: 547–552.
6. Smilkstein MJ, Knapp GL, Kulig KW, Rumack B.

Efficacy of oral N-acetylcysteine in the treatment of acetaminophen overdose. Analysis of the National Multicentre Study (1976–1985). N Engl J Med 1988;319:1557–1562.
7. Prescott LF. Paracetamol overdosage. Pharmacological considerations and clinical management. Drugs 1983;25:290–314.
8. Pond SM, Lewis-Driver DJ, Williams GM, Green AC, Stevenson NW. Gastric emptying in acute overdose: a prospective randomised controlled trial. Med J Aust 1995;163:345–349.
9. Krenzelok EP, McGuigan M, Lheur P. Position statement: ipecac syrup. American Academy of Clinical Toxicology and European Association of Poisons Centres and Clinical Toxicologists. J Toxicol Clin Toxicol 1997;35:699–709.
10. Vale JA. Position statement: gastric lavage. American Academy of Clinical Toxicology and European Association of Poisons Centres and

Clinical Toxicologists. J Toxicol Clin Toxicol 1997; 35:711–719.

11. Buckley NA, Whyte IM, O'Connell DL, Dawson AH. Activated charcoal reduces the need for N-acetylcysteine treatment after acetaminophen (paracetamol) overdose. J Toxicol Clin Toxicol 1999;37:753–757.

12. Chyka PA, Seger D. Position statement: single-dose activated charcoal. American Academy of Clinical Toxicology; European Association of Poisons Centres and Clinical Toxicologists. J Toxicol Clin Toxicol 1997;35:721–741.

13. Rose SR, Gorman RL, Oderda GM, Klein-Schwartz W, Watson WA. Simulated acetaminophen overdose: pharmacokinetics and effectiveness of activated charcoal. Ann Emerg Med 1991;20: 1064–1068.

14. Keays R, Harrison PM, Wendon JA, Forbes A, Gove C, Alexander GJ, Williams R. Intravenous acetylcysteine in paracetamol induced fulminant hepatic failure: a prospective controlled trial. BMJ 1991;303:1026–1029.

15. Buckley NA, Whyte IM, O'Connell DL, Dawson AH. Oral or intravenous N-acetylcysteine: which is the treatment of choice for acetaminophen (paracetamol) poisoning? J Toxicol Clin Toxicol 1999;37:759–767.

16. Chan TY, Critchley JA. Adverse reactions to intravenous N-acetylcysteine in Chinese patients

with paracetamol (acetaminophen) poisoning. Hum Exp Toxicol 1994;13:542–544.

17. Schmidt LE, Dalhoff KP. Side-effects of N-acetylcysteine treatment in patients with paracetamol poisoning (in Danisih). Ugeskri Laeger 1999;161:2669–2672.

18. Wright RO, Anderson AC, Lesko SL, Woolf AD, Linakis JG, Lewander WJ. Effect of metoclopramide dose on preventing emesis after oral administration of N-acetylcysteine for acetaminophen overdose. J Toxicol Clin Toxicol 1999;37:35–42.

19. Perry HE, Shannon MW. Efficacy of oral versus intravenous N-acetylcysteine in acetaminophen overdose: results of an open-label, clinical trial. J Pediatr 1998;132:149–152.

20. Mant TG, Tempowski JH, Volans GN, Talbot JC. Adverse reactions to acetylcysteine and effects of overdose. BMJ 1984;289:217–219.

21. Hamlyn AN, Lesna M, Record CO, et al. Methionine and cysteamine in paracetamol (acetaminophen) overdose; prospective controlled trial of early therapy. J Int Med Res 1981;9:226–231.

22. Vale JA, Meredith TJ, Goulding R. Treatment of acetaminophen poisoning. The use of oral methionine. Arch Intern Med 1981;141:394–396.

Michael Eddleston
Research Fellow
Centre for Tropical Medicine
University of Oxford
Oxford
UK

Nick Buckley
Consultant Clinical Pharmacologist
and Toxicologist
Royal Adelaide Hospital
Adelaide
Australia

Competing interests: None declared.

FIGURE 1 Nomograms used to determine acetylcysteine or methionine treatment, based on the blood concentrations between 4 and 24 hours after ingestion of paracetamol. Published with permission (see text, p 776).[11]

Updated this issue

Leanne Bricker, Patricia Crowley, James Neilson and Tom O'Dowd

Key Messages

- A systematic review of RCTs has found that routine ultrasound screening before 24 weeks' gestation leads to earlier diagnosis of multiple pregnancies but has not been shown to have an important positive impact on the outcome of multiple pregnancies.

- A systematic review of RCTs has found that routine ultrasound screening before 24 weeks' gestation is associated with fewer inductions of labour for "post-term" pregnancy.

- One large RCT found that routine ultrasound screening before 24 weeks' gestation reduced perinatal mortality if detection of fetal malformation was an important objective, there was a high level of diagnostic expertise, and termination of pregnancy for fetal abnormality was widely accepted in the population screened.

- Routine ultrasound screening in the first trimester for increased nuchal translucency, fetal abnormalities, or both has not yet been evaluated in controlled trials.

- A systematic review of RCTs and primary observational studies has found that detection rates of fetal abnormality by screening ultrasound examinations vary with the organ system affected, with generally high rates of detection of abnormalities of the central nervous system, and low rates for skeletal and cardiac abnormalities. Similar variations are seen at both second and third trimester examinations.

- A systematic review of RCTs has found no evidence that routine ultrasound after 24 weeks confers clear benefit to mother or baby, except that assessment of placental appearances may, as an adjunct to fetal measurement, help reduce perinatal mortality.

- In a systematic review of RCTs, Doppler ultrasound in pregnancy has not been shown to be of benefit, and may even increase the risk of adverse outcome.

DEFINITION   A low risk pregnancy is one in which a rate of perinatal and maternal mortality and morbidity lower than that in the overall population can be achieved without a high rate of obstetric or paediatric intervention.

INCIDENCE/   In England, Wales, and Northern Ireland in 1995 the stillbirth rate
PREVALENCE was 5.48 per 1000 deliveries and the neonatal death rate was 4.04 per 1000 deliveries.[1] In the UK during the same period, the maternal death rate was 12.2 per 100 000,[2] the caesarean section rate was 17%,[3] and the rate of induction of labour was 27%.[3]

AETIOLOGY/   Obstetric factors associated with an increased risk of perinatal
RISK FACTORS morbidity or mortality include pre-eclampsia, prematurity, antepartum and postpartum haemorrhage, and intrauterine growth retardation. Perinatal morbidity and mortality are higher if the fetus is congenitally abnormal. Obstetric factors associated with maternal mortality and morbidity are pre-eclampsia, haemorrhage, and venous thromboembolism.

AIMS   To prevent avoidable maternal and perinatal mortality and morbidity; to enhance satisfaction with pregnancy, childbirth, and parenting; to avoid unnecessary intervention; and to improve convenience of care.

OUTCOMES   Perinatal death; maternal death; incidence and detection of fetal malformation; incidence of termination of pregnancy for medical reasons; rates of normal and uncomplicated birth; quality of experience of pregnancy and childbirth including feeling worried or not feeling relaxed about the pregnancy. Some intermediate outcomes (such as incidence of undiagnosed multiple pregnancy at 26 weeks, low birth weight, and rates of induction of labour for post-term pregnancy) have also been used.

METHODS   We searched the Cochrane Controlled Trials Register and the Cochrane Pregnancy and Childbirth Group's Register in May 2000. We included only randomised and quasi-randomised trials (e.g. those using allocation by date of birth). Primary studies assessing the detection of fetal anomalies by routine ultrasound before 1995 were taken from Chitty;[4] for subsequent primary studies we searched Medline from 1995 to May 2000 using the terms: pregnancy, ultrasound, prenatal and abnormalities. Predefined quality criteria were: population based study of unselected or low risk population; clearly stated study aim, setting, participants and time period; ultrasound intervention fully described, including gestation at the time of ultrasound, diagnostic approach, quality control, operators and skills, equipment used, anomalies sought, method of postnatal ascertainment (including description of false positives and false negatives), anomalies detected reported per fetus or per system. A few other good quality studies are quoted in the text to demonstrate particular issues.

QUESTION What are the effects of routine ultrasound screening?

Leanne Bricker, James P Neilson

Updated this issue

OPTION ROUTINE ULTRASOUND SCREENING BEFORE 24 WEEKS' GESTATION TO ESTABLISH GESTATIONAL AGE, DETECT FETAL HEART ACTIVITY AND MULTIPLE PREGNANCY, AND DETERMINE CHORIONICITY (IF APPROPRIATE)

One systematic review of RCTs has found better gestational age assessment and earlier detection of multiple pregnancy with routine than with selective early ultrasound screening (before 24 weeks' gestation). The effects on substantive clinical outcomes are unclear.

Benefits:
We found one systematic review of routine versus selective ultrasound in pregnancy before 24 weeks (search date 1998, 9 RCTs, 34 245 pregnancies),[5] and one subsequent RCT.[6] Routine ultrasound examination before 24 weeks' gestation was associated with earlier detection of multiple pregnancies (twins undiagnosed at 26 weeks 2/116 [1.7%] of screened group v 41/104 [39%] of control group; OR 0.08, 95% CI 0.04 to 0.16; three twin pregnancies need scanning in early pregnancy to diagnose one additional twin pregnancy), but with no demonstrable improvement in perinatal outcome of twin pregnancies (perinatal mortality of twins: 12/228 [5.2%] for screened group v 13/262 [5.0%] for controls; pooled RRI 6%, 95% CI –51% to +123%), and reduced rates of induction of labour for post-term pregnancy (220/12 149 [1.8%] for screened group v 357/12 046 [3.0%] for controls; OR 0.61, 95% CI 0.52 to 0.72; 87 women would need ultrasound screening in early pregnancy to prevent one induction for post-term pregnancy, 95% CI 70 to 121), presumably because of more accurate gestational dating. There were no differences detected for substantive clinical outcomes, such as perinatal mortality (111/17 192 [0.65%] for screened group v 127/17 053 [0.74%] for controls; OR 0.86, 95% CI 0.67 to 1.12). The subsequent RCT (648 women) assessed the efficacy of an ultrasound assessment of gestational age at the first antenatal visit (≤ 17 weeks' gestation) as an adjunct to the routine second trimester anomaly scan (18–20 weeks' gestation).[6] Fewer women needed adjustment of their expected date of delivery at their second trimester anomaly scan (9% v 18%; RR 0.52, 95% CI 0.34 to 0.79). The number of women who had a repeat blood sample taken for maternal serum screening was similar in the ultrasound and control groups (AR 6% v 6%). Fewer women in the ultrasound group reported feeling worried (AR 32% v 40%; RR 0.80, 95% CI 0.65 to 0.99) or not feeling relaxed about their pregnancy compared with the control group (AR 22% v 30%; RR 0.73, 95% CI 0.56 to 0.96). The pregnancy outcomes were similar in the two groups, including rates of induction of labour, but the numbers are too small to draw conclusions about effects on substantive outcomes relating to maternal and perinatal morbidity and mortality.

Harms:
At present there is no clear evidence that ultrasound examination during pregnancy is harmful. Long term follow up of children in

Norway who, as fetuses, were entered into the Alesund and Trondheim trials found no adverse influence on school performance or neurobehavioural function as a consequence of prenatal exposure to ultrasound. Fewer of the ultrasound exposed children were right handed. Similar follow up of a subset of children from the Sweden trial found no evidence of an adverse effect on vision or hearing. This study found no overall effect on non-right handedness, although there may have been an effect if boys were considered separately.[5]

Comment: A 1996 survey found that in the UK virtually all women were offered at least one routine scan during pregnancy, and the majority were offered two.[7] This may be an underestimate of current UK use of routine ultrasound. It was not possible to determine from published reports the extent or effect of ultrasound screening performed to date the pregnancy to allow interpretation of antenatal serum screening tests for Down's syndrome. Routine ultrasound is difficult to evaluate because it is a relatively new technology and an individual study may have little relevance within a few years as technical advances expand clinical application. The immediacy of seeing the fetal image has made the procedure popular with pregnant women. The Norwegian finding about ultrasound exposure and hand preference is difficult to interpret, and may have been a chance observation that emanated from the large number of outcome measures assessed, or from the method of ascertainment. Alternatively, it could imply that diagnostic ultrasound alters developmental pathways of the brain.

OPTION   NUCHAL TRANSLUCENCY SCREENING

We found no RCTs evaluating screening for increased fetal nuchal translucency.

Benefits: We found no systematic review and no RCTs. We found a non-systematic review of 13 studies comprising 56 896 women that assessed nuchal translucency screening for fetal chromosomal abnormalities.[8] Only six studies, comprising 8840 women, described screening in unselected or low risk populations. The overall detection rates in these routine screening populations for all chromosomal abnormalities was 70% (range 40–100%), the overall detection rate of trisomy 21 was 62% (range 33–100%), and the overall false positive rate was 4% (range 0.9–6.3%). The gestational age at screening and the cut off value for normal versus abnormal nuchal translucency measurement varied among studies. A large longitudinal prospective study of nuchal translucency screening described the outcome of 96 127 pregnancies screened in 22 centres by 306 ultrasonographers.[9] Based on an algorithm that included maternal age, gestational age related prevalence of Down's syndrome, and nuchal translucency thickness compared with crown–rump length, 8.3% of women with normal pregnancies were considered to be at high risk of a fetus with Down's syndrome (risk ≥ 1 : 300). The technique identified 82% of Down's syndrome pregnancies and 78% of pregnancies with other chromosomal abnormalities. Thirty women underwent invasive diagnostic procedures to detect one additional chromosomally abnormal fetus.

Harms: We found two systematic reviews (search dates 1996 and 1998), each of three RCTs evaluating invasive procedures for prenatal diagnosis in 9067 and 1832 pregnancies.[10,11] One systematic review found that spontaneous miscarriage was more likely after early chorionic villus sampling than after second trimester amniocentesis (455/5037 [9.0%] v 299/4030 [7.4%]; OR of miscarriage 1.37, 95% CI 1.18 to 1.60; NNH 62, 95% CI 34 to 228).[10] The second systematic review found that early amniocentesis (performed before 14 weeks' gestation) versus early chorionic villus sampling (also performed before 14 weeks' gestation) resulted in more spontaneous miscarriages (40/915 [4.4%] v 21/917 [2.3%]; OR 1.92, 95% CI 1.15 to 3.20; NNH 48, 95% CI 20 to 318).[11] Routine first trimester ultrasound screening to include nuchal translucency measurement may therefore be associated with the miscarriage of normal pregnancies after early invasive procedures. We found no evidence on the anxiety generated by ultrasound findings or of any increased pregnancy loss because of planned termination associated with that anxiety. We found no RCTs that evaluated the acceptability of transvaginal scanning, which may be required if ultrasound features are not clear on transabdominal examination.

Comment: Theoretically, the benefit of the early detection of fetal chromosomal abnormalities is to allow earlier termination of pregnancy if this is the woman's preferred option. Some studies of screening unselected/low risk populations found a high rate of failure to measure nuchal translucency, questioning the feasibility and reproducibility of the examination. The UK based Serum Ultrasound and Urine Screening Study (SURUSS) is currently in progress and may provide insights into the generalisability of the technique. Small, preliminary studies have reported other sonographic features associated with chromosomal abnormalities, including variation of fetal heart rate, smaller than expected crown–rump length, and structural anomalies such as exomphalos or urinary tract obstruction, but the value of screening for these features remains unknown.[8]

OPTION	ULTRASOUND SCREENING FOR FETAL ANOMALIES IN THE FIRST TRIMESTER

We found insufficient evidence to support the use of detailed ultrasound visualisation to screen for fetal anomalies in the first trimester.

Benefits: We found no systematic review and no RCTs or other studies of routine first trimester anomaly screening that fulfilled our quality criteria.

Harms: Insufficient data.

Comment: First trimester anomaly screening may be affected by the same problems as second trimester anomaly screening (see comment under ultrasound screening for fetal anomalies in the second trimester, p 787). Furthermore little is known about the natural history of ultrasonographic abnormalities detected in the first trimester and some may be variants of normal.[8] In a non-systematic review, preliminary results of one ongoing study were reported. Of 5664 unselected pregnancies, 32/47 [68%] anomalies were detected at first trimester anomaly scan and a further 10/47 [17%]

at second trimester anomaly scan with a false positive rate of 1 : 3000. The authors concluded that if first trimester anomaly screening was to be introduced it may need to be supplemented with a further scan in the second trimester.[12]

| OPTION | ULTRASOUND SCREENING FOR FETAL ANOMALIES IN THE SECOND TRIMESTER |

Leanne Bricker, James P Neilson

We found that no easily generaliseable conclusions could be drawn from the available evidence. One RCT found that second trimester ultrasound screening performed specifically to detect fetal abnormality was associated with increased rates of planned termination of pregnancy and fewer perinatal deaths. Another RCT found conflicting results.

Benefits: We found no systematic review of RCTs, but found two large RCTs.[13,14] We also found one unpublished systematic review (L Bricker et al, unpublished data, 2000) mainly of observational studies (see comment below). The two RCTs compared screening for fetal abnormalities by routine ultrasound before 24 weeks versus selective ultrasound in 24 017 pregnancies.[13,14] The findings of these trials were conflicting. In one RCT,[13] in which detection of fetal abnormality was a specific aim of ultrasound screening, the number of planned terminations of pregnancy increased (11/4353 [0.25%] for the screened group, 0/4309 for the control group; for every 415 women screened there was one additional termination of pregnancy, 95% CI 24 to 30 508 women) and there were fewer perinatal deaths (20/4389 [0.46%] for the screened group v 39/4347 [0.90%] for controls; OR 0.51, 95% CI 0.30 to 0.87; NNT 227, 95% CI 158 to 853). There were large differences in the detection rates between the two hospitals involved in this study (36% v 77% of babies with fetal abnormalities). In the other RCT,[14] only 17% of babies with abnormalities were identified in the ultrasound screened group before 24 weeks of pregnancy, and there was minimal impact on perinatal mortality (52/7685 [0.68%] for the screened group v 41/7596 [0.54%] for controls; OR 1.25, 95% CI 0.83 to 1.88). We found no RCTs that addressed the psychological impact or long term maternal and childhood outcomes associated with prenatal detection of fetal abnormalities. We found no RCTs evaluating the overall long term effect of fetal abnormality detection. However, prior knowledge of the presence of some abnormalities associated with possible survival and long term handicap may alter the management of the pregnancy, with regard to mode of delivery or place of delivery, in an attempt to improve outcome. We found several studies suggesting that the outcome of conditions such as gastroschisis[15] and cardiac abnormalities[16] may be improved by prenatal detection.

Harms: There is a risk of pregnancy loss from invasive procedures to investigate positive ultrasound results, and a risk of psychological sequelae. Available evidence does not allow quantification of the risk of increased intervention and hence the risk of maternal morbidity in pregnancies where abnormalities are diagnosed prenatally, or of any subsequent improvement in long term outcome. One non-randomised study found that prenatal diagnosis of congenital diaphragmatic hernia, abdominal wall defects, meningomyelocele, or bladder exstrophy resulted in all diagnosed fetuses being delivered by caesarean section in a hospital attached to a neonatal surgical unit, but it found no obvious difference in neonatal outcome between fetuses diagnosed and fetuses not diagnosed prenatally.[17] The gestational age at birth was significantly lower in the prenatally diagnosed group. The absence of randomisation makes comparison difficult because diagnosed cases may have been more severe or serious.

Comment: Many factors affect detection rates for fetal abnormalities: technical difficulties such as maternal obesity and fetal position at the time of scanning; the fact that sonographic signs for some anomalies are subtle or absent at the particular gestation of scanning; the anatomical system affected; and the equipment used. There was a difference in detection rates between different centres and between the two RCTs. The findings of studies may not generalise. One explanation is that experience and skill in performing ultrasonography affects detection rates. The detection rate of major fetal malformation was low in the RCT[14] undertaken in 109 centres where staff may have had different levels of skill. The limit of less than 24 weeks' gestation for legal termination of pregnancy in this trial may have contributed to the lack of impact on perinatal outcomes. Some studies report number of anomalies and not number of anomalous fetuses, thus overestimating sensitivity, as a fetus with multiple anomalies would be included more than once. Some exclude minor anomalies, or anomalies not detectable by ultrasound scan, or both. We found one unpublished systematic review (L Bricker et al, unpublished data, 2000) of 11 primary studies[18–28] that included one RCT, four prospective observational studies and six retrospective studies. The review assessed in 96 633 pregnancies the overall detection of fetal abnormalities by routine ultrasound (L Bricker et al, unpublished data, 2000). Overall the sensitivity for detection of fetal anomalies was 45% (range 15–85%). Detection rates by routine second trimester ultrasound for different anatomical systems were: central nervous system 76%, urinary tract 67%, pulmonary 50%, gastrointestinal 42%, skeletal 24%, and cardiac 17%. Overall detection rates for chromosomal abnormalities was 19%. Only one termination of pregnancy occurred as a result of false positive diagnosis (L Bricker et al, unpublished data, 2000). All studies reviewed had high specificity, confirming that normal ultrasound examinations may be reassuring. Only one study in the review addressed the role of ultrasonographic soft markers in improving detection of chromosomal abnormalities; it found that for a 4% increase in the detection rate of congenital abnormalities (from 51% to 55%) there was a 12-fold increase in false positives.[26]

OPTION   **ROUTINE ULTRASOUND AFTER 24 WEEKS' GESTATION**

One systematic review of routine late pregnancy ultrasound (> 24 weeks' gestation) in low risk or unselected populations found no significant benefit for mother or baby. We found no evidence about the psychological effects of routine ultrasound in late pregnancy, or about the effects on neonatal and childhood outcomes. One RCT found that placental grading in the third trimester may be beneficial.

Antenatal care of low risk pregnancies: ultrasound

Benefits:
We found one systematic review (search date 1999, seven RCTs, 25 036 unselected or low risk pregnancies) comparing routine ultrasound after 24 weeks' gestation versus concealed or selective ultrasound after 24 weeks gestation.[29] One of the seven trials combined repeated ultrasound scan for fetal biometry and amniotic fluid assessment with Doppler ultrasound, and its data were analysed separately. **Routine ultrasound after 24 weeks:** Meta-analysis of the results of six trials comprising 22 202 unselected or low risk pregnancies found no difference between the screened and control groups in the following outcomes: antenatal admissions or other tests of fetal wellbeing; obstetric interventions such as induction of labour, instrumental delivery and caesarean section; preterm delivery rates and birthweight; neonatal interventions such as resuscitation, ventilation, admission to special care; and neonatal morbidity such as Apgar score at 5 minutes. One RCT found no difference between screened and unscreened groups in the rates of moderate and severe neonatal morbidity. Overall, there was no difference between the groups in perinatal mortality, including congenital abnormalities (77/11199 [0.69%] v 74/11079 [0.67%]; OR 1.03, 95% CI 0.75 to 1.42) or in perinatal mortality excluding congenital abnormalities (50/9924 [0.50%] v 44/9812 [0.45%]; OR 1.12, 95% CI 0.75 to 1.68). There was also no difference in perinatal mortality of twins (6/168 [3.6%] v 8/146 [5.5%] for controls; OR 0.60, 95% CI 0.20 to 1.76). One of the RCTs found reduced stillbirth rate when placental grading was incorporated into routine third trimester ultrasound scan (1/1014 [0.10%] with placental assessment v 12/1011 [1.2%] for controls; OR 0.13, 95% CI 0.04 to 0.50; NNT 92 to prevent one additional stillbirth, 95% CI 85 to 231). Psychological and other maternal outcomes were not reported in any of the studies. **Intensive ultrasound screening including Doppler:** The review identified one RCT (2834 unselected pregnancies) comparing the combination of repeated ultrasound scanning for fetal biometry, amniotic fluid assessment plus Doppler ultrasound (intensive screening) with selective ultrasound. It found no significant difference between the two groups in other tests of fetal wellbeing, obstetric interventions, neonatal interventions, or perinatal mortality. **Routine ultrasound after 24 weeks to detect fetal abnormalities:** We found one systematic review (11 primary studies, 96 633 pregnancies) assessing the differential performance associated with different anatomical systems. Four of these primary studies (35 834 screened fetuses) included a routine third trimester ultrasound scan.[19,22,23,25] One of these studies was an RCT, two were prospective studies, and one was a retrospective study. However, all included second trimester scans and some anomalies were detected before routine scans in the third trimester. At routine third trimester ultrasound, the overall detection rate for fetal abnormalities was 19% (range 16–40%).

Harms:
The trial of intensive ultrasound screening unexpectedly found significantly more babies in the intensive screening group had birthweight under the 10th centile (179/1415 [12.7%] v 132/1419 [9.3%]; OR 1.41, 95% CI 1.11 to 1.78; NNH 30, 95% CI 16 to 106), and under the third centile (58/1415 [4.1%] v 35/1419 [2.5%]; OR 1.67, 95% CI 1.11 to 2.53; NNH 61, 95% CI 27 to

402).[30] This may have arisen by chance or frequent exposure to ultrasound may reduce fetal growth. There was no association with increased perinatal morbidity or mortality (perinatal mortality: 13/1415 [0.92%] v 22/1419 [1.55%] for controls; OR 0.60, 95% CI 0.31 to 1.17). Follow up of 2222 (81%) of these children at 1 year of age found no difference between those given intensive as opposed to selective screening (J Newnham, Australian Perinatal Society in conjunction with the New Zealand Perinatal Society, 1996).

Comment: Routine ultrasound in late pregnancy (after 24 weeks' gestation) is aimed at assessing some of the following: fetal size, amniotic fluid volume, placental site, placental grading, fetal structural abnormality, or fetal presentation. The trials used different ultrasound examination options and evaluated different outcomes. Some offered the control group no routine scans at any time in pregnancy. Some offered routine scans to all participants earlier in pregnancy (that is, before 24 weeks' gestation), whereas others offered routine scan at all stages of the trial, but only revealed results of late pregnancy ultrasound (after 24 weeks' gestation) for the study groups. It is unclear whether the specific nature of the ultrasound regimens affected the outcome measures.

| OPTION | ROUTINE DOPPLER ULTRASOUND OF THE UMBILICAL OR UTERINE ARTERIES IN UNSELECTED OR LOW RISK PREGNANCIES |

One systematic review of RCTs has found that routine Doppler ultrasound in low risk or unselected pregnancies benefits neither mother nor baby, and may be harmful. One systematic review of primary observational diagnostic studies has found that routine Doppler ultrasound of the uterine artery has limited diagnostic accuracy in predicting pre-eclampsia, intrauterine growth retardation, and perinatal death. We found no evidence to assess the effect on long term outcomes such as childhood neurological development and maternal outcomes, particularly psychological effects.

Benefits: We found two systematic reviews.[31,32] The first systematic review (search date 1999; 5 RCTs, 14 338 unselected or low risk pregnancies) compared routine Doppler ultrasound of the umbilical artery or a combination of the umbilical and uterine arteries versus control (no, concealed, or selective Doppler ultrasound).[31] Meta-analysis found no difference between groups in antenatal admissions, obstetric interventions, neonatal interventions, or overall perinatal mortality (perinatal mortality: 27/5853 [0.46%] v 29/5522 [0.53%] for controls; OR 0.88, 95% CI 0.52 to 1.48). In one trial, the screened group was more likely to have further Doppler ultrasound examinations (296/1950 [15.2%] v 198/1948 [10.2%] for controls; OR 1.57, 95% CI 1.30 to 1.90). Another trial found increased perinatal mortality among congenitally normal fetuses/neonates in the screened group (16/1246 [1.3%] v 4/1229 [0.3%]; OR 3.31, 95% CI 1.37 to 7.97; NNH 104, 95% CI 29 to 941) (see harms below). The second systematic review (search date not clearly specified, last included reference published 1998; 27 primary observational diagnostic studies comprising 12 994 women in low and high risk populations) evaluated Doppler ultrasound of the uterine artery in the prediction of pre-eclampsia, intrauterine growth retardation and perinatal death.[32] The predictive value of this test in low risk populations (9806 people) was poor with pooled likelihood ratios for both positive and negative tests all falling below 5.0 (see table 1, p 792). **Intensive screening including Doppler:** See benefits of routine ultrasound after 24 weeks' gestation, p 788.

Harms: The higher perinatal mortality among normal fetuses or neonates in the screened group in one trial raised fears that routine Doppler ultrasound in unselected pregnancies may do more harm than good. However, this was an unexpected finding that may have occurred by chance. The trial was not powered to test the ability of routine Doppler ultrasound examinations to reduce perinatal mortality. In the systematic review,[31] meta-analysis of perinatal outcome in normal fetuses included data from 9359 pregnancies, and no such effect was found (perinatal mortality of normal fetuses: 21/4838 [0.43%] v 18/4521 [0.40%]; OR 1.10, 95% CI 0.59 to 2.07) (See also harms under routine ultrasound after 24 weeks' gestation, p 788).

Comment: The five RCTs included in the first systematic review had different designs. Two trials studied unselected populations and three studied low risk populations. No trials included a standardised management protocol for abnormal Doppler results. The type of Doppler ultrasound differed; two trials evaluated umbilical and uterine artery Doppler and three trials evaluated umbilical artery Doppler alone.

Substantive changes since last issue

Non-ultrasound options Omitted from this issue, pending update.
Routine ultrasound New RCT of ultrasound assessment of gestational age at the first antenatal visit; conclusions unchanged.[6]
Doppler ultrasound in low risk pregnancies New systematic review in prediction of pre-eclampsia, intrauterine growth retardation and perinatal death; conclusions limited diagnostic accuracy.[32]

REFERENCES

1. Maternal and Child Health Consortium. *Confidential enquiry into stillbirths and deaths in infancy, 4th annual report.* London: Maternal and Child Health Consortium, 1997:8.
2. Department of Health. Why mothers die. *Report on confidential enquiries into maternal deaths in the United Kingdom 1994–1996.* London: The Stationery Office, 1998.
3. Audit Commission. *First class delivery. Improving maternity services in England and Wales.* London: Audit Commission, 1997.
4. Chitty LS. Ultrasound screening for fetal abnormalities. *Prenat Diagn* 1995;15:1241–1257.
5. Neilson JP. Ultrasound for fetal assessment in early pregnancy. In: The Cochrane Library, Issue 4, 1999. Oxford: Update Software. Search date July 1998; primary sources Cochrane Pregnancy and Childbirth Groups Trials Register, and the Cochrane Controlled Trials Register.
6. Crowther CA, Kornman L, O'Callaghan S, George K, Furness M, Willson K. Is an ultrasound assessment of gestational age at the first antenatal visit of value? A randomised clinical trial. *Br J Obstet Gynaecol* 1999;106:1273–1279.
7. Royal College of Obstetricians and Gynaecologists. *Ultrasound screening for fetal abnormalities: report of the RCOG Working Party.* London: RCOG, 1997.
8. Chitty LS, Pandya PP. Ultrasound screening for fetal abnormalities in the first trimester. *Prenat Diagn* 1997;17:1269–1281.
9. Snijders RJM, Noble P, Sebire N, Souka A, Nicolaides KN. UK multicentre project on assessment of risk of trisomy 21 by maternal age and fetal nuchal-translucency thickness at 10–14 weeks of gestation. *Lancet* 1998;351:343–346.
10. Alfirevic Z, Gosden C, Neilson JP. Chorion villus sampling versus amniocentesis for prenatal diagnosis. In: The Cochrane Library, Issue 4, 1999. Oxford: Update Software. Search date 1996; primary sources Cochrane Pregnancy and Childbirth Groups Trials Register and the Cochrane Controlled Trials Register.
11. Alfirevic Z. Early amniocentesis versus transabdominal chorion villus sampling for prenatal diagnosis. In: The Cochrane Library, Issue 4, 1999. Oxford: Update Software. Search date

October 1998; primary sources Cochrane Pregnancy and Childbirth Groups Trials Register and the Cochrane Controlled Trials Register.

12. Economides DL, Whitlow BJ, Braithwaite JM. Ultrasonography in the detection of fetal anomalies in early pregnancy. Br J Obstet Gynaecol 1999;106:516–523.

13. Saari-Kemppainen A, Karjalainen O, Ylostalo P, Heinonen OP. Fetal anomalies in a controlled one-stage ultrasound screening trial. A report from the Helsinki ultrasound group. J Perinat Med 1994; 22:279–289.

14. Ewigman BG, Crane JP, Frigoletto FD, LeFevre ML, Bain RP, McNellis D, and the RADIUS study group. Effect of prenatal ultrasound screening on perinatal outcome. N Engl J Med 1993;329:821–827.

15. Roberts JP, Burge DM. Antenatal diagnosis of abdominal wall defects: a missed opportunity? Arch Dis Child 1990;65(7 Spec No):687–689.

16. Cohen DM. Surgical management of congenital heart disease in the 1990s. Am J Dis Child 1992; 146:1447–1452.

17. Skari H, Bjornland K, Bjornstad Ostensen A, Haugen G, Emblem R. Consequences of prenatal ultrasound diagnosis: a preliminary report on neonates with congenital malformations. Acta Obstet Gynecol Scand 1998;77:635–642.

18. Chitty LS, Hunt GH, Moore J, Lobb MO. Effectiveness of routine ultrasonography in detecting fetal structural abnormalities in a low risk population. BMJ 1991;303:1165–1169.

19. Levi S, Hyjazi Y, Schaaps JP, Defoort P, Coulon R, Buekens P. Sensitivity and specificity of routine antenatal screening for congenital anomalies by ultrasound: the Belgian multicentric study. Ultrasound Obstet Gynecol 1991;1:366–371.

20. Shirley IM, Bottomley F, Robinson VP. Routine radiographer screening for fetal abnormalities by ultrasound in an unselected low risk population. Br J Radiol 1992;65:564–569.

21. Luck CA. Value of routine ultrasound scanning at 19 weeks: a four year study of 8849 deliveries. BMJ 1992;304:1474–1478.

22. Crane JP, LeFevre ML, Winborn RC, et al. A randomized trial of prenatal ultrasonographic screening: impact on the detection, management, and outcome of anomalous fetuses. Am J Obstet Gynecol 1994;171:392–399.

23. Levi S, Schaaps JP, De Havay P, Coulon R, Defoort P. End-result of routine ultrasound screening for congenital anomalies: the Belgian multicentric study 1984–92. Ultrasound Obstet Gynecol 1995; 5:366–371.

24. Skupski DW, Newman S, Edersheim T, et al. The impact of routine obstetric ultrasonographic screening in a low-risk population. Am J Obstet Gynecol 1996;175:1142–1145.

25. Lee K, Kim SY, Choi SM, et al. Effectiveness of prenatal ultrasonography in detecting fetal anomalies and perinatal outcome of anomalous fetuses. Yonsei Med J 1998;39:372–382.

26. Boyd P, Chamberlain P, Hicks N. Six-year experience of prenatal diagnosis in an unselected population in Oxford, UK. Lancet 1998;352: 1577–1581.

27. Van Dorsten JP, Hulsey TC, Newman RB, Menard MK. Fetal anomaly detection by second-trimester ultrasonography in a tertiary center. Am J Obstet Gynecol 1998;178:742–749.

28. Magriples U, Copel JA. Accurate detection of anomalies by routine ultrasonography in an indigent clinic population. Am J Obstet Gynecol 1998;179:978–981.

29. Bricker L, Neilson JP. Routine ultrasound in late pregnancy (> 24 weeks gestation). In: The Cochrane Library, Issue 1, 2000. Oxford: Update Software. Search date 1999; primary sources Cochrane Pregnancy and Childbirth Groups Trials Register, and the Cochrane Controlled Trials Register.

30. Newnham JP, Evans SF, Michael CA, Stanley FJ, Landau LI. Effects of frequent ultrasound during pregnancy: a randomised controlled trial. Lancet 1993; 342: 887–891.

31. Bricker L, Neilson JP. Routine Doppler ultrasound in pregnancy. In: The Cochrane Library, Issue 2, 2000. Search date 1999; primary sources Cochrane Pregnancy and Childbirth Groups Trials Register, and the Cochrane Controlled Trials Register.

32. Chien PF, Arnott N, Gordon A, Owen P, Khan KS. How useful is uterine artery Doppler flow velocimetry in the prediction of pre-eclampsia, intrauterine growth retardation and perinatal death? An overview. Br J Obstet Gynaecol 2000; 107:196–208. Search date 1997; primary sources Medline, hand searches of bibliographies and known unpublished studies

Leanne Bricker
Clinical Lecturer in Obstetrics
University Department of Obstetrics
and Gynaecology
Liverpool Women's Hospital
Liverpool
UK

James Neilson
Professor of Obstetrics and
Gynaecology
University of Liverpool
Liverpool
UK

Patricia Crowley
Consultant Obstetrician and
Gynaecologist
Coombe Women's Hospital
Dublin
Ireland

Tom O'Dowd
Professor of General Practice
Trinity College
Dublin
Ireland
Competing interests: None declared.

Pregnancy and childbirth

TABLE 1 Operative characteristics of Doppler ultrasound of the uterine artery in the prediction of three outcomes (see benefits of Doppler ultrasound, p 790).[32]

Predicted outcome	Abnormal test result (true positive/all positive)	Normal test result (false negative/all negative)	Sensitivity (95% CI)*	Specificity (95% CI)*	LR+ (95% CI)*	LR– (95% CI)*
Pre-eclampsia	150/891	117/6724	56% (50% to 62%)	90% (89% to 91%)	5.57 (4.9 to 6.3)	0.49 (0.43 to 0.56)
Intrauterine growth retardation	303/1076	665/8730	31% (29% to 34%)	91% (91% to 92%)	3.58 (3.19 to 4.02)	0.75 (0.72 to 0.79)
Perinatal death	12/607	43/3795	22% (13% to 34%)	86% (85% to 87%)	1.59 (0.96 to 2.60)	0.91 (0.79 to 1.04)

LR+ is the positive likelihood ratio (see main glossary); LR– is the negative likelihood ratio (see main glossary). Sensitivity and specificity are defined in the main glossary.

Pregnancy and childbirth

INTERVENTIONS

© *Clinical Evidence* 2000;4:793–803.

Intrapartum surgical interventions

- One systematic review of RCTs has found that restricting episiotomy to specific fetal and maternal indications reduces rates of posterior perineal trauma but slightly increases the rates of anterior vaginal and labial trauma.

- We found no evidence that midline episiotomy incision improves outcome compared with mediolateral incision. Limited evidence suggests that midline incision may increase the risk of third and fourth degree tears.

- One systematic review of RCTs found no direct evidence about the effect of epidural anaesthesia on rates of perineal trauma. However, epidural anaesthesia is associated with an increased risk of instrumental delivery, which in turn is associated with an increased risk of perineal trauma.

- One systematic review of RCTs has found that the use of the vacuum extractor reduces the rate of perineal trauma compared with forceps delivery but increases the incidence of neonatal cephalhaematoma and retinal haemorrhage. One additional case of severe perineal trauma was prevented for every nine occasions that vacuum extraction was used instead of forceps.

Intrapartum non-surgical interventions

- One systematic review of RCTs has found that providing continuous support for women during childbirth versus usual care reduces the rate of instrumental delivery. Two RCTs found no significant difference in the risk of perineal trauma. The trials, however, were too small to rule out a clinically important difference.

- One systematic review comparing an upright position versus the recumbent position during delivery found no significant difference in overall rates of perineal trauma. A subsequent RCT found a reduced episiotomy rate in women who delivered in an upright position. There was a slight increase in labial trauma and a slight reduction in third degree tears in women delivering in an upright position.

- A systematic review of controlled trials has found no significant difference in the extent or rate of perineal trauma when sustained breath holding (Valsalva) or spontaneous exhalatory methods of pushing are used during the second stage of labour.

- One RCT found that the "hands poised" method (not touching the baby's head or supporting the mother's perineum) versus the conventional "hands on" method (applying pressure to the baby's head during delivery and supporting the mother's perineum) increased short term perineal pain. However, it found no evidence of an effect on the risk of perineal trauma or third/fourth degree tears.

Methods and materials for primary repair

- Two systematic reviews of RCTs have found that use of absorbable synthetic suture materials with a continuous subcuticular stitch to appose the skin reduces short term pain. The effects on long term pain and other complications remain uncertain.

- One large RCT found no evidence that leaving the perineal skin unsutured altered short term pain, but dyspareunia was reduced at 3 months postpartum.

- We found no good evidence on the best method or material for repairing third and fourth degree tears and major vaginal lacerations.

DEFINITION	Perineal trauma is any damage to the genitalia during childbirth that occurs spontaneously or intentionally by surgical incision (episiotomy). Anterior perineal trauma is injury to the labia, anterior vagina, urethra or clitoris and is usually associated with little morbidity. Posterior perineal trauma is any injury to the posterior vaginal wall, perineal muscles, or anal sphincter. Depending on severity, posterior perineal trauma is associated with increased morbidity. First degree spontaneous tears involve only skin; second degree involve perineal muscles; third degree partially or completely disrupt the anal sphincter; and fourth degree tears completely disrupt the external and internal anal sphincter and epithelium.[1]
INCIDENCE/ PREVALENCE	Over 85% of women having a vaginal birth sustain some form of perineal trauma,[2] and 60–70% receive stitches — equivalent to 400 000 women per year in the UK in 1997.[2,3] There are wide variations in rates of episiotomy: 8% in the Netherlands, 26–67% in the UK, 50% in the USA, and 99% in east European countries.[4–8] Sutured spontaneous tears are reported in about a third of women in the USA[4] and the UK,[6] but this is probably an underestimate because of inconsistency of reporting and classification of perineal trauma. The incidence of anal sphincter tears varies between 0.5% in the UK, 2.5% in Denmark, and 7% in Canada.[9]
AETIOLOGY/ RISK FACTORS	Perineal trauma occurs during spontaneous or assisted vaginal delivery and is usually more extensive after the first vaginal delivery.[1] Associated risk factors include parity, size of baby, mode of delivery, malpresentation, and malposition of the fetus. Other maternal factors that may contribute to the extent and degree of trauma are ethnicity, age, tissue type, and nutritional state.[10] Clinicians' practices or preferences in terms of intrapartum interventions may influence the severity and rate of perineal trauma.
PROGNOSIS	Perineal trauma affects women's physical, psychological, and social wellbeing in the immediate postnatal period as well as the long term. It can also disrupt breast feeding, family life, and sexual relations. In the UK, about 23–42% of women will continue to have pain and discomfort for 10–12 days postpartum, and 7–10% of women will continue to have long term pain (3–18 months after delivery);[2,3,11] 23% of women will experience superficial dyspareunia at 3 months; 3–10% will report faecal incontinence,[12,13] and up to 24% will have urinary problems.[2,3] Complications depend on severity of perineal trauma and on effectiveness of treatment.
AIMS	To reduce the rate and severity of trauma; to improve the short and long term maternal morbidity associated with perineal injury and repair.
OUTCOMES	Quality of life, incidence and severity of perineal trauma, psychological trauma, short and long term perineal pain, blood loss, infection, wound dehiscence, superficial dyspareunia, stress incontinence, faecal incontinence, adverse effects of treatment.
METHODS	*Clinical Evidence* update search and appraisal May 2000, supplemented by a detailed hand search of relevant journals. All relevant trials were assessed and included, depending on their methodological quality and value.

QUESTION What effects do intrapartum surgical interventions have on the risk of perineal trauma?

OPTION RESTRICTIVE VERSUS ROUTINE USE OF EPISIOTOMY

One systematic review of RCTs has found that restricting the use of episiotomy to specific fetal and maternal indications reduces rates of posterior perineal trauma, need for suturing, and healing complications. Rates of anterior vaginal and labial trauma are slightly increased.

Benefits: We found one systematic review (updated in 1999), which identified six RCTs comparing restricted versus routine episiotomy in 4850 women having a vaginal birth.[14] In the routine episiotomy group, 1752/2409 [73%] had an episiotomy compared with 673/2441 [28%] in the restricted group. Restricted use of episiotomy was associated with lower risk of posterior perineal trauma (AR 72% for restricted v 82% for routine; ARR 10%, 95% CI 6% to 14%; RRR 12%, 95% CI 7% to 18%; NNT 10, 95% CI 7 to 17); less perineal pain at discharge from hospital (AR 31% for restricted v 42% for routine; ARR 12%, 95% CI 8% to 15%; RRR 27%, 95% CI 19% to 36%; NNT 9, 95% CI 7 to 12); less suturing (AR 64% v 86%; ARR 22%, 95% CI 19% to 26%; RRR 26%, 95% CI 22% to 30%; NNT 4, 95% CI 4 to 5); and fewer healing complications (AR 21% v 30%; ARR 9%, 95% CI 4% to 13%; RRR 31%, 95% CI 15% to 45%; NNT 11, 95% CI 7 to 23). There were no significant differences in the two groups in overall rates of severe vaginal or perineal trauma (AR 4% v 4%; ARI 0%, 95% CI −1% to +2%; RRI 11%, 95% CI % −11% to +50%); dyspareunia (AR 52% v 51%; ARI 1%, 95% CI −6% to +7%; RRI 2%, 95% CI −11% to +15%); and urinary incontinence (AR 18% v 19%; ARR 1%, 95% CI −4% to +4%; RRR 2%, 95% CI −20% to +21%).

Harms: We found no reports of serious harms associated with restricted use of episiotomy apart from higher rates of anterior perineal trauma, which carries minimal morbidity (AR 20% for restricted v 11% for routine; ARI 9%, 95% CI 6% to 12%; RRI 79%, 95% CI 56% to 105%; NNH 11, 95% CI 9 to 16).[14]

Comment: The six trials included in the review varied in quality. The method of randomisation was not clear in one trial. All trials performed intention to treat analysis. The trials took place in the UK, Canada, and Argentina. The types of episiotomy performed were mediolateral in five of the trials and midline in the sixth.

OPTION TYPE OF EPISIOTOMY INCISION

We found no evidence that midline episiotomy incision improves outcome compared with mediolateral incision. Limited evidence suggests that midline incision may increase the risk of third and fourth degree tears.

Benefits: We found no systematic review comparing mediolateral versus midline episiotomy incisions. However, stratified analysis of data from the systematic review of routine versus restricted episiotomy[14] found no difference in the overall results between midline and mediolateral episiotomies. We found two published RCTs comparing midline versus mediolateral episiotomies. These were of poor quality and found no evidence of a difference in perineal pain or wound dehiscence.[15,16] Women who had a midline episiotomy experienced significantly less perineal bruising and resumed intercourse earlier.

Harms: One of the RCTs found an increased risk of third or fourth degree tears with midline episiotomies (RRI 126%, 95% CI 64% to 330%).[15] Two retrospective cohort studies, including 5376 primiparous and 341 multiparous women, also found that midline episiotomies were associated with a fourfold increased risk of third and fourth degree tears after allowing for multiple confounders (CI not available).[17,18]

Comment: It has been claimed that midline incision causes less blood loss, easier repair, better healing, less pain, and earlier resumption of sexual intercourse, but at an increased risk of anal sphincter trauma. We found no good evidence to support these claims. One of the trials had an increased risk of selection bias owing to a quasi random method of treatment allocation and because analysis was not by intention to treat.[15] The other trial did not describe the method of treatment allocation.[16]

OPTION EPIDURAL ANAESTHESIA

One systematic review of RCTs found no direct evidence about the effect of epidural anaesthesia on rates of perineal trauma. However, epidural anaesthesia is associated with an increased risk of instrumental delivery, which in turn is associated with an increased risk of perineal trauma.

Benefits: We found one systematic review (updated in 1999, 11 RCTs comparing epidural anaesthesia versus other forms of analgesia, 3157 women).[19] The RCTs did not report the incidence of perineal trauma. Six trials provided data on rates of instrumental delivery when the epidural block was maintained beyond the first stage of labour (n = 1252). The women who had epidurals had increased risk of instrumental delivery (AR 27% for epidural v 16% for no epidural; ARI 10%, 95% CI 5% to 16%; RRI 64%, 95% CI 33% to 99%; NNH 10, 95% CI 6 to 19).

Harms: Analysis of observational evidence found that epidural block was associated with an increased incidence of chronic backache, chronic headache, bladder problems, tingling and numbness, and "sensory confusion".[20]

Comment: The quality of the trials was variable.

OPTION VACUUM EXTRACTOR VERSUS FORCEPS

One systematic review of RCTs has found that the use of the vacuum extractor reduces the rate of perineal trauma compared with forceps delivery but increases the incidence of neonatal cephalhaematoma and retinal haemorrhage. One additional case of severe perineal trauma was prevented for every nine occasions that vacuum extraction was used instead of forceps.

Benefits: We found one systematic review (updated in 1999, 10 RCTs comparing vacuum extraction v forceps, 2885 women).[21] Women allocated to vacuum extraction sustained significantly less perineal trauma (AR 9.8% for vacuum extraction v 20.3% for forceps; ARR 11%, 95% CI 8% to 12%; RRR 52%, 95% CI 41% to 61%; NNT to prevent one case of severe perineal trauma 10, 95% CI 8 to 12), and suffered less short term pain (AR 9% for vacuum extraction, 15% for forceps; ARR 6%, 95% CI 0.8% to 10%; RRR 43%, 95% CI 6% to 67%; NNT 16, 95% CI 10 to 119).

Harms: The systematic review found that babies delivered by vacuum extraction were at higher risk of cephalhaematoma (AR 10% v 4%; ARI 6%, 95% CI 3% to 10%; RRI 139%, 95% CI 69% to 234%; NNH 17, 95% CI 10 to 35) and retinal haemorrhage (AR 49% v 33%; ARI 15%, 95% CI 6% to 25%; RRI 45%, 95% CI 17% to 74%; NNH 7, 95% CI 4 to 17).[21]

Comment: The trials in the review varied in quality, some using quasi random methods of treatment allocation. None of the trials attempted to "blind" the allocated intervention during the postnatal assessments. The trials took place in different countries (UK, USA, South Africa, Denmark, Sweden, and Greece), and the procedures in the studies were comparable to everyday practice when an assisted delivery is required. Although some studies were performed in teaching hospitals, they were pragmatic, with wide inclusion criteria. The evidence is likely to be generaliseable.[21]

QUESTION What effect do intrapartum non-surgical interventions have on the risk of perineal trauma?

OPTION CONTINUOUS SUPPORT DURING LABOUR

One systematic review of RCTs has found that providing continuous support for women during childbirth versus usual care reduces the rate of instrumental delivery. Two small RCTs found no significant difference in the risk of perineal trauma but could not rule out a clinically important difference.

Benefits: We found one systematic review (updated in 1999, 14 RCTs, over 5000 women) comparing usual care versus continuous support from a professional nurse, midwife, or lay person.[22] Women given continuous support versus usual care were less likely to have instrumental delivery (AR 14% v 17%; ARR 2%, 95% CI 0.4% to 4%; RRR 14%, 95% CI 3% to 25%; NNT 41, 95% CI 24 to 239) or episiotomy (data from one RCT; AR 42% v 62%; ARR 21%, 95% CI 5% to 36%; RRR 34%, 95% CI 8% to 57%; NNT 5, 95% CI 3 to 21), but there was no overall reduction in the risk of perineal trauma (data from two RCTs; AR 224/281, [80%] for continuous care, 233/277 [84%] for usual care; ARR 4%, 95% CI −2% to +12%; RRR 5%, 95% CI −2% to +15%).

Harms: We found no evidence of harmful effects. The trials in the review examined a wide range of outcomes but none revealed harmful effects.[22]

Comment: The trials were of reasonable quality, with 11 using sequentially numbered sealed opaque envelopes for treatment allocation. Only one trial "blinded" the participants to the experimental intervention before randomisation and maintained this throughout the study. Although the experimental intervention was always described as one to one support, the timing and duration varied between trials. The pragmatic trials took place in a wide variety of settings (Europe, Scandinavia, South Africa, and the USA) and found similar results, which suggests that the results are generaliseable.[22]

| OPTION | POSITION DURING DELIVERY |

One systematic review comparing an upright position during delivery versus the recumbent position found no significant difference in overall rates of perineal trauma. A subsequent RCT found a reduced episiotomy rate in women who delivered in an upright position. There was a slight increase in labial trauma, and a slight reduction in third degree tears in women delivering in an upright position.

Benefits: We found one systematic review (updated in 1994), which identified 16 RCTs comparing upright position for delivery (birthing chairs, cushions, and squatting) versus conventional recumbent position.[23] Only eight of the trials from the review and a more recent South African RCT[24,25] (total n = 3627) provided data regarding perineal trauma. Analysis of the combined data[23,24] found no significant difference between groups in the number of women with perineal trauma requiring suturing (AR 61% for upright, 64% for recumbent; ARR 3%, 95% CI −0.2% to +6%; RRR 5%, 95% CI −0.3% to +95%). There were only eight third degree tears, and there was no significant difference in rate between groups (AR 0.2% for upright, 1.5% for recumbent; ARR 1.3%, 95% CI −0.2% to +1.5%; RRR 86%, 95% CI −15% to +98%). The more recent RCT found a small reduction in the episiotomy rate in women who delivered in an upright (squatting) position (AR 17% v 25%; ARR 8%, 95% CI 1% to 14%; RRR 33%, 95% CI 6% to 54%; NNT 12, 95% CI 7 to 73).

Harms: Women in the upright group suffered more labial tears, which are thought to be associated with minimal long term morbidity (AR 37% v 28%; ARI 9%, 95% CI 2% to 17%; RRI 33%, 95% CI 7% to 61%; NNH 11, 95% CI 6 to 52). The combined data suggest an increased risk in rate of postpartum haemorrhage with upright delivery, mainly in women delivering on the birthing chair (RRI 78%, 95% CI 35% to 136%). However, this was not supported by the more objective measurement of haemoglobin (RRI for haemoglobin < 11 g/dl 7%, 95% CI −13% to +31%) or the small numbers of women requiring blood transfusions (RRI 93%, 95% CI −17% to +349%).

Comment: The South African RCT was of high quality, including full compliance with the allocated intervention,[24] but the other 16 RCTs included in the systematic review varied in quality.[23] It is difficult to interpret the results of some of the trials because of non-compliance and diversity of the treatment interventions (squatting, kneeling, Gardosi cushion, birthing chair). The published report of the South African trial[24] contained incorrect data regarding the total number of episiotomies in each intervention group; the corrected data have been published and are included here.[25]

OPTION   ALTERNATIVE METHODS OF BEARING DOWN (PUSHING)

A systematic review that compared sustained breath holding (Valsalva) with spontaneous exhalatory methods of pushing during the second stage of labour has found no significant difference in the extent or rate of perineal trauma.

Benefits:
We found one systematic review (amended in 1993, 5 trials, 471 women) comparing bearing down by sustained breath holding (Valsalva) versus exhalatory or spontaneous pushing.[26] Only two of the trials provided data on perineal trauma requiring suturing, and they found no significant difference between the two interventions (AR 33% for Valsalva method, 40% for exhalatory method; ARR 7%, 95% CI −4% to +16%; RRR 16%, 95% CI −10% to +40%).

Harms:
It is unclear whether the rate of adverse perineal outcomes is affected by different types of bearing down during the second stage of labour.

Comment:
The review included published and unpublished trials. Three of the trials were small and of very poor quality. Two of these trials found reduced rates of perineal trauma in the spontaneous bearing down group but this was not supported by data from the two subsequent, more robust controlled trials.[26]

OPTION   "HANDS ON" VERSUS "HANDS POISED"

One RCT found that the "hands poised" method (not touching the baby's head or supporting the mother's perineum) versus the conventional "hands on" method (applying pressure to the baby's head during delivery and supporting the mother's perineum) increased short term perineal pain. It found no evidence of an effect on the risk of perineal trauma or third/fourth degree tears.

Benefits:
We found no systematic review. We found one multicentre RCT, which compared the "hands poised" to the "hands on" method of delivery in 5471 women.[2] There was no significant difference between groups in the risk of perineal trauma requiring suture (AR 60% for "hands poised", 59% for "hands on"; ARI 1%, 95% CI −1.7% to +3.5%; RRI 1.6%, 95% CI −3% to +6%) or third/fourth degree tears (AR 1% in each group; ARI 0.3%, 95% CI −0.2% to +1.2%; RRI 28%, 95% CI −19% to +104%). In the "hands poised" group, the episiotomy rate was reduced (AR 10% v 13%; ARR 3%, 95% CI 1% to 4%; RRR 20%, 95% CI 8% to 32%; NNT 38, 95% CI 25 to 100) and perineal pain at day 10 was increased (AR 34% v 31%; ARI 3%, 95% CI 0.5% to 6%; RRI 10%, 95% CI 1.5% to 18%; NNH 33, 95% CI 18 to 212).

Harms:
There was a significant increase in manual removal of placenta in the "hands poised" group (AR 2.6% v 1.5%; ARI 1.1%, 95% CI 0.2% to 2.2%; RRI 69%, 95% CI 16% to 145%; NNH 95, 95% CI 45 to 417).[2]

Comment: This was the only identified trial comparing "hands poised" with "hands on." It was a large, robust multicentred pragmatic trial, and the results are likely to be generaliseable.

QUESTION **What are the effects of different methods and materials for primary repair of perineal trauma, including non-suturing?**

OPTION   IN FIRST AND SECOND DEGREE TEARS AND EPISIOTOMIES

Two systematic reviews have found that use of absorbable synthetic suture materials with a continuous subcuticular stitch to appose the skin reduces short term pain. The effects on long term pain and other complications remain uncertain. One large RCT found no evidence that leaving the perineal skin unsutured altered short term pain, but dyspareunia was reduced at 3 months postpartum.

Benefits: We found two systematic reviews (updated 1999, 12 RCTs of different suture methods). The reviews compared absorbable synthetic versus catgut suture material for repair of episiotomies and second degree tears,[27] and continuous subcuticular versus interrupted sutures to appose the perineal skin.[28] The trials involved 5506 primiparous and multiparous women and were conducted in Europe and the USA. **Absorbable synthetic versus catgut sutures:** Absorbable synthetic material was associated with less analgesia use within 7 days (AR 38% v 49% with catgut; ARR 11%, 95% CI 5% to 17%; RRR 22%, 95% CI 10% to 34%; NNT 9, 95% CI 6 to 20) and less suture dehiscence, resuturing, and short term pain. There was no clear difference in long term pain with different materials (data from two RCTs; AR perineal pain at 3 months 92/1061 [8.7%] with absorbable synthetic sutures, 112/1068 [10.5%] with catgut). **Continuous subcutaneous versus interrupted transcutaneous suture:** Short term pain was also reduced when a continuous subcutaneous suture was used compared with the interrupted, transcutaneous method of repairing perineal skin (AR 20% with continuous, 27% with interrupted; ARR 7%, 95% CI 3% to 11%; RRR 26%, 95% CI 11% to 39%; NNT 14, 95% CI 10 to 34), but there was no clear difference in long term pain (data from one RCT; AR of pain at 3 months 58/465 [12.5%] with continuous, 51/451 [11.3%] with interrupted; ARI 1.2%, 95% CI –3% to +6%; RRI 10%, 95% CI –23% to +55%). Sutures were removed less frequently (up to 3 months postpartum) in the continuous subcuticular group compared with the interrupted group (AR 26% v 37%; ARR 11%, 95% CI 5% to 16%; RRR 29%, 95% CI 14% to 43%; NNT 9, 95% CI 6 to 20), probably as a result of them being less accessible. **Non-suturing of perineal skin:** We found no systematic review. We found one RCT carried out in a single centre in the UK in 1780 primiparous and multiparous women who sustained perineal trauma (first and second degree tears or episiotomies) after spontaneous or assisted vaginal delivery.[29] It compared a two stage method of repair (the vagina and perineal muscle was sutured, leaving the perineal skin unsutured but apposed) versus a conventional three stage method (the vagina, perineal muscle, and skin were sutured). It found no significant difference between the two and three stage groups in terms of pain at 10 days post partum (AR 25% v 28%; RR 0.90, 95% CI 0.77 to 1.06), but at 3 months fewer women reported dyspareunia in the two stage group (AR 15% v 19%; RR 0.80, 95% CI 0.65 to 0.99; NNT to avoid one additional woman developing dyspareunia 25). **Non-suturing of perineal muscle:** We found one small RCT, which compared non-suturing to suturing of minor perineal trauma (first and second degree tears) in 78 primiparous women in Sweden (two women of the sutured group were excluded; n = 38 sutured v 40 unsutured). Outcomes were assessed after 2 to 3 days and 8 weeks.[30] It found that the type of pain was different between the two groups (burning sensation 9/40 v 1/38; soreness 3/40 v 1/38, but there was no significant difference in healing.[30]

Harms: Up to 3 months postpartum, suture removal was more common in the absorbable synthetic group than in the catgut group (AR 191/1061 [18%] v 108/1068 [10%] for catgut; RRI 78%, 95% CI 43% to 122%).[27] We found no reliable evidence that qualifies the harms of leaving perineal muscle unsutured.

Comment: The trials varied in quality and in operator skills and training. It was not possible to "blind" outcome assessment because of the obvious differences in method and materials used. Most of the trials used "intention to treat" as the method of analysis. A study is currently carrying out a 1 year follow up of 1540 women who participated in an RCT comparing a traditional method to a loose continuous technique of perineal repair using two types of absorbable synthetic suture material (C Kettle, personal communication, 2000). Another study is investigating two different methods of obstetric anal sphincter repair for third and fourth degree tears (R Fernando, personal communication, 2000). The RCT comparing "non-suturing of perineal skin to suturing of perineal skin" was a pragmatic study, and the results are likely to be generaliseable.[29] An RCT is in progress evaluating short term outcomes of non-suturing and suturing in 300 women (V Fleming, personal communication, 2000). We found no reliable evidence to support a policy of leaving minor perineal trauma unsutured (first or second degree tears). The findings of the small RCT on non-suturing of perineal muscle are difficult to interpret: published data are inconsistent with reported conclusions.[30]

OPTION   IN THIRD AND FOURTH DEGREE TEARS

We found no good evidence on the effects of different methods and materials for repair of third and fourth degree tears.

Benefits: We found no systematic review or RCTs.

Harms: Insufficient data.

Comment: None.

REFERENCES

1. Sultan AH, Kamm MA, Bartram CI, Hudson CN. Perineal damage at delivery. *Contemp Rev Obstet Gynaecol* 1994;6:18–24.
2. McCandlish R, Bowler U, van Asten H, et al. A randomised controlled trial of care of the perineum during second stage of normal labour. *Br J Obstet Gynaecol* 1998;105:1262–1272.
3. Sleep J, Grant A, Garcia J, et al. West Berkshire perineal management trial. *BMJ* 1984;298:587–690.
4. Graves EJ. 1993 summary: National hospital discharge survey. *Advance Data* 1995;264:1–11.
5. Graham ID, Graham DF. Episiotomy counts: trends and prevalence in Canada, 1981/1982 to 1993/1994. *Birth* 1997;24:141–147.
6. Audit Commission. First class delivery: improving maternity services in England and Wales. London: Audit Commission Publications, 1997.
7. Wagner M. *Pursuing the birth machine: the search for appropriate technology.* Camperdown: ACE Graphics, 1994;165–174.
8. Williams FL, du V Florey C, Mires GJ, Ogston SA. Episiotomy and perineal tears in low-risk UK primigravidae. *J Pub Health Med* 1998;20;422–427.
9. Sultan AH, Monga AK, Kumar D, et al. Primary repair of anal sphincter using the overlap technique. *Br J Obstet Gynaecol* 1999;106:318–323.
10. Renfrew MJ, Hannah W, Albers L, et al. Practices that minimize trauma to the genital tract in childbirth: a systematic review of the literature. *Birth* 1998;25:143–160. Search date May 1997; primary Sources Cochrane Database of Systematic Reviews, Medline, Cinahl, Miriad, Midirs, Index Medicus plus hand searches of current textbooks of obstetrics, midwifery and nursing.
11. Glazener CMA, Abdalla M, Stroud P, et al. Postnatal maternal morbidity: extent, causes, prevention and treatment. *Br J Obstet Gynaecol* 1995;102:286–287.
12. Sleep J, Grant A. Pelvic floor exercises in postnatal care. *Br J Midwifery* 1987;3:158–164.
13. Sultan AH, Kamm MA, Hudson CN. Anal sphincter disruption during vaginal delivery. *N Engl J Med* 1993;329:1905–1911.
14. Carroli G, Belizan J, Stamp G. Episiotomy for vaginal birth. In: The Cochrane Library, Issue 4, 1999. Oxford; Update Software. Search date not given: review updated May 1999; primary source Cochrane Pregnancy and Childbirth Group Trials Register.
15. Coats PM, Chan KK, Wilkins M, et al. A comparison between midline and mediolateral episiotomies. *Br J Obstet Gynaecol* 1989;87:408–412.
16. Werner CH, Schuler W, Meskendahl I. Midline episiotomy versus mediolateral episiotomy: a randomised prospective study. *Int J Gynaecol Obstet.* Proceedings of 13th World Congress of Gynaecology and Obstetrics (FIGO), Singapore 1991;Book 1:33.
17. Shiono P, Klebanof MD, Carey JC. Midline episiotomies: more harm than good? *Obstet Gynacol* 1990;75:756–770.
18. Klein MC, Gauthier MD, Robbins JM, et al.

Relationship of episiotomy to perineal trauma and morbidity, sexual function, and pelvic floor relaxation. *Am J Obstet Gynecol* 1994;17:591–598.
19. Howell CJ. Epidural vs non-epidural analgesia for pain relief in labour. In: The Cochrane Library, Issue 4, 1999. Oxford: Update Software. Search date not given; primary source Cochrane Pregnancy and Childbirth Group Trials Register.
20. Howell CJ, Chalmers I. A review of prospectively controlled comparisons of epidural with non-epidural forms of pain relief during labour. *Int J Obstet Anaesth* 1992;1:93–110.
21. Johanson RB, Menon VJ. Vacuum extraction vs forceps delivery. In: The Cochrane Library, Issue 4, 1999. Oxford: Update Software. Search date February 1999; primary source Cochrane Pregnancy and Childbirth Group trials register.
22. Hodnett ED. Caregiver support for women during childbirth. In: The Cochrane Library, Issue 4, 1999. Oxford: Update Software. Search date April 1999; primary sources Cochrane Pregnancy and Childbirth Group trials register; Cochrane Controlled Trials Register.
23. Nikodem VC. Upright vs recumbent position during the second stage of labour. In: Enkin MW, Keirse MJNC, Renfrew MJ, et al, eds. *Pregnancy and childbirth module.* In: The Cochrane Library, Issue 2. Oxford: Update Software. Search date not given; primary sources not given.
24. De Jong PR, Johanson RB, Baxen P, et al. Randomised trial comparing the upright and supine positions for the second stage of labour. *Br J Obstet Gynaecol* 1997;104:567–571.
25. Eason E, de Jong P. Randomised trial comparing the upright and supine positions for the second stage of labour. *Br J Obstet Gynaecol* 1999;106:291–292.
26. Nikodem VC. Sustained (Valsalva) vs exhalatory bearing down in 2nd stage of labour. In: Enkin MW, Keirse MJNC, Renfrew MJ, et al, eds. *Pregnancy and childbirth module.* In: The Cochrane Library, Issue 2, 1994. Oxford: Update Software. Search date October 1993; primary sources Cochrane Pregnancy and Childbirth Database, Medline plus handsearch of specialist journals, conference proceedings.
27. Kettle C, Johanson RB. Absorbable synthetic vs catgut suture material for perineal repair. In: The Cochrane Library, Issue 4, 1999. Oxford: Update Software. Search date not given; primary source Cochrane Pregnancy and Childbirth Group trials register.
28. Kettle C, Johanson RB. Continuous versus interrupted sutures for perineal repair. In: The Cochrane Library, Issue 4, 1999. Oxford: Update Software. Search date not given; primary source Cochrane Pregnancy and Childbirth Group Specialised Register of Controlled Trials.
29. Gordon B, Mackrodt C, Fern E, et al. The Ipswich Childbirth Study: 1. A randomised evaluation of two stage postpartum perineal repair leaving the skin unsutured. *Br J Obstet Gynaecol* 1998;105:435–440.
30. Lundquist M, Olsson A, Nissen E, Norman M. Is it necessary to suture all lacerations after a vaginal delivery? *Birth* 2000;27:79–85.

Chris Kettle
Midwifery Research Fellow
North Staffordshire Hospital (NHS Trust) and Keele University, Stoke-on-Trent, UK

Competing interests: The author has received a grant from the Iolanthe Midwifery Research Trust and support from Ethicon Ltd, which enabled her to carry out a randomised controlled trial of perineal management — The Methods or Materials Study (MOMS).

Pregnancy and childbirth

Updated this issue

Lelia Duley

INTERVENTIONS

See glossary, p 813

Key Messages

- One systematic review of RCTs has found that antiplatelet drugs (mainly aspirin) reduce the risk of pre-eclampsia. One systemic review of RCTs has found that calcium supplementation reduces the relative risk of pre-eclampsia by about a third.

- We found insufficient evidence on the effects of fish oil, or of evening primrose oil plus fish oil or calcium on the risk of pre-eclampsia and preterm birth.

- It is unclear whether women with mild to moderate hypertension during pregnancy derive benefit from antihypertensive drugs.

- For women with severe hypertension during pregnancy, antihypertensive drugs will lower blood pressure, but we found no reliable evidence that any one agent is substantially better than another.

- We found insufficient evidence to assess the effect of hospital admission, bed rest, or day care compared with outpatient care.

- We found promising evidence that magnesium sulphate may reduce the risk of developing eclampsia, but other possible benefits and harms are unclear. These are being addressed by an ongoing trial.

- One large systematic review has found that magnesium sulphate is the best choice of anticonvulsant for treatment of eclampsia.

- More efficient systems need to be developed to assess severe adverse events (likely to be rare), particularly for drugs widely used during pregnancy. They should include monitoring of events for both the woman and child.

DEFINITION	Hypertension during pregnancy may be associated with one of several conditions. **Pregnancy induced hypertension** is a rise in blood pressure, without proteinuria, during the second half of pregnancy. **Pre-eclampsia** is a multisystem disorder, unique to pregnancy, which is usually associated with raised blood pressure and proteinuria. It rarely presents before 20 weeks' gestation. **Eclampsia** is one or more convulsions in association with the syndrome of pre-eclampsia. **Pre-existing hypertension** is known hypertension before pregnancy, or raised blood pressure before 20 weeks' gestation. It may be essential hypertension or, less commonly, secondary to underlying disease.[1]
INCIDENCE/ PREVALENCE	Pregnancy induced hypertension affects 10% of pregnancies, and pre-eclampsia complicates 2–8%.[2] Eclampsia occurs in about 1 in 2000 deliveries in developed countries.[3] In developing countries, estimates of the incidence of eclampsia vary from 1 in 100 to 1 in 1700.[4,5]
AETIOLOGY/ RISK FACTORS	Aetiology of pre-eclampsia is unknown. It is likely to be multifactorial and may result from deficient placental implantation during the first half of pregnancy.[6] Pre-eclampsia is more common among women likely to have a large placenta, such as those with multiple pregnancy, and among women with medical conditions associated with microvascular disease, such as diabetes, hypertension, and collagen vascular disease.[7,8] Other risk factors include genetic susceptibility, increased parity, and older maternal age.[9] Cigarette smoking seems to be associated with a lower risk of pre-eclampsia, but this potential benefit is outweighed by an increase in adverse outcomes such as low birth weight, placental abruption and perinatal death.[10]
PROGNOSIS	The outcome of pregnancy in women with pregnancy induced hypertension alone is at least as good as that for normotensive pregnancies.[7,11] However, once pre-eclampsia develops, morbidity and mortality rise for both mother and child. For example, perinatal mortality for women with severe pre-eclampsia is double that for normotensive women.[7] Perinatal outcome is worse with early gestational hypertension.[7,9,11] Perinatal mortality also increases in women with severe essential hypertension.[12]
AIMS	To delay or prevent the development of pre-eclampsia and eclampsia, and to improve outcomes for women and their children. Once pre-eclampsia has occurred, to minimise morbidity and mortality for

the woman and her child, and to ensure that health service resources are used appropriately.

OUTCOMES **For the woman:** rates of pre-eclampsia (proteinuria and hypertension), eclampsia, death, severe morbidity (such as renal failure, coagulopathy, cardiac failure, liver failure, and stroke), placental abruption, and caesarean section; use of health service resources (such as dialysis, ventilation, admission to intensive care, or length of stay); adverse effects of treatment. **For the child:** rates of death, intrauterine growth restriction, prematurity, and severe morbidity (such as intraventricular haemorrhage, respiratory distress syndrome, or asphyxia); measures of infant and child development (such as cerebral palsy or significant learning disability); use of health service resources (such as admission to special care nursery, ventilation, length of stay in hospital, and special needs in the community); adverse effects of treatment.

METHODS *Clinical Evidence* update search and appraisal May 2000. Trials were included if they met *Clinical Evidence* criteria. Most of the evidence presented here is included in the relevant Cochrane reviews, where the methods are described in greater detail.

QUESTION **What are the effects of preventive interventions in women at high risk of pre-eclampsia?**

OPTION **ANTIPLATELET DRUGS**

One systematic review of large RCTs has found that antiplatelet drugs (mainly aspirin) are associated with reduced relative risk of pre-eclampsia (15%), death of the baby (14%), and prematurity (8%), with no significant difference in other important outcomes. Two large aspirin trials that followed children to age 12–18 months have found that aspirin is safe in the short to medium term.

Benefits: We found one systematic review of antiplatelet agents (search date 1999, 41 RCTs, over 32 000 women) and one subsequent RCT.[13,14] **Versus placebo/no antiplatelet:** The systematic review found that antiplatelet agents were associated with a 15% reduction in pre-eclampsia (RR 0.85, 95% CI 0.78 to 0.92) but a smaller reduction in premature delivery (before 37 completed weeks; RR 0.92, 95% CI 0.88 to 0.97). There were fewer baby deaths associated with antiplatelet agents (RR 0.86, 95% CI 0.77 to 0.98). There were no clear effects on other important outcomes. There was no apparent effect of starting treatment before 20 weeks, or differences between women at high and low risk. The effect seemed to be greatest for women given more than 75 mg aspirin daily. The subsequent small RCT compared ozagrel hydrochloride with placebo, but was too small for any reliable conclusions.[14] **Versus each other:** Trials comparing one antiplatelet agent with another were too small for reliable conclusions.[13]

Harms: The systematic review found no evidence of aspirin being associated with an increased risk of bleeding for mother or baby.[13] Two large trials that followed up children to age 12–18 months found no differences between the two groups.[15,16]

Comment: Almost all studies used low dose aspirin (50–75 mg), and most were placebo controlled. The trials included women with a variety of risk factors, including a history of previous early onset disease, diabetes, or chronic hypertension, and were conducted in different countries in the developed and developing world.

OPTION CALCIUM SUPPLEMENTATION

One systematic review of RCTs, and one subsequent RCT, have found a 30% relative reduction in the risk of pre-eclampsia and a 17% relative reduction in the risk of having a baby with birthweight under 2500 g associated with calcium supplementation ($\geq$ 1 g/day). There was no significant effect on caesarean delivery, preterm delivery, or death of the baby.

Benefits: We found one systematic review of calcium supplementation (search date 1997, 9 RCTs, over 6000 women)[17] and one subsequent RCT (including 456 women) that met the inclusion criteria for the systematic review.[18] **Versus placebo:** In the 10 RCTs, calcium (mainly 2 g daily) was associated with a 30% relative reduction in the risk of pre-eclampsia (RR 0.70, 95% CI 0.58 to 0.83; NNT 40, 95% CI 28 to 77). The effect seemed strongest for high risk women and for those with low dietary calcium. There was also a 17% relative reduction in the risk of having a baby with birthweight under 2500 g (RR 0.83, 95% CI 0.71 to 0.98; NNT 67, 95% CI 36 to 1000). There was little evidence of effect on caesarean delivery, preterm delivery, or death of the baby. **Calcium and primrose oil versus placebo:** One small trial (48 women) did not provide sufficient evidence for reliable conclusions.[19]

Harms: No adverse events were reported in these trials. One large study that followed children for 7 years provided additional reassurance about the long term safety of calcium supplementation.

Comment: Most trials in the systematic review were of good quality and included a wide range of women. They were conducted largely in the USA and South America. They mainly included women at low risk with adequate dietary calcium, so the numbers of women in the more promising categories were small. Several studies reported that adherence to treatment usually lay between 60–90%. The proportion of women taking 90–100% of all allocated treatment was low (20% in one study).

OPTION OTHER DIETARY INTERVENTIONS

We found insufficient evidence on the effects of fish oil, or of evening primrose oil plus fish oil or calcium, on the risk of pre-eclampsia and preterm birth. One RCT found that fish oil was associated with increased risk of post-term delivery and postpartum haemorrhage. Reduced salt intake (to 20–50 mmol/day) or supplementation with magnesium does not apparently influence the risk of pre-eclampsia or its complications. One RCT found that supplementation with vitamins C and E reduced the risk of pre-eclampsia.

Benefits: **Fish and evening primrose oil:** We found no systematic review. We found six trials of fish and primrose oil that were too small to draw reliable conclusions.[20–25] **Reduced salt versus normal or high salt:** We found one systematic review (2 RCTs, 600 women) comparing reduced salt with normal dietary salt.[26] Although these trials were too small for reliable conclusions, together they did not provide any substantive evidence that reducing salt intake during pregnancy affected pre-eclampsia (RR 1.11, 95% CI 0.46 to 2.66). **Magnesium:** We found one systematic review, which included two RCTs (474 women) reporting pre-eclampsia. These were too small for reliable conclusions.[27] **Vitamins C and E:** We found one RCT in 283 high risk women that found a reduced risk of pre-eclampsia with vitamin C (1000 mg/day) and vitamin E (400 IU/day) compared with placebo (11/141 [8%] with vitamins v 24/142 [17%] with placebo; RR 0.46, 95% CI 0.24 to 0.91; NNT 11, 95% CI 8 to 61).[28] The study was too small to provide reliable evidence about effects on other important outcomes.

Harms: **Fish oil:** One trial (533 women) found that fish oil compared with either olive oil or no supplement produced an insignificant increase in post-term delivery (RR 1.19, 95% CI 0.73 to 1.93) and postpartum haemorrhage (RR 1.21, 95% CI 0.76 to 1.92).[29] These outcomes were not reported in the other smaller studies. **Fish oil and primrose oil:** Vomiting was more commonly reported in the oil treated group, but numbers were not given.[24] No other adverse events were reported. **Primrose oil:** These studies were too small for reliable conclusions. **Reduced salt:** We found no evidence of harmful effects in the trials.[26] **Magnesium:** There was no significant difference between the groups in reported adverse effects (RR 0.84, 95% CI 0.65 to 1.08).[25] **Vitamins C and E:** We found little information about the safety of these agents at the high doses used in the RCT.[28]

Comment: The fish oil trials may have suffered from the difficulty of getting a true placebo, because of the distinctive taste of fish oil. One study found that olive oil provided better masking than a no-oil placebo.[29] The trials of salt restriction were conducted in the Netherlands, where advice to restrict salt intake during pregnancy has been routine for many years. Such advice is no longer widespread elsewhere. An updated systematic review of fish oil for prevention of pre-eclampsia will be available in 2001.

<hr>

QUESTION What are the effects of interventions in women who develop hypertension during pregnancy?

<hr>

OPTION BED REST/HOSPITAL ADMISSION OR DAY CARE

We found limited evidence from which it was not possible to demonstrate benefit for hospital admission, bed rest, or day care compared with outpatient care.

Benefits: **Bed rest/hospital admission:** We found two systematic reviews of hospital admission.[30,31] The first compared hospital admission with outpatient clinic assessment for non-proteinuric hypertension (search date 1993, 3 trials, 408 women) and found no significant difference for any major outcome.[30] The second review (search date 1993) compared bed rest in hospital with normal ambulation in hospital for proteinuric hypertension (2 trials, 145 women), but the trials were too small for any reliable conclusions.[31] **Day care versus outpatient clinic assessment:** We found one trial (54 women) but again this study was too small for reliable conclusions.[32]

Harms:
Although it is plausible that hospital admission may promote venous stasis and increase the risk of thromboembolic disease, we found no data on these rarer outcomes. In the trial of day care units, women preferred not to be admitted to hospital. We found no information from the other trials about the views of women and their families, or the costs to them and to the health services.

Comment:
Trials of hospital admission and bed rest in hospital were conducted before widespread introduction of day care assessment units. Women with hypertension during pregnancy are now often seen in day care units, but only one small trial has compared day care assessment with assessment in an outpatient clinic.

| OPTION | ANTIHYPERTENSIVE AGENTS |

Two systematic reviews found evidence from small trials that antihypertensive agents may reduce the chance of developing severe hypertension by more than half. The effects of antihypertensive agents on pre-eclampsia and on perinatal death are unclear. We found insufficient evidence for reliable conclusions about any other important outcomes, and few trials reported on hospital admission and use of health service resources.

Benefits:
We found two systematic reviews. The first systematic review included 23 small trials (search date 1994, over 2600 women).[33] The second systematic review of eight trials (search date 1997, 991 women) included only studies that compared β blockers with no antihypertensive.[34] **Versus placebo or no antihypertensive:** The only effect was reduced risk of developing severe hypertension (RR 0.40, 95% CI 0.27 to 0.58), which was not reflected in other, more substantive outcomes (pre-eclampsia: RR 0.81, 95% CI 0.58 to 1.14; perinatal death: RR 0.59, 95% CI 0.31 to 1.10). **Versus other antihypertensive agents:** The trials comparing one drug with another were too small for reliable conclusions.

Harms:
Although antihypertensive drugs seem to be well tolerated during pregnancy, adverse effects have not been reported in many trials. All antihypertensive drugs cross the placenta, but few trials reported possible adverse effects for the baby. The baby's risk of being small for its gestational age was increased if a β blocker was used to control the mother's hypertension (RR 1.34, 95% CI 1.01 to 1.79; 13 trials, 1382 women).[35] Meta regression within a systematic review has suggested that lowering blood pressure for women with mild or moderate hypertension may be associated with an increased risk of having a baby that is small for its gestational age.[36]

Comment:
The trials were too small to exclude beneficial effects of antihypertensive agents on substantive outcomes. The trials were not of good quality. Many were not placebo controlled, and few attempted to blind blood pressure measurement. In addition, many important

outcomes were reported by only a small number of studies. We found little information about adherence to treatment. One systematic review of six trials in women with pre-existing chronic hypertension found that the effects of antihypertensive agents were similar to those for women with pregnancy induced hypertension.[33] An updated systematic review of antihypertensive drugs for mild to moderate hypertension will be available early in 2001.

QUESTION What are the effects of interventions in women who develop severe pre-eclampsia or very high blood pressure during pregnancy?

OPTION ANTIHYPERTENSIVE DRUGS FOR VERY HIGH BLOOD PRESSURE

One systematic review has found no evidence of a difference between the various antihypertensive drugs in terms of their ability to control blood pressure, with the possible exceptions of diazoxide and ketanserin, which seem to be less effective. Studies were too small for any further conclusions about relative effects of different agents.

Benefits: We found one systematic review (search date 1998, 14 trials, 1200 women), which compared many agents (including hydralazine, labetalol, nifedipine, diazoxide, and ketanserin) mainly with hydralazine.[37] All reduced blood pressure, but there was no significant evidence that any one was better than another.

Harms: The use of ketanserin is associated with more persistent high blood pressure than hydralazine (RR 8.44, 95% CI 2.05 to 34.7), and diazoxide is associated with more hypotension requiring treatment than labetalol (RR 0.06, 95% CI 0.00 to 0.99).[37] Hypotension may compromise fetoplacental blood flow. Only four studies reported adverse effects, and frequency varied from 5–50%. These drugs cross the placenta, but we found little information about possible effects on the baby.

Comment: Women in these studies had blood pressures high enough to merit immediate treatment, and many also had proteinuria or "severe pre-eclampsia". The trials were small and reported few outcomes other than control of blood pressure. Also, there is potential for bias, as in most trials there was no blinding after trial entry.

OPTION PLASMA VOLUME EXPANSION

One systematic review of small RCTs has found insufficient evidence for reliable conclusions, although the results suggest that benefit is unlikely.

Benefits: We found one systematic review (search date 1999, 3 RCTs, 61 women) evaluating colloid solutions compared with placebo or no infusion. The trials were too small for reliable conclusions but suggest that plasma volume expansion is not beneficial.[38]

Harms: Trials found a non-significant increased risk of caesarean section (RR 1.46, 95% CI 0.75 to 2.85) and a non-significant increased need for additional treatment (RR 1.51, 95% CI 0.73 to 3.11) associated with the use of plasma volume expansion compared with placebo or no infusion.

Comment: These three trials all used a colloid rather than crystalloid solution. Evidence from systematic reviews of plasma volume expansion in critically ill men and non-pregnant women has shown an increase in mortality associated with albumin (a colloid) when compared with either no expansion or crystalloid.[39,40]

OPTION ANTIOXIDANTS

We found insufficient evidence on the effects of antioxidants.

Benefits: We found no systematic review. We found one placebo controlled RCT (56 women) evaluating a combination of vitamin E, vitamin C, and allopurinol.[41] It was too small for reliable conclusions to be drawn.

Harms: We found insufficient data for reliable conclusions.

Comment: Women in this study had severe pre-eclampsia at 24–32 weeks' gestation.

OPTION PROPHYLACTIC ANTICONVULSANTS FOR WOMEN WITH SEVERE PRE-ECLAMPSIA

One systematic review has found that prophylactic anticonvulsants may reduce the risk of eclampsia, but it provides little information about possible effects on other important outcomes. Limited evidence from case control studies suggests that _in utero_ exposure to magnesium sulphate may reduce the risk of cerebral palsy, but it is also possible that such exposure may increase infant mortality.

Benefits: We found one systematic review (search date 1999, 10 trials, 3747 women).[42] **Magnesium sulphate versus placebo or no anticonvulsant:** Four trials (1249 women) found reduction in the risk of eclampsia that did not quite reach significance (RR 0.33, 95% CI 0.11 to 1.02). There were no clear effects on other reported outcomes. Limited evidence from case control studies suggests that magnesium sulphate may reduce the risk of cerebral palsy for babies weighing less than 1500 g by as much as 80%.[43,44] One small trial (59 women) compared diazepam with no anticonvulsant; it was too small for any reliable conclusions. **Magnesium sulphate versus phenytoin or diazepam:** Five trials (2439 women) found that magnesium sulphate was better than phenytoin for preventing eclampsia (RR 0.05, 95% CI 0.00 to 0.84), but there was insufficient evidence for reliable conclusions about the differential effect compared with diazepam.[42]

Harms: We found only one trial (135 women) that reported maternal adverse effects, in this case slurred speech (RR 3.04, 95% CI 0.13 to 73.4) and flushing (RR 3.81, 95% CI 2.22 to 6.53).[42] Compared with phenytoin, magnesium sulphate was associated with an increased risk of caesarean section (RR 1.21, 95% CI 1.05 to 1.41; NNH 29, 95% CI 12 to 84). One small trial evaluated magnesium sulphate for preventing and treating preterm labour in women who did not have pre-eclampsia. It reported an increase in infant mortality for babies born to these women, many of whom had very low birthweight.[45]

Comment: The quality of these trials was average to poor. Most trials included women with severe pre-eclampsia. One small study recruited women with mild pre-eclampsia. A large international trial (the Magpie trial) comparing magnesium sulphate with placebo for women with pre-eclampsia is under way (L Duley, personal communication, 2000).

OPTION   AGGRESSIVE MANAGEMENT FOR SEVERE EARLY ONSET PRE-ECLAMPSIA

Two trials found that a policy of expectant, or conservative, management for severe early onset pre-eclampsia may have substantive benefits for the baby. There was insufficient evidence for reliable conclusions about possible effects for the woman.

Benefits: We found two small trials (133 women) that, taken together, found expectant management to be associated with reduced risk of respiratory distress syndrome in the baby (RR 2.30, 95% CI 1.39 to 3.81). The trials were too small for any reliable conclusions on the effect on perinatal mortality or on maternal morbidity.[46,47]

Harms: Additional time *in utero* for the baby should not be at the expense of increased morbidity for the women. There is insufficient evidence for reliable conclusions about possible effects of expectant management on maternal morbidity.

Comment: The women in these trials were at 28–34 weeks' gestation. A systematic review is in preparation (D Churchill, personal communication, 2000).

QUESTION   What is the best choice of anticonvulsant for women with eclampsia?

Systematic reviews have found that magnesium sulphate is better than phenytoin, diazepam, or lytic cocktail for the prevention of further fits in women with eclampsia. Although the effects on maternal mortality are not statistically significant, all three reviews found trends towards a reduced risk associated with magnesium sulphate.

Benefits: **Versus diazepam:** We found one systematic review (search date 1999, 5 trials, 1236 women).[48] Magnesium sulphate reduced maternal mortality (RR 0.59, 95% CI 0.36 to 1.00) and prevented further fits (RR 0.45, 95% CI 0.35 to 0.58) more than diazepam. There was no evidence of any differential effects on any other reported outcome. **Versus phenytoin:** We found one systematic review (search date 1999, 4 trials, 845 women).[49] Magnesium sulphate reduced the risks of further fits (RR 0.32, 95% CI 0.20 to 0.49), pneumonia (RR 0.44, 95% CI 0.24 to 0.79), requiring ventilation (RR 0.66, 95% CI 0.49 to 0.90), and admission to intensive care (RR 0.67, 95% CI 0.50 to 0.89) more than phenytoin.[49] Fewer babies died or stayed in a special baby care unit for more than 7 days (RR 0.77, 95% CI 0.63 to 0.95). The lower maternal death rate with magnesium sulphate compared with phenytoin was not significant, but the confidence interval was wide and a clinically important effect could not be excluded (RR 0.50, 95% CI 0.24 to 1.05). **Versus lytic cocktail:** See glossary, below. We found two trials comparing magnesium sulphate with lytic cocktail (198 women).[50,51] Magnesium sulphate was better than lytic cocktail for preventing further fits (RR 0.09, 95% CI 0.03 to 0.24). It was also associated with a lower risk of pneumonia (RR 0.08, 95% CI 0.02 to 0.42) and of respiratory depression (RR 0.12, 95% CI 0.02 to 0.91).

Harms: **Versus diazepam:** We found no evidence that magnesium sulphate has more harmful effects than diazepam. **Versus phenytoin:** Clinical experience suggests that magnesium sulphate is safer than phenytoin. **Versus lytic cocktail:** Magnesium sulphate seems to be considerably safer than lytic cocktail.

Comment: Most information about the comparisons with diazepam and phenytoin comes from one large multicentre trial, in which adherence to treatment was 99%. The lytic cocktail trials were conducted in India. Women with both antepartum and postpartum eclampsia were included.

GLOSSARY

Lytic cocktail A mixture of pethidine, chlorpromazine, and promethazine.

REFERENCES

1. Gifford RW, August P, Chesley LC, et al. National high blood pressure education program working group report on high blood pressure in pregnancy. *Am J Obstet Gynecol* 1990;163(5 Pt 1):1691–1712.
2. WHO international collaborative study of hypertensive disorders of pregnancy. Geographic variation in the incidence of hypertension in pregnancy. *Am J Obstet Gynecol* 1988;158:80–83.
3. Douglas K, Redman C. Eclampsia in the United Kingdom. *BMJ* 1994;309:1395–1400.
4. Crowther CA. Eclampsia at Harare maternity hospital. An epidemiological study. *S Afr Med J* 1985;68:927–929.
5. Bergström S, Povey G, Songane F, et al. Seasonal incidence of eclampsia and its relationship to meteorological data in Mozambique. *J Perinat Med* 1992;20:153–158.
6. Roberts JM, Redman CWG. Pre-eclampsia: more than pregnancy-induced hypertension. *Lancet* 1993;341:1447–1451.
7. Taylor DJ. The epidemiology of hypertension during pregnancy. In: Rubin PC, ed. *Hypertension in Pregnancy.* Amsterdam: Elsevier Science, 1988: 223–240.
8. Sibai BM, Caritis S, Hauth J. Risks of preeclampsia and adverse neonatal outcomes among women with pregestational diabetes mellitus. National Institute of Child Health and Human Development Network of Maternal-Fetal Medicine Units. *Am J Obstet Gynecol* 2000;182: 364–369.
9. MacGillivray I. *Pre-eclampsia. The hypertensive disease of pregnancy.* London: WB Saunders, 1983.
10. Conde-Agudelo A, Althabe F, Belizan JM, Kafury-Goeta AC. Cigarette smoking during pregnancy and risk of preeclampsia: a systematic review. *Am J Obstet Gynecol* 1999;181:1026–1035. Search date 1998; primary sources Medline, Embase, Popline, Cinahl, Lilacs, and hand searches of proceedings of international meetings on pre-eclampsia and reference lists of retrieved articles.
11. Chamberlain GVP, Philip E, Howlett B, Masters K. *British births.* London: Heinemann, 1970.
12. Sibai B, Lindheimer M, Hauth J, et al. Risk factors for preeclampsia, abruptio placentae, and adverse neonatal outcomes among women with chronic hypertension. *N Engl J Med* 1998;339:667–671.
13. Knight M, Duley L, Henderson-Smart D, et al. The effectiveness and safety of antiplatelet agents for the prevention and treatment of pre-eclampsia. In: Cochrane Library, Issue 3. Oxford: Update software, 2000. Search date 1999; primary sources Cochrane Pregnancy and Childbirth Group Trials Register; conference proceedings.
14. Seki H, Kuromaki K, Takeda S, Kinoshita K, Satoh K. Trial of prophylactic administration of TXA2 synthetase inhibitor, ozagrel hydrochloride, for pre-eclampsia. *Hypertens Pregnancy* 1999;18:157–164.
15. Grant A, Farrell B, Heineman J, et al. Low dose aspirin in pregnancy and early childhood development: Follow up of the collaborative low dose aspirin study in pregnancy. *Br J Obstet Gynaecol* 1995;102:861–868.
16. Parazzini F, Bortolus R, Chatenoud L, Restelli S, Benedetto C. Follow-up of children in the Italian study of aspirin in pregnancy. *Lancet* 1994;343: 1235.
17. Atallah AN, Hofmeyr GJ, Duley L. Calcium supplementation during pregnancy to prevent hypertensive disorders and related adverse outcomes. In: Cochrane Library, Issue 3. Oxford: Update software, 2000. Search date 1997; primary sources Cochrane Pregnancy and Childbirth Group Trials Register.
18. Crowther CA, Hiller JE, Pridmore B, Bryce R, et al. Calcium supplementation in nulliparous women for the prevention of pregnancy-induced hypertension, preeclampsia and preterm birth: an Australian randomized trial. *Aust NZ J Obstet Gynaecol* 1999; 39:12–18.

19. Herrera JA, Arevalo-Herrera M, Herrera S. Prevention of pre-eclampsia by linoleic acid and calcium supplementation: a randomized controlled trial. *Obstet Gynecol* 1998;91:585–590.

20. Salvig JD, Olsen SF, Secher NJ. Effects of fish oil supplementation in late pregnancy on blood pressure: a randomised controlled trial. *Br J Obstet Gynaecol* 1996;103:529–533.

21. Onwude JL, Lilford RJ, Hjartardottir H, et al. A randomised double blind placebo controlled trial of fish oil in high risk pregnancy. *Br J Obstet Gynaecol* 1995;102:95–100.

22. Bulstra-Ramakers MTE, Huisjes HJ, Visser GHA. The effects of 3 g eicosapentaenoic acid daily on recurrence of intrauterine growth retardation and pregnancy induced hypertension. *Br J Obstet Gynaecol* 1994;102:123–126.

23. Laivuori H, Hovatta O, Viinikka L, et al. Dietary supplementation with primrose oil or fish oil dose not change urinary excretion of prostacyclin and thromboxane metabolites in pre-eclamptic women. *Prostaglandins Leukot Essent Fatty Acids* 1993;49:691–694.

24. D'Almeida A, Carter JP, Anatol A, Prost C. Effects of a combination of evening primrose oil (gamma linolenic acid) and fish oil (eicosapentaenoic + docahaxaenoic acid) versus magnesium, and versus placebo in preventing pre-eclampsia. *Women Health* 1992;19:117–131.

25. Moodley J, Norman RJ. Attempts at dietary alteration of prostaglandin pathways in the management of pre-eclampsia. *Prostaglandins Leukot Essent Fatty Acids* 1989;37:145–147.

26. Duley L, Henderson-Smart D. Reduced salt intake compared to normal dietary salt, or high intake, during pregnancy. In: Cochrane Library, Issue 3. Oxford: Update software, 2000. Search date 1999; primary sources Cochrane Pregnancy and Childbirth Group Trials Register.

27. Makrides M, Crowther C. Magnesium supplementation during pregnancy. In: Cochrane Library, Issue 3. Oxford: Update software, 2000. Search date 1998; primary sources Cochrane Pregnancy and Childbirth Group Trials Register.

28. Chappell LC, Seed PT, Briley AL, et al. Effect of antioxidants on the occurrence of pre-eclampsia in women at increased risk: a randomised trial. *Lancet* 1999;354:810–816.

29. Olsen SF, Sorensen JD, Secher NJ, et al. Randomised controlled trial of effect of fish oil supplementation on pregnancy duration. *Lancet* 1992;339:1003–1007.

30. Duley L. Hospitalisation for non-proteinuric pregnancy hypertension. In: Keirse MJNC, Renfrew MJ, Neilson JP, et al, eds. *Pregnancy and childbirth module.* In: Cochrane Library, Issue 2. Oxford: Update software, 1995. Search date 1993; primary sources Cochrane Pregnancy and Childbirth Group Trials Register.

31. Duley L. Strict bed rest for proteinuric hypertension in pregnancy. In: Keirse MJNC, Renfrew MJ, Neilson JP, et al, eds. *Pregnancy and childbirth module.* In: Cochrane Library, Issue 4. Oxford: Update software, 1995. Search date 1993; primary sources Cochrane Pregnancy and Childbirth Group Trials Register.

32. Tuffnell DJ, Lilford RJ, Buchan PC, et al. Randomised controlled trial of day care for hypertension in pregnancy. *Lancet* 1992;339: 224–227.

33. Duley L. Any antihypertensive therapy for pregnancy hypertension. In: Keirse MJNC, Renfrew MJ, Neilson JP, et al, eds. *Pregnancy and childbirth module.* In: Cochrane Library, Issue 2. Oxford: Update software, 1995. Search date 1994; primary sources Cochrane Pregnancy and Childbirth Group Trials Register.

34. Magee LA, Elran E, Bull SB, Logan A, Koren G. Risks and benefits of beta-receptor blockers for pregnancy hypertension: Overview of the randomized trials. *Eur J Obstet Gynecol Reprod Biol* 2000; 88:15–26. Search date 1997; primary sources Medline, Embase, hand searches of reference lists, *Hypertension and Pregnancy* journal 1992–1997, and a standard toxicology text.

35. Magee L, Duley L. Oral beta-blockers for mild to moderate hypertension during pregnancy. In: The Cochrane Library, Oxford: Update software [In press].

36. von Dadelszen P, Ornstein MP, Bull SB, Logan AG, Koren G, Magee LA. Fall in mean arterial pressure and fetal growth restriction in pregnancy hypertension: a meta-analysis. *Lancet* 2000;355: 87–92. Search date 1997; primary sources Medline, Embase, hand searches of reference lists, *Hypertension and Pregnancy* 1992–1997, and a standard toxicology text.

37. Duley L, Henderson-Smart D. Drugs for rapid treatment of very high blood pressure during pregnancy. In: Cochrane Library, Issue 3. Oxford: Update software, 2000. Search date 1998; primary sources Cochrane Pregnancy and Childbirth Group Trials Register.

38. Duley L, Williams J, Henderson-Smart D. Plasma volume expansion for severe pre-eclampsia. In: Cochrane Library, Issue 3. Oxford: Update Software, 2000. Search date 1999; primary sources Cochrane Pregnancy and Childbirth Group Trials Register.

39. The Albumin Reviewers (Alderson P, Bunn F, Li Wan Po L, Roberts I, Schierhout I). Human albumin solution for resuscitation and volume expansion in critically ill patients. In: Cochrane Library, Issue 3. Oxford: Update software, 2000. Search date 1999; primary sources Cochrane Injuries Group trials register, Cochrane Controlled Trials Register, Medline, Embase, Bids Scientific and Technical Proceedings, hand searches of reference lists of trials and review articles, and personal contacts with authors of identified trials.

40. Alderson P, Schierhout G, Roberts I, Bunn F. Colloids versus crystalloids for fluid resuscitation in critically ill patients. In: The Cochrane Library, Issue 3, Oxford: Update software, 2000. Search date 1999; primary sources Cochrane Clinical Trials Register, Medline, Embase, Bids Index to Scientific and Technical Proceedings, and reference lists of trials and review articles.

41. G Imezoglu AM, Hofmeyr GJ, Oosthuizen MMJ. Antioxidants in the treatment of severe preeclampsia: a randomized explanatory study. *Br J Obstet Gynaecol* 1997;104:689–696.

42. Duley L, G Imezoglu AM, Henderson-Smart D. Anticonvulsants for women with pre-eclampsia. In: Cochrane Library, Issue 2. Oxford: Update software, 1999. Search date 1998; primary sources Cochrane Pregnancy and Childbirth Group Trials Register.

43. Nelson K, Grether JK. Can magnesium sulfate reduce the risk of cerebral palsy in very low birthweight infants? *Pediatrics* 1995;95:263–269.

44. Schendel DE, Berg CJ, Yeargin-Allsopp M, et al. Prenatal magnesium sulfate exposure and the risk of cerebral palsy or mental retardation among very low-birth-weight children aged 3 to 5 years. *JAMA* 1996;276:1805–1810.

45. Mittendorf R, Covert R, Boman J, et al. Is tocolytic magnesium sulphate associated with increased total paediatric mortality? *Lancet* 1997;350: 1517–1518.

46. Odendaal HJ, Pattinson RC, Bam R, et al. Aggressive or expectant management for patients

with severe preeclampsia between 28–34 weeks gestation: a randomized controlled trial. *Obstet Gynecol* 1990;76:1070–1075.

47. Sibai BM, Mercer BM, Schiff E, et al. Aggressive versus expectant management of severe preeclampsia at 28–32 weeks' gestation: a randomized controlled trial. *Am J Obstet Gynecol* 1994;171:818–822.

48. Duley L, Henderson-Smart D. Magnesium sulphate versus diazepam for eclampsia. In: Cochrane Library, Issue 3. Oxford: Update software, 2000. Search date 1999; primary sources Cochrane Pregnancy and Childbirth Group Trials Register.

49. Duley L, Henderson-Smart D. Magnesium sulphate versus phenytoin for eclampsia. In: Cochrane Library, Issue 3. Oxford: Update software, 2000. Search date 1999; primary sources Cochrane Pregnancy and Childbirth Group Trials Register.

50. Bhalla AK, Dhall GI, Dhall K. A safer and more effective treatment regimen for eclampsia. *Aust NZ J Obstet Gynaecol* 1994;34:144–148.

51. Jacob S, Gopalakrishnan K, Lalitha K. Standardised clinical trial of magnesium sulphate regime in comparison with M K K. Menon's lytic cocktail regime in the management of eclampsia. Presented at the 27th British Congress of Obstetrics and Gynaecology, 4–7 July 1995, abstract number 303. London: Royal College of Obstetrics and Gynaecology, 1995.

Lelia Duley
Obstetric Epidemiologist
Institute of Health Sciences
Oxford
UK

Competing interests: None declared.

Preterm birth

Last updated Issue 3

John Morrison

INTERVENTIONS

Key Messages

In women at high risk of preterm delivery

- One systematic review of placebo controlled RCTs has found that antibiotic treatment of bacterial vaginosis during pregnancy decreases the incidence of preterm delivery, especially in women who have had a previous preterm delivery.

- RCTs, carried out in a range of countries, have found no evidence that enhanced antenatal care reduces the risk of preterm delivery.

- One large RCT found that, in women presumed to have cervical incompetence, prophylactic cervical cerclage was associated with a significant reduction in preterm births (less than 33 weeks' gestation). It found that 25 women would need to undergo cerclage to prevent one additional preterm delivery.

In threatened preterm labour

- One systematic review of RCTs has found that tocolytics are associated with a significant prolongation of pregnancy but with no evidence of improved perinatal mortality or neonatal morbidity. Tocolytics are associated with a significant increase in adverse maternal events.

In preterm delivery

- Systematic reviews of RCTs have found:
  - Antenatal treatment with glucocorticoids reduces the risk of respiratory distress syndrome, neonatal mortality, infant mortality, and intraventricular haemorrhage in preterm infants.
  - Treatment with thyrotropin releasing hormone and corticosteroids before preterm delivery is not associated with better neonatal outcomes than corticosteroids alone. There were significantly more maternal adverse events with thyrotropin releasing hormone.
  - No evidence of benefit from antibiotics in women in preterm labour with intact membranes, but that antibiotics are associated with increased perinatal mortality.

In women with preterm premature rupture of membranes

- One systematic review of RCTs has found that, in women with preterm premature rupture of membranes, antibiotics prolong pregnancy and reduce the risk of neonatal infection. The review found no significant reduction in perinatal mortality, but this may have been because most trials did not include administration of antenatal corticosteroids.

- One systematic review found limited evidence from one small RCT that amnioinfusion was associated with improved neonatal outcomes.

DEFINITION Preterm or premature birth is defined by the World Health Organization as delivery of an infant before 37 completed weeks of gestation.[1] There is no set lower limit to this definition, but 23–24 weeks' gestation is widely accepted,[1] which approximates to an average fetal weight of 500 g.

INCIDENCE/ PREVALENCE Preterm birth occurs in about 5–10% of all births in developed countries,[2–4] but in recent years the incidence seems to have increased in some countries, particularly the USA.[5] We found little reliable evidence for less developed countries that used the exact definition of premature birth. The rate in northwestern Ethiopia has been reported to vary between 11.3–21.8% depending on the age group studied, being highest in teenagers.[6]

AETIOLOGY/ RISK FACTORS About 30% of preterm births are unexplained and spontaneous.[4,7,8] The two strongest risk factors for idiopathic preterm labour are low socioeconomic status and previous preterm delivery. Multiple pregnancy accounts for about another 30% of cases.[4,7] Other known risk factors include genital tract infection, preterm premature rupture of the membranes, antepartum haemorrhage, cervical incompetence, and congenital uterine abnormalities, which collectively account for about 20–25% of cases. The remaining cases (15–20%) are attributed to elective preterm delivery secondary to hypertensive disorders of pregnancy, intrauterine fetal growth restriction, congenital abnormalities, and medical disorders of pregnancy.[4,5,7,8]

PROGNOSIS Preterm labour usually results in preterm birth. One systematic review of tocolysis versus placebo found that about 27% of preterm labours spontaneously resolved, and around 70% progressed to preterm delivery (search date not stated).[9] Observational studies have found that one preterm birth significantly raises the risk of another in a subsequent pregnancy.[10]

AIMS To prevent preterm birth, to prolong the interval between threatened preterm labour and delivery, and to optimise the condition of the fetus in preparation for delivery in order to improve neonatal outcome.

OUTCOMES The main clinical outcome is improved neonatal outcome, as indicated by perinatal mortality, neonatal mortality and morbidity (incidence of respiratory distress syndrome, intraventricular haemorrhage, necrotising enterocolitis, neonatal sepsis, and neonatal convulsions). Proxy outcomes include duration of pregnancy, number of hours or days between onset of labour and delivery, and number of deliveries before 37 completed weeks of gestation. An additional clinical outcome is incidence of maternal adverse effects.

METHODS *Clinical Evidence* search and appraisal January 2000. In addition, the author performed a detailed search of the Cochrane Library and Medline from 1966 using the terms preterm delivery, preterm labour, perinatal mortality, respiratory distress syndrome, thyrotropin releasing hormone, corticosteroids, tocolysis, and cervical cerclage. All relevant trials were assessed and included depending on the quality of their methods and relevance. Ideally, trials should state their definition of preterm labour, which should include uterine contractions, change in cervical condition, cervical dilatation or cervical effacement.

QUESTION What are the effects of preventive interventions in women at high risk of preterm delivery?

OPTION ANTIBIOTIC TREATMENT OF BACTERIAL VAGINOSIS IN PREGNANCY

One systematic review of placebo controlled RCTs found a reduced incidence of preterm delivery after antibiotic treatment of bacterial vaginosis during pregnancy, but the difference was not significant. Limited evidence from a subgroup analysis of women who had had a

previous preterm delivery found significantly less risk of preterm delivery after treatment for bacterial vaginosis than after placebo.

Benefits: We found one systematic review (updated July 1998, 5 RCTs, 1508 women) comparing one or more antibiotic regimens versus placebo.[11] It found fewer cases of preterm delivery after treatment for bacterial vaginosis than after placebo, but the difference was not significant (OR 0.78, 95% CI 0.60 to 1.02). In the subgroup of women who had had a previous preterm birth, the reduced risk of preterm birth was significant (OR 0.37, 95% CI 0.23 to 0.60).

Harms: Adverse effects occurred in 4% of women receiving antibiotics for bacterial vaginosis. However, loss to follow up varied between 1–17% for the various treatment and placebo groups in the five trials.

Comment: The quality of the trials was generally good; all trials provided data on losses to follow up.[11]

OPTION   **ENHANCED ANTENATAL CARE FOR SOCIALLY DEPRIVED WOMEN AND OTHER HIGH RISK GROUPS**

RCTs, carried out in a range of countries, have found no evidence that enhanced antenatal care (see glossary, p 824) reduces the risk of preterm delivery.

Benefits: We found no systematic review. We found eight RCTs. All RCTs (carried out in Europe, USA, and Latin America; number of high risk women ranging from 150–2200) found no significant difference between enhanced and normal antenatal care.[12–19]

Harms: No adverse effects were reported.

Comment: The definition of enhanced prenatal care varied.[12–18] Examples of enhanced prenatal care include increased number of antenatal visits, a bed rest programme, including rest periods three times daily, home visits by midwives, fortnightly social worker counselling sessions, nutritional education, and counselling by a psychologist. We found no evidence of superiority of one particular intervention.

OPTION   **PROPHYLACTIC CERVICAL CERCLAGE IN WOMEN AT RISK OF CERVICAL INCOMPETENCE**

One large RCT found that, in women presumed to have cervical incompetence, prophylactic cervical cerclage (see glossary, p 824) was associated with a significant reduction in preterm births (less than 33 weeks' gestation). Twenty five women would need to undergo cerclage to prevent one additional preterm delivery.

Benefits: We found no systematic review. We found one multicentre RCT. It reported the incidence of delivery before 33 weeks' gestation and before 37 weeks' gestation, and the vital status of the baby after delivery, in 647 women who underwent cerclage and 645 women who did not.[20] All women had a history of early delivery or cervical surgery, and their obstetrician was uncertain whether to advise cerclage or not. Cerclage was associated with a reduced rate of delivery before 33 weeks' gestation (83/647 [13%] with cerclage v

110/645 [17%]; ARR 4%, 95% CI 0.4% to 7.3%; RR 0.75, 95% CI 0.57 to 0.98; NNT 24, 95% CI 14 to 275). There was no significant difference in the rate of deliveries occurring between weeks 33 and 36.

Harms: Insertion of cervical sutures was associated with a doubling of the risk of puerperal pyrexia (24/415 [6%] with cerclage *v* 11/405 [3%] with no cerclage; ARI 3%, 95% CI 0.2% to 8.6%; RR 2.13; 95% CI 1.06 to 4.15; NNT 33, 95% CI 12 to 607).[20] Information about puerperal pyrexia was collected only after 360 women had been recruited to the trial.

Comment: The commonest indication for entry to the trial was having had a previous preterm delivery or second trimester miscarriage (74% of the cerclage group, 70% of the controls).[20]

QUESTION **What are the effects of interventions to improve outcome after preterm premature rupture of the membranes?**

OPTION **ANTIBIOTICS**

One systematic review of RCTs has found that, in women with preterm premature rupture of membranes (see glossary, p 825), antibiotics prolong pregnancy and reduce the risk of neonatal infection. The review found no significant reduction in perinatal mortality (see glossary, p 826), but this may have been due to the fact that most trials did not include administration of antenatal corticosteroids.

Benefits: We found one systematic review (updated January 1998, 12 RCTs, 1599 women with preterm premature rupture of membranes) comparing antibiotics versus placebo (see table 1, p 826).[21] Antibiotics reduced the number of babies born within 48 hours of rupture, the number of babies born within 7 days, the risk of chorioamnionitis, and the risk of neonatal infection. However, there was no significant reduction in risk of perinatal death or necrotising enterocolitis (see comment below). Pooled data from the trials found lower risk of abnormal brain scan and respiratory distress syndrome among babies exposed to antibiotics, but these also did not reach significance.

Harms: Adverse effects were looked for in the trials, and none were reported.[21]

Comment: Most of the trials did not include antenatal administration of corticosteroids, which may explain the lack of beneficial effect on neonatal mortality. All but one of the trials gave data on loss to follow up, which was always less than 20%. Various different antibiotic regimens were used in the different studies, including use of one of the following: erythromycin, benzylpenicillin, ampicillin, piperacillin, and clindamycin.[21]

OPTION **AMNIOINFUSION**

One systematic review found limited evidence from one small RCT that amnioinfusion (see glossary, p 824) is associated with improved neonatal outcomes after preterm premature rupture of the membranes.

Benefits: We found one systematic review (updated October 1997, 1 RCT, 61 women) (see table 2, p 827).[22] No significant difference in rates of caesarean section, low Apgar scores, neonatal death, or endometritis were detected. Ammioinfusion was associated with fewer severe fetal heart rate decelerations per hour during the first stage of labour (mean difference −1.20, 95% CI −1.83 to −0.57) and higher mean umbilical artery pH values (difference 0.11, 95% CI 0.077 to 0.14).

Harms: Adverse effects were looked for in the trials, and none were reported.

Comment: The trial was too small to detect clinically important changes of some of the outcomes (rates of Caesarean section, neonatal death, and infectious morbidity) and had shortcomings in methods used (unspecified method of random assignment of women; blinding of treatment not possible).

QUESTION What are the effects of treatments in threatened preterm labour?

OPTION TOCOLYTICS AND β-MIMETICS

One systematic review of RCTs has found that tocolytics are associated with a significant prolongation of pregnancy for women in threatened preterm labour (see glossary, p 825) but with no evidence of improved perinatal mortality or neonatal morbidity. Tocolytics are associated with a significant increase in adverse events in women with preterm labour.

Benefits: **Tocolytics:** We found one systematic review (search date December 1999, 18 RCTs, 2785 women in preterm labour) comparing a tocolytic drug versus placebo or no tocolytic.[23] Three trials included women with ruptured membranes. The most frequently evaluated tocolytic was ritodrine (5 RCTs); others included isoxuprine, ethanol, terbutaline, magnesium sulfate, indomethacin, and atosiban. Tocolytics were associated with a significant decrease in the likelihood of delivery within 24 hours (OR 0.47, 95% CI 0.29 to 0.77), 48 hours (OR 0.57, 95% CI 0.38 to 0.83), and 7 days (OR 0.60, 95% CI 0.38 to 0.95). Tocolytics were not associated with significant reduction in births before 30 weeks' gestation (OR 1.33, 95% CI 0.53 to 3.33), before 32 weeks' gestation (OR 0.81, 95% CI 0.61 to 1.07), or before 37 weeks' gestation (OR 0.17, 95% CI 0.02 to 1.62). Tocolytics were not associated with significantly reduced rates of perinatal deaths (OR 1.22, 95% CI 0.84 to 1.78), respiratory distress syndrome (OR 0.82, 95% CI 0.64 to 1.07), intraventricular haemorrhage (OR 0.73, 95% CI 0.46 to 1.15), necrotising enterocolitis (OR 0.96, 95% CI 0.35 to 2.65), patent ductus arteriosus (OR 1.05 95% CI 0.52 to 1.30), neonatal sepsis (OR 1.09, 95% CI 0.70 to 1.68), neonatal seizures (OR 0.81, 95% CI 0.36 to 3.14), hypoglycaemia (OR 1.36, 95% CI 0.87 to 2.14), or birth weight under 2500 g (OR 0.62, 95% CI 0.35 to 1.09). **β Mimetics:** The review identified seven RCTs and concluded that β mimetics were associated with less respiratory distress syndrome but the difference was not quite significant (OR 0.76, 95% CI 0.57 to 1.01).

Harms: Tocolytics were associated with an increased risk of maternal palpitations (200/420 v 19/423 on control; OR 10.2, 95% CI 7.4 to 13.9), tremor (138/352 v 13/356 on control; OR 8.30, 95% CI 5.8 to 11.9), and nausea (72/352 v 42/356 on control; OR 1.90, 95% CI 1.27 to 2.83). There was also an increased risk of chorioamnionitis (OR 2.88, 95% CI 1.13 to 7.33), hyperglycaemia (OR 3.39, 95% CI 2.35 to 4.90), hypokalaemia (OR 6.43, 95% CI 4.53 to 9.14), and the need to discontinue treatment (OR 10.1, 95% CI 4.91 to 20.7). There was no significant increase in rates of pulmonary oedema, chest pain, cardiac arrythmias, dyspnoea, vomiting, headaches, endometritis, or hypotension, all of which have been reported with tocolytics. None of the trials reported any maternal deaths.[23]

Comment: Spurious preterm labour presents a problem in analysis of effects of tocolytic agents. However, in 15 of the 17 trials included in the systematic review, the definition of preterm labour used for entry into the study included cervical dilatation, effacement, or change in the cervical condition in addition to uterine contractions. This would minimise the potential confounding effect of spurious preterm labour. Combining results for all tocolytics was reasonable based on the lack of evidence of the merits of one tocolytic over another.[24] The confidence intervals for delivery before 37 weeks' gestation were wide and included the possibility of a large positive effect.[23]

<hr>

QUESTION What are the effects of interventions to improve outcome in preterm delivery?

<hr>

OPTION CORTICOSTEROIDS BEFORE PRETERM DELIVERY

One systematic review of RCTs has found that antenatal treatment with glucocorticoids reduces the risk of respiratory distress syndrome, neonatal mortality, infant mortality, and intraventricular haemorrhage in preterm infants.

Benefits: We found one systematic review (updated January 1996, 18 RCTs, > 3700 babies).[25] The RCTs compared corticosteroids (betamethasone, dexamethasone, or hydrocortisone) versus placebo or no treatment in women before anticipated preterm delivery (elective or after spontaneous onset of preterm labour). The review found that treatment with antenatal corticosteroids was associated with lower rates of respiratory distress syndrome (292/1885 v 439/1850 on control; OR 0.53, 95% CI 0.44 to 0.63). In the subgroup of neonates delivered before 28 weeks' gestation, no significant effect was seen (7/17 v 18/31 on control; OR 0.64, 95% CI 0.16 to 2.50). There was a clinically significant lower rate of respiratory distress syndrome in babies delivered within less than 24 hours (45/176 v 57/173 on control; OR 0.70, 95% CI 0.43 to 1.16) or less than 48 hours (3/23 v 6/19 on control; OR 0.34, 95% CI 0.08 to 1.47), but a statistically significant effect was not seen until after this time. For babies born between 24 hours and 7 days after treatment, there was a significant reduction in respiratory distress syndrome (44/382 v 87/346 on control; OR 0.38, 95% CI 0.25 to 0.57). A significant reduction in respiratory distress syndrome was seen only 48 hours after receiving corticosteroids. There was no significant effect in neonates delivered more than 7 days after treatment. Significant reductions in respiratory distress were seen with both betamethasone and dexamethasone but not with hydrocortisone. The sex of the neonate had no effect. The small numbers of evaluable neonates from twin pregnancies did not allow a confident statement about the effects in multiple pregnancy. Antenatal corticosteroids were associated with reduced neonatal mortality, infant mortality, and risk of intraventricular haemorrhage. No effect on rates of necrotising enterocolitis (17/587 v 27/567 on control; OR 0.59, 95% CI 0.32 to 1.09) or chronic lung disease (38/204 v 25/207 on control; OR 1.57, 95% CI 0.87 to 2.84).

Harms: There was no strong evidence of any adverse effects of corticosteroids in these trials. Subgroup analysis in one trial suggested that corticosteroids might predispose to fetal death in hypertensive women. No deaths were observed in this subgroup in the other three trials for which data were available.[25]

Comment: The fact that the beneficial effect of corticosteroids on respiratory distress syndrome was not significant at less than 28 weeks' gestation may be due to the tiny numbers available for analysis at this gestation. No trials addressed the potentially harmful effects of repeated doses of antenatal corticosteroids, or whether one form of corticosteroid was more harmful than another, as a recent retrospective cohort study involving 883 babies delivered between 24 and 31 weeks' gestation suggests.[26]

OPTION   THYROTROPIN RELEASING HORMONE BEFORE PRETERM DELIVERY

One systematic review of RCTs has found that treatment with thyrotropin releasing hormone and corticosteroids before preterm delivery is not associated with better neonatal outcomes than corticosteroids alone. There were significantly more maternal adverse events with thyrotropin releasing hormone.

Benefits: We found one systematic review (updated May 1997, 7 RCTs, in > 3358 women).[27] The trials compared thyrotropin releasing hormone versus placebo before preterm delivery in women who all received antenatal corticosteroids. The three trials that reported clinical neonatal outcome data in full found no significant effect on neonatal mortality (95/963 v 84/976 with placebo; OR 1.17, 95% CI 0.86 to 1.59), risk of respiratory distress syndrome (306/963 v 304/976 with placebo; OR 1.03, 95% CI 0.85 to 1.24), or chronic oxygen dependence (the need for oxygen at 28 days) (183/963 v 185/976 with placebo; OR 1.00, 95% CI 0.80 to 1.26). There was no evidence of an effect on gestational age at delivery, need for admission to neonatal intensive care unit, or incidence of periventricular or intraventricular haemorrhage, air leak syndrome, necrotising enterocolitis, or patent ductus arteriosus, although pulmonary haemorrhage was less likely in neonates born to women who received antenatal thyrotropin releasing hormone (3/699 v 11/698 with placebo; OR 0.32, 95% CI 0.11 to 0.90).

Harms: Antenatal thyrotropin releasing hormone was associated with a significant rise in maternal diastolic blood pressure (> 15 mmHg)

(115/506 v 71/505 with placebo; OR 1.78, 95% CI 1.30 to 2.45) and a rise in systolic blood pressure (> 25 mmHg: 36/506 v 20/505 with placebo; OR 1.83, 95% CI 1.07 to 3.13). Other maternal adverse effects were nausea, vomiting, lightheadedness, urgency of micturition, and facial flushing.[27]

Comment: Two further multicentre, double blind, placebo controlled RCTs of antenatal thyrotropin releasing hormone were stopped early because previously analysed evidence suggested that benefit was unlikely.[28] Too few data are available from these trials to allow reliable conclusions.

OPTION ANTIBIOTICS IN PRETERM LABOUR WITH INTACT MEMBRANES

One systematic review of RCTs found no evidence of benefit from antibiotics in women in preterm labour with intact membranes but found that antibiotics are associated with increased perinatal mortality (see glossary, p 824).

Benefits: We found one systematic review (updated October 1997, 8 RCTs, 707 women) investigating the value of treatment with antibiotics in preterm labour with intact membranes.[29] The trials all used similar definitions of preterm labour, including uterine contractions and cervical dilatation, and compared antibiotics (single agent in 2 trials, combinations in 6 trials) versus placebo or no antibiotic.[29] The antibiotics were ampicillin, erythromycin, metronidazole, sulbactam, mezlocillin, clavulonic acid, clindamycin, and ceftizoxime. Antibiotics were associated with significantly lower rates of maternal infection (chorioamnionitis/endometritis) (29/353 v 43/354 on control; OR 0.50, 95% CI 0.28 to 0.88) and neonatal necrotising enterocolitis (4/261 v 12/269 on control; OR 0.36, 95% CI 0.13 to 0.97). No significant difference was found in mean days of prolongation of pregnancy, mean gestational age at delivery, frequency of preterm birth, mean birthweight, or rates of neonatal sepsis, respiratory distress syndrome, or intraventricular haemorrhage.

Harms: Antibiotics were associated with increased perinatal mortality (9/344 v 2/345 on control; OR 3.47, 95% CI 1.05 to 11.4), including postnatal deaths because of complications of prematurity.[29]

Comment: Multiple pregnancies were excluded from most of the trials. Seven of the eight trials were double blind and placebo controlled. The outcome assessment was not blinded in one of the trials.[29]

GLOSSARY

Amnioinfusion Infusion of physiological saline or Ringers lactate via a catheter transabdominally or transcervically into the amniotic cavity.

Cervical cerclage Insertion of a cervical suture, using non-absorbable suture material, circumferentially around the cervix. May be done transvaginally or transabdominally.

Enhanced antenatal care Includes various programmes of increased medical, midwifery, psychological, social, and nutritional support during pregnancy.

Perinatal Refers to the period after 24 weeks' gestation and includes the first 7 days of postnatal life for the neonate.

Preterm labour Onset of labour (regular uterine contractions with cervical efface-ment and dilatation) in the preterm period.

Preterm premature rupture of membranes Leakage of amniotic fluid from the amniotic cavity during the preterm period due to rupture of the fetal membranes.

REFERENCES

1. Morrison JJ, Rennie JM. Clinical, scientific and ethical aspects of fetal and neonatal care at extremely preterm periods of gestation. *Br J Obstet Gynaecol* 1997;104:1341–1350.
2. Rush RW, Keirse MJNC, Howat P, et al. Contribution of preterm delivery to perinatal mortality. *BMJ* 1976;2:965–968.
3. Creasy RK. Preterm birth prevention: Where are we? *Am J Obstet Gynecol* 1993;168:1223–1230.
4. Burke C, Morrison JJ. Perinatal factors and preterm delivery in an Irish obstetric population. *J Perinat Med* 2000;28:49–53.
5. Goldenberg RL, Rouse DJ. Prevention of premature birth. *N Engl J Med* 1998;339:313–320.
6. Kumbi S, Isehak A. Obstetric outcome of teenage pregnancy in northwestern Ethiopia. *East Afr Med J* 1999;76:138–140.
7. Iannucci TA, Tomich PG, Gianopoulos JG. Etiology and outcome of extremely low-birth-weight infants. *Am J Obstet Gynecol* 1996;174:1896–1902.
8. Main DM, Gabbe SG, Richardson D, et al. Can preterm deliveries be prevented? *Am J Obstet Gynecol* 1985;151:892–898.
9. King JF, Grant A, Keirse MJNC, et al. Beta-mimetics in preterm labour: an overview of the randomised controlled trials. *Br J Obstet Gynaecol* 1988;95:211–222. Search date not stated; primary sources Oxford Database of Perinatal Trials, hand searches of reference lists, and personal contacts.
10. Keirse MJNC, Rush RW, Anderson AB, et al. Risk of preterm delivery and/or abortion. *Br J Obstet Gynaecol* 1978;85:81–85.
11. Brocklehurst P, Hannah M, McDonald H. Interventions for treating bacterial vaginosis in pregnancy. In: The Cochrane Library, Issue 1, 2000. Oxford: Update software. Search date July 1998; primary sources Cochrane Pregnancy and Childbirth Group Trials Register, Cochrane Controlled Trial Registers.
12. Spencer B, Thomas H, Morris J. A randomized controlled trial of the provision of a social support service during pregnancy; the South Manchester Family Worker project. *Br J Obstet Gynaecol* 1989; 96:281–288.
13. Mueller-Heubach E, Reddick D, Barrett B, et al. Preterm birth prevention: Evaluation of a prospective controlled randomized trial. *Am J Obstet Gynecol* 1989;160:1172–1178.
14. Goldenberg R, Davis R, Copper R, et al. The Alabama birth prevention project. *Obstet Gynecol* 1990;75:933–939.
15. Blondel B, Breart G, Glado J, et al Evaluation of the home-visiting system for women with threatened preterm labour. Results of a randomized controlled trial. *Eur J Obstet Gynaecol Reprod Biol* 1990;34:47–58.
16. Villar J, Farnot U, Barros F, et al. A randomized trial of psychosocial support during high-risk pregnancies. *N Engl J Med* 1992;327:1266–1271.
17. Collaborative Group on Preterm Birth Prevention. Multicenter randomized controlled trial of a preterm birth prevention program. *Am J Obstet Gynecol* 1993;169:352–366.
18. Moore ML, Meis PJ, Ernest JM, et al. A randomized trial of nurse intervention to reduce preterm and low birth weight births. *Obstet Gynecol* 1998;91:656–661.
19. Olds DL, Henderson CR Jr, Tatelbaum R, et al. Improving the delivery of prenatal care and outcomes of pregnancy: a randomized trial of nurse home visitation. *Pediatrics* 1986;77:16–28.
20. MRC/RCOG Working Party on Cervical Cerclage. Final report of the Medical Research Council/Royal College of Obstetricians and Gynaecologists Multicentre Randomised Trial of Cervical Cerclage. *Br J Obstet Gynaecol* 1993;100:516–523.
21. Kenyon S, Boulvain M. Antibiotics for preterm premature rupture of membranes. In: The Cochrane Library, Issue 1, 2000 Oxford: Update software. Search date 1998; primary sources all randomised trials identified by the Cochrane Pregnancy Childbirth Group Trials Register.
22. Hofmeyr GJ. Amnioinfusion for preterm rupture of membranes. In: The Cochrane Library, Issue 1, 2000 Oxford: Update software. Search date 1998; primary sources Cochrane Pregnancy and Childbirth Group Trials Register, Cochrane Register of Controlled Trials.
23. Gyetvai K, Hannah ME, Hodnett ED, et al. Tocolytics for preterm labor: A systematic review. *Obstet Gynecol* 1999;94:869–877. Search date 1998; primary sources Medline, Cochrane Register of Controlled Trials.
24. Hannah M, Amankwah K, Barret J, et al. The Canadian consensus on the use of tocolytics for preterm labour. *J SOGC* 1995;17:1089–1115.
25. Crowley P. Corticosteroids prior to preterm delivery. In: The Cochrane Library, Issue 1, 2000. Oxford: Update software. Search date 1996; primary sources Cochrane Pregnancy and Childbirth Group Trials Register.
26. Baud O, Foix-L'Helias L, Kaminski M, et al. Antenatal glucocorticoid treatment and cyctic periventricular leokomalacia in very premature infants. *N Engl J Med* 1999;341:1190–1196.
27. Crowther CA, Alfirevic Z, Haslam RR. Antenatal thyrotropin-releasing hormone (TRH) prior to preterm delivery. In: The Cochrane Library, Issue 1, 2000 Oxford: Update software. Search date 1997; primary source Cochrane Pregnancy and Childbirth Group Trials Register.
28. Alfirevic Z, Boer K, Brocklehurst P, et al. Two trials of antenatal thyrotropin-releasing hormone for fetal maturation: stopping before the due date. *Br J Obstet Gynaecol* 1999;106:898–906.
29. King J, Flenady V. Antibiotics in preterm labour with intact membranes. In: The Cochrane Library, Issue 1, 2000 Oxford: Update software. Search date 1997; primary sources Cochrane Pregnancy and Childbirth Group Trials Register; personal contacts and hand searches of reference lists.

John Morrison

Professor of Obstetrics and Gynaecology
Clinical Science Institute, University College Hospital, Galway, Ireland

Competing interests: None declared.

TABLE 1 The effects of antibiotics after premature preterm rupture of membranes: results of placebo controlled RCTs (see text, p 820).[21]

Outcome	Absolute risks		ARR (95% CI)	OR (95% CI)	NNT (95% CI)
	Antibiotic	Control			
Born within 48 hours of rupture	140/513 (27%)	207/545 (38%)	11% (6% to 16%)	0.6 (0.46 to 0.77)	9 (6 to 17)
Born within 7 days of rupture	283/483 (59%)	364/508 (72%)	14% (8% to 21%)	0.54 (0.41 to 0.70)	7 (5 to 13)
Chorioamnionitis	122/736 (17%)	188/763 (25%)	8% (4% to 11%)	0.61 (0.47 to 0.79)	12 (9 to 24)
Neonatal infection	86/775 (11%)	127/799 (16%)	5% (2% to 8%)	0.62 (0.45 to 0.86)	18 (12 to 52)
Perinatal death	50/700 (7%)	53/732 (7%)	0.1% (−3% to +2%)	0.98 (0.66 to 1.47)	–
Necrotising enterocolitis	43/611 (7.0%)	48/644 (7.5%)	0.4% (−2.9% to +2.7%)	0.93 (0.61 to 1.44)	–

TABLE 2 | Effects of amnioinfusion after premature preterm rupture of membranes: results of RCT (see text, p 821).[22]

Outcome	Absolute risks		OR (95% CI)
	Antibiotic	Control	
Caesarean section	2/29	7/32	0.31 (0.08 to 1.26)
Low Apgar scores	1/29	4/32	0.31 (0.05 to 1.88)
Neonatal death	1/29	2/32	0.55 (0.06 to 5.56)
Endometritis	2/29	3/32	0.03 (0.05 to 2.89)

Respiratory disorders

Asthma

Last updated Issue 3

Christopher Cates and Mark FitzGerald

INTERVENTIONS

*No direct randomised evidence available, but highly likely to be effective. Trials unlikely to be conducted.

Key Messages

In people with chronic asthma

- RCTs have found that regular use of short acting inhaled β_2 agonists provides no additional clinical benefits and may worsen asthma control in people with mild intermittent asthma.
- RCTs have found that low doses of inhaled corticosteroids control asthma more than placebo or regular β_2 agonists in people with mild persistent asthma.

© *Clinical Evidence* 2000;4:828–842.

- In people with asthma which is poorly controlled on inhaled corticosteroids, RCTs have found that adding long acting, inhaled β_2 agonists improves symptoms and lung function, improves quality of life, and has not been linked to deterioration in asthma control when used regularly.

In people with acute exacerbations of asthma

- There is a strong consensus that oxygen should be a key component of acute treatment. We found no RCTs of oxygen therapy. Clinical monitoring and case control studies have found that people with near fatal asthma suffer from significant hypoxaemia.

- One systematic review of RCTs has found no difference in outcomes when β_2 agonists are delivered by spacer device/holding chamber versus nebulisers.

- One systematic review of RCTs has found that taking oral corticosteroids at the start of an acute exacerbation reduces rates of admission and relapse. We found no good evidence about optimal duration of treatment.

- Limited, small RCTs have found that bronchodilatation, primarily with short acting β-agonists, is associated with improved peak flow and reduced hospital admission.

- We found conflicting evidence from RCTs of intravenous salbutamol versus nebulised salbutamol in acute exacerbations. Intravenous salbutamol was associated with more adverse effects.

- One large RCT found that continuous treatment with β_2 agonists was associated with greater improvement in lung capacity compared with as needed treatment. Other smaller RCTs found no significant difference.

- Two systematic reviews have found that addition of ipratropium bromide to β_2 agonist improves lung function and significantly reduces hospital admission rates.

- One non-systematic review has found that specialist care for people with acute exacerbations of asthma is more effective than generalist care.

- Sub-group analysis from a recent systematic review suggested that intravenous magnesium might reduce hospital admission rates in people with severe, acute asthma.

- We found no RCT but clinical experience, historical cohort studies, and case-series suggests that mechanical ventilation is likely to reduce death rates in near fatal asthma.

- One systematic review has found that asthma self management involving asthma education reduces hospital admission, unscheduled visits to physicians and days off work.

DEFINITION	Asthma is characterised by dyspnoea, cough, chest tightness, wheezing, variable airflow obstruction, and airway hyperresponsiveness. **Chronic asthma** is defined here as disease requiring maintenance treatment. Asthma is classified differently in the US and UK (see table 1, p 842): where necessary, the text specifies the system of classification used.[1,2] **Acute asthma** is defined here as an exacerbation of underlying disease requiring urgent or emergency treatment.
INCIDENCE/ PREVALENCE	Reported prevalence is increasing worldwide. Up to 10% of people have suffered an attack of asthma.[3,4]
AETIOLOGY/ RISK FACTORS	Most people with asthma are atopic; exposure to certain stimuli initiates inflammation and structural changes in airways, causing airway hyperresponsiveness and variable airflow obstruction, which

in turn cause most asthma symptoms. Stimuli include environmental allergens, occupational sensitising agents, and respiratory viral infections.[5,6]

PROGNOSIS **Chronic asthma:** In people with mild asthma, prognosis is good and progression to severe disease rare. However, as a group, people with asthma lose lung function faster than those without asthma, although less quickly than people with asthma who smoke.[7] People with persistent asthma can improve with current treatment. However, for reasons not clearly understood, some people (possibly up to 5%) have severe disease that responds poorly to treatment. These people are most at risk of morbidity and death from asthma. **Acute asthma:** About 10–20% of people presenting to the emergency department with asthma are admitted to hospital. Of these, fewer than 10% receive mechanical ventilation, although previous ventilation is associated with a 19-fold increased risk of ventilation for the current episode.[8] It is unusual for people who reach emergency care to die unless they have suffered respiratory arrest before reaching hospital.[9] One prospective study of 939 people discharged from emergency care found that 17% (95% CI 14% to 20%) relapsed by 2 weeks.[10]

AIMS To minimise or eliminate symptoms; to maximise lung function; to prevent exacerbations; to minimise the need for medication; to minimise adverse effects of treatment; and to educate people about their asthma.

OUTCOMES Symptoms (daytime and nocturnal); lung function (peak expiratory flow rate [PEFR] and forced expiratory volume in one second [FEV1]); need for rescue medication such as inhaled β_2 agonists; variability of flow rates; activities of daily living; adverse effects of treatment.

METHODS *Clinical Evidence* search and appraisal November 1999. We reviewed all identified systematic reviews and double blind, placebo controlled RCTs. We used the following key words for the acute sections: acute asthma, therapy, β agonists, oxygen, corticosteroids, anticholinergics, mechanical ventilation, magnesium sulphate, and asthma education. Personal files on acute asthma management were also reviewed.

QUESTION What are effects of treatments for chronic asthma?

Christopher Cates

OPTION REGULAR VERSUS AS NEEDED USE OF SHORT ACTING, INHALED β_2 AGONISTS IN ADULTS WITH MILD INTERMITTENT ASTHMA

RCTs have found that regular use of short acting inhaled β_2 agonists in people with mild, intermittent asthma provides no additional clinical benefits, compared with as needed use, and may worsen asthma control.

Benefits: We found no systematic review. We found several RCTs comparing regular versus as needed inhaled salbutamol. The most recent included 255 people with mild, intermittent asthma taking inhaled β agonists only.[11] At 16 weeks, there was no significant difference between the groups in symptoms, quality of life, airflow obstruction, or frequency of exacerbations. However, people taking regular salbutamol used more medication than those taking it as needed (total salbutamol 9.3 v 1.6 puffs/day), and experienced significantly worse variability in peak expiratory flow rate (PEFR) and methacholine responsiveness. An earlier placebo controlled, double blind crossover trial in 64 people (continuing inhaled or oral corticosteroids and/or inhaled cromoglycate if usually required) found that of the 57 people who had better control during active treatment periods, most did better with as needed versus regular treatment (40 v 17). Furthermore, most people using regular fenoterol suffered deterioration in asthma control and increased frequency of exacerbations compared with those on as needed treatment.[12] Inhaled corticosteroids did not seem to protect against deterioration.

Harms: Two case control studies found increased asthma mortality with overuse of inhaled short acting β_2 agonists.[13,14] However, there was insufficient evidence to attribute causality, as overusing β_2 agonists to treat frequent symptoms may simply indicate severe, uncontrolled asthma in high risk individuals. Other RCTs found that regular use of inhaled β_2 agonists was associated with transient rebound deterioration in airway hyperresponsiveness after stopping the medication,[15] and increased allergen induced bronchoconstriction.[16] Finally, tremor is commonly reported, although tolerance develops with more frequent use.[17]

Comment: None.

OPTION **LOW DOSES OF INHALED CORTICOSTEROIDS IN PEOPLE WITH MILD, PERSISTENT ASTHMA**

RCTs have found that low doses of inhaled corticosteroids (250–500 µg of beclomethasone dipropionate or equivalent) are more effective than placebo or regular β_2 agonists in people with mild, persistent asthma. We found no evidence of clinically important adverse effects in adults.

Benefits: **Versus placebo:** We found no systematic review. We found seven placebo controlled RCTs evaluating low doses of inhaled budesonide,[18–21] beclomethasone,[22,23] and triamcinolone[23–25] in a total of over 1000 adults and adolescents with mild, persistent asthma (using US classification; see table 1, p 842). They all found significant improvement in lung function, symptoms, and short acting bronchodilator usage compared with placebo. **Versus β_2 agonists:** We found one systematic review (no search date given) which identified five small RCTs in 141 adults with mild persistent asthma (regular use of inhaled corticosteroids, but not more than two drugs to control asthma).[26] The review found that inhaled corticosteroids significantly improved lung function (overall weighted effect size for PEFR 0.59, 95% CI 0.32 to 0.84). One RCT not included in the review compared inhaled budesonide 1200 µg/day versus inhaled β_2 agonists in 103 adults with mild asthma (diagnosed within 12 months, not using oral corticosteroids). The trial found that those taking budesonide had persistent, significant improvements in all outcomes over a 2 year period (no CI available).[27]

Harms: We found no published evidence that low doses of inhaled corticosteroids (< 1000 µg/day of beclomethasone dipropionate or equivalent) cause important systemic effects in adults.[28] Although posterior subcasular cataracts occur more frequently in people taking oral corticosteroids,[29] most studies in adults provide no evidence that inhaled corticosteroids increase the risk once the confounding effect of oral corticosteroids is removed.[30] However, a recent population based, case control study suggested that, in older people, inhaled high dose beclomethasone dipropionate was associated with a slightly greater risk of nuclear cataracts (RR 1.5, 95% CI 1.2 to 1.9) and posterior subcapsular cataracts (RR 1.9, 95% CI 1.3 to 2.8).[31] We found no published reports of an increased risk of osteoporosis or fractures. Inhaled corticosteroids can cause oral candidiasis, dysphonia, and bruising, but these are troublesome in less than 5% of people.[32,33]

Comment: The results of the systematic review should be interpreted with caution as the few small RCTs included neither consistently measured PEFR at the same time of the day nor reported morning and evening PEFRs.[26] The case control study on cataract formation did not stratify for the confounding effect of allergy,[31] which is also a risk factor for cataract development.[34]

OPTION **ADDITION OF LONG ACTING INHALED β_2 AGONISTS IN PEOPLE WHOSE ASTHMA IS POORLY CONTROLLED BY INHALED CORTICOSTEROIDS**

RCTs have found that, in people with poorly controlled asthma, adding regular doses of long acting, inhaled β_2 agonists to inhaled corticosteroids improves symptoms and lung function. Unlike regular use of short acting β_2 agonists, regular use of long acting β_2 agonists has not been linked to deterioration in asthma control. We found no good evidence relating to their effect on mortality.

Benefits: **Versus placebo:** We found no systematic review. We found two RCTs [35,36] (506 and 217 people, respectively) of regular, long acting inhaled β_2 agonists versus placebo in people with moderate, persistent asthma, which was not controlled on inhaled corticosteroids (250–2000 µg/day). These trials found that twice daily salmeterol or formoterol improved quality of life scores, PEFR, and FEV_1 more than placebo. Exacerbation rates were not significantly different between the two groups in either trial. **Versus increased use of inhaled corticosteroids:** We found six RCTs of regular use of long acting inhaled β_2 agonists. Four were in people whose asthma symptoms were poorly controlled on inhaled corticosteroids (176–1000 µg/day; total n = 1878).[37–40] These four trials found that adding twice daily salmeterol had a significantly greater beneficial effect on PEFR, FEV_1, symptom free days and nights, and rescue free days and nights than doubling the dose of inhaled corticosteroid, although the trials did not find significant differences in exacerbation rates. The fifth trial, in 852 people taking low to moderate dose inhaled corticosteroids, found that twice daily formoterol plus terbutaline as needed, in addition to low or moderate doses of inhaled budesonide, significantly improved symptoms, and lung function, and reduced exacerbations.[41] Exacerbations were reduced further by a fourfold increase in daily dosage of inhaled corticosteroid, and further still by combined, higher dose of budesonide plus formoterol. The sixth RCT, in 233 people with mild persistent asthma in primary care taking lower doses of inhaled corticosteroids (200–400 µg/day), found that salmeterol reduced symptoms more rapidly than additional beclomethasone.[42] At 2 and 7 weeks, PEFRs measured in general practice were better in the salmeterol group, but by 12 weeks there was no significant difference between the two groups. No significant differences were found in symptom scores, overall quality of life, or exacerbation rates.

Harms: Several studies have found that people taking regular doses of long acting, inhaled β_2 agonists develop tolerance to protection against bronchoconstriction[43–45] and may develop a tremor. Short acting inhaled β_2 agonists are associated with deterioration in asthma control and increased risk of death.[12–14] Regular use of long acting inhaled β_2 agonists has not been linked to deterioration in asthma control.

Comment: We found no RCTs or other studies with sufficient power to assess the effect of regular use of long acting inhaled β_2 agonists on death rates.[46]

QUESTION What are the effects of treatments for acute asthma?

Mark FitzGerald

OPTION SPACER DEVICES/HOLDING CHAMBERS VERSUS NEBULISERS FOR DELIVERING β_2 AGONISTS

One systematic review of RCTs has found no difference in efficacy between nebulisers and holding chambers with metered dose inhalers for delivering β_2 agonists in people with acute but not life threatening asthma.

Benefits: We found one systematic review (updated 1999, 13 RCTs) comparing holding chambers plus metered dose inhalers versus nebulisation for delivering β_2 agonists. Participants were non-hospitalised adults and children with acute asthma.[47] Results in adults and children were analysed separately (see asthma in children, p 173). In adults, there was no significant difference in rates of hospital admission (OR 1.12, 95% CI 0.45 to 2.76), length of time spent in the emergency department (WMD 0.02 hours, 95% CI −0.40 to +0.44 hours), or in PEFR or FEV_1. There was still no significant difference when the three studies involving the most severely affected people (FEV_1 < 30% predicted) were included (WMD for FEV_1 holding chamber v nebuliser −1.5% predicted, 95% CI −8.3% to +5.3%). Symptoms were measured on different scales and findings could not be combined.

Harms: The review found no significant difference in pulse rates between the two methods (WMD with holding chamber v nebuliser 1.6% of baseline, 95% CI −2.4% to +5.5% of baseline).

Comment: The review found no evidence of publication bias and was confined to studies that used multiple treatment doses, which can be titrated against the individual patient response to overcome possible dose confounding. As studies excluded people with life threatening asthma, results cannot be generalised to such people.

| OPTION | WHAT ARE THE EFFECTS OF ORAL CORTICOSTEROIDS, AND WHAT IS THE OPTIMAL DOSE AND DURATION OF TREATMENT IN ACUTE ASTHMA? |

One systematic review of RCTs has found that taking a short course of systemic corticosteroids at the start of an acute exacerbation reduces rates of admission and relapse, and reduces β_2 agonist use, without increasing adverse effects. We found no good evidence on the optimal dose or duration of treatment. The review found no significant difference between intramuscular and oral corticosteroids.

Benefits: **Rates of admission:** We found two systematic reviews. The first (search date 1997, 7 RCTs in about 320 people) compared oral corticosteroids versus placebo (4 trials), oral versus intramuscular corticosteroids (2 trials), and intramuscular corticosteroids versus placebo (1 trial).[48] It found that systemic corticosteroids given at the time of an acute asthma exacerbation reduced the number of relapses requiring additional care (first week RR v placebo 0.39, 95% CI 0.21 to 0.74; NNT 10, first 21 days RR 0.47, 95% CI 0.25 to 0.89). It also found fewer admissions to hospital (RR 0.35, 95% CI 0.13 to 0.95). People receiving corticosteroids also had less need for β_2 agonists (WMD −3.3 activations/day, 95% CI −5.5 to −1.0). The review found no clear difference between intramuscular and oral corticosteroids. The second, earlier systematic review (search date 1991, 5 RCTs, 422 people) compared systemic corticosteroids versus placebo.[49] It also found that early use of systemic corticosteroids reduced hospital admissions and relapses in both adults and children (OR of admission in adults v placebo 0.47, 95% CI 0.27 to 0.79). **Stopping treatment:** We found no systematic review. One RCT compared tapering of prednisolone over a week versus abrupt cessation in 35 people who were admitted to hospital with acute asthma. It found that a daily dose of 0.5–1 mg/kg for 10 days was effective when administered once daily for 10 days, and could be stopped without tapering off once asthma control was re-established.[50] **Optimal dose and duration of treatment:** We found no systematic review or RCTs. The optimal duration of treatment is likely to depend on the individual, the severity of the exacerbation, and use of concomitant medications.

Harms: Systemic corticosteroids can cause the same adverse effects in asthma as in other diseases, even when administered for a short time (see asthma in children, p 173).

Comment: We found no reliable evidence about the role of oral corticosteroids in acute asthma after admission to hospital, nor is it likely that a placebo controlled RCT would be conducted in acute severe asthma. One RCT found no difference in rates of treatment failure between a short course of oral steroids and a high dose of inhaled fluticasone in 413 adults presenting to general practitioners with acute asthma.[51]

OPTION	CONTINUOUS VERSUS AS NEEDED SHORT ACTING β_2 AGONISTS FOR ACUTE ASTHMA

One RCT found that continuous delivery of β_2 agonists in acute asthma was associated with greater improvement in FEV_1. Other smaller RCTs found no significant difference. RCTs consistently found that continuous nebulised treatment improved outcome more than intermittent treatment in adults with more severe airflow obstruction.

Benefits:
We found no systematic review. We found five RCTs.[52–56] The first, larger RCT (n = 99) found that in a sugroup of 69 people with more severe asthma, continuous aerosol delivery was associated with a PEFR at 120 minutes of 296 l/minute (95% CI 266 to 329) compared with 244 l/minute (95% CI 216 to 272) for as needed delivery.[52] Hospital admissions were also significantly lower in the continuous delivery group (11/35 [28%] v 19/34 [57%], P = 0.03). However, the post hoc nature of the analysis weakens these results. Another RCT (n = 38) found no significant difference in improvement in FEV_1 between continuous and as needed salbutamol. Subgroup analysis found that, in people with lower initial FEV_1, continuous treatment was associated with a greater improvement in FEV_1.[54] One RCT (n = 165) randomised people to four regimens of salbutamol: as needed high dose (1.5 mg), as needed standard dose (0.5 mg), continuous high dose (1.5 mg), continuous standard dose (0.5 mg). It found at 2 hours that both continuous treatments were associated with greater improvement in FEV_1 than as needed treatment.[51]

Harms:
Commonly reported, mild adverse effects associated with frequent dosing include tachycardia, tremor, and headache. Metabolic upsets are less common, and include hypokalemia. One RCT found the highest rate of adverse effects with high dose as needed treatment. The most common adverse effect was tremor (24% as needed high dose, 20% continuous high dose, 9.3% hourly standard dose, and 2.5% continuous standard dose).[57]

Comment:
We also found one RCT in 46 adult inpatients, which addressed the slightly different, but related question of regular salbutamol (5 mg every 4 hours) versus on demand salbutamol (2.5–5 mg).[58] This trial found that on demand dosage was significantly associated with shorter hospital stay (3.7 days v 4.7 days), reduced number of nebulisations (geometric mean 7.0 v 14, P = 0.003), and fewer palpitations (P = 0.049).

OPTION	INTRAVENOUS VERSUS NEBULISED DELIVERY OF SHORT ACTING β_2 AGONISTS FOR ACUTE ASTHMA

RCTs found conflicting evidence. Intravenous salbutamol was associated with more adverse effects.

Benefits:
We found no systematic review, and conflicting results from three RCTs comparing intravenous versus nebulised salbutamol.[57,59,60] The largest trial (n = 76) randomised only people who had not responded after 30 minutes to nebulised salbutamol. Nebulised treatment was given at 30 minutes and 2 hours. The trial found greater bronchodilation in the intravenous group, (FEV_1 improved by

25% in the intravenous group v 14% in the nebuliser group, 95% CI for difference 2.4% to 19.1%).[60] The second, multicentre trial (n = 47) found that nebulised salbutamol (total 10 mg) was more effective than intravenous salbutamol (0.5 mg) over 1 hour (19/22 responded successfully to nebuliser, 12/25 responded successfully to intravenous salbutamol, P = 0.006).[57] The third trial (n = 16) found no difference in FEV_1, but greater self reported improvement in symptoms among those treated with inhaled salbutamol.[59]

Harms: All trials found adverse effects to be more common with intravenous delivery.[57,59,60] In the largest trial, 2/39 people in the intravenous group withdrew due to tachyardia. In the nebulised salbutamol group none withdrew because of adverse effects, but three people withdrew due to lack of effect.[60]

Comment: None.

OPTION ADDITION OF IPRATROPIUM BROMIDE TO β_2 AGONISTS IN ACUTE ASTHMA

One systematic review of RCTs found that combining short acting β_2 agonists with ipratropium bromide was associated with significant reductions in admission to hospital and improvements in lung function in people with more severe acute asthma.

Benefits: We found one systematic review of published RCTs (search date 1999) comparing salbutamol plus inhaled ipratropium bromide versus salbutamol alone.[61] The review identified five RCTs that evaluated hospital admissions, and found ipratropium treatment to be associated with a significant reduction in admissions (OR 0.62, 95% CI 0.44 to 0.88; NNT 18, 95% CI 11 to 77). Meta-analysis of the four trials that evaluated people with severe airflow obstruction ($FEV_1 < 35\%$) found that additional treatment with ipratropium bromide was associated with substantial improvement in FEV_1 over 90 minutes (effect size 0.38, 95% CI 0.05 to 0.67).

Harms: Addition of ipratropium bromide had no significant effect on adverse effects.[61]

Comment: None.

OPTION OXYGEN

We found no systematic review or RCTs of oxygen in acute asthma. However, experience and pathophysiology suggest that its role is vital in acute asthma. Small RCTs found mixed evidence that combining oxygen with helium may improve PEFR.

Benefits: **Oxygen alone:** We found no systematic review and no RCTs. **Oxygen with helium:** We found three RCTs of combined helium (70% or 80%) and oxygen (30% or 20%) in adults with acute asthma.[62–64] One trial included 27 people whose peak flow rate remained below 250 l/minute despite treatment, with a pulsus paradoxus greater than 15 mm. Breathing a helium–oxygen mixture of 80 : 20 was associated with reduced pulsus paradoxus and improved peak flow compared with breathing room air alone (no numerical data, results presented as a graph).[62] The second trial (n = 23) found the helium–oxygen combination to be associated with a greater increase in PEFR rate than 30% oxygen (58%, P < 0.001 v 10%, P < 0.1).[63] The third trial found no evidence of benefit from helium plus oxygen. However, although large (n = 205), it was limited by short duration of intervention (15 minutes), single blinding, and inclusion of people with mild to moderate acute asthma.[64]

Harms: We found no evidence of adverse effects associated with oxygen alone or oxygen with helium in acute asthma.

Comment: The final common pathway in acute asthma is respiratory failure and cardiopulmonary arrest.[8,9] Studies assessing pathophysiology of near fatal asthma suggest that hypoxia rather than arrhythmias account for asthma deaths. Therefore it seems reasonable that supplemental oxygen continue to form a critical part of management even though we found no RCTs that provide direct evidence for this. Peak flow readings vary depending on the viscosity of the gas being delivered (helium is less dense than oxygen, so non-standardised measures of peak flow will increase relative to air, even if the mixture has no effect on airway narrowing). It was not clear in all studies whether peak flow readings were standardised for air and helium–oxygen mixtures.

OPTION	INTRAVENOUS MAGNESIUM SULPHATE

Valid subgroup analysis from one systematic review of RCTs suggests that, in people with more severe acute asthma, adding intravenous magnesium sulphate to usual treatment may reduce rates of hospital admission.

Benefits: We found one systematic review (search date 1999) of five adult and two child RCTs (total n = 665) comparing intravenous magnesium sulphate versus placebo, both combined with usual treatment.[65] Overall admission to hospital was not significantly reduced (OR 0.31 95% CI, 0.09 to 1.02). Prespecified subgroup analysis of adults with more severe airflow obstruction (sample size not given; FEV_1 < 30% at presentation, failure to respond to initial treatment, or failure to improve beyond 60% in FEV_1 after 1 hour) found that those receiving adjunct magnesium sulphate had better PEFR and reduced rates of admission to hospital.

Harms: We found no significant adverse effects associated with treatment.

Comment: Further studies are needed to clarify the role of intravenous magnesium sulphate in acute asthma. Two of the studies involved treatment with aminophylline and one with ipratropium, both of which have been found to affect hospital admission rates without affecting the degree of airflow obstruction.[66] The subgroup analysis involved intergroup and intragroup analyses specified before the trial was conducted, and so provides reasonably strong evidence of an effect.

Asthma

OPTION   MECHANICAL VENTILATION

We found no RCTs comparing mechanical ventilation versus no ventilation for severe acute asthma. Evidence from cohort studies and case series support its use, despite a high level of morbidity related to the intervention.

Benefits: We found no systematic reviews or RCTs.

Harms: Mechanical ventilation is associated with hypotension, barotrauma, infection, and myopathy, especially when prolonged paralysis is required with muscle relaxants and systemic corticosteroids.[67] Adverse effects reported in one retrospective study of 88 episodes of mechanical ventilation were hypotension (20%), pulmonary barotrauma (14%), and arrhythmias (10%).[68]

Comment: Experience suggests that mechanical ventilation is a life saving intervention needed by a small minority of people with severe acute asthma. Cohort studies[69,70] and one case series[71] found fewer deaths with controlled hypoventilation compared with historical cohorts and case series in which carbon dioxide levels were normalised, which report mortality in the range of 7.5–23%.[68,72–74] Non-invasive ventilation has been used in people with acute exacerbations of chronic obstructive lung disease,[75] but requires prospective validation in people with acute asthma. Future research should focus on the role of non-invasive mechanical ventilation to prevent the need for intubation and improvement of management strategies during ventilation, including potential benefits of controlled hypoventilation, delivery of bronchodilators, optimal use of muscle relaxants, and dose of corticosteroids.

OPTION   SPECIALIST VERSUS GENERALIST CARE

Non-randomised trials suggest that specialist care is more effective that generalist care.

Benefits: We found no systematic review and no RCTs. One non-systematic review of controlled trials (search date November 1999) found that "expert based" care was associated with improved outcomes.[76] One trial quasi-randomised people (based on day of attendance) referred from the emergency department to specialist care versus routine general medical follow up.[77] It found that people receiving specialist care were significantly less likely to wake at night (OR 0.24, 95% CI 0.11 to 0.52); suffer relapse requiring emergency admission by 6 months (for one admission RR 0.56, 95% CI 0.34 to 0.95; for two admissions RR 0.3, 95% CI 0.16 to 0.6); suffer multiple relapses; and were more likely to use inhaled corticosteroids (OR 3.6, 95% CI 1.9 to 6.6) and cromolyn (RR 2.2, 95% CI 1.9 to 2.5). A second prospective, non-randomised trial prospectively assessed people with asthma admitted to a respiratory ward (n = 64) versus a general medical ward (n = 86).[78] Those receiving expert care were less likely to be admitted in the following year (2% v 20%).

Harms: We found no harms associated with specialist versus generalist care.

Comment: None.

OPTION ASTHMA EDUCATION FOR PEOPLE WITH ACUTE ASTHMA

One systematic review of RCTs has found that education to facilitate self management of asthma in adults reduces hospital admission, unscheduled visits to the doctor, and days off work.

Benefits: We found one systematic review of 22 RCTs (search date 1999) of adult self management of asthma.[78] The review found that education about asthma to facilitate self management, whether initiated from a specialist or generalist setting, significantly reduced the risk of hospital admission (RRR 38%, 95% CI 6% to 59%; NNT 38, 95% CI 20 to 382), unscheduled visits to the doctor (RRR 26%, 95% CI 10% to 37%; NNT 12, 95% CI 8 to 36), and days off work (RRR 25%, 95% CI 10% to 37%; NNT 7, 95% CI 5 to 13). Best results were achieved in people who had written care plans.

Harms: None reported.

Comment: None.

REFERENCES

1. National Heart, Blood and Lung Institute. National Asthma Education and Prevention Program. Expert Panel Report 2. Guidelines for the Diagnosis and Management of Asthma. NIH Publication No. 97–4051;July 1997:20.
2. British Thoracic Society Guidelines. *Thorax* 1997; 52:S1–S2.
3. Kaur B, Anderson HR, Austin J, et al. Prevalence of asthma symptoms, diagnosis, and treatment in 12–14 year old children across Great Britain (international study of asthma and allergies in childhood, ISAAC UK). *BMJ* 1998;316:118–124.
4. Woolcock AJ, Peat JK. Evidence for an increase in asthma world-wide. *Ciba Found Symp* 1997;206: 122–134.
5. Duff AL, Platts-Mills TA. Allergens and asthma. *Pediatr Clin North Am* 1992;39:1277–1291.
6. Chan-Yeung M, Malo JL. Occupational asthma. *N Engl J Med* 1995;333:107–112.
7. Lange P, Parner J, Vestbo J, Schnohr P, Jensen G. A 15-year follow-up study of ventilatory function in adults with asthma. *N Engl J Med* 1998;339: 1194–1200.
8. Turner MT, Noertjojo K, Vedal S, Bai T, Crump S, FitzGerald JM. Risk factors for near-fatal asthma: a case control study in patients hospitalised with acute asthma. *Am J Respir Crit Care Med* 1998; 157:1804–1809.
9. Molfino NA, Nannimi A, Martelli AN, Slutsky AS. Respiratory arrest in near fatal asthma. *N Engl J Med* 1991;324:285–288.
10. Emmerman CL, Woodruff PG, Cydulka RK, Gibbs MA, Pollack CV, Camargo Jr. CA. Prospective multi-center study of relapse following treatment for acute asthma among adults presenting to the emergency department. *Chest* 1999;115:919–927.
11. Drazen JM, Israel E, Boushey HA, et al. Comparison of regularly scheduled with as-needed use of albuterol in mild asthma. Asthma clinical research network. *N Engl J Med* 1996;335:841–847.
12. Sears MR, Taylor DR, Print CG, et al. Regular inhaled β-agonist treatment in bronchial asthma. *Lancet* 1990;336:1391–1396.
13. Spitzer WO, Suissa S, Ernst P, et al. The use of β-agonists and the risk of death and near death from asthma. *N Engl J Med* 1992;326:501–506.
14. Crane J, Pearce N, Flatt A, et al. Prescribed fenoterol and death from asthma in New Zealand, 1981–1983: case-control study. *Lancet* 1989;1: 917–922.
15. Kerrebijn KF, van Essen-Zandvliet EE, Neijens HJ. Effect of long-term treatment with inhaled corticosteroids and β-agonists on the bronchial responsiveness in children with asthma. *J Allergy Clin Immunol* 1987;79:653–659.
16. Cockcroft DW, McParland CP, Britto SA, Swystun VA, Rutherford BC. Regular inhaled salbutamol and airway responsiveness to allergen. *Lancet* 1993;342:833–837.
17. Ahrens RC. Skeletal muscle tremor and the influence of adrenergic drugs. *J Asthma* 1990,27: 11–20.
18. O'Byrne PM, Cuddy L, Taylor DW, Birch S, Morris J, Syrotiuk J. The clinical efficacy and cost benefit of inhaled corticosteroids as therapy in patients with mild asthma in primary care practice. *Can Respir J* 1996;3:169–175.
19. Kemp J, Wanderer AA, Ramsdell J, Southern DL, et al. Rapid onset of control with budesonide turbuhaler in patients with mild-to-moderate asthma. *Ann Allergy Asthma Immunol* 1999;82: 463–471.
20. Busse WW, Chervinsky P, Condemi J, et al. Budesonide delivered by Turbuhaler is effective in a dose-dependent fashion when used in the treatment of adult patients with chronic asthma. *J Allergy Clin Immunol* 1998;101:457–463.
21. McFadden ER, Casale TB, Edwards TB, et al. Administration of budesonide once daily by means of turbuhaler to subjects with stable asthma. *J Allergy Clin Immunol* 1999;104:46–52.
22. Nathan RA, Pinnas JL, Schwartz HJ, Grossman J, et al. A six-month, placebo-controlled comparison of the safety and efficacy of salmeterol or beclomethasone for persistent asthma. *Ann Allergy Asthma Immunol* 1999;82:521–529.
23. Bronsky E, Korenblat P, Harris AG, and Chen R. Comparative clinical study of inhaled beclomethasone dipropionate and triamcinolone acetonide in persistent asthma. *Ann Allergy* 1998; 80:295–302.
24. Bernstein DI, Cohen R, Ginchansky E, Pedinoff AJ, Tinkelman DG. A multicenter, placebo-controlled study of twice daily triamcinolone acetonide (800 µg per day) for the treatment of patients with

mild-to-moderate asthma. *J Allergy Clin Immunol* 1998;101:433–438.

25. Ramsdell JW, Fish L, Graft D, et al. A controlled trial of twice daily triamcinolone oral inhaler in patients with mild-to-moderate asthma. *Ann Allergy* 1998;80:385–390.

26. Hatoum HT, Schumock GT, Kendzierski DL. Meta-analysis of controlled trials of drug therapy in mild chronic asthma: the role of inhaled corticosteroids. *Ann Pharmacother* 1994;28:1285–1289. Search date not given; primary sources Medline.

27. Haahtela T, Jarvinen M, Tuomo K, et al. Comparison of a β_2 antagonist, terbutaline, with an inhaled corticosteroid, budesonide, in newly detected asthma. *N Engl J Med* 1991;325:388–392.

28. Barnes PJ, Pedersen S, Busse WW. Efficacy and safety of inhaled corticosteroids: new developments. *Am J Respir Crit Care Med* 1998;157:1–53.

29. Weusten BL, Jacobs JW, Bijlsma JW. Corticosteroid pulse therapy in active rheumatoid arthritis. *Semin Arthritis Rheum* 1993;23:183–192.

30. Toogood JH, Markov AE, Baskerville JC, Dyson C. Association of ocular cataracts with inhaled and oral steroid therapy during long-term treatment of asthma. *J Allergy Clin Immunol* 1993;91:571–579.

31. Cumming RG, Mitchell P, Leeder SR. Use of inhaled corticosteroids and the risk of cataracts. *N Engl J Med* 1997;337:8–14.

32. Toogood JH, Jennings B, Greenway RW, Chuang L. Candidiasis and dysphonia complicating beclomethasone treatment of asthma. *J Allergy Clin Immunol* 1980;65:145–153.

33. Roy A, Levlanc C, Paquette L, Ghezzo H, Cote J, Malo JL. Skin bruising in asthmatic subjects treated with high doses of inhaled steroids: frequency and association with adrenal function. *Eur Respir J* 1996;9:226–231.

34. Eckerskorn U, Hockwin O, M ller-Breitenkamp R, Chen TT, Knowles W, Dobbs RE. Evaluation of cataract-related risk factors using detailed classification systems and multivariate statistical methods. *Dev Ophthalmol* 1987;15:82–91.

35. Kemp JP, Cook DA, Incaudo GA, et al. Salmeterol improves quality of life in patients with asthma requiring inhaled corticosteroids. *J Allergy Clin Immunol* 1998;101:188–195.

36. FitzGerald JM, Chapman KR, Della Cioppa G, et al. Sustained bronchoprotection, bronchodilatation, and symptom control during regular formoterol use in asthma of moderate or greater severity. *J Allergy Clin Immunol* 1999;103:427–435

37. Greening AP, Ind PW, Northfield M, Shaw G. Added salmeterol versus higher-dose corticosteroid in asthma patients with symptoms on existing inhaled corticosteroid. *Lancet* 1994;344:219–224.

38. Woolcock AJ, Lundback B, Ringdal N, Jacques LA. Comparison of addition of salmeterol to inhaled steroids with doubling of the dose of inhaled steroids. *Am J Respir Crit Care Med* 1996;153:1481–1488.

39. Van Noord JA, Schreurs AJM, Mol SJM, Mulder PGH. Addition of salmeterol versus doubling the dose of fluticasone propionate in patients with mild to moderate asthma. *Thorax* 1999;54:207–212.

40. Condemi JJ, Goldstein S, Kalberg C, et al. The addition of salmeterol to fluticasone propionate versus increasing the dose of fluticasone propionate in patients with persistent asthma. *Ann Allergy* 1999;82:383–389.

41. Pauwels RA, Lofdahl C-G, Postma DS, O'Byrne PM, Barnes PJ, Ullman A. Effect of inhaled formoterol and budesonide on exacerbations of asthma. *N Engl J Med* 1997;337:1405–1411.

42. Vermetten FAAM, Boermans AJM, Luiten WDVF, Mulder PGH, Vermue NA. Comparison of salmeterol with beclomethasone in adult patients with mild persistent asthma who are already on low-dose inhaled steroids. *J Asthma* 1999;36:97–106.

43. Cheung D, Timmers MC, Zwinderman AH, Bel EH, Dijkman JH, Sterk PJ. Long-term effects of a long-acting β_2-adrenoceptor agonist, salmeterol, on airway hyperresponsiveness in patients with mild asthma. *N Engl J Med* 1992;327:1198–1203.

44. O'Connor BJ, Aikman SL, Barnes PJ. Tolerance to the nonbronchodilating effects of inhaled β_2-agonists in asthma. *N Engl J Med* 1992;327:1204–1208.

45. Nelson JA, Strauss L, Skowronski M, Ciufo R, Novak R, McFadden ER, Jr. Effect of long-term salmeterol treatment on exercise-induced asthma. *N Engl J Med* 1998;339:141–146.

46. Castle W, Fuller R, Hall J, Palmer J. Serevent nationwide surveillance study: comparison of salmeterol with salbutamol in asthmatic patients who require regular bronchodilator treatment. *BMJ* 1993;306:1034–1037.

47. Cates C. Holding chambers versus nebulisers for β agonist treatment of acute asthma. In: The Cochrane Library, Issue 1, 2000. Search date February 1999; primary sources Cochrane Airways Review Group Register of Trials; bibliographies of all included papers; authors of included studies; and the Cochrane Controlled Trials Register.

48. Rowe BH, Spooner CH, Duchrame FM, Bratzlaff JA, Bota GW. Corticosteroids for preventing relapse following acute exacerbations of asthma. In: The Cochrane Library, Issue 1, 2000. Oxford: Update software. Search date 1997; primary sources Cochrane Airways Review Group Asthma and Wheeze RCT register.

49. Rowe BH, Keller JL, Oxman AD. Effectiveness of steroid therapy in acute exacerbations of asthma: a meta-analysis. *Am J Emerg Med* 1992;10:301–310. Search date 1991; primary sources Medline 1966 to 1991; Science Citation Index 1980 to 1990; review articles; textbooks; experts and primary authors.

50. O'Driscoll BR, Kalra S, Wilson M, Pickering CA, Carroll KB, Woodcock AA. Double-blind trial of steroid tapering in acute asthma. *Lancet* 1993;341:324–327.

51. Levy ML, Stevenson C, Maslen T. Comparison of a short course of oral prednisone and fluticasone propionate in the treatment of adults with acute exacerbations of asthma in primary care. *Thorax* 1996;51:1087–1092.

52. Rudnitsky GS, Eberlein RS, Schoffstall JM, Mazur JE, Spivey WH. Comparison of intermittent and continuously nebulized albuterol for treatment of asthma in an urban emergency department. *Ann Emerg Med* 1993;22:1842–1846.

53. Resiner C, Kotch A, Dworkin G. Continuous versus frequent intermittent nebulisations of albuterol in acute asthma: a randomized, prospective study. *Ann Allergy Asthma Immunol* 1995;75:41–47.

54. Lin RY, Sauter D, Newman T, Sirleaf J, Walters J, Tavakol M. Continuous versus intermittent nebulization in the treatment of acute asthma. *Ann Emerg Med* 1993;22:1847–1853.

55. Khine H, Fuchs SM, Saville AL. Continuous vs intermittent nebulized albuterol for emergency management of asthma. *Acad Emerg Med* 1969;3:1019–1024.

56. Shrestha M, Bidadi K, Gourlay S, Hayes J. Continuous vs intermittent albuterol, at high and low doses, in the treatment of severe acute asthma in adults. *Chest* 1996;110:42–47.

57. Salmeron S, Brochard L, Mal H, et al Nebulized versus intravenous albuterol in hypercapnoeic acute asthma. A multi-center, double blind, randomized study. *Am J Respir Crit Care Med* 1994;149:1466–1470.

58. Bradding P, Rushby I, Scullion J, Morgan MDL. As required versus regular nebulized salbutamol for the treatment of acute severe asthma. *Eur Respir J* 1999;13:290–294.

59. Lawford P, Jones BJM, Milledge JS. Comparison of intravenous and nebulized salbutamol in the initial treatment of severe asthma. *BMJ* 1978;1:84.

60. Cheong B , Reynolds SR, Rajan G, Ward MJ. Intravenous β-agonist in acute severe asthma. *BMJ* 1988;297:448 –50.

61. Rodrigo G, Rodrigo C, Burschtin O. Ipratropium bromide in acute adult severe asthma:a meta-analysis of randomized controlled trials. *Am J Med* 1999;107:363–370. Search date April 1999; primary sources Medline 1978 to 1999; Current Contents; Science Citation Index; review articles; experts; pharmaceutical manufacturer; Medical Editor's Trial Amnesty register and hand searched references

62. Manthous CA, Hall JB, Caputo MA, et al. Heliox improves pulsus paradoxus and peak expiratory flow in non-intubated patients with severe asthma. *Am J Respir Care Crit Care Med* 1995;151:310–314.

63. Kass JE, Terregino CA. The effect of heliox in acute severe asthma: a randomized controlled trial. *Chest* 1999;116:296–300.

64. Henderson SO, Acharay P, Kilaghbian T, Perez J, Kom CS, Chan LS. Use of heliox-driven nebulized therapy in the treatment of acute asthma. *Ann Emerg Med* 1999;33:141–146.

65. Rowe BH, Bretzlaff JA, Bourdon C, Bota GW, Camargo CA Jr. Magnesium sulphate treatment for acute asthmatic exacerbations treated in the emergency department. In: The Cochrane Library, Issue 1, 2000. Oxford: Update software. Search date 1999; primary sources Cochrane Airways Review Group trials register; review articles; textbooks; experts; primary authors of included studies and hand searched references.

66. FitzGerald JM. Commentary: Intravenous magnesium in acute asthma. *Evid Based Med* 1999;Sept/Oct:138.

67. Behbehani NA, Al-Mane FD, Yachkova Y, Pare PD, FitzGerald JM. Myopathy following mechanical ventilation for acute severe asthma: the role of muscle relaxants and corticosteroids. *Chest* 1999;115:1627–1631.

68. Williams TJ, Tuxen DV, Sceinkestel CD, Czarny D, Bowes G. Risk factors for morbidity in mechanically ventilated patients with acute severe asthma. *Am Rev Respir Dis* 1992;146:607–615.

69. Darioli R, Perret C. Mechanical controlled hypoventilation in status asthmaticus. *Am Rev Respir Dis* 1984;129:385–387.

70. Menitove SM, Godring RM. Combined ventilator and bicarbonate strategy in the management of status asthmaticus. *Am J Med* 1983;74:898–901.

71. Higgins B, Greening AP, Crompton GK. Assisted ventilation in severe acute asthma. *Thorax* 1986;41:464–467.

72. Lam KN, Mow BM, Chew LS. The profile of ICU admissions for acute severe asthma in a general hospital. *Singapore Med J* 1993;34:460–462.

73. Mansel JK, Stogner SW, Petrini MF, Norman JR. Mechanical ventilation in patients with acute severe asthma. *Am J Med* 1990;89:42–48.

74. Lim TK. Status asthmaticus in a medical intensive care unit. *Singapore Med J* 1989;30:334–338.

75. Keenan SP, Brake D. An evidence based approach to non invasive ventilation in acute respiratory failure. *Crit Care Clin* 1998;14:359–372.

76. Bartter T, Pratter MR. Asthma: better outcome at a lower cost? The role of the expert in the care system. *Chest* 1996;110:1589–1596.

77. Zeiger RS, Heller S, Mellon MH, Wald J, Falkoff R, Schatz M. Facilitated referral to asthma specialist reduces relapses in asthma emergency room visits. *J Allergy Clin Immunol* 1991;87:1160–1168.

78. Gibson PG, Coughlan J, Wilson AJ, et al. Self-management education and regular practitioner review of adults with asthma. The Cochrane Library, Issue 4, 1999:1–12. Search date 1999; primary sources Cochrane Airways Group trials register and hand searched references.

Christopher Cates
General Practitioner
Manor View Practice
Bushey
UK

Mark FitzGerald
Respiratory Clinic
Vancouver General Hospital
Vancouver
Canada

Competing interests: CC, none declared. MF has received honoraria for lectures and research funds from GlaxoWellcome, Merck, AstraZeneca, Novartis, Boehringer Ingelheim and 3M.

Asthma

TABLE 1	Classification of severity for chronic asthma (see text, p 829).

In the USA[1]

Asthma is classified by symptoms of severity. Using this system, even people with mild, intermittent asthma can develop severe exacerbations if exposed to appropriate stimuli.

Mild intermittent asthma	Symptoms less than weekly with normal or near normal lung function.
Mild persistent asthma	Symptoms more than weekly but less than daily with normal or near normal lung function.
Moderate persistent asthma	Daily symptoms with mild to moderate variable airflow obstruction.
Severe asthma	Daily symptoms and frequent night symptoms, and moderate to severe variable airflow obstruction.

In the UK[2]

Chronic asthma in ambulatory settings is graded according to the amount of medication required to keep symptoms controlled. People are classified according to whether, for symptom control, they need:

Step 1	Occasional β agonists for symptomatic relief.
Step 2	In addition, regular, inhaled anti-inflammatory agents (such as inhaled corticosteroids, cromoglycate, or nedocromil).
Step 3	In addition, high-dose inhaled corticosteroids or low dose inahled steroids plus long-acting inhaled β_2 bronchodilator.
Step 4	In addition, high-dose inhaled corticosteroids plus regular bronchodilators.
Step 5	In addition, regular oral corticosteroids.

Updated this issue

Huib Kerstjens and Dirkje Postma

QUESTIONS

INTERVENTIONS

Key Messages

Short term effects of treatment

- RCTs have found evidence of short term benefit from oral steroids, inhaled anticholinergic drugs, and inhaled β$_2$ agonists. The short term benefits of anticholinergic drugs and β$_2$ agonists are not seen in all people with chronic obstructive pulmonary disease (COPD). RCTs found that the two agents combined are slightly more effective than either alone.

- RCTs have found no evidence of short term benefit from inhaled corticosteroids.

- Small, short term RCTs of theophyllines found some evidence of benefit, but the usefulness of these drugs is limited by adverse effects and the need for frequent monitoring of blood concentrations.

Long term effects of treatment

- One systematic review has found some evidence of reduction in mortality in people with hypoxaemia from long term treatment with oxygen.

- We found insufficient evidence on the long term effects of maintenance treatment with antibiotics, oral steroids, inhaled β$_2$ agonists, or theophyllines.

Chronic obstructive pulmonary disease

- RCTs of inhaled anticholinergic drugs or inhaled steroids provide no clear evidence of an effect on disease course.
- Two systematic reviews of RCTs have found evidence that mucolytics reduce the frequency of exacerbations.

DEFINITION   Chronic obstructive pulmonary disease (COPD) is characterised by airflow obstruction caused by chronic bronchitis or emphysema. Emphysema is abnormal permanent enlargement of the air spaces distal to the terminal bronchioles, accompanied by destruction of their walls and without obvious fibrosis. Chronic bronchitis is chronic cough or mucus production for at least 3 months in at least 2 successive years when other causes of chronic cough have been excluded.[1]

INCIDENCE/ COPD mainly affects middle aged and elderly people. It is one of the
PREVALENCE leading causes of morbidity and mortality worldwide. In the USA, it affects about 14 million people and is the fourth leading cause of death. Both morbidity and mortality are rising. Estimated prevalence in the USA has risen by 41% since 1982, and age adjusted death rates rose by 71% between 1966 and 1985. All cause age adjusted mortality declined over the same period by 22% and mortality from cardiovascular diseases by 45%.[1]

AETIOLOGY/ COPD is largely preventable. The main cause is exposure to ciga-
RISK FACTORS rette smoke. COPD is rare in lifetime non-smokers (estimated incidence 5% in three large representative US surveys from 1971 to 1984), in whom exposure to environmental tobacco smoke will explain at least some disease.[2,3] Other proposed causes include airway hyperresponsiveness, air pollution, and allergy.[4–6]

PROGNOSIS   The airway obstruction is usually progressive in those who continue to smoke. Progression results in early disability and shortened survival. Smoking cessation reverts decline in lung function to values of non-smokers.[7] Many people will use medication chronically for the rest of their lives, with the need for increased doses and additional drugs during exacerbations.

AIMS   To alleviate symptoms, to prevent exacerbations, to preserve optimal lung function, and to improve activities of daily living, quality of life, and survival.[8]

OUTCOMES   Short and long term changes in lung function, including changes in forced expiratory volume in one second (FEV_1); exercise tolerance; peak expiratory flow rate (PEF); frequency, severity, and duration of exacerbations; symptom scores for dyspnoea; quality of life; and survival.

METHODS   This review deals only with treatment of stable COPD and not with treatment of acute exacerbations. *Clinical Evidence* update search and appraisal May 2000. Because we were interested in the maintenance treatment of stable COPD, we did not include single dose or single day cumulative dose response trials.

OPTION INHALED ANTICHOLINERGIC DRUGS

RCTs using a range of methods found that anticholinergic drugs achieved short term bronchodilation and symptomatic relief in people with COPD. One large RCT found no evidence that long term treatment with inhaled anticholinergic drugs improved long term prognosis in COPD.

Benefits: We found no systematic review comparing anticholinergic drugs with placebo. **Short term treatment:** We found many small placebo controlled RCTs using different methods and end points. Most included at least some measure of airways obstruction and found a significant effect of ipratropium bromide.[9-12] We found one large (n = 276) 12 week RCT comparing ipratropium bromide 36 μg four times daily versus placebo or versus salmeterol xinafoate.[13] The FEV_1 for people using ipratropium bromide improved significantly from baseline but results against placebo were only presented graphically. **Long term treatment:** We found one RCT in 5887 men and women smokers aged 35–60 with spirometric signs of early COPD (FEV_1 75% predicted).[7] Three interventions were compared over a 5 year period: usual care; an intensive 12 session smoking cessation programme combining behaviour modification and use of nicotine gum; and the same smoking intervention programme plus ipratropium bromide three times daily. The addition of ipratropium bromide had no significant effect on decline in FEV_1. Decline in FEV_1 was significantly slower in people in the smoking cessation group (5 year mean cumulative decline in prebronchodilator FEV_1: usual care 249 ml, 95% CI 236 to 262 ml; smoking programme and ipratropium bromide 188 ml, 95% CI 175 to 200 ml; smoking programme and placebo 172 ml, 95% CI 159 to 185 ml).

Harms: In the RCT of long term treatment, serious adverse events (cardiac symptoms, hypertension, skin rashes, and urinary retention) occurred in 1.2% of people taking ipratropium bromide versus 0.8% taking placebo.[7] Dry mouth was the most common mild adverse event. One RCT (233 people with asthma or COPD) found that continuous (as opposed to as needed) treatment with bronchodilators (both ipratropium bromide and fenoterol) resulted in faster decline in lung function.[14] This result has not been found in other trials.

Comment: Over a 5 year period, there was no evidence that people developed tachyphylaxis to the bronchodilating effect of ipratropium bromide.[7]

OPTION INHALED β₂ AGONISTS

Short term RCTs found that short and long acting inhaled β_2 agonists achieved bronchodilation and symptomatic relief in many people. The effects of long term treatment with β_2 agonists on the disease progression have not yet been adequately evaluated.

Benefits: **Short term treatment with short acting β_2 agonists:** We found no systematic review. We found over 100 placebo controlled RCTs.

In general these found improved symptoms and some bronchodilatory effect, the magnitude of which depended partly on whether participants were selected on the basis of having irreversible airways obstruction. One RCT (985 people with severe COPD) found a significant increase in lung function in up to half of participants.[15] Ten out of 17 trials assessing walking distance as a measure of exercise capacity found a significant improvement with short acting β_2 agonists. **Short term treatment with long acting β_2 agonists:** We found one systematic review (search date 1998, 3 RCTs of salmeterol)[16] and two subsequent RCTs.[13,17] All found significant improvements in either symptoms, lung function, or quality of life. The first RCT in the systematic review (n = 674) compared salmeterol 50 µg and 100 µg doses twice daily for 16 weeks and found a significant increase in FEV_1 in both treatment groups (50 µg: WMD 0.10 litre, 95% CI 0.05 to 0.15 litre; 100 µg: WMD 0.12 litre, 95% CI 0.06 to 0.17 litre).[18] Quality of life improved significantly in the group taking the lower but not the higher dose compared with placebo.[19] The second RCT, a crossover trial in 63 smokers, found significant increases in morning FEV_1 after 4 weeks of treatment with salmeterol 50 µg twice daily compared with placebo (mean treatment difference 12 ml, 95% CI 6 ml to 17 ml). Evening values were not significantly different from placebo.[20] The third RCT (29 people) found that significantly fewer people taking salmeterol 50 µg daily were scored as moderately dyspnoeic or worse (OR 0.60, 95% CI 0.40 to 0.88). There was no significant difference in the mean change from baseline in the 6 minute walking distance (WMD +1.9 m, 95% CI −15.4 m to +19.3 m).[21] The systematic review found no trials of formoterol.[16] The first subsequent RCT compared salmeterol 42 µg twice daily versus placebo over 12 weeks (n = 278).[13] It found a significant improvement of average FEV_1 for salmeterol compared with placebo. The second subsequent RCT in 97 people compared salmeterol 50 µg twice daily versus placebo over 12 weeks.[17] There was a significant improvement with salmeterol in morning and evening peak flow rates and in FEV_1 (mean improvement as a percentage of the predicted FEV_1: 5% v 1%, P < 0.01), and day time but not night time symptoms. In the same study, no improvement in quality of life was found with salmeterol compared with placebo.[22] **Long term treatment:** We found no systematic review or RCTs looking at reduction of decline in lung function with inhaled β_2 agonists compared with placebo.

Harms: In people with asthma, β_2 agonists have been linked to increased risk of death, worsened asthma control, and deterioration in lung function.[23] We found no evidence for people with COPD. One RCT (223 people with asthma or COPD) found that continuous (as opposed to as needed) treatment with bronchodilators (ipratropium bromide as well as fenoterol) resulted in faster decline in lung function.[14] We found no other studies of β_2 agonists in COPD addressing this possibility. We found no systematic review on frequency of adverse effects of β_2 agonists in COPD. The most common immediate adverse effect is tremor, which is usually worse in the first few days of treatment. High doses of β_2 agonists can cause a fall in plasma potassium, dysrhythmias, and reduced arterial oxygen tension.[24] Extra caution is warranted for use in people with pre-existing cardiac arrhythmias and hypoxaemia.[25]

One trial comparing salmeterol versus placebo over 12 weeks found no increase in any adverse events, but allowed rescue salbutamol.[13]

Comment: The measured improvement in lung function does not seem to reflect the symptomatic improvement that can occur in some people when taking β_2 agonists. Long term placebo controlled RCTs of β_2 agonists, looking at adverse effects such as decline in lung function or worsened COPD control, are ethically difficult because of their beneficial effects in the short term.

| OPTION | ANTICHOLINERGICS PLUS INHALED β_2 AGONISTS |

RCTs found that combining a β_2 agonist with an anticholinergic drug provided small additional bronchodilation compared with either drug alone.

Benefits: We found no systematic review. **With short acting inhaled β_2 agonists:** We found six RCTs (one article combined the results from two RCTs, n = 705, 195, 652, 863, and 357) comparing the addition of ipratropium versus standard dose short acting inhaled β_2 agonists for 2 weeks to 3 months in people with stable COPD.[26–30] All found significant improvements in FEV_1 of about 25% with the combination compared with either drug alone. **With long acting inhaled β_2 agonists:** One RCT evaluated a long acting β_2 agonist, salmeterol 50 µg twice daily versus salmeterol 50 µg twice daily plus ipratropium bromide 40 µg four times daily in 94 people over 12 weeks.[17] It found the combination versus the β_2 agonist alone significantly improved FEV_1 (mean improvement as a percentage of predicted FEV_1 8% v 5%, P < 0.01) and evening but not morning peak flow rates. It found no significant difference in day time or night time symptoms. Quality of life was found to improve more with the combination than with salmeterol alone.[22]

Harms: The trials found no significant differences in adverse effects between the groups.

Comment: None.

| OPTION | INHALED β_2 AGONISTS VERSUS ANTICHOLINERGICS |

One non-systematic review of RCTs has found greater bronchodilator response with inhaled anticholinergic drugs than β_2 agonists in people with COPD.

Benefits: We found no systematic review. **Short term treatment:** Several RCTs with different methods and outcomes have compared ipratropium bromide versus a β_2 agonist. They used different methods and found conflicting results. **Long term treatment:** One non-systematic review pooled data from seven RCTs (n = 1445) of ipratropium bromide versus various short acting β_2 agonists for 90 days.[31] Lung function measurements were performed after withholding bronchodilators for at least 12 hours. There was a significantly greater mean improvement in FEV_1 with ipratropium bromide than with the β_2 agonists (28 ml increase v 1 ml decrease, P < 0.05). We found one additional trial comparing the long acting

β_2 agonist salmeterol (42 µg) twice daily versus ipratropium (36 µg) four times daily during 12 weeks' treatment.[13] It found a significant effect on average FEV_1 with salmeterol treatment compared with ipratropium at weeks 4 and 8, but not at weeks 0 and 12.

Harms: Although adverse clinical events associated with β_2 agonists such as tremor and dysrhythmias seem to be more frequent than the adverse clinical events associated with anticholinergics, the review provides no evidence.[31] The RCT comparing salmeterol versus ipratropium versus placebo found no significant difference in adverse events.[13]

Comment: A residual effect of the anticholinergic drugs cannot be ruled out, limiting the interpretation of a favourable effect of anticholinergic drugs compared with β_2 agonists. It has been suggested that older people experience greater bronchodilator response with anticholinergic drugs than with β_2 agonists, but we found no evidence for this.

OPTION THEOPHYLLINES

We found limited evidence from small RCTs of a small bronchodilatory effect of theophyllines in people with COPD. Adverse effects are frequent.

Benefits: We found no systematic review. **Short term treatment:** We found one non-systematic review (published in 1995), which identified 11 small RCTs of theophyllines in people with COPD.[32] These evaluated treatment periods ranging from 1 week to 2 months and found changes in FEV_1 ranging from 0–20%, with equally varied effects on exercise capacity and symptoms. **Long term treatment:** We found no RCTs.

Harms: The RCTs did not report adverse effects. The therapeutic range for theophyllines is small with blood concentrations of 10–15 mg/l required for optimal effects. Well documented adverse effects include nausea, diarrhoea, headache, irritability, seizures, and cardiac arrhythmias. These may occur within the therapeutic range.[33]

Comment: Non-bronchodilator effects of theophylline have been found in laboratory settings, including effects on respiratory muscles and improved right ventricular function. Clinical significance has not been established. Anti-inflammatory effects have been claimed in asthma, especially at lower dosages, but have not been measured in COPD. One RCT found little value from the use of "n of 1" trials to determine objective individualised treatment effects.[34]

OPTION ORAL CORTICOSTEROIDS

One systematic review of short term RCTs has found a significant effect on lung function of oral steroids compared with placebo. We found no RCT of the effects of long term treatment on lung function. We found evidence of potentially serious adverse effects.

Benefits: **Short term treatment:** We found one systematic review (search date 1989), which identified 15 RCTs of oral steroids in stable COPD.[35] Treatment usually lasted 2–4 weeks. Data pooling from the 10 RCTs that met all inclusion criteria found that a 20% or greater improvement in baseline FEV_1 occurred significantly more often in people taking oral corticosteroids than those on placebo (WMD 10%, 95% CI 2% to 18%). When the other five RCTs were included, the difference in effect size was 11% (95% CI 4% to 18%). **Long term treatment:** We found no long term RCTs examining the effects of oral steroids on decline in lung function.

Harms: Many reviews have described the considerable harms of systemic corticosteroids, including osteoporosis and induction of diabetes.[36]

Comment: None.

OPTION	INHALED CORTICOSTEROIDS

Short term RCTs have found no evidence of benefit of inhaled corticosteroids. Large RCTs of at least 6 months have found that inhaled steroids increase FEV_1 during the first 3–6 months of use, but found no subsequent effect on decline of lung function. Two studies also found a reduction in exacerbation frequency and an improvement in health status.

Benefits: **Short term treatment:** We found no systematic review. We found 10 placebo controlled RCTs shorter than 6 months summarised in one non-systematic review.[37] Nine short term trials (10 days to 10 weeks, n = 10–127) found no significant benefit in lung function (FEV_1) with inhaled steroids. None of the trials measuring airway hyperresponsiveness to histamine found a change. **Long term treatment:** We found one systematic review (search date 1996, 3 long term placebo controlled RCTs of inhaled steroids, n = 197 people treated for 2–2.5 years)[38] and four large subsequent RCTs.[39–42] The systematic review found that, at 2 years, people on inhaled steroids experienced a significantly greater rate of improvement in prebronchodilator FEV_1 compared with placebo (WMD 34 ml/year, 95% CI 5 to 63 ml/year). There was no significant difference in rate of improvement of postbronchodilator FEV_1 (WMD +39 ml/year, 95% CI −6 to +84 ml/year) or in the frequency of exacerbations. The first subsequent RCT compared 6 months' treatment with fluticasone (n = 281) or placebo and found a significant reduction in moderate and severe exacerbations (86% v 60%, P < 0.001) but not mild exacerbations. It found improvement in lung function (adjusted baseline daily peak expiratory flow 15 litres/minute v 2 litres/minute on placebo, P < 0.001) and 6 minute walking distance (adjusted mean change in distance walked 27 m v 8 m, P = 0.03).[39] The second RCT (290 people with mild airways obstruction, FEV_1 86% of predicted) found no effect of budesonide (800 µg plus 400 µg daily for 6 months followed by 400 µg twice daily for 30 months) on decline in lung function or exacerbation frequency.[40] The third RCT (n = 1277, mean FEV_1 77% of predicted; 912 completed the trial) compared 800 µg budesonide daily versus placebo for 3 years.[41] In the first 6 months of the study, FEV_1 improved at the rate of 17 ml per year in the budesonide group compared with a decline of 81 ml per year in the placebo group (P < 0.001). However, there was no effect on subsequent decline. The fourth RCT compared fluticasone 500 µg twice daily for 3 years versus placebo in 751 more severely affected people (FEV_1 50% of predicted).[42] It found no effect on decline in lung function but there was a 25% reduction in exacerbation rate (from 1.32 per year on placebo to 0.99 on fluticasone). It also found a significant reduction in the deterioration of quality of life with fluticasone compared to placebo.[42]

Harms: Extrapolation from studies in people with asthma is of limited value, as people with COPD are generally at higher risk for osteoporosis because of age, menopausal status, inactivity, and cigarette smoking.[36] One RCT (n = 1277) reported skin bruising in 10% of people in the budesonide group and 4% in the placebo group.[41] Newly diagnosed hypertension, bone fractures, postcapsular cataracts, myopathy, and diabetes occurred in less than 5% of people, with no significant difference between the groups.[41]

Comment: The findings of improved quality of life in one trial are preliminary.[42] A large North American RCT is underway (AS Buist, personal communication, 1999).

OPTION   ORAL VERSUS INHALED STEROIDS

We found limited evidence from RCTs suggesting that oral prednisolone is more effective than inhaled beclomethasone in people with mild to moderate COPD.

Benefits: We found no systematic review. **Short term treatment:** We found three RCTs comparing oral prednisolone versus inhaled beclomethasone (n = 12, 83, 107).[43–45] All were double blind placebo controlled crossover trials, with treatment periods of 2 weeks. One small RCT found no significant difference between the number of people responding to either or both treatments.[43] The other two trials found greater benefit with oral than inhaled steroids. One found that FEV_1 rose from 0.65 to 1 litre on prednisolone compared with 0.63 to 0.81 litres on beclomethasone dipropionate (P < 0.01). The other found that the proportion of participants responding to oral treatment was significantly higher (39/107 v 26/107, P < 0.05).[44,45] **Long term treatment:** We found no RCTs.

Harms: None of the RCTs reported adverse effects.

Comment: The smallest RCT only recruited people known to be responsive to oral steroids, and did not report severity of COPD.[44] The other two RCTs included people with COPD of more than 5 years' duration and FEV_1 less than 70% predicted.[43,45] All trials excluded people with evidence of reversible airflow obstruction.

OPTION   MUCOLYTIC DRUGS

Two systematic reviews of RCTs have found that long term treatment with mucolytics compared with placebo has a beneficial effect on frequency and duration of exacerbations.

Benefits: **Long term treatment:** We found two systematic reviews.[46,47] The first systematic review (updated in 1999) identified 15 double blind placebo controlled RCTs.[46] Mucolytics were associated with a significant reduction in the average number of exacerbations (WMD 0.105 exacerbations per month, 95% CI 0.10 to 0.11), days of disability (WMD 0.65 days per month, 95% CI 0.61 to 0.69), and days on antibiotics (WMD 0.68 days per month, 95% CI 0.64 to 0.71). Most of the trials were in people with mild COPD. Two trials in people with severe COPD ($FEV_1 < 50\%$) found greater reductions in exacerbation frequency (WMD compared with placebo 0.142, CI not given). The review found a small but significant improvement in lung function compared with placebo (WMD in FEV_1 compared with mucolytics 0.057 litres, 95% CI 0.075 litres to 0.039 litres; WMD in forced vital capacity 0.040 litres, 95% CI 0.063 litres to 0.017 litres). However, this finding should be interpreted with caution since it was based on only three trials which reported FEV_1 and four trials which reported vital capacity, and there was considerable heterogeneity in the studies. There was no significant difference between N-acetylcysteine and other mucolytics as a group. The second systematic review (search date 1995) identified nine RCTs of N-acetylcysteine,[47] seven of which were included in the first review.[46] It found an overall weighted effect size of 1.37 (95% CI 1.25 to 1.5), corresponding to a 23% reduction in exacerbations compared with placebo.

Harms: The first systematic review found no differences between mucolytics and placebo in the total number of adverse events.[46] Adverse effects of N-acetylcysteine were mainly mild gastrointestinal complaints.

Comment: In both reviews there was significant heterogeneity between the RCTs, and symptom scores could not be pooled.[46,47] The effect of N-acetylcysteine in slowing the decline in lung function is being examined in a large European multicentre study (PNR Dekhuijzen, personal communication, 1999).

OPTION   ANTIBIOTICS

We found no RCTs evaluating the effects of antibiotics in long term treatment of stable COPD.

Benefits: **Long term treatment:** We found one systematic review (search date 1994), which identified no RCTs on the use of antibiotics as long term treatment in stable COPD.[48]

Harms: The adverse effects of antibiotics vary between agents and individuals.

Comment: None.

OPTION   DOMICILIARY OXYGEN TREATMENT

We found limited evidence suggesting that domiciliary oxygen treatment improves survival in people with COPD and hypoxaemia. One RCT found that continuous treatment was more effective than nocturnal treatment.

Benefits: **Long term treatment:** We found one systematic review (search date 1999, 4 RCTs) and one additional RCT comparing domiciliary oxygen treatment versus a control treatment.[49] Results could not be aggregated because of differences in trial design and participant selection. One 5 year trial (87 people) compared oxygen for at least 15 hours versus no oxygen. Domiciliary oxygen treatment was associated with reduced mortality (OR 0.42, 95% CI 0.18 to 0.98).[50] The second RCT (38 people) compared nocturnal domiciliary oxygen versus room air in people with arterial desaturation at night. It found no difference in mortality at 3 years (figures not given).[51] The third trial (135 people) compared oxygen versus no oxygen in people with moderate hypoxaemia and found no effect on survival at 3 years (HR 0.92, 95% CI 0.57 to 1.47).[52] The fourth RCT (203 people) compared continuous versus nocturnal domiciliary oxygen treatment. Continuous oxygen was associated with a significant reduction in mortality over 24 months (OR 0.45, 95% CI 0.25 to 0.81).[53] The additional RCT compared 2 years of nocturnal oxygen therapy with placebo in 76 people with moderate daytime hypoxaemia (7.4–9.2 kPa) and significant nocturnal desaturation.[54] There was no difference in survival.

Harms: No adverse effects of domiciliary oxygen have been reported. Administration is cumbersome.

Comment: Only one of the studies was double blinded. Domiciliary oxygen treatment seems to be more effective in people with severe hypoxaemia (arterial $Po_2 < 8.0$ kPa) than in people with moderate hypoxaemia or those who have arterial desaturation only at night.

Substantive changes since last issue

Inhaled β_2 agonists: New RCT found that salmeterol improved FEV1 and peak flow rate compared with placebo.[17]

Inhaled β_2 agonists + anticholinergics: New RCT found that salmeterol plus ipratropium bromide improved FEV_1 and quality of life compared with salmeterol alone.[17]

Inhaled corticosteroids: New RCT found that fluticasone reduced exacerbation frequency and deterioration in quality of life, but had no effect on decline in lung function.[42]

Mucolytic drugs: New systemic review found that N-acetylcysteine reduced exacerbation frequency compared with placebo.[47]

Domiciliary oxygen: New RCT found no difference in survival between nocturnal oxygen and placebo in people with moderate hypoxaemia.[54]

REFERENCES

1. American Thoracic Society. Standards for the diagnosis and care of patients with chronic obstructive pulmonary disease: ATS statement. *Am J Respir Crit Care Med* 1995;152 (5 pt 2) (suppl): S77–120.

2. Whittemore AS, Perlin SA, DiCiccio Y. Chronic obstructive pulmonary disease in lifelong nonsmokers: results from NHANES. *Am J Public Health* 1995;85:702–706.

3. Brunekreef B, Fischer P, Remijn B, van der Lende R, Schouten JP, Quanjer PH. Indoor air pollution and its effects on pulmonary function of adult non-smoking women: III passive smoking and pulmonary function. *Int J Epidemiol* 1985;14: 227–230.

4. Rijcken B, Weiss ST. Longitudinal analyses of airway responsiveness and pulmonary function decline. *Am J Respir Crit Care Med* 1996;154 (6 pt 2) (suppl):S246–249.

5. Dockery DW, Brunekreef B. Longitudinal studies of air pollution effects on lung function. *Am J Respir Crit Care Med* 1996;154 (6 pt 2) (suppl):S250–256.

6. O'Connor GT, Sparrow D, Weiss ST. The role of allergy and non-specific airway hyperresponsiveness in the pathogenesis of chronic obstructive pulmonary disease: state of

the art. *Am Rev Respir Dis* 1989;140:225–252.

7. Anthonisen NR, Connett JE, Kiley JP, et al. Effects of smoking intervention and the use of an inhaled anticholinergic bronchodilator on the rate of decline of FEV1: the lung health study. *JAMA* 1994;272:1497–1505.

8. Siafakas NM, Vermeire P, Pride NB, et al. Optimal assessment and management of chronic obstructive pulmonary disease (COPD): a consensus statement of the European Respiratory Society. *Eur Respir J* 1995;8:1398–1420.

9. Braun SR, McKenzie WN, Copeland W, Kingman L, Ellersieck M, Knight GJ. A comparison of the effect of ipratropium bromide and albuterol in the treatment of chronic obstructive pulmonary airway disease. *Arch Intern Med* 1989;149:544–547.

10. Higgins BG, Powell RM, Cooper S, Tattersfield AE. Effect of salbutamol and ipratropium bromide on airway calibre and bronchial reactivity in asthma and chronic bronchitis. *Eur Respir J* 1991;4:415–420.

11. Ikeda A, Nishimura K, Koyama H, Izumi T. Bronchodilating effects of combined therapy with clinical dosages of ipratropium bromide and salbutamol for stable COPD: comparison with ipratropium bromide alone. *Chest* 1995;107:401–405.

12. Ikeda A, Nishimura K, Koyama H, Izumi T. Comparative dose-response study of three anticholinergic agents and fenoterol using a metered dose inhaler in patients with chronic obstructive pulmonary disease. *Thorax* 1995;50: 62–66.

13. Mahler DA, Donohue JF, Barbee RA, et al. Efficacy of salmeterol xinafoate in the treatment of COPD. *Chest* 1999;115:957–965.

14. Van Schayck CP, Dompeling E, van Herwaarden CLA, et al. Bronchodilator treatment in moderate asthma or chronic bronchitis: continuous or on demand? A randomised controlled study. *BMJ* 1991;303:1426–1431.

15. Anthonisen NR, Wright EC, IPPB Trial Group. Bronchodilator response in chronic obstructive pulmonary disease. *Am Rev Respir Dis* 1986;133: 814–819.

16. Appleton S, Smith B, Veale A, Bara A. Regular long-acting beta-2 adrenoceptor agonists in stable chronic obstructive airways disease. In: The Cochrane Library, Issue 1, 2000. Oxford: Update Software. Search date October 1998; primary sources Cochrane Airways Group Register to October 1998; hand searched references; and pharmaceutical companies contacted for unpublished studies.

17. Van Noord JM, de Munck DR, Bantje TA, Hop WC, Akveld ML, Bommer, AM. Long-term treatment of chronic obstructive pulmonary disease with salmeterol and the additive effect of ipratropium. *Eur Respir J* 2000;15:878–885.

18. Boyd G, Morice AH, Pounsford JC, Siebert M, Peslis N, Crawford C. An evaluation of salmeterol in the treatment of chronic obstructive pulmonary disease (COPD). *Eur Respir J* 1997;10:815–821.

19. Jones PW, Bosh TK. Quality of life changes in COPD patients treated with salmeterol. *Am J Respir Crit Care Med* 1997;155:1283–1289.

20. Ulrik CS. Efficacy of inhaled salmeterol in the management of smokers with chronic obstructive pulmonary disease: a single centre randomised, double blind, placebo controlled, crossover study. *Thorax* 1995;50:750–754.

21. Grove A, Lipworth BJ, Reid P, et al. Effects of regular salmeterol on lung function and exercise capacity in patients with chronic obstructive airways disease. *Thorax* 1996;51:689–693.

22. Rutten van Molken M, Roos B, van Noord JA. An empirical comparison of the St George's Respiratory Questionnaire (SGRQ) and the Chronic Respiratory Disease Questionnaire (CRQ) in a clinical trial setting. *Thorax* 1999;54:995–1003.

23. O'Byrne PM, Kerstjens HAM. Inhaled β_2-agonists in the treatment of asthma. *N Engl J Med* 1996; 335:886–888.

24. Hall IP, Tattersfield AE. Beta-agonists. In: Clark TJH, Godfrey S, Lee TH, eds. *Asthma*. 3rd ed. London: Chapman and Hall Medical, 1992:341–365.

25. Cazzola M, Imperatore F, Salzillo A, et al. Cardiac effects of formoterol and salmeterol in patients suffering from COPD with preexisting cardiac arrhythmias and hypoxemia. *Chest* 1998;114: 411–415.

26. Friedman M, Serby C, Menjoge S, Wilson JD, Hilleman DE, Witek TJ Jr. Pharmoeconomic evaluation of a combination of ipratropium plus albuterol compared with ipratropium alone and albuterol alone in COPD. *Chest* 1999:115:635–641.

27. Levin DC, Little KS, Laughlin KR, et al. Addition of anticholinergic solution prolongs bronchodilator effect of beta 2 agonists in patients with chronic obstructive pulmonary disease. *Am J Med* 1996; 100(1A) supplement:40S–48S.

28. Combivent Inhalation Solution Study Group. Routine nebulized ipratropium and albuterol together are better than either alone in COPD. *Chest* 1997;112:1514–1521.

29. Gross N, Tashkin D, Miller R, Oren J, Coleman W, Linberg S. Inhalation by nebulization of albuterol-ipratropium combination (Dey combination) is superior to either agent alone in the treatment of chronic obstructive pulmonary disease. Dey combination solution study group. *Respiration* 1998;65:354–362.

30. Campbell S. For COPD a combination of ipratropium bromide and albuterol sulfate is more effective than albuterol base. *Arch Intern Med* 1999;159:156–160.

31. Rennard SI, Serby CW, Ghafouri M, Johnson PA, Friedman M. Extended therapy with ipratropium is associated with improved lung function in patients with COPD: a retrospective analysis of data from seven clinical trials. *Chest* 1996;110:62–70.

32. Calverley PMA. Symptomatic bronchodilator treatment. In: Calverley PMA, Pride N, eds. *Chronic obstructive pulmonary disease*. London: Chapman and Hall, 1995:419–446.

33. Ramsdell J. Use of theophylline in the treatment of COPD. *Chest* 1995;107(suppl):206S–209S.

34. Mahon JL, Laupacis A, Hodder RV, et al. Theophylline for irreversible chronic airflow limitation: a randomized study comparing n of 1 trials to standard practice. *Chest* 1999;115:38–48.

35. Callahan CM, Dittus RS, Katz BP. Oral corticosteroid therapy for patients with stable chronic obstructive pulmonary disease: a meta-analysis. *Ann Intern Med* 1991;114:216–223. Search date 1989; primary sources Medline 1966 to 1989.

36. McEvoy CE, Niewoehner DE. Adverse effects of corticosteroid therapy for COPD: a critical review. *Chest* 1997;111:732–743.

37. Postma DS, Kerstjens HAM. Are inhaled glucocorticosteroids effective in chronic obstructive pulmonary disease? *Am J Respir Crit Care Med* 1999;160 (5 pt 2):S66–S71.

38. Van Grunsven PM, van Schayck CP, Derenne JP, et al. Long term effects of inhaled corticosteroids in chronic obstructive pulmonary disease: a meta-analysis. *Thorax* 1999;54:714–729. Search date 1996; primary sources Medline 1983 to 1996, Biosis 1991 to 1996; Online Contents 1993 to 1996; GLin 1982 to 1996; Cochrane Library; Embase 1993 to 1996.

39. Paggiaro PL, Dahle R, Bakran I, Frith L, Hollingworth K, Efthimou J. Multicentre randomised placebo-controlled trial of inhaled fluticasone propionate in patients with chronic obstructive pulmonary disease. *Lancet* 1998;351: 773–780.

40. Vestbo J, Sorensen T, Lange P, Brix A, Torre P, Viskum K. Long-term effect of inhaled budesonide in mild and moderate chronic obstructive pulmonary disease: a randomised controlled trial. *Lancet* 1999; 353:1819–1823.

41. Pauwels RA, Lofdahl CG, Laitinen LA, et al. Long-term treatment with inhaled budesonide in persons with mild chronic obstructive pulmonary disease who continue smoking. European Respiratory Society study on chronic obstructive pulmonary disease. *N Engl J Med* 1999;340: 1948–1953.

42. Burge PS, Calverley PM, Jones PW, Spencer S, Anderson JA, Maslen TK. Randomised, double blind, placebo controlled study of fluticasone propionate in patients with moderate to severe chronic obstructive pulmonary disease: the ISOLDE trial. *BMJ* 2000;320:1297–1303

43. Robertson AS, Gove RI, Wieland GA, Burge PS. A double-blind comparison of oral prednisolone

40 mg/day with inhaled beclomethasone dipropionate 1500 g/day in patients with adult onset chronic obstructive airways disease. *Eur J Respir Dis* 1986;69(suppl 146):565–569.

44. Shim CS, Williams MH. Aerosol beclomethasone in patients with steroid-responsive chronic obstructive pulmonary disease. *Am J Med* 1985; 78:655–658.

45. Weir DC, Gove RI, Robertson AS, Burge PS. Corticosteroid trials in non-asthmatic chronic airflow obstruction: a comparison of oral prednisolone and inhaled beclomethasone dipropionate. *Thorax* 1990;45:112–117.

46. Poole PJ, Black PN. Mucolytic agents for chronic bronchitis or chronic obstructive pulmonary disease. In: The Cochrane Library, Issue 1, 2000. Oxford: Update Software. Search date May 1999; primary sources Cochrane Airways Group Register to May 1999; and hand searched references.

47. Grandjean EM, Berthet P, Ruffmann R, Leuenberger P. Efficacy of oral long-term N-acetylcysteine in chronic bronchopulmonary disease: a meta-analysis of published double-blind, placebo-controlled clinical trials. *Clin Ther* 2000;22:209–221. Search date 1999; primary sources Medline and hand searches of reference list, and personal contact with two experts.

48. Saint S, Bent S, Vittinghoff E, Grady D. Antibiotics in chronic obstructive pulmonary disease exacerbations: a meta-analysis. *JAMA* 1995;273: 957–960. Search date 1994; primary sources Medline 1966 to May 1994; hand searched Index Medicus up to 1966.

49. Crockett AJ, Moss JR, Cranston JM, Alpers JH. Domiciliary oxygen in chronic obstructive pulmonary disease. In: The Cochrane Library, Issue 1, 2000. Oxford: Update Software. Search date April 1999; primary sources Cochrane Airways Group Register.

50. Medical Research Council Working Party. Long term domiciliary oxygen therapy in chronic hypoxic cor pulmonale complicating chronic bronchitis and emphysema. *Lancet* 1981;1:681–686.

51. Fletcher EC, Luckett RA, Goodnight-White S, Miller CC, Qian W, Costarangos-Galarza C. A double-blind trial of nocturnal supplemental oxygen for sleep desaturation in patients with chronic obstructive pulmonary disease and a daytime PaO_2 above 60 mm Hg. *Am Rev Respir Dis* 1992; 145:1070–1076.

52. Gorecka D, Gorzelak K, Sliwinski P, Tobiasz M, Zielinski J. Effect of long-term oxygen therapy on survival in patients with chronic obstructive pulmonary disease with moderate hypoxaemia. *Thorax* 1997;52:674–679.

53. Nocturnal Oxygen Therapy Trial Group. Continuous or nocturnal oxygen therapy in hypoxemic chronic obstructive lung disease: a clinical trial. *Ann Intern Med* 1980;93:391–398.

54. Chaouat A, Weitzenblum E, Kessler R, Charpentier C, Enrhart M, Schott R, et al. A randomized trial of nocturnal oxygen therapy in chronic obstructive pulmonary disease patients. *Eur Respir J* 1999; 14:1002–1008.

Huib Kerstjens

Dirkje Postma
Professor of Pulmonary Medicine

University Hospital Groningen
Groningen
The Netherlands

Competing interests: Both authors have received funding from the following manufacturers: AstraZeneca, the manufacturer of budesonide, terbutaline, formoterol; Glaxo–Wellcome, the manufacturer of beclomethasone, salbutamol, salmeterol, and fluticasone; Boehringer Ingelheim, the manufacturer of fenoterol and ipratropium bromide: and Novartis, the manufacturer of formoterol. DSP has also received funding from Zambon, the manufacturer of N-acetylcysteine.

Updated this issue

Thomas Marrie

INTERVENTIONS

TREATMENT
Likely to be beneficial
Prompt administration of antibiotics
   in vulnerable people. 859

Unknown effectiveness
Bottle blowing. 859
Specific combinations of antibiotics
   in intensive care settings . . .859
Guidelines for treating pneumonia
   (for clinical outcomes) 860

Unlikely to be beneficial
New antibiotics over older agents,
   unless microbes are resistant to
   older drugs 857
Intravenous antibiotics over oral
   antibiotics in immunocompetent
   people in hospital without life
   threatening illness 858

PREVENTION
Beneficial
Pneumococcal vaccine in young,
   fit adults 861

Likely to be beneficial
Influenza vaccine in elderly
   people 860

Unknown effectiveness
Pneumococcal vaccine in
   chronically ill,
   immunosuppressed, or elderly
   people 861

To be covered in future issues of
Clinical Evidence
Antiviral treatments

Key Messages

Treatment

- One systematic review has found no evidence of a difference between most oral antibiotics in people with community acquired pneumonia, when local microbial sensitivities are taken into account.

- We found no strong evidence supporting new over older antibiotics for people admitted to hospital, nor of any particular combination of antibiotics for use in intensive care.

- RCTs in immunocompetent people in hospital found no evidence of a difference in effectiveness between intravenous antibiotics and oral antibiotics. Intravenous antibiotics were associated with longer hospital stays.

- We found no evidence that critical pathways improve clinical outcomes in community acquired pneumonia. One multicentre RCT found that critical pathways improved process outcomes: more people treated at home, fewer hospital bed days for people managed, fewer days on intravenous antibiotics, and more frequent use of one class of antibiotics.

Prevention

- One systematic review of cohort studies, and several subsequent RCTs, have found evidence that influenza vaccine reduces risk of pneumonia and death in elderly people.

- RCTs of pneumococcal vaccine have found mixed results. One systematic review of RCTs found evidence that vaccination with currently available pneumococcal vaccines did not protect against death. It also found that pneumococcal vaccine was associated with increased protection in young, fit adults (but not older adults at high risk) against pneumococcal pneumonia. Subsequent RCTs found no evidence of benefit in older adults. Subgroup analysis suggested a benefit in older adults at high risk of pneumonia.

DEFINITION Community acquired pneumonia is pneumonia contracted in the community rather than in hospital.

INCIDENCE/ PREVALENCE In the northern hemisphere, community acquired pneumonia affects about 12/1000 people per year, particularly during winter and at the extremes of age (incidence: < 1 year old 30–50/1000 per year; 15–45 years 1–5/1000 per year; 60–70 years 10–20/1000 per year; 71–85 years 50/1000 per year).[1–6]

AETIOLOGY/ RISK FACTORS Over 100 microorganisms have been implicated, but most cases are caused by *Streptococcus pneumoniae* (see table 1, p 864).[4–7] Smoking is probably an important risk factor.[8]

PROGNOSIS Severity varies from mild to life threatening illness within days of the onset of symptoms. One systematic review of prognosis studies for community acquired pneumonia found overall mortality to be 13.7%, ranging from 5.1% for ambulant people to 36.5% for people requiring intensive care.[9] The following prognostic factors were significantly associated with mortality: male sex (OR 1.3, 95% CI 1.2 to 1.4); pleuritic chest pain (OR 0.5, 95% CI 0.3 to 0.8, i.e. lower mortality); hypothermia (OR 5, 95% CI 2.4 to 10.4); systolic hypotension (OR 4.8, 95% CI 2.8 to 8.3); tachypnoea (OR 2.9, 95% CI 1.7 to 4.9); diabetes mellitus (OR 1.3, 95% CI 1.1 to 1.5); neoplastic disease (OR 2.8, 95% CI 2.4 to 3.1); neurologic disease (OR 4.6, 95% CI 2.3 to 8.9); bacteraemia (OR 2.8, 95% CI 2.3 to 3.6); leukopenia (OR 2.5, 95% CI 1.6 to 3.7); and multilobar radiographic pulmonary infiltrates (OR 3.1, 95% CI 1.9 to 5.1).

AIMS **Treatment:** To cure infection; to prevent death in seriously ill people; to alleviate symptoms; to enable a return to normal activities; and to prevent recurrence. **Prevention:** To prevent infection and death.

OUTCOMES Clinical cure (defined as return to premorbid health status); relief of symptoms; admission to hospital; complications (empyema, endocarditis, lung abscess); death; adverse effects of antibiotics (allergy, diarrhoea, colitis); adverse effects of procedures (endotracheal intubation, central vascular lines).

METHODS *Clinical Evidence* update search and appraisal May 2000.

| QUESTION | Which antibiotics should be used in outpatient settings? |

| OPTION | NEW VERSUS OLD ANTIBIOTICS |

One systematic review has found no evidence that newer antibiotics have an advantage over older antibiotics, such as broad spectrum penicillins, in outpatient settings.

Benefits: We found one systematic review (published in 1994), which identified nine RCTs of oral antibiotics in outpatient settings.[10] Five trials had fewer than 100 participants, the other trials included between 118 to 267 people, (total n = 1164). Antibiotics tested were amoxycillin with and without clavulanate; macrolides; first, second, and third generation cephalosporins; and quinolones. Cure or improvement was reported in over 90% of trial participants.

Harms: Antibiotics can cause allergic reactions (including anaphylaxis), rash, gastrointestinal intolerance (nausea, vomiting, diarrhoea), vaginal or oral candidiasis, and *Clostridium difficile* diarrhoea (including pseudomembranous colitis). Frequency of adverse effects varies with the antibiotic used.

Comment: None.

| QUESTION | Which treatments should be used in people admitted to hospital? |

| OPTION | NEW VERSUS OLD ANTIBIOTICS |

RCTs found no evidence of a significant difference in effectiveness between new and older antibiotics in people with community acquired pneumonia admitted to hospital. However, most trials were small and were designed to show equivalence between treatments rather than superiority of one over another.

Benefits: We found no systematic review. **Second generation cephalosporin versus broad spectrum penicillin:** We found several RCTs, all too small, too old, or both, to be reliable, given the changing sensitivity of organisms to antibiotics. **Quinolones versus high dose amoxycillin:** We found one multicentre double blind RCT comparing sparfloxacin versus amoxycillin in 329 people in hospital in France, South Africa, and Switzerland.[11] Early discontinuation of the drug (days 3, 4, or 5) occurred in 2.4% of people treated with sparfloxacin compared with 7.9% of those treated with amoxycillin (no CIs given). It found no significant difference in clinical cure rates (84% with sparfloxacin v 85% with amoxycillin). **Quinolones versus second and third generation cephalosporins:** We found one double blind RCT comparing levofloxacin versus intravenous ceftriaxone followed by oral cefuroxime in 226 participants, half of whom had been admitted to hospital. Clinical cure was greater with levofloxacin compared with cephalosporins (96.5% v 90.4%, ARR 6.1%, 95% CI 1.3% to 10.7%).[12]

Harms: See new versus old antibiotics in outpatient settings above.

Comment: Although penicillin resistant and multidrug resistant *S pneumoniae* is commonly reported, it is hard to enrol people with this infection in randomised studies. One of the studies was carried out in areas with high prevalence of penicillin resistant *S pneumoniae*.[11] However, only 8 of 135 isolates tested were resistant to penicillin and none showed high level resistance. The trials in uncomplicated pneumonia may not apply in people with comorbidities such as meningitis.[13] There are also concerns about macrolide-resistant *S pneumoniae*, but so far treatment failure in ambulatory people with community acquired pneumonia is uncommon.[14] We found one retrospective review of 12 945 hospitalised people (≥ 65 years old) with community acquired pneumonia. It found that initial treatment with a second generation cephalosporin plus a macrolide, a non-pseudomonal third generation cephalosporin plus a macrolide, or a fluoroquinolone alone, was associated with lower mortality at 30 days than treatment with beta-lactam/beta-lactamase inhibitor plus a macrolide, and an aminoglycoside plus another agent.[15] However, the results should be interpreted with caution as they may not account for potential confounding factors.

OPTION   **INTRAVENOUS VERSUS ORAL ANTIBIOTICS**

RCTs found evidence that, in immunocompetent people admitted to hospital who were not suffering life threatening illness, intravenous antibiotics were no more effective than oral antibiotics and were associated with increased length of hospital stay.

Benefits: We found no systematic review. We found two RCTs comparing oral with intravenous antibiotics in people admitted to hospital with community acquired pneumonia. The first included 541 participants with lower respiratory tract infections, two fifths of whom had chest radiographs that were compatible with pneumonia.[16] People were excluded if they had life threatening infection or were immunocompromised. Participants were randomised to 7 days of treatment with oral co-amoxiclav, intravenous co-amoxiclav for 3 days followed by oral co-amoxiclav, or intravenous cefotaxime for 3 days followed by oral cefuroxime. At discharge there was no difference in cure rates or mortality among the three groups, but hospital stay was significantly shorter in those on oral treatment than in those on intravenous treatment (P < 0.001). The second RCT (no intention to treat analysis) compared intravenous versus oral cefuroxime in 73 people.[17] Participants were randomised to 2 days of intravenous followed by 8 days of oral treatment, 5 days of each treatment, or 10 days of intravenous treatment. The only significant difference was in the length of hospital stay (6, 8, and 11 days, no CI or P values given).

Harms: None reported.

Comment: Intravenous antibiotics are needed in people who cannot take oral medication because of severe nausea or vomiting, or who are bacteraemic or in septicaemic shock. A follow up study in 96 people admitted to hospital with community acquired pneumonia found that people could be switched from intravenous to oral antibiotics when they had been afebrile for 8 hours, symptoms of cough and shortness of breath were improving, white blood counts were returning to normal, and they could tolerate oral medication.[18]

OPTION **BOTTLE BLOWING**

One RCT found slightly faster recovery with bottle blowing physiotherapy.

Benefits: We found no systematic review. We found one RCT in 145 people in hospital with community acquired pneumonia.[19] People were randomised to three groups: early mobilisation; early mobilisation and encouragement to sit up 10 times a day and take 20 deep breaths; and early mobilisation and encouragement to sit up 10 times a day and blow bubbles through a plastic tube for 20 breaths into a bottle containing 10 cm water. Mean hospital stay in the three groups was 5.3, 4.6, and 3.9 days (P = 0.01 for early mobilisation compared with bottle blowing).

Harms: None reported.

Comment: Neither study participants nor clinicians could be blinded to the intervention.

QUESTION **Which treatments should be used in people with community acquired pneumonia receiving intensive care?**

OPTION **DIFFERENT COMBINATIONS OF ANTIBIOTICS**

We found no good evidence supporting any particular antibiotic combination in this setting.

Benefits: We found no systematic review and no RCTs comparing one combination of antibiotics with another in intensive care units.

Harms: We found no good evidence.

Comment: Using a combination of antibiotics is regarded as current best practice.

OPTION **PROMPT VERSUS DELAYED ANTIBIOTIC TREATMENT**

Retrospective studies found that prompt administration of antibiotics improved survival.

Benefits: We found no systematic review and no prospective studies. One multicentre retrospective review examined the medical records of over 14 000 people aged 65 years or older who were severely ill with community acquired pneumonia. It found that administering antibiotics within 8 hours of admission to hospital was associated with lower 30 day mortality (OR 0.90, 95% CI 0.75 to 0.96).[20] Another retrospective study examined outcome and time to start of treatment in 39 people with serologically confirmed legionnaires' disease.[21] For the 10 people who died, the median delay between diagnosis of pneumonia and start of erythromycin was 5 days (range 1–10 days), and for those who survived it was 1 day (range 1–5 days, P < 0.001).

Harms: None reported.

Comment: It would probably be regarded as unethical to perform an RCT of delayed antibiotic treatment.

QUESTION **What are the effects of guidelines on the treatment of community acquired pneumonia?**

We found no evidence that guidelines improve clinical outcomes in community acquired pneumonia. One multicentre RCT found that a critical pathway guideline improved process outcomes: more people treated at home; fewer hospital bed days for people managed; fewer days on intravenous antibiotics; and more frequent use of one class of antibiotics.

Benefits: We found one multicentre trial with cluster randomisation involving nine teaching and ten community hospitals in Canada.[22] It included 1743 people presenting to emergency rooms at participating hospitals. People who were immunosuppressed, people with active tuberculosis, people with cystic fibrosis, pregnant or lactating women, people with alcohol addiction, and people with chronic renal failure were excluded. Intervention hospitals (n = 9) used a critical pathway for treating pneumonia consisting of an admission guideline based on a severity of illness scoring system, a guideline for switching from intravenous to oral antibiotic therapy, a discharge guideline, and treatment with the antibiotic levofloxacin. Treatment at control hospitals (n = 10) consisted of usual care. The two groups did not significantly differ in quality of life (short form 36 physical component score), occurrence of complications, readmission, or mortality. Intervention hospitals admitted fewer people at low risk (31% v 49%, P = 0.01), used fewer bed days per person managed (4.4 v 6.1, P = 0.04), administered 1.7 fewer days of intravenous antibiotic therapy (4.6 v 6.3 days, P = 0.01), and were more likely to use only one class of antibiotic (64% v 27%, P < 0.001).

Harms: None identified.

Comment: The effects might be larger than observed because people admitted with the critical pathway were at higher risk, so might have been expected to spend longer in hospital. The trial did not identify which components of the pathway were likely to be beneficial.

QUESTION **What are the effects of preventive interventions?**

OPTION **INFLUENZA VACCINE**

One systematic review of cohort studies, and several recent RCTs, have found that influenza vaccination reduces the risk of influenza and death in elderly people.

Benefits: We found one systematic review (published in 1995, 20 cohort studies).[23] The pooled estimate for prevention of pneumonia was an absolute risk reduction of 53% (95% CI 35% to 66%) and for prevention of death 68% (95% CI 56% to 76%). Analysis of data from an administrative database of over 25 000 people aged 64 or over suggested that influenza vaccination reduced the rate of admission to hospital for pneumonia and influenza by 48%–57% (P < 0.01).[24] We found one double blind RCT comparing split viron vaccine versus saline solution in over 1800 people aged 60 years or over.[25] At 5 months' follow up, the incidence of clinical influenza was significantly lower with vaccine than placebo (2% v 3%, RR 0.53, 95% CI 0.39 to 0.73). One double blind RCT compared trivalent inactivated parenteral vaccine with or without intranasal live attenuated cold adapted vaccine in 324 elderly residents of nursing homes. It found that live vaccine provided additional protection against influenza A (rates of documented influenza 5.5% v 14.8%; RRR 60%, 95% CI 18% to 82%).[26] One RCT found that vaccination of healthcare workers in geriatric long term care facilities reduced total mortality of elderly residents from 17% to 10% during one winter (OR compared with no vaccination 0.56, 95% CI 0.40 to 0.80).[27]

Harms: Local adverse effects included pain and tenderness at the site of injection. Guillain-Barré syndrome was rare. It complicated 1 in 100 000 vaccinations during the national immunisation programme against swine influenza in the USA in 1976, during which 45 million people were vaccinated.[28]

Comment: None.

OPTION	PNEUMOCOCCAL VACCINE

RCTs of pneumococcal vaccine have found mixed results. One systematic review of RCTs found evidence that vaccination with currently available pneumococcal vaccines did not protect against death. It also found evidence that pneumococcal vaccine protected young fit adults (but not older adults at high risk) against pneumococcal pneumonia. Subsequent RCTs found no evidence of benefit in older adults. Subgroup analysis suggested a benefit in older adults at high risk of pneumonia.

Benefits: We found one systematic review (search date 1991), which identified nine RCTs with a total of 12 direct comparisons between vaccine and control, including 40 431 people.[29] In adults at low risk (immunocompetent, aged < 55 years, no other chronic medical conditions), vaccination was associated with protection against definitive pneumococcal pneumonia (positive S pneumoniae cultures) (OR compared with no vaccine 0.32, 95% CI 0.22 to 0.46). Meta-analysis found no evidence of benefit in adults at high risk (people aged > 55 years, with one or more chronic medical condition) or immunosuppresssed people (OR 1.23, 95% CI 0.28 to 5.43). It found no evidence of significant protection against other outcomes (all cause pneumonia, bronchitis, or death). We found two subsequent double blind RCTs. The first compared a 23-valent pneumococcal capsular polysaccharide vaccine with placebo in 691 middle aged and elderly people who had been admitted to hospital with community acquired pneumonia. It found no evidence of a significant protective effect against pneumococcal pneumonia (RR 0.78, 95% CI 0.40 to 1.51) or all cause pneumonia (RR 0.83, 95% CI 0.58 to 1.12).[30] The second RCT (2837 nursing home residents) compared pneumococcal and influenza vaccines with influenza vaccine only.[27] All participants were followed for 3 years for development of radiologically confirmed pneumonia. Pneumococcal cause was defined serologically. No significant protection from pneumococcal pneumonia was found in the study group as a whole (RR *v* influenza vaccine alone 0.85, 95% CI −0.57 to 1.50). However, there was evidence of significant protection in people with risk factors for contracting pneumonia: those who were immunocompromised; had received immunosuppressive treatment within 1 year before vaccination; had cancer, systemic connective tissue diseases, alcohol dependence, heart or lung disease; or were institutionalised or permanently bedridden (RR 0.41, 95% CI 0.18 to 0.94).[31] Independent risk factors for a poor response to pneumococcal vaccine were malignancy (RR 2.64, P = 0.01) and daily use of angiotensin converting enzyme inhibitors (RR 4.16, P = 0.0002).

Harms: Discomfort at the site of the injection. No other harms reported.

Comment: A fifth of healthy elderly adults (mean age 71 years) do not mount an antibody response after vaccination.[32] New conjugate pneumococcal vaccines are being evaluated. These have been shown to be immunogenic in infants and have decreased the rate of carriage of resistant strains of *S pneumoniae*.[33,34] One recent retrospective cohort study among 1898 elderly members of a staff health care organisation found that pneumococcal vaccination was associated with lower risks of admission to hospital for pneumonia (adjusted RR 0.57, 95% CI 0.38 to 0.84) and for death (adjusted RR 0.71, 95% CI 0.56 to 0.91).[35] The study found evidence of an additive effect for people who received both pneumococcal and influenza vaccinations during the influenza season (RR 0.28, 95% CI 0.14 to 0.58 for admission to hospital for pneumonia and influenza; RR 0.18, 95% CI 0.11 to 0.31 for death).

Substantive changes since last issue

New versus old antibiotics in hospital New retrospective study.[15]

REFERENCES

1. Foy HM, Cooney MK, Allan I, Kenny GE. Rates of pneumonia during influenza epidemics in Seattle, 1964–1975. *JAMA* 1979;241:253–258.
2. Murphy TF, Henderson FW, Clyde WA, Collier AM, Denny FW. Pneumonia: an 11 year study in a pediatric practice. *Am J Epidemiol* 1981;113:12–21.
3. McConnochie KM, Hall CB, Barker WH. Lower respiratory tract illness in the first two years of life: epidemiologic patterns and costs in a suburban pediatric practice. *Am J Public Health* 1988;78:34–39.
4. Porath A, Schlaeffer F, Lieberman D. The epidemiology of community-acquired pneumonia among hospitalized adults. *J Infect* 1997;34:41–48.
5. Jokinen C, Heiskanen L, Juvonen H, et al. Incidence of community-acquired pneumonia in the population of four municipalities in eastern Finland. *Am J Epidemiol* 1993;137:977–988.
6. Houston MS, Silverstein MD, Suman VJ. Risk factors for 30-day mortality in elderly patients with lower respiratory tract infection. *Arch Intern Med* 1997;157:2190–2195.
7. Bartlett JG, Mundy LM. Community-acquired pneumonia. *N Engl J Med* 1995;333:1618–1624.
8. Almirall J, Gonzalez CA, Balanco X, Bolibar I. Proportion of community-acquired pneumonia attributable to tobacco smoking. *Chest* 1999;116:375–379.
9. Fine MJ, Smith MA, Carson CA, et al. Prognosis and outcomes of patients with community-acquired pneumonia: a meta-analysis. *JAMA* 1995;274:134–141.
10. Pomilla PV, Brown RB. Outpatient treatment of community-acquired pneumonia in adults. *Arch Intern Med* 1994;154:1793–1802. Search date not given; primary sources Medline from 1966.
11. Aubier M, Verster R, Regamey C, Geslin, Vercken J-B, and the Sparfloxacin European Study Group. Once-daily sparfloxacin versus high-dosage amoxicillin in the treatment of community-acquired, suspected pneumococcal pneumonia in adults. *Clin Infect Dis* 1998;26:1312–1320.
12. File TM Jr, Segreti J, Dunbar L, et al. A multicenter, randomized study comparing the efficacy and safety of intravenous and/or oral levofloxacin versus ceftriaxone and/or cefuroxime axetil in treatment of adults with community-acquired

pneumonia. *Antimicrob Agents Chemother* 1997; 41:1965–1972.

13. Friedland IR, McCracken GH Jr. Management of infections caused by antibiotic-resistant *Streptococcus pneumoniae*. *N Engl J Med* 1994; 331:377–382.

14. Siegel RE. The significance of serum vs. tissue levels of antibiotics in the treatment of penicillin-resistant *Streptococcus pneumoniae* and community-acquired pneumonia. Are we looking in the wrong place? *Chest* 1999;116:535–538.

15. Gleason PP, Meehan TP, Fine JM, et al. Associations between initial antimicrobial therapy and medical outcomes for hospitalized elderly patients with pneumonia. *Arch Intern Med* 1999; 159:2562–2572.

16. Chan R, Hemeryck L, O'Regan M, Clancy C, Feely J. Oral versus intravenous antibiotics for community-acquired lower respiratory tract infection in a general hospital: open randomised controlled trial. *BMJ* 1995;310:1360–1362.

17. Siegel RE, Halperin NA, Almenoff PL, Lee A, Greene JG. A prospective randomized study of inpatient IV antibiotics for community-acquired pneumonia: the optimal duration of therapy. *Chest* 1996;110:965–971.

18. Ramirez JA, Ahkee S. Early switch from intravenous antimicrobials to oral clarithromycin in patients with community acquired pneumonia. *Infect Med* 1997;14:319–323.

19. Bjorkqvist M, Wiberg B, Bodin L, Barany M, Holmberg H. Bottle-blowing in hospital-treated patients with community-acquired pneumonia. *Scand J Infect Dis* 1997;29:77–82.

20. Meehan TP, Fine MJ, Krumholz HM, et al. Quality of care, process, and outcomes in elderly patients with pneumonia. *JAMA* 1997;278:2080–2084.

21. Heath CH, Grove DI, Looke DFM. Delay in appropriate therapy of Legionella pneumonia associated with increased mortality. *Eur J Clin Microbiol Infect Dis* 1966;15:286–290.

22. Marrie TJ, Lau CY, Wheeler SL, et al. A controlled trial of a critical pathway for treatment of community-acquired pneumonia. *JAMA* 2000; 283:749–755.

23. Gross PA, Hermogenes AW, Sacks HS, Lau J, Levandowski RA. The efficacy of influenza vaccine in elderly persons: a meta-analysis and review of the literature. *Ann Intern Med* 1995;123:518–527. Search date not stated; primary source Medline.

24. Nichol KL, Margolis KL, Wuorenma J, Von Sternberg T. The efficacy and cost effectiveness of vaccination against influenza among elderly persons living in the community. *N Engl J Med* 1994;331:778–784.

25. Govaert TM, Thijs CT, Masurel N, Sprenger MJW, Dinant GJ, Knottnerus JA. The efficacy of influenza vaccination in elderly individuals: a randomized double-blind placebo-controlled trial. *JAMA* 1994; 272:1661–1665.

26. Treanor JJ, Mattison HR, Dumyati G, et al. Protective efficacy of combined live intranasal and inactivated influenza A virus vaccines in the elderly. *Ann Intern Med* 1992;117:625–633.

27. Potter J, Stott DJ, Roberts MA, et al. Influenza vaccination of health care workers in long-term-care hospitals reduces the mortality of elderly patients. *J Infect Dis* 1997;175:1–6.

28. Betts RF. Influenza virus. In: Mandell GL, Bennett JE, Dolin R, eds. *Principles and practice of infectious diseases.* 4th edn. New York: Churchill Livingstone, 1995.

29. Fine MJ, Smith MA, Carson CA, et al. Efficacy of pneumococcal vaccination in adults: a meta-analysis of randomized controlled clinical trials. *Arch Intern Med* 1994;154:2666–2677. Search date 1991; primary source Medline; bibliographies of retrieved articles; and search for unpublished material by contact with key researchers and manufacturers.

30. Ortqvist A, Hedlund J, Burman L-A, et al, and Swedish Pneumococcal Vaccination Study Group. Randomised trial of 23-valent penumococcal capsular polysaccharide vaccine in prevention of pneumonia in middle-aged and elderly people. *Lancet* 1998;351:399–403.

31. Koivula I, Sten M, Leinonen M, Makela PH. Clinical efficacy of par pneumococcal vaccine in the elderly: a randomized, single-blind population-based trial. *Am J Med* 1997;103:281–290.

32. Rubins JB, Puri AKG, Loch J, et al. Magnitude, duration, quality and function of pneumococcal vaccine responses in elderly adults. *J Infect Dis* 1998;178:431–440.

33. Mbelle N, Wasas A, Huebner R, Kimura A, Chang I, Klugman K. Immunogenicity and impact on carriage of 9-valent pneumococcal conjugate vaccine given to infants in Soweto, South Africa. *Proceedings of the 37th Interscience Conference on Antimicrobial Agents and Chemotherapy; 1997 September.* Toronto, Herndon VA: ASM Press, 1997.

34. Gesner M, Desidero D, Kim M, et al. Streptococcus pneumoniae in human immunodeficiency virus type 1 infected children. *Pediatr Infect Dis J* 1994;13:697–703.

35. Nichol KL, Baken L, Wuorenma J, Nelson A. The health and economic benefits associated with pneumococcal vaccination in elderly people with chronic lung disease. *Arch Intern Med* 1999;159: 2437–2442.

Thomas Marrie
Professor and Chair
Department of Medicine
University of Alberta
Edmonton
Canada

Competing interests: The author has received a research grant from Janssen Ortho, and honoraria for scientific talks from Janssen Ortho, Pfizer, and Glaxo Wellcome.

TABLE 1 Causes of community acquired pneumonia (see text, p 856).

	USA (% of participants)*	UK (% of participants)†	Susceptibility (laboratory results)‡
Streptococcus pneumoniae	20–60	60–75	25% penicillin resistant, sensitive to quinolones
Haemophilus influenzae	3–10	4–5	30% ampicillin resistant, sensitive to cephalosporins or amoxycillin/clavulanic acid
Staphylococcus aureus	3–5	1–5	Methicillin resistant S aureus rare as cause of community acquired pneumonia
Chlamydia pneumoniae	4–6	–	Sensitive to macrolides, tetracyclines, quinolones
Mycoplasma pneumoniae	1–6	5–18	Sensitive to macrolides, tetracyclines, quinolones
Legionella pneumophila	2–8	2–5	Sensitive to macrolides, tetracyclines, quinolones
Gram-negative bacilli	3–10	Rare	
Aspiration	6–10	–	
Viruses	2–15	8–16	

*Pooled data from 15 published reports from North America[7]; †Data from British Thoracic Society[7]; ‡Susceptibility data from recent studies.

Respiratory disorders

INTERVENTIONS

NON-SMALL CELL LUNG CANCER
Beneficial
Adding thoracic irradiation to
  chemotherapy in unresected
  stage 3 disease 867
Palliative chemotherapy with
  cisplatin or docetaxel containing
  regimens in stage 4 disease .867

Unknown effectiveness

Newer single drug or combined
  drug regimens in stage 4 disease
  (not clearly better than cisplatin
  or docetaxel based
  regimens) 867

To be covered in future issues of
Clinical Evidence

Continuous hyperfractionated
  accelerated radiotherapy for
  unresectable stage 3 non-small
  cell lung cancer
Palliative chemotherapy for stage 4
  non-small cell lung cancer

SMALL CELL LUNG CANCER
Beneficial
Adding thoracic irradiation to
  chemotherapy in limited stage
  disease 869

Trade off between benefits and
harms
Prophylactic cranial irradiation in
  people in complete remission
  with limited stage disease. . .870
Oral etoposide in extensive stage
  disease (less effective but also
  less toxic than combination
  chemotherapy) 871

Unknown effectiveness
Comparative effects of standard
  chemotherapy compared with
  other chemotherapy
  regimens. 868

See glossary, p 871
*available at
  http://clicicalevidence.org
  from December 2000

Key Messages

Non-small cell lung cancer

- Systematic reviews of RCTs have found that regimens based on cisplatin are effective for non-small cell lung cancer. Other promising new drug treatments require further evaluation.

- Systematic reviews of RCTs have found that the combination of thoracic irradiation plus chemotherapy is associated with improved survival compared with radiotherapy alone in people with unresectable stage 3 non-small cell lung cancer.

- Four systematic reviews of RCTs have found survival benefit with cisplatin chemotherapy regimens compared with best supportive care in people with stage 4 non-small cell lung cancer. Limited evidence suggests that chemotherapy may improve quality of life. Limited evidence suggests that docetaxel improves survival of people with stage 3B or 4 lung cancer, who had previously received cisplatin based chemotherapy.

Small cell lung cancer

- We found no good data on standard cisplatin or doxorubicin based chemotherapy versus other chemotherapy regimens.

- Systematic reviews of RCTs have found that adding thoracic irradiation improves survival in people with limited stage small cell lung cancer. The best timing, dose, and fractionation of radiation remain uncertain.

- One meta-analysis of RCTs has found that prophylactic cranial irradiation reduces the incidence of brain metastases in people in complete remission with limited stage small cell lung cancer, with a small improvement in survival but uncertain effects on neuropsychological function.

- RCTs have found that oral etoposide is associated with worse survival than combination chemotherapy. Etoposide is less toxic in the short term but we found no evidence that it offers significantly better quality of life.

DEFINITION	Lung cancer or bronchogenic carcinoma is an epithelial cancer arising from the bronchial surface epithelium or bronchial mucous glands (see table 1, p 873).
INCIDENCE/ PREVALENCE	Lung cancer is the leading cause of cancer death in both men and women, affecting about 100 000 men and 80 000 women annually in North America, and about 40 000 men and women in the UK. Small cell lung cancer constitutes about 20–25% of all lung cancers, the remainder being non-small cell lung cancers, of which adenocarcinoma is now the most prevalent form.[1]
AETIOLOGY/ RISK FACTORS	Smoking remains the major preventable risk factor, accounting for about 80–90% of all cases.
PROGNOSIS	Lung cancer has an overall 5 year survival rate of 10–12%.[2] At the time of diagnosis, 10–15% of people with lung cancer have localised disease. Of these, half will have died at 5 years despite potentially curative surgery. Over half of people have metastatic disease at the time of diagnosis. For those with initially unresectable non-small cell lung cancer, combined treatment with radiotherapy and chemotherapy followed by surgery has achieved modest improvements in 5 year survival.[2] Prognosis depends on the stage of disease. In people with small cell cancer, those with limited stage disease who undergo combined chemotherapy and mediastinal irradiation have a median survival of 18–24 months, whereas those with extensive stage disease who are given palliative chemotherapy have a median survival of 10–12 months. About 5–10% of people with small cell lung cancer present with central nervous system involvement, and half develop symptomatic brain metastases by 2 years. Of these, only half respond to palliative radiation, and their median survival is less than 3 months. People with non-small cell cancer who undergo surgery have a 5 year survival of 60–80% for stage 1 disease and 25–50% for stage 2 disease.[2]
AIMS	To cure disease, to prolong life, to improve quality of life and to provide palliation, with minimum adverse effects of treatment.
OUTCOMES	Survival, clinical response rates, disease related symptoms, adverse effects of treatment, quality of life. Despite recent progress

in the development of valid instruments, measuring quality of life in people with lung cancer remains a serious challenge.[3,4]

METHODS   *Clinical Evidence* update search and appraisal May 2000.

QUESTION   **What are the effects of treatments for non-small cell lung cancer?**

OPTION   **THORACIC RADIATION ADDED TO CHEMOTHERAPY FOR UNRESECTABLE STAGE 3 NON-SMALL CELL LUNG CANCER**

Systematic reviews of RCTs have found that combining thoracic irradiation with chemotherapy is associated with improved survival compared with radiotherapy alone in people with unresectable stage 3 non-small cell lung cancer. We found insufficient evidence about effects on quality of life.

Benefits: We found three systematic reviews comparing thoracic irradiation plus chemotherapy versus radiotherapy alone in people with unresected stage 3 non-small cell lung cancer. The first review (search date 1995, 22 RCTs, n = 3033, range 48–353) found a pooled hazard ratio for mortality of 0.90 (95% CI 0.83 to 0.97), with an absolute survival benefit associated with combined treatment of 3% at 2 years.[5] The second review (search date 1995, 14 RCTs, n = 1887) found that adding a cisplatin based regimen to radiotherapy was associated with a significant reduction in mortality at 1 and 2 years (pooled OR at 1 year 0.76, 95% CI 0.6 to 0.9; at 2 years 0.7, 95% CI 0.5 to 0.9).[6] The third review (search date 1995, 14 RCTs, n = 2589) found similar results.[7]

Harms: The reviews gave no information on long term adverse effects of treatment.

Comment: We found insufficient evidence about effects on quality of life.

OPTION   **PALLIATIVE CHEMOTHERAPY IN STAGE 4 NON-SMALL CELL LUNG CANCER**

Four systematic reviews of RCTs have found a survival benefit with chemotherapy regimens containing cisplatin compared with best supportive care in people with stage 4 non-small cell lung cancer. One RCT found that cisplatin based therapy improved lung cancer related symptoms. Limited evidence suggests that chemotherapy may improve quality of life. We found limited evidence from one RCT that docetaxel improves survival of people with stage 3B or 4 lung cancer, who had previously received cisplatin based chemotherapy.

Benefits: **First line chemotherapy:** We found four systematic reviews,[4,5,8,9] and two subsequent RCTs[10,11] that addressed survival in people with stage 4 non-small cell lung cancer. Three found a significant benefit from chemotherapy. The largest and most recent review (search date 1995, 11 RCTs, n = 1190) found that chemotherapy regimens containing cisplatin were associated with improved survival at 1 year (pooled hazard ratio for death 0.73, 95% CI 0.62 to 0.85), although combined results of all chemotherapy regimens, including long term alkylating agents, found no advantage at 1 year or beyond 1 year (HR 0.87, 95% CI 0.64 to 1.20).[5] We found two subsequent RCTs of palliative care with chemotherapy versus palliative care without chemotherapy. Both RCTs found a small improvement in quality of life in the chemotherapy group. The first RCT (n = 351) found median survival was greater for people treated with cisplatin based chemotherapy (6.7 months v 4.8 months). The trial also found that quality of life improved over the first 6 weeks with chemotherapy treatment compared with deterioration with palliative care alone (P = 0.007).[10] The second RCT (n = 287) compared supportive care versus supportive care plus two chemotherapy regimens. It found that median survival was longer in both chemotherapy regimens (4.1 v 5.9 v 8.1 months). Improvements in quality of life scores were found in both chemotherapy arms up to 2 months after treatment, but not with supportive care.[11] **Second line chemotherapy:** We found no systematic review but found one RCT of 104 people with stage 3B or 4 lung cancer who had previously received cisplatin based chemotherapy, been given docetaxel (second line chemotherapy), or had been given best supportive care (median survival 7.0 months [docetaxel] v 4.6 months [control]; log rank test, P = 0.047).[12]

Harms: Some studies have reported improvement in lung cancer symptoms with chemotherapy, but over 50% of advanced lung cancer patients treated with chemotherapy reported alopecia, and gastrointestinal and haematological toxicity.[13] One non-systematic review found greater toxicity in patients with Eastern Cooperative Oncology Group performance status 3 or 4 (see glossary, p 871).[14]

Comment: People with Eastern Cooperative Oncology Group performance status 3 or 4 have usually been excluded from RCTs of lung cancer chemotherapy. Carboplatin has comparable activity to, but a better toxicity profile than, cisplatin in patients with stage 4 non-small cell lung cancer.[15] Newer agents such as vinorelbine, gemcitabine, irinotecan, paclitaxel, and docetaxel produce objective responses in more than 20% of patients with advanced lung cancer and are being studied prospectively alone or in combination with cisplatin or carboplatin in RCTs.[15] For people with stage 4 non-small cell lung cancer, treatment options consist of either chemotherapy or symptomatic care, including palliative radiation. Measuring quality of life in people with lung cancer remains a serious challenge.

QUESTION What are the effects of treatments for small cell lung cancer?

OPTION STANDARD CHEMOTHERAPY VERSUS OTHER REGIMENS

We found no good evidence comparing standard cisplatin or doxorubicin based chemotherapy with other drug regimens.

Benefits: We found no systematic review and no large scale RCT. One RCT (n = 229) comparing dose intense treatment versus standard chemotherapy found no significant difference in progression free survival or overall survival (0.98 v 0.91 years).[16]

Harms: Except in people with widespread extensive stage disease, adverse effects of chemotherapy were of short duration. One RCT found evidence that dose intense treatment increased toxic deaths (deaths related to toxicity AR 9/110 [8%] with dose intense treatment v 1/109 [1%] with standard chemotherapy; ARI 7%, 95% CI 2% to 14%; RR 8.9, 95% CI 1.1 to 69.2; NNH 14; 95% CI 7 to 60).[16]

Comment: Standard chemotherapy for both limited and extensive stage disease comprises four to six cycles of etoposide plus cisplatin, or a regimen that alternates three cycles of etoposide plus cisplatin with three cycles of cyclophosphamide, doxorubicin, and vincristine.[17] Thoracic irradiation was given to people responding to high dose treatment and by discretion to people on standard dose treatment.

OPTION   ADDING THORACIC IRRADIATION TO CHEMOTHERAPY IN LIMITED STAGE SMALL CELL LUNG CANCER

Two systematic reviews of RCTs have found that adding thoracic irradiation to chemotherapy is associated with improved survival in people with limited stage small cell lung cancer. The best timing, dose, and fractionation of radiation remain uncertain.

Benefits: We found two systematic reviews of adding thoracic irradiation to chemotherapy in people with limited stage small cell lung cancer. The first review (search date 1992, 13 RCTs, n = 2573, range 52–426 people) found 3 year survival was 15% with radiation v 10% with chemotherapy alone (P = 0.001).[18] The second review (search date not given, 11 RCTs, n = 1911) pooled data from nine of the RCTs (n = 1521) and found that local control was achieved in 50% with radiation versus 25% with chemotherapy alone (ARR 25%, 95% CI 17% to 34%).[19] **Timing of radiation:** We found no systematic review but found five RCTs[20-24] addressing the timing of radiation (concurrent radiotherapy early or late in the chemotherapy, sequential or alternating). We found three RCTs comparing early versus late concurrent radiotherapy. The first RCT (n = 270) delivered the most intensive radiotherapy treatment and found a non-significant survival advantage for chest irradiation at week 9 versus chest irradiation at week 1 (P = 0.08), and no difference in local disease control in the chest.[20] The second RCT (n = 308) of people given chest irradiation at 4 weeks (early) compared with chest irradiation at 15 weeks (late) found a significant survival advantage for early irradiation (progression free survival at 3 years: 26% early v 19% late, P = 0.036; survival at 5 years: 20% early v 11% late, P = 0.008).[21] The third RCT (n = 199) found no difference in survival or local disease control between week 1 (early) and week 18 (late) irradiation.[22] One large RCT (n = 228) compared concurrent versus sequential radiotherapy; 2 year survival favoured concurrent radiotherapy (50% v 40%).[23] One RCT (n = 156) compared alternating versus concurrent radiotherapy. The trial found that 3 year survival was greater with alternating radiotherapy (7% v 4%)[24] **Dose and fractionation:** One RCT (n = 417) compared twice daily thoracic irradiation over 3 weeks versus once daily irradiation over 5 weeks in people given cisplatin and etoposide. Survival rates were 47% at 2 years and 26% at 5 years in the twice daily group, and 41% at 2 years and 16% at 5 years among those given once daily irradiation (P = 0.04).[25]

Harms: The risk of treatment related death was more than twice as high in people given thoracic irradiation compared with those receiving chemotherapy alone (29/884 [3.3%] v 12/841 [1.4%]; OR 2.54, 95% CI 1.90 to 3.18).[19] The incidence of oesophagitis was also higher in those treated with twice daily irradiation.[25]

Comment: Interest in adding thoracic irradiation derives from the observation that local recurrence in the chest is a major cause of first treatment failure and carries an extremely poor prognosis. A non-systematic review found that median survival in limited stage disease has improved over the past 10 years from 14–16 months to 20–24 months.[26] The causes of this improvement have not been established but may include the early use of radiation plus chemotherapy rather than improvements in either modality alone.[21] The RCTs of timing used different methods and do not provide strong evidence. The different results from the three RCTs on early versus late concurrent radiotherapy may be explained by different rates of early toxicity from treatment and different rates of relapse in the central nervous system.

OPTION **PROPHYLACTIC CRANIAL IRRADIATION IN LIMITED STAGE SMALL CELL LUNG CANCER**

One systematic review of RCTs of irradiation in people in complete remission found that prophylactic cranial irradiation reduces the risk of developing brain metastases. Long term cognitive dysfunction following cranial irradiation has been described, but longer follow up studies are needed to assess its significance and importance.

Benefits: We found one systematic review (search date not given, 7 RCTs, n = 987) of cranial irradiation for people with small cell lung cancer in complete remission.[27] The review identified RCTs that used individual participant data. Of the people studied, 12% in the irradiation group and 17% in the control group had extensive stage disease at presentation. Meta-analysis found that cranial irradiation was associated with improved survival (RR of death at 3 years 0.84, 95% CI 0.73 to 0.97, corresponding to a 5.4% increase in survival) and increased disease free survival (RR of recurrence or death at 3 years 0.75, 95% CI 0.65 to 0.86). Subgroup analysis identified survival benefit only for men and not for women, but the difference in survival was not significant (P = 0.07). The cumulative incidence of brain metastases was decreased (RR 0.46, 95% CI 0.38 to 0.57). Larger doses of radiation led to a greater decrease in brain metastases (P = 0.02) but did not influence survival significantly (P = 0.89).

Harms: Whether prophylactic cranial irradiation leads to neuropsychological sequelae could not be addressed in the meta-analysis because adequate assessments were carried out in only two of the seven trials. These and other studies found that 24–60% of participants may have neuropsychological problems before treatment,[27] and other studies have not accounted for potential confounding factors such as age, tobacco use, paraneoplastic syndromes, and neurotoxic chemotherapy effects.[27]

Comment: The clinical significance of cognitive impairment after prophylactic cranial irradiation remains unclear.

OPTION	ORAL ETOPOSIDE IN EXTENSIVE STAGE SMALL CELL LUNG CANCER

RCTs have found evidence that survival is worse with oral etoposide than with combination chemotherapy. Etoposide is less toxic in the short term, but we found no evidence that it offers significantly better quality of life.

Benefits: We found no systematic review. Several RCTs have compared oral etoposide versus chemotherapy. One RCT (n = 155) in people with extensive stage disease compared oral etoposide 100 mg daily for 5 days versus combination chemotherapy. Survival at 1 year was significantly higher with combination chemotherapy than with etoposide (19.3% v 9.8%, P < 0.05). There was no significant difference in median survival (5.9 v 4.8 months) and there were conflicting results on quality of life. Nausea was worse with combination chemotherapy (P < 0.01), but pain, appetite, general wellbeing, and mood were worse with oral etoposide (P < 0.001). Palliation of lung cancer symptoms was of shorter duration with etoposide (P < 0.01).[28]

Harms: Acute nausea and vomiting were worse with combined intravenous chemotherapy, but there was no significant difference in overall quality of life.[28] Treatment related symptoms were worse with combination chemotherapy (P < 0.01).

Comment: Because treatment of extensive stage disease is palliative, and because age has been identified as a prognostic factor in small cell lung cancer, studies have looked at outcomes in elderly people with limited and extensive stage disease, and in people of all ages with a poor prognosis. Although small cell lung cancer is relatively sensitive to chemotherapy, extensive stage disease remains incurable. Median survival with treatment is 10–12 months, and as yet has been unaffected by high dose combination chemotherapy. Because of its lower toxicity, etoposide may be considered for elderly people with extensive stage disease or people with a poor prognosis.

GLOSSARY

Performance status Expression used to describe functional status or wellness of participants in studies of cancer. There are two widely accepted scales: the Eastern Cooperative Oncology Group scale (0 = no symptoms; 1 = symptomatic but no extra time in bed; 2 = in bed less than 50% of the day, no work, can care for self; 3 = in bed more than 50% of day, not bedridden, minimal self care; 4 = completely bedridden), and the Karnofsky Scale of symptoms and disability (from 100% = no symptoms to 0% = dead).

Substantive changes since last issue

Palliative chemotherapy in stage 4 non-small cell lung cancer One new RCT of docetaxel in people with stage 3B or 4 lung cancer.[12]
Palliative chemotherapy in stage 4 non-small cell lung cancer One review found that toxicity is greater in patients with Eastern Cooperative Oncology Group performance status 3 or 4.[14]
Adding thoracic irradiation to chemotherapy in limited stage small cell lung cancer, timing of radiation Two new RCTs; no change in conclusion.[20,22]

REFERENCES

1. Travis WD, Travis LB, Devesa SS. Lung cancer. *Cancer* 1995;75(suppl 1):191–202.
2. Ihde DC, Pass HI, Glatstein E. Lung cancer. In: DeVita VT Jr, Hellman S, Rosenberg SA, eds. *Cancer, principles and practice of oncology*, 5th ed. Philadelphia: Lippincott-Raven, 1997;849–959.
3. Montazeri A, Gillis CR, McEwen J. Quality of life in people with lung cancer: a review of literature from 1970 to 1995. *Chest* 1998;113:467–481.
4. Grilli R, Oxman AD, Julian JA. Chemotherapy for advanced non-small-cell lung cancer: how much benefit is enough? *J Clin Oncol* 1993;11:1866–1872. Search date 1991; primary source Medline 1970–1991.
5. Non-Small Cell Lung Cancer Collaborative Group. Chemotherapy in non-small cell lung cancer: a meta-analysis using update individual patient data from 52 randomized clinical trials. *BMJ* 1995; 311:899–909. Search date 1995; primary sources Medline; Cancer CD; hand search of meetings abstracts, bibliographies of books and specialist journals; consultation of trials registers of National Cancer Institute, UK Coordinating Committee for Cancer Research, and the Union Internationale Contre le Cancer.
6. Marino P, Preatoni A. Randomized trials of radiotherapy alone versus combined chemotherapy and radiotherapy in stages IIIa and IIIb non small cell lung cancer. *Cancer* 1995;76: 593–601. Search date 1995; primary sources Medline; manual search of references of review articles and abstracts.
7. Pritchard RS, Anthony SP. Chemotherapy plus radiotherapy compared with radiotherapy alone in the treatment of locally advance, unresectable, non-small-cell lung cancer. *Ann Intern Med* 1996; 125:723–729. Search date 1995; primary sources Medline, plus manual search of references of review articles and abstracts.
8. Souquet PJ, Chauvin F, Boissel JP, et al. Polychemotherapy in advanced non small cell lung cancer: a meta-analysis. *Lancet* 1993;342:19–21. Search date not given; manual and computerised search of medical journals.
9. Marino P, Pampallona S, Preatoni A, et al. Chemotherapy versus supportive care in advanced non-small-cell lung cancer: results of a meta-analysis of the literature. *Chest* 1994;106:861–865. Search date not given; primary sources Medline, and manual search of references from review articles and abstracts.
10. Cullen MH, Billingham CM, Woodroffe AD, et al. Mitomycin, ifosfamide, and cisplatin in unresectable non-small cell lung cancer: effects on survival and quality of life. *J Clin Oncol* 1999; 17:3188–3194.
11. Thongprasert S, Sanguanmitra P, Juthapan W, Clinch J. Relationship between quality of life and clinical outcomes in advanced non-small cell lung cancer: best supportive care (BSC) versus BSC plus chemotherapy. *Lung Cancer* 1999;24:17–24.
12. Shepherd FA, Dancey J, Ramlau, et al. Prospective randomized trial of docetaxel versus best supportive care in patients with non-small-cell lung cancer previously treated with platinum-based chemotherapy. *J Clin Oncol* 2000;18: 2095–2103.
13. Le Chevalier T, Brisgand D, Douillard J-Y, et al. Randomized study of vinorelbine and cisplatin versus vindesine and cisplatin versus vinorelbine alone in advanced non-small-cell lung cancer: results of a European multicenter trial including 612 people. *J Clin Oncol* 1994;12:360–367.
14. Bunn PA Jr, Kelly K. New chemotherapeutic agents prolong survival and improve quality of life in non-small cell lung cancer: a review of literature and future directions. *Clin Cancer Res* 1998;16:27–33.
15. Bunn PA Jr. Review of therapeutic trials of carboplatin in lung cancer. *Semin Oncol* 1989;16: 27–33.
16. Murray N, Livingston RB, Shepherd FA, et al. Randomised study of CODE versus alternating CAV/EP for extensive-stage small-cell lung cancer: an intergroup study of the National Cancer Institute of Canada clinical trials group and the Southwest oncology group. *J Clin Oncol* 1999;17: 2300–2308.
17. Murray N. New drugs for small cell lung cancer. *Oncology* 1997;11:38–42.
18. Pignon JP, Arriagada R, Ihde DC, et al. A meta-analysis of thoracic radiotherapy for small-cell lung cancer. *N Engl J Med* 1992;327:1618–1624. Search date 1992; primary sources Medline; and hand search of proceedings of key oncology meetings.
19. Warde P, Payne D. Does thoracic irradiation improve survival and local control in limited-stage small cell carcinoma of the lung? A meta-analysis. *J Clin Oncol* 1992;10:890–895. Search date not given; primary sources Medline; Cancerline.
20. Perry MC, Eaton WL, Propert KJ, et al. Chemotherapy with or without radiation therapy in limited small-cell carcinoma of the lung. *N Engl J Med* 1987;316:912–918.
21. Murray N, Coy P, Pater JL, et al. Importance of timing for thoracic irradiation in the combined modality treatment of limited-stage small cell lung cancer. *J Clin Oncol* 1993;11:336–344.
22. Work E, Steen Nielsen O, Bentzen SM, et al. Randomised study of initial versus late chest irradiation combined with chemotherapy in limited-stage small-cell lung cancer. *J Clin Oncol* 1997; 15:3030–3037.
23. Takada M, Fukuoka M, Furuse K, et al. A phase III study of concurrent versus sequential thoracic radiotherapy in combination with cisplatin and etoposide for limited-stage small-cell lung cancer: preliminary results of the Japan clinical oncology group [abstract 1103]. *Proc Am Soc Clin Oncol* 1996;15:372.
24. Lebeau B, Chastang C, Urban T, et al. A randomized clinical trial comparing concurrent and alternating thoracic irradiation in limited small cell lung cancer (SCLC) [abstract]. *Proc Am Soc Clin Oncol* 1996;15:383.
25. Turrisi AT, Kim K, Blum R, et al. Twice-daily compared with once-daily thoracic radiotherapy in limited small-cell lung cancer treated concurrently with cisplatin and etoposide. *N Engl J Med* 1999; 340:265–271.
26. Kumar P. The role of radiotherapy in the management of limited-stage small cell lung cancer: past, present, and future. *Chest* 1997; 112(suppl):259–265.
27. Auperin A, Arriagada R, Pignon J-P, et al. Prophylactic cranial irradiation for people with small-cell lung cancer in complete remission. *N Engl J Med* 1999;341:476–484. Search date not given; primary sources Medline, CancerLit, Excerpta Medica, and Biosis.
28. Souhami RL, Spiro SG, Rudd RM, et al. Five day oral etoposide treatment for advanced small cell lung cancer: randomized comparison with intravenous chemotherapy. *J Natl Cancer Inst* 1997;89:577–580.

Alan Neville
Professor
McMaster University
Hamilton
Canada

Competing interests: None declared.

Respiratory disorders

TABLE 1	Staging lung cancer (see text, p 866).

Non-small cell lung cancer

Stage	Definition*	5 year survival (%)
1	T1–T2, N0, M0	55–75
2	T1–T2, N1, M0	25–50
3A	T3, N0–N1, M0 or T1–T3, N2, M0	20–40
3B	T4, any N, M0 or any T, N3, M0	≤5
4	Any M1	≤5

Small cell lung cancer

Stage	Definition	Median survival
Limited stage disease	Tumour confined to the same side of the chest, supraclavicular lymph nodes, or both	18–24 months†
Extensive stage disease	Defined as anything beyond limited stage	10–12 months‡

*M, metastases; N, nodes; T, tumor; †with combined chemotherapy and mediastinal irradiation; ‡with palliative chemotherapy.

Respiratory disorders

Updated this issue

John Cunnington

QUESTIONS
Effects of treatments 875
Effects of interventions to prevent recurrence 878

INTERVENTIONS	
TREATMENT **Likely to be beneficial** One way valves on chest tubes versus bottles with underwater seal . . . . .877 **Trade off between benefits and harms** Small versus standard sized chest tubes . . . . .876 **Unknown effectiveness** Needle aspiration . . . . .875 Chest tube drainage 876	**Unlikely to be beneficial** Chest tube drainage plus suction . . . . .877 **PREVENTING RECURRENCE** **Trade off between benefits and harms** Chemical pleurodesis . . . . . .878 **Unknown effectiveness** Optimal timing of pleurodesis (after first, second, or third spontaneous pneumothorax).878 Surgical pleurodesis 878

Key Messages

Treatment

- We found insufficient evidence to determine whether any intervention is more effective than none for spontaneous pneumothorax.

- Two small RCTs found that resolution was more rapid with chest tube drainage than needle aspiration, but people treated with needle aspiration required less analgesia and spent less time in hospital.

- One small RCT found no difference in duration of tube drainage between small and standard sized chest tubes, but for people with larger pneumothoraces successful resolution was more likely with larger tubes.

- One small RCT found no difference in rate of resolution when one way valves were compared with drainage bottles with an underwater seal, but people treated with one way valves required less analgesia and spent less time in hospital.

- One small RCT found no difference in rate of resolution whether chest tube drainage bottles were connected to suction or not.

Preventing recurrence

- Two RCTs and one non-randomised trial found that chemical pleurodesis reduced the rate of recurrence of spontaneous pneumothorax. The studies found that pleurodesis can be painful and may increase time spent in hospital.

- We found insufficient evidence to inform decisions on whether pleurodesis should take place after the first, second, or subsequent episodes of spontaneous pneumothorax.

■ We found insufficient evidence to compare the effects of chemical pleurodesis, thoracotomy, and video assisted thoracoscopic surgery.

DEFINITION	A pneumothorax is air in the pleural space. A spontaneous pneumothorax occurs when there is no provoking factor, such as trauma, surgery, or diagnostic intervention. It implies a leak of air from the lung parenchyma through the visceral pleura into the pleural space.
INCIDENCE/ PREVALENCE	Incidence is about 7/100 000 for men and 1/100 000 for women.[1] Smoking increases the likelihood of spontaneous pneumothorax by 22 times for men and 8 times for women. A dose response relationship has been observed.[2]
AETIOLOGY/ RISK FACTORS	Spontaneous pneumothorax can be primary (generally occurring in young fit people and thought to be due to a congenital abnormality of the pleura, a subpleural apical bleb) or secondary (owing to underlying lung disease, typically occurring in older people with emphysema or pulmonary fibrosis).
PROGNOSIS	Death from spontaneous pneumothorax is rare and in some cases a consequence of tension pneumothorax. Morbidity with pain and dyspnoea is common. Published recurrence rates vary, but one cohort study found that, after a first episode of primary spontaneous pneumothorax, 23% of people suffered a recurrence within 5 years, most within a year.[3] Recurrence rates had been thought to increase substantially after the first recurrence, but one case control study of military personnel found that 28% of men with a first spontaneous pneumothorax had a recurrence; 23% of the 28% had a second recurrence; and only 14% of that 23% had a third recurrence, giving a total recurrence rate of 35%.[4]
AIMS	To reduce morbidity; to restore normal function as quickly as possible; to prevent recurrence and mortality, with minimum adverse effects.
OUTCOMES	Rate of successful resolution of spontaneous pneumothorax; time to full expansion; duration of hospital stay; time off work; harmful effects of treatments (pain, surgical emphysema, wound and pleural space infection); and rate of recurrence.
METHODS	*Clinical Evidence* update search and appraisal May 2000. Most of the literature comprised uncontrolled case series. We found no systematic reviews and seven RCTs.

QUESTION What are the effects of treatments?

OPTION NEEDLE ASPIRATION

Limited data from one small RCT provided no good evidence of a difference between needle aspiration and observation. Two small RCTs found faster resolution with chest tube drainage than with needle aspiration, but no evidence of a difference in recurrence rate, mortality, or rate of return to normal function. One of the trials found that people treated with needle aspiration experienced less pain and spent less time in hospital than those treated with chest tube drainage.

Benefits: We found no systematic review. **Versus observation:** We found one small RCT (n = 21) comparing needle aspiration versus no treatment.[5] It found that there may have been more rapid re-expansion in the treatment group (3.2 weeks v 1.6 weeks; insufficient information for reliable statistical analysis). **Versus chest tube drainage:** We found two small RCTs, both reporting higher success rates with chest tube drainage. In the first, all 38 people treated with chest tube drainage had resolution of the pneumothorax (time frame not given), compared with 28/35 people treated with needle aspiration. The other seven people required subsequent chest tube drainage.[6] There was no significant difference in recurrence rate at 1 year. The second RCT reported success (resolution of the pneumothorax within 24 hours) in 26/28 people treated with chest tube drainage, and 22/33 treated with needle aspiration (93% v 67%, P = 0.01).[7] There was no significant difference in recurrence rate. The study was not designed to show a difference in duration of hospital stay because chest tube drainage was done on admission whereas in most cases needle aspiration was performed after 3 days of observation in hospital.

Harms: We found no reports of harmful effects of needle aspiration. **Versus chest tube drainage:** In one RCT, people treated with needle aspiration experienced significantly less pain on daily total pain scores during their hospital stay, compared with those treated with chest tube drainage (total pain with needle aspiration 2.7, 95% CI 1.6 to 3.8; with chest tube drainage 6.7, 95% CI 5.5 to 7.9) and spent an average of 2 days less in hospital (3.2 v 5.3, P = 0.005).[6]

Comment: The RCT of needle aspiration versus simple observation[5] is consistent with a large case series in which 74% (88/119) of spontaneous pneumothoraces presenting to an outpatient chest clinic were managed successfully without intervention or hospital admission.[8]

OPTION   CHEST TUBE DRAINAGE

We found insufficient evidence on the effects of chest tube drainage compared with observation. Two small RCTs found faster resolution with chest tube drainage than needle aspiration but no evidence of a difference in recurrence rate, mortality, or rate of return to normal function. Chest tube drainage caused more pain and longer hospital stay. Limited data provided no evidence that larger tubes reduce duration of drainage, but suggested that they increase success rates in people with large pneumothoraces.

Benefits: We found no systematic review. **Versus observation:** We found no sufficiently large RCTs. **Versus needle aspiration:** See option, p 875. **Different sized tubes:** We found no RCTs. One non-randomised trial in 44 people compared small gauge (8 French) catheters (n = 21) versus standard chest tubes (n = 23).[9] There was no significant difference in duration of drainage between groups. In people with large pneumothoraces (> 50% lung volume), successful resolution was more likely with standard chest tubes than catheters (100% v 57%, P < 0.05). No such difference was reported in people with small (< 50%) pneumothoraces.

Harms: **Versus needle aspiration:** In one RCT, people treated with chest tube drainage experienced significantly more pain on daily and total pain scores during their hospital stay (total pain with needle aspiration 2.7, 95% CI 1.6 to 3.8; with chest tube drainage 6.7, 95% CI 5.5 to 7.9) and spent an average of 2 days less in hospital (3.2 *v* 5.3, P = 0.005).[6] Small gauge chest tubes are easier to insert and may cause less pain and morbidity. Subcutaneous emphysema was reported in 9/23 people treated with conventional chest tubes compared with 0/21 treated with catheters (P < 0.05).[9]

Comment: None.

OPTION   **ONE WAY VALVES ON CHEST TUBES**

One small RCT found no evidence of a difference in rates of resolution between one way valves and drainage bottles with underwater seals, but the trial was too small to rule out a clinically important difference. People treated with one way valves required less analgesia and spent less time in hospital.

Benefits: We found no systematic review. We found one RCT in 30 people with spontaneous pneumothorax and respiratory distress, comparing a 13 French chest tube connected to a one way valve (n = 17) versus a 14 French chest tube connected to a drainage bottle with an underwater seal (n = 13).[10] There was no significant difference in rates of resolution between the groups, but there was significantly lower need for analgesia in people treated with a one way valve (29% *v* 77%, P = 0.027).

Harms: The RCT found that, compared with drainage using an underwater seal, there was no evidence of a difference in the rate of complications.[10]

Comment: One way valves often allow people to be treated at home. All people treated with drainage bottles were treated in hospital compared with only 30% of those treated with one way valves (P < 0.01).[10]

OPTION   **CHEST TUBE DRAINAGE PLUS SUCTION**

One RCT found no evidence of a difference in rate of resolution regardless of whether chest tube drainage bottles were connected to suction or not. However, the trial was too small to rule out a clinically important difference.

Benefits: We found no systematic review. We found one RCT comparing chest tube drainage using an underwater seal only (n = 30) versus drainage with suction (n = 23). Suction pressures ranged from 8–20 cm H_2O.[11] There was no significant difference in rate of success, defined as full lung expansion within 10 days (57% with suction *v* 50% without).

Harms: We found no reports of adverse effects due to suction.

Comment: We found one RCT comparing suction versus no suction in 80 people with traumatic pneumothorax, but because the mechanism of injury is different the results should not be extrapolated to spontaneous pneumothorax.[12]

Spontaneous pneumothorax

| QUESTION | What are the effects of interventions to prevent recurrence? |

| OPTION | CHEMICAL PLEURODESIS |

Two RCTs found that chemical pleurodesis reduced the rate of recurrence of spontaneous pneumothorax. RCTs found that treatment can be painful. We found conflicting evidence about the effect of pleurodesis on the duration of hospital stay compared with chest tube drainage alone. We found no reliable evidence about the optimal timing of pleurodesis.

Benefits:
We found no systematic review. We found two RCTs. One unblinded RCT (229 men) compared chest tube insertion plus intrapleural instillation of tetracycline (n = 113, mean follow up 34 months) versus chest tube insertion alone (n = 116, mean follow up 29 months).[13] The recurrence rate was 25% in the tetracycline group and 41% in the control group (P = 0.02). There was no significant difference in length of hospital stay or 5 year survival (40 deaths in the tetracycline group and 42 in the control group). The other RCT (96 people treated with a chest tube) compared three groups: no further treatment; tetracycline pleurodesis; and talc pleurodesis.[14] Mean follow up was 4.6 years. The recurrence rate in the control group was 36%, compared with 8% in the talc group (P < 0.05), and 13% in the tetracycline group. **Versus surgical pleurodesis:** See option, below. **Optimal timing of pleurodesis:** We found no systematic reviews, RCTs, or high quality cohort studies comparing pleurodesis undertaken at different times (after the first, second, or subsequent episodes of spontaneous pneumothorax).

Harms:
In the first unblinded RCT, 58% of people reported intense chest pain on injection of tetracycline.[13] The trial found no effect on pulmonary function at 2 years' follow up.[13] In a similar prospective, controlled, but not randomised, study, the duration of hospital stay was significantly longer for the tetracycline group than for the other two groups (mean 10 days v 4 days, P < 0.01).[15]

Comment:
If the 5 year recurrence rate after a first pneumothorax is around 28%, there may be little reason to undertake pleurodesis with the first episode.[4] Although it has generally been thought that pleurodesis is warranted after the second or third episode, this convention may be questionable if only 23% of this 28% will have a second recurrence and only 14% of that 23% will have a third recurrence.[4] Even though the probability of success with pleurodesis is high, clinicians will have to weigh the likelihood of recurrence against the morbidity associated with the procedure.

| OPTION | SURGICAL PLEURODESIS |

We found insufficient evidence on the effects of surgical pleurodesis, or surgical compared with chemical pleurodesis.

Benefits:
We found no systematic review or RCTs. **Versus chemical pleurodesis:** We found one non-randomised prospective study that compared tetracycline pleurodesis (n = 78) versus thoracotomy (n = 28).[15] The mean follow up was 45 months. There was no

significant difference in recurrence rate (chemical pleurodesis 9%, 8 treatment failures, 4 lost to follow up; thoracotomy 0%, $P = 0.13$). **Video assisted thorascopic surgery:** We found no good studies comparing video assisted thorascopic surgery versus conventional thoracotomy or chemical pleurodesis.

Harms: We found no good information on harms.

Comment: Compared with chemical pleurodesis, thoracotomy is likely to increase morbidity and time lost from work, although this may change with the advent of video assisted thoracoscopic surgery.

REFERENCES

1. Melton LJ, Hepper NG, Offord KP. Incidence of spontaneous pneumothorax in Olmsted County, Minnesota: 1950–1974. *Am Rev Respir Dis* 1979;120:1379–1382.
2. Bense L, Eklung G, Wiman LG. Smoking and the increased risk of contracting spontaneous pneumothorax. *Chest* 1987;92:1009–1012.
3. Lippert HL, Lund O, Blegvad S, et al. Independent risk factors for cumulative recurrence rate after first spontaneous pneumothorax. *Eur Respir J* 1991;4:324–331.
4. Voge VM, Anthracite R. Spontaneous pneumothorax in the USAF aircrew population: a retrospective study. *Aviat Space Environ Med* 1986;57:939–949.
5. Flint K, Al-Hillawi AH, Johnson NM. Conservative management of spontaneous pneumothorax. *Lancet* 1984;1:687–688.
6. Harvey J, Prescott RJ. Simple aspiration versus intercostal tube drainage for spontaneous pneumothorax in patients with normal lungs. British Thoracic Society Research Committee. *BMJ* 1994;309:1338–1339.
7. Andrivet P, Djedaini K, Teboul JL, et al. Spontaneous pneumothorax. Comparison of thoracic drainage vs immediate or delayed needle aspiration. *Chest* 1995;108:335–339.
8. Stradling P, Poole G. Conservative management of spontaneous pneumothorax. *Thorax* 1966;21:145–149.
9. Kang YJ, Koh HG, Shin JW, et al. The effect of 8 French catheter and chest tube on the treatment of spontaneous pneumothorax. *Tuber Respir Dis* 1996;43:410–419.
10. Roggla M, Wagner A, Brunner C, et al. The management of pneumothorax with the thoracic vent versus conventional intercostal tube drainage. *Wien Klin Wochenschr* 1996;108:330–333.
11. So SY, Yu DYC. Catheter drainage of spontaneous pneumothorax: suction or no suction, early or late removal? *Thorax* 1982;37:46–48.
12. Davis JW, Mackersie RC, Hoyt DB, et al. Randomized study of algorithms for discontinuing tube thoracostomy drainage. *J Am Coll Surg* 1994;179:553–557.
13. Light RW, O'Hara VS, Moritz TE, et al. Intrapleural tetracycline for the prevention of recurrent spontaneous pneumothorax. Results of a Department of Veterans Affairs cooperative study. *JAMA* 1990;264:2224–2230.
14. Almind M, Lange P, Viskum K. Spontaneous pneumothorax: comparison of simple drainage, talc pleurodesis, and tetracycline pleurodesis. *Thorax* 1989;44:627–630.
15. Alfageme I, Moreno L, Huertas C, Vargas A, Hernandez J, Beiztegui A. Spontaneous pneumothorax. Long-term results with tetracycline pleurodesis. *Chest* 1994;106:347–350.

John Cunnington
Associate Professor, Medicine
McMaster University
Hamilton, Ontario
Canada

Competing interests: None declared.

Upper respiratory tract infection

Updated and expanded this issue

Paul Glasziou and Chris Del Mar

INTERVENTIONS

Key Messages

- We found no evidence that antibiotics have a clinically important effect on colds uncomplicated by secondary infection. Systematic reviews have found a minimal to modest effect of antibiotics in acute bronchitis, pharyngitis, and sinusitis. Antibiotics can prevent non-suppurative complications of β haemolytic streptococcal pharyngitis, but in developed societies such complications are rare.

- RCTs have found that β agonists reduce the duration of cough in acute bronchitis.

- One systematic review of RCTs has found that vitamin C reduces duration of symptoms in undifferentiated colds. However, the beneficial effect is small and may be explained by publication bias.

- One systematic review found inconsistent evidence on the effects of zinc gluconate.

- We found limited evidence from one systematic review of RCTs that some preparations of echinacea may be superior to placebo for treatment and prevention of cold, but we found insufficient evidence to recommend a specific product.

- One systematic review of RCTs found conflicting evidence for the efficacy of steam inhalation.
- One systematic review of RCTs found evidence for limited short term benefit of decongestants but no evidence of benefit with longer term use.
- One systematic review of RCTs found evidence that antihistamines reduce runny nose and sneezing.

DEFINITION	Upper respiratory tract infection involves inflammation of the respiratory mucosa from the nose to the lower respiratory tree, not including the alveoli. In addition to malaise, it causes localised symptoms that constitute several overlapping syndromes: sore throat (pharyngitis); rhinorrhoea (common cold); facial fullness and pain (sinusitis); and cough (bronchitis).
INCIDENCE/ PREVALENCE	Upper respiratory tract infections, nasal congestion, throat complaints, and cough are responsible for 11% of general practice consultations in Australia.[1] Each year, children suffer about five such infections, and adults two to three.[1]
AETIOLOGY/ RISK FACTORS	Infective agents include over 200 viruses (with 100 rhinoviruses) and several bacteria. Transmission is mostly through hand to hand contact with subsequent passage to the nares or eyes, rather than, as commonly perceived, through droplets in the air.[2]
PROGNOSIS	Upper respiratory tract infections are usually self limiting. Although they cause little mortality or serious morbidity, upper respiratory tract infections are responsible for considerable discomfort, lost work, and medical costs. Clinical patterns vary and overlap between infective agents. In addition to nasal symptoms, half of sufferers experience sore throat and 40% experience cough. Symptoms peak within 1–3 days and generally clear by 1 week, although cough often persists.[2]
AIMS	To relieve symptoms and to prevent suppurative and non-suppurative complications of bacterial infection, with minimal adverse effects from treatments.
OUTCOMES	Cure rate, duration of symptoms, incidence of complications, incidence of adverse effects of treatment.
METHODS	*Clinical Evidence* update search and appraisal May 2000.

QUESTION What are the effects of treatments?

OPTION ANTIBIOTICS

We found no evidence that antibiotics have a clinically important effect on undifferentiated colds. Systematic reviews have found a minimal to modest effect of antibiotics in acute bronchitis, pharyngitis, and sinusitis. Antibiotics can prevent non-suppurative complications of β haemolytic streptococcal pharyngitis, but in industrialised countries, such complications are rare.

Benefits: **Colds:** We found two systematic reviews. The first, identifying seven RCTs in acute upper respiratory infections without complications, found no effect of antibiotics on general improvement or cure (RR 0.95; 95% CI 0.70 to 1.25).[3] The second (identifying 12 RCTs of antibiotics in children) found no change in clinical outcomes in the six trials with adequate data (RR 1.01; 95% CI 0.90 to 1.13) or in complications or progression (RR 0.71; 95% CI 0.45 to 1.12).[4] Similarly, one recent RCT in 314 adults comparing co-amoxiclav (375 mg three times daily) versus placebo found no overall difference in "cure" rates.[5] However, in the 61 people (20%) who were found to have positive sputum cultures for *Haemophilus influenzae, Moraxella catarrhalis,* or *Streptococcus pneumoniae,* there was a significant difference in recovery of 27% with co-amoxiclav versus 4% with placebo at 5 days. If such people could be identified at first consultation, then treating four of these people with antibiotic rather than placebo would result in one more recovery at 5 days (NNT 4, no CI given). **Cough:** We found one systematic review (updated in 1997), which identified eight RCTs comparing doxycycline (4 RCTs), erythromycin (3 RCTs), and trimethoprim/sulfamethoxazole (1 RCT) versus placebo in 750 people (aged 8 to >65 years).[6] People receiving antibiotics were less likely to report feeling unwell at a follow up visit (OR for reporting feeling unwell at follow up antibiotics *v* placebo 0.42, 95% CI 0.22 to 0.82), although the review reported only significant results, which may have led to optimistic bias. There was a small but significant difference in time to return to work or usual activities (WMD 0.74 days earlier with antibiotics *v* placebo; 95% CI 0.16 to 1.32). **Sore throat:** We found one systematic review (updated in 1998), which identified 18 controlled trials in 9189 people with sore throat.[7] The combined effects from six trials found that antibiotics reduced the risk of rheumatic fever compared with no antibiotic (RR 0.28, 95% CI 0.19 to 0.40). There were too few events to detect any possible protective effect of antibiotics against acute glomerulonephritis (2/1459 cases among controls *v* 0/1625 treated with antibiotics). Suppurative complications were also significantly reduced (otitis media RR 0.23, 95% CI 0.12 to 0.45; quinsy RR 0.19, 95% CI 0.08 to 0.47). Acute sinusitis was not significantly reduced (RR 0.33, 95% CI 0.07 to 1.65). To prevent one case of otitis media, 30 children or 145 adults suffering from sore throat would need to be treated. Antibiotics shortened symptom duration but by a mean of only about 8 hours overall. **Sinusitis:** We found one systematic review, published in 1998, which identified six RCTs comparing antibiotics versus placebo in 761 people with sinusitis.[8] It found that antimicrobial agents (amoxicillin in 3 trials, other agents in 3 trials) were effective in treating uncomplicated acute sinusitis. Symptoms improved or disappeared in 69% of people on placebo, compared with nearly 84% with antibiotics (RRR for symptoms not improving or disappearing compared with placebo 46%, 95% CI 21% to 63%). The same review analysed head to head trials of different antibiotics and found no advantage for other antibiotics over amoxicillin.

Harms: Adverse effects such as nausea, vomiting, headache, skin rash, or vaginitis were more common on antibiotics than placebo. For example, in the bronchitis review the absolute risk increase for adverse effects was 6% (95% CI 0.1% to 12%), or a rate of one extra adverse effect per 16 people treated. We found no evidence of the size of the risk of antibiotic resistance or pseudomembranous colitis.

Comment: Since most upper respiratory tract infections are viral, the potential benefit from antibiotics is limited. Until rapid identification of those likely to benefit is possible, the modest effects seen in trials must be weighed against the adverse effects of antibiotics, costs, and potential for inducing antibiotic resistance.

OPTION β AGONISTS

We found that β agonists reduce the duration of cough in acute bronchitis compared with placebo or erythromycin, although we found limited evidence that this beneficial effect may only be in people with bronchial hyperresponsiveness, wheeze, or airflow limitation.

Benefits: We found no systematic review. Two RCTs in people with acute bronchitis have compared erythromycin versus the β agonist, salbutamol, and one RCT compared fenoterol versus placebo.[9–11] In the first study, 59% on liquid salbutamol compared with 12% on erythromycin were not coughing at 7 days.[9] In the second study, 39% on inhaled salbutamol compared with 9% on erythromycin were not coughing.[10] These absolute risk reductions of 47% and 30% mean two to three people need to be treated for one less person to be coughing at the end of 1 week. A subgroup analysis of the fenoterol trial found that benefits may be confined to people with bronchial hyperresponsiveness, wheezes, or baseline $FEV_1 < 80\%$ of predicted.[11]

Harms: Short term use of a β agonist may cause tachycardia and anxiety.

Comment: The cough associated with acute bronchitis is self limiting, so treatment is for symptomatic relief. Hence it is important to consider the degree of disturbance caused and people's preferences and interpretation of cough.

OPTION VITAMIN C

One systematic review of RCTs has found evidence that vitamin C reduces the duration of symptoms in people with upper respiratory tract infections. However, the beneficial effect is small and may be explained by publication bias.

Benefits: We found one systematic review, updated in 1998.[12–14] This identified 30 RCTs comparing vitamin C with placebo for prophylaxis and treatment of colds. Three RCTs used 1 g or more daily of vitamin C taken at symptom onset. Duration of symptoms was half a day less (WMD 0.55 days per cold episode, 95% CI 0.17 to 0.92), representing about 15% fewer symptomatic days per episode.

Harms: The studies of treatment found no difference in adverse effects potentially caused by vitamin C.

Comment: The beneficial effect reported in the review was small and might be explained by publication bias.

OPTION ZINC

One systematic review of RCTs has found no clear evidence that zinc gluconate or acetate is beneficial in people with upper respiratory tract infections.

Benefits: We found one systematic review, which identified seven RCTs comparing zinc (gluconate or acetate) versus placebo for the treatment of colds.[15] Symptoms were unchanged at 3 and 5 days, but there was a relative reduction of 31% at 7 days (NNT 7, 95% CI 5 to 15). However the 7 day results showed statistically significant heterogeneity, which may be due to the zinc formulation, the type of virus, or to other, unknown factors.

Harms: Adverse outcomes were not systematically reviewed, but individual trials found that nausea, altered taste, dry mouth, abdominal pain, and headache were increased in the zinc group.

Comment: None.

OPTION	ECHINACEA

One recent systematic review of RCTs suggests that some preparations of echinacea may be better than placebo for cold treatment and prevention, but we found insufficient evidence to recommend a specific echinacea product for treating or preventing common colds.

Benefits: **Treatment:** We found one systematic review (search data 1998, 8 RCTs).[16] All trials were double blind except one, which was single blind. The review found most trials to be of poor quality. Quantitative data could only be extracted for two trials on duration of illness, for three trials for runny nose, and for five trials for a summary symptom score. Data pooling was not possible because of trial heterogeneity. There were nine comparisons (8 versus placebo and, in 1 trial, an additional comparison of high versus low dose treatment) from the eight trials. Six comparisons found significantly better results associated with echinacea. One trial found significant results for a subgroup only and two trials found no difference after treatment.[16]
Prevention: The systematic review identified eight trials, with a total of almost 4000 participants.[16] The trials varied considerably in quality of methods and preparation used and so results were not combined. Of the five placebo controlled treatment trials, two found a significantly lower incidence of infection in the treatment group. One of these had large loss to follow up. The other trials found a non-significant reduction in the rate of infection. Data pooling found that significantly fewer people had one infection episode after taking echinacea (167/571 v 292/566; OR 0.36, 95% CI 0.28 to 0.46). The three uncontrolled trials all found a significant benefit, but were not randomised or blinded.

Harms: Three of the eight treatment trials and four of the eight prevention trials reported adverse events. These were generally infrequent and not significantly different between echinacea and placebo. However, outside the trials, anaphylaxis has been reported with echinacea.[17]

Comment: Echinacea is not a single product. There are more than 200 different preparations based upon different plants, different parts of the plant (roots, herbs, whole plant), and different methods of extraction. None of the trials were published in a Medline listed journal. The weakness of trial methods and differences in interventions make drawing conclusive evidence of effectiveness impossible. Large studies may not be done because echinacea is not patentable and each producer controls a small share of the market. The authors of the systematic review received personal information about several unpublished studies that they were not able to include.

| OPTION | STEAM INHALATION | New |

One systematic review of six RCTs found conflicting evidence for the efficacy of steam inhalation.

Benefits: Steam inhalation at 40–47° has been evaluated in several trials, with conflicting results. Six RCTs (n = 319 were included in a systematic review (search dates 1966–1998).[18] Some suggest benefit, and none found any harm. Benefits included increased patency of the nose following exposure to hot, humid steam.

Harms: The trials found no evidence of harms. There may be a danger from spilling very hot water and from nosocomial infections related to humidifier units.

Comment: None.

| OPTION | DECONGESTANTS | New |

One systematic review of four RCTs found evidence for limited short term benefit following a single dose but no evidence of benefit with longer use of decongestants for symptomatic relief.

Benefits: We found one systematic review (search dates 1966 to 1999, four RCTs, 246 adults).[19] It found that in the common cold a single dose of nasal decongestant was only moderately effective (reducing subjective symptom scores by 13%) for the short term relief of congestion in adults. We found no evidence of benefit after repeated use over several days.

Harms: Information about harms was not sought actively or reported in RCTs.

Comment: There were no trials undertaken in children.

| OPTION | ANTIHISTAMINES | New |

One systematic review of nine RCTs in adults found evidence that antihistamines produce small clinical benefits for the symptoms of runny nose and sneezing.

Benefits: One well conducted systematic review of previously unpublished individual patient data from nine RCTs (n = 1757) of antihistamines against placebo found antihistamines reduced the symptoms of runny nose and sneezing for the first 2 days of both natural and experimentally induced colds.[20] The effects were small. On a severity scale ranging from 0 (no symptoms) to 3.0 or 4.0 (severe symptoms), antihistamines reduced the score by 0.25 (95% CI 0.12 to 0.73) for runny nose on days 1 and 2, and 0.14 (95% CI 0.0 to 0.3) for sneezing on day 1 and 0.3 (95% CI 1.5 to 4.5) on day 2.

Harms: Harms were not actively sought in RCTs, but are known to include drowsiness and dry mouth.

Comment: None.

REFERENCES

1. Fry J, Sandler G. *Common diseases. Their nature, prevalence and care.* Dordrecht, The Netherlands: Kluwer Academic, 1993.
2. Lauber B. The common cold. *J Gen Intern Med* 1996;11:229–236.
3. Arroll B, Kenealy T. The use of antibiotics versus placebo in the common cold. In: The Cochrane Library, Issue 1, 2000. Oxford: Update software. Search date 1998; primary sources Cochrane Controlled Trials Register; Medline; Embase; Family Medicine Database; reference lists in articles; principal investigators.
4. Fahey T, Stocks N, Thomas T. Systematic review of the treatment of upper respiratory tract infection. *Arch Dis Child* 1998;79:225–230. Search date not given; primary sources Medline; Embase; Science Citation Index; Cochrane Controlled Trials Register; authors of published RCTs; drug manufacturers, and hand search references.
5. Kaiser L, Lew D, Hirschel B, et al. Effects of antibiotic treatment in the subset of common-cold patients who have bacteria in nasopharyngeal secretions. *Lancet* 1996;347:1507–1510.
6. Becker L, Glazier R, McIsaac W, Smucny J. Antibiotics for acute bronchitis. In: The Cochrane Library, Issue 1, 2000. Oxford: Update software. Search date 1997; primary sources Medline 1966 to 1996; Embase 1974 to 1996; Science Citation Index 1989 to 1996; hand search of reference lists of relevant trials, textbooks, and review articles.
7. Del Mar CB, Glasziou PP. Antibiotics for the symptoms and complications of sore throat. In: The Cochrane Library, Issue 1, 2000. Oxford: Update software. Search date 1998; primary sources Index Medicus 1945 to 1965; Medline 1966 to 1997; Cochrane Library 1997 issue 4; hand search of reference lists of relevant articles.
8. De Ferranti SD, Ioannidis JPA, Lau J, et al. Are amoxycillin and folate inhibitors as effective as other antibiotics for acute sinusitis? A meta-analysis. *BMJ* 1998;317:632–637. Search date May 1998; primary sources Medline 1966 to May 1998; manual search of Excerpta Medica; recent abstracts for Interscience Conference on Antimicrobial Agents and Chemotherapy 1993 to 1997; and references of all trials, review articles, and special issues for additional studies.
9. Hueston WJ. A comparison of albuterol and erythromycin for the treatment of acute bronchitis. *J Fam Pract* 1991;33:476–480.
10. Hueston WJ. Albuterol delivered by metered-dose inhaler to treat acute bronchitis. *J Fam Pract* 1994;39:437–440.
11. Melbye H, Aasebo U, Straume B. Symptomatic effect of inhaled fenoterol in acute bronchitis: a placebo-controlled double-blind study. *Fam Pract* 1991;8:216–222.
12. Douglas RM, Chalker EB, Treacy B. Vitamin C for preventing and treating the ommon cold. In: The Cochrane Library, Issue 2, 1998. Oxford: Update Software. Search date not given; primary sources reviews by Kleinjen and Hemila.[13,14]
13. Kleijnen J, ter Riet G, Knipschild PG. Vitamin C and the common cold; review of a megadoses literature (in Dutch). *Ned Tijdschr Geneeskd* 1989;133:1532–1535. Search date 1998; primary sources Medline 1963 to 1988, and hand searched references.
14. Hemila H. Vitamin C and the common cold. *Br J Nutr* 1992;67:3–16. Search date not given; primary sources not given.
15. Marshall I. Zinc in the treatment of the common cold. In: The Cochrane Library, Issue 1, 2000. Oxford: Update software. Search date December 1997; primary sources Medline, Embase, The Cochrane Library, hand searched journals.
16. Melchart D, Linde K, Fischer P, Kaesmayr J. Echinacea for the prevention and treatment of the common cold. In: The Cochrane Library, Issue 1, 2000. Oxford: Update software. Search date 1998; primary sources Medline 1966 to 1998; Embase 1991 to 1998; database of the Cochrane Acute Respiratory Infections Group; database of the Cochrane Field Complementary Medicine; database Phytodok; bibliographies of existing reviews, personal communications.
17. Mullins RJ. Echinacea associated anaphylaxis. *Med J Aust* 1998;168:170–171.
18. Singh M. Heated, humidified air for the common cold. In: The Cochrane Library, Issue 2, 2000. Oxford: Update Software. Search date 1999; primary sources Medline; Embase; Current Contents and hand search of review articles and reference lists and contact with manufacturers.
19. Taverner D, Bickford L, Draper M. Nasal decongestants for the common cold. In: The Cochrane Library, Issue 2, 2000. Oxford: Update Software. Search date 1999; primary sources Medline; Embase; Current Contents; Cochrane Acute Respiratory Infectious Group's trials register, and hand search of reference lists and personal contacts with known investigators and pharmaceutical companies.
20. D'Agostino RB Sr, Weintraub M, Russell HK, et al. The effectiveness of antihistamines in reducing the severity of runny nose and sneezing: a meta-analysis. *Clin Pharmacol Ther* 1998;64:579–96. Search date not given; primary sources Medline, FDA unpublished clinical trials.

Paul Glasziou
Professor of Evidence-Based Medicine
University of Queensland Medical
School
Brisbane
Australia

Chris Del Mar
Professor of General Practice
University of Queensland
Brisbane
Australia
Competing interests: None declared.

INTERVENTIONS

TREATMENT
Beneficial
Antianaerobic treatment in
  symptomatic non-pregnant
  women 889

Likely to be beneficial
Antianaerobic treatment in
  pregnant women who have had a
  previous preterm birth 890
Oral antianaerobic treatment before
  surgical abortion 892

Unknown effectiveness
Antianaerobic treatment in low risk
  pregnancy 890
Antianaerobic treatment before
  gynaecological procedures . .892

PREVENTING RECURRENCE
Likely to be ineffective or harmful
Treating a woman's one steady
  male sexual partner 891

To be covered in future issues of
Clinical Evidence
Screening in pregnancy

Key Messages

- Bacterial vaginosis may resolve spontaneously.

In non-pregnant women

- RCTs have found no evidence of a difference in effectiveness between oral and intravaginal antianaerobic treatment in non-pregnant women with symptoms caused by bacterial vaginosis. Intravaginal treatment causes fewer adverse effects. Limited evidence suggests that 1 week of oral metronidazole may be more effective than a single dose.

In pregnant women

- In high risk pregnant women (those who have previously delivered prematurely) we found limited evidence suggesting that oral antianaerobic treatment for bacterial vaginosis reduces the risk of premature delivery.

- RCTs provide no evidence of benefit from antianaerobic treatment for bacterial vaginosis in low risk pregnant women (those with no history of premature delivery).

Before procedures

- We found limited evidence suggesting that antianaerobic treatment for bacterial vaginosis in women about to undergo surgical abortion reduces the risk of pelvic inflammatory disease.

- We found no evidence on the effects of treatment in women about to undergo other gynaecological procedures, including abdominal hysterectomy, caesarean section, or insertion of an intrauterine contraceptive device.

Preventing recurrence

- Infection recurs in about one third of women. RCTs have found that in women with one steady male sexual partner, treating the partner with an oral anti-anaerobic agent does not reduce the woman's risk of recurrence.

DEFINITION	Bacterial vaginosis is a microbial disease characterised by an alteration in the bacterial flora of the vagina, from a predominance of *Lactobacillus* species to high concentrations of anaerobic bacteria. Diagnosis requires three out of four features: the presence of clue cells; a homogenous discharge adherent to the vaginal walls; pH of vaginal fluid > 4.5; and a "fishy" amine odour of the vaginal discharge before or after addition of 10% potassium hydroxide. The condition is asymptomatic in 50% of women. Those with symptoms have an excessive white to grey, or malodorous, vaginal discharge; the odour may be particularly noticeable during sexual intercourse.
INCIDENCE/ PREVALENCE	Bacterial vaginosis is the most common infectious cause of vaginitis, being about twice as common as candidiasis.[1] Prevalences of 10–61% have been reported among unselected women from a range of settings.[2] Data on incidence are limited, but one study found that over a 2 year period, 50% of women using an intrauterine contraceptive device had at least one episode, as did 20% of women using oral contraceptives.[3] Bacterial vaginosis is particularly prevalent in lesbians.[4]
AETIOLOGY/ RISK FACTORS	The cause is not fully understood. Risk factors include new or multiple sexual partners[1,3,5] and early age of sexual debut,[6] but no causative microorganism has been shown to be transmitted between partners. Use of an intrauterine contraceptive device[3] and douching[5] have also been reported as risk factors. Infection seems to be most common around the time of menstruation.[7]
PROGNOSIS	The course of bacterial vaginosis varies and is poorly understood. Without treatment, symptoms may persist or resolve, in both pregnant and non-pregnant women. Recurrence after treatment occurs in about one third of women. The condition is associated with complications of pregnancy: low birth weight; preterm birth; preterm labour; premature rupture of membranes (occurring in 6.3% of women with bacterial vaginosis v 4.2% of women without bacterial vaginosis; OR 1.4, 95% CI 1.1 to 1.8,[6] OR in other studies ranged from 1.5 to 6.9); late miscarriage; chorioamnionitis (48% v 22%; OR 2.6, 95% CI 1.0 to 6.6); endometritis (8.2% v 1.5%; OR 5.6, 95% CI 1.8 to 17.2); endometritis after normal delivery; caesarean section (55% v 17%; OR 5.8, 95% CI 3.0 to 10.9); and surgery to the genital tract.[6,8] Women who have had a previous premature delivery are especially at risk of complications in pregnancy, with a 36% increased risk of preterm birth (AR 5.6% [24/428] in all women v 41.7% [10/24] in women with a previous preterm birth).[9] Bacterial vaginosis may also enhance HIV acquisition and transmission.[10]
AIMS	To alleviate symptoms and to prevent complications relating to childbirth, termination of pregnancy, and gynaecological surgery, with minimal adverse effects. To reduce adverse neonatal outcomes.

OUTCOMES Preterm delivery. Puerperal and neonatal morbidity and mortality. Clinical or microbiological cure rates, usually at 1–2 weeks or 4 weeks after completing treatment.

METHODS We searched Medline (bacterial vaginosis, non-specific vaginosis, clindamycin, metronidazole) from 1988 to September 1998. We also used information from drug manufacturers. For each study, we assessed study design, study population, treatment, outcome measures, reported findings, and potential biases. *Clinical Evidence* update search and appraisal December 1999.

QUESTION **What are the effects of different antianaerobic regimens in non-pregnant women with symptomatic bacterial vaginosis?**

A systematic review of RCTs found no evidence of a difference in effectiveness between oral and intravaginal antianaerobic drugs. Intravaginal administration causes fewer systemic adverse effects. A systematic review of RCTs found that a 7 day course of twice daily oral metronidazole is more effective than a single 2 g dose. Limited evidence suggests no difference between oral clindamycin and oral metronidazole, and no difference between once and twice daily dosing with intravaginal metronidazole gel. Symptoms recur after treatment in over a third of women regardless of route or type of antianaerobic agent.

Benefits: **Oral versus intravaginal antianaerobic treatment:** We found one systematic review (search date 1996, 5 RCTs) comparing oral and intravaginal formulations of metronidazole and clindamycin.[11] Three trials were in symptomatic non-pregnant women, and two were in symptomatic and asymptomatic non-pregnant women. There was no significant difference in cumulative cure rates 5–10 days after completing treatment; (86% for oral metronidazole 500 mg twice a day for 7 days; 85% for clindamycin vaginal cream 5 g at bedtime for 7 consecutive days; and 81% for metronidazole vaginal gel 5 g twice a day for 5 days). Four weeks after completing treatment, the cumulative cure rates were 78% for oral metronidazole, 82% for clindamycin vaginal cream, and 71% for metronidazole vaginal gel. **Different oral antianaerobic regimens:** We found one systematic review (search date 1992), which identified four RCTs comparing metronidazole 500 mg twice daily for 7 days versus a single 2 g dose of metronidazole.[9] Cumulative cure rates 3 to 4 weeks after completing treatment were 82% and 62% (P < 0.05). We found one RCT comparing oral metronidazole 500 mg twice daily for 7 days versus oral clindamycin 300 mg twice daily for 7 days in 144 symptomatic non-pregnant women.[12] It found no evidence of a difference (cure rates within 7–10 days of starting treatment 94% v 96%), but one third of women were lost to follow up. **Different intravaginal antianaerobic regimens:** One RCT found no difference in effectiveness between once daily dosing (n = 252) and twice daily dosing (n = 262) of intravaginal metronidazole gel.[13] **Recurrence:** This occurred in 30% of women after 12 weeks' treatment with clindamycin vaginal cream.[14] We found no good studies of maintenance regimens for recurrent bacterial vaginosis.

Harms: A quarter to two thirds of women in the trials experienced adverse effects from oral metronidazole including mild to moderate nausea/

dyspepsia, unpleasant metallic taste, headache, and dizziness.[9] Infrequent adverse effects from oral clindamycin included heartburn, nausea, vomiting, diarrhoea, constipation, headache, dizziness, and vertigo; the trials gave no data on frequency. Intravaginal clindamycin has been associated, rarely, with mild to severe colitis,[15] and with vaginal candidiasis. The RCT of once versus twice daily intravaginal metronidazole gel found no difference in frequency of adverse effects.[13] Yeast vulvovaginitis may be less common with intravaginal than with oral metronidazole (4% for intravaginal[16] v 8–22% for oral[17]).

Comment: Intravaginal administration reduces systemic absorption and systemic adverse effects. Some women may prefer oral medication because it is more convenient.[18]

QUESTION   **What are the effects of treatments in pregnant women with bacterial vaginosis?**

A systematic review of placebo controlled RCTs found a reduced incidence of preterm delivery after antianaerobic treatment of bacterial vaginosis during pregnancy, but the difference was not significant. Limited evidence from a subgroup analysis of women who had had a previous preterm delivery found no significant effect on the risk of preterm delivery of treatment for bacterial vaginosis.

Benefits: We found one systematic review (updated 1998, 5 RCTs, 1508 women) and three subsequent RCTs comparing one or more antibiotic regimens versus placebo.[19–22] The systematic review found fewer cases of preterm delivery after treatment for bacterial vaginosis than after placebo, but the difference was not significant (144/985 [14.6%] with antibiotics v 136/891 [15.3%] with placebo; OR 0.78, 95% CI 0.6 to 1.02). In the subgroup of women who had had a previous preterm birth, the reduced risk of preterm birth was significant (57/187 [30%] with antibiotics v 58/116 [50%] with placebo; OR 0.37, 95% CI 0.23 to 0.60; NNT 4, 95% CI 3 to 8).[19] One subsequent large RCT of oral metronidazole treatment of asymptomatic bacterial vaginosis in pregnant women found no difference in preterm birth between the metronidazole group and the placebo group (116/953 [12.2%] with metronidazole v 121/966 [12.5%] with placebo; RR 0.97, 95% CI 0.76 to 1.23). A subgroup analysis of women with previous preterm birth in this study also found no difference in preterm birth between metronidazole and placebo groups (30/101 [30%] with metronidazole v 26/109 [24%] with placebo; RR 1.24, 95% CI 0.78 to 1.84).[20] One RCT comparing intravaginal clindamycin cream (5 g at bedtime for 7 days) versus placebo in 129 pregnant women with bacterial vaginosis reported no difference in preterm birth (9/60 [15%] with clindamycin v 5/69 [7%] with placebo; RR 2.1, 95% CI 0.7 to 5.0) or in low birth weight (8/59 [14%] with clindamycin v 3/69 [4%] with placebo; RR 3.1, 95% CI 0.9 to 11.2).[21] A subgroup analysis of a previous trial did not find differences in rates of preterm birth (before 37 weeks' gestation) in women without bacterial vaginosis (1/11 [9.1%] with clindamycin cream v 1/11 [9.1%] with placebo).[22]

Harms: Adverse effects occurred in 4% of women receiving antibiotics for bacterial vaginosis. **In women without bacterial vaginosis:** Two trials[22,23] found an increase in preterm birth (before 34 weeks' gestation) in a subgroup of women without bacterial vaginosis who received intravaginal clindamycin cream[22] or oral metranidazole and erythromycin.[23] For the first trial differences between groups did not reach statistical significance (AR 6/62 [9.7%] with clindamycin v 1/64 [1.6%] with placebo; recalculation by *Clinical Evidence*: ARI 8.1%, 95% CI −0.3% to +46%; RR 6.2, 95% CI 0.79 to 31).[22] The second trial found no significant increase in preterm birth in the subgroup before 37 weeks' gestation (AR 56/254 [22%] with metronidazole and erythromycin v 26/104 [25%] with placebo; ARI 3%, 95% CI 0.8 to 1.7; RR 0.88, 95% CI 0.57 to 1.3), but found a significant difference for preterm delivery before 34 weeks' gestation (AR 34/254 [13%] with metronidazole and erythromycin v 5/104 [5%] with placebo; ARI 9%, 95% CI 0.7% to 24%; RR 2.8, 95% CI 1.2 to 6.0; NNH 12, 95% CI 4 to 136).[23]

Comment: The average quality of the trials in the systematic review was good; all trials reported loss to follow up between 1–17% for the various treatment groups.[19] Results from the two additional RCTs conflict with those of the systematic review.

QUESTION   **Does treating male partners prevent recurrence?**

RCTs have found that in women with one steady male sexual partner, treating the partner with an oral antianaerobic agent does not reduce the woman's risk of recurrence.

Benefits: We found no systematic review. We found four RCTs on treating the partners of women who had one steady male partner.[14,24–26] Two RCTs (348 couples) used two single 2 g doses of oral metronidazole or placebo given to the male partner at 1 and 3 days and found no evidence of a difference in recurrence rates among the women.[25,26] The third RCT (140 couples) compared a single 2 g dose of oral metronidazole versus placebo.[24] There was no significant difference in clinical cure or recurrence rates. The fourth RCT (139 couples) compared treating the partner with clindamycin hydrochloride capsules (150 g 4 times a day for 7 days) versus placebo.[14] It found no significant difference in recurrence rates within 3 months of diagnosis.

Harms: No harmful effects were reported in the trials.

Comment: The lack of evidence of effectiveness of both metronidazole and clindamycin suggests that anaerobes are unlikely to be the sole pathogenic agents linking bacterial vaginosis with sexual intercourse.

QUESTION   **What are the effects of treatment before gynaecological procedures?**

In women with bacterial vaginosis who are about to undergo surgical abortion, one RCT found that oral antianaerobic treatment reduced the risk of pelvic inflammatory disease. We found no RCTs on the effects of treatment before other gynaecological procedures, including insertion of intrauterine contraceptive devices.

Bacterial vaginosis

Benefits: We found no systematic review. **Before surgical abortion:** We found one RCT. This compared oral metronidazole 500 mg three times daily for 10 days versus placebo in 174 women with bacterial vaginosis who were about to undergo surgical abortion.[27] Fewer women in the metronidazole group developed pelvic inflammatory disease than in the placebo group (3.8% v 12.2%, P < 0.05, RR and CI not calculable from report). **Before gynaecological surgery:** Bacterial vaginosis is associated with an increased risk of endometritis after caesarean section and vaginal cuff cellulitis after abdominal hysterectomy,[28,29] but we found no RCTs of antianaerobic treatment in women before such surgery. **Before insertion of an intrauterine contraceptive device:** Bacterial vaginosis has been associated with pelvic inflammatory disease (see pelvic inflammatory disease, p 934) in women using intrauterine contraceptive devices,[3] but we found no RCTs of antianaerobic treatment in women with bacterial vaginosis before insertion of these devices.

Harms: The trial gave no information on harmful effects.[27]

Comment: None.

Substantive changes since last issue

Treatment in pregnant women Two additional RCTs provide more information, but overall conclusion is unaltered.[22,23]

REFERENCES

1. Barbone F, Austin H, Louv WC, et al. A follow-up study of methods of contraception, sexual activity, and rates of trichomoniasis, candidiasis, and bacterial vaginosis. Am J Obstet Gynecol 1990; 163:510–514.

2. Mead PB. Epidemiology of bacterial vaginosis. Am J Obstet Gynecol 1993;169:446–449.

3. Avonts D, Sercu M, Heyerick P, et al. Incidence of uncomplicated genital infections in women using oral contraception or an intrauterine device: a prospective study. Sex Transm Dis 1990;17:23–29.

4. Berger BJ, Kolton S, Zenilman JM, et al. Bacterial vaginosis in lesbians: a sexually transmitted disease. Clin Infect Dis 1995;21:1402–1405.

5. Hawes SE, Hillier SL, Benedetti J, et al. Hydrogen peroxide-producing lactobacilli and acquisition of vaginal infections. J Infect Dis 1996;174:1058–1063.

6. Hillier SL, Nugent RP, Eschenbach DA, et al. Association between bacterial vaginosis and preterm delivery of a low-birth-weight infant. N Engl J Med 1995;333:1737–1742.

7. Schwebke JR, Morgan SC, Weiss HL. The use of sequential self-obtained vaginal smears for detecting changes in the vaginal flora. Sex Transm Dis 1997;24:236–239.

8. McDonald HM, O'Loughlin JA, Vigneswaran R, et al. Impact of metronidazole therapy on preterm birth in women with bacterial vaginosis flora (Gardnerella vaginalis): a randomised, placebo controlled trial. Br J Obstet Gynaecol 1997;104: 1391–1397.

9. Joesoef MR, Schmid GP. Bacterial vaginosis: review of treatment options and potential clinical indications for therapy. Clin Infect Dis 1995; 20(suppl 1):S72–79. Search date 1996; primary sources Medline 1989 to 1996; textbooks about sexually transmitted diseases and information from drug manufacturers relevant pre 1989 material, identified through above search methods.

10. Taha TE, Hoover DR, Dallabetta GA, et al. Bacterial vaginosis and disturbances of vaginal flora: association with increased acquisition of HIV. AIDS 1998;12:1699–1706.

11. Joesoef MR, Schmid GP, Hillier SL. Bacterial vaginosis: review of treatment options and potential clinical indications for therapy. Clin Infect Dis 1999;28(suppl 1):S57–S65. Search date 1992; primary sources Medline 1989 to 1992, textbooks about sexually transmitted diseases and information from drug manufacturers relevant pre-1989 material, identified through above search methods.

12. Greaves WL, Chungafung J, Morris B, et al. Clindamycin versus metronidazole in the treatment of bacterial vaginosis. Obstet Gynecol 1988;72: 799–802.

13. Livengood CH, Soper DE, Sheehan KL, et al. Comparison of once-daily and twice daily dosing of 0.75% metronidazole gel in the treatment of bacterial vaginosis. Sex Transm Dis 1999;26:137–142.

14. Colli E, Landoni M, Parazzini F. Treatment of male partners and recurrence of bacterial vaginosis: a randomised trial. Genitourin Med 1997;73:267–270.

15. Trexler MF, Fraser TG, Jones MP. Fulminant pseudomembranous colitis caused by clindamycin phosphate vaginal cream. Am J Gastroenterol 1997;92:2112–2113.

16. Hillier SL, Lipinski C, Briselden AM, et al. Efficacy of intravaginal 0.75% metronidazole gel for the treatment of bacterial vaginosis. Obstet Gynecol 1993;81:963–967.

17. Schmitt C, Sobel JD, Meriwether C. Bacterial vaginosis: treatment with clindamycin cream versus oral metronidazole. Obstet Gynecol 1992; 79:1020–1023.

18. Ransom SB, McComish JF, Greenberg R, et al. Oral metronidazole vs. Metrogel vaginal for treating bacterial vaginosis. Cost-effectiveness evaluation. J Reprod Med 1999;44:359–362.

19. Brocklehurst P, Hannah M, McDonald H. The management of bacterial vaginosis in pregnancy. In: The Cochrane Library, Issue 1, 2000. Oxford: Update software. Most recent substantive amendment/ search date July 1998; primary sources Cochrane Pregnancy and Childbirth Group Trials Register.

20. Carey JC, Klebanoff MA, Hauth JC, et al. Metronidazole to prevent preterm delivery in pregnant women with asymptomatic bacterial vaginosis. N Eng J Med 2000;342:534–540.

21. McGregor JA, French JI, Jones W, et al. Bacterial vaginosis is associated with prematurity and vaginal fluid mucinase and sialidase: results of a controlled trial of topical clindamycin cream. Am J Obstet Gynecol 1994; 170:1048–1059.

22. Vermeulen GM, Bruinse HW. Prophylactic administration of clindamycin 2% vaginal cream to reduce the incidence of spontaneous preterm birth in women with an increased recurrence risk: a randomized placebo-controlled double-blind trial. Br J Obstet Gynaecol 1999;106:652–657.

23. Hauth JC, Goldberg RL, Andrews WW, et al. Reduced incidence of preterm delivery with metronidazole and erythromycin in women with bacterial vaginosis. N Engl J Med 1995;333: 1732–1736.

24. Mengel MB, Berg AO, Weaver CH, et al. The effectiveness of single-dose metronidazole therapy for patients and their partners with bacterial vaginosis. J Fam Pract 1989;28:163–171.

25. Vejtorp M, Bollerup AC, Vejtorp L, et al. Bacterial vaginosis: a double-blind randomized trial of the effect of treatment of the sexual partner. Br J Obstet Gynecol 1988;95:920–926.

26. Moi H, Erkkola R, Jerve F, et al. Should male consorts of women with bacterial vaginosis be treated? Genitourin Med 1989;65:263–268.

27. Larsson PG, Platz-Christensen JJ, Thejls H, et al. Incidence of pelvic inflammatory disease after first-trimester legal abortion in women with bacterial vaginosis after treatment with metronidazole: a double-blind, randomized study. Am J Obstet Gynecol 1992;166:100–103.

28. Soper DE, Bump RC, Hurt WG. Bacterial vaginosis and trichomoniasis vaginitis are risk factors for cuff cellulitis after abdominal hysterectomy. Am J Obstet Gynecol 1990;163:1016–1021.

29. Watts D, Krohn M, Hillier S, et al. Bacterial vaginosis as a risk factor for postcesarean endometritis. Obstet Gynecol 1990;75:52–58.

M Joesoef
Medical Epidemiologist

George Schmid
Medical Epidemiologist

National Center for HIV, STD
and TB Prevention
Atlanta
USA

Competing interests: None declared.

Genital chlamydial infection

Updated this issue

Nicola Low and Frances Cowan

QUESTIONS

INTERVENTIONS

Key Messages

- Short term microbiological cure is the outcome used in most trials, but this may not mean eradication of *Chlamydia trachomatis*. Long term cure rates have not been studied extensively because of high default rates and difficulty in distinguishing persistent infection from reinfection due to re-exposure.

In men and non-pregnant women

- Evidence, mostly from small RCTs with short term follow up and high withdrawal rates, suggests that multiple dose regimens of tetracyclines (doxycycline, tetracycline) and macrolides (rosaramicin) achieve microbiological cure in at least 95% of people with genital chlamydia. Erythromycin (daily dose 2 g) is likely to be beneficial. Ciprofloxacin is unlikely to be beneficial. We found limited evidence on the effectiveness of other antibiotics. We found no differences in microbiological cure rates between men and women or between those with proven or presumed infection.

- A meta-analysis of short term RCTs has found that a single dose of azithromycin may be as effective in achieving microbiological cure of *C trachomatis* as a 7 day course of doxycycline. Rates of adverse effects were similar.

In pregnant women

- Two systematic reviews of RCTs have found that both amoxicillin and erythromycin are likely to be effective in achieving microbiological cure.

- One small RCT found that clindamycin and erythromycin had a similar effect on cure rates.

- One systematic review of RCTs has found that a single dose of azithromycin is more effective in achieving microbiological cure of C trachomatis than a 7 day course of erythromycin.

DEFINITION	Uncomplicated genital chlamydia is a sexually transmitted infection of the urethra in men and of the endocervix, urethra, or both, in women that has not ascended to the upper genital tract. Infection is asymptomatic in up to 80% of women, but may cause non-specific symptoms, including vaginal discharge and intermenstrual bleeding. Infection in men causes urethral discharge and urethral irritation or dysuria, but may also be asymptomatic in up to half of cases.
INCIDENCE/ PREVALENCE	Genital chlamydia is the commonest bacterial sexually transmitted infection in developed countries. In the USA, over 590 000 cases of chlamydia were reported in 1999.[1] The prevalence of uncomplicated genital chlamydia in women attending general practice surgeries in the UK is reported to be 3–5%.[2] Prevalence is highest in young adults. Reported rates in 15–19 year old women are around 600 per 100 000 in the UK[3] (accessed 10/01/00), 1000 per 100 000 in Sweden[4] and 2000 per 100 000 in the USA.[5]
AETIOLOGY/ RISK FACTORS	Infection is caused by the bacterium Chlamydia trachomatis serotypes D-K. It is transmitted primarily through sexual intercourse.
PROGNOSIS	Untreated chlamydial infection may persist asymptomatically in women for at least 15 months[6] and for an unknown period in men. In women, untreated chlamydial infection that ascends to the upper genital tract causes pelvic inflammatory disease in an estimated 30–40% of women[7] (see pelvic inflammatory disease, p 934). Tubal infertility has been found to occur in about 11% of women after a single episode of pelvic inflammatory disease, and the risk of ectopic pregnancy is increased six- to sevenfold.[8] Ascending infection in men causes epididymitis, but evidence that this causes male infertility is limited.[9] Maternal to infant transmission can lead to neonatal conjunctivitis and pneumonitis in 30–40% of cases.[4] Chlamydia may coexist with other genital infections and may facilitate transmission and acquisition of HIV infection.
AIMS	To eradicate C trachomatis in order to prevent the development of upper genital tract infection, and to prevent further sexual transmissionb with minimal adverse effects of treatment.
OUTCOMES	Microbiological cure rate (calculated as the percentage of people attending a follow up visit at least 1 week after the end of antibiotic treatment who had a negative test for C trachomatis); adverse effects of treatment, including effects on the fetus. Short term microbiological cure may not mean eradication of C trachomatis but long term cure rates have not been studied extensively because of high default rates and difficulty in distinguishing persistent infection from reinfection due to re-exposure.

METHODS   *Clinical Evidence* update search and appraisal May 2000. We considered trials comparing any antibiotic regimen against another antibiotic or placebo in the treatment of laboratory proven *C trachomatis* and of symptoms suggestive of infection if data for participants with proven *C trachomatis* could be extracted. We included all trials reported to be randomised and double blinded, or with blinded outcome assessment. We present the range of cure rates (with exact binomial confidence intervals) or, if there was no evidence of statistical heterogeneity, the summary cure rate (95% confidence intervals) weighted by the standard error. Summary rates do not include cure rates of 100% because the standard error cannot be computed if there are no treatment failures. Where two or more trials compared the same regimens with no evidence of statistical heterogeneity we used a fixed effects model to calculate the summary odds ratio with 95% confidence intervals. Trial quality was assessed in terms of randomisation, blinding, and numbers of withdrawals from analysis.[10] Trials with methodological limitations have been included but relevant problems are mentioned in the text. **Categorising interventions:** We considered a regimen beneficial if the summary cure rate from two or more RCTs was 95% or greater, as previously suggested,[11] and if the lower confidence limit was also above 90%. There were insufficient data to differentiate reinfections from persistent infections. We considered regimens to be likely (or unlikely) to be beneficial based on positive (or negative) results from two or more RCTs, and of unknown effectiveness if there was only one RCT or if results were conflicting.

QUESTION   **What are the effects of antibiotic treatment for men and non-pregnant women with uncomplicated genital chlamydial infection?**

OPTION   MULTIPLE DOSE REGIMENS

Evidence, mostly from small RCTs with short term follow up and high withdrawal rates, suggests that tetracyclines (doxycycline, tetracycline) and macrolides (rosaramicin) achieve microbiological cure in 95% or more cases of genital chlamydia. We found no differences in microbiological cure rates between men and women or between those with proven or presumed infection. We found limited evidence on the effectiveness of other macrolides, quinolones, and penicillins.

Benefits: We found no systematic review. We found 22 RCTs reported to be double blind or with blinded outcome assessment comparing 19 different antibiotic regimens (see table on website www.clinicalevidence.org).[12–33] Results were similar in men and women and in populations with proven and presumed infection, so data were combined. **Doxycycline:** We found 11 RCTs (1434 men and women) comparing doxycycline with another antibiotic.[12–14,16–23] The cure rate was 100% in six trials and the weighted average 98% (96%–99%) in the other five. We found no trials comparing different regimens for doxycycline but the most frequent schedule (in 6 trials) was 100 mg twice daily for 7 days. **Tetracycline:** The summary cure rate in four trials (201 men and women) comparing tetracycline hydrochloride 500 mg four times daily for 7 days versus another antibiotic was 97% (95% CI 94% to 99%).[24–27] Meta-analysis of three trials[25–27] found no significant difference in rates of treatment failure between rosaramicin and tetracycline (OR 1.5, 95% CI 0.5 to 4.4). **Erythromycin:** Cure rates with erythromycin stearate 1 g daily for 7 days (3 trials, 191 participants) ranged from 77–95%,[30–32] and with erythromycin 2 g daily for 7 days (2 trials, 40 participants) from 94–100%.[29–32] **Ciprofloxacin:** In two trials (190 men and women) the cure rate for ciprofloxacin ranged from 63–92%.[20,21] Meta-analysis found that failure of microbiological cure was more frequent with ciprofloxacin than doxycycline (OR 5.0, 95% CI 1.2 to 10.0). A variety of other antibiotics were studied in single trials (see table on website www.clinicalevidence.org).

Harms: Reported adverse effects varied widely between trials but were mostly gastrointestinal (see table on website www.clinicalevidence.org).

Comment: Most trials were conducted in sexually transmitted diseases clinics where follow up is difficult; in 7/14 trials with available data, more than 15% of randomised participants were not included in the analysis.[15,22,29–33] Most trials were small (three had fewer than 40 participants with chlamydia[16,24,29]) and many antibiotic regimens were compared so it is difficult to draw conclusions about relative efficacy. Only five trials reported that sexual partners of participants were offered treatment. Amoxicillin and ampicillin have not been adequately assessed in the treatment of genital chlamydia infection (see table on website www.clinicalevidence.org) because in vitro studies suggest that amoxicillin does not eradicate *C trachomatis*,[34] raising the concern that infection may persist and recrudesce *in vivo*.

| OPTION | SINGLE DOSE VERSUS MULTIPLE DOSE REGIMENS |

A meta-analysis of short term RCTs has found that a single dose of azithromycin may be as effective in achieving microbiological cure of *C trachomatis* as a 7 day course of doxycycline. Rates of adverse effects were similar.

Benefits: We found one systematic review (search date 1990–1996, 9 blinded and unblinded RCTs, n = 1800) comparing azithromycin 1 g as a single dose versus doxycycline 100 mg twice daily for 7 days in participants with proven or presumed genital chlamydia.[35] Data about laboratory diagnosed infection were available for five trials (554 men and women). Cure rates for azithromycin ranged from 90–100% and for doxycycline from 93–100%. Microbiological failure tended to be more frequent with azithromycin than with doxycycline but this did not reach statistical significance (22/301 v 10/253, OR recalculated from data in the paper 1.8, 95% CI 0.9 to 3.9).

Harms: Short term adverse effects of both azithromycin and doxycycline were reported to be mild.

Comment: Azithromycin can be given in a single dose as directly observed therapy. More comparisons of azithromycin and doxycycline are needed to rule out a clinically important difference between them.

QUESTION	What are the effects of treatment for pregnant women with uncomplicated genital chlamydial infection?

OPTION	MULTIPLE DOSE REGIMENS

Two systematic reviews of RCTs have found that both amoxicillin and erythromycin are likely to be effective in achieving microbiological cure of genital chlamydia in pregnant women. One small RCT found that clindamycin and erythromycin had a similar effect on cure rates.

Benefits: We found two systematic reviews (search date 1998),[36] (search date not stated) [37] the most recent of which[36] (11 blinded and unblinded trials, n = 1449) included all studies in the earlier review. **Erythromycin and amoxicillin:** Both achieved high rates of microbiological cure. Greater benefit from amoxicillin did not quite reach significance (cure rates 182/199 [91%] with amoxicillin 500 mg three times daily for seven days, 163/191 [85%] with erythromycin 500 mg four times daily for 7 days, OR for failure of cure with amoxicillin compared with erythromycin 0.54, 95% CI 0.28 to 1.02; with any antibiotic v placebo 0.06, 95% CI 0.03 to 0.12). **Clindamycin:** One small RCT found no significant difference in cure rates between clindamycin and erythromycin (38/41 [93%] v 31/37 [84%]).

Harms: Rates of adverse effects were similar for clindamycin and erythromycin, but adverse effects sufficient to stop treatment were less frequent with amoxicillin than erythromycin (OR 0.16, 95% CI 0.09 to 0.30). None of the trials gave information on adverse clinical outcomes in the offspring.

Comment: We found no long term follow up data.

OPTION	SINGLE VERSUS MULTIPLE DOSE REGIMENS

One systematic review of RCTs has found that, in pregnant women, a single dose of azithromycin is as effective in achieving microbiological cure of C trachomatis as a 7 day course of erythromycin.

Benefits: We found one systematic review (search date 1999, 4 non-blinded RCTs, 290 pregnant women) comparing a single dose of azithromycin 1 g versus erythromycin 500 mg four times daily for 7 days. Failure of microbiological cure was less frequent with azithromycin than erythromycin (11/145 [8%] v 27/145 [19%], OR 0.38, 95% CI 0.19 to 0.74).[36]

Harms: There was no significant difference in the rate of premature delivery (OR 0.73, 95% CI 0.24 to 2.20). Fetal anomaly was reported in one infant in each group. Effects of azithromycin in pregnancy have not been extensively studied. The RCTs found that azithromycin was associated with fewer adverse effects.

Comment: None.

REFERENCES

1. Anonymous. Notifiable diseases/deaths in selected cities weekly information. *MMWR Morb Mortal Wkly Rep* 2000;489510:1183–90.
2. Stokes T. Screening for chlamydia in general practice: a literature review and summary of the evidence [review]. *J Public Health Med* 1997;19: 222–232.
3. http://www.phls.co.uk/facts/chla-inf.htm
4. Holmes KK, Sparling PF, Mardh PA, et al, eds. *Sexually Transmitted Diseases*. 3rd edition. New York: McGraw Hill Inc, 1999.
5. Division of STD Prevention. Sexually Transmitted Disease Surveillance, 1997. U.S. Department of Health and Human Services, Public Health Service. Atlanta. Centers for Disease Control and Prevention (CDC), September 1998.
6. McCormack WM, Alpert S, McComb DE, Nichols RL, Semine DZ, Zinner SH. Fifteen-month follow-up study of women infected with *Chlamydia trachomatis. N Engl J Med* 1979;300:123–125.
7. Cates W, Jr, Rolfs RT, Jr, Aral SO. Sexually transmitted diseases, pelvic inflammatory disease, and infertility: an epidemiologic update. *Epidemiol Rev* 1990;12:199–220.
8. Westrom L, Bengtsson LP, Mardh PA. Incidence, trends, and risks of ectopic pregnancy in a population of women. *BMJ* 1981;282:15–18.
9. Ness RB, Markovic N, Carlson CL, Coughlin MT. Do men become infertile after having sexually transmitted urethritis? An epidemiologic examination [review]. *Fertil Steril* 1997;68:205–213.
10. Chalmers I, Adams M, Dickersin K, et al. A cohort study of summary reports of controlled trials. *JAMA* 1990;263:1401–1405.
11. Clinical Effectiveness Group. National guideline for the management of *Chlamydia trachomatis* genital tract infection. *Sex Transm Infect* 1999;75(suppl 1):4–8
12. Nilsen A, Halsos A, Johansen A, et al. A double blind study of single dose azithromycin and doxycycline in the treatment of chlamydial urethritis in males. *Genitourin Med* 1992;68:325–327.
13. Steingrimsson O, Olafsson JH, Thorarinsson H, Ryan RW, Johnson RB, Tilton RC. Single dose azithromycin treatment of gonorrhea and infections caused by *C trachomatis* and *U urealyticum* in men. *Sex Transm Dis* 1994;21:43–46.
14. Stamm WE, Hicks CB, Martin DH, et al. Azithromycin for empirical treatment of the nongonococcal urethritis syndrome in men. A randomized double-blind study. *JAMA* 1995;274:545–549.
15. Brihmer C, Mardh PA, Kallings I, et al. Efficacy and safety of azithromycin versus lymecycline in the treatment of genital chlamydial infections in women. *Scand J Infect Dis* 1996;28:451–454.
16. Stein GE, Mummaw NL, Havlichek DH. A preliminary study of clarithromycin versus doxycycline in the treatment of nongonococcal urethritis and mucopurulent cervicitis. *Pharmacotherapy* 1995;15:727–731.
17. Romanowski B, Talbot H, Stadnyk M, Kowalchuk P, Bowie WR. Minocycline compared with doxycycline in the treatment of nongonococcal urethritis and mucopurulent cervicitis. *Ann Intern Med* 1993; 119:16–22.
18. Boslego JW, Hicks CB, Greenup R, et al. A prospective randomized trial of ofloxacin vs. doxycycline in the treatment of uncomplicated male urethritis. *Sex Transm Dis* 1988;15:186–191.
19. Phillips I, Dimian C, Barlow D, et al. A comparative study of two different regimens of sparfloxacin versus doxycycline in the treatment of non-gonococcal urethritis in men. *J Antimicrob Chemother* 1996;37(suppl A):123–134.
20. Hooton TM, Rogers ME, Medina TG, et al. Ciprofloxacin compared with doxycycline for nongonococcal urethritis. Ineffectiveness against *Chlamydia trachomatis* due to relapsing infection. *JAMA* 1990;264:1418–1421.
21. Jeskanen L, Karppinen L, Ingervo L, Reitamo S, Happonen HP, Lassus A. Ciprofloxacin versus doxycycline in the treatment of uncomplicated urogenital *Chlamydia trachomatis* infections. A double-blind comparative study. *Scand J Infect Dis Suppl* 1989;60:62–65.
22. McCormack WM, Dalu ZA, Martin DH, et al. Double-blind comparison of trovafloxacin and doxycycline in the treatment of uncomplicated Chlamydial urethritis and cervicitis. Trovafloxacin Chlamydial Urethritis/Cervicitis Study Group. *Sex Transm Dis* 1999;26:531–536.
23. Lassus AB, Virrankoski T, Reitamo SJ, et al. Pivampicillin versus doxycycline in the treatment of chlamydial urethritis in men. *Sex Transm Dis* 1990;17:20–22.
24. Lassus A, Juvakoski T, Kanerva L. Comparison between rifampicin and tetracycline in the treatment of nongonococcal urethritis in males with special reference to *Chlamydia trachomatis. Eur J Sex Transm Dis* 1984;2:15–7.
25. Lassus A, Allgulander C, Juvakoski T. Efficacy of rosaramicin and tetracycline in chlamydia-positive and -negative nongonococcal urethritis. *Eur J Sex Transm Dis* 1982;1:29–31.
26. Juvakoski T, Allgulander C, Lassus A. Rosaramicin and tetracycline treatment in *Chlamydia trachomatis*-positive and -negative nongonococcal urethritis. *Sex Transm Dis* 1981;8:12–15.
27. Brunham RC, Kuo CC, Stevens CE, Holmes KK. Therapy of cervical chlamydial infection. *Ann Intern Med* 1982;97:216–219.
28. Batteiger BE, Zwickl BE, French ML, Jones RB. Women at risk for gonorrhea: comparison of rosaramicin and ampicillin plus probenecid in the eradication of *Neisseria gonorrhoeae, Chlamydia trachomatis* and genital mycoplasmas. *Sex Transm Dis* 1985;12:1–4.
29. Robson HG, Shah PP, Lalonde RG, Hayes L, Senikas VM. Comparison of rosaramicin and erythromycin stearate for treatment of cervical infection with *Chlamydia trachomatis. Sex Transm Dis* 1983;10:130–134.
30. Worm AM, Hoff G, Kroon S, Petersen CS, Christensen JJ. Roxithromycin compared with erythromycin against genitourinary chlamydial infections. *Genitourin Med* 1989;65:35–38.
31. Worm AM, Avnstorp C, Petersen CS. Erythromycin against Chlamydia trachomatis infections. A double blind study comparing 4- and 7-day treatment in men and women. *Dan Med Bull* 1985;32:269–271.
32. Linnemann CCJ, Heaton CL, Ritchey M. Treatment of *Chlamydia trachomatis* infections: comparison of 1- and 2-g doses of erythromycin daily for seven days. *Sex Transm Dis* 1987;14:102–106.
33. Paavonen J, Kousa M, Saikku P, Vartiainen E, Kanerva L, Lassus A. Treatment of nongonococcal urethritis with trimethoprim-sulphadiazine and with placebo. A double-blind partner-controlled study. *Br J Venereal Dis* 1980;56:101–104.
34. Kuo CC, Wang SP, Grayston JT. Antimicrobial activity of several antibiotics and a sulfonamide against *Chlamydia trachomatis* organisms in cell culture. *Antimicrob Agents Chemother* 1977;12: 80–83.

35. Chlamydial STD treatment. *Bandolier* 1996;28: 4–6. Search date 1996; primary source Medline 1990 to 1996. http://www.jr2.ox.ac.uk/bandolier/band28/b28-4.html

36. Brocklehurst P, Rooney G. Interventions for treating genital *Chlamydia trachomatis* infection in pregnancy. In: The Cochrane Library. Issue 4, 1999. Oxford: Update Software. Search date 1998; primary sources Cochrane Pregnancy and Childbirth Review Group Specialised Register of Controlled Trials, and Cochrane Controlled Trials Register.

37. Turrentine MA, Newton ER. Amoxicillin or erythromycin for the treatment of antenatal chlamydial infection: a meta-analysis. *Obstet Gynecol* 1995;86:1021–1025. Search date not stated; primary sources Medline and Cochrane Pregnancy and Childbirth Database.

Nicola Low
Department of Social Medicine
University of Bristol
Bristol
UK

Frances Cowan
Department of Sexually Transmitted
Diseases, Royal Free and University
College Medical School
London
UK

Competing interests: None declared.

Sexual health

INTERVENTIONS

Key Messages

Treating first and recurrent episodes of genital herpes

- RCTs have found that oral antiviral treatment reduces the duration of symptoms, lesions, and viral shedding in first and recurrent episodes of genital herpes, and that daily treatment reduces rates of recurrence and may improve quality of life.

- RCTs have found no evidence of significant differences in effectiveness or adverse events between aciclovir, valaciclovir, and famciclovir.

- We found only limited evidence of an effect of antiviral treatment versus placebo for genital herpes in people with HIV infection.

Preventing transmission of HSV

- Limited evidence from a prospective cohort study suggests that condom use may decrease the risk of sexual transmission of HSV-2. Other interventions aimed at preventing transmission (antiviral treatment and immunisation) have not been adequately studied.

Genital herpes

- The highest risk of mother to baby transmission is in women newly infected with genital herpes in late pregnancy. We found inadequate evaluation of interventions to prevent infection in late pregnancy (such as serological screening and counselling).

- We found that the effect of abdominal delivery on mother to baby transmission has not been adequately evaluated. The procedure carries the risk of increased maternal morbidity and mortality.

- Limited evidence from RCTs suggests that antiviral treatment may reduce the number of pregnant women with genital lesions at term. Since women with genital lesions at term are usually offered abdominal deliveries, antiviral treatment may reduce the rate of abdominal delivery.

DEFINITION	Genital herpes is an infection with herpes simplex virus (HSV) type 1 or 2 (HSV-1 or HSV-2), causing ulceration in the genital area. HSV infections can be defined on the basis of virological and serological findings. Types of infection include: **first episode primary infection**, which is HSV in a person without prior HSV-1 or HSV-2 antibodies; **first episode non-primary infection**, which is HSV-2 in a person with prior HSV-1 antibodies or vice-versa; **first recognised recurrence**, which is HSV-2 (or HSV-1) in a person with prior HSV-2 (or HSV-1) antibodies; and **recurrent genital herpes**, which is caused by reactivation of latent HSV.
INCIDENCE/ PREVALENCE	Genital herpes infections are among the most common sexually transmitted diseases. Seroprevalence studies show that 22% of adults in the USA have HSV-2 antibodies.[1] A UK study found that 23% of adults attending sexual medicine clinics and 7.6% of blood donors in London had antibodies to HSV-2.[2]
AETIOLOGY/ RISK FACTORS	Both HSV-1 and HSV-2 can cause a first episode of genital infection, but HSV-2 is more likely to cause recurrent disease.[3] Most people with HSV-2 infection are not aware that they have genital herpes, as their symptoms are mild. However, these people can pass on the infection to sexual partners and newborns.[4,5]
PROGNOSIS	Sequelae of HSV infection include neonatal HSV, opportunistic infections in immunocompromised people, recurrent genital ulceration, and psychosocial morbidity. HSV-2 infection is associated with an increased risk of HIV transmission and acquisition. The most common neurological complications are aseptic meningitis (reported in about one quarter of women during primary infection) and urinary retention. The absolute risk of neonatal infection is high (41%, 95% CI 26% to 56%) in babies born to women who acquire infection near the time of labour[6,7] and low (< 3%) in women with established infection, even in those who have a recurrence at term. About 15% of neonatal infections result from postnatal transmission from oral lesions.
AIMS	To reduce the morbidity of the first episode, to reduce the risk of recurrent disease after a first episode, and to prevent further transmission, with minimal adverse effects of treatment.
OUTCOMES	Severity and duration of symptoms; healing time; duration of viral shedding; recurrence rates; psychosocial morbidity; rates of transmission; and adverse effects of treatment.

METHODS   *Clinical Evidence* update search and appraisal May 2000, using the terms herpes simplex virus, aciclovir, valaciclovir, famciclovir, cidofovir, trifluridine, and neonatal herpes. We also included preliminary results of clinical trials published in the abstracts of the Interscience Conference on Antimicrobial Agents and Chemotherapy and International Society for STD Research. We also contacted experts in the field and manufacturers of antiviral drugs to identify completed studies that were undergoing peer review, but which had not yet been published.

QUESTION   What are the effects of antiviral treatment in people with a first episode of genital herpes?

RCTs have found that oral antiviral treatment decreases the duration of lesions, symptoms, and viral shedding, and prevents neurological complications in people with first episode genital herpes. Oral treatment is more convenient than intravenous and more effective than topical treatment. Limited data provide no evidence that oral antiviral treatment reduces the rate of recurrence compared with placebo. RCTs have found no evidence of a significant difference between aciclovir, valaciclovir, and famciclovir.

Benefits: We found no systematic review. **Immediate effects:** We found several RCTs (350 men and women) of oral aciclovir for the treatment of first episode genital herpes. Compared with placebo, aciclovir (200 mg five times daily) decreased the duration of viral shedding (2 *v* 10 days), pain (5 *v* 7 days), time to healing of lesions (8 *v* 14 days), and prevented formation of new lesions. Neurological complications (aseptic meningitis and urinary retention) were also reduced. Numbers were small so no firm estimates of effectiveness were available.[8–12] **Different regimens:** In one international trial of 643 healthy adults with first episode genital herpes, oral valaciclovir (1000 mg twice daily) was compared with oral aciclovir (200 mg five times daily) for 10 days.[13] No significant differences were noted between the two medications in terms of any clinical or virological variables. Another RCT evaluated three different doses of oral famciclovir (125 mg, 250 mg, or 500 mg three times daily) versus oral aciclovir (200 mg five times daily) in 951 adults with first episode genital herpes.[14] No significant differences were found. **Recurrence rates:** A meta-analysis review of two small placebo controlled RCTs (61 people) found no significant difference in time to recurrence or frequency of recurrence between those given oral aciclovir and those given placebo.[15] **Systemic versus topical treatment:** We found no direct randomised comparisons of oral, intravenous, or topical antiviral treatment. Comparison of results from different trials performed at one institution suggests that systemic treatment is more effective than topical.[16]

Harms: Adverse effects (mostly headache and nausea) were rare and frequency was similar for aciclovir, valaciclovir, famciclovir, and placebo.

Comment: Oral aciclovir has the advantage of convenience over intravenous aciclovir.[16]

QUESTION What interventions reduce the impact of recurrence?

OPTION ANTIVIRAL TREATMENT AT THE START OF RECURRENCE

RCTs have found that oral antiviral treatment taken at the start of a recurrence reduces the duration of lesions, symptoms, and viral shedding in people with recurrent genital herpes.

Benefits: We found one systematic review (search date 1997; 4 RCTs; 3393 people).[17] **Famciclovir versus placebo:** One trial (467 people with recurrent genital herpes) found that oral famciclovir (125–500 mg twice daily) significantly reduced the duration of lesions (5 v 4 days) and viral shedding (3 v 2 days) compared with placebo. **Valaciclovir versus placebo:** Another trial (987 people with recurrent genital herpes) found that self initiated oral valaciclovir (500 mg or 1000 mg twice daily) for 5 days decreased the episode duration (4 v 6 days) and viral shedding (2 v 4 days), and increased the rate of aborted recurrences (31% v 21%) compared with placebo. **Valaciclovir versus aciclovir:** The other two RCTs (1939 people) found no significant difference between oral valaciclovir and aciclovir. **Aciclovir versus placebo:** Several RCTs on more than 650 healthy adults with recurrent genital herpes were identified in a non-systematic review published in 1990.[18] These evaluated 5 days of oral aciclovir (200 mg five times daily or 800 mg twice daily), started at the first sign of recurrence. Compared with placebo, treatment decreased the period of viral shedding (1 v 2 days) and duration of lesions (5 v 6 days).

Harms: Adverse effects (mostly headache and nausea) were rare and frequency was similar for aciclovir, valaciclovir, famciclovir, and placebo.

Comment: The benefit was found to be greater if the person with recurrent herpes initiated treatment at the first symptom or sign of a recurrence.[19] People can learn to recognise recurrences early on and should have an adequate supply of medication at home.

OPTION DAILY MAINTENANCE ANTIVIRAL TREATMENT

RCTs have found that daily maintenance treatment with oral antiviral agents reduces the frequency of recurrences and viral shedding in people with genital herpes. Daily treatment may also improve psychosocial function.

Benefits: **Recurrence rates:** We found one systematic review (search date 1997; 4 RCTs).[17] Two trials evaluated treatment for 1 year. In one trial (1479 people), freedom from recurrence was reported in 40–50% of people who received valaciclovir (500 mg or 1000 mg once daily), valaciclovir (250 mg twice daily), or aciclovir (400 mg twice daily) compared with 5% who received placebo.[20] In the other trial (455 people), the median time to first recurrence was 11 months with famciclovir (250 mg twice daily) and 1.5 months with placebo.[21] One non-systematic review (published in 1990) identified several placebo controlled RCTs of aciclovir.[18] Most participants had a history of frequent recurrence (six or more a year). Daily aciclovir was associated with reduced recurrence rate (74–93%) and duration of recurrences (3.5 v 5 days).[18] Of 210 adults in one trial who completed 5 years of continuous treatment with aciclovir (400 mg twice daily), 53–70% were free of recurrence each year.[22] The first year of this trial was a double blind placebo controlled RCT in 1146 adults. Those on aciclovir had significantly fewer recurrences during the first year (1.7 v 12.5, P < 0.0001). **Viral shedding:** We found one RCT that evaluated the effect of daily maintenance treatment on viral shedding in women with recently acquired genital HSV-2 infection. Participants obtained swabs for viral cultures daily for 70 days while receiving aciclovir (400 mg twice daily) or placebo.[23] Viral shedding was reduced by 95% with aciclovir on days with reported lesions and by 94% on days without lesions. **Psychosocial morbidity:** We found one RCT (1479 people) that evaluated the effect of daily oral antiviral treatment on a genital herpes quality of life scale.[24] Participants receiving daily aciclovir or valaciclovir had significantly greater mean improvements from baseline than those receiving placebo.[25]

Harms: Daily treatment with aciclovir, famciclovir, and valaciclovir was well tolerated. People taking aciclovir have been followed for up to 7 years, and those taking famciclovir and valaciclovir for up to 1 year. Nausea and headache were infrequent, and participants rarely discontinued treatment because of adverse effects. We found no studies evaluating whether daily maintenance treatment increases high risk sexual behaviour. We found no evidence that daily treatment with aciclovir results in emergence of aciclovir resistant HSV during or after cessation of treatment in healthy adults.[26]

Comment: Viral shedding is an intermediate outcome, but may be important to people with herpes as it reflects the risk of transmitting infection.

| OPTION | PSYCHOTHERAPY |

We found that the effects of psychotherapy on the rate of genital herpes recurrence have not yet been adequately studied.

Benefits: We found one systematic review (search date 1991), which identified six poor quality studies of psychotherapeutic interventions in 69 participants (4 studies had < 10 participants).[27] Interventions varied from hypnotherapy and progressive muscle relaxation to cognitive therapy and multifaceted intervention. In the largest study, 31 people with four or more recurrences a year were randomly assigned to psychosocial intervention, social support, or waiting list. Participants receiving psychosocial intervention had significantly lower recurrence rates (6 recurrences a year) compared with the pretreatment frequency (11 a year), and with the other groups (11 a year).

Harms: No adverse effects were noted.

Comment: Small numbers of people, inadequate controls, and subjective and retrospective assessment of recurrence frequency at baseline, limit the usefulness of these studies. Controlled studies that include prospective clinical evaluation of disease activity are needed.

QUESTION   What interventions prevent transmission of HSV?

OPTION   CONDOMS, ANTIVIRAL TREATMENT, IMMUNISATION

Limited evidence from a non-randomised study suggests that condom use may decrease the risk of sexual transmission of HSV-2. Other interventions have not been adequately studied.

Benefits: **Condoms:** We found no RCTs. In a prospective study of 528 couples discordant for HSV-2 infection, the use of condoms was associated with lower risk of HSV-2 acquisition (adjusted RR of acquiring HSV infection when using condoms in less than versus more than 25% of sexual acts was 3.9, 95% CI 1.1 to 13.6). Only 61% of couples ever used condoms during the study and only 7.6% used them consistently. One person acquired HSV-2 despite consistent condom use (A Wald et al, personal communication, 1999).[28] **Antiviral treatment:** We found no direct evidence that treatment reduces HSV transmission in serologically discordant couples. However, RCTs have shown that daily antiviral treatment decreases the frequency of clinical and subclinical viral shedding (see text, p 904). **Immunisation:** No effective vaccines are currently available.

Harms: As for individual interventions.

Comment: Controlled trials of condoms for prevention of HSV-2 transmission are unlikely to be done. Even with routine counselling, many couples do not regularly use condoms.

OPTION   ABDOMINAL DELIVERY TO PREVENT NEONATAL HERPES

We found insufficient evidence for the effect of abdominal delivery on the risk of neonatal herpes. The procedure carries the risk of increased maternal morbidity and mortality.

Benefits: We found no systematic review and no RCTs that assessed the effects of abdominal delivery on the risk of mother to child transmission of HSV. In the Netherlands, women with recurrent genital herpes at delivery have been allowed vaginal birth since 1987. This policy has not resulted in an increase of neonatal herpes: 26 cases from 1981–1986, and 19 cases from 1987–1991.[7]

Harms: Abdominal delivery is associated with significant maternal morbidity and mortality. It has been estimated that, for every two neonatal deaths from HSV infection prevented by abdominal delivery, one maternal death may be caused.[29]

Comment: Countries vary in their approach to obstetric management of women with recurrent genital herpes at term. In the USA and the UK, these women are advised to undergo abdominal delivery, with its attendant risks to the mother. The absolute risk of neonatal infection is high (AR 41%, 95% CI 26% to 56%) in babies born to women who acquire infection near the time of labour[6,7] and low (AR < 3%) in women with established infection, even in those who have recurrence at term. Most women who acquire infection towards the end of pregnancy are undiagnosed and most cases of neonatal HSV infection are acquired from women without a history of genital herpes. The available evidence suggests that efforts to prevent neonatal HSV infection should focus on preventing the acquisition of infection in late pregnancy.

OPTION ANTIVIRAL TREATMENT DURING PREGNANCY

We found limited evidence from a systematic review of RCTs suggesting that aciclovir reduces the rate of genital lesions at term in women with first or recurrent episodes of genital HSV during pregnancy. We found that adverse effects have not been adequately studied.

Benefits: We found one systematic review (published 1998). This identified three studies, including two RCTs, of daily aciclovir versus placebo in 210 pregnant women near term with genital herpes.[7] The studies differed in terms of the dose and duration of aciclovir and the populations enrolled. Abdominal delivery was performed in women with genital lesions at term. All three studies found lower rates of abdominal delivery in women treated with aciclovir, although in one study this effect was not significant (8% v 34%, P = 0.02; 13% v 33%, P = 0.03; and 13% v 25%, P = 0.2).

Harms: No adverse effects for women or newborns were reported, but the number of women was small. Rare adverse events, such as an increase in asymptomatic viral shedding or aciclovir related obstructive uropathy in the newborns, would be difficult to detect.

Comment: None.

OPTION SEROLOGICAL SCREENING AND COUNSELLING TO PREVENT ACQUISITION OF HSV DURING PREGNANCY

We found insufficient evidence about the effects of serological screening and counselling during pregnancy on infection rates.

Benefits: We found no systematic review or RCTs that assessed either serological screening with type specific assays to identify women at risk for HSV acquisition in late pregnancy, or counselling to avoid genital–genital and oral–genital contact in late pregnancy.

Harms: We found insufficient evidence.

Comment: None.

QUESTION What are the effects of treatments in people with genital herpes and HIV infection? New

OPTION ANTIVIRAL TREATMENTS

We found only limited evidence of the effect of antiviral treatment for genital herpes in people with HIV infection. However, evidence from other settings suggests that antivirals may be effective treatment of genital herpes in immunocompromised people.

Benefits: We found no systematic review and no RCTs on the treatment of the first episode of genital herpes in people with HIV infection. **Treatment of recurrence:** We found two RCTs. One (193 people on stable anti-retroviral therapy) compared famciclovir (500 mg twice daily) with aciclovir (400 mg five times daily) for 1 week.[30] No difference was found between the two drugs in mucocutaneous recurrence of HSV. The other (467 people) compared valaciclovir (1 g twice daily) to aciclovir (200 mg five times daily) for 5 days.[31] No differences between the two drugs were found. **Prevention of recurrence:** We found two RCTs. One crossover RCT (48 people with antibodies to HIV and HSV; 38 with a history of genital herpes) compared famciclovir with placebo over 8 weeks.[32] The conclusions of this study are difficult to interpret (see comment below). The other RCT (1062 people with a median CD4 count of 320/mm^3) compared valaciclovir (500 mg twice daily) versus valaciclovir (1000 mg once daily) versus aciclovir (400 mg twice daily) over one year.[33] Neither valaciclovir dose differed significantly from aciclovir, but recurrence was less likely with valaciclovir (500 mg twice daily) than with the valaciclovir (1000 mg once daily) group (82% v 71% recurrence free at 48 weeks, P < 0.05).

Harms: Adverse effects (mostly headache and nausea) occurred with similar frequency with aciclovir, valaciclovir, and famciclovir. Thrombotic microangiopathy, which has been reported in patients receiving valaciclovir (8 g daily), has not been reported among 713 HIV-infected persons who received oral valaciclovir in daily doses ranging from 250 to 1000 mg for up to 1 year (A Wald, 2000, personal communication).

Comment: Three of the four RCTs did not have a placebo control. Most studies to date have compared new treatments with aciclovir, rather than placebo. The crossover trial of famciclovir versus placebo is difficult to interpret because the dropout rate was high. Although we found only limited evidence of an effect of antivirals for treatment of genital herpes in people with HIV infection, there is a consensus that antiviral treatment may be helpful, based on evidence from immunocompromised people who do not have HIV. Aciclovir has been found effective in immunocompromised populations. With the availability of effective treatments for HIV, trials of antiviral (anti-HSV) versus placebo may now be done. A trial of valaciclovir versus placebo is now in progress (A Wald, 2000, personal communication). In HIV infected people, there is a markedly increased rate of HSV viral shedding.[34] HIV has been recovered from genital herpes lesions.[35] We found no evidence about the effect of daily antiviral therapy on transmission of HIV to sexual partners.

REFERENCES

1. Fleming DT, McQuillan GM, Johnson RE, et al. Herpes simplex virus type 2 in the United States, 1976 to 1994. N Engl J Med 1997;337:1105–1111.

2. Cowan FM, Johnson AM, Ashley R, et al. Antibody to herpes simplex virus type 2 as serological marker of sexual lifestyle in populations. BMJ 1994;309:1325–1329.

3. Benedetti J, Corey L, Ashley R. Recurrence rates in genital herpes after symptomatic first-episode infection. Ann Intern Med 1994;121:847–854.

4. Mertz GJ, Schmidt O, Jourden JL, et al. Frequency of acquisition of first-episode genital infection with herpes simplex virus from symptomatic and asymptomatic source contacts. Sex Transm Dis 1985;12:33–39.

5. Whitley RJ, Kimberlin DW, Roizman B. Herpes simplex viruses. Clin Infect Dis 1998;26:541–553.

6. Brown ZA, Selke SA, Zeh J, et al. Acquisition of herpes simplex virus during pregnancy. N Engl J Med 1997;337:509–515.

7. Smith J, Cowan, FM, Munday P. The management of herpes simplex virus infection in pregnancy. Br J Obstet Gynaecol 1998;105:255–268. Search date 1996; primary source Medline.

8. Nilsen AE, Aasen T, Halsos AM, et al. Efficacy of oral acyclovir in treatment of initial and recurrent genital herpes. Lancet 1982;2:571–573.

9. Corey L, Fife K, Benedetti JK, et al. Intravenous acyclovir for the treatment of primary genital herpes. Ann Int Med 1983;98:914–921.

10. Mertz G, Critchlow C, Benedetti J, et al. Double-blind placebo-controlled trial of oral acyclovir in the first episode genital herpes simplex virus infection. *JAMA* 1984;252:1147–1151.

11. Mindel A, Adler MW, Sutherland S, et al. Intravenous acyclovir treatment for primary genital herpes. *Lancet* 1982;2:697–700.

12. Bryson YJ, Dillon M, Lovett M, et al. Treatment of first episodes of genital herpes simplex virus infections with oral acyclovir: a randomized double-blind controlled trial in normal subjects. *N Engl J Med* 1983;308:916–1920.

13. Fife KH, Barbarash RA, Rudolph T, et al. Valaciclovir versus acyclovir in the treatment of first-episode genital herpes infection: results of an international, multicenter, double-blind randomized clinical trial. *Sex Trans Dis* 1997;24: 481–486.

14. Loveless M, Harris W, Sacks S. Treatment of first episode genital herpes with famciclovir. *Programs and abstracts of the 35th Interscience Conference on Antimicrobial Agents and Chemotherapy.* San Francisco, California, 1995.

15. Corey L, Mindel A, Fife KH, et al. Risk of recurrence after treatment of first episode genital herpes with intravenous acyclovir. *Sex Trans Dis* 1985;12:215–218.

16. Corey L, Benedetti J, Critchlow C, et al. Treatment of primary first-episode genital herpes simplex virus infections with acyclovir: results of topical, intravenous and oral therapy. *J Antimicrob Chemother* 1983;12(suppl B):79–88.

17. Wald A. New therapies and prevention strategies for genital herpes. *Clin Infect Dis* 1999;28:S4–13. Search date not stated; primary source Medline.

18. Stone K, Whittington W. Treatment of genital herpes. *Rev Infect Dis* 1990;12(suppl 6):610–619.

19. Reichman RC, Badger GJ, Mertz GJ, et al. Treatment of recurrent genital herpes simplex infections with oral acyclovir: a controlled trial. *JAMA* 1984;251:2103–2107.

20. Reitano M, Tyring S, Lang W, et al. Valaciclovir for the suppression of recurrent genital herpes simplex virus infection: a large-scale dose range finding study. *J Infect Dis* 1998;178:603–610.

21. Diaz-Mitoma F, Sibbald RG, Shafran SD. Oral famciclovir for the suppression of recurrent genital herpes: a randomized controlled trial. *JAMA* 1998; 280:887–892.

22. Goldberg L, Kaufman R, Kurtz T, et al. Continuous five-year treatment of patients with frequently recurring genital herpes simplex virus infection with acyclovir. *J Med Virol* 1993(suppl 1);45–50.

23. Wald A, Zeh J, Barnum G, et al. Suppression of subclinical shedding of herpes simplex virus type 2 with acyclovir. *Ann Intern Med* 1996;124:8–15.

24. Doward LC, McKenna SP, Kohlmann T, et al. The international development of the RGHQoL: a quality of life measure for recurrent genital herpes. *Qual Life Res* 1998;7:143–153.

25. Patel R, Tyring S, Strand A, et al. Impact of suppressive antiviral therapy on the health related quality of life of patients with recurrent genital herpes infection. *Sex Trans Infect* 1999;75:398–402.

26. Fife KH, Crumpacker CS, Mertz GJ. Recurrence and resistance patterns of herpes simplex virus following cessation of ≥ 6 years of chronic suppression with acyclovir. *J Infect Dis* 1994;169: 1338–1341.

27. Longo D, Koehn K. Psychosocial factors and recurrent genital herpes: a review of prediction and psychiatric treatment studies. *Int J Psychiatry Med* 1993;23:99–117. Search date 1991; primary sources Psychological Abstracts, Medline and hand searches of referee lists.

28. Corey L, Langenberg AG, Ashley R, et al. Recombinant glycoprotein vaccine for the prevention of genital HSV-2 infection: two randomized controlled trials. Chiron HSV Vaccine Study Group. *JAMA* 1999;282:331–340.

29. Randolph A, Washington A, Prober C. Cesarean delivery for women presenting with genital herpes lesions. *JAMA* 1993;270:77–82.

30. Romanowski B. Efficacy and safety of famciclovir for the treatment of HSV infections in HIV+ patients. Update '98: Clinical Management of Viral Infections. Whistler, BC Canada, 1998.

31. Schacker T, International Valaciclovir Study Group. Valaciclovir as acute treatment for recurrent ano-genital herpes in immunocompromised (HIV positive) individuals. 13th International Society for STD Research. Denver, Colorado, 1999.

32. Schacker T, Hu HL, Koelle DM et al. Famciclovir for the suppression of symptomatic and asymptomatic herpes simplex virus reactivation in HIV-infected persons. A double-blind, placebo-controlled trial. *Ann Intern Med* 1998;128(1):21–28.

33. Gold J, Bell A, and the Valaciclovir International HSV Study Group. Valaciclovir prevents herpes simplex virus recurrences in HIV-infected individuals – a double-blind controlled trial. *Programs and abstracts of the 20th International Congress of Chemotherapy.* Sydney, Australia, 1997.

34. Schacker T, Zeh J, Hu HL, et al. Frequency of symptomatic and asymptomatic HSV-2 reactivations among HIV-infected men. *J Infect Dis* 1998;178:1616–1622.

35. Schacker T, Ryncarz A, Goddard J, et al. Frequent recovery of HIV from genital herpes simplex virus lesions in HIV infected persons. *JAMA* 1998;280: 61–66.

Anna Wald
Assistant Professor of Medicine and
Epidemiology
University of Washington
Seattle
USA

Competing interests: The author has received a fee from Glaxo Wellcome, SmithKline Beecham, Wyeth Lederle Vaccines and Paediatrics, Bristol Myers Squibb for research support, and from Glaxo Wellcome for consultancy.

Updated this issue

DJ Wiley and Karl Beutner

INTERVENTIONS

Key Messages

- We found five treatments that were compared with placebo. Podophyllotoxin, imiquimod, and intralesional interferon have been found to be significantly more effective in the clearance of warts compared with placebo, but data on recurrence are lacking. Placebo controlled RCTs of topical interferon give conflicting results, and those of systemic interferon show no evidence of benefits.

- We found no RCTs comparing placebo with cryotherapy, electrosurgery, surgical excision, or laser surgery.

- We found no clear evidence that one treatment is superior to another.

- Topical 5-fluorouracil, and bi- and trichloroacetic acid have not been adequately evaluated.

- We found no evidence that treatment of external genital warts decreases infectivity, and the preventive effects of condoms have not been adequately evaluated.

DEFINITION	External genital warts are benign epidermal growths on the external perianal and perigenital region. There are four morphological types: condylomatous, keratotic, papular, and flat warts.
INCIDENCE/ PREVALENCE	In 1996, external and internal genital warts accounted for over 180 000 initial visits to private physicians' offices in the USA, about 60 000 fewer than were reported for 1995.[1] In the USA, 1% of sexually active men and women aged 18–49 years are estimated to have external genital warts.[2]
AETIOLOGY/ RISK FACTORS	External genital warts are caused by the human papillomavirus (HPV). Although more than 70 types of HPV have been identified, most external genital warts in immunocompetent people are caused by HPV types 6 and 11.[3,4] HPV infections and, more specifically, external genital warts are sexually transmissible.
PROGNOSIS	Clinical trials found that recurrences are frequent and may necessitate repeated treatment. Without treatment, external genital warts may remain unchanged, may increase in size or number, or may completely resolve. They rarely, if ever, progress to cancer.[5] Juvenile laryngeal papillomatosis, a rare and sometimes life threatening condition, occurs in children of women with a history of genital warts. Its rarity makes it hard to design studies that can evaluate whether treatment in pregnant women alters the risk.[6,7]
AIMS	To eliminate symptomatic warts from the external genitalia, to prevent recurrence, and to avoid sequelae, with minimal adverse effects.
OUTCOMES	Wart clearance (generally accepted as complete eradication of warts from the treated area); recurrence; sequelae; adverse effects of treatment; quality of life; transmission.
METHODS	*Clinical Evidence* update search and appraisal from 1985 to May 2000. We also performed selected Medline searches for papers published before 1985. Other data came from abstract booklets, conference proceedings, references identified from bibliographies of pertinent articles and books, and manufacturers of therapeutic agents. This review is limited to systematic reviews of RCTs and subsequent RCTs, unless no RCTs were found for a particular treatment. This limitation may have biased the review in favour of newer and heavily marketed treatments.

QUESTION   What are the effects of non-surgical treatments?

OPTION   PODOPHYLLOTOXIN

RCTs have found that podophyllotoxin is more effective than placebo.

Benefits: We found no systematic review. **Versus placebo:** Data from eight placebo controlled RCTs in a total of 1035 people found that, within 16 weeks of treatment, podophyllotoxin was more effective than placebo (wart clearance occurred in 45–77% of people on treatment; RR of clearance v placebo between 2.0, 95% CI 0.9 to 4.3,[8] and 48, 95% CI 3.0 to 773).[9–15] **Recurrence rates:** RCTs of 0.5% cream or solution found recurrence rates ranging from 4%[15] to 33%.[9] One RCT in 57 people of 0.5% podophyllotoxin solution as prophylaxis against recurrence of external genital warts (initially treated in an open label study) found fewer recurrences among people taking placebo.[16] **Versus podophyllin:** Five RCTs compared podophyllotoxin versus podophyllin.[17–21] They found no significant difference in wart clearance (RRs for podophyllin v podophyllotoxin between 0.7, 95% CI 0.4 to 1.12 and 1.7, 95% CI 0.9 to 3.2[20]). One RCT used a 2% solution in a limited study of self treatment for penile warts and found no significant difference with podophyllotoxin versus podophyllin (RR for podophyllin v podophyllotoxin 0.6, 95% CI 0.3 to 1.3).[21]

Harms: Safety during pregnancy is unknown. Podophyllotoxin does not contain the mutagenic flavonoid compounds, quercetin and kaempherol, that are contained in podophyllin resin preparations.[22] Local inflammation or irritation, erosion, burning, pain, and itching are reported in most trials. Balanoposthitis,[23,24] dyspareunia, bleeding, scarring, and insomnia are reported rarely.[8] One large RCT reported burning and inflammation in 75% and bleeding in 25% of treated people.[12] Although rare, preputial tightening has been reported.[17]

Comment: RCTs examined the efficacy of podophyllotoxin solutions more often than cream preparations, but cream or gel preparations may be easier to apply than solutions. This and other differences may cause variable efficacy.

OPTION   IMIQUIMOD

RCTs have found that imiquimod is more effective at clearing warts than placebo.

Benefits: We found no systematic review. **Versus placebo:** We found two RCTs in a total of 968 people. Wart clearance within 3 months occurred twice as often with 1% cream as placebo (clearance rate 37–56% with imiquimod v 0–56% with placebo; RR 1.9, 95% CI 1.1 to 3.3).[25,26] For 5% cream, clearance was 13 times greater than with placebo (RR 13, 95% CI 4.2 to 40.2.[26] **Recurrence:** No recurrences were reported in people using 1% cream, but recurrences were reported in 13–19% of participants treated with 5% cream.[25,26] This compared to 10% among placebo treated participants in one study.[25]

Harms: One RCT reported local itching, erythema, and burning in more than 15% of people, and irritation, tenderness, ulceration, and pain in less than 10%.[26]

Comment: None.

OPTION   CRYOTHERAPY

RCTs have found that cryotherapy is as effective as podophyllin at clearing warts, trichloroacetic acid, and electrosurgery. We found no trials comparing cryotherapy with placebo. One RCT found that recurrence rates were similar after cryotherapy and electrosurgery. Cryotherapy has been used successfully in pregnancy.

Benefits: We found no systematic review. **Versus placebo:** We found no RCTs. **Versus other treatments:** We found six comparative RCTs:

two compared cryotherapy plus interferon versus cryotherapy alone;[27,28] the other four compared cryotherapy versus podophyllin,[29] trichloroacetic acid,[30,31] or electrosurgery.[29,32] **Clearance:** Four RCTs reported 63–88% clearance 3 months or more after cryotherapy.[29–32] Although one trial found cryotherapy was more effective than podophyllin after six treatments (RR of wart clearance compared with podophyllin 1.9, 95% CI 1.4 to 2.6), there was no significant difference in wart clearance 3 months after treatment (RR 1.4, 95% CI 0.9 to 2.2), suggesting merely a difference in speed of effect.[29] Two of the trials found no significant difference between cryotherapy and trichloroacetic acid at the end of treatment or 3 months later (RRs 1.1, 95% CI 0.8 to 1.5,[30] and 0.9, 95% CI 0.8 to 1.1[31]). Two trials found that electrosurgery was slightly more effective than cryotherapy (RRs of wart clearance with electrosurgery v cryotherapy at the end of treatment: 1.2, 95% CI 1.1 to 1.3, and after 3 months 1.4, 95% CI 1.0 to 2.0).[29,32] **Recurrence:** One trial found no significant difference in recurrence rates between cryotherapy and electrosurgery (21% v 22%).[29]

Harms: Discomfort, ulceration, and scabbing were reported in nearly a fifth of people after cryotherapy.[29,32] One RCT reported local infection in one of 86 people taking cryotherapy versus none of 149 people taking podophyllin resin or electrosurgery.[29]

Comment: One case series of 34 pregnant women who received three or fewer treatments of cryotherapy found no subsequent infection or premature rupture of membranes.[33]

OPTION	PODOPHYLLIN

RCTs have found that podophyllin resin is as effective as most other treatments, but is less effective than surgical excision. We found no trials comparing podophyllin with placebo.

Benefits: We found no systematic review. **Versus placebo:** We found no RCTs. **Versus other treatments:** We found 13 RCTs: four compared podophyllin versus podophyllotoxin,[17–20] one versus cryotherapy,[28] one versus electrosurgery,[29] three with and without interferon,[34–36] one with and without trichloroacetic acid,[37] two versus surgical excision,[37,38] and two compared alternative doses of podophyllin.[39] **Clearance:** None of the four trials comparing podophyllin with podophyllotoxin found a significant difference in wart clearance (RRs ranging between 0.7, 95% CI 0.4 to 1.1[18] and 1.7, 95% CI 0.9 to 3.2[20]). The trials comparing cryotherapy or electrosurgery versus podophyllin found no significant difference 3 months after treatment (RR for both comparison treatments 1.4, 95% CI 0.9 to 2.1).[29] One RCT found that podophyllin and intralesional interferon together were more effective than podophyllin alone for clearance 3 weeks after treatment (RR 2.0, 95% CI 1.1 to 3.6), however, it found no significant difference at 11 weeks (RR 2.3 95% CI 0.9 to 5.8).[35] Two RCTs found that podophyllin was less effective than surgical excision (RRs 0.3, 95% CI 0.2 to 0.7; and 0.5, 95% CI 0.2 to 0.9).[37,38] **Recurrence:** Two RCTs found that recurrence was more frequent with podophyllin versus surgical excision (60–65% v 19–29% after surgery).[37,38]

Harms: Eight RCTs reported pain, erythema, irritation, and tenderness in 3–17% of participants treated with podophyllin.[17,18,20,29,34,35,37,38] Skin burns (1–3%[37,38]), bleeding (4%[38]), and erosion or ulcerations (1%[18]–11%[34]) were also reported. Faecal incontinence (4%[38]) and preputial tightening (1%[17]) were reported rarely.

Comment: Safety during pregnancy is unknown. Podophyllin may contain the mutagenic flavonoid compounds, quercetin and kaempherol.[22]

OPTION BI- AND TRICHLOROACETIC ACID

We found inadequate evidence to evaluate the efficacy of bi- and trichloroacetic acid.

Benefits: We found no systematic review. **Versus placebo:** We found no RCTs. **Versus other treatments:** We found two RCTs comparing trichloroacetic acid versus cryotherapy in 192 participants. These found no significant difference in wart clearance (RRs of trichloroacetic acid v cryotherapy 1.1, 95% CI 0.8 to 1.5 and 0.9, 95% CI 0.8 to 1.1).[30,31] We also reviewed one RCT in 73 people comparing trichloroacetic acid plus podophyllin versus podophyllin alone.[40] Participants were followed for 3 months. The trial found no significant difference in wart clearance between the two groups.

Harms: Insufficient data are available to comment on possible harms.

Comment: Small numbers of participants and inadequate study designs make it difficult to evaluate effectiveness. In pregnant women, only case series are available: 31 of 32 pregnant women treated with trichloroacetic acid showed wart clearance, and 2 of 31 showed recurrence.[41] The evidence is inadequate to evaluate adverse effects of trichloroacetic acid in pregnancy.

OPTION TOPICAL INTERFERON

Three RCTs found increased wart clearance with topical interferon versus placebo.

Benefits: We found no systematic review. **Versus placebo:** We found three RCTs in 223 men and women. Complete wart clearance 4 weeks after treatment occurred in more people using interferon versus placebo (6% v 3%, no P value given;[42] 73% v 10%, P < 0.0001;[43] 90% v 20%, no P value given[11]). About a third of each group in the first study had cleared their warts by 16 weeks.[42] Recurrence rates were not evaluated. **Versus podophyllotoxin:** One of the trials also compared topical interferon versus podophyllotoxin, and found that interferon was significantly more effective than podophyllotoxin about 4 weeks after treatment (RR compared with podophyllotoxin 1.5, 95% CI 1.03 to 1.63).[11] **As adjuvant to other treatment:** One RCT compared recombinant β interferon at two doses plus CO_2 laser versus CO_2 laser alone, electrotherapy, and liquid nitrogen. Recurrences occurred in 62% of participants (21/36) treated with 1 million IU interferon, in 54% (19/35) treated with 150 000 IU interferon, and 75% (27/36) treated with placebo.[44]

Harms: One placebo controlled study reported local burning and itching in 39% of treated people.[42] Another RCT reported fever, headache, and itching in 18% of people treated with interferon.[11]

Comment: Differences in the RCTs' findings may be attributable to the preparations used; one preparation was incorporated into a methyl cellulose aqueous base[42] and the other was instilled into a cream base.[11]

OPTION INTRALESIONAL INJECTION OF INTERFERON

RCTs have found that intralesional injection of interferon is more effective than placebo.

Benefits: We found no systematic review. We found eight placebo controlled trials,[45–53] and one RCT comparing interferon plus podophyllin versus podophyllin alone (1000 people).[35] Doses and follow up intervals varied. Two of the placebo controlled RCTs randomised treatment to lesions rather than to people.[48,50] Complete wart clearance was reported in 17–63% of participants on intralesional interferon within 8–20 weeks of treatment. **Versus placebo:** In studies using 1 MU/ml, intralesional interferon was between twofold (95% CI 0.8 to 4.6)[49] and 3.5 fold (95% CI 1.4 to 8.8)[46] more likely to achieve complete wart clearance than placebo. One RCT found no significant difference for complete wart clearance between 1 MU/ml intralesional interferon and placebo. However, it found a twofold improvement if complete and partial responders were grouped together for analysis (RR of clearance 2.3, 95% CI 1.2 to 4.3).[53] **Added to podophyllin:** One RCT found that podophyllin and intralesional interferon together were more effective than podophyllin alone 3 weeks after treatment (RR 2.0, 95% CI 1.1 to 3.6), however, no significant difference was observed at 11 weeks (RR 2.3, 95% CI 0.9 to 5.8).[35]

Harms: Flu like symptoms (dizziness, fever, malaise, myalgia, nausea and vomiting, headache, and pain) were reported in 0–100% of participants. Eight of nine studies reported local irritation and one reported hypopigmentation among treated individuals.[53] Several studies reported a fall in white cell counts,[35,45–47,49–52] thrombocytopenia (1%),[45] and raised serum aspartate transaminase concentrations (6%)[35] in people on interferon.

Comment: None.

OPTION SYSTEMIC INTERFERON

RCTs have found no evidence that systemic interferon is more effective than placebo, and it is associated with a range of adverse effects.

Benefits: We found no systematic review. We found 16 RCTs in 1992 men and women: six placebo controlled trials, two trials that compared systemic interferon versus podophyllin or diathermocoagulation, and eight trials that evaluated its use with one or more adjunct therapies.[27,28,54–67] **Clearance:** Fourteen of the trials reported wart clearance within 3 months of treatment in 17–67% of participants. However, four trials comparing systemic interferon with placebo found no significant difference in rates of wart clearance.[55–60] One study found that people taking systemic interferon showed greater wart clearance than placebo treated people, which was significant at 8 weeks of follow up (51% v 29%, P < 0.05), but no difference was detected 12 months after treatment.[59] **Recurrence:** Recurrence rates varied from 9–69%.[27,55,57,67]

Harms: Flu like symptoms were reported at variable frequencies; headache, fatigue and malaise, myalgia, nausea and vomiting, fever, chills, and dizziness were reported in 0.5–100% of participants on interferon.[27,28,54–62,64,65,67–69] Anaphylactic reaction occurred in 2% of participants in one RCT,[62] leukopenia in 6–28%,[57,64,65] thrombocytopenia in 3–4%,[57,65] and raised liver enzymes in 3%.[57,68] Bronchospasm and depression were rarely reported (in 1 of 97 participants for each symptom in one trial).[27]

Comment: None.

OPTION TOPICAL 5-FLUOROURACIL

Topical 5-fluorouracil has not yet been adequately evaluated in the treatment of external genital warts.

Benefits: We found no systematic review or RCTs.

Harms: One case series of 1% solution reported minor local erosions (48%), urinary meatus erosions (5%), vulvar irritation (10%), burning (10%), and dysuria (4%).[70]

Comment: We found three case series in 224 men and women treated with 1% and 5% cream and solution preparations in various doses.[70–72] Wart clearance was reported in 10–50% of participants within 3 months of treatment. Only one study reported recurrence rates based on data from only 20 of its 49 participants; recurrences were noted in 10.[71] 5-fluorouracil has teratogenic and mutagenic properties. Safety in pregnancy is not known. Exposure to 5-fluorouracil during pregnancy has been reported rarely, with no untoward outcomes.[73,74]

QUESTION What are the effects of surgical treatments?

OPTION ELECTROSURGERY

Limited evidence from RCTs suggests that electrosurgery is more effective than intramuscular and subcutaneous interferon. We found no trials comparing electrosurgery with no treatment.

Benefits: We found no systematic review. **Clearance:** We found no RCTs versus no or sham treatment and found three RCTs comparing electrosurgery versus interferon, cryotherapy, or podophyllin resin in 482 men and women.[29,32,62] Complete wart clearance was reported in 61–94% of participants 3–6 weeks after treatment. Electrosurgery was more effective than intramuscular interferon (RR v intramuscular 3.3, 95% CI 1.8 to 5.9), or subcutaneous interferon (RR v subcutaneous 6.9, 95% CI 2.8 to 17.1).[62] One RCT found that electrosurgery was more effective than podophyllin resin 4 weeks after treatment (RR 2.3, 95% CI 1.7 to 3.0), but this difference ceased to be significant after 3 months (RR 1.4, 95% CI 0.9 to 2.1).[29] Two studies found that electrosurgery was slightly more effective than cryotherapy within 3–4 weeks of treatment (RRs

1.2, 95% CI 1.1 to 1.3[29]; and 1.4, 95% CI 1.0 to 2.0[32]). One of these trials followed people for 3 months, after which time this difference ceased to be significant (RR 1.0, 95% CI 0.8 to 1.2).[29]
Recurrence: One trial found recurrence in 22% of participants after electrosurgery versus 21% after cryotherapy and 44% using podophyllin resin.[29]

Harms: Pain and local irritation were reported in 17% of treated participants.[29]

Comment: None.

OPTION   SURGICAL EXCISION

RCTs have found that surgical (scissor) excision is as effective as laser surgery and more effective than podophyllin. We found no trials comparing surgical excision with no treatment.

Benefits: We found no systematic review. **Clearance:** We found no RCTs versus no treatment or sham treatment, but found three RCTs comparing surgical excision versus CO_2 laser[75] or podophyllin.[38,37] Within 1 year of treatment, complete wart clearance occurred in 35–72% of people treated with surgical excision. Two studies found that podophyllin was less effective than surgery for clearance (RRs of clearance 0.3, 95% CI 0.2 to 0.7[38]; and 0.5, 95% CI 0.2 to 0.9[37]). One trial found no significant difference in clearance between laser and conventional surgery (RR 1.2, 95% CI 0.6 to 2.4).[75] **Recurrence:** Recurrence occurred in 19–29% of excision treated participants versus 60–65% of those treated with podophyllin.[38,37] The trial comparing conventional and laser surgery found no significant difference in recurrence rates between the two treatments.[75]

Harms: All surgically treated participants experienced pain. Scar formation (9%)[75] and bleeding (37%)[38] were less frequent.

Comment: None.

OPTION   LASER SURGERY

One RCT found limited evidence of a difference in wart clearance or recurrence rates between laser and conventional surgery. We found no trials comparing laser surgery with no treatment.

Benefits: We found no systematic review. We found no RCT versus no or sham treatment, three RCTs in 285 people evaluating laser surgery plus interferon versus laser alone,[64–66] and one RCT in 50 people comparing laser surgery versus conventional surgical excision.[75] **Clearance:** Complete wart clearance was reported in 23–52% of participants within 36 months of laser surgery. This was not significantly different from clearance after conventional surgery (RR for laser v conventional surgery 1.2, 95% CI 0.6 to 2.4).[75] **Recurrence:** Recurrence was reported in 60–77% of participants after laser surgery.[64,66,75] This did not differ significantly from recurrence rates with conventional surgery.[75]

Genital warts

Harms: The RCT comparing laser with conventional surgery found no significant difference in the rate of local scar formation (28% after laser surgery v 9% after conventional surgery, P > 0.2).[75] Postoperative pain was reported equally in both groups.

Comment: We found two case series of laser surgery, which included 47 pregnant women.[41,76] These reported premature rupture of membranes in 2 of 32 women, prolonged rupture of membranes in 1 of 32, the need for postoperative suprapubic catheterisation in 7 of 32, pyelonephritis in 1 of 32, prolonged healing time in 1 of 52, and rectal perforation with secondary abscess in 1 of 52.

QUESTION   **Does treatment of external genital warts or the use of barrier contraceptives prevent transmission of HPV?**

We found insufficient evidence about barrier contraceptives or treatment of external genital warts to prevent transmission of human papillomavirus (HPV).

Benefits: We found no controlled studies about the effects of barrier contraceptives or treatment of external genital warts on the rate of transmitting HIV.

Harms: None reported.

Comment: Penetrative intercourse may not be required for transmission of HPV infection, and it is unclear whether sexual contact with any infected and uninfected perigenital tissues is sufficient to cause external genital warts.

REFERENCES

1. US Department of Health and Human Services, Public Health Service. Division of STD Prevention. *Sexually transmitted disease surveillance.* Atlanta: Centers for Disease Control and Prevention, 1996.
2. Koutsky LA, Galloway DA, Holmes KK. Epidemiology of genital human papillomavirus infection. *Epidemiol Rev* 1988;10:122–163.
3. Gissmann L, zur Hausen H. Partial characterization of viral DNA from human genital warts (condylomata acuminata). *Int J Cancer* 1980;25:605–609.
4. Gissmann L, Boshart M, Durst M, Ikenberg H, Wagner D, zur Hausen H. Presence of human papillomavirus in genital tumors. *J Invest Dermatol* 1984;83(suppl 1):26–28.
5. IARC Working Group on Evaluation of Carcinogenic Risks to Humans. *IARC monographs on the evaluation of carcinogenic risks to humans: human papillomaviruses.* Lyon, France: World Health Organization, International Agency for Research on Cancer, 1995.
6. Bonnez W, Kashima HK, Leventhal B, et al. Antibody response to human papillomavirus (HPV) type 11 in children with juvenile-onset recurrent respiratory papillomatosis (RRP). *Virology* 1992;188:384–387.
7. Hallden C, Majmudar B. The relationship between juvenile laryngeal papillomatosis and maternal condylomata acuminata. *J Reprod Med* 1986;31:804–807.
8. Greenberg MD, Rutledge LH, Reid R, Berman NR, Precop SL, Elswick RK, Jr. A double-blind, randomized trial of 0.5% podofilox and placebo for the treatment of genital warts in women. *Obstet Gynecol* 1991;77:735–739.
9. Beutner KR, Conant MA, Friedman-Kien AE, et al. Patient-applied podofilox for treatment of genital warts. *Lancet* 1989;i:831–834.
10. Kirby P, Dunne King D, Corey L. Double-blind randomized clinical trial of self-administered podofilox solution versus vehicle in the treatment of genital warts. *Am J Med* 1990;88:465–469.
11. Syed TA, Khayyami M, Kriz D, et al. Management of genital warts in women with human leukocyte interferon-α vs podophyllotoxin in cream: a placebo-controlled, double-blind, comparative study. *J Mol Med* 1995;73:255–258.
12. Tyring S, Edwards L, Cherry LK, et al. Safety and efficacy of 0.5% podofilox gel in the treatment of anogenital warts. *Arch Dermatol* 1998;134:33–38.
13. Von Krogh G, Hellberg D. Self-treatment using a 0.5% podophyllotoxin cream of external genital condylomata acuminata in women. A placebo-controlled, double-blind study. *Sex Transm Dis* 1992;19:170–174.
14. Von Krogh G, Szpak E, Andersson M, Bergelin I. Self-treatment using 0.25%–0.50% podophyllotoxin-ethanol solutions against penile condylomata acuminata: a placebo-controlled comparative study. *Genitourin Med* 1994;70:105–109.
15. Syed TA, Lundin S, Ahmad SA. Topical 0.3% and 0.5% podophyllotoxin cream for self-treatment of condylomata acuminata in women: a placebo-controlled, double-blind study. *Dermatology* 1994;189:142–145.
16. Bonnez W, Elswick RK, Jr, Bailey-Farchione A, et al. Efficacy and safety of 0.5% podofilox solution in the treatment and suppression of anogenital warts. *Am J Med* 1994;96:420–425.
17. Edwards A, Atma-Ram A, Thin RN. Podophyllotoxin

0.5% v podophyllin 20% to treat penile warts. *Genitourin Med* 1988;64:263–265.

18. Hellberg D, Svarrer T, Nilsson S, Valentin J. Self-treatment of female external genital warts with 0.5% podophyllotoxin cream (Condyline) vs weekly applications of 20% podophyllin solution. *Int J STD AIDS* 1995;6:257–261.

19. Kinghorn GR, McMillan A, Mulcahy F, Drake S, Lacey C, Bingham JS. An open, comparative, study of the efficacy of 0.5% podophyllotoxin lotion and 25% podophyllotoxin solution in the treatment of condylomata acuminata in males and females. *Int J STD AIDS* 1993;4:194–199.

20. Lassus A, Haukka K, Forsstrom S. Podophyllotoxin for treatment of genital warts in males: a comparison with conventional podophyllin therapy. *Eur J Sex Transm Dis* 1984;2:31–33.

21. White, DJ, Billingham C, Chapman S, et al. Podophyllin 0.5% or 2.0% v podophyllotoxin 0.5% for self treatment of penile warts: a double blind randomised study. *Genitourin Med* 1997;73:184–187.

22. Petersen CS, Weismann K. Quercetin and kaempherol: an argument against the use of podophyllin? *Genitourin Med* 1995;71:92–93.

23. Von Krogh G. Topical self-treatment of penile warts with 0.5% podophyllotoxin in ethanol for four or five days. *Sex Transm Dis* 1987;14:135–140.

24. Von Krogh G. Penile condylomata acuminata: an experimental model for evaluation of topical self-treatment with 0.5–1.0% ethanolic preparations of podophyllotoxin for three days. *Sex Transm Dis* 1981;8:179–186.

25. Edwards L, Ferenczy A, Eron L, et al. Self-administered topical 5% imiquimod cream for external anogenital warts. *Arch Dermatol* 1998; 134:25–30.

26. Beutner KR, Spruance SL, Hougham AJ, Fox TL, Owens ML, Douglas JM, Jr. Treatment of genital warts with an immune-response modifier (imiquimod). *J Am Acad Dermatol* 1998;38(2 pt 1):230–239.

27. Eron LJ, Alder MB, O'Rourke JM, Rittweger K, DePamphilis J, Pizzuti DJ. Recurrence of condylomata acuminata following cryotherapy is not prevented by systemically administered interferon. *Genitourin Med* 1993;69:91–93.

28. Handley JM, Horner T, Maw RD, Lawther H, Dinsmore WW. Subcutaneous interferon α 2a combined with cryotherapy vs cryotherapy alone in the treatment of primary anogenital warts: a randomised observer blind placebo controlled study. *Genitourin Med* 1991;67:297–302.

29. Stone KM, Becker TM, Hadgu A, Kraus SJ. Treatment of external genital warts: a randomised clinical trial comparing podophyllin, cryotherapy, and electrodesiccation. *Genitourin Med* 1990;66:16–19.

30. Abdullah AN, Walzman M, Wade A. Treatment of external genital warts comparing cryotherapy (liquid nitrogen) and trichloroacetic acid. *Sex Transm Dis* 1993;20:344–345.

31. Godley MJ, Bradbeer CS, Gellan M, Thin RN. Cryotherapy compared with trichloroacetic acid in treating genital warts. *Genitourin Med* 1987;63:390–392.

32. Simmons PD, Langlet F, Thin RN. Cryotherapy versus electrocautery in the treatment of genital warts. *Br J Venereal Dis* 1981;57:273–274.

33. Bergman A, Bhatia NN, Broen EM. Cryotherapy for treatment of genital condylomata during pregnancy. *J Reprod Med* 1984;29:432–435.

34. Condylomata International Collaborative Study Group. A comparison of interferon alfa-2a and podophyllin in the treatment of primary condylomata acuminata. *Genitourin Med* 1991; 67:394–399.

35. Douglas JM Jr, Eron LJ, Judson FN, et al. A randomized trial of combination therapy with intralesional interferon α 2b and podophyllin versus podophyllin alone for the therapy of anogenital warts. *J Infect Dis* 1990;162:52–59.

36. Potkul RK, Lancaster WD, Kurman RJ, Lewandowski G, Weck PK, Delgado G. Vulvar condylomas and squamous vestibular micropapilloma. Differences in appearance and response to treatment. *J Reprod Med* 1990;35:1019–1022.

37. Khawaja HT. Podophyllin versus scissor excision in the treatment of perianal condylomata acuminata: a prospective study. *Br J Surg* 1989;76:1067–1068.

38. Jensen SL. Comparison of podophyllin application with simple surgical excision in clearance and recurrence of perianal condylomata acuminata. *Lancet* 1985;2:1146–1148.

39. Simmons PD. Podophyllin 10% and 25% in the treatment of ano-genital warts: a comparative double-blind study. *Br J Venereal Dis* 1981;57:208–209.

40. Gabriel G, Thin RN. Treatment of anogenital warts. Comparison of trichloroacetic acid and podophyllin versus podophyllin alone. *Br J Venereal Dis* 1983;59:124–126.

41. Schwartz DB, Greenberg MD, Daoud Y, Reid R. Genital condylomas in pregnancy: use of trichloroacetic acid and laser therapy. *Am J Obstet Gynecol* 1988;158(6 pt 1):1407–1416.

42. Keay S, Teng N, Eisenberg M, Story B, Sellers PW, Merigan TC. Topical interferon for treating condyloma acuminata in women. *J Infect Dis* 1988;158:934–939.

43. Syed TA, Ahmadpour OA: Human leukocyte derived interferon-α in a hydrophilic gel for the treatment of intravaginal warts in women: a placebo-controlled, double-blind study. *Int J STD AIDS* 1998;9:769–772.

44. Gross G, Rogozinski T, Schofer H, et al. Recombinant interferon β gel as an adjuvant in the treatment of recurrent genital warts: results of a placebo-controlled double blind study of 120 patients. *Dermatology* 1998;196:330–334.

45. Eron LJ, Judson F, Tucker S, et al. Interferon therapy for condylomata acuminata. *N Engl J Med* 1986;315:1059–1064.

46. Friedman-Kien AE, Eron LJ, Conant M, et al. Natural interferon alfa for treatment of condylomata acuminata. *JAMA* 1988;259:533–538.

47. Friedman-Kien A. Management of condylomata acuminata with Alferon N injection, interferon alfa-n3 (human leukocyte derived). *Am J Obstet Gynecol* 1995;172(4 pt 2):1359–1368.

48. Monsonego J, Cessot G, Ince SE, Galazka AR, Abdul-Ahad AK. Randomised double-blind trial of recombinant interferon-β for condyloma acuminatum. *Genitourin Med* 1996;72:111–114.

49. Reichman RC, Oakes D, Bonnez W, et al. Treatment of condyloma acuminatum with three different interferons administered intralesionally: a double-blind, placebo-controlled trial. *Ann Intern Med* 1988;108:675–679.

50. Scott GM, Csonka GW. Effect of injections of small doses of human fibroblast interferon into genital warts: a pilot study. *Br J Venereal Dis* 1979;55:442–445.

51. Vance JC, Bart BJ, Hansen RC, et al. Intralesional recombinant α-2 interferon for the treatment of patients with condyloma acuminatum or verruca plantaris. *Arch Dermatol* 1986;122:272–277.

52. Welander CE, Homesley HD, Smiles KA, Peets EA. Intralesional interferon alfa-2b for the treatment of genital warts. *Am J Obstet Gynecol* 1990;162:348–354.

53. Bornstein J, Pascal B, Zarfati D, et al. Recombinant human interferon-β for condylomata acuminata: a randomized, double-blind, placebo controlled study of intralesional therapy. *Int J STD AIDS* 1997;8:614–621.

54. Armstrong DK, Maw RD, Dinsmore WW, et al. A randomised, double-blind, parallel group study to compare subcutaneous interferon α-2a plus podophyllin with placebo plus podophyllin in the treatment of primary condylomata acuminata. *Genitourin Med* 1994;70:389–393.

55. Armstrong DK, Maw RD, Dinsmore WW, et al. Combined therapy trial with interferon α-2a and ablative therapy in the treatment of anogenital warts. *Genitourin Med* 1996;72:103–107.

56. Condylomata International Collaborative Study Group. Recurrent condylomata acuminata treated with recombinant interferon alfa-2a: a multicenter double-blind placebo-controlled clinical trial. *JAMA* 1991;265:2684–2687.

57. Condylomata International Collaborative Study Group. Recurrent condylomata acuminata treated with recombinant interferon α-2a: a multicenter double-blind placebo-controlled clinical trial. *Acta Derm Venereol* 1993;73:223–226.

58. Gall SA, Constantine L, Koukol D. Therapy of persistent human papillomavirus disease with two different interferon species. *Am J Obstet Gynecol* 1991;164(1 pt 1):130–134.

59. Olmos L, Vilata J, Rodriguez Pichardo A, Lloret A, Ojeda A, Calderon MD. Double-blind, randomized clinical trial on the effect of interferon-β in the treatment of condylomata acuminata. *Int J STD AIDS* 1994;5:182–185.

60. Reichman RC, Oakes D, Bonnez W, et al. Treatment of condyloma acuminatum with three different interferon-α preparations administered parenterally: a double-blind, placebo-controlled trial. *J Infect Dis* 1990;162:1270–1276.

61. Condylomata International Collaborative Study Group. A comparison of interferon alfa-2a and podophyllin in the treatment of primary condylomata acuminata. *Genitourin Med* 1991; 67:394–399.

62. Benedetti Panici P, Scambia G, Baiocchi G, Perrone L, Pintus C, Mancuso S. Randomized clinical trial comparing systemic interferon with diathermocoagulation in primary multiple and widespread anogenital condyloma. *Obstet Gynecol* 1989;74(3 pt 1):393–397.

63. Bonnez W, Oakes D, Bailey-Farchione A, et al. A randomized, double-blind, placebo-controlled trial of systemically administered interferon-α, -β, or -γ in combination with cryotherapy for the treatment of condyloma acuminatum. *J Infect Dis* 1995; 171:1081–1089.

64. Condylomata International Collaborative Study Group. Randomized placebo-controlled double-blind combined therapy with laser surgery and systemic interferon-α 2a in the treatment of anogenital condylomata acuminatum. *J Infect Dis* 1993;167:824–829.

65. Petersen C, Bjerring P, Larson J, et al. Systemic interferon α-2b increases the cure rate in laser treated patients with multiple persistent genital warts: a placebo-controlled study. *Genitourin Med* 1991;67:99–102.

66. Reid R, Greenberg MD, Pizzuti DJ, Omoto KH, Rutledge LH, Soo W. Superficial laser vulvectomy. V. Surgical debulking is enhanced by adjuvant systemic interferon. *Am J Obstet Gynecol* 1992; 166:815–820.

67. Bonnez W, Oakes D, Bailey-Farchione A, et al. A randomized, double blind trial of parenteral low dose versus high dose interferon β in combination with cryotherapy for treatment of condylomata acuminatum. *Antiviral Res* 1997;35:41–52.

68. Kirby PK, Kiviat N, Beckman A, Wells D, Sherwin S, Corey L. Tolerance and efficacy of recombinant human interferon γ in the treatment of refractory genital warts. *Am J Med* 1988;85:183–188.

69. Reichman RC, Micha JP, Weck PK, et al. Interferon α-n1 (Wellferon) for refractory genital warts: efficacy and tolerance of low dose systemic therapy. *Antiviral Res* 1988;10(1–3):41–57.

70. Von Krogh G. The beneficial effect of 1% 5-fluorouracil in 70% ethanol on therapeutically refractory condylomas in the preputial cavity. *Sex Transm Dis* 1978;5:137–140.

71. Krebs H. Treatment of extensive vulvar condylomata acuminata with topical 5-fluorouracil. *South Med J* 1990;83:761–764.

72. Haye KR. Treatment of condyloma acuminata with 5 per cent 5-fluorouracil (5-FU) cream [letter]. *Br J Vener Dis* 1974;50:466.

73. Dreicer R, Love RR. High total dose 5-fluorouracil treatment during pregnancy. *Wis Med J* 1991;90: 582–583.

74. Van Le L, Pizzuti DJ, Greenberg M, Reid R. Accidental use of low-dose 5-fluorouracil in pregnancy. *J Reprod Med* 1991;36:872–874.

75. Duus BR, Philipsen T, Christensen JD, Lundvall F, Sondergaard J. Refractory condylomata acuminata: a controlled clinical trial of carbon dioxide laser versus conventional surgical treatment. *Genitourin Med* 1985;61:59–61.

76. Kryger-Baggesen N, Falck Larsen J, Hjortkjaer Pedersen P. CO_2 laser treatment of condylomata acuminata. *Acta Obstet Gynecol Scand* 1984;63: 341–343.

DJ Wiley
Assistant Professor in Residence
School of Nursing, Primary Care
University of California
Los Angeles, California
USA

Karl Beutner
Associate Clinical Professor
Department of Dermatology University
of California
San Francisco, California
USA

Competing interests: KB has been reimbursed for speaking at symposia, paid a fee for speaking and organising education, performing clinical trials, and consulting by Oclassem Dermatologics, a division of Watson Pharmaceuticals, 3M Pharmaceuticals, Epitome Pharmaceuticals, Matrix Pharmaceuticals, Puntose Pharmaceuticals, and ISIS Pharmaceuticals. DJW has been a consultant to 3M Pharmaceuticals and has received research funding from Merck and Co.

Updated this issue

John Moran

INTERVENTIONS

Beneficial
Single-dose regimens using
  selected fluoroquinolones,
  selected cephalosporins, or
  spectinomycin in uncomplicated
  infection 923
Single-dose regimens using
  selected cephalosporins or
  spectinomycin in uncomplicated
  infection in pregnant women .923
Selected injectable
  fluoroquinolones or selected

injectable cephalosporins in
  disseminated infection* 924

Unknown effectiveness
Dual treatment for gonorrhoea and
  chlamydia infections in all
  patients diagnosed with
  gonorrhoea 924

*Based only on non-RCT evidence
  and consensus.

Key Messages

- One systematic review of RCTs in people with uncomplicated gonococcal infection has found that single-drug regimens using selected fluoroquinolones, selected cephalosporins, or spectinomycin are highly effective and safe. Resistance to penicillins, sulphonamides, and tetracyclines is now widespread.

- We found little evidence on treatment in pregnant women. Two RCTs found that antibiotics were effective in pregnant women. We found no reports of serious adverse effects.

- We found no trials evaluating injectable cephalosporins or quinolones in gonococcal infection, but found no reports of treatment failures.

- Dual treatment for gonorrhoea and chlamydia infections is based on theory and expert opinion rather than on evidence from clinical trials. The balance between benefits and harms varies with the prevalence of co-infection in each population.

Gonorrhoea

DEFINITION Gonorrhoea is caused by infection with *Neisseria gonorrhoeae*. In men, uncomplicated urethritis is the most common manifestation, with dysuria and urethral discharge. Less typically, signs and symptoms are mild and indistinguishable from chlamydial urethritis. In women, the most common manifestation is cervicitis, which produces symptoms (e.g. vaginal discharge, lower abdominal discomfort, and dyspareunia) in only half of cases. Co-infection with chlamydia is reported in 20–40% of people.[1]

INCIDENCE/ PREVALENCE Between 1975 and 1997, the incidence of reported gonorrhoea in the USA fell by 74%, reaching a level in 1997 of 122/100 000 people, but it increased by 9% in 1998 to 133/100 000.[2] In England and Wales, 8511 males (33/100 000 population) and 4115 females (15/100 000) presented to genitourinary medicine clinics with uncomplicated gonorrhoea in 1998.[3] In poor communities, rates may be higher: the estimated incidence in people aged 15–59 living in three inner London boroughs in 1994–1995 was 138/100 000 women and 292/100 000 men.[4] Rates are highest in younger people. In the USA in 1998, incidence was highest in women aged 15–19 (780/100 000) and men aged 20–24 (575/ 100 000).[2]

AETIOLOGY/ RISK FACTORS Most infections result from penile-vaginal, penile-rectal, or penile-pharyngeal contact. An important minority of infections are transmitted from mother to child during birth, which can cause ophthalmia neonatorum. Less common are ocular infections in older children and adults as a result of sexual exposure, poor hygiene, or the medicinal use of urine.

PROGNOSIS Symptoms in most men are severe enough to cause them to seek treatment, but an estimated 1–3% of infected men remain asymptomatic. These men, and men who are infectious but not yet symptomatic, are largely responsible for spread of the disease. In many women, the lack of readily discernible signs or symptoms of cervicitis means that infections go unrecognised and untreated. An unknown proportion of untreated infections causes local complications. These include lymphangitis, periurethral abscess, bartholinitis, and urethral stricture; epididymitis in men; and in women involvement of the uterus, fallopian tubes, or ovaries causing pelvic inflammatory disease (see pelvic inflammatory disease, p 934). It is the association of gonorrhoea with pelvic inflammatory disease — a major cause of secondary infertility, ectopic pregnancy, and chronic pelvic pain — that makes gonorrhoea an important public health issue. Manifestations of disseminated infection are petechial or pustular skin lesions; asymmetrical arthropathies, tenosynovitis or septic arthritis; and, rarely, meningitis or endocarditis.

AIMS To relieve symptoms, avoid complications, and prevent further transmission, with minimal adverse effects of treatment.

OUTCOMES Microbiological cure rates (percentage of positive cultures 3–7 days after treatment) or rates of treatment failure

METHODS *Clinical Evidence* update search and appraisal May 2000 (key words gonorrhoea and *N gonorrhoeae* infections), plus search of references of key articles and books. Studies were excluded if they defined possible treatment failures as "reinfections", if they did not use end points based on microbiological cure, or if they were based on drug regimens unlikely to be of general use (e.g. those using antibiotic regimens that are toxic, or to which resistance is now widespread).[5]

QUESTION **What are the effects of treatments for uncomplicated infections in men and non-pregnant women?**

One systematic review has found that modern antimicrobial agents other than penicillin and tetracycline achieve cure rates of 97% or higher. Cure rates are lower (≤80%) for pharyngeal infection. Most regimens cause few adverse effects. Resistance is now widespread to penicillins, tetracyclines, and sulphonamides.

Benefits: **Uncomplicated urogenital, rectal, and pharyngeal infections:** We found one systematic review (search date 1993). It identified studies published from 1981 to 1993 that used a single dose regimen based on an antimicrobial other than a β lactamase sensitive penicillin or a tetracycline.[5] The data comprised 24 383 evaluable patients or infections, of which 96.7% were cured based on culture results. Sites of infection, when specified, included the cervix, urethra, rectum, and pharynx. Comparison of cure rates by site of infection found that cure rates were over 95% for all sites except the pharynx, for which they were about 80%.[6] **Eye infections:** We found no systematic review or RCTs. In the only recent published study of the treatment of gonococcal conjunctivitis, all 12 participants responded well to a single 1 g dose of ceftriaxone.[7]

Harms: Single dose regimens using fluoroquinolones, third generation and extended spectrum cephalosporins, or spectinomycin are generally safe and well tolerated. The most important adverse effects are rare hypersensitivity reactions. Minor adverse effects are most troublesome for the 800 mg cefixime regimen,[8,9] and the 2 g azithromycin regimen;[10] both cause frequent gastrointestinal upset. The ceftriaxone and spectinomycin regimens require intramuscular injection. One large observational cohort study of azithromycin, cefixime, ciprofloxacin, and ofloxacin "in everyday use" found few serious adverse effects.[11] Quinolones may cause arthropathy in animals. No evidence of joint toxicity has been observed in clinical use, even with prolonged, multiple dose regimens used for the management of children with cystic fibrosis.[12–16] Resistance is now widespread for all penicillins, sulphonamides, and tetracyclines, but has not been reported widely for fluoroquinolones, third generation and extended spectrum cephalosporins, or spectinomycin (see table 1, p 926).

Comment: There is good agreement between antigonococcal activity of antimicrobials *in vitro* and their efficacy in clinical trials. The large number of patients evaluated in a range of settings means the results can be generalised. Single dose regimens may make adherence more likely.

QUESTION **What are the effects of treatments for uncomplicated infections in pregnant women?**

Two RCTs found that antibiotic treatment in pregnancy was effective. We found no reports of serious adverse effects.

Benefits: We found no systematic review. We found two RCTs of the treatment of gonococcal infection during pregnancy,[17,18] only one of which has been published in full.[17] The first RCT allocated 62 women with endocervical gonorrhoea to ceftriaxone intramuscularly or cefixime orally. It found that eradication rates were similar in the two groups (28/30 [93%] with ceftriaxone, 31/32 [97%] with cefixime; RR 2.1, 95% CI 0.2 to 14).[18] The second RCT compared amoxycillin with probenecid, spectinomycin, and ceftriaxone regimens in 267 pregnant women with positive cultures for gonorrhoea.[17] Eradication rates ranged from 89% to 97%. Single dose ceftriaxone 250 mg cured 95.2% (95% CI 89.2% to 98.5%) of rectal and cervical infections and 100% (95% CI 54.1% to 100%) of pharyngeal infections; spectinomycin 2 g cured 97.0% (95% CI 91.5% to 99.4%) of rectal and cervical infections and 83.3% (95% CI 35.9% to 99.6%) of pharyngeal infections.[17]

Harms: The second trial reported vomiting after treatment in only one of the 267 women.[17] Little information on other adverse effects was available. Because quinolones cause arthropathy in animals, their use is not recommended in pregnancy, although we found no reports of adverse effects of quinolones on pregnancy outcome in humans. A single, multicentre, prospective, controlled study of 200 exposed women found no evidence of adverse effects.[19] We found no evidence that the non-quinolone regimens listed above are less safe or less well tolerated by pregnant women than by men or non-pregnant women.

Comment: None.

QUESTION **What are the effects of treatments for disseminated gonococcal infection?**

We found no recent trials evaluating treatment for disseminated gonococcal infection. However, we found no reports of treatment failure with accepted treatment using injectable cephalosporins or quinolones.

Benefits: We found no systematic review and no studies of the treatment of disseminated gonococcal infection published in the last 10 years.

Harms: We found no reports of adverse effects of these drugs in this context.

Comment: Widespread consensus suggests that the most effective treatment is injectable cephalosporins or quinolones. Although we found no published data establishing the efficacy of this treatment, we found no reports of treatment failures.

QUESTION **What are the effects of dual treatment for gonorrhoea and chlamydia infection?**

Dual treatment with an antimicrobial effective against *Chlamydia trachomatis* is based on theory and expert opinion rather than evidence. The balance between benefits and harms from controlled trials will vary with the prevalence of co-infection in each population.

Benefits: We found no systematic review or RCTs.

Harms: We found no good evidence on the harms of dual treatment. Treatment for chlamydia can cause mild gastrointestinal distress, and there is the possibility that using a second drug could stimulate the emergence or spread of resistance in *Neisseria* or other bacteria.

Comment: Routine dual treatment has been advocated and implemented for the last 10 years, and is believed to have two potential benefits. First, it is believed to have contributed to the decline in the prevalence of chlamydia infection observed in some populations. We found no evidence for any direct effect of dual treatment on chlamydia prevalence. Other factors may have contributed to reduced chlamydia prevalence (including widespread screening for asymptomatic chlamydia infection and changes in sexual behaviour), making it difficult to attribute decreases in the prevalence of chlamydia infection to any specific cause. Secondly, routine dual treatment is believed to retard the spread of resistant gonococcal strains. Limited data from case reports support this belief. In the past, chlamydia testing was often unavailable, expensive, time consuming, and not highly sensitive, whereas dual treatment with a tetracycline such as doxycycline was safe and inexpensive. Chlamydia testing has now become more widely available, more affordable, quicker, and more sensitive, and the prevalence of chlamydia has fallen in some populations. Nevertheless, chlamydia is still found in 20–40% of people with gonorrhoea in many clinics.[1]

REFERENCES

1. Centers for Disease Control and Prevention. 1998 Guidelines for the treatment of sexually transmitted diseases. *Morb Mortal Wkly Rep* 1998;47(RR-1):60.

2. Division of STD Prevention, Centers for Disease Control and Prevention. *Sexually transmitted diseases surveillance, 1998.* Atlanta: US Department of Health and Human Services. 1999. http://www.cdc.gov/nchstp/dstd/Stats_Trends/1998_Surv_Rtp_main_pg.htm.

3. Sexually transmitted disease quarterly report: gonorrhoea in England and Wales. *Commun Dis Rep CDR Wkly* 1999;9:270–271.

4. Low N, Daker-White G, Barlow D, Pozniak AI. Gonorrhoea in inner London: results of a cross-sectional study. *BMJ* 1997;314:1719–1723.

5. Moran JS, Levine WC. Drugs of choice for the treatment of uncomplicated gonococcal infections. *Clin Infect Dis* 1995;20(suppl 1):47–65. Search date 1993; primary sources Medline 1981 to 1993; reference lists from retrieved articles; abstracts from the annual Interscience Conference on Antimicrobial Agents and Chemotherapy and the meeting of the International Society for Sexually Transmitted Disease Research 1990 to 1993.

6. Moran JS. Treating uncomplicated *Neisseria gonorrhoeae* infections: is the anatomic site of infection important? *Sex Transm Dis* 1995;22:39–47.

7. Haimovici R, Roussel TJ. Treatment of gonococcal conjunctivitis with single-dose intramuscular ceftriaxone. *Am J Ophthalmol* 1989;107:511–514.

8. Handsfield HH, McCormack WM, Hook EW III, et al. The Gonorrhea Treatment Study Group. A comparison of single-dose cefixime with ceftriaxone as treatment for uncomplicated gonorrhea. *N Engl J Med* 1991;325:1337–1341.

9. Megran DW, LeFebvre K, Willets V, Bowie WR. Single-dose oral cefixime versus amoxicillin plus probenecid for the treatment of uncomplicated gonorrhea in men. *Antimicrob Agents Chemother* 1990;34:355–357.

10. Handsfield HH, Dalu ZA, Martin DH, et al. Azithromycin Gonorrhea Study Group. Multicenter trial of single-dose azithromycin vs. ceftriaxone in the treatment of uncomplicated gonorrhea. *Sex Transm Dis* 1994;21:107–111.

11. Wilton LV, Pearce GL, Mann RD. A comparison of ciprofloxacin, norfloxacin, ofloxacin, azithromycin and cefixime examined by observational cohort studies. *Br J Clin Pharmacol* 1996;41:277–284.

12. Green SD. Indications and restrictions of fluoroquinolone use in children. *Br J Hosp Med* 1996;56:420–423.

13. Grenier B. Use of fluoroquinolones in children. An overview. *Adv Antimicr Antineopl Chemother* 1992; 11–2:135–140.

14. Schaad UB. Use of quinolones in children and articular risk. *Arch Pediatr* 1996;3:183–184.

15. Hampel B, Hullmann R, Schmidt H. Ciprofloxacin in pediatrics: worldwide clinical experience based on compassionate use. Safety report. *Pediatr Infect Dis J* 1997;16:127–129.

16. Warren RW. Rheumatologic aspects of pediatric cystic fibrosis patients treated with fluoroquinolones. *Pediatr Infect Dis J* 1997;16:118–122.

17. Cavenee MR, Farris JR, Spalding TR, Barnes DL, Castaneda YS, Wendel GD. Treatment of gonorrhea in pregnancy. *Obstet Gynecol* 1993;81:33–38.

18. Ramus R, Mayfield J, Wendel G. Evaluation of the current CDC recommended treatment guidelines for gonorrhea in pregnancy [abstract]. *Am J Obstet Gynecol* 1996;174:409.

19. Loebstein R, Addis A, Ho E, et al. Pregnancy outcome following gestational exposure to fluoroquinolones: a multicenter prospective controlled study. *Antimicrob Agents Chemother* 1998;42:1336–1339.

John Moran
STD Advisor
US Agency for International Development
Jakarta
Indonesia

Competing interests: None declared.

Sexual health

TABLE 1	Reported resistance of *N gonorrhoeae* to antimicrobials HARMS (see text, p 923).

Drug	Resistance
Sulphonamides	Widespread
Penicillins	Widespread
Tetracyclines	Widespread
Third-generation cephalosporins (e.g. ceftriaxone, cefixime)	None reported
Spectinomycin	Rare
Quinolones	Parts of Asia and Australia: widespread USA: in 1998, decreased susceptibility to ciprofloxacin was reported in 0.6% of isolates, and resistance in 0.1%[2] No increase since 1995 UK: rare reports of imported fluoroquinolone resistant *N gonorrhoeae*

Updated this issue

Catherine Mathews, Nicol Coetzee, Merrick Zwarenstein and Sally Guttmacher

INTERVENTIONS

Key Messages

- We found little evidence on acceptability of different strategies of partner notification.

- We found no good evidence on the effects of partner notification on relationships between patients and partners and, in particular, on the rate of violence, abuse, and abandonment of patient or partner.

- We found no studies comparing the effects of an intervention across different groups, such as people with different diseases or combinations of diseases, or people from different settings.

- RCTs comparing different partner notification strategies found that provider referral was more effective than patient referral in HIV and chlamydia infections, and that in people with syphilis there was no significant difference between provider and contract referral.

- One RCT found that adding telephone reminders and contact cards improved patient referral compared with counselling alone. We found insufficient evidence about other methods, such as educational videos.

- We found insufficient evidence on the effects of giving people choice about which type of partner notification should be used.

| DEFINITION | Partner notification is a process whereby the sexual partners of people with a diagnosis of sexually transmitted infection are informed of their exposure to infection. The main methods are patient referral, provider referral, contract referral, and outreach assistance (see glossary, p 932). |

INCIDENCE/ PREVALENCE A large proportion of people infected with sexually transmitted infections will have neither symptoms nor signs of infection. For example, 22–68% of men with gonorrhoea who were identified through partner notification were asymptomatic.[1] Partner notification is one of the two strategies to reach such individuals, the other strategy being screening. Managing infection in people with more than one current sexual partner is likely to have the greatest impact on the spread of sexually transmitted infections.[2]

AIMS To prevent complications of infection in the partner; to prevent transmission to others; to prevent reinfection; and to identify social networks of people practising risky sexual behaviours.

OUTCOMES Partners identified; partners notified; partners presenting for care; partners testing positive; partners treated; rates of reinfection in the patient; incidence of sexually transmitted diseases in the population; harms to patient or partner, such as domestic violence and abuse; ethical outcomes (patient autonomy versus beneficence).

METHODS *Clinical Evidence* update search and appraisal May 2000. We included RCTs that compared at least two alternative partner notification strategies and in which randomisation was appropriate, patient follow up was greater than 80%, participants were analysed in the groups to which they were assigned, and the groups were similar at the start of the trial. The outcome used in this summary was the absolute difference between the ratio of partners identified, notified, presenting for care, testing positive, or treated per index case.

QUESTION What are the effects of different partner notification strategies in different groups of people?

OPTION IN PEOPLE WITH HIV INFECTION

One RCT found that, for people with HIV infection, provider referral results in more partners being notified than patient referral.

Benefits: We found one RCT.[3] **Provider versus patient referral:** The RCT compared provider referral (see glossary, p 932) with patient referral (see glossary, p 932). It was conducted at three public health departments in North Carolina, USA, with 162 people who had tested positive for HIV. Of those approached, the 46% who agreed to participate in the study were mostly men (69%), of whom most were homosexual or bisexual (76%). Provider referral significantly increased the likelihood that partners would be notified (AR 78/157 [50%] for the provider referral group *v* 10/153 [7%] for the patient referral group; RR 7.6, 95% CI 6.3 to 8.9; NNT 3 CI 95% 2 to 3). Thus, three patients would have to be offered provider referral, compared with using patient referral, for one additional partner to be notified. One group in the USA tried to compare contract referral (see glossary, p 932) with provider referral, but contamination between comparison groups made this impossible.[4] The results were therefore analysed as a cohort study without comparison groups, where all patients were assigned to provider referral. The study included 1070 people, who reported having had 8633 partners in the past year. Of these partners, 1035 were successfully located of whom 248 had previously tested positive for HIV, 560 were tested by the disease intervention specialist, 69 refused testing, and 158 were located by record search only. Of the 560 partners tested, 122 tested positive. **Contract referral:** We found no RCTs evaluating contract referral in people with HIV infection. **Outreach assistance:** See glossary, p 932. We found one RCT comparing patient referral with outreach assistance in 63 people with HIV who were injecting drug users.[5] The full results have yet to be reported.

Harms: People's reluctance to disclose their HIV status to partners (see comment below) suggests expectation of harms from doing so. These and other potential harms are poorly understood.

Comment: The number of partners notified is an intermediate outcome. The number of infections in partners that are prevented or treated has not been evaluated. Thus, the true benefits and harms of HIV partner notification are unknown. **Rates of disclosure:** A descriptive study of 276 people attending for initial primary care for HIV infection in the USA found that 40% of the respondents had not disclosed their HIV status to all partners over the preceding 6 months.[6] Individuals with more than one partner were significantly less likely to disclose to all partners. Only 42% of the non-disclosers reported that they used condoms all the time, which indicates that many partners were at risk of HIV infection. Another descriptive study conducted in the USA found that, even after repeated individual counselling of people with HIV infection, and a 6 month opportunity to disclose HIV status, 30% had not informed any of their past partners, and 29% had not informed any of their present partners.[7]

OPTION   IN PEOPLE WITH GONORRHOEA AND CHLAMYDIA

Two RCTs have found that, for people with gonorrhoea, contract referral is no better at identifying partners with positive culture than patient referral. For people with chlamydia, one RCT found that provider referral increases the proportion of partners notified and of positive partners detected per patient compared with patient referral.

Benefits: We found one systematic review (published in 1994), which identified two RCTs of partner notification in people with gonorrhoea and one in people with non-gonococcal urethritis.[8] We found no subsequent studies that met our inclusion criteria. **Gonorrhoea:** The two RCTs compared patient referral with contract referral in 2085 people with gonorrhoea. A meta-analysis found no significant difference in the proportion of partners with positive gonorrhoea culture per patient (ARR 5%, 95% CI −10% to +21%).[8] **Chlamydia:** The RCT in people with non-gonococcal urethritis compared patient referral with provider referral in 678 patients. It found that provider referral significantly increased the proportion of partners assessed per patient (ARR for non-assessment 52%, 95% CI 44% to 59%). In this study, provider referral also significantly increased the proportion of partners with positive culture per index patient (ARR 6%, 95% CI 2% to 10%). Provider referral was six times as costly per partner with positive culture. Provider referral would have to be offered to two index patients with non-gonococcal urethritis for one additional partner to be assessed (NNT 2, 95% CI 1 to 2) and to 17 index patients to identify one additional partner with a positive culture (NNT 17, 95% CI 10 to 50). These findings are likely to underestimate the effectiveness of patient referral, as partners referred by index patients may have been assessed elsewhere.[8]

Harms: These are poorly understood.

Comment: A cohort study in 265 urban, adolescent girls attending a clinic in Alabama, USA, found that, given the choice, people with gonorrhoea or chlamydia are about as likely to choose provider referral as patient referral.[9]

OPTION IN PEOPLE WITH SYPHILIS

One large RCT found that provider referral was no more effective than contract referral, when people receiving the contract referral option were given only 2 days in which to notify their partners. We found no RCTs evaluating patient referral.

Benefits: We found no systematic review. We found one RCT in 1966 people diagnosed with syphilis in three American states.[10] It compared the proportion of partners per patient who were located, tested, tested positive, and treated, using three types of referral process: contract referral (patients were given 2 days to notify partners themselves, before disease intervention specialists would notify them); provider referral (immediate notification by an intervention specialist); and provider referral with the option of a blood test (immediate notification by an intervention specialist who had the option of performing a blood test if he or she thought that the partner would not seek medical attention despite being notified of exposure). In the three groups: 1.2, 1.1, and 1.1 partners per patient were located; 0.92, 0.87, and 0.86 were tested; and 0.67, 0.61, and 0.62 were treated (confidence intervals not reported).

Harms: These are poorly understood.

Comment: In this trial, the investigators had no way of determining whether disease intervention specialists began actively seeking partners in the contract referral group before waiting 2 days.[10] The use of disease intervention specialists is an approach that may not be generalisable outside the USA.

QUESTION   What can be done to improve the effectiveness of patient referral?

One RCT found that adding telephone reminders and contact cards improved patient referral compared with counselling alone. One RCT found no difference between different kinds of healthcare professional. We found insufficient evidence about other methods, such as educational videos.

Benefits: We found one systematic review (published in 1994), which identified two published RCTs and one unpublished RCT. All were in people with gonococcal or chlamydial infections.[8] We found no subsequent studies that met our inclusion criteria. **Counselling plus referral cards and telephone follow up:** One RCT compared the use of counselling plus referral cards and telephone follow up of the index case with counselling alone in 65 people from a university clinic in the USA. The referral card was to be given to the partner or to be used in preparing to speak to the partner. It contained the patient's diagnosis to facilitate treatment of the partner and a message exhorting the partner to seek treatment. The addition of referral cards and telephone follow up significantly increased the number of partners presenting for care per patient identified (ARR for failure to present 34%, 95% CI 13% to 56%). A referral card and telephone follow up would have to be offered to only three patients for one additional partner to present for care (NNT 3, 95% CI 2 to 8). The trial also evaluated adding a $3 incentive to the referral card. Charges for clinic visits for patients and partners would be waived following successful recruitment of partners for treatment. This had no effect on the number of partners presenting for care.[8] **Different health professionals:** One RCT found that there was no difference between patient referral using nurses who did not ask for partners' names and gave referral letters, and disease intervention specialists who took partners' names but no contact details, in terms of the number of partners with positive cultures who were identified (ARR 0.1%, 95% CI −3% to +3%).[8] **Information pamphlets:** One unpublished RCT, conducted in the USA, investigated the use of information pamphlets compared with a routine counselling interview. Providing patients with information pamphlets was slightly less effective than the interview and significantly reduced the number of partners presenting for care per index patient (ARR for failing to present −5%, 95% CI −7% to −3%). The two strategies were equally effective (and costly) in terms of the number of partners identified with a positive culture per patient. However, the RCT combined two interventions: different health professionals and asking for partners' names, either of which may have affected the results.[8] **Optional outreach assistance:** We found one RCT comparing patient referral with a choice between patient referral and outreach assistance.[5] The full results have yet to be published. The 60 patients who returned for their test results named an average of 2.4 partners each, and no differences were found in the ratio of partners named per patient by treatment group. Of those in the outreach assisted group, 82% chose to have the outreach team notify at least one partner, and the team was asked to notify 71% of all partners named by this group. **Educational videos:** We found no RCTs.

Harms: None reported.

Comment: Contact cards seem to be easily generalised to other settings. Telephone reminders may not be possible in countries with poorly developed telecommunication systems.

QUESTION   **What are the effects of allowing people to choose the type of partner notification?**

We found insufficient evidence on the effects of giving people choice about which type of partner notification should be used compared with assigning them to one or other type.

Benefits: We found no systematic review. We found one RCT comparing patient referral with a choice between patient referral and outreach assistance.[5] The full results have not yet been published.

Harms: These are poorly understood.

Comment: None.

GLOSSARY

Contract referral (also referred to as conditional referral) Index patients are encouraged to inform their partners, with the understanding that health service personnel will notify those partners who do not visit the health service within a contracted time period.

Outreach assistance At the request of patients, partners are notified by members of an outreach team indigenous to the community, who do not disclose the name of the patient to the partners.

Patient referral Health service personnel encourage index patients to inform partners directly of their possible exposure to sexually transmitted infections.

Provider referral Third parties (usually health service personnel) notify partners identified by index patients.

REFERENCES

1. Holmes KK, Mardh PA, Sparling PF, Weisner PJ, eds. Sexually Transmitted Diseases, 2nd edn. New York: McGraw-Hill, 1990:1083.
2. Fenton KA, Peterman TA. HIV partner notification: taking a new look. AIDS 1997;11:1535–1546.
3. Landis SE, Schoenbach VE, Weber DJ, et al. Results of a randomized trial of partner notification in cases of HIV infection in North Carolina. N Engl J Med 1992;326:101–106.
4. Toomey KE, Peterman TA, Dicker LW, Zaidi AA, Wroten JE, Carolina J. Human immunodeficiency virus partner notification. Sex Transm Dis 1998; 25:310–316.
5. Levy JA, Fox SE. The outreach-assisted model of partner notification with IDUs. Public Health Rep 1998;113(suppl 1):160–169.
6. Stein MD, Freedberg KA, Sullivan LM, et al. Sexual ethics: disclosure of HIV-positive status to partners. Arch Intern Med 1998;158:253–257.
7. Perry SW, Card CAL, Moffatt M, Ashman T, Fishman B, Jacobsberg LB. Self-disclosure of HIV infection to sexual partners after repeated counseling. AIDS Educ Prev 1994;6:403–411.
8. Oxman AD, Scott EAF, Sellors JW, et al. Partner notification for sexually transmitted diseases: an overview of the evidence. Can J Public Health 1994;85:127–132. Search date not provided; primary sources Medline, Embase, SciSearch, hand searching of five key journals, personal contact with 80 key experts.
9. Oh MK, Boker JR, Genuardi FJ, Cloud GA, Reynolds J, Hodgens JB. Sexual contact tracing in adolescent chlamydial and gonococcal cervicitis cases. J Adolesc Health 1996;18:4–9.
10. Peterman TA, Toomey KE, Dicker LW, Zaidi AA, Wroten JE, Carolina J. Partner notification for syphilis: a randomized, controlled trial of three approaches. Sex Transm Dis 1997;24:511–518.

Catherine Mathews
Senior Scientist
Health Systems Unit, South African
Medical Research Council and
Department of Public Health, University
of Cape Town

Nicol Coetzee
Senior Lecturer and Consultant
Department of Public Health, University
of Cape Town
Cape Town
South Africa

Merrick Zwarenstein
Head of Health Systems
Research Division
South African Medical Research Council
Centre for Epidemiological Research
South African Medical Research Council
Tygerberg
South Africa

Sally Guttmacher
Professor
Department of Health Studies
New York University
New York
USA

Competing interests: None declared.

Sexual health

Pelvic inflammatory disease

Updated this issue

Jonathan Ross

INTERVENTIONS

Unknown effectiveness

To be covered in future issues of Clinical Evidence

Prevention

Outpatient versus inpatient treatment

Key Messages

- We found no good evidence comparing empirical treatment with antibiotics (before receiving results of microbiological tests) versus delaying treatment until test results are available.

- One systematic review has found that several regimens of parenteral followed by oral antibiotic treatment are effective in relieving the short term symptoms and signs of pelvic inflammatory disease (PID).

- We found no good evidence on the optimal duration of treatment, or on oral versus parenteral treatment.

DEFINITION	Pelvic inflammatory disease (PID) is inflammation and infection of the upper genital tract in women, typically involving the fallopian tubes, ovaries, and surrounding structures.
INCIDENCE/ PREVALENCE	The exact incidence of PID is unknown because the disease cannot be diagnosed reliably from clinical symptoms and signs.[1–3] Direct visualisation of the fallopian tubes by laparoscopy is the best single diagnostic test, but it is invasive and not used routinely in clinical practice. PID is the most common gynaecological reason for admission to hospital in the USA, accounting for 49 per 10 000 recorded hospital discharges. However, since most PID is asymptomatic, this figure almost certainly underestimates true prevalence.[1,4]
AETIOLOGY/ RISK FACTORS	Factors associated with PID mirror those for sexually transmitted infections: young age, reduced socioeconomic circumstances, African/Afro-Caribbean ethnicity, lower educational attainment, and recent new sexual partner.[2,5,6] Most cases seem to result from ascending infection from the cervix. Initial epithelial damage caused by bacteria (especially *Chlamydia trachomatis* and *Neisseria gonorrhoeae*) allows the opportunistic entry of other organisms. Isolates from the upper genital tract are polymicrobial, including *Mycoplasma hominis* and anaerobes.[7] The spread of infection to the upper genital tract may be influenced by vaginal douching, instrumentation of the cervix, and using contraceptives.[8–11]
PROGNOSIS	PID has high morbidity; about 20% of affected women become infertile, 20% develop chronic pelvic pain, and 10% of those who conceive have an ectopic pregnancy.[2] We found no placebo controlled trials of antibiotic treatment. Uncontrolled observations suggest that clinical symptoms and signs resolve in a significant number of untreated women.[12] Repeated episodes of PID are associated with a four to sixfold increase in the risk of permanent tubal damage.[13]
AIMS	To alleviate the pain and systemic malaise associated with infection; to achieve microbiological cure; to prevent development of permanent tubal damage with associated sequelae, such as chronic pelvic pain, ectopic pregnancy and infertility; and to prevent the spread of infection to others.
OUTCOMES	Incidence and severity of acute symptoms and signs; microbiological cure of the upper genital tract; incidence of chronic pelvic pain, ectopic pregnancy, and infertility; rate of transmission to others.
METHODS	*Clinical Evidence* update search and appraisal May 2000.

QUESTION	Should suspected PID be treated empirically or should treatment be delayed until the results of microbiological investigations are known?

OPTION	EMPIRICAL ANTIBIOTIC TREATMENT

We found no evidence to support or refute empirical treatment for suspected PID.

Benefits:	We found no systematic review or RCTs comparing empirical versus delayed treatment.

Harms: We found no reliable evidence on harms of empirical treatment.

Comment: Because there are no reliable clinical diagnostic criteria for PID, early empirical treatment is common.[3] The positive predictive value of a clinical diagnosis is 65–90% compared with laparoscopy.[1–3] The absence of infection from the lower genital tract, where samples are usually taken, does not exclude PID,[2] and so may not influence the decision to treat.

QUESTION How do different antimicrobial regimens compare?

One systematic review has found that several regimens of parenteral followed by oral antibiotic treatment are effective in resolving the acute symptoms and signs associated with PID (see table 1, p 938). We found no good evidence on the optimal duration of treatment, or comparing oral versus parenteral treatment.

Benefits: We found one systematic review (search dates 1966 to 1992),[14] which was subsequently updated (search date 1992 to 1997).[15] These reviews identified 26 studies of 16 antimicrobial regimens in 1925 women with PID. The identified studies included case series, and it is not possible from the aggregated data published in the reviews to ascertain how many studies were RCTs. Inclusion criteria were a diagnosis of PID (clinical, microbiological, laparoscopic, or by endometrial biopsy) and microbiological testing for *C trachomatis* and *N gonorrhoeae*. The reviews found antibiotics to be effective in relieving the symptoms associated with PID, with clinical and microbiological cure rates of 90–100% (see table 1, p 938). **Duration of treatment:** The duration of treatment was not addressed, although the most common treatment period was 14 days. **Oral versus parenteral treatment:** The reviews did not analyse outcomes by oral or parenteral route of administration. Most regimens started with parenteral treatment and continued with oral treatment at different points. Two RCTs (n = 249, n = 72) compared oral ofloxacin versus parenteral cefoxitin and doxycycline. The trials found no significant difference in cure rates among groups (clinical cure rates about 95% for all treatments).[16,17]

Harms: The harms associated with treatment were not specifically addressed by the systematic reviews.[14,15] In two RCTs reporting adverse effects, withdrawal from treatment was uncommon (2/20 for doxycycline/metronidazole; 0/20 for perfloxacin/metronidazole; 0/16 for ciprofloxacin).[18,19]

Comment: We found little evidence about long term sequelae of PID, adverse effects of treatment, treatment of PID of differing severity, the effect of ethnicity, or the relevance of tracing sexual contacts. The risks of tubal occlusion and subsequent infertility relate to the severity of PID prior to starting therapy,[20] and clinical improvement may not translate into preserved fertility.[21,22]

Substantive changes since last issue

Oral versus parenteral treatment Two RCTs comparing oral ofloxacin versus parenteral doxycycline and cefoxitin. Found no significant difference for cure rates.[16,17]

Antibiotic treatments Two RCTs found that withdrawal from treatment was rare for a range of antibiotics.[18,19]

REFERENCES

1. Morcos R, Frost N, Hnat M, Petrunak A, Caldito G. Laparoscopic versus clinical diagnosis of acute pelvic inflammatory disease. *J Reprod Med* 1993; 38:53–56.
2. Metters JS, Catchpole M, Smith C, et al. *Chlamydia trachomatis: summary and conclusions of CMO's expert advisory group.* London: Department of Health, 1998.
3. Centers for Disease Control. *1998 guidelines for treatment of sexually transmitted diseases.* Bethesda, Maryland: CDC, 1998. http://www.cdc.gov/epo/mmwr/preview/mmwrhtml/00050909.htm.
4. Velebil P, Wingo PA, Xia Z, Wilcox LS, Peterson HB. Rate of hospitalization for gynecologic disorders among reproductive-age women in the United States. *Obstet Gynecol* 1995;86:764–769.
5. Simms I, Catchpole M, Brugha R, Rogers P, Mallinson H, Nicoll A. Epidemiology of genital Chlamydia trachomatis in England and Wales. *Genitourin Med* 1997;73:122–126.
6. Grodstein F, Rothman KJ. Epidemiology of pelvic inflammatory disease. *Epidemiology* 1994;5:234–242.
7. Bevan CD, Johal BJ, Mumtaz G, Ridgway GL, Siddle NC. Clinical, laparoscopic and microbiological findings in acute salpingitis: report on a United Kingdom cohort. *Br J Obstet Gynaecol* 1995;102:407–414.
8. Wolner-Hanssen P, Eschenbach DA, Paavonen J, et al. Association between vaginal douching and acute pelvic inflammatory disease. *JAMA* 1990; 263:1936–1941.
9. Jacobson L, Westrom L. Objectivized diagnosis of acute pelvic inflammatory disease. Diagnostic and prognostic value of routine laparoscopy. *Am J Obstet Gynecol* 1969;105:1088–1098.
10. Kelaghan J, Rubin GL, Ory HW, Layde PM. Barrier-method contraceptives and pelvic inflammatory disease. *JAMA* 1982;248:184–187.
11. Wolner-Hanssen P, Eschenbach DA, Paavonen J, et al. Decreased risk of symptomatic chlamydial pelvic inflammatory disease associated with oral contraceptive use. *JAMA* 1990;263:54–59.
12. Curtis AH. Bacteriology and pathology of fallopian tubes removed at operation. *Surg Gynecol Obstet* 1921;33:621.
13. Hillis SD, Owens LM, Marchbanks PA, Amsterdam LF, MacKenzie WR. Recurrent chlamydial infections increase the risks of hospitalization for ectopic pregnancy and pelvic inflammatory disease. *Am J Obstet Gynecol* 1997;176:103–107.
14. Walker CK, Kahn JG, Washington AE, Peterson HB, Sweet RL. Pelvic inflammatory disease: metaanalysis of antimicrobial regimen efficacy. *J Infect Dis* 1993;168:969–978. Search date 1992; primary sources Medline 1966–1992, and bibliographies from reviews, textbooks, and references.
15. Walker CK, Workowski KA, Washington AE, Soper DE, Sweet RL. Anaerobes in pelvic inflammatory disease: implications for the Centers for Disease Control and Prevention's guidelines for treatment of sexually transmitted diseases. *Clin Infect Dis* 1999;28:S29–36. Search date 1997; primary sources Medline 1966–1997, and bibliographies from reviews, textbooks, and references.
16. Martens MG, Gordon S, Yarborough DR, Faro S, Binder D, Berkeley A. Multicenter randomized trial of ofloxacin versus cefoxitin and doxycycline in outpatient treatment of pelvic inflammatory disease. Ambulatory PID Research Group. *South Med J* 1993; 86:604–610.
17. Wendel GD, Cox SM, Bawdon RE, Theriot SK, Heard MC, Nobles BJ. A randomized trial of ofloxacin versus cefoxitin and doxycycline in the outpatient treatment of acute salpingitis. *Am J Obstet Gynecol* 1991;164:1390–1396.
18. Witte EH, Peters AA, Smit IB, et al. A comparison of pefloxacin/metronidazole and doxycycline/metronidazole in the treatment of laparoscopically confirmed acute pelvic inflammatory disease. *Eur J Obstet Gynecol Reprod Biol* 1993;50:153–158.
19. Heinonen PK, Teisala K, Miettinen A, Aine R, Punnonen R, Gronroos P. A comparison of ciprofloxacin with doxycycline plus metronidazole in the treatment of acute pelvic inflammatory disease. *Scand J Infect Dis Suppl* 1989;60:66–73.
20. Soper DE, Brockwell NJ, Dalton HP. Microbial etiology of urban emergency department acute salpingitis: treatment with ofloxacin. *Am J Obstet Gynecol* 1992;167:653–660.
21. Buchan H, Vessey M, Goldacre M, Fairweather J. Morbidity following pelvic inflammatory disease. *Br J Obstet Gynaecol* 1993;100:558–562.
22. Brunham RC, Binns B, Guijon F, et al. Etiology and outcome of acute pelvic inflammatory disease. *J Infect Dis* 1988;158:510–517.

Jonathan Ross
Honorary Senior Lecturer
University of Birmingham
Birmingham
UK

Competing interests: None declared.

TABLE 1	**Cure rates for the antibiotic treatment of acute PID: aggregated data from systematic reviews of RCTs and case series (see text, p 936).[14,15]**		

Drug regimen	Number of studies	Number of women	Cure rate (%) Clinical/ microbiological*
Inpatient treatment (initially parenteral switching to oral)			
Clindamycin + aminoglycoside	11	470	91/97
Cefoxitin + doxycycline	8	427	91/98
Cefotetan + doxycycline	3	174	95/100
Ceftizoxime + tetracycline	1	18	88/100
Cefotaxime + tetracycline	1	19	94/100
Ciprofloxacin	4	90	94/96
Ofloxacin	1	36	100/97
Sulbactam/ampicillin + doxycycline	1	37	95/100
Amoxicillin/clavulanic acid	1	32	93/-
Metronidazole + doxycycline	2	36	75/71
Outpatient treatment (oral unless indicated otherwise)			
Cefoxitin (im) + probenecid + doxycycline	3	219	89/93
Ofloxacin	2	165	95/100
Amoxicillin/clavulanic acid	1	35	100/100
Sulbactam/ampicillin	1	36	70/70
Ceftriaxone (im) + doxycycline	1	64	95/100
Ciprofloxacin + clindamycin	1	67	97/94

im, intramuscular; *N gonorrhoeae, C trachomatis, or both, when detected in lower genital tract.

Updated this issue

*Fay Crawford, Rachel Hart, Sally EM Bell-Syer, David J Togerson
Philip Young and Ian Russell*

QUESTIONS

INTERVENTIONS

Beneficial

Likely to be beneficial

Unknown effectiveness

**To be covered in future issues of
*Clinical Evidence***
Oral antifungal treatments

Key Messages

- Systematic reviews of RCTs have found strong evidence that topical treatments, including allylamines, azoles, undecenoic acid, and tolnaftate, increase cure rates in fungal skin infections of the foot compared with placebo (NNT 2).

- We found no evidence of significant differences in efficacy between individual allylamines or individual azoles.

- One systematic review of RCTs has found that topical allylamines produce a faster response than azoles but the cure rates are similar.

- Single RCTs found that topical ciclopiroxolamine and griseofulvin were more effective than placebo.

- We found no evidence about the effectiveness of topical treatments for fungal nail infections.

DEFINITION	Athlete's foot is a cutaneous fungal infection that causes the skin to itch, flake, and fissure. Nail involvement is characterised by ungual thickening and discolouration.
INCIDENCE/ PREVALENCE	In the UK, athlete's foot is present in about 15% of the general population,[1] and 1.2 million people have fungally infected toe nails.[2]
AETIOLOGY/ RISK FACTORS	Swimming pool users and industrial workers may have increased risk of fungal foot infection. However, one survey found fungal foot infection in only 8.5% of swimmers, with the highest incidence (20%) in men aged 16 years and over.[1]
PROGNOSIS	Fungal infections of the foot are not life threatening in people with normal immunity, but in some people they cause persistent symptoms. Others are apparently oblivious of persistent infection. The infection can spread to other parts of the body and to other individuals.
AIMS	To control symptoms and prevent recurrence, with minimal adverse effects.
OUTCOMES	Rates of fungal eradication, shown by negative microscopy and culture, and resolution of clinical signs and symptoms at follow up.
METHODS	We searched Medline, Embase, and the Cochrane Controlled Trials Register to May 2000 for systematic reviews and subsequent RCTs (all languages). Studies were excluded if foot specific data could not be extracted. We excluded studies that did not use microscopy and culture (skin infections) or culture (nail infections) for diagnosis and as an outcome measure.

QUESTION **What are the effects of topical antifungals for athlete's foot?**

OPTION **TOPICAL ALLYLAMINES**

A systematic review of RCTs has found that allylamines are more effective than placebo in curing fungal skin infections. It found insufficient evidence comparing different allylamines with one another. Allylamines produce a faster response than azoles but the cure rates are similar.

Benefits: We found one systematic review (search date May 1999).[3,4] **Versus placebo:** The review identified 12 RCTs comparing topical allylamines versus placebo for 1–4 weeks in 1433 people with fungal infections of the foot.[3,4] Follow up was 6–8 weeks. Topical allylamines reduced the risk of treatment failure assessed by culture or microscopy (AR 27% v 80% for placebo; ARR 54%, 95% CI 48% to 58%; RRR 67%, 95% CI 61% to 73%; NNT 2 at 6 weeks). **Different allylamines:** The systematic review identified one small RCT that compared different allylamines (n = 60).[3] It found no significant difference between naftifine versus terbinafine (AR of treatment failure 75% v 81% for terbinafine; ARR 5%, 95% CI –17% to +21%). **Versus topical azoles:** See topical azoles, p 941.

Harms: The systematic review did not report frequency of adverse effects.[3] We found few reports of local irritation in any of the trials.

Comment: The systematic review assessed the quality of reporting in the trials. Out of a possible 12 points, the mean quality score for all 72 included studies was 6.3. Few demographic details of participants were reported.[3]

OPTION TOPICAL AZOLES

A systematic review of RCTs has found that azole creams administered for 4–6 weeks increase cure rate compared with placebo. We found no evidence of differences in efficacy between individual azoles. Allylamines produce a faster response than azoles but the cure rates are similar.

Benefits: We found one systematic review (search date May 1999).[3,4] **Versus placebo:** The review identified 17 placebo controlled RCTs in 1259 people with fungal skin infections of the foot. Intervention lasted for 4–6 weeks and follow up ranged from 6–10 weeks. Azoles reduced the risk of failure to cure, determined by culture or microscopy (AR 126/664 [19%] with azoles, 362/595 [61%] with placebo; ARR 42%, 95% CI 38% to 48%; RRR 69%, 95% CI 62% to 75%; NNT 2 to achieve one extra cure, 95% CI 2 to 3). **Different azoles:** The systematic review identified 12 RCTs in 584 people with fungal infection of the foot comparing one azole against another over 3–4 weeks and with follow up over 3–10 weeks. No consistent difference was found. **Versus topical allylamines:** The systematic review identified 12 RCTs (n = 1487) that compared at least 4 weeks of azole treatment with 1–6 weeks of topical allylamine treatment in people with fungal infections of the foot. It found that after 3–12 weeks of follow up, allylamines reduced the risk of treatment failure compared with azoles (AR of treatment failure with allylamines 146/773 [19%] v 224/714 [31%] for azoles; ARR 13%, 95% CI 9% to 16%; RRR 40%, 95% CI 27% to 51%; NNT 8, 95% CI 6 to 12). Four included RCTs found that a 1 week course of allylamines produced similar cure rates as a 4 week course of azoles (AR of treatment failure 53/464 [11%] for 1 week allylamine, 71/448 [16%] for 4 weeks azole; ARR 4.4%, 95% CI 0% to 8%).[3,4]

Harms: The systematic review did not report frequency of adverse effects with topical azoles. We found few reports of local irritation of the feet.

Comment: The trials comparing allylamines and azoles were not consistent in their results; four non-English language RCTs found no evidence of a difference between allylamines and azoles.

OPTION OTHER TOPICAL AGENTS

A systematic review of RCTs has found that topical undecenoic acid and tolnaftate are more effective than placebo (NNT 2). Single RCTs found that topical ciclopiroxolamine and griseofulvin cured more than placebo.

Benefits: We found one systematic review (search date May 1999).[3,4] **Topical ciclopiroxolamine versus placebo:** The review identified one RCT comparing ciclopiroxolamine with placebo in 144 people with fungal skin infection of the foot for 4 weeks, with 6 weeks' follow up. Ciclopiroxolamine reduced the risk of treatment failure (AR 31/71 [44%] for ciclopiroxolamine, 67/73 [92%] for placebo; ARR 48%, 95% CI 25% to 69%; RRR 52%, 95% CI 27% to 75%; NNT 2, 95% CI 1 to 4). **Topical griseofulvin versus placebo:** The review identified one RCT in 94 people, which found that griseofulvin reduced the risk of treatment failure compared with placebo (AR 9/47 [19%] for griseofulvin, 31/47 [66%] for placebo; ARR 47%, 95% CI 28% to 58%; RRR 71%, 95% CI 43% to 87%; NNT 2, 95% CI 2 to 4). **Topical undecenoic acid versus placebo:** The review identified four RCTs in 223 people, which found that undecenoic acid reduced the risk of treatment failure compared with placebo (AR 40/123 [33%] with undecenoic acid, 81/103 [79%] with placebo; ARR 46%, 95% CI 32% to 58%; RRR 59%, 95% CI 40% to 73%; NNT 2, 95% CI 2 to 3). **Topical tolnaftate versus placebo:** The review identified three RCTs in 148 people, which found that tolnaftate for 4 weeks was more effective than placebo at 5–8 weeks' follow up (AR 20/78 [26%] for tolnaftate v 49/70 [70%] for placebo; ARR 44%, 95% CI 29% to 56%; RRR 63%, 95% CI 41% to 79%; NNT 2, 95% CI 2 to 4).

Harms: The systematic review did not report frequency of adverse effects.

Comment: None.

QUESTION What are the effects of topical antifungals for nail infections?

We found insufficient evidence on the effects of topical antifungal agents in people with frequently infected toenails.

Benefits: We found one systematic review (search date May 1999, 2 RCTs, n = 36 and n = 117) comparing topical treatments for toenail infections. The review found insufficient evidence to draw conclusions.[3,4]

Harms: We found no evidence.

Comment: Neither trial included in the systematic review reported blinding of outcome assessment. The smaller trial did not report the method of randomisation.[3,4]

REFERENCES

1. Gentles JC, Evans EGV. Foot infections in swimming baths. *BMJ* 1973;3:260–262.
2. Roberts DT. Prevalence of dermatophyte onychomycosis in the UK: results of an omnibus survey. *Br J Dermatol* 1992;126(suppl 39):23–27.
3. Crawford F, Hart R, Bell-Syer S, Torgerson D, Young P, Russell I. Topical treatments for fungal infections of the skin and nails of the foot. In: The Cochrane Library, Issue 1, 2000. Oxford: Update Software. Search date May 1999; primary sources Medline 1966 to May 1999; Embase 1980 to May 1999; Cinahl to May 1999; Cochrane Controlled Trials Register 1966 to May 1999; Science Citation Index (no search dates given); Biosis (no search dates given); CAB-Health to 1997; Healthstar to 1997; DARE to 1997; the NHS Economic Evaluation Database to 1997; Econlit to 1997; hand searched references and key journals, and pharmaceutical companies contacted.
4. Hart R, Bell-Syer EM, Crawford F, Torgerson DJ, Young P, Russell I. Systematic review of topical treatments for fungal infections of the skin and nails of the feet. *BMJ* 1999;319:79–82. Search date 1997; primary sources Medline to 1997; Embase to 1997; Cinahl to 1997; Cochrane Controlled Trials Register to 1997; CAB—Health to 1997; Healthstar to 1997; BIDS to 1997; DARE to 1997; the NHS Economic Evaluation Database to 1997; Econlit to 1997; hand searched references and key journals, and pharmaceutical companies contacted.

Fay Crawford
MRC Fellow

University of York
York
UK

Rachel Hart
Research Podiatrist

University of Wales Institute
Cardiff
UK

Sally EM Bell-Syer
Research Fellow

David J Torgerson
Senior Research Fellow

Philip Young
Lecturer

Ian Russell
Professor of Health Sciences

University of York
York
UK

Competing interests: None declared.

Updated this issue

Carolyn Charman

Key Messages

Treatments

- Small RCTs have found that topical corticosteroids provide symptomatic relief and are safe in the short term. We found little good information on their long term adverse effects or on effects (if any) on the natural history of atopic eczema.

- Three RCTs provide no evidence that routinely adding antimicrobial agents to topical steroid preparations provides additional benefit. However, only two of the trials studied people with clinically infected eczema.

- We found limited evidence suggesting that adding emollients to topical steroid treatment improves symptoms and signs more than topical steroids alone.

- We found insufficient evidence on the effects of wet wrap or other forms of bandaging.

- We found limited evidence suggesting that controlling house dust mite reduces severity of symptoms, especially in people with positive mite radioallergosorbent test (RAST) scores and in children, but only if very low levels are achieved. Bedding covers were found to be the most effective method of control.

- We found insufficient evidence that dietary manipulation in adults or children reduces symptom severity.

Prevention in predisposed infants

- We found insufficient evidence that either prolonged breast feeding or maternal dietary manipulation during lactation protects against eczema in infants with a family history of atopy.

Avoidance of provoking factors

- We found no evidence that avoidance of animals, detergents containing enzymes, all washing detergents, or vaccinations is beneficial in atopic eczema.

- We found limited evidence suggesting that the roughness of clothing textiles is a more important factor for skin irritation than the type of fabric (cotton or polyester).

DEFINITION	Atopic eczema (atopic dermatitis) is an inflammatory skin disease characterised by an itchy erythematous poorly demarcated skin eruption with a predilection for skin creases.[1]
INCIDENCE/ PREVALENCE	Atopic eczema affects 15–20% of school children in the UK and 2–3% of adults.[2] Prevalence has increased substantially over the past 30 years,[3] possibly because of environmental and lifestyle changes.
AETIOLOGY/ RISK FACTORS	Aetiology is believed to be multifactorial. Recent interest has focused on airborne allergens (house dust mites, pollen, animal dander), outdoor pollution, climate, diet, and prenatal/early life factors such as infections.
PROGNOSIS	Although there is currently no cure, several interventions can help to control symptoms. Atopic eczema clears in 60–70% of children by their early teens, although relapses may occur.
AIMS	To reduce the risk of atopic eczema in predisposed infants and children; to minimise the impact of the disease on quality of life.
OUTCOMES	Severity of symptoms (pruritus, sleep disturbance) and signs (erythema, oozing/crusting, lichenification, cracking, oedema/ papulation, excoriation, and dryness); quality of life; area of skin involvement. Trials used a range of atopic eczema scoring systems, including SCORAD (scoring of atopic dermatitis), SASSAD (six area six sign atopic dermatitis severity score), Rajka and Langeland scoring system, and the dermatology life quality index.
METHODS	Systematic reviews and controlled clinical trials were located by searching the Cochrane Library (1998), Best Evidence (1998), Medline (1966 to 1998), and Embase (1988 to 1998). *Clinical Evidence* update search and appraisal May 2000. We included all RCTs that met *Clinical Evidence* quality criteria. Because of the limited studies available for many questions, we included some with shortcomings in methods, which we mention in the text.

QUESTION What are the effects of treatments in adults and children?

OPTION TOPICAL STEROIDS

Small, short term, placebo controlled RCTs have found that topical corticosteroids applied for 1–4 weeks improve atopic eczema. We found little good information on their long term effects. No systemic effects have been reported in short term RCTs or in one longer term cohort study. Volunteer studies found that potent topical steroid preparations cause skin thinning after twice daily application for up to 6 weeks, although skin thickness returns to normal within 4 weeks of stopping treatment. Topical steroids provide symptomatic relief while used, but their effect on the natural history of atopic eczema is unknown.

Benefits: We found no systematic review. **Versus placebo:** We found 10 double blind RCTs comparing topical steroids versus placebo cream (vehicle) in children and adults with atopic eczema.[4–13] All the studies found significant improvement with steroid compared with placebo (see table 2, p 956). **Versus each other:** We found 35 additional double blind RCTs in children and adults with atopic eczema which compared a variety of topical steroids with each other. These found significant improvements in 22–100% of people after 1–6 weeks of treatment. **Prevention of relapse:** One RCT included 54 adults with atopic eczema that had "completely healed" with a 4 week course of a potent topical steroid. It found that application of fluticasone propionate on two consecutive days per week for 16 weeks resulted in significant maintenance of improvement, compared with clinical deterioration in people receiving only the placebo.[14]

Harms: No serious systemic effects or cases of skin atrophy were reported in these short term RCTs, nor in a longer cohort study in 14 prepubertal children (median treatment 6.5 years with mild to moderate potency topical steroids). Minor adverse effects such as burning, stinging, irritation, folliculitis, hypertrichosis, contact dermatitis, and pigmentary disturbances occurred in less than 10% of patients. **Skin thinning:** In the RCT examining prevention of relapse in people with atopic eczema, no histological evidence of skin atrophy was noted after 16 weeks of applying a potent steroid compared with placebo twice weekly to healed lesions.[14] We found no further RCTs looking at skin thinning in people with atopic eczema. Four small RCTs in healthy volunteers (n = 12) used ultrasound to evaluate skin thickness.[15–18] Significant skin thinning occurred after 1 week with clobetasol 17-propionate 0.05% twice daily, and after 3 weeks with twice daily triaminolone acetate 0.1%, and betamethasone 17-valerate 0.1%. All preparations were used for up to 6 weeks, and skin thinning reversed within 4 weeks of stopping treatment. No significant thinning was reported with hydrocortisone prednicarbate twice daily, or mometasone furoate once daily after 6 weeks.

Comment: Studies that did not specify the type of eczema, or those which included other dermatoses in the overall analysis, were excluded. The RCTs used different clinical scoring systems, making it difficult to compare results.

Three RCTs found no evidence that combinations of topical antimicrobial agents and steroids are better than topical steroids alone in improving the clinical signs and symptoms of atopic eczema. Only two of the trials studied people with clinically infected eczema.

Benefits: We found no systematic review. **Versus topical steroid alone:** We found three RCTs comparing topical antimicrobial/steroid combinations versus topical steroid alone in people with atopic dermatitis.[19-21] The RCTs found no significant improvement in clinical signs and symptoms after betamethasone valerate/fusidic acid,[20] hydrocortisone acetate/fusidic acid,[19] or betamethasone valerate/gentamicin[21] compared with topical steroid alone. **Versus each other:** We found five further RCTs (34–207 people) comparing different topical steroid/antimicrobial preparations with each other in people with clinically infected eczema (atopic eczema not specified).[22-26] These found clinical improvement in 54–95% of participants, with no significant difference between the various preparations with respect to improvement in clinical signs and symptoms. People treated with fusidic acid/hydrocortisone showed a more rapid clinical response than those treated with miconazole/hydrocortisone, and bacteriological responses to betamethasone/fusidic acid and fucidic acid/hydrocortisone were superior to those with betamethasone/clioquinol and miconazole/hydrocortisone, respectively.

Harms: Overall, the trials reported minor adverse effects comprising itching, stinging, burning, and irritation in fewer than 2% of patients.

Comment: Only two of the studies specified a degree of infection in most participants at recruitment.[20,21] One of these also included people with contact dermatitis in the overall analysis, and the use of left/right comparisons within individual participants may have reduced the difference between groups because of systemic absorption of the antimicrobial agent.[20]

OPTION   EMOLLIENTS

One RCT found that adding an emollient to a topical corticosteroid regimen further improved clinical signs and symptoms of atopic eczema. One comparative study also found improvements in atopic eczema when emollients were used in combination with topical steroids.

Benefits: We found no systematic review. **As adjunct to topical steroids:** One RCT (n = 80) assessed adding moisturising cream three times daily to a topical corticosteroid regimen (desonide 0.05%) applied twice daily to children and adults with mild to moderate atopic eczema.[27] It found additional significant improvement in people receiving the emollient after 3 weeks (70% v 55%), with 96% of people preferring treatment with the emollient and topical steroid than with topical steroid alone. One further controlled clinical trial (25 children, randomisation not mentioned) found no significant difference between once daily emollient cream plus once daily hydrocortisone 2.5% cream, and twice daily hydrocortisone 2.5% cream; both treatment regimens produced no significant difference in signs and symptoms after 3 weeks.[28] One RCT compared the efficacy of two different emollients (cream and lotion) applied once daily as an adjunct to once daily 2.5% hydrocortisone cream in people with atopic eczema (n = 50). After 3 weeks, a significant improvement in signs and symptoms was noted with both treatment regimens.[29]

Harms: Minor adverse effects, such as a burning sensation, were reported in fewer than 2% of people.

Comment: Many of the studies located in our search did not specify the type of eczema, or included people with other forms of eczema, so were excluded from this review. We have not included studies looking at bath additives.

OPTION WET WRAP DRESSINGS AND BANDAGING

We found insufficient evidence on the effects of wet wrap or other forms of bandaging in people with atopic eczema.

Benefits: We found no systematic review or RCTs.

Harms: Enhanced topical steroid absorption and adverse effects have been found with earlier forms of wet wrap dressings (see glossary, p 953). Mean serum cortisol concentrations were depressed significantly after treatment in the 30 erythrodermic children described (see comment below) returning to normal after 2 weeks.[30]

Comment: One uncontrolled study used wet wrap dressings in 30 children with acute erythrodermic eczema.[30] All children responded well to treatment after 2–5 days, with no relapses 2 weeks later (no quantitative results given). One uncontrolled study in 21 children with chronic severe atopic eczema treated with wet wrap dressings twice per week or less for 3 months found that in all children the eczema improved after starting treatment and sleep disturbance was reduced. Most parents reported a reduction in topical steroid requirements (no quantitative results given).[31] As both studies were uncontrolled, the improvement may have been attributable to the additional medical or nursing input during the study rather than to an effect of the wet wraps.

OPTION CONTROL OF HOUSE DUST MITE

One small RCT found that extreme reduction in dust levels (achieved by synthetic mattress covers, acaricidal spraying, and high filtration vacuuming) reduced eczema severity score. It is impossible to tell from this evidence how many people might benefit and for how long. The clinical relevance of the reduced severity score is uncertain. Bedding covers seem to be the most effective intervention for reducing levels in the home (see table 1, p 955).

Benefits: We found no systematic review. We found three controlled trials, one of which did not mention randomisation. One double blind RCT in 48 atopic people (24 adults and 24 children > 7 years old, skin prick and RAST status not specified) compared bed covers made of a breathable synthetic material plus benzyltannate spray and high filtration vacuuming, versus cotton bedcovers plus placebo spray and standard vacuum cleaners. After 6 months there was a significantly greater reduction in eczema severity scores on active treatment compared with placebo (mean difference in severity score [maximum 108 units] 4.3 units, 95% CI 1.3 to 7.3). This was associated with a 98% reduction in mean mattress dust load compared with 16% in the placebo group (P = 0.002) and a 91% and 76% reduction in the concentration of mite allergen Der p1 on bedroom and living room carpet, compared with 89% (P = 0.94) and 38% (P = 0.27) in the placebo group.[34] One double blind RCT using natamycin or placebo spray with or without vacuuming in 20 atopic dermatitis patients (aged 12–47 years with positive skin prick and RAST tests to house dust mite) showed no correlation between improvement in clinical score and lowered mite numbers. The study was small, however, and the maximum reduction in mite numbers in mattresses was only 68%.[35] One controlled trial (randomisation not mentioned) in people with atopic eczema showed induction of an itch free period and prolonged remission in 30 people with positive mite RAST scores after 3 weeks in a "clean room" with reduced dust levels (Der p1 levels were not measured). Neither an itch free period nor prolonged remission were seen in the 11 people with negative RAST scores treated in a similar environment, or in the 10 controls with positive mite RAST scores treated in a common hospital room.[36]

Harms: No harmful effects were reported in the trials.

Comment: Additional, small, uncontrolled studies have suggested a beneficial effect of mite reduction measures on symptoms, although mite or allergen levels were not quantified. The use of bedding covers seems to be the simplest and most effective measure to reduce house dust mite levels in the home (see table 1, p 955).

OPTION	DIETARY MANIPULATION

We found insufficient evidence for dietary manipulation such as exclusion of egg and cow's milk in children with atopic eczema. We found no good evidence that dietary manipulation alters the severity of eczema in adults.

Benefits: **In infants:** We found one systematic review (search date 1995), which identified one small RCT in 17 breast fed infants with atopic eczema. This looked at the effect of excluding allergenic foods, such as cow's milk and eggs, from the mother's diet. It found no effect on eczema severity.[37] However, soya milk, which is potentially allergenic itself, was used as a cow's milk substitute in this trial. **In children:** We found no systematic review. We found two double blind crossover RCTs evaluating the effects of an egg and milk exclusion diet in unselected children with eczema. Both used potentially allergenic soya based milk substitute during the trial period.[38,39] One (20 children aged 2–8 years) found a significant improvement in eczema severity (14/20 treated children improved v 1/20 controls).[38] The other trial (40 children and young adults) found no significant effect.[40] One further RCT evaluated the effect of an egg exclusion diet in 55 children with proven sensitivity to eggs (positive RAST). The mean reduction in surface area affected by eczema was significantly greater in the group receiving dietary advice (from 19.6% to 10.9%) than in controls (from 21.9% to 18.9%). The mean improvement in severity score in the diet group (from 33.9 to 24) was also significantly greater than in controls (from 36.7 to 33.5).[40] Double blind placebo controlled food challenges have been used to identify people with food allergy, but the clinical relevance of positive reactions (which may include gastrointestinal, respiratory, or cutaneous symptoms) to subsequent eczema control is unclear. One retrospective diagnostic study examined hypersensitivity reactions up to 48 hours after double blind, placebo controlled food challenges in 107 children aged 5 months to 12 years with moderate to severe atopic dermatitis and a history suggestive of food allergy. This study found positive reactions in 81% of children, with 70% of reactions occurring within 2 hours. Egg and cow's milk accounted for 83% of the positive reactions.[41] In three further studies, double blind, placebo controlled food challenges caused hypersensitivity reactions (all within 2 hours of the challenge) in 63% of children with moderate to severe atopic eczema (n = 320), and in 33–39% of children with mild to severe atopic eczema (n = 211). Egg, milk, and peanut accounted for 67–78% of the reactions. The effect of subsequent dietary elimination was studied in only 27 of these children. This showed a greater improvement in children on exclusion diets than in non-randomly selected controls, using a crude scoring system.[42] We found one RCT in 85 children (46 evaluable) that looked at a "few foods diet", in which all but a handful of foods were excluded. It did not find a significant benefit on eczema severity.[43] **In adults:** We found no systematic review but found two RCTs.[39,44] One double blind, crossover RCT studied adults and children separately. It found no significant improvement in eczema severity with an egg and cow's milk exclusion diet in 18 adults, although potentially allergenic soya milk was used as a cow's milk substitute.[39] One further RCT (33 adults, 25 evaluable) found no significant benefit of an elemental diet (containing amino acids, essential fatty acids, glucose, trace elements, sorbic acid, and vitamins) on eczema severity.[44]

Harms: Calcium, protein, and calorie deficiency are risks of dairy free diets in children.

Comment: The clinical relevance of changes in severity scores obtained in many studies is unknown. We have not included studies looking at the role of food additives, fatty acid supplementation, or trace elements in eczema.

QUESTION   **What are the effects of preventive interventions in predisposed infants?**

OPTION   PROLONGED BREAST FEEDING IN PREDISPOSED INFANTS

We found limited observational evidence suggesting that exclusive breast feeding for at least 5 months reduces the risk of eczema in infants with a family history of atopy.

Benefits: We found no systematic review or RCTs. One 17 year prospective cohort study of 236 healthy infants found that those who were breast fed exclusively for more than 6 months had a significantly lower prevalence of eczema at 1 year (all infants) and 3 years (infants with a family history of atopy) than those breast fed for less than 1 month and weaned onto cow's milk formula.[45] There was no reduction in the prevalence of eczema in infants who were intermittently breast fed for 2–6 months. Two prospective studies compared prevalence of eczema in exclusively breast fed infants and in non-breast fed infants (non-breast fed infants were randomised to different formulae).[46,47] In infants with a family history of atopy, those who were exclusively breast fed for an average of 5 months had a significantly lower prevalence of eczema at 18 months compared with non-breast fed infants randomised to soya or cow's milk, but not compared with those randomised to whey hydrolysate or casein hydrolysate. One further prospective study that randomised non-breast fed infants to different formulae found a significantly lower incidence of eczema at 3 years in infants breast fed for 6–13 months (8.1%) compared with those fed conventional adapted formula (23.7%) but a comparable incidence to those fed hydrolysed milk formula (10%). All infants were given hypoantigenic weaning diet.[48]

Harms: We found no evidence of harms associated with prolonged breast feeding.

Comment: Some additional studies found no beneficial effect of breast feeding, but all were methodologically poor. Much of the available evidence was methodologically flawed, for example by selection and information bias, short duration of breast feeding, and inadequate control for confounding factors such as introducing supplemental milk or solid foods. Prolonged self selected breast feeding may be associated with unknown protective factors, leading to bias.

OPTION MATERNAL DIETARY RESTRICTION DURING LACTATION

We found limited evidence from one systematic review of poor quality trials that maternal dietary restriction during lactation may protect against the development of eczema in infants with a family history of atopy.

Benefits: We found one systematic review (search date 1995, 3 RCTs).[49] The trials found a lower prevalence of eczema in breast fed infants whose mothers took antigen avoidance diets compared with those on normal diets during lactation.

Harms: None reported.

Comment: Shortcomings in method in all three trials argue for caution in applying these results.[49]

QUESTION **What are the effects of avoidance of provoking factors in adults and children?**

OPTION CLOTHING TEXTILES

Two small RCTs found that, in people with atopic eczema, the roughness of clothing textiles is a more important factor for skin irritation than the

type of textile fibre (synthetic or natural). Polyester and cotton of similar textile fineness seem to be equally well tolerated. We found no evidence on the long term effect of different textiles on the severity of atopic eczema.

Benefits: We found no systematic review but found two small RCTs. The first double blind RCT (20 people with atopic eczema and 20 healthy controls; mean age 25 years) compared cotton and polyester shirts of different fabric structure and coarseness at rest and after exercise to induce sweating.[50] All fabrics were tolerated less well when sweating, in people with eczema and in healthy controls. Comfort ratings for the fabrics did not differ significantly between the two groups. Knitted fabrics (polyester or cotton) were better tolerated than woven fabrics (all polyester). Of the knitted fabrics, polyester was as well tolerated by people with eczema as the comparable cotton shirt of similar textile fineness. At rest, people with eczema tolerated the less course knitted polyester better than the other polyester knitted fabrics, although there was no significant difference during exercise. Of the woven fabrics, the finer polyester was better tolerated by people with eczema than the coarser fabrics, both at rest and during exercise, although controls showed no significant difference. The second randomised crossover trial (24 women with atopic eczema, aged 15–20 years, with a history of wool irritation) compared the effects of two different wool fibres on itching.[51] Wool induced itching was more frequent after 12 hours with the coarser $36\,\mu$m wool fibre (16 women) than with the $20\,\mu$m wool fibre (9 women). Visible skin changes were seen in six women as a result of the thin fibre wool and 11 women with the thick fibre wool, disappearing within 24 hours in all cases.

Harms: With the exception of short term skin irritation, no harmful effects were reported in these trials.

Comment: None.

OPTION   **WASHING DETERGENTS**

One RCT found no evidence that washing detergents containing enzymes had a significant provoking effect on eczema severity compared with washing detergents without enzymes. We found no studies looking at the effect of avoidance of all contact with washing detergents.

Benefits: We found no systematic review. **Biological versus non-biological detergents:** We found one double blind crossover RCT (25 people with atopic eczema, aged 17–59 years), which compared washing detergents with or without enzymes.[52] It found no significant difference in clinical disease severity (using SCORAD scale), subjective symptoms, or corticosteroid use between the two groups after using each detergent for 1 month. **Avoidance of all washing detergents:** We found no RCTs.

Harms: No harmful effects were reported in this trial.

Comment: None.

OPTION   VACCINATION/IMMUNISATION

We found no studies of the effects of vaccination on atopic eczema severity.

Benefits: We found no systematic reviews or RCTs.

Harms: One observational study in 134 allergic children reported transient mild generalised urticaria and fever in two children with atopic eczema within 24 hours of vaccination.[53]

Comment: The study found that the lowest rate of positive skin prick tests to measles, mumps, and rubella vaccine was in the 68 children with atopic eczema (4% positive), compared with the 47 children with asthma (9% positive), and the 11 children with cow's milk allergy (18% positive).[53] The 64 children with atopic eczema who were subsequently vaccinated had no serious reactions, although the long term effect on eczema severity was not studied.

OPTION   ANIMAL CONTACT

We found no good evidence on the effects of avoiding animal contact on the severity of atopic eczema.

Benefits: We found no systematic review, RCTs, or cohort studies of the effects of avoiding animals or removing the family pet on the severity of atopic eczema.

Harms: We found no evidence.

Comment: Observational studies have suggested that keeping pets is associated with an increased prevalence of atopic eczema. Following removal of animals from the home it may take many months for the allergen load to decrease because of widespread distribution in carpets and soft furnishings.

GLOSSARY

Wet wrap dressings Are wet occlusive tubifast dressings which are applied over topical steroid or emollient.

REFERENCES

1. Williams HC, Burney PGJ, Pembroke AC, Hay RH. The UK working party's diagnostic criteria for atopic dermatitis. III. Independent hospital validation. Br J Dermatol 1994;131:406–417.

2. Kay J, Gawkrodger DJ, Mortimer MJ, Jaron AG. The prevalence of childhood atopic eczema in a general population. J Am Acad Dermatol 1994;30:35–39.

3. Williams HC. Is the prevalence of atopic dermatitis increasing? Clin Exp Dermatol 1992;17:385–391.

4. Lawlor F, Black AK, Greaves M. Prednicarbate 0.25% ointment in the treatment of atopic dermatitis: A vehicle-controlled double-blind study. J Dermatol Treat 1995;6:233–235.

5. Roth HL, Brown EP. Hydrocortisone valerate. Double-blind comparison with two other topical steroids. Cutis 1978;21:695–698.

6. Maloney JM, Morman MR, Stewart DM, et al. Clobetasol propionate emollient 0.05% in the treatment of atopic dermatitis. Int J Dermatol 1998;37:128–144.

7. Sears HW, Bailer JW, Yeadon A. Efficacy and safety

of hydrocortisone buteprate 0.1% cream in patients with atopic dermatitis. Clin ther 1997;19:710–719.

8. Vanderploeg DE. Betamethasone dipropionate ointment in the treatment of psoriasis and atopic dermatitis: a double-blind study. South Med J 1976;69:862–863.

9. Lupton ES, Abbrecht MM, Brandon ML. Short-term topical corticosteroid therapy (halcinonide ointment) in the management of atopic dermatitis. Cutis 1982;30:671–675.

10. Stalder JF, Fleury M, Sourisse M, et al. Local steroid therapy and bacterial skin flora in atopic dermatitis. Br J Dermatol 1994;131:536–540.

11. Sefton J, Loder JS, Kyriakopoulos AA. Clinical evaluation of hydrocortisone valerate 0.2% ointment. Clin ther 1984;6:282–293.

12. Wahlgren CF, H germark O, Bergström R, Hedin B. Evaluation of a new method of assessing pruritus and antipruritic drugs. Skin Pharmacol 1988;1:3–13.

13. Sudilovsky A, Muir JG, Bocobo FC. A comparison

of single and multiple applications of Halcinonide cream. *Int J Dermatol* 1981;20:609–613.

14. Van der Meer JB, Glazenburg EJ, Mulder PGH, et al. The management of moderate to severe atopic dermatitis in adults with topical fluticasone propionate. *Br J Dermatol* 1999;140:1114–1121.

15. Kerscher MJ, Hart H, Korting HC, Stalleicken D. In vivo assessment of the atrophogenic potency of mometasone furoate, a newly developed chlorinated potent topical glucocorticoid as compared to other topical glucocorticoids old and new. *Int J Clin Pharmacol ther* 1995;33:187–189.

16. Kerscher MJ, Korting HC. Comparative atrophogenicity potential of medium and highly potent topical glucocorticoids in cream and ointment according to ultrasound analysis. *Skin Pharmacol* 1992;5:77–80.

17. Kerscher MJ, Korting HC. Topical glucocorticoids of the non-fluorinated double-ester type. *Acta Derm Venereol* 1992;72:214–216.

18. Korting HC, Vieluf D, Kerscher M. 0.25% prednicarbate cream and the corresponding vehicle induce less skin atrophy than 0.1% betamethasone-17-valerate cream and 0.05% clobetasol-17-propionate cream. *Eur J Clin Pharmacol* 1992;42:159–161.

19. Ramsay CA, Savoie JM, Gilbert M, et al. The treatment of atopic dermatitis with topical fusidic acid and hydrocortisone acetate. *J Eur Acad Dermatol Venereol* 1996;7(suppl 1):15–22.

20. Hjorth N, Schmidt H, Thomsen K. Fusidic acid plus betamethasone in infected or potentially infected eczema. *Pharmatherapeutica* 1985;4:126–131.

21. Wachs GN, Maibach HI. Co-operative double-blind trial of an antibiotic/corticoid combination in impetiginized atopic dermatitis. *Br J Dermatol* 1976;95:323.

22. Hill VA, Wong E, Corbett MF, Menday AP. Comparative efficacy of betamethasone/clioquinol (Betnovate-C) cream and betamethasone/fusidic acid (Fucibet) cream in the treatment of infected hand eczema. *J Dermatol Treat* 1998;9:15–19.

23. Poyner TF, Dass BK. Comparative efficacy and tolerability of fusidic acid/hydrocortisone cream (Fucidin H cream) and miconazole/hydrocortisone cream (Daktacort cream) in infected eczema. *J Eur Acad Dermatol Venereol* 1996;7(suppl 1):23–30.

24. Meenan FOC. A double-blind comparative study to compare the efficacy of Locoid C with Tri-Adcortyl in children with infected eczema. *Br J Clin Pract* 1988;42:200–202.

25. Jaffe GV, Grimshaw JJ. A clinical trial of hydrocortisone/potassium hydroxyquinolone sulphate (Quinocort) in the treatment of infected eczema and impetigo in general practice. *Pharmatherapeutica* 1986;4:628–636.

26. Wilkinson JD, Leigh DA. Comparative efficacy of betamethasone and either fusidic acid or neomycin in infected or potentially infected eczema. *Curr Ther Res* 1985;38:177–182.

27. Hanifin JM, Hebert AA, Mays SR, et al. Effects of a low-potency corticosteroid lotion plus a moisturizing regimen in the treatment of atopic dermatitis. *Curr Ther Res* 1998;59:227–233.

28. Lucky AW, Leach AD, Laskarzewski P, Wenck H. Use of an emollient as a steroid-sparing agent in the treatment of mild to moderate atopic dermatitis in children. *Pediatr Dermatol* 1997;14:321–324.

29. Kantor I, Milbauer J, Posner M, et al. Efficacy and safety of emollients as adjunctive agents in topical corticosteroid therapy for atopic dermatitis. *Today Ther Trend* 1993;11:157–166.

30. Goodyear HM, Spowart K, Harper JI. 'Wet wrap' dressings for the treatment of atopic eczema in

children. *Br J Dermatol* 1991;125:604.

31. Mallon E, Powell S, Bridgman A. 'Wet-wrap' dressings for the treatment of atopic eczema in the community. *J Dermatol Treat* 1994;5:97–98.

32. Owen S, Morganstern M, Hepworth J, Woodcock A. Control of house dust mite antigen in bedding. *Lancet* 1990;335:396–397.

33. Nishioka K, Yasueda H, Saito H. Preventative effect of bedding encasement with microfine fibers on mite sensitization. *J Allergy Clin Immunol* 1998;101:28–32.

34. Tan B, Weald D, Strickland I, Frieman PS. Double-blind controlled trial of effect of house dust-mite allergen avoidance on atopic dermatitis. *Lancet* 1996;347:15–18.

35. Colloff MJ, Lever RS, McSharry C. A controlled trial of house dust mite eradication using natamycin in homes of patients with atopic dermatitis: effect on clinical status and mite populations. *Br J Dermatol* 1989;121:199–208.

36. Sanda T, Yasue T, Oohashi M, Yasue A. Effectiveness of house dust-mite allergen avoidance through clean room therapy in patients with atopic dermatitis. *J Allergy Clin Immunol* 1992;89:653–657.

37. Kramer MS. Maternal antigen avoidance during lactation for infants with atopic eczema. In: Neilson JP, Crowther CA, Hodnett ED, Hofmeyr GJ, eds. *Pregnancy and childbirth module*. The Cochrane Library, Issue 4, 1999. Oxford: Update Software. Search date 1995; primary sources the Cochrane Pregnancy and Childhood Review Group strategy; Medline; hand search selected journals; conference proceedings, survey of unpublished trials.

38. Atherton DJ, Sewell M, Soothill JF, Wells RS, Chilvers CE. A double-blind controlled crossover trial of an antigen avoidance diet in atopic eczema. *Lancet* 1978;1:401–403.

39. Neild VS, Marsden RA, Bailes JA, Bland JM. Egg and milk exclusion diets in atopic eczema. *Br J Dermatol* 1986;114:117–123.

40. Lever R, MacDonald C, Waugh P, Aitchison T. Randomised controlled trial of advice on an egg exclusion diet in young children with atopic eczema and sensitivity to eggs. *Pediatr Allergy* 1998;9:13–19.

41. Niggemann B, Sielaff B, Beyer K, Binder C, Wahn U. Outcome of double-blind, placebo-controlled food challenge tests in 107 children with atopic dermatitis. *Clin Exp Allergy* 1999;29:91–96.

42. Sampson HA, McCaskill CM. Food hypersensitivity and atopic dermatitis: evaluation of 113 patients. *J Pediatr* 1985;107:669–675.

43. Mabin DC, Sykes AE, David TJ. Controlled trial of a few foods diet in severe atopic dermatitis. *Arch Dis Child* 1995;73:202–207.

44. Munkvad M, Danielsen L, Høj L, et al. Antigen-free diet in adult patients with atopic dermatitis. *Acta Derm Venereol* 1984;64:524–528.

45. Saarinen UM, Kajosaari M. Breast-feeding as prophylaxis against atopic disease: prospective follow-up study until 17 years old. *Lancet* 1995;346:1065–1069.

46. Chandra RK. Five year follow up of high risk infants with a family history of allergy. *J Pediatr Gastroenterol Nutr* 1997;24:380–388.

47. Chandra RK, Shakuntla P, Hamed A. Influence of maternal diet during lactation and use of formula feeds on development of atopic eczema in high risk infants. *BMJ* 1989;299:228–230.

48. Marini A, Agostoi M, Motta G, Mosca F. Effects of a dietary and environmental prevention programme on the incidence of allergic symptoms in high atopic risk infants: three years follow-up. *Acta Paediatr* 1996;414(suppl):1–22.

49. Kramer MS. Maternal antigen avoidance during

lactation in women at high risk for atopic offspring. In: Neilson JP, Crowther CA, Hodnett ED, Hofmeyr GJ, eds. *Pregnancy and childbirth module*. In: The Cochrane Library, Issue 4, 1999. Oxford: Update Software. Search date 1995; primary sources the Cochrane Pregnancy and Childhood Review Group strategy; Medline; hand search selected journals; conference proceedings; survey of unpublished trials.

50. Diepgen TL, Salzer B, Tepe A, Hornstein OP. A study of skin irritations caused by textiles under standardized sweating conditions in patients with atopic eczema. *Dermatosen in Beruf und Umwelt (Occup Environ Dermatoses)* 1994;42:226–230.

English translation in Melliand English 1995;12: E268–E269.

51. Bendsöe N, Björnberg A, snes H. Itching from wool fibres in atopic dermatitis. *Contact Dermatitis* 1987;17:21–22.

52. Andersen PH, Bindslev-Jensen C, Mosbech H, et al. Skin symptoms in patients with atopic dermatitis using enzyme-containing detergents. *Acta Derm Venereol* 1998;78:60–62.

53. Juntunen-Backman K, Peltola H, Backman A, Salo OP. Safe immunisation of allergic children against measles, mumps and rubella. *Am J Dis Child* 1987;141:1103–1105.

Carolyn Charman
Research Fellow in Dermatology
Queen's Medical Centre
Nottingham
UK

Competing interests: None declared.

TABLE 1 **Methods for reducing house dust mite levels: results of controlled trials (see text, p 948).**

Methods	Results*
Mattress, pillow and duvet covers (micro-porous or polyurethane coated)	Very effective (3 RCTs).[33–35] Dust mite allergen levels 1–25% of control levels after 3–12 months; 44–98% reduction in dust load after 3 months.
Washing bedding at 55°C	Effective (2 RCTs). Reduces levels of dust mite allergen by > 95% and kills 100% of mites.
Removal of carpets and curtains	Unknown.
Acaricides (e.g. benzyl benzoate)	Conflicting results from RCTs — better when used on carpets than on mattresses. Effect may be short lived.
Intensive vacuuming	Small effect on mite levels in mattresses (1 RCT, 1 crossover trial) but not correlated with improvement in symptoms, possibly because conventional rather than high filtration cleaners may increase levels of airborne mite allergens, which may aggravate atopic disease (1 RCT in 16 rooms).
Air filters and dehumidifiers	Conflicting results from RCTs.

*Trials have tended to use a combination of control measures, making it difficult to see which measures were responsible for beneficial effects.

TABLE 2 Topical steroids versus placebo in atopic eczema: results of RCTs* (see text, p 946).[4-13]

	Number of participants (age in years)	Outcome
Prednicarbate ointment, 0.25% twice daily for 4 weeks.[4]	51 (18–60)	Reduced dermatitis: 87% active treatment, 8% controls. Significantly reduced patient-assessed pruritis on active treatment.
Hydrocortisone valerate cream, 0.2% three times daily for 2 weeks.[5]	20 (2–75)	Excellent or better: 75% active treatment, 20% controls.
Clobetasol propionate cream, 0.05% twice daily for 4 weeks.[6]	81 (≥ 12)	Good, excellent, or clear: 82% active treatment, 29% controls.
Hydrocortisone buteprate cream, 0.1% once daily for 2 weeks.[9]	194 (17–76)	Excellent or good: 69% active treatment, 26% controls.
Betamethasone dipropionate ointment, 0.05% twice daily for 3 weeks.[8]	36 (2–63)	Good or excellent: 94% active treatment, 13% controls.
Halcinonide ointment 0.1% three times daily for 2 weeks.[7]	233 (2–67)	Good or excellent: 85% active treatment, 44% controls.
Desonide cream once daily for 1 week.[10]	40 (0.4–15)	Improvement or resolution: 67% active treatment, 16% controls.
Hydrocortisone valerate 0.2% ointment twice daily for 2 weeks.[11]	64 (> 12)	Disease severity score: 70% reduction with active treatment, 15% controls.
Betamethasone dipropionate twice daily for 4 days.[12]	30 (19–57)	Itch free on days 3–4: 36% active treatment, 22% controls.
Halcinonide cream 0.1% twice daily for 3 weeks.[13]	58 (0.8–86)	57% of people achieved a better response with active treatment than control treatment ("better response" was not defined).

*Confidence intervals not reported.

New topic

Andrew Morris

QUESTIONS

INTERVENTIONS

Likely to be beneficial
Flucloxacillin, penicillin, ceftriaxone
and roxithromycin 959

Unknown effectiveness
Microbiological investigations . .958
Short versus long courses of
antibiotics 959

Oral versus intravenous
antibiotics 959

To be covered in future issues of
Clinical Evidence
Role of prophylactic antibiotics in
reducing risk of recurrent disease

Key Messages

- We found little RCT evidence on the treatment of cellulitis and erysipelas.
- We found no evidence on the effect of routine microbiological investigations on clinical outcomes.
- We found no placebo controlled trials of antibiotics.
- We found no good evidence on the effects of oral versus intravenous antibiotics, on combinations of antibiotics, on optimal duration of treatment, or on the effects of treating predisposing factors on recurrence.

DEFINITION	Cellulitis is a spreading bacterial infection of the dermis and subcutaneous tissues. It manifests as local signs of inflammation such as warmth, erythema, pain, and lymphangitis, and frequently, systemic upset with fever and leucocytosis. Erysipelas differs from cellulitis in that it tends to be more superficial, with a clearly demarcated edge. The lower limb is by far the commonest site, but any area can be affected.
INCIDENCE/ PREVALENCE	We found no specific data on the incidence of cellulitis. However, in the UK in 1991, cellulitis and abscess infections were responsible for 158 consultations per 10 000 person years at risk. In 1985, skin and subcutaneous tissue infections resulted in 29 820 hospital admissions and a mean occupancy of 664 hospital beds each day.[1,2]
AETIOLOGY/ RISK FACTORS	The commonest infective organisms in adults are Streptococci (particularly S. pyogenes) and Staphylococcus aureus.[3] In children, Haemophilus influenzae is a frequent cause. Several risk factors for erysipelas/cellulitis have been identified in a case control study (167 cases and 294 controls): lymphoedema (OR 71.2, 95% CI 5.6 to 908), leg ulcer (OR 62.5, 95% CI 7.0 to 556), toe web intertrigo (OR 13.9, 95% CI 7.2 to 27.0), and traumatic wounds (OR 10.7, 95% CI 4.8 to 23.8).[4]
PROGNOSIS	Cellulitis can spread via the blood stream and lymphatics. A retrospective case note study of people admitted to hospital with cellulitis found that systemic symptoms such as fever and leucocytosis were present in up to 42% of cases at presentation.[5] Lymphatic involvement can lead to obstruction and damage that predisposes to recurrent cellulitis. Recurrence can occur rapidly or after months or years. One study found that 29% of people with erysipelas had a recurrent episode within 3 years.[6] Local necrosis and abscess formation can also occur. It is not known whether the prognosis of erysipelas differs from that of cellulitis. We found no evidence about factors that predict recurrence, or a better or worse outcome. We found no good evidence on the prognosis of untreated cellulitis.
AIMS	To reduce the severity and duration of infection; to relieve pain and systemic symptoms; to restore the skin to its premorbid state; to prevent recurrence; and to minimise adverse effects of treatment.
OUTCOMES	Duration and severity of symptoms (pain, swelling, erythema, fever); clinical cure (defined as the absence of pain, swelling, and erythema); recurrence rate; adverse effects of treatment. We found no standard scales of severity in cellulitis or erysipelas.
METHODS	Clinical Evidence search and appraisal May 2000. Where we found no RCTs we included observational studies.

QUESTION What are the effects of routine microbiological investigations?

We found no good evidence.

Benefits: We found no systematic reviews, RCTs, or observational studies that addressed the impact of routine microbiological investigations on clinical outcomes.

Harms: Two small prospective studies reported no adverse effects.[7,8]

Comment: Two small prospective studies found that routine microbiological investigations had low diagnostic yields except where a primary lesion (e.g. leg ulcer) was present.[7,8]

QUESTION What are the effects of antibiotics?

We found no good evidence evaluating antibiotics versus placebo, oral versus intravenous antibiotics, different combinations of antibiotics, or different durations of treatment. Small RCTs found cure rates of about 70% for all antibiotics evaluated (penicillin, flucloxacillin, ceftriaxone, and roxithromycin).

Benefits: We found no systematic review. **Antibiotics versus placebo:** We found no placebo controlled RCTs. **Oral versus intravenous antibiotics:** We found one small quasi randomised trial (people assigned alternately to each group) of oral versus intravenous penicillin in 73 people in hospital with erysipelas. Inclusion criteria were no suspected septicemia and a temperature greater than 38.5 °C on admission. It found no significant difference in clinical efficacy.[9] However, clinical efficacy was assessed by indirect measures (temperature fall, length of hospital stay, and absence from work), and no data were provided on relapse rates. **Combinations of antibiotics:** We found no RCTs of combinations of antibiotics. **Different antibiotic regimens:** We found two RCTs comparing different antibiotic regimens. One small unblinded RCT compared intravenous flucloxacillin (1 g every 6 hours for a mean of 9 days) versus ceftriaxone (1 g daily for 7 days), in people with moderate to severe cellulitis (defined as cellulitis requiring parenteral antibiotics).[10] Data were evaluated on 45 of the initial 58 participants. The trial found no significant difference in the rate of clinical cure (complete resolution of all signs and symptoms). More people achieved clinical success (cure or improvement) with ceftriaxone, but the difference did not quite reach significance (16/22 [72%] with flucloxacillin v 22/23 [96%] with ceftriaxone; ARR 23%, 95% CI −0.4% to +73%). The trial provided no data on relapse rates. One RCT in 69 people with erysipelas compared oral roxithromycin versus intravenous followed by oral penicillin.[11] Inclusion criteria were a white blood cell count greater than $10 \times 10^9/l$ and a body temperature greater than 38 °C. Mean treatment duration in both groups was 13 days (range 2–29). It found no significant difference in cure rates between the treatment arms (29/38 [76%] with penicillin v 26/31 [84%] with roxithromycin; ARR 7.6%, 95% CI −7.7% to +35%). **Short versus long courses of antibiotics:** We found no RCTs comparing different durations of treatment.

Harms: Out of 22 people treated with flucloxacillin, three had nausea and vomiting, two had diarrhoea, and one had abdominal pain.[10] Out of 23 people treated with ceftriaxone, two had diarrhoea and vomiting and one had vaginal candidosis.[10] Drug related exanthem occurred in two out of 38 people receiving penicillin, although no adverse effects were reported in 31 people receiving roxithromycin.[11] Adverse events occurred in 15 people taking oral penicillin (exanthem 4, diarrhoea 7, abscess 4) and in 10 people taking intravenous penicillin (exanthem 2, diarrhoea 4, cannula phlebitis 4).[9]

Comment: We found several RCTs of antibiotics in people with a range of skin infections, including cellulitis, but none analysed the subgroup with cellulitis separately.[12-16] The trials of different antibiotics were too small to detect clinically important differences.[10,11] The first trial defined moderate to severe cellulitis as cellulitis requiring parenteral antibiotics.[10] It gave no information on what factors were used to assess the need for parenteral antibiotics.

QUESTION Does the treatment of predisposing factors reduce disease recurrence?

We found no reliable evidence on the effects of treatment of predisposing factors on disease recurrence.

Benefits: We found no systematic reviews, RCTs, or observational studies answering this question.

Harms: We found no good evidence.

Comment: Although there is a consensus that successful treatment of the predisposing factors (see aetiology, p 958) reduces the risk of developing erysipelas/cellulitis, we found no evidence to support this.

REFERENCES

1. Office of Population Censuses and Surveys. *Morbidity statistics from general practice.* Fourth National Study. HMSO 1992 (series MB5):272.
2. Hospital in-patient inquiry. HMSO 1985 (series MB4):16,28.
3. Bernard P, Bedane C, Mounier M, et al. Streptococcal cause of erysipelas and cellulitis in adults. *Arch Dermatol* 1989;125:779–782.
4. Dupuy A, Benchikhi H, Roujeau J-C, et al. Risk factors for erysipelas of the leg (cellulitis): case-control study. *BMJ* 1999;318:1591–1594.
5. Aly AA, Roberts NM, Seipol K, MacLellan DG. Case survey of management of cellulitis in a tertiary teaching hospital. *Med J Aust* 1996;165:553–556.
6. Jorup-Ronstrom C, Britton S. Recurrent erysipelas: predisposing factors and costs of prophylaxis. *Infection* 1987;15:105–106.
7. Hook EW, Hooton TM, Horton CA, et al. Microbiologic evaluation of cutaneous cellulitis in adults. *Arch Intern Med* 1986;146:295–297.
8. Leppard BJ, Seal DV, Colman G, Hallas G. The value of bacteriology and serology in the diagnosis of cellulitis and erysipelas. *Br J Dermatol* 1985; 112:559–567.
9. Jorup-Ronstrom C, Britton A, Gavlevik K, et al. The course, costs and complications of oral versus intravenous penicillin therapy of erysipelas. *Infection* 1984;12:390–394.
10. Vinen J, Hudson B, Chan B, Fernandes C. A randomized comparative study of once-daily ceftriaxone and 6-hourly flucloxacillin in the treatment of moderate to severe cellulitis. Clinical efficacy, safety and pharmacoeconomic implications. *Clin Drug Invest* 1996;12:221–225.
11. Bernard P, Plantin P, Roger H, et al. Roxithromycin versus penicillin in the treatment of erysipelas in adults: a comparative study. *Br J Dermatol* 1992; 127:155–159.
12. Neldner KH. Double-blind randomized study of oral Temafloxacin and Cefadroxil in patients with mild to moderately severe bacterial skin infections. *Am J Med* 1991;91(suppl 6A):111–114.
13. Nolen TM, Conetta BJ, Durham SJ, Wilber RB. Treatment of mild to moderate skin and skin-structure infections. *Infect Med* 1992;9(suppl C):56–67.
14. Wachs G, Rogan MP, Cefprozil Multicentre Study Group. Cefprozil vs. Erythromycin for mild to moderate skin and skin-structure infections. *Infect Med* 1992;9(suppl E):57–65.
15. Nolen TM. Clinical trials of cefprozil for treatment of skin and skin structure infections: review. *Clin Infect Dis* 1992;14(suppl 2):255–263.
16. Perez-Ruvalcaba JA, Quintero-Perez NP, Morales-Reyes JJ, et al. Double-blind comparison of Ciprofloxacin with Cefotaxime in the treatment of skin and skin structure infections. *Am J Med* 1987;82(suppl 4A):242–246.

Andrew Morris
Specialist Registrar in Dermatology
University Hospital
Nottingham
UK

Competing interests: None declared.

Updated this issue

Luigi Naldi

INTERVENTIONS

Key Messages

- We found no good evidence on the effects of heliotherapy, lifestyle change, dietary supplements, stress reduction, or antistreptococcal treatments.

- We found that topical treatments have been evaluated only in the short term, with few comparative RCTs. We found no good evidence on the value of maintenance treatment with topical treatments or on methods for assessing patients' preferences and satisfaction.

- RCTs have found that ultraviolet B (UVB) phototherapy and psoralen plus ultraviolet A (PUVA) are effective in clearing psoriasis and in its long term maintenance. Long term treatment with PUVA carries a risk of squamous cell carcinoma.

- RCTs have found that cyclosporin clears psoriasis, but we found little evidence of its value as maintenance treatment. Toxicity makes treatment unacceptable to many people.

- We found limited evidence on the long term effects of other systemic treatments (etretinate, acitretin, methotrexate, and fumaric acid derivatives) and no comparative RCTs.

DEFINITION Chronic plaque psoriasis is a chronic inflammatory skin disease characterised by well demarcated erythematous scaly patches on the extensor surfaces of the body and scalp. The lesions may itch, sting, and occasionally bleed. Dystrophic nail changes are found in more than a third of people with chronic plaque psoriasis, and psoriatic arthropathy occurs in 1–3%. The condition waxes and wanes with wide variations between and within individuals. Other varieties of psoriasis include guttate, inverse, pustular, and erythrodermic psoriasis. This review deals only with treatments for chronic plaque psoriasis.

INCIDENCE/ PREVALENCE Psoriasis affects 1–2% of the general population. It is believed to be less frequent in people from Africa and Asia, but we found no convincing epidemiological data.[1]

AETIOLOGY/ RISK FACTORS Genetic and environmental factors are both important. About a third of people with psoriasis have a family history of psoriasis, but physical trauma, acute infection, and selected medications (e.g. lithium salts and β blockers) are commonly viewed as triggers. A few observational studies have linked the onset or relapse of psoriasis with stressful life events and personal habits, including cigarette smoking and, less consistently, alcohol consumption. Others have found an association of psoriasis with body mass index and an inverse association with the intake of fruit and vegetables.

PROGNOSIS We found no long term prognostic studies. With the exception of erythrodermic and acute generalised pustular psoriasis (severe conditions affecting less than 1% of people with psoriasis and requiring intensive hospital care), psoriasis is not known to affect mortality. Psoriasis may substantially affect quality of life.[2] At present there is no cure for psoriasis.

AIMS To achieve short term suppression of symptoms and long term modulation of disease severity; to improve quality of life with minimal adverse effects of treatment.

OUTCOMES State of lesions over time; use of routine treatments; duration of remission; patient satisfaction and autonomy; disease related quality of life; adverse effects of treatment. We found no documented evidence that clinical activity scores, such as the Psoriasis Area Severity Index (PASI), are reliable proxies for these outcomes. Many clinical studies provide no explicit criteria for severity.[3]

METHODS *Clinical Evidence* update search and appraisal May 2000. In addition, we hand searched a number of dermatological and medical journals for the years 1976–1996 as a project of the European Dermatoepidemiology Network. These were the *Journal of Investigative Dermatology, British Journal of Dermatology, Dermatology, Acta Dermo-Venereologica, Archives of Dermatology, Journal of the American Academy of Dermatology, Annales de Dermatologie et de Vénéréologie, Giornale Italiano di Dermatologia e Venereologia, Hautarzt, British Medical Journal, Lancet, Journal of the American Medical Association,* and *New England Journal of Medicine.*

As several trigger and perpetuating factors for psoriasis have been recognised, including physical trauma, acute infections, smoking, diet, and stress, there is good reason to believe that disease severity could be modulated by non-drug treatments. However, we found no good evidence on the effects of non-drug treatments. A few interventions have been tested in small RCTs.

Benefits: We found no systematic review. **Heliotherapy:** We found one RCT (2 year crossover design, n = 95), which compared 4 weeks of supervised heliotherapy versus no intervention.[4] Heliotherapy significantly improved psoriasis and reduced use of routine treatment in the year after heliotherapy by 30%. **Fish oil supplementation:** We found six RCTs, which reported conflicting results. The largest RCT (n = 145) found no evidence of benefit from fish oil compared with corn oil.[5] **Oral Vitamin D:** One RCT (n = 50) found no significant difference in effectiveness between oral cholecalciferol and placebo.[6] **Stress reduction:** We found two small RCTs, which found that psychological interventions to reduce stress improved psoriasis. The largest trial, in 51 people, found slight but significant changes in psoriasis activity scores.[7] **Lifestyle change:** We found no RCTs of smoking cessation or dietary change in people with psoriasis. **Antistreptococcal treatments:** We found one systematic review of antistreptococcal interventions for guttate and chronic plaque psoriasis (search date 1999, 1 RCT, n = 20).[8] The review found no evidence that tonsillectomy (or antibiotics) versus placebo is beneficial. **Thermal baths:** We found no RCTs. **Acupuncture:** We found one RCT in 56 people. This found no significant difference between classic acupuncture and sham (placebo) acupuncture.[9]

Harms: Inadequate data available.

Comment: None.

OPTION   EMOLLIENTS AND KERATOLYTICS

Emollients and keratolytics are well established in the treatment of psoriasis, but we found only a few small RCTs.

Benefits: We found two systematic reviews of emollients and keratolytics.[10,11] One systematic review (search date 1994, 4 RCTs, n = 245) found that capsaicin versus other treatments had a beneficial effect on itching, scaling, and erythema.[11] However, there was significant unexplained heterogeneity in the results from individual trials. Another systematic review (search date 1999, 10 RCTs) evaluated *aloe vera* for a large variety of conditions, including psoriasis. The review found no clear evidence of effectiveness, but did not exclude the possibility of a clinically important effect.[12] We found five RCTs. The largest (n = 43) found that emollients temporarily improved psoriasis when they were combined with UVB radiation.[12]

Harms: Local irritation and contact dermatitis have been reported with emollients and keratolytics.

Comment: Emollients and keratolytics are usually used as adjuncts to other treatments.

OPTION   TARS

Tars are well established in the treatment of psoriasis, but we found only a few small RCTs.

Benefits: We found no systematic review. We found one small RCT in 18 people, which found that tar was more effective than the emollient base in improving disease activity scores.[13] Four small RCTs found conflicting results on the added efficacy of coal tar when combined with UVB exposure and dithranol (see Ingram regimen, p 968).

Harms: Smell, staining, and burning are the main adverse effects of coal tar.

Comment: None.

OPTION   DITHRANOL

Small RCTs have found that dithranol improves chronic plaque psoriasis more than placebo. The best evidence on its effects relates to its use in the Ingram regimen (see Ingram regimen, p 968).

Benefits: **Versus placebo:** We found no systematic review. We found two small RCTs, which reported that dithranol was better than placebo in improving psoriasis. **Conventional versus short contact treatment:** A survey of published studies (search date 1989) identified 22 small RCTs comparing conventional dithranol treatment versus dithranol short contact treatment (shorter contact time at higher concentrations).[14] These found no evidence of differences, but the trials were too small to rule out clinically important differences.

Harms: Smell, staining, and burning are the main adverse effects of dithranol.

Comment: Few trials examined patient satisfaction, so it remains unclear whether short contact treatment is easier and more convenient for people at home compared with conventional dithranol treatment.

OPTION   TOPICAL STEROIDS

RCTs have found that topical steroids improve psoriasis in the short term.

Benefits: We found no systematic review. **Clearance:** More than 30 short term, mainly small, vehicle controlled RCTs, often involving within-person comparisons, found that topical mid to high potency steroids temporarily improved psoriatic lesions. The study duration was usually no longer than 8 weeks and improvement was judged mainly in terms of reduced erythema and scaling. The largest parallel group RCTs have evaluated the more recently developed molecules (such as mometasone). **Maintenance:** One RCT (in 90 people with one target area cleared or nearly cleared of psoriasis by betamethasone dipropionate) found better control at 6 months by topical steroids applied once a week than by placebo (AR for maintenance of clearance in the target area 60% v 20%).[15] **Occlusive dressings:** Twelve small RCTs, mostly using people as their own controls, found that occlusive polyethylene or hydrocolloid dressings enhanced clinical activity.

Harms: Topical steroids may cause striae and atrophy, which increase with clinical potency and use of occlusive dressings. Continuous use may lead to adrenocortical suppression,[16] and case reports suggest that severe flares of the disease may occur on withdrawal. Diminishing clinical response with repeated use (tachyphylaxis) has been described, but we found no estimates of its frequency.

Comment: As the RCT assessed only maintenance value within the target area, the results may not generalise to clinical practice.[15]

OPTION   VITAMIN D DERIVATIVES

One systematic review of RCTs and long term uncontrolled studies have found that calcipotriol improves plaque psoriasis compared with placebo and is at least as effective as topical steroids, coal tars, and dithranol. The review found that calcipotriol monotherapy causes more irritation than potent topical steroids. Only limited evidence is available for other vitamin D derivatives, including tacalcitol and maxacalcitol.

Benefits: We found one systematic review (search date 1999, 37 RCTs, 6038 people)[17] and an additional 7 RCTs of calcipotriol. **Versus placebo:** The review identified eight RCTs, which found benefit in people with mild to moderately severe plaque psoriasis (mean difference in the percentage change in severity index was 44%, 95% CI 28% to 60%). Long term uncontrolled studies found that treatment gains were maintained in about 70% of people for as long as the treatment was continued.[18] **Versus each other:** We found six RCTs comparing calcipotriol versus another vitamin D derivative. Five were of tacalcitol, the largest of which (n = 287) found that tacalcitol once daily was slightly less effective than calcipotriol twice daily in clearing psoriasis.[19] The other RCT (n = 144) found that maxacalcitol once daily compared favourably with calcipotriol once daily (55% v 46% of patients reporting large improvement or clearance). However, the established dosage of calcipotriol is twice daily.[20] **Versus topical steroids:** In four short term comparative RCTs, the largest one involving 345 people, calcipotriol was either as effective or slightly more effective than topical steroids.[21] **Versus dithranol short contact treatment:** Four RCTs, the largest one involving 478 people,[22] found that calcipotriol was either as effective or slightly more effective than dithranol short contact treatment. However, one additional RCT (n = 171) found that of those people who initially improved on treatment, more stayed in remission with dithranol than with calcipotriol.[23] **Versus coal tar:** Two RCTs, the largest one involving 122 people,[24] found that calcipotriol was more effective than coal tar. **With other treatments:** Four RCTs, the largest one involving 169 people, found that a combination of calcipotriol with topical steroids provided better clearance and maintenance.[25]

Harms: The review found that calcipotriol monotherapy caused more irritation than potent topical steroids (NNH 10, 95% CI 6 to 34).[17]

Perilesional irritation from calcipotriol has been reported in as many as 25% of people, the face and intertriginous areas being more susceptible. In the short term, the combination of a topical steroid may reduce the incidence of skin irritation.[26] Hypercalcaemia and hypercalciuria are dose related adverse effects.

Comment: There is a consensus that the dosage of calcipotriol should be limited to 100 g per week.

OPTION **TOPICAL RETINOIDS (TAZAROTENE)**

RCTs have found that tazarotene improves chronic plaque psoriasis in the short term compared with placebo.

Benefits: We found no systematic review. Three vehicle controlled RCTs found that tazarotene was effective in chronic plaque psoriasis. In the largest RCT (318 evaluable people), clinical response was judged after 12 weeks of treatment to be good, excellent, or completely cleared in 60% on tazarotene 0.1%, 50% on tazarotene 0.05%, and 30% on vehicle control (RRR for tazarotene 0.1% compared with placebo 43%, 95% CI 30% to 60%).[27] One RCT in 275 evaluable people found that tazarotene was nearly as effective in clearing psoriasis as the high potency topical steroid flucinonide.[28]
Plus steroids: Three RCTs, the largest one involving 398 people, found that topical mid or high potency steroids added to tazarotene, or alternated on a daily basis with tazarotene, increased the response rate compared with tazarotene alone.[29,30]

Harms: Some perilesional irritation was reported in most people. The RCTs found that addition of steroids reduced the incidence of patient withdrawals and treatment related adverse effects.[29,30]

Comment: Tazarotene is contraindicated in women who are, or intend to become, pregnant as it is potentially teratogenic.

QUESTION **What are the effects of treatments with ultraviolet light?**

OPTION **PHOTOTHERAPY**

RCTs have found that phototherapy improves psoriasis in the short term and when used as maintenance treatment. We found no good evidence that narrow band phototherapy is better than broad band.

Benefits: We found no systematic review. **Clearance:** We found two RCTs comparing UVB with PUVA.[31-32] The first RCT in 183 people with moderate to severe psoriasis found no significant difference in clearance rates between PUVA and UVB radiation (88% for PUVA v 80% for UVB; RRR for non-clearance with PUVA compared with broad band UVB radiation 38%, 95% CI −22% to +71%).[31] Sub-group analysis found that UVB radiation was significantly less effective in people with more than 50% body involvement. The second RCT (n = 100) found that clearance was achieved in more people treated with PUVA compared with narrow band UVB (84% v 63%).[32] **Maintenance:** One RCT examined the maintenance value of weekly treatment with UVB phototherapy after initial clearance.

Of the 165 people enrolled, 104 (63%) were cleared of their symptoms. More than 50% of people in the maintenance group were still clear 181 days after initial clearance compared with 28% in the control group (RRR for relapsing at 181 days 33%, 95% CI 8% to 59%).[33] **Narrow versus broad band phototherapy:** We found only three small, short term, self controlled RCTs, the largest one involving 23 people.[34]

Harms: UVB radiation may increase photoageing and the risk of skin cancer. A recent systematic review (search date 1996) concluded that it was unlikely that the excess risk of non-melanoma skin cancer associated with UVB radiation exceeded 2% per year.[35]

Comment: None.

OPTION **PUVA**

RCTs have found effective clearance and long term maintenance with conventional PUVA treatment (i.e. oral 8-methoxypsoralen plus ultraviolet A [UVA] radiation). Long term treatment carries the risk of squamous cell carcinoma, reported in a quarter of people.

Benefits: We found no systematic review. We found 17 RCTs. **Clearance:** One RCT (n = 224) compared PUVA treatment versus an inpatient Ingram regimen in people with at least 10% of body surface area involved.[36] The trial found clearance rates of 91% with PUVA compared with 82% with the Ingram regimen. One RCT (n = 85), in people with skin types (see glossary, p 972) I and II, found that the clearance rate was lower with the minimal phototoxic dose regimen compared with the skin type regimen (see glossary, p 972) (67.5% v 95%).[37] **Maintenance:** The largest RCT, in 1005 people whose psoriasis had been cleared by PUVA, found that maintenance treatment reduced relapse at 18 months (AR of flares: 27% with treatment once a week, 34% with treatment once every 3 weeks, and 62% with no treatment; RRR for relapse with once weekly treatment v no treatment 56%, 95% CI 44% to 68%).[38] **Different regimens:** At least eight small RCTs have looked at different combinations of ultraviolet radiation and systemic or topical treatments, including UVA plus 5-methoxypsoralen, UVA plus bath water delivered psoralen (bath PUVA), and psoralen plus UVB. The trials found no significant difference from conventional PUVA treatment, but they were probably too small to exclude a clinically important difference.

Harms: The best evidence on chronic toxicity comes from an ongoing study of more than 1300 people who first received PUVA treatment in 1975.[39,40] The study found a dose dependent increased risk of squamous cell carcinoma, basal cell carcinoma, and possibly malignant melanoma compared with the risk in the general population. The findings concerning non-melanoma skin cancer have been repeated by a recent systematic review of eight additional studies (search date 1998).[41] Premature photoageing is another expected adverse effect. After less than 15 years, about a quarter of people exposed to 300 or more treatments of PUVA had at least one squamous cell carcinoma of the skin, with particularly high risk for people with skin types I and II. In patients who wear UVA opaque glasses for 24 hours after psoralen ingestion, the risk of cataract development seems negligible. A combined analysis of two cohort studies including a total of 944 people treated with bath PUVA excluded a threefold excess risk of squamous cell carcinoma after a mean follow up of 14.7 years, suggesting that bath PUVA is possibly safer than conventional PUVA.[42]

Comment: People receiving PUVA need close monitoring for acute toxicity and cutaneous carcinogenic effects.

OPTION   COMBINATION REGIMENS

Of the two most established combination regimens, the Ingram regimen has been found in one RCT to be nearly as effective as PUVA in clearing moderate to severe psoriasis. We found no good evidence on effectiveness of the Goeckerman treatment (see glossary, p 972).

Benefits: We found no systematic review. **Ingram regimen:** See glossary, p 972. One RCT (n = 224) compared an in-patient Ingram regimen (dithranol concentration 0.01–1.0%) versus PUVA in people with at least 10% of body surface involvement. It found that clearance rates were 82% (95% CI 77% to 89%) with the Ingram regimen compared with 91% (95% CI 86% to 96%) with PUVA.[36] Five small RCTs, the largest one involving 53 people,[43] gave conflicting results on the added efficacy of dithranol when combined with UVB exposure. However, the trials were too small to rule out a clinically important difference. **Goeckerman treatment:** See glossary, p 972. We found no good evidence on the effects of combining coal tar and UVB radiation. **Other combinations:** We found five RCTs that assessed the combination of calcipotriol with UVB radiation or PUVA, but the results were conflicting.[44–47] The largest RCT (n = 164) found that fewer UVB treatments were required to achieve clearance in people receiving calcipotriol plus UVB compared with UVB alone (median number of UVB treatments required with calcipotriol plus UVB was 22 v 25 with UVB alone; no statistical analysis for a continuous variable was reported).[44]

Harms: Adverse effects vary with the treatments being combined. Local irritation often occurs.

Comment: None.

QUESTION   What are the effects of systemic treatments?

OPTION   ORAL RETINOIDS (ETRETINATE AND ACITRETIN)

We found limited evidence that oral retinoids may achieve complete clearance in a small proportion of people with plaque psoriasis. We found no good evidence about the effects of oral retinoids as maintenance treatment. Adverse effects and the risk of teratogenicity make retinoids unacceptable to some people.

Benefits: We found no systematic review (although there has been one of oral retinoids in psoriatic arthropathy).[48] **Versus placebo:** We found eight RCTs, the largest one involving 291 people,[49] comparing etretinate (0.2–1.2 mg/kg per day) versus placebo or conventional treatment in people with severe psoriasis. These trials reported wide differences in treatment effects, with clearance in 15–90% of participants. Differences may be explained by different entry criteria, outcome measures, or treatment schedules. The high withdrawal rates in most RCTs called for an intention to treat analysis, which was rarely performed. **Versus each other:** Etretinate and acitretin (0.5–1.0 mg/kg per day) have been compared in four RCTs. The largest, in 168 people, reported similar benefits but a higher rate of mucocutaneous adverse effects with acitretin.[50] **With other treatments:** Nine RCTs, the largest one involving 82 people,[51] found that the combination of PUVA or UVB and retinoids speeded up the response and, by doing so, reduced the cumulative ultraviolet exposure or retinoid dosage. One RCT in 135 people found a higher clearance rate from the combination of calcipotriol with acitretin compared with acitretin alone.[52] **Different types of psoriasis:** In subgroup analyses of the above mentioned RCTs and two further small RCTs,[53,54] pustular and erythrodermic psoriasis seemed to be more responsive to etretinate and acitretin than plaque psoriasis. **Maintenance:** We found only one small RCT (n = 36) of 1 year's duration supporting the maintenance value of etretinate over placebo, after clearance by PUVA.[55]

Harms: Most people experience mucocutaneous adverse effects, such as dry skin, cheilitis, and conjunctivitis. Increased serum cholesterol and triglyceride concentrations occurred in about half of the people. Low grade hepatotoxicity was observed in about 1% of people treated with etretinate.[56] Occasionally, acute hepatitis occurred as a purported idiosyncratic hypersensitivity reaction. Radiographic evidence of extraspinal tendon and ligament calcifications has been documented. In one cohort study, a quarter of 956 people treated with etretinate attributed a joint problem or its worsening to the drug.[56] Etretinate is a known teratogen and may be detected in the plasma for 2–3 years after treatment stops. Acitretin can undergo esterification to etretinate.

Comment: Women of childbearing age are given effective contraception for 1 month before starting etretinate, throughout treatment, and after stopping treatment for at least 3 years because it is potentially teratogenic. Etretinate is no longer available in many countries.

OPTION | **METHOTREXATE**

Limited evidence from one small RCT suggests that methotrexate improves skin lesions in psoriasis. Non-randomised data suggest that clearance can be maintained as long as treatment is continued. About half of people relapse within 6 months of stopping treatment. Long term treatment carries the risk of serious adverse effects, especially liver fibrosis, reported in about a third of people.

Benefits: We found no systematic review (although there has been one in psoriatic arthropathy).[48] **Clearance:** We found two small RCTs, dealing primarily with psoriatic arthropathy. One of the trials provided data on skin lesions and documented improvement compared with placebo.[57] **Maintenance:** We found no RCTs. In an uncontrolled series of 113 people with severe psoriasis, maintenance treatment with low dose methotrexate (weekly dose not to exceed 15 mg) provided satisfactory control of skin lesions in 81% of people (mean treatment duration 8 years). When treatment was stopped, 45% of people experienced a full relapse within 6 months.[58]

Harms: In the uncontrolled case series mentioned above, treatment was stopped in 33/113 people because of adverse effects.[58] The most serious acute reaction, particularly in elderly people, is dose related myelosuppression. In the long term, major adverse events included liver fibrosis and pulmonary toxicity. One systematic review found that about 28% (95% CI 24% to 32%) of people on chronic methotrexate for psoriasis and rheumatoid arthritis developed liver fibrosis of histological grade 1 or higher on liver biopsy, while 5% developed advanced liver disease (histological grade IIIB or IV).[59] The risk was dose related and increased with increased alcohol consumption. A limitation of the systematic review was the lack of untreated control groups. Pulmonary disease associated with methotrexate has been described as an acute or chronic interstitial pneumonitis.[60] Adverse pulmonary effects of treatment are considered much rarer in psoriasis than in rheumatoid arthritis, but we found no published evidence to support this claim. Several drug interactions that increase methotrexate toxicity have been described (e.g. with sulphonamides). Methotrexate seems to double the risk of developing squamous cell carcinoma in people exposed to PUVA and may be an independent risk factor for this cancer.[39] A higher risk of lymphoproliferative diseases in long term users has been suggested by a few case reports. On the basis of data from a large case series (n = 248), the cumulative incidence of lymphoma is not expected to be much higher than 1%.[61]

Comment: People using methotrexate are closely monitored for liver toxicity,[62] and advised to limit their consumption of alcohol. The most reliable test of liver damage remains needle biopsy of the liver. It is rare for life threatening liver disease to develop with the first 1.0–1.5 g of methotrexate.

OPTION CYCLOSPORIN AND OTHER IMMUNOSUPPRESSIVE DRUGS

RCTs have found that cyclosporin clears psoriasis, especially at higher doses, although toxicity is high and causes many people to withdraw from continuous long term treatment. We found little evidence about the effects of other immunosuppressive drugs, such as tacrolimus.

Benefits: We found no systematic review. **Clearance:** Six dose-finding, placebo controlled RCTs found that cyclosporin temporarily controlled psoriasis. A pooled analysis based on five European dose-finding studies used individual data from 457 people. Success (defined as activity score reduction ≥ 75%) was more likely with higher initial daily doses of cyclosporin (24% achieved success with 1.25 mg/kg per day; 52% with 2.5–3 mg/kg per day; 88% with 5 mg/kg per day).[63] Most people relapsed within weeks after stopping treatment. One RCT (n = 309) found a more rapid response with a microemulsion formulation than with the usual oil-in-water emulsion.[64] **Maintenance:** Three RCTs have assessed different maintenance schedules.[65–67] In one study, 61 people who had achieved clearance during an induction phase were randomised to 1.5 mg or 3.0 mg per kg per day cyclosporin or placebo.[65] At 4 months' follow up there had been no relapse in 57% of the 3 mg/kg group compared with 21% of the 1.5 mg/kg group and 5% of the placebo group (RRR for relapse in the 3 mg/kg group compared with placebo 55%, 95% CI 30% to 80%). **Speed of discontinuation:** Another RCT (n = 400) compared abrupt versus tapered discontinuation of a microemulsion formulation of cyclosporin (starting dose 2.5 mg/kg per day) after clearance was achieved or after a maximum of 12 weeks' treatment (short course treatment). The median time to relapse was 109 days among people stopping abruptly and 113 days among those reducing the dose gradually (P = 0.04). Participants were followed up for at least 1 year during which time they were allowed to use as many treatment courses as necessary (intermittent short course treatment). 259 people (65%) received two treatment courses and 117 (29%) three treatment courses.[67] **Versus other treatments:** One RCT compared cyclosporin 2.5 mg/kg per day versus etretinate 0.5 mg/kg per day in 210 people. After 10 weeks, 47% of the people taking cyclosporin and 10% taking etretinate showed a reduction of more than 80% in skin involvement.[68] **Different types of psoriasis:** One small RCT (n = 58) found that low dose (1–2 mg/kg per day) cyclosporin was effective maintenance treatment in palmoplantar pustulosis.[69]

Harms: In a follow up study of 122 consecutive people treated for 3–76 months at a dose not exceeding 5 mg/kg per day, 104 people discontinued treatment.[70] Of these, 55 stopped treatment because of adverse effects, which included renal dysfunction in 34 people (28%) and hypertension in 23 people (19%). One RCT in 400 people found that intermittent treatment with a microemulsion formulation for 1 year was well tolerated and produced no clinically significant change of blood pressure or creatinine concentration.[67] Long term follow up studies are needed to confirm this finding.

Comment: Renal function should be monitored. The long term safety profile has yet to be defined. Evidence about the effects of other immunosuppressive drugs remains inconclusive.

| OPTION | FUMARIC ACID DERIVATIVES |

We found limited evidence of short term effectiveness but high rates of acute adverse effects. We found no evidence on the value of fumaric acid derivatives as maintenance treatment.

Benefits: We found no systematic review. We found five RCTs. The largest RCT (n = 100) found a response, ranging from slight improvement to complete clearance, in 71% of those treated with esters of fumaric acid (maximum dose 1290 mg ester mixture per day) compared with 18% in the placebo group.[71]

Harms: The safety profile is poorly defined. Acute adverse effects, including flushing and gastrointestinal symptoms, have been reported in as many as 75% of people.[71] Eosinophilia is often observed, and we found a few case reports of drug induced tubular nephropathy.[72]

Comment: The largest RCT had a high withdrawal rate (48%).[71]

GLOSSARY

Goeckerman treatment A daily application of coal tar followed by UVB irradiation.

Ingram regimen A daily coal tar bath, UVB irradiation, and dithranol.

Skin types A clinical classification of an individual's burning and tanning tendencies. Usually ranges from skin phototype I (which always burns and never tans) to skin phototype VI (marked constitutive pigmentation).

Skin type regimen and minimal phototoxic dose regimen The four parameters of PUVA are the dose of psoralen, the frequency of treatment, the initial dose of UVA, and the incremental UVA dose. The initial and incremental UVA doses are described by at least two regimens. In the minimal phototoxic dose regimen, the initial UVA dose is a fraction of the minimal phototoxic dose. Weekly increments in dose occur until a maximum dose is reached. In the skin type regimen the initial dose is based on skin phototype. Weekly dose increments are decreased if erythema develops.

Substantive changes since last issue

Oral vitamin D One RCT found no difference in effectiveness between oral vitamin D and placebo.[6]

Antistreptococcal treatments One systematic review found no evidence that tonsillectomy (or antibiotics) is beneficial compared with placebo.[8]

Vitamin D derivatives One systematic review found that calcipotriol improves plaque psoriasis compared with placebo.[17]

Vitamin D derivatives One RCT found that more people who initially improved taking dithranol stayed in remission compared with calcipotriol.[23]

Phototherapy One RCT found that more people treated with PUVA achieved clearance compared with narrow band UVB.[32]

PUVA One RCT found that the clearance rate was lower with the minimal phototoxic dose regimen compared with the skin type regimen.[37]

Combination therapy One RCT found that less UVB treatments were required to achieve clearance in people receiving calcipotriol plus UVB compared with UVB alone.[44]

REFERENCES

1. Naldi L. Psoriasis. In: Williams HC, Strachan DP, eds. *The challenge of dermato-epidemiology*. Boca Raton: CRC Press, 1997;175–190.

2. O'Neill P, Kelly P. Postal questionnaire of disability in the community associated with psoriasis. *BMJ* 1996;313:919–921.

3. Petersen LI, Kristensen JK. Selection of patients for psoriasis clinical trials: a survey of the recent dermatological literature. *J Dermatol Treat* 1992; 3:171–176.

4. Snellman E, Aromaa A, Jansen CT, et al. Supervised four-week heliotherapy alleviates the long-term course of psoriasis. *Acta Derm Venereol* 1993;73:388–392.

5. Soyland E, Funk J, Rajka G, et al. Effect of dietary supplementation with very-long-chain n-3 fatty acids in patients with psoriasis. *N Engl J Med* 1993;328:1812–1816.

6. Siddiqui MA, Al Khawajah MM. Vitamin D and psoriasis: a randomised double-blind placebo-controlled study. *J Dermatol Treat* 1990;1:243–245.

7. Zachariae H, Oster H, Bjerring P, Kragballe K. Effects of psychologic intervention on psoriasis: a preliminary report. *J Am Acad Dermatol* 1996;34: 1008–1015.

8. Owen CM, Chalmers RJG, O'Sullivan T, Griffiths CEM. Antistreptococcal interventions for guttate and chronic plaque psoriasis. In: The Cochrane Library, Issue 2, 2000. Oxford: Update software. Search date November 1999; primary sources Cochrane Clinical Trials Register, Medline, Embase, Salford Database of Psoriasis Trials, European Dermato-Epidemiology Network Psoriasis Trials Database.

9. Jerner B, Skogh M, Vahlquist A. A controlled trial of acupuncture in psoriasis: no convincing effect. *Acta Derm Venereol* 1997;77:154–156.

10. Zhang WY, Li Wan Po A. The effectiveness of topically applied capsaicin. a meta-analysis. *Eur J Clin Pharmacol* 1994;46:517–522. Search date 1994; primary sources BIDS, Medline.

11. Vogler BK, Ernst E. Aloe vera: a systematic review of its clinical effectiveness. *Br J Gen Pract* 1999; 49:823–828. Search date May 1998; primary sources Medline 1966 to May 1998; Embase 1980 to May 1998; Biosis 1985 to May 1998 and Cochrane Library, Issue 2, 1998.

12. Berne B, Blom I, Spangberg S. Enhanced response of psoriasis to UVB therapy after pretreatment with a lubrificating base. *Acta Derm Venereol* 1990;70:474–477.

13. Kanzler MH, Gorsulowsky DC. Efficacy of topical 5% liquor carbonis detergens vs. its emollient base in the treatment of psoriasis. *Br J Dermatol* 1993;129:310–314.

14. Naldi L, Carrel CF, Parazzini F, et al. Development of anthralin short-contact therapy in psoriasis: survey of published clinical trials. *Int J Dermatol* 1992;31:126–130. Search date 1989; primary sources Medline, Index Medicus, Excerpta Medica.

15. Katz HI, Prawer SE, Medansky RS, et al. Intermittent corticosteroid treatment of psoriasis: a double-blind multicenter trial of augmented betamethasone dipropionate ointment in a pulse dose treatment regimen. *Dermatologica* 1991; 183:269–274.

16. Wilson L, Williams DI, Marsh SD. Plasma corticosteroid levels in outpatients treated with topical steroids. *Br J Dermatol* 1973;88:373–380.

17. Ashcroft DM, Li Wan Po A, Williams HC, Griffiths CEM. Systematic review of comparative efficacy and tolerability of calcipotriol in treating chronic plaque psoriasis. *BMJ* 2000;320:963–967.

18. Ramsay CA, Berth-Johnes J, Brundin J, et al. Long-term use of topical calcipotriol in chronic plaque psoriasis. *Dermatology* 1994;189:260–264.

19. Veien NK, Bjerke JR, Rossmann-Ringdahl I, Jakobsen HB. Once daily treatment of psoriasis with tacalcitol compared with twice daily treatment with calcipotriol. a double-blind trial. *Br J Dermatol* 1997;137:581–586.

20. Barker JN, Ashton RE, Marks R, et al. Topical maxacalcitol for the treatment of psoriasis vulgaris: a placebo controlled, double-blind, dose-finding study with active comparator. *Br J Dermatol* 1999;141:274–278.

21. Kragballe K, Gjertsen BT, De Hoop D, et al. Double-blind, right/left comparison of calcipotriol and betamethasone valerate in treatment of psoriasis vulgaris. *Lancet* 1991;337:193–196.

22. Berth-Jones J, Chu AC, Dodd WAH, et al. A multicentre, parallel-group comparison of calcipotriol ointment and short-contact therapy in chronic plaque psoriasis. *Br J Dermatol* 1992; 127:266–271.

23. Christensen OB, Mork NJ, Ashton R, Daniel F, Anehus S. Comparison of a treatment phase and a follow-up phase of short contact dithranol and calcipotriol in outpatients with chronic plaque psoriasis. *J Dermatol Treat* 1999;10:261–265.

24. Pinheiro N. Comparative effects of calcipotriol ointment (50 micrograms/g) and 5% coal tar/2% allantoin/0.5% hydrocortisone cream in treating plaque psoriasis. *Br J Clin Pract* 1997;51:16–19.

25. Ruzicka T, Lorenz B. Comparison of calcipotriol monotherapy and a combination of calcipotriol and betamethasone valerate after 2 weeks' treatment with calcipotriol in the topical therapy of psoriasis vulgaris: a multicentre, double-blind, randomized study. *Br J Dermatol* 1998;138:254–258.

26. Kragballe K, Barnes L, Hamberg K, et al. Calcipotriol cream with or without concurrent topical corticosteroid in psoriasis: tolerability and efficacy. *Br J Dermatol* 1998;139:649–654.

27. Weinstein GD, Krueger GG, Lowe NJ, et al. Tazarotene gel, a new retinoid, for topical therapy of psoriasis: vehicle-controlled study of safety, efficacy, and duration of therapeutic effect. *J Am Acad Dermatol* 1997;37:85–92.

28. Lebwohl M, Ast E, Callen JP, et al. Once-daily tazarotene gel versus twice-daily fluocinonide cream in the treatment of plaque psoriasis. *J Am Acad Dermatol* 1998;38:705–711.

29. Lebwohl MG, Breneman DL, Goffe BS, et al. Tazarotene 0.1% gel plus corticosteroid cream in the treatment of plaque psoriasis. *J Am Acad Dermatol* 1998;39:590–596.

30. Gollnick H, Menter A. Combination therapy with tazarotene plus a topical corticosteroid for the treatment of plaque psoriasis. *Br J Dermatol* 1999;140(suppl):18–23.

31. Boer J, Hermans J, Schothorst AA, Suurmond D. Comparison of phototherapy (UVB) and photochemotherapy (PUVA) for clearing and maintenance therapy of psoriasis. *Arch Dermatol* 1984:120:52–57.

32. Gorden PM, Diffey BL, Mathews JN, Farr PM. A randomised comparison of narrow-band TL-01 phototherapy for psoriasis. *J Am Acad Dermatol* 1999;41:728–732.

33. Stern RS, Armstrong RB, Anderson TF, et al. Effect of continued ultraviolet B phototherapy on the duration of remission of psoriasis. A randomized study. *J Am Acad Dermatol* 1986;15:546–552.

34. Storbeck K, Holzle E, Schurer N, et al. Narrow-band UVB (311 nm) versus conventional broad-band UVB with and without dithranol in phototherapy for psoriasis. *J Am Acad Dermatol* 1993;28:227–231.

35. Pieternel CM, Pasker-de-Jong M, Wielink G, et al. Treatment with UV-B for psoriasis and nonmelanoma skin cancer. A systematic review of the literature. *Arch Dermatol* 1999;135:834–840. Search date 1996; primary sources Medline, Biosis, Online Contents.

36. Rogers S, Marks J, Shuster S, et al. Comparison of photochemotherapy and dithranol in the treatment of chronic plaque psoriasis. *Lancet* 1979;i:455–458.

37. Kirby B, Buckley DA, Rogers S. Large increments in psoralen-ultraviolet A (PUVA) therapy are unsuitable for fair skinned individuals with psoriasis. *Br J Dermatol* 1999;336:661–666.

38. Melski JW, Tanenbaum L, Parrish JA, et al. Oral methoxsalen photochemotherapy for the treatment of psoriasis. A cooperative clinical trial. *J Invest Dermatol* 1977;68:328–324.

39. Stern RS, Laird N. The carcinogenic risk of treatments for severe psoriasis. Photochemotherapy follow-up study. *Cancer* 1994;73:2759–2764.

40. Stern RS, Nichols KT, Vakeva LH. Malignant melanoma in patients treated for psoriasis with methoxsalen (psoralen) and ultraviolet A radiation. *N Engl J Med* 1997;336:1041–1045.

41. Stern RS, Lunder EJ. Risk of squamous cell carcinoma and methoxsalen (psoralen) and UV-A radiation (PUVA). A meta-analysis. *Arch Dermatol* 1998;134:1582–1585. Search date 1998; primary sources Medline, Healthstar, Aidsline, Cancerlit.

42. Hannuksela-Svahn A, Sigurgeirsson B, Pukkala E, et al. Trioxsalen bath PUVA did not increase the risk of squamous cell skin carcinoma and cutaneous malignant melanoma in a joint analysis of 944 Swedish and Finnish patients with psoriasis. *Br J Dermatol* 1999;141:497–501.

43. Paramsothy Y. Effect of UVB therapy and a coal tar bath on short contact dithranol treatment for psoriasis. *Br J Dermatol* 1988;118:783–789.

44. Ramsay CA, Schwartz BE, Lowson D, et al. Calcipotriol cream combined with twice weekly broad-band UVB phototherapy: a safe, effective and UVB-sparing antipsoriatic combination treatment. The Canadian Calcipotriol and UVB Study Group. *Dermatology* 2000;200:17–24.

45. Kragballe K. Combination of topical calcipotriol (MC 903) and UVB radiation for psoriasis vulgaris. *Dermatologica* 1990;181:211–214.

46. Frappaz A, Thivolet J. Calcipotriol in combination with PUVA: a randomized double-blind placebo study in severe psoriasis. *Eur J Dermatol* 1993;3:351–354.

47. Molin L. Topical calcipotriol with phototherapy for psoriasis. The results of two randomized trials and a review of the literature. Calcipotriol-UVB Study

Chronic plaque psoriasis

Group. *Dermatology* 1999;198:375–381.

48. Jones G, Crotty M, Brooks P. Psoriatic arthritis. An overview of therapy and toxicity. In: The Cochrane Library, Issue 4, 1999. Oxford: Update Software. Search date 1995; Primary sources Medline, Excerpta Medica.

49. Orfanos CED, Goerz A. Orale Psoriasis-therapie mit einem neuen aromatischen Retinoid (Ro 10–9359). Eine multizentrische kontrollierte Studie an 291 Patienten in der Bundesrepublik. *Dtsch Med Wochenschr* 1978;103:195–199.

50. Kragballe K, Jansen CT, Bjerke JR, et al. A double-blind comparison of acitretin and etretinate in the treatment of severe psoriasis. Results of a Nordic multicentre study. *Acta Derm Venereol* 1989;69: 35–40.

51. Ruzicka T, Sommerburg C, Braun-Falco O, et al. Efficiency of acitretin in combination with UV-B in the treatment of severe psoriasis. *Arch Dermatol* 1990;126:482–486.

52. Van de Kerkhof PC, Cambazard F, Hutchinson PE, et al. The effect of addition of calcipotriol ointment (50 micrograms/g) to acitretin therapy in psoriasis. *Br J Dermatol* 1998;138:84–89.

53. Lassus A, Lauharanta J, Juvakoski T, Kanerva L. Efficacy of etretinate (Tigason) in clearing and prevention of relapse of palmoplantar pustulosis. *Dermatologica* 1983;166:215–219.

54. White SI, Puttick L, Marks JM. Low-dose etretinate in the maintenance of remission of palmoplantar pustular psoriasis. *Br J Dermatol* 1986;115:577–582.

55. Dubertret L, Chastang C, Beylot C, et al. Maintenance treatment of psoriasis by Tigason: a double-blind randomized clinical trial. *Br J Dermatol* 1985;113:323–330.

56. Stern RS, Fitzgerald E, Ellis CN, et al. The safety of etretinate as long-term therapy for psoriasis. Results of the etretinate follow-up study. *J Am Acad Dermatol* 1995;33:44–52.

57. Wilkens RF, Williams HJ, Ward JR, et al. Randomized, double-blind, placebo controlled trial of low-dose pulse methotrexate in psoriatic arthritis. *Arthritis Rheum* 1984;27:376–381.

58. Van Dooren-Greebe RJ, Kuijpers AL, Mulder J, et al. Methotrexate revisited: effects of long-term treatment of psoriasis. *Br J Dermatol* 1994;130: 204–210.

59. Whiting-O'Keefe QE, Fye KH, Sack KD. Methotrexate and histologic hepatic abnormalities. *Am J Med* 1991;90:711–716. Search date 1989 and primary sources not stated.

60. Cottin V, Tebib J, Souquet PJ, Bernard JP, Pulmonary function in patients receiving long-term low-dose methotrexate. *Chest* 1996;109:933–938.

61. Nyfors A, Jensen H. Frequency of malignant neoplasms in 248 long-term methotrexate-treated psoriatics. A preliminary study. *Dermatologica* 1983;167:260–261.

62. Roenigk HH, Auerbach R, Maibach H, Weinstein G, Lebwohl M. Methotrexate in psoriasis: consensus conference. *J Am Acad Dermatol* 1998;38:478–485.

63. Timonen P, Friend D, Abeywickrama K, et al. Efficacy of low-dose cyclosporin A in psoriasis: results of dose finding studies. *Br J Dermatol* 1990;122(suppl 36):33–39.

64. Koo J. A randomized double-blind study comparing the efficacy, safety and optimal dose of two formulations of cyclosporin, Neoral and Sandimmun in patients with severe psoriasis. OLP302 Study Group. *Br J Dermatol* 1998;139: 88–95.

65. Shupack J, Abel E, Bauer E, et al. Cyclosporin as maintenance therapy in patients with severe psoriasis. *J Am Acad Dermatol* 1997;36:423–432.

66. Ellis CN, Fradin MS, Hamilton TA, Voorhees JJ. Duration of remission during maintenance cyclosporin therapy for psoriasis. *Arch Dermatol* 1995;131:791–795.

67. Ho V, Griffiths CEM, Albrecht G, et al. Intermittent short courses of cyclosporin (Neoral) for psoriasis unresponsive to topical therapy: a 1-year multicentre, randomized study. *Br J Dermatol* 1999;141:283–291.

68. Mahrle G, Schulze HJ, Fraber L, et al. Low-dose short-term cyclosporin versus etretinate: improvement of skin, nail, and joint involvement. *J Am Acad Dermatol* 1995;32:78–88.

69. Erkko P, Granlund H, Remitz A, et al. Double-blind placebo-controlled study of long-term low-dose cyclosporin in the treatment of palmoplantar pustulosis. *Br J Dermatol* 1998;139:997–1004.

70. Grossman RM, Chevret S, Abi-Rached J, Blanchet F, Dubertret L. Long-term safety of cyclosporin in the treatment of psoriasis. *Arch Dermatol* 1996; 132:623–629.

71. Altmeyer PJ, Matthes U, Pawlak F, et al. Antipsoriatic effect of fumaric acid derivatives. Results of a multicenter double-blind study in 100 patients. *J Am Acad Dermatol* 1994;30:977–981.

72. Mrowietz U, Christophers E, Altmeyer P. Treatment of psoriasis with fumaric acid esters: Results of a prospective multicentre study. *Br J Dermatol* 1998;138:456–460.

Luigi Naldi
Dermatologist
Ospedali Riuniti Bergamo
Bergamo
Italy

Competing interests: The research activities of the Italian Group for Epidemiological Research in Dermatology, which is coordinated by the author, have been supported partly by grants from GlaxoWellcome, Roche, Novartis, Schering, and Schering-Plough.

INTERVENTIONS

Key Messages

- We found limited evidence from two systematic reviews of RCTs that chemical insecticides are effective.
- We found no good evidence on combing or alternative treatments.

© *Clinical Evidence* 2000;4:975–978.

DEFINITION	Head lice are obligate ectoparasites of socially active humans. They infest the scalp, causing itching, and attach their eggs to the hair shafts. Infestation can be diagnosed only by finding living lice. Eggs glued to hairs, whether hatched (nits) or unhatched, are not proof of active infection, because eggs may retain a viable appearance for weeks after death.
INCIDENCE/ PREVALENCE	We found no data on incidence and no recent published prevalence data from any developed country. Anecdotal reports suggest that prevalence has increased in the last 4–5 years in most communities in the UK and USA.
AETIOLOGY/ RISK FACTORS	Observational studies indicate that infections occur most frequently in school children, although there is no proof of a link with school attendance. We found no evidence that lice prefer clean hair to dirty hair.
PROGNOSIS	The infection is essentially harmless. Sensitisation reactions to louse saliva and faeces may result in localised irritation and erythema. Secondary infection of scratches may occur. Lice have been identified as primary mechanical vectors of scalp pyoderma caused by streptococci and staphylococci usually found on the skin.[1]
AIMS	To eliminate infestation by killing or removing all head lice and their eggs.
OUTCOMES	Treatment success is given as the percentage of people completely cleared of head lice. A clinically important difference between treatments might be a more than 20% difference in the numbers of people successfully treated. There are no standard criteria for judging treatment success. Trials used different methods, and in many cases the method was not stated.
METHODS	The initial search was performed by the Cochrane Infectious Diseases Group at the Liverpool School of Tropical Medicine for a systematic review compiled in July 1998.[2] *Clinical Evidence* update search and appraisal June 2000.

QUESTION What are the effects of treatment for head lice?

OPTION INSECTICIDE BASED PHARMACEUTICAL PRODUCTS

We found two systematic reviews of small, poor quality RCTs of insecticide based pharmaceutical products. One review of three RCTs found that permethrin and malathion were more effective than placebo, and synergised pyrethrins and permethrin were of similar effectiveness. An earlier systematic review found permethrin more effective than lindane. All RCTs had methodological flaws.

Benefits: We found two systematic reviews.[2,3] The first (search date, March 1995) identified 7 RCTs (1808 people) of 11 insecticide products, including lindane, carbaryl, malathion, permethrin, and other pyrethroids in various vehicles.[3] Two RCTs found that only permethrin produced clinically significant differences in the rate of treatment success; both compared lindane (1% shampoo) against permethrin (1% cream rinse). Permethrin was found to be more effective (lindane v permethrin; OR for not clearing head lice 15.2, 95% CI 8.0 to 28.8). The subsequent systematic review (search date, April/May 1998) set stricter criteria for RCTs and rejected all but three trials.[2] It excluded both studies on which the earlier review was based. One RCT (n = 63 found that after 7 days, permethrin (1% cream rinse) was more effective against headlice than placebo (29/29 people with permethrin v 3/34; RR 11.3, 95% CI 3.9 to 33.4). Two weeks after permethrin treatment 28/29 people had no headlice versus 2/24 for placebo (RR 16.4, 95% CI 4.3 to 63.1). One RCT (n = 115 people) compared malathion (0.5% alcoholic lotion) with the vehicle base as placebo. At one week, more people treated with malathion had no headlice versus 21/47 for placebo; RR 2.1, 95% CI 1.6 to 3.0). One RCT (22 people) of synergised pyrethrin (0.16% mousse) versus permethrin (1% cream rinse) found that at six days, 17/19 people treated with pyrethrin had no lice, against 3/3 treated with permethrin (RR 0.89, 95% CI 0.8 to 1.0).

Harms: Only minor adverse effects have been reported for most insecticides. The exception is lindane, where there are extensive reports of effects related to overdosing (treatment of scabies), and absorption (treatment of head lice). Transdermal passage of lindane occurs during treatment of headlice,[4] but we found no reports of adverse effects in this setting. We found no confirmed reports of adverse effects from the organophosphate, malathion, when used therapeutically. One study (n = 32 people) of four different head louse preparations, investigated transdermal absorption of malathion and its effect on plasma and erythrocyte cholinesterase.[5] After application of 0.1–0.2 g malathion, between one third and two thirds was washed off the hair. About 0.2–3.2% of applied malathion was excreted in urine as metabolites. No effect was observed on cholinesterase activity.

Comment: Six day follow up is inadequate, as the eggs take at least 7 days to hatch. The three trials included in the most recent systematic review were conducted in developing countries, where insecticide treatments were not regularly available.[3] This may have resulted in greater efficacy, because the insects have not been subjected to any kind of selection pressure. No RCT has yet considered that a pediculicide's formulation might affect its activity. Studies in vitro suggest that other components of products (e.g. terpenoids and solvents) may be more effective pediculicides than the insecticide itself.[6] Resistance to one or more insecticides is now common.[7–9]

OPTION	MECHANICAL REMOVAL OF LICE OR VIABLE EGGS BY COMBING

We found insufficient evidence on the effects of combing.

Benefits: We found no systematic reviews that evaluated lice removal by combing, or nit combing to remove eggs. We found one new pragmatic RCT (72 people), comparing "Bug-busting" (wet combing with conditioner) with two applications of 0.5% malathion, 7 days apart. Seven days after treatment, more people taking malathion had no lice compared with "Bug-busting" (31/40 v 12/32; RR 2.8, 95% CI 1.5 to 5.2).[10] We found two RCTs comparing different pediculicides in combination with nit combing, but neither included a non-combing control group.[11,12]

Harms: We found no evidence of harms apart from discomfort.

Comment: None.

OPTION   HERBAL TREATMENTS AND AROMATHERAPY

We found no good evidence on the effects of these alternative treatments.

Benefits: We found no systematic reviews, RCTs, or cohort studies evaluating herbal treatments or aromatherapy.

Harms: We found no evidence of harms.

Comment: None.

Substantive changes since last issue

Mechanical removal of lice or viable eggs by combing One new RCT comparing insecticide use against wet combing with conditioner; no change in conclusion.[10]

REFERENCES

1. Taplin D, Meinking TL. Infestations. In: Schachner LA, Hansen RC, eds. *Pediatric dermatology*, vol 2. New York: Churchill Livingstone, 1988:1465–1493.
2. Dodd C. Head lice treatment. In: The Cochrane Library, Issue 4, 1999. Oxford: Update Software. Search date April/May 1998; primary sources CCTR, Medline, Embase, BIDS SC, BIOSIS, Toxline.
3. Vander Stichele RH, Dezeure EM, Bogaert MG. Systematic review of clinical efficacy of topical treatments for head lice. *BMJ* 1995;311:604–608. Search date March 1995; primary sources Medline, International Pharmaceutical Abstracts, Science Citation Index.
4. Ginsburg CM, Lowry W. Absorption of gamma benzene hexachloride following application of Kwell shampoo. *Pediatr Dermatol* 1983;1:74–76.
5. Dennis GA, Lee PN. A phase I volunteer study to establish the degree of absorption and effect on cholinesterase activity of four head lice preparations containing malathion. *Clin Drug Invest* 1999;18:105–115.
6. Burgess I. Malathion lotions for head lice: a less reliable treatment than commonly believed. *Pharm J* 1991;247:630–632.
7. Burgess IF, Brown CM, Peock S, et al. Head lice resistant to pyrethroid insecticides in Britain [letter]. *BMJ* 1995;311:752.
8. Pollack RJ, Kiszewski A, Armstrong P, et al. Differential permethrin susceptibility of head lice sampled in the United States and Borneo. *Arch Pediatr Adolesc Med* 1999;153:969–973.
9. Lee SH, Yoon KS, Williamson M, et al. Molecular analyses of *kdr*-like resistance in permethrin-resistant strains of head lice, *Pediculus capitis*. *Pestic Biochem Physiol* 2000;66:130–143.
10. Roberts RJ, Casey D, Morgan DA, et al. Pragmatic randomised controlled trial comparing "Bug Busting" with malathion for the treatment of head lice in the UK. *Lancet* (in press).
11. Bainbridge CV, Klein GI, Neibart SI, et al. Comparative study of the clinical effectiveness of a pyrethrin-based pediculicide with combing versus a permethrin-based pediculicide with combing. *Clin Pediatr (Phila)* 1998;37:17–22.
12. Clore ER, Longyear LA. A comparative study of seven pediculicides and their packaged nit combs. *J Pediatr Health Care* 1993;7:55–60.

Ian Burgess
Director
Medical Entomology Centre
Cambridge
UK

Competing interests: The author has received consultancy fees from all major producers of pediculicides and several smaller companies.

Updated and expanded this issue

Graham Worrall

INTERVENTIONS

Key Messages

Prevention

- Limited evidence from RCTs suggests that prophylactic oral aciclovir may reduce the frequency and severity of attacks, but the optimal timing and duration of treatment is uncertain.
- We found no good evidence on the effects of topical antiviral agents used as prophylaxis.
- One small RCT found that ultraviolet sunscreen reduced the rate of herpes recurrence.

Treatment

- RCTs have found that oral aciclovir marginally reduces the duration of symptoms and pain of first time and recurrent herpes labialis.
- We found limited evidence of benefit from RCTs for the use of topical antiviral agents early in an attack.
- One RCT found that topical tetracaine used early in an attack reduced time to scab loss.

DEFINITION	Herpes labialis is a mild self limiting infection with herpes simplex virus type 1 (HSV-1). It causes pain and blistering on the lips and perioral area (cold sores); fever and constitutional symptoms are rare. Most people have no warning of an attack, but some experience a recognisable prodrome.
INCIDENCE/ PREVALENCE	Herpes labialis accounts for about 1% of primary care consultations in the UK each year; 20–40% of people have experienced cold sores at some time.[1]
AETIOLOGY/ RISK FACTORS	Herpes labialis is caused by HSV-1. After the primary infection, which usually occurs in childhood, the virus is thought to remain latent in the trigeminal ganglion.[2] A variety of factors, including exposure to bright sunlight, fatigue, or psychological stress, can precipitate a recurrence.
PROGNOSIS	In most people, herpes labialis is a mild, self limiting illness. Recurrences are usually shorter and less severe than the initial attack. Healing is usually complete in 7–10 days without scarring.[3] Rates of reactivation are unknown. Herpes labialis can cause serious illness in immunocompromised patients.
AIMS	To reduce the frequency and severity of recurrent attacks, to speed healing of lesions, and to reduce pain, with minimal adverse effects.
OUTCOMES	Severity of symptoms, time to healing, rate of recurrence, adverse effects of treatment.
METHODS	*Clinical Evidence* update search and appraisal May 2000. Medline and FAMLI databases were searched from 1980 to 1998. Keywords were "herpes labialis", "treatment", "prevention", "prophylaxis", "controlled trial", and "effectiveness".

QUESTION **What are the effects of antiviral treatment for the first attack of herpes labialis?**

We found no good evidence on the effects of topical agents on the duration or severity of symptoms of the first attack of herpes labialis. Limited evidence from small RCTs in children suggests that oral aciclovir may marginally reduce duration of pain and time to healing.

Benefits: We found no systematic review. **Topical antiviral agents:** We found no RCTs. **Oral antiviral agents:** We found two small RCTs, both of which found a beneficial effect.[4,5] One double blind RCT in 20 children having their first attack compared oral aciclovir 200 mg five times a day versus placebo.[4] Mean duration of pain was reduced from 5.0 to 4.3 days, and mean duration of excess salivation was reduced from 5.0 to 3.3 days (P < 0.05). The second RCT, in 72 children aged 1–6 years with gingivostomatitis of less than 3 days duration, compared oral aciclovir 15 mg/kg five times a day for 7 days versus placebo. Time to healing was reduced from 10 to 4 days, a mean reduction of 6 days (95% CI 4 to 8 days).[5] We found no RCTs in adults.

Harms: Topical aciclovir causes rash, pruritus, and irritation in some people, but no more frequently in trials than placebo.[6–8] It has also caused head and tail abnormalities in fetal rats, but we found no recorded cases of teratogenicity in humans. Oral aciclovir is excreted in breast milk. Aciclovir has been used to treat pregnant women with genital herpes, and one systematic review of three studies found no evidence of adverse effects in women or newborn children[8] (see antiviral treatment during pregnancy under genital herpes, p 901). However, the evidence is limited, and clinically significant adverse effects cannot be ruled out.

Comment: Research in this area is difficult because people do not usually consult clinicians until after they have had several attacks of herpes labialis.

QUESTION   Do treatments taken at the beginning or during a recurrent attack reduce the duration or severity of symptoms?

OPTION   ORAL/TOPICAL ANTIVIRAL AGENTS

We found limited evidence of benefit from RCTs for the use of topical antiviral agents early in an attack.

Benefits: We found no systematic review. **Topical antiviral agents:** We found several trials of antiviral cream, which reported mixed results.[6,7,9–14] The largest RCT (double blind) compared penciclovir cream 2 hourly for 4 days versus placebo in 2209 people.[12] Penciclovir cream reduced healing times by 0.7 days and duration of pain by 0.6 days (CIs could not be calculated from the published report). One small RCT with three parallel arms compared 5% aciclovir cream (n = 10) versus 5% aciclovir in a liposomal carrier (n = 12) versus the drug free vehicle (n = 9) in 31 people aged over 17 years with recurrent herpes labialis. The mean time to crusting of the lesions was significantly reduced for aciclovir in liposomal carrier versus drug free carrier (1.6 days for aciclovir in liposomes v 4.8 days for control, $P < 0.05$) but not for aciclovir cream versus the drug free carrier (4.3 days for aciclovir cream v 4.8 days for control).[14] Fifteen of the participants then participated in a crossover study in which they received the two forms of aciclovir (in random order) separated by a washout period of at least 1 month. Again, the time to crusting of lesions was shorter with aciclovir in liposomes than for aciclovir cream (1.8 v 3.5 days, $P < 0.05$). Too few people experienced pain to analyse the impact of the preparations on discomfort. A further double blind RCT compared 1% penciclovir cream versus placebo in 534 people.[15] It found that penciclovir reduced the mean healing time of lesions from 8.8 to 7.6 days ($P < 0.01$). **Oral antiviral agents:** We found two RCTs. One double blind RCT in 174 adults with recurrent herpes labialis compared oral aciclovir 400 mg five times a day for 5 days versus placebo.[16] Taken early in the attack (when the patient first experienced tingling), oral aciclovir led to a reduction in duration of symptoms from 12.5 to 8.1 days (CIs could not be calculated from the published report). If treatment was initiated later (when the vesicular rash appeared), there was no benefit compared with placebo. A second double blind RCT in 149 people compared oral aciclovir within 12 hours of onset of symptoms versus placebo.[17] It found a significant but clinically small effect; oral aciclovir reduced healing time by 0.98 days and duration of pain by 0.04 days ($P < 0.05$).

Harms: See harms under the effects of antiviral treatment for the first attack of herpes labialis, p 980.

Comment: We found no RCTs comparing early versus delayed intervention, so no firm conclusions regarding timing of treatment can be drawn.

OPTION   TOPICAL ANAESTHETIC AGENTS   New

One RCT of topical tetracaine found that use early in an attack reduced time to scab loss. We found insufficient evidence on the effects of other agents.

Benefits: We found no systematic review. A double blind RCT (n = 72) found that 1.8% tetracaine cream compared with placebo, applied six times daily until scab loss occurred, reduced mean time to scab loss from 7.2 to 5.1 days (P = 0.002), and increased a composite symptom benefit index from 5.9 to 7.3 (P = 0.036).[18]

Harms: None reported.

Comment: See comment under antiviral agents for recurrent attacks above.

QUESTION   What are the effects of interventions aimed at preventing attacks?

OPTION   ORAL/TOPICAL ANTIVIRAL AGENTS

We found limited evidence from RCTs that prophylactic oral aciclovir reduced the frequency and severity of attacks. It is not clear whether prophylaxis should be continuous or restricted to high risk periods. We found no good evidence on the effects of topical antiviral agents.

Benefits: We found no systematic review. **Topical antiviral agents:** We found no good quality RCTs. **Oral antiviral agents:** We found four double blind placebo controlled RCTs. The first, in 147 American skiers with a history of herpes labialis precipitated by ultraviolet (UV) light, concluded that those given prophylactic oral aciclovir (200 mg five times a day for 5 days beginning 7 days before UV exposure) suffered fewer attacks and shorter duration of symptoms (P < 0.05).[19] The second, in 239 Canadian skiers, found no significant difference between aciclovir 800 mg twice a day, starting on the day before exposure to ultraviolet light for 37 days, compared with placebo.[20] The third, in 20 people with recurrent herpes labialis, found that aciclovir 400 mg twice a day for 4 months led to 53% fewer clinical recurrences and 71% fewer virus culture positive recurrences (P = 0.05).[21] The fourth trial compared three different dosages of famciclovir (125 mg, 250 mg, and 500 mg) versus placebo in 248 adults with a history of sun induced recurrent herpes labialis.[22] Treatment was given three times a day for 5 days beginning 48 hours after exposure to artificial UV light. There was no significant difference in the number of lesions in the four groups, but increasing the dose of famciclovir significantly reduced the mean size (P = 0.04) and duration of lesions, in a dose response relation. Compared with placebo, the 500 mg dose reduced the mean time to healing by 2 days (P ≤ 0.01).

Harms: See harms under the effects of antiviral treatment for the first attack of herpes labialis, p 980.

Comment: None.

| OPTION | SUNSCREEN |

Two small RCTs found that sunscreen reduced the rate of herpes recurrence.

Benefits: We found no systematic review. We found two small randomised double blind crossover trials,[23,24] both of which found that sunscreen significantly reduced the rate of recurrence. Of 38 people with a history of recurrent herpes, 71% suffered recurrence with placebo compared with 0% with sunscreen.[23] Of the 19 people in the second trial, 11 suffered recurrence with placebo compared with one with sunscreen ($P < 0.01$).[24]

Harms: None reported.

Comment: None.

Substantive changes since last issue
Topical antivirals for recurrent attacks New RCT; found that topical penciclovir reduced healing time of lesions.[15]

REFERENCES

1. Hodgkin K. *Towards earlier diagnosis: a guide to general practice*. London: Churchill Livingstone 1973:129.
2. Baringer SR, Swoveland P. Recovery of herpes simplex virus from human trigeminal ganglions. *N Engl J Med* 1973;288:648–650.
3. Baker C, Crumpacker CS, Schnipner LE. The natural history of recurrent facial-oral infections with the herpes simplex virus. *J Infect Dis* 1978; 138:897–905.
4. Ducoulombier H, Cousin J, DeWilde A. La stomato-gingivite herpétique de l'enfant: essai a contolle aciclovir versus placebo [in French]. *Ann Pediatr* 1988;35:212–216.
5. Amir J, Harel L, Smetana Z, Varsano I. Treatment of herpes simplex gingivostomatitis with aciclovir in children: a randomised double blind placebo controlled trial. *BMJ* 1997;314:1800–1803.
6. Raborn GW, Martel WT, Grace M, Percy UJ, Samuels S. Herpes labialis treatment with acyclovir modified aqueous cream: a double-blind randomized trial. *Oral Surg Oral Med Oral Pathol* 1989;67:676–679.
7. Fiddian AP, Ivanyi L. Topical acyclovir in the management of recurrent herpes labialis. *Br J Dermatol* 1983;109:321–326.
8. Smith J, Cowan FM, Munday P. The management of herpes simplex virus infection in pregnancy. *Br J Obstet Gynaecol* 1998;105:255–268. Search date 1996; primary sources Medline 1983 to 1996, and hand searched references.
9. Van Vloten WA, Swart RNJ, Pot F. Topical acyclovir therapy in patients with recurrent orofacial herpes simplex infections. *J Antimicrob Chemother* 1993; 12(suppl B):89–93.
10. Shaw M, King M, Best JM. Failure of acyclovir ointment in treatment of recurrent herpes labialis. *BMJ* 1985;291:79.
11. Spruance SL, Schnipper LE, Overcall JC. Treatment of herpes simplex labialis with topical acyclovir in polyethylene glycol. *J Infect Dis* 1982; 146:85–90.
12. Spruance SL, Rea TL, Thoming C, Tucker R, Saltzman R, Boon R. Penciclovir cream for the treatment of herpes simplex labialis. *JAMA* 1997; 277:1374–1379.
13. Raborn GW, McGraw WT, Grace MG, Houle L. Herpes labialis treatment with acyclovir 5 per cent ointment. *Sci J* 1989;55:135–137.
14. Horwitz E, Pisanty S, Czerninski R, Helser M, Eliav E, Touitou E. A clinical evaluation of a novel liposomal carrier for acyclovir in the topical treatment of recurrent herpes labialis. *Oral Surg Oral Med Oral Pathol* 1999;87:700–705.
15. Boon R, Goodman JJ, Martinez J, Marks GL, Gamble M, Welch C. Penciclovir cream for the treatment of sunlight-induced herpes simplex labialis: a randomized, double-blind, placebo-controlled trial. Penciclovir Cream Herpes Labialis Study Group. *Clin Ther* 2000;22:76–90.
16. Spruance SL, Hammil ML, Hoge WS, Davis G, Mills J. ACV prevents reactivation of herpes labialis in skiers. *JAMA* 1988;260:1597–1599.
17. Rooney JF, Strauss SE, Mannix ML, et al. Oral acyclovir to suppress frequently recurrent herpes labialis: a double-blind, placebo controlled trial. *Ann Intern Med* 1993;118:268–272.
18. Kaminester LH, Pariser RJ, Pariser DM, Weiss JS, Shavin JS, Landsman L, Haines HG, Osborne DW. A double-blind, placebo-controlled study of topical tetracaine in the treatment of herpes labialis. *J Am Acad Dermatol* 1999;41:996–1001.
19. Raborn GW, Martel AY, Grace MG, McGaw WT. Oral acyclovir in prevention of herpes labialis: a randomized, double-blind, placebo controlled trial. *Oral Surg Oral Med Oral Pathol Oral Radiol Endod* 1998;85:55–59.
20. Spruance SL, Stewart JC, Rowe NH, et al. Treatment of recurrent herpes simplex labialis with oral acyclovir. *J Infect Dis* 1990;161:185–190.
21. Raborn WG, McGraw WT, Grace M, Tyrell LD, Samuels SM. Oral acyclovir and herpes labialis: a randomized, double-blind, placebo-controlled study. *J Am Dental Assoc* 1987;115:38–42.

22. Spruance SL, Rowe NH, Raborn GW, et al. Peroral famciclovir in the treatment of experimental ultraviolet radiation-induced herpes simplex labialis: a double-blind, dose-ranging, placebo-controlled, multicenter trial. *J Infect Dis* 1999; 179:303–310.

23. Rooney JF, Bryson Y, Mannix ML, Dillon M, et al. Prevention of ultraviolet-light-induced herpes labialis by sunscreen. *Lancet* 1991;338:1419–1421.

24. Duteil L, Queille-Roussel C, Loesche C, Verschoore M. Assessment of the effect of a sunblock stick in the prevention of solar-simulating ultraviolet light-induced herpes labialis. *J Dermatol Treat* 1998;9:11–14.

Graham Worrall
Associate Professor of Family Medicine
Memorial University of Newfoundland
Whitbourne
Canada

Competing interests: None declared.

Updated this issue

Thomas Crosby, Malcolm Mason and David Crosby

INTERVENTIONS

Key Messages

- We found insufficient evidence on the preventive effect of sunscreens.
- RCTs have found narrow primary excision to be as effective as wide excision in terms of overall survival and probably local recurrence. Narrow excision reduces the need for skin grafting.
- RCTs have found that elective lymph node dissection offers no advantage in overall survival compared with surgery deferred until clinical recurrence.
- We found insufficient evidence on the effects of adjuvant treatments, although limited evidence from one RCT suggests that alfa-2_b interferon may improve survival in high risk people.

DEFINITION   Cutaneous malignant melanoma is a tumour derived from melanocytes in the basal layer of the epidermis. After undergoing malignant transformation, it becomes invasive by penetrating into and beyond the dermis.

INCIDENCE/ PREVALENCE   Incidence in developed countries has increased by 50% in the past 20 years. Incidence varies in different populations (see table 1, p 991), and is about 10-fold higher in white than in non-white populations. Despite the rise in incidence, mortality has plateaued and even fallen in some populations (e.g. in women and young men in Australia).[1,2] During the same period there has been a sixfold increase in the incidence of melanoma *in situ,* suggesting earlier detection.

AETIOLOGY/ RISK FACTORS   The number of common, atypical, and dysplastic naevi on a person's body correlates closely with the risk of developing malignant melanoma. A genetic predisposition probably accounts for 5–10% of all cases. Although the risk of developing malignant melanoma is higher in fair skinned white populations living close to the equator, the relation between sun exposure, sunscreen use, and skin type is not clear cut. Exposure to excessive sunlight and severe sunburn in childhood are associated with an increased risk of developing malignant melanoma in adult life. However, people do not necessarily develop tumours at sites of maximum exposure to the sun.

PROGNOSIS   The prognosis of early malignant melanoma (stages I–III) (see table 2, p 992) relates to the depth of invasion of the primary lesion, the presence of ulceration, and involvement of the regional lymph nodes, the prognosis worsening with the number of nodes involved.[3] A person with a thin lesion (Breslow depth < 0.75 mm) and without lymph node involvement has a 3% risk of developing metastases and a 95% chance of surviving 5 years.[4] If regional lymph nodes are macroscopically involved there is a 20–50% chance of surviving 5 years. Most studies have shown a better prognosis in women and in people with lesions on the extremities compared with those with lesions on the trunk.

AIMS   To prevent melanoma; to detect melanoma earlier; to minimise mutilating surgical treatment while still achieving cure of local disease; to optimise quality of life; and to eradicate occult micrometastatic disease, with minimum adverse effects.

OUTCOMES   **Prevention:** Rates and severity of sunburn (proxy measure); incidence of malignant melanoma; mortality from malignant melanoma. **Primary excision:** Local recurrence; overall survival; requirement for skin grafting. **Lymph node dissection and adjuvant treatment:** Overall survival; disease free survival; quality of life; morbidity of disease treatment, or both.

METHODS   *Clinical Evidence* update search and appraisal May 2000, plus search of reference lists of all review articles found, and the main oncological and dermatological textbooks.

QUESTION **Does the use of sunscreens help to prevent malignant melanoma?**

OPTION SUNSCREENS

We found no RCTs assessing the effect of sunscreens on the incidence of, or mortality from, malignant melanoma. The correct use of sunscreen, however, seems a sensible measure to avoid excessive exposure to sunlight.

Benefits: We found no systematic review. Although one RCT found that sunscreens reduced the incidence or progression of solar keratosis,[5] we found no similar evidence for malignant melanoma. Retrospective case control studies and questionnaire based surveys, all of which have potential biases and confounding factors, have found conflicting results.[6–8] One case control study found that adults with melanoma were less likely to have been protected from sunlight as children,[7] whereas some questionnaire based surveys found no such effect.[6,8]

Harms: Sunscreens can irritate the skin and cause allergic contact dermatitis. Some questionnaire based surveys have suggested that sunscreen may have contributed to the development of malignant melanoma.[6,8] A possible mechanism for this suggestion may be that since some sunscreens protect predominantly against ultraviolet B (UVB, which induces sunburn), people may spend more time exposed to higher doses of ultraviolet A (UVA). One placebo controlled RCT found that a sunscreen with a high sun protection factor (SPF 30) was associated with significantly longer recreational sun exposure.[9]

Comment: Although we found no prospective evidence, it would seem reasonable to take sensible precautions to avoid excessive exposure to sunlight, particularly in children and fair skinned individuals. Sunscreens may have a role if used appropriately (sun protection factor of at least 15 and a star rating for UVA protection of 3–4), rather than being used to prolong the time spent in direct sunlight.

QUESTION **Is there an optimal margin for primary excision of melanoma of different Breslow thicknesses?**

RCTs have found that more radical local surgery (4–5 cm excision margins) provides no greater benefit than less radical surgery (1–2 cm excision margins).

Benefits: **Radical local surgery versus less radical surgery:** We found no systematic review. We found three RCTs in people with thin (< 1 mm) and intermediate thickness (1–4 mm) malignant melanoma.[10–12] The first trial randomised 612 people with lesions < 2 mm thick to surgical excision with either 1 or 3 cm margins.[10] The second trial randomised 486 people with intermediate thickness lesions (1–4 mm) to either 2 or 4 cm margins. The remaining trial randomised 769 people with lesions 0.8–2.0 mm to either 2 or 5 cm margins.[12] None of the trials found that wide margins reduced local recurrence rates or increased overall survival compared with narrow excision margins.

Harms: Narrower excision margins reduced skin grafting (in one RCT by 75%), anaesthetic requirements, and inpatient stay.[10] Narrow margin surgery can usually be performed on outpatient day surgery lists. Of concern is the possibility of higher local recurrence rates using 1 cm margins for tumours 1–2 mm. One RCT in 612 people comparing narrow margin with wide margin surgery reported three local recurrences, all in people with tumours 1–2 mm treated with narrow (1 cm) margin excision; local cure was achieved in two people with further surgery.[10] Although not measured, there is potential for psychological and physical morbidity associated with further surgery after local recurrence.

Comment: The evidence relating to survival is good but we found no good evidence relating to quality of life or physical and psychological morbidity caused by extent of surgery or local recurrence.

QUESTION **Does elective lymph node dissection improve outcomes in people with clinically uninvolved lymph nodes?**

RCTs found no benefit from elective lymph node dissection in people with clinically uninvolved lymph nodes, although an effect within particular subgroups cannot be ruled out.

Benefits: We found no systematic review. We found four RCTs comparing elective lymph node dissection with surgery deferred until the time of clinical recurrence in a total of 1718 people with no clinical evidence of lymph node metastases.[13–16] None of the studies showed a significant overall survival benefit for people receiving elective lymph node dissection. Retrospective subgroup analyses found non-significant trends in favour of elective lymph node dissection in certain groups of people (those with intermediate thickness tumours, especially those under 60 years of age), but such analyses are subject to bias.

Harms: Lymph node dissection has several complications. In one retrospective case series, these included temporary seroma (17%), wound infection (9%), wound necrosis (3%), and lymphoedema (20%).[17]

Comment: In about 20% of people who do not have clinically apparent lymph node involvement, the lymph nodes will contain occult micrometastases. None of the RCTs gave data on morbidity and quality of life in people undergoing lymph node dissection. An alternative to elective lymph node dissection, sentinel lymph node excision, which can accurately determine the specific nodes draining the primary lesion and their involvement with metastatic disease,[18] is currently being evaluated in clinical trials.

QUESTION **Does adjuvant treatment improve prognosis after curative surgery of cutaneous malignant melanoma and at what stage?**

OPTION ALFA-2$_b$ INTERFERON

RCTs have found that alfa-2$_b$ interferon extends the time to relapse and, in high doses, may improve survival in high risk people. However, toxicity and withdrawal rates are high. Less toxic regimens for interferon treatment are being evaluated.

Benefits: We found no systematic review. **High dose:** We found one RCT comparing high dose alfa-2_b interferon (20 MIU/m^2 per day intravenously for 1 month, followed by 10 MIU/m^2 three times a week subcutaneously for 11 months) versus observation in 287 people with primary lesions greater than 4 mm or resectable stage III disease.[19] At a median of 6.9 years of follow up, an intention to treat analysis found a significant improvement in disease free survival (median 1.7 v 1.0 years) and overall survival (median 3.8 v 2.8 years, CIs not given in the report). A retrospective analysis of this study by the authors showed prolonged quality of life-adjusted survival in people receiving interferon alfa. The significance of this gain varied with the values assigned by people for the impact of treatment toxicity and time with relapsed disease.[20] Preliminary results at a median of 4.3 years of follow up of a larger study of 642 people failed to confirm a survival benefit for high or low dose adjuvant alfa interferon.[21] **Low dose:** We found two RCTs. Both of these studies were performed in people with stage II melanoma (primary tumours > 1.5 mm and lymph node negative). One RCT compared low dose interferon (3 MIU three times a week for 18 months) versus surgery alone in 499 people. It showed a significant extension of the relapse free interval and a trend towards extension of overall survival (HR for relapse free survival 0.75, 95% CI 0.57 to 0.98, P = 0.038; HR for overall survival 0.72, 95% CI 0.51 to 1.0, P = 0.059).[22] The second trial randomised 311 people to receive interferon alfa-2_b (3 MIU given daily for 3 weeks and three times per week for 12 months) or observation after excision of their primary tumour. At 41 months follow up there was a prolonged relapse free survival (P = 0.02, CIs not reported) but no effect on overall survival.[23]

Harms: Interferons commonly cause malaise, fevers, and flu-like symptoms. In the RCT described above, high dose alfa interferon also caused significant (> grade 3) myelosuppression in 24% of people, hepatotoxicity in 15% (including 2 deaths), and neurotoxicity in 28%. At 11 months, only 25% of participants were receiving more than 80% of the planned dose.[19] In the trial of low dose interferon, 10% of people suffered significant toxicity.[22]

Comment: RCTs investigating the effects of more tolerable alfa interferon regimens are underway.

OPTION OTHER ADJUVANT TREATMENTS

We found no evidence of benefit in terms of survival with other adjuvant treatments (non-specific immunotherapy and chemotherapy); surveillance, specific immunotherapy, hormones, coumarin, retinoids have not been evaluated adequately.

Benefits: We found no systematic review. We found 60 RCTs of adjuvant systemic treatment. Most were too small or too short term to detect a clinically significant benefit, and involved heterogeneous groups of participants (see table 3, p 992). **Non-specific immunostimulation:** A total of 24 RCTs (mainly small, ranging from 26 to 400 people) evaluated non-specific immunostimulation with agents such as bacille Calmette-Guérin and *Corynebacterium parvum*.

These found no beneficial effect on survival, although most trials were too small to exclude a beneficial effect. **Active specific immunostimulation:** Results from RCTs are awaited, but small pilot studies in single institutions found encouraging results compared with historical controls, especially from allogeneic tumour cell vaccines, viral oncolysates, gangliosides, or melanoma associated peptide vaccines. **Chemotherapy:** About 15 RCTs (mostly small, ranging from 15 to 258 people) compared single agent cytotoxic agents, especially dacarbazine, chemo-immunotherapy, and multi-agent cytotoxic treatments versus placebo. No beneficial effect on survival was found. The regimen believed to be most powerful in advanced disease—cisplatin, bischloroethylnitrosourea, dacarbazine, and tamoxifen (the Dartmouth regimen)—has not yet been tested in RCTs. **Hormones, coumarins, retinoids:** Several small RCTs of hormones (megesterol acetate) and coumarins found mixed results. Several small RCTs all found no benefit from retinoids. **Surveillance:** We found no RCTs. Retrospective studies found that people presented with symptomatic recurrent disease regardless of whether they were taking part in an intensive follow up programme.[24] Thinner lesions (< 0.76 mm) may require longer surveillance as recurrences peak between 5 and 10 years.[25]

Harms:
Certain types of immunostimulation may be associated with flu-like symptoms such as fevers, arthralgias, and rigors. Chemotherapy toxicities are well known and include nausea and vomiting, myelosuppression, and alopecia, depending on the cytotoxic agents used. Hormonal therapy can cause weight gain and lead to an increased risk of thromboembolism. Long term adverse effects of retinoids are less well known, but they may possibly be carcinogenic in certain circumstances. Although surveillance can do little physical harm, the possibility of inducing anxiety has not been excluded.

Comment: None.

REFERENCES

1. Giles GG, Armstrong BK, Burton RC, et al. Has mortality from melanoma stopped rising in Australia? Analysis of trends between 1931 and 1994. *BMJ* 1996;312:1121–1125.
2. Armstrong BK, Kricker A. Cutaneous melanoma. *Cancer Surv* 1994;19–20:219–240.
3. Balch CM, Soong SJ, Shaw HM, et al. An analysis of prognostic factors in 8500 patients with cutaneous melanoma. In: Balch CM, Houghton Anilton GW, Sober AJ, Soong SJ, eds. *Cutaneous melanoma*, 2nd ed. New York: Ellis Horwood, 1992.
4. Balch CM, Smalley RV, Bartolucci AA, et al. A randomised prospective clinical trial of adjuvant *C. parvum* immunotherapy in 260 patients with clinically localized melanoma (stage I): prognostic factor analysis and preliminary results of immunotherapy. *Cancer* 1982;49:1079–1084.
5. Thompson SC, Jolley D, Marks R. Reduction of solar keratoses by regular sunscreen use. *N Engl J Med* 1993;329;1147–1151.
6. Autier P, Dore J-F, Lejeune FJ, et al. Sun protection in childhood or early adolescence and reduction of melanoma risk in adults: an EORTC case-control study in Germany, Belgium and France. *J Epidemiol Biostat* 1996;1:51–57.
7. Holly EA, Aston DA, Cress RD, et al. Cutaneous melanoma in women. *Am J Epidemiol* 1995;141: 923–933.
8. Wolf P, Quehenberger F, Mullegger R, et al. Phenotypic markers, sunlight-related factors and sunscreen use in patients with cutaneous melanoma: an Austrian case-control study. *Melanoma Res* 1998;8:370–378.
9. Autier P, Dore JF, Negrier S, et al. Sunscreen use and duration of sun exposure: a double-blind, randomized trial. *J Natl Cancer Inst* 1999;91: 1304–1309.
10. Veronesi U, Cascinelli N, Adamus J, et al. Thin stage I primary cutaneous malignant melanoma: comparison of excision with margins of 1 or 3 cm. *N Engl J Med* 1988;318:1159–1162.
11. Balch CM, Urist MM, Karakousis, CP, et al. Efficacy of 2 cm surgical margins for intermediate-thickness melanomas (1 to 4 mm): results of a multi-institutional randomized surgical trial. *Ann Surg* 1993;218:262–267.
12. Ringborg U, Anderron R, Eldh J, et al. Resection margins of 2 versus 5 cm for cutaneous malignant melanoma with a tumour thickness of 0.8 to 2.0 mm: randomized study by the Swedish melanoma study group. *Cancer* 1996;77:1809–1814.
13. Balch CM, Soong SJ, Bartolucci AA, et al. Efficacy of an elective regional lymph node dissection of 1–4 mm thick melanomas for patients 60 years of age and younger. *Ann Surg* 1996;224:255–263.
14. Cascinelli N, Morabito A, Santinami M, et al.

Immediate or delayed dissection of regional nodes in patients with melanoma of the trunk: a randomised trial. WHO Melanoma Programme. *Lancet* 1998;351:793–796.

15. Sim FH, Taylor WF, Ivins JC, et al. A prospective randomized study of the efficacy of routine elective lymphadenectomy in management of malignant melanoma: preliminary results. *Cancer* 1978;41:948–956.

16. Veronesi U, Adamus J, Bandiera DC, et al. Inefficacy of immediate node dissection in stage I melanoma of the limbs. *N Engl J Med* 1977;297:627–630.

17. Baas PC, Schraffordt KH, Koops H, et al. Groin dissection in the treatment of lower-extremity melanoma: short-term and long-term morbidity. *Arch Surg* 1992;127:281–286.

18. Ross MI. Surgical management of stage I and II melanoma patients: approach to the regional lymph node basin. *Semin Surg Oncol* 1996;12:394–401.

19. Kirkwood JM, Strawderman MH, Erstoff MS, et al. Interferon alfa-2_b adjuvant therapy of high-risk resected cutaneous melanoma: The eastern cooperative oncology group trial EST 1684. *J Clin Oncol* 1996;14:7–17.

20. Cole BF, Gelber RD, Kirkwood JM, et al. Quality-of-life-adjusted survival analysis of high-risk resected cutaneous melanoma: the eastern cooperative oncology group study. *J Clin Oncol* 1996;14:2666–2673.

21. Kirkwood JM, Ibrahim J, Sondak V, et al. Preliminary analysis of the E1690/S9111/C9190 intergroup postoperative adjuvant trial of high- and low-dose IFN-2_b (HDI and LDI) in high risk primary or lymph node metastatic melanoma. *Proc ASCO* 1999;18 (abstract 2072)

22. Grob JJ, Dreno B, de la Salmoniere P, et al. Randomised trial of interferon alpha-2_a as adjuvant therapy in resected primary melanoma thicker than 1.5 mm without clinically detectable node metastases. French cooperative group on melanoma. *Lancet* 1998;351:1905–1910.

23. Pehamberger H, Peter Soyer H, Steiner A, et al. Adjuvant interferon alfa-2_a treatment in resected primary stage II cutaneous melanoma. *J Clin Oncol* 1998;16:1425–1429.

24. Shumate CR, Urist MM, Maddox WA. Melanoma recurrence surveillance: patient or physician based? *Ann Surg* 1995;221:566–559.

25. Rogers GS, Kopf AW, Rigel DS, et al. Hazard-rate analysis in stage I malignant melanoma. *Arch Dermatol* 1986;122:999–1002.

Thomas Crosby
Consultant Clinical Oncologist

Malcolm Mason
Professor of Clinical Oncology

Velindre Hospital
Cardiff
UK

David Crosby
Consultant Surgeon
Cardiff Community Healthcare Trust
Cardiff
UK

Competing interests: None declared.

TABLE 1	Melanoma incidence and mortality in different populations (see text, p 986).[2]		
Population	**Incidence (per 100 000 people)**	**New cases per year**	**Deaths per year**
Asian/Oriental	0.2	NA	NA
United Kingdom	8	4000	1500
United States	12	32 000	6700
Caucasians in Queensland, Australia	40	NA	NA

NA, not available.

TABLE 2 Stage of malignant melanoma and 5 year survival (see text, p 986).[3]

Stage	Description	Approx 5 year survival (%)
I	Primary tumour < 0.75 mm (T1) or > 0.75–1.5 mm (T2). No lymphadenopathy (N0).	95
II	Primary tumour > 1.5–4 mm (T3). No lymphadenopathy (N0).	50–70
III	Primary tumour > 4 mm or satellite(s) within 2 cm, lymphadenopathy < 3 cm (N1) or > 3 cm/in transit metastasis (N2). No metastases (M0).	20–50
IV	Presence of metastases (M1).	0–5

TABLE 3 Effects of non-cytokine adjuvant treatment (see text, p 989).

Intervention	Example	Evidence
Non-specific immunotherapy	BCG Corynebacterium parvum	Many RCTs have found no evidence of improved overall or disease free survival
Active specific immunotherapy	Melanoma cell vaccines Viral oncolysates Defined antigen vaccines Dendritic cells	No evidence from RCTs (although some are under way)
Chemotherapy	Single agents Combination treatments	RCTs reported no evidence of benefit. The most powerful regimen (DTIC, cisplatin, BCNU, and tamoxifen) has not been evaluated in RCTs
Others	Hormones (megesterol acetate) Coumarin Retinoids	Small RCTs reported survival benefit from hormones and coumarin, but not from retinoids. Findings have not yet been replicated in larger studies
Surveillance	Follow up programme (e.g. every 3 months for first 2 years)	Standard management for stage I (thin lesions < 0.76 mm). Thinner lesions may require longer follow up to detect later relapses. Has not been evaluated in RCTs

BCG, Bacille Calmette-Guérin; BCNU, bischloroethylnitrosourea; DTIC, dimethyltriazeno-imidazole carboxamide (dacarbazine).

Updated this issue

Godfrey Walker and Paul Johnstone

INTERVENTIONS

Key Messages

- One systematic review of mainly small RCTs has found that topical permethrin and gamma benzene hexachloride are effective in the treatment of scabies. However, gamma benzene hexachloride has been linked to rare reports of serious adverse effects.

- We found limited evidence from two RCTs suggesting that crotamiton is safe but less effective than permethrin.

- We found insufficient evidence on the effects of other topical agents (malathion, benzyl benzoate, and sulphur compounds). Case series have found that malathion achieves cure rates of over 80%, but its safety has not been assessed adequately.

- We found insufficient evidence on the effects of oral ivermectin. It is known to be safe in young adults from its use in onchocerciasis, but its safety in children and elderly people is uncertain.

Scabies

DEFINITION Scabies is an infestation of the skin by the mite *Sarcoptes scabiei*.[1] Typical sites of infestation are skin folds and flexor surfaces. In adults, the most common sites are between the fingers and on the wrists, although infection may manifest in elderly people as a diffuse truncal eruption. In infants and children, the face, scalp, palms, and soles are also often affected.

INCIDENCE/ PREVALENCE Scabies is a common public health problem with an estimated prevalence of 300 million cases worldwide, mostly affecting people in developing countries where prevalence can exceed 50%.[2] In industrialised countries, it is most common in institutionalised communities. Case studies suggest that epidemic cycles occur every 7–15 years and that these partly reflect the population's immune status.

AETIOLOGY/ RISK FACTORS Scabies is particularly common where there is social disruption, overcrowding with close body contact, and limited access to water.[3] Young children, immobilised elderly people, people with HIV/AIDS, and other medically and immunologically compromised people are predisposed to infestation and have particularly high mite counts.[4]

PROGNOSIS Scabies is not life threatening, but the severe, persistent itch and secondary infections may be debilitating. Occasionally, crusted scabies develops. This form of the disease is resistant to routine treatment and can be a source of continued reinfestation and spread to others.

AIMS To eliminate the scabies mites and ova from the skin; to cure pruritus (itching); to prevent reinfestation; to prevent spread to other people.

OUTCOMES Number of visible burrows and papular and vesicular eruptions; presence of mites, ova, or faecal pellets in skin scrapings under a magnifying lens or microscope; pruritus. Outcomes should be assessed 28–30 days after start of treatment, which is the time it takes for lesions to heal and for any eggs and mites to reach maturity if treatment fails.

METHODS In preparing a systematic review,[5] we searched for all RCTs of pharmaceutical preparations, both topical and oral, using the Cochrane Controlled Trials Register, Medline and Embase, using standardised search strategies, and by direct approaches to pharmaceutical companies and experts in the field. A *Clinical Evidence* update search and appraisal was performed in May 2000. Of the five trials of different topical treatments that we identified, four used gamma benzene hexachloride (lindane) as one of the comparators. Gamma benzene hexachloride has been off the market in the UK since 1995 because of concern about possible adverse effects.

QUESTION What are the effects of topical treatments?

OPTION PERMETHRIN

One systematic review of RCTs has found that permethrin is effective in the treatment of scabies, with a parasitic cure rate of about 90%. Two small trials found that it was more effective than crotamiton. A larger trial

found no difference compared with gamma benzene hexachloride, although non-trial data suggest that permethrin is less toxic.

Benefits:
We found one systematic review (search date 1997),[5] which identified four RCTs.[6–9] **Permethrin versus crotamiton:** Two RCTs in a total of 194 adults and children compared topical permethrin versus crotamiton.[6,7] Permethrin was associated with significantly higher clinical cure rates in both trials (OR for failed clinical cure with permethrin v crotamiton 0.21, 95% CI 0.10 to 0.47).[5] Only one of the RCTs evaluated parasitic cure rates.[7] It also found permethrin to be significantly more effective (OR for failed parasitic cure with permethrin v crotamiton 0.21, 95% CI 0.08 to 0.53). The same RCT found no significant difference in patients' reports of pruritus (OR for itch persistence with permethrin v with crotamiton 0.38, 95% CI 0.12 to 1.19).[7] **Permethrin versus gamma benzene hexachloride:** The systematic review[5] found three RCTs comparing permethrin versus gamma benzene hexachloride, all using the same drug concentrations.[6,8,9] Two trials in a total of 152 adults and children found permethrin to be more effective than gamma benzene hexachloride.[6,9] The largest trial, with 467 participants,[8] found no significant difference between the two treatments (OR for failed parasitic cure with permethrin v gamma benzene hexachloride 0.68, 95% CI 0.34 to 1.36). This trial also reported patient assessed outcome, with a result in favour of permethrin (OR for itch persistence with permethrin v gamma benzene hexachloride 0.65, 95% CI 0.44 to 0.96). **Permethrin versus ivermectin:** We found one additional RCT that compared topical permethrin with ivermectin, but details were insufficient to report results in this issue. The RCT will be reported fully in a subsequent issue.[10]

Harms:
One RCT reported five serious adverse effects, two in the permethrin group (rash and possible diarrhoea) and three in the gamma benzene hexachloride group (pruritic rash, papules, and diarrhoea).[8] During 1990–1995, six adverse events were reported per 100 000 units distributed in the USA (one central nervous system adverse effect reported per 500 000 units of permethrin distributed).[11] Resistance to permethrin seems to be rare.[11]

Comment:
None.

| OPTION | GAMMA BENZENE HEXACHLORIDE |

One systematic review of RCTs has found that gamma benzene hexachloride is effective in the treatment of scabies, but we found rare reports of convulsions and other adverse effects.

Benefits:
We found one systematic review,[5] which identified three RCTs comparing gamma benzene hexachloride versus other topical agents.[6,8,9] We also found one subsequent RCT comparing gamma benzene hexachloride versus ivermectin.[12] **Gamma benzene hexachloride versus crotamiton:** One RCT in 100 adults and children found no significant difference in clinical cure rates (OR for failed clinical cure with crotamiton v gamma benzene hexachloride 0.41, 95% CI 0.15 to 1.10).[6] **Gamma benzene hexachloride versus permethrin:** See permethrin. **Gamma benzene hexachloride versus ivermectin:** One RCT in 53 adults referred to hospital

with scabies found no significant difference in clinical cure rates at 15 days (risk of being cured AR 14/26 [54%] with ivermectin v 13/27 [48%] with gamma benzene hydrochloride; ARI 6%, 95% CI −20% to +31%; RR 1.1, 95% CI 0.7 to 1.9) or at 29 days (risk of being cured AR 18/26 [69%] with ivermectin v 23/27 [85%] with gamma benzene hexachloride; ARI 16%, 95% CI −7% to +37%; RR 0.8, 95% CI 0.6 to 1.1).[12]

Harms: The RCTs reported no severe adverse effects. Case reports and data from the WHO collaborating Centre for International Drug Monitoring included reports of rare severe adverse effects (e.g. convulsions and aplastic anaemia), particularly when gamma benzene hexachloride was applied to people with extensive skin disease and to children.[13,14] Summary reports from 47 countries suggest that gamma benzene hexachloride is more toxic than other preparations. Four convulsions were reported in people on benzyl benzoate, one on crotamiton, 38 on gamma benzene hexachloride, two on malathion, and six on permethrin. Deaths reported on benzyl benzoate were nil, crotamiton one, gamma benzene hexachloride one, malathion nil, and permethrin five.[15] Resistance has been reported in many countries.[16]

Comment: Gamma benzene hexachloride has been off the market in the UK since 1995 because of concern about possible adverse effects. The evidence linking gamma benzene hexachloride with convulsions is suggestive but not conclusive. Summary reports are influenced by how much the products are used for the treatment of scabies and other infestations, and the quality of reporting. Safety data from trials and observational studies need to be summarised, particularly regarding additional risks in infants and pregnant women.

OPTION   CROTAMITON

One systematic review of RCTs found no evidence of a difference between crotamiton and gamma benzene hexachloride, but found crotamiton to be less effective than permethrin.

Benefits: We found one systematic review,[5] which identified two RCTs comparing crotamiton versus other topical agents.[6,7] **Crotamiton versus permethrin:** See benefits of permethrin, p 995. **Crotamiton versus gamma benzene hexachloride:** See benefits of permethrin, p 995.

Harms: We found limited data on the toxicity of crotamiton, but reports of serious adverse effects are rare.[13] There have been a few reports of resistance (see above).[13]

Comment: None.

OPTION   MALATHION

We found insufficient evidence. Cure rates of over 80% have been reported in case series.

Benefits: We found one systematic review, which identified no RCTs comparing malathion with any other drug treatments.[5] Case series suggest that malathion is effective in curing infestation with scabies, with a cure rate at 4 weeks of over 80%.[17,18]

Harms: No important adverse events have been reported.

Comment: The safety data from trials and observational studies need to be summarised, particularly with regard to additional risks in infants and pregnant women.

OPTION BENZYL BENZOATE

We found insufficient evidence from RCTs. Cure rates of about 50% have been reported in non-randomised trials.

Benefits: We found one systematic review and one additional RCT. **Benzyl benzoate versus ivermectin:** The review (search date 1997)[5] identified one small RCT in 44 adults and children that compared benzyl benzoate versus oral ivermectin.[19] This found no significant difference between the two treatments (see text, p 998). **Benzyl benzoate versus sulphur ointment:** One RCT compared benzyl benzoate and sulphur ointment in 158 adults and children identified in a house to house survey of a semi-urban area of India.[20] There was no significant difference between the number with apparently cured lesions by 8 days (AR 68/89 [76%] with benzyl benzoate v 45/69 [65%] with sulphur ointment; RR cure 1.17, 95% CI 0.95 to 1.33) or by 14 days (AR 81/89 [91%] v 67/69 [97%]; RR 0.94, 95% CI 0.86 to 1.01).

Harms: About one quarter of people treated with benzyl benzoate reported a transient increase in pruritus and dermatitis.[19]

Comment: Non-randomised trials suggest benzyl benzoate has variable effectiveness (as low as 50%).[21–23] The low cure rate may be related to concentration of the preparation and resistance of the mite to benzyl benzoate.

OPTION SULPHUR COMPOUNDS

We found insufficient evidence.

Benefits: We found one RCT comparing sulphur ointment with benzyl benzoate (see benzyl benzoate above).[20]

Harms: Use of sulphur was associated with increased local irritation in about a quarter of cases.[13]

Comment: None.

QUESTION What are the effects of systemic treatments?

OPTION IVERMECTIN

We found inadequate evaluation of ivermectin in RCTs. Experience of its use in onchocerciasis suggests that it is safe in younger adults, but no such experience exists for children, and there have been reports of increased risk of death in elderly people.

Scabies

Benefits: We found one systematic review,[5] which identified two RCTs comparing ivermectin with other topical agents.[19,24] We also found one subsequent RCT comparing ivermectin with gamma benzene hexachloride.[12] **Ivermectin versus placebo:** One RCT in 55 young adults and children aged over 5 years found oral ivermectin significantly more effective than placebo (clinical cure after 7 days AR 23/29 [79%] with ivermectin v 4/26 [15%] with placebo; ARI 64%, 95% CI 39% to 78%; RR 5.2, 95% CI 2.1 to 12.9; NNT 2, 95% CI 1 to 3).[24] **Ivermectin versus benzyl benzoate:** One RCT in 44 adults and children found no significant difference in clinical cure rates at 30 days (clinical cure AR 16/23 [70%] with ivermectin v 10/21 [48%] with benzyl benzoate; ARI 22%, 95% CI −7% to +46%; RR 1.5, 95% CI 0.9 to 2.5).[19] **Ivermectin versus gamma benzene hexachloride:** See benefits of gamma benzene hexachloride, p 995. **Ivermectin versus permethrin:** See benefits of permethrin, p 995.

Harms: The three RCTs were too small to give adequate data on harms.[12,19,24] Ivermectin has been used widely in adults with onchocerciasis; even with repeated doses, serious adverse effects have been rare.[25,26] There are no good data on its safety in children. An increased risk of death has been reported among elderly people taking ivermectin for scabies in a long term care facility.[27] It is not clear whether this was caused by ivermectin, or interactions with other scabicides (including gamma benzene hexachloride and permethrin) or other treatments such as psychoactive drugs. Other studies reported no such complications from its use in elderly people.[28]

Comment: Case series suggest that ivermectin may be effective when included in the treatment of hyperkeratotic crusted scabies (also known as Norwegian scabies),[29,30] and in people with concomitant HIV disease.[4]

Substantive changes since last issue

Permethrin versus ivermectin Additional RCT. Results will be reported in a subsequent issue.[10]

REFERENCES

1. Meinking TL, Taplin D. Infestations. In: Schachner LA, Hansen RC, eds. *Pediatric dermatology*. New York: Churchill Livingston, 1995.
2. Stein DH. Scabies and pediculosis. *Curr Opin Pediatr* 1991;3:660–666.
3. Green M. Epidemiology of scabies. *Epidemiol Rev* 1989;11:126–150.
4. Meinking TL, Taplin D, Hermida JL, Pardo R, Kerddel FA. The treatment of scabies with ivermectin. *N Engl J Med* 1995;333:26–30.
5. Walker GJA, Johnstone PW. Treating scabies. In: The Cochrane Library, Issue 4, 1999. Oxford: Update Software. Search date 1997; primary sources Medline 1966 to 1997; Embase 1974 to 1997; records of military trials from UK, USA, Russia; and specialist register of the Cochrane Diseases Group.
6. Amer M, El-Gharib I. Permethrin versus crotamiton and lindane in the treatment of scabies. *Int J Dermatol* 1992;31:357–358.
7. Taplin D, Meinking TL, Chen JA, Sanchez R. Comparison of crotamiton 10% cream (Eurax) and permethrin 5% cream (Elimite) for the treatment

8. of scabies in children. *Pediatr Dermatol* 1990;7:67–73.
9. Schultz MW, Gomez M, Hansen RC, et al. Comparative study of 5% permethrin cream and 1% lindane lotion for the treatment of scabies. *Arch Dermatol* 1990;126:167–170.
10. Taplin D, Meinking TL, Porcelain SL, Castilero PM, Chen JA. Permethrin 5% dermal cream: a new treatment for scabies. *J Am Acad Dermatol* 1986;15:995–1001.
10. Usha, V. and Gopalakrishnan Nair, TV. A comparative study of oral ivermectin and topical permethrin cream in the treatment of scabies. *J Am Acad Dermatol* 2000;42:236–240.
11. Meinking TL, Taplin D. Safety of permethrin vs lindane for the treatment of scabies. *Arch Dermatol* 1996;132:959–962.
12. Chouela EN, Abeldano AM, Pellerano G, et al. Equivalent therapeutic efficacy and safety of ivermectin and lindane in the treatment of human scabies. *Arch Dermatol* 1999;135:651–655.
13. Elgart ML. A risk-benefit assessment of agents

used in the treatment of scabies. *Drug Saf* 1996; 14:386–393.

14. McLeod WA. Acute lindane poisoning [letter]. *Can Med Assoc J* 1978;118:123–125.

15. WHO Collaborating Centre for International Drug Monitoring. Reported adverse reactions to ectoparasiticodes, including scabicides, insecticides and repellents. Uppsala, Sweden. January 1998.

16. Brown S, Belcher J, Brady W. Treatment of ectoparasitic infections: review of the English-language literature. *Clin Infect Dis* 1995;20(suppl 1):104–109.

17. Hanna NF, Clay JC, Harris JRW. *Sarcoptes scabiei* infestation treated with malathion liquid. *Br J Vener Dis* 1978;54:354.

18. Thianprasit M, Schuetzenberger R. Prioderm lotion in the treatment of scabies. *Southeast Asian J Trop Med Public Health* 1984;15:119–120.

19. Glaziou P, Cartel JL, Alzieu P, Moulia-Pelat JP, Martin PMV. Comparison of ivermectin and benzyl benzoate for treatment of scabies. *Trop Med Parasitol* 1993;44:331–332.

20. Gulati PV, Singh KP. A family based study on the treatment of scabies with benzyl benzoate and sulphur ointment. *Indian J Dermatol Venereol Lepr* 1978;44:269–273.

21. Burgess I, Robinson RJF, Robinson J, Maunder JW, Hassan Z. Aqueous malathion 0.5% as a scabicide: clinical trial. *BMJ* 1986;292:1172.

22. Kaur GA, Nadeswary K. Field trials on the management of scabies in Jengka Triangle, Pahang. *Med J Malaysia* 1980;35:14–21.

23. Haustein UF, Hlawa B. Treatment of scabies with permethrin versus lindane and benzyl benzoate. *Acta Derm Venereol* 1989;69:348–351.

24. Macotela-Ruiz E, Pena-Gonzalez G. Tratamiento de la escabiasis con ivermectina por via oral. *Gac Med Mex* 1993;129:201–205.

25. Pacque M, Munoz B, Greene BM, et al. Safety of and compliance with community-based ivermectin therapy. *Lancet* 1990;335:1377–1380.

26. De Sole G, Remme J, Awadzi K, et al. Adverse reactions after large-scale treatment of onchocerciasis with ivermectin: combined results from eight community trials. *Bull World Health Organ* 1989;67:707–719.

27. Barkwell R, Shields S. Deaths associated with ivermectin treatment of scabies. *Lancet* 1997; 349:1144–1145.

28. Diazgranados JA, Costa JL. Deaths after ivermectin treatment. *Lancet* 1997;349:1698.

29. Sullivan JR, Watt G, Barker B. Successful use of ivermectin in the treatment of endemic scabies in a nursing home. *Australas J Dermatol* 1997;38: 137–140.

30. Aubin F, Humbert P. Ivermectin for crusted (Norwegian) scabies. *N Engl J Med* 1995;332: 612.

Godfrey Walker
WHO Adviser in Reproductive Health
UNFPA Country Support Team for
Central and South Asia
Kathmandu
Nepal

Paul Johnstone
Director of Public Health, Visiting
Professor in Public Health
University of Teeside
Middlesborough
UK
Competing interests: None declared.

Women's health

Breast cancer: metastatic

Updated this issue

Stephen Johnston and Justin Stebbing

INTERVENTIONS

Key Messages

RCTs have found:

- Overall survival benefit from tamoxifen in the first line treatment of women with oestrogen receptor positive metastatic breast cancer.

- No good evidence of increased benefit (compared with tamoxifen) from ovarian ablation in premenopausal women with oestrogen receptor positive disease, or from progestins in first or second line treatment.

- Survival benefit (and acceptable toxicity profile) from selective aromatase inhibitors in women who have relapsed during or after treatment with tamoxifen.

- Overall survival benefit with combination chemotherapy regimens (particularly those containing an anthracycline, such as doxorubicin) compared with single drug regimens or hormonal treatment.

- No evidence that high dose chemotherapy confers additional survival benefit compared with standard dose chemotherapy.

- Limited survival benefit from second line chemotherapy, but no good evidence on its impact on quality of life compared with best supportive care.

- Benefit from bisphosphonates in terms of reduced skeletal complications with minimal toxicity in women with bone metastases secondary to metastatic breast cancer.

- Benefit from radiotherapy in women with symptoms from bone or spinal metastases, and probable benefit in those with cerebral or choroidal metastases.

DEFINITION Metastatic or advanced breast cancer is the presence of disease at distant sites such as the bone, liver, or lung. It is not treatable by primary surgery and is currently considered incurable. Symptoms may include pain from bone metastases, breathlessness from spread to the lung, and nausea or abdominal discomfort from liver involvement.

INCIDENCE/ PREVALENCE Metastatic breast cancer causes up to 500 000 deaths worldwide per year (46 000 in the USA and 15 000 in the UK).[1] The true prevalence of metastatic disease is much higher because some women live with the disease for many years.

AETIOLOGY/ RISK FACTORS The risk of metastatic disease relates to known prognostic factors in the original primary tumour. These factors include oestrogen receptor negative disease, early breast cancer (see glossary, p 1014), primary tumours 3 cm or more in diameter, and axillary node involvement — recurrence occurred within 10 years of adjuvant chemotherapy for early breast cancer in 60–70% of node positive women and 25–30% of node negative women in one large systematic review.[2]

PROGNOSIS Most women who develop metastatic breast cancer will ultimately die of their disease. Prognosis depends on age, extent of disease, and oestrogen receptor status. There is also evidence that overexpression of the product of the HER2/neu oncogene, which occurs in about a third of women with metastatic breast cancer, is associated with a worse prognosis.[3] A short disease free interval (e.g. less than 1 year) between surgery for early breast cancer and developing metastases suggests that the recurrent disease is likely to be resistant to the drug used for adjuvant treatment.[4] In women who receive no treatment for metastatic disease, the median survival from diagnosis of metastases is 12 months.[5] The choice of first line treatment (hormonal or chemotherapy) is based on a variety of clinical factors (see glossary, p 1014 and table 1, p 1017.[6-9]

AIMS	To relieve symptoms, prolong life, and improve quality of life, with minimal adverse effects.
OUTCOMES	Symptoms; progression free survival; overall objective response rate; complete response; partial response; duration of response; disease stabilisation; time to progression of disease (progression defined as more than a 25% increase in lesion size or the appearance of new lesions); quality of life[10]; improvement in performance status (according to validated scales of daily functioning/activity[11]); adverse effects and toxicity of treatment[12]; and overall survival (see glossary, p1013). Response to treatment is a surrogate outcome measure for assessing the effects of treatment on survival or quality of life. The link between clinical and proxy outcomes has not been clearly validated. Women who respond to treatment are more likely to experience improved symptomatic relief, performance status, and survival.[13-15] One recent prospective study of 300 women with metastatic breast cancer showed that there was a significant relationship between improvement and objective response for three symptoms in particular: cancer pain, shortness of breath, and abnormal mood. Symptom improvement was greatest in those patients who had a complete or partial response.[16]
METHODS	*Clinical Evidence* update search and appraisal May 2000. We looked for good systematic reviews of RCTs that used the outcome measures listed above. Where we found no good systematic reviews, we selected relevant randomised phase III trials using these outcomes. Data presented only in abstract form were discarded. A complete evaluation of the literature is made difficult by varied treatment regimens, patient populations, end points, and follow up times.[17] Response to treatment is often assessed in an unblinded fashion, introducing the possibility of bias. Few trials of acceptable quality reported data on symptoms or quality of life.

QUESTION What are the effects of first line treatments?

OPTION ANTIOESTROGENS (TAMOXIFEN)

RCTs have found that antioestrogens such as tamoxifen (see glossary, p 1014) are effective in prolonging remission and survival in women with oestrogen receptor positive metastatic breast cancer.

Benefits: We found no systematic review. Non-systematic reviews published in 1987 and 1991 identified 86 RCTs in 5353 women with metastatic breast cancer unselected for oestrogen receptor status. The overall objective response rate to tamoxifen was 34%. Disease stabilisation was achieved in a further 20%, and overall the median duration of response was 12–18 months.[6,7] The likelihood of responding to tamoxifen was highest (60–70%) in postmenopausal women with oestrogen receptor positive disease (see comment below).[8,9] **Versus ovarian ablation in premenopausal women:** See ovarian ablation in premenopausal women, p 1004.

Harms:

Minor adverse effects: Tamoxifen is well tolerated in women with metastatic breast cancer; fewer than 3% of women discontinued tamoxifen as a result of toxicity.[17] Reported adverse effects included minor gastrointestinal upset (8%), hot flushes (27%), and menstrual disturbance in premenopausal women (13%).[18] **Tumour flare:** During the first few weeks of treatment, tumour flare occurred in fewer than 5% of women. For those with bone metastases, this may result in increased pain or symptomatic hypercalcaemia. **Relapse:** Most women who initially respond to tamoxifen eventually progress and develop acquired resistance to tamoxifen, although they may still respond to further hormonal interventions.[19]

Comment:

The choice of first line treatment (hormonal or chemotherapy) is based on a variety of clinical factors (see table 1, p 1017).[6–9] **Tamoxifen resistance:** An emerging problem is that many women have already received adjuvant tamoxifen for early breast cancer, or have developed metastatic disease while still on tamoxifen, and are thus considered resistant to it. Effective second line hormonal drugs such as selective aromatase inhibitors are now used after tamoxifen failure (see selective aromatase inhibitors in postmenopausal women, p 1005), and RCTs are in progress comparing these drugs with tamoxifen as first line treatment. **Oestrogen receptor status:** Tamoxifen is a competitive oestrogen receptor antagonist, and adjuvant tamoxifen has been found to have no effect in women with early breast cancer that is oestrogen receptor negative (systematic review of 55 RCTs in 37 000 women).[20] We found no RCTs comparing outcomes in women with oestrogen receptor positive disease versus those whose oestrogen receptor status was unknown (oestrogen receptor negative women were excluded from most trials). **Selective oestrogen receptor modulators:** New nonsteroidal antioestrogens (toremifene, idoxifene, raloxifene) and steroidal antioestrogens (faslodex) may have fewer long term adverse effects owing to reduced agonist effects on the breast and endometrium, while maintaining the agonist effects that reduce osteoporosis and lipid concentrations. RCTs comparing some of these drugs with tamoxifen as first line hormonal treatment in metastatic breast cancer are in progress. So far, one RCT in 658 women has found no evidence of clear clinical superiority of toremifene over tamoxifen.[21]

| OPTION | PROGESTINS (MEDROXYPROGESTERONE ACETATE; MEGESTROL ACETATE) |

RCTs have found that progestins (see glossary, p 1014) are as effective as tamoxifen in first line treatment of metastatic breast cancer, but they are not as well tolerated. Specific beneficial effects can make progestins useful in women with bone pain or anorexia.

Benefits:

We found one systematic review (7 RCTs, 801 women with metastatic breast cancer) comparing medroxyprogesterone acetate versus tamoxifen. This found no significant difference in response rates (35–54%), remission rates, or survival between the two groups.[22] Benefits of progestins included an analgesic effect especially on painful bone metastases,[23] increased appetite, weight gain, and a feeling of wellbeing. A more recent RCT (166 women) found that the rate of response of bone metastases was significantly higher with medroxyprogesterone than with tamoxifen (33% v 13%, P = 0.01), although there was no significant difference in survival.[24]

Harms: Women taking medroxyprogesterone acetate experienced more adverse effects than women taking tamoxifen.[25] These were more common at higher doses and included nausea (14%), weight gain (56%), vaginal bleeding (10%), and exacerbation of hypertension.[26] In women with lymphangitis carcinomatosis, progestins may exacerbate symptoms of breathlessness.[27]

Comment: In view of the lack of evidence of greater benefit, and the evidence of greater harm, synthetic progestins are reserved for second or third line hormonal treatment in women with advanced breast cancer who have not responded to tamoxifen. Specific groups of women may benefit from earlier use, such as those with painful bone metastases and anorexia.

OPTION OVARIAN ABLATION IN PREMENOPAUSAL WOMEN

RCTs have found no evidence in premenopausal women that ovarian ablation is more effective than tamoxifen in response to treatment or survival. It is associated with substantial adverse effects.

Benefits: **Versus tamoxifen:** We found one systematic review (published in 1997, 4 RCTs, 220 premenopausal women) comparing tamoxifen versus ovarian ablation carried out by either surgery or irradiation.[27] There was no significant difference between treatments in terms of response rate, response duration, or survival. A subsequent RCT comparing initial treatment with tamoxifen or ovarian ablation in 39 premenopausal women confirmed these findings (OR for progressive disease (see glossary, p 1014) 0.71, 95% CI 0.37 to 1.38; median survival 2.35 years with tamoxifen, 2.46 years with ovarian ablation, P = 0.98; OR for death 1.07, 95% CI 0.55 to 2.06).[28] **Different methods of ovarian ablation:** We found no good systematic review. We found two RCTs comparing luteinising hormone releasing hormone (LHRH) analogues versus surgical ovariectomy or irradiation. They found no significant difference in survival between treatments.[29,30] Adding tamoxifen improved the response rate for the LHRH analogue (45% v 27% with LHRH analogues alone) but worsened the response rate for surgical ovariectomy (11% v 46% with ovariectomy alone).[30]

Harms: Adverse effects include hot flashes (75% with LHRH analogues, 46% with surgical ovariectomy) and "tumour flare" (16% with LHRH analogues).[29] In addition, surgical ovariectomy requires an operation and anaesthetic in someone with an incurable disease.

Comment: None.

QUESTION	What are the effects of second line hormonal treatments in women who have not responded to tamoxifen?

OPTION	PROGESTINS

RCTs have found that progestins are less effective in second line treatment than selective aromatase inhibitors and have more adverse effects (see glossary).

Benefits: **Versus selective aromatase inhibitors:** See selective aromatase inhibitors in postmenopausal women below.

Harms: **Versus selective aromatase inhibitors:** See selective aromatase inhibitors in postmenopausal women, p 1006.

Comment: In women who are not responding to tamoxifen, progestins may have a role in increasing feelings of wellbeing and relieving anorexia.

OPTION	SELECTIVE AROMATASE INHIBITORS IN POSTMENOPAUSAL WOMEN

RCTs have found that, in postmenopausal women with metastatic breast cancer who have relapsed on adjuvant tamoxifen or progressed during first line treatment with tamoxifen, the triazole class of selective and potent non-steroidal aromatase inhibitors (anastrozole, letrozole, vorozole) prolong survival with minimal adverse effects. The evidence suggests that they are significantly more effective and better tolerated than previous standard second line hormonal treatments (progestins or non-selective aromatase inhibitors), and that they are most effective in oestrogen receptor positive women.

Benefits: We found no systematic review. **Anastrozole versus progestins:** A meta-analysis of the only two randomised phase III trials (anastrozole versus megestrol acetate, 764 postmenopausal women with metastatic breast cancer unresponsive to tamoxifen, median age 65 years, 70% oestrogen receptor positive, 30% oestrogen receptor status unknown) found no significant difference in objective response rates (10.3% v 7.9%) or in the proportion of women whose disease was stabilised for 6 months (25.1% v 26.1%).[31] A subsequent analysis after a median of 31 months' follow up found a significant improvement in overall survival with anastrozole (HR 0.78, P = 0.02), with an absolute improvement in 2 year survival from 46.3% to 56.1% (P = 0.02) and an improvement in median survival of 4 months (from 22.5 to 26.7 months).[32] **Exemestane versus progestins:** Exemestane is a new irreversible steroidal aromatase inhibitor, currently being evaluated in phase II trials.[33] One RCT (769 women, 67% oestrogen receptor positive, the remainder unknown) found that median survival time was significantly longer with exemestane than progestins (P = 0.039). Median time to tumour progression was longer (20.3 v 16.6 weeks, P = 0.037) and time to treatment failure was increased (16.3 v 15.7 weeks, P = 0.042).[34] **Letrozole versus progestins or less potent aromatase inhibitor:** Two large RCTs compared letrozole 0.5 mg or 2.5 mg versus standard second line hormonal treatments (megestrol acetate, n = 551[35] and the non-selective and less potent aromatase inhibitor, aminoglutethimide, n = 555[36]). Both trials were in postmenopausal women with metastatic breast cancer unresponsive to tamoxifen (median age 64–65 years, 55% oestrogen receptor positive, 45% oestrogen receptor status unknown). Letrozole was significantly more effective than either of the standard drugs; compared with megestrol acetate, letrozole 2.5 mg was associated with a significantly higher response rate (HR 1.82, 95% CI 1.02 to 3.25, P = 0.04), longer duration of response (HR 0.42, 95% CI 0.2 to 0.86, P = 0.02), and longer time to treatment failure (HR 0.77, 95% CI 0.61 to 0.99, P = 0.04).[35] Compared with the progestins aminoglutethimide, letrozole achieved better overall survival (HR 0.64, 95% CI 0.49 to 0.85, P = 0.002) and time to progression (HR 0.72, 95% CI 0.57 to 0.92, P = 0.008).[36] **Vorozole versus progestins:** One RCT (452 women) found no significant difference in survival or duration of response between vorozole 2.5 mg daily and progestins (18.2 v 12.5 months, P = 0.074).[37]

Harms: The selective aromatase inhibitors were generally well tolerated and associated with fewer adverse events than standard second line hormonal treatments. **Anastrozole:** In the RCTs, anastrozole 1 mg was associated with a higher incidence of minor gastrointestinal disturbance (nausea or change in bowel habit) than megestrol acetate (29% v 21%, P = 0.005) but a significantly lower incidence of greater than 5% gain in weight (13% v 34%, P < 0.0001).[31] **Exemestane:** In the RCTs, more progestins treated women had adverse events (45.8% v 39.1%). The most frequently reported adverse events in the women treated with exemestane were low grade hot flashes (12.6%), nausea (9.2%), and fatigue (7.5%). **Letrozole:** Compared with megestrol acetate, letrozole 2.5 mg was associated with a significantly lower incidence of serious cardiovascular adverse events (2% v 11%) and greater than 5% weight gain (19% v 30%).[33] Compared with aminoglutethimide, letrozole 2.5 mg had a significantly lower incidence of skin rash (3% v 11%) and serious drug related adverse events (0% v 3%).[36] **Vorozole:** Women taking vorozole discontinued treatment because of adverse events less frequently than those taking progestins (3.1% v 6.2%).[37]

Comment: The greater efficacy and tolerability of anastrozole, letrozole, and vorozole over existing second line treatments (megestrol acetate or aminoglutethimide) means that they are now considered the agents of choice as second line hormonal treatment in postmenopausal women no longer responding to tamoxifen. An ongoing RCT is comparing anastrozole versus letrozole in this context (C Rose et al, personal communication, 1999).

QUESTION What are the effects of first line chemotherapy?

OPTION COMBINATION CHEMOTHERAPY

We found no RCTs comparing combination chemotherapy versus no chemotherapy in women with metastatic breast cancer (see comment). Trials comparing one type of chemotherapy versus another found that first line chemotherapy was associated with an objective tumour response in 40–60% of women, with a median response duration of 6–12 months irrespective of menopausal or oestrogen receptor status. A small proportion of women achieve complete remission, which may persist for an extended length of time (see high dose chemotherapy, p 1008).

Benefits: **Versus best supportive care:** We found no systematic review and no RCTs comparing first line chemotherapy versus palliative (best supportive) care in women with metastatic breast cancer. **Different chemotherapy regimens:** We found one systematic review (189 RCTs, 31 510 women) evaluating different chemotherapy and endocrine regimens.[17] **"Classical" versus modified CMF:** In the largest RCT in 254 postmenopausal women with metastatic breast cancer who had received no prior chemotherapy, the classical CMF (see glossary, p 1014) regimen was more effective than a modified version in which all three drugs were given intravenously every 3 weeks (response rate 48% v 29%, P = 0.03; median survival 17 v 12 months, P = 0.016).[38] An RCT in 133 women who had received no prior chemotherapy found that standard dose CMF was also significantly more effective than low dose CMF, both in response rate (30% v 11%, P = 0.03) and symptom control.[39] **CAF versus CMF:** One systematic review of RCTs (published in 1993), found that regimens containing doxorubicin versus other regimens had better off response rate, time to progression, and survival.[40] However, two RCTs comparing CAF versus non-anthracycyline based regimens (CMF) found no evidence of improved survival.[41,42] **Standard versus modified CAF regimens:** Two large multicentre trials of CAF (containing doxorubicin) versus FEC (see glossary, p 1014), a modified anthracycline based regimen containing epirubicin found no significant difference in response rates (n = 263, response rate 52% v 50%[43]; n = 497, response rate 56% v 54%[41]). An RCT in 249 women comparing standard CAF (containing doxorubicin) versus a modified better tolerated anthracycline based regimen containing mitoxantrone found that the regimen containing doxorubicin was associated with significantly longer time to progression (3.2 v 5.3 months, P = 0.03) and longer median survival (10.9 v 15.2 months, P = 0.003).[44]

Harms: The toxicity profiles of different combination chemotherapy regimens vary. In RCTs, anthracycline based regimens (CAF) and non-anthracycline based regimens (CMF) are equally associated with haematological toxicity,[42] but CAF is more likely to be associated with alopecia (34% v 22%) and severe nausea and vomiting (17% v 7%, P = 0.05). Other studies reported the incidence of greater than grade 3 alopecia to be 55–61% with CAF, which is significantly higher than with either mitoxantrone or epirubicin (FEC).[44,45] In one of the trials comparing CAF versus FEC, FEC was associated with fewer episodes of ≥ grade 2 neutropenia (10% v 13.1%), significantly lower rates of nausea and greater than vomiting (7.8% v 13.3%, P < 0.01), and no cardiotoxicity (8 women taking CAF discontinued treatment because of cardiac dysfunction compared with none taking FEC).[45]

Comment: The choice of first line treatment (see glossary, p 1014) (hormonal or chemotherapy) is based on a variety of clinical factors (see table

1, p 1017).[6-9] In one RCT, 231 women undergoing first line treatment (60% oestrogen receptor positive, remainder unknown) were randomised to receive either chemotherapy (CAF) or chemo-hormonal therapy (CAF plus tamoxifen and fluoxymesterone). The response rates were similar, although time to treatment failure was slightly longer for women who received chemohormonal therapy compared with chemotherapy alone (13.4 months v 10.3 months, P = 0.087). The effect on time to treatment failure was just significant for women who were oestrogen receptor positive compared with those who were negative (17.4 v 10.3 months, P = 0.048).The oestrogen receptor status had no effect on overall survival.[46]The choice of a specific drug or regimen is based on what drugs have already been given as adjuvant treatment, together with the likelihood of benefit balanced against a given drug's adverse effects and tolerability profile. Retrospective series in sequential decades (from 1950 to 1980) have compared the survival of women from the time of diagnosis with metastatic breast cancer. They suggest that the introduction of chemotherapy has improved median survival by about 9 months (from 12 months without treatment to 21 months with treatment).[5,47] This median survival conceals a bimodal distribution of benefit, with the 40–60% of women who respond to treatment achieving survival of 1 year or greater, and the non-responders experiencing little or no survival benefit. Fifteen year follow up of women with metastatic breast cancer treated with standard dose FAC (see glossary, p 1014) chemotherapy found that 263/1581 achieved complete remission and had a median time to progression of 2 years, and that 19% of these women remained free of disease at 5 years.[15] With the increasing use of adjuvant chemotherapy,[48] more women who develop metastatic disease will have received combination chemotherapy. This may influence the likelihood of response to further treatment.[4,49] An emerging problem is a subgroup of women with good performance status who have not responded to anthracycline based combination chemotherapy as first line treatment for metastatic disease or have relapsed within a few months of adjuvant chemotherapy.

OPTION   HIGH DOSE VERSUS STANDARD DOSE CHEMOTHERAPY

One RCT provides no evidence that high dose chemotherapy improves time to progression or overall survival.

Benefits: We found no systematic review. We found one RCT (n = 533, women aged 18–60 who had complete or partial response to induction chemotherapy). It compared high dose chemotherapy (single course of high doses of carboplatin, thiotepa, and cyclo-phosphamide) plus hematopoietic stem cell rescue versus prolonged course of monthly conventional dose chemotherapy (cyclo-phosphamide, methotrexate, and fluorouracil). It found no significant difference in overall survival at 3 years (32%, 95% CI 21% to 42% v 38%, 95% CI 26% to 50%) or in median progression free survival (9.6 months v 9.0 months, CI not given).[50]

Harms: Although haematological support with colony stimulating growth factors has lessened complications from high dose chemotherapy, non-haematological toxicity to the gastrointestinal tract and nervous system remain dose limiting. There is a recognised mortality with high dose chemotherapy (3%), although this is lower than in the early days of this approach.

Comment: Fifteen year follow up of women with metastatic breast cancer treated with standard dose FAC chemotherapy found that 263/1581 achieved a complete response and had a median time to progression of 2 years, and that 19% of these women remained free of disease at 5 years.[15] Any long term remissions associated with high dose chemotherapy in metastatic disease must be interpreted in the context of these figures. Five RCTs are in progress and full results from RCTs published as abstracts are awaited. It remains to be seen if certain women, for example those with a complete response after standard dose chemotherapy, may benefit from high dose treatment as a "coup de grace" for any remaining cancer cells. Several RCTs have found that inadequate doses of chemotherapy produce an inadequate response, and that once adequate doses are achieved, further dose escalation within the limits of haematological toxicity produces no further benefit.[51,52]

QUESTION What are the effects of second line chemotherapy?

The response rates to further chemotherapy when women relapse after standard dose chemotherapy are generally poor, with objective response rates of only 20–30%, and median durations of response ranging from 3–6 months. New cytotoxic drugs, in particular the taxanes and semi-synthetic vinca alkaloids, are associated with higher response rates, especially in anthracycline resistant disease.

Benefits: We found no systematic review and no RCTs comparing treatment with no treatment. **Taxanes:** One non-systematic review of RCTs and other studies concluded that, in women with anthracycline resistant disease, second line treatment with paclitaxel was associated with response rates ranging from 6–48%.[53] One RCT compared the taxane docetaxel ($100 \, mg/m^2$ intravenously every 3 weeks) versus a standard relapse treatment of mitomycin C $12 \, mg/m^2$ plus vinblastine $6 \, mg/m^2$ in 392 women with anthracycline resistant metastatic disease.[54] Docetaxel was associated with a significantly higher response rate (30% v 11.6%, P < 0.001), longer time to progression (median 19 weeks v 11 weeks, P = 0.001), and longer overall survival (11.4 v 8.7 months, P = 0.0097). Another RCT, comparing docetaxel versus methotrexate and 5-fluorouracil in 283 women with anthracycline resistant metastatic disease, found a similar improvement for docetaxel both in response rate (42% v 19%, P < 0.001) and time to progression (median 6 months v 3 months, P = 0.006).[55] In a separate RCT in 326 women who had not responded to an alkylating regimen (CMF) either in the adjuvant setting or as first line treatment, docetaxel was associated with a significantly higher response rate than single drug doxorubicin (43% v 21%, P = 0.003).[56] **Semi-synthetic vinca alkaloids:** We found no RCTs comparing vinorelbine versus a taxane for second line treatment. One RCT (303 women, first or second line treatment, no previous vinca alkaloid or anthracycline) compared doxorubicin combined with vinorelbine versus doxorubicin alone. The response rates, quality of life scores, and overall survival were not significantly improved with combined chemotherapy in this setting.[57]Vinorelbine has single agent antitumour activity with response rates of 20–33%, including in women with anthacycline resistant metastatic disease.[53] An RCT in 183 women with anthracycline resistant disease found improved time to progression and survival with vinorelbine 30 mg/m^2 weekly compared with intravenous melphalan (median survival 35 v 31 weeks, $P < 0.001$).[58]

Harms: **Taxanes:** Docetaxel is associated with moderate to severe haematological toxicity; 89% of women experienced grade III/IV neutropenia in the phase III study compared with 69% given mitomycin plus vinblastine,[54] although the incidence of febrile neutropenia with docetaxel was only 9%. Other specific toxicities associated with docetaxel include alopecia, neurotoxicity, arthralgia, and occasionally fluid retention. Hypersensitivity reactions can be avoided by premedication with corticosteroids and H$_2$ blockers. **Semisynthetic vinca alkaloids:** Vinorelbine is associated with minimal toxicity compared with anthracycline based chemotherapy (FAC/FEC), with considerably lower rates of nausea (8% v 16%, $P = 0.03$) and grade 3 alopecia (7% v 30%, $P = 0.0001$), although haematological toxicity that delayed treatment was more frequent (27% v 17%).[59]

Comment: Docetaxel seems to be the most active taxane and has become the single drug of choice in anthracycline resistant disease. Trials are in progress to determine the efficacy and tolerability of taxanes in combination with anthracyclines as first line treatment, although there are concerns about cardiac toxicity. At present the indication for docetaxel remains as a single drug for second line treatment, especially in anthracycline resistant disease, although definitive data on improvement in quality of life are awaited. Vinorelbine seems to have a favourable toxicity profile, but data from phase III trials are awaited.

QUESTION What are the effects of treatments for bone metastases?

OPTION BISPHOSPHONATES

RCTs have found that bisphosphonates (see glossary, p 1013) are associated with reduced bone pain and fewer skeletal complications such as fracture, spinal cord compression, and hypercalcaemia in women with breast cancer and bone metastases. Although these effects are likely to improve quality of life, this outcome has not been formally evaluated. We found no evidence that bisphosphonates improve survival.

Benefits: We found no systematic review. **Versus placebo:** Three double blind RCTs in women with metastatic breast cancer who had bone involvement compared bisphosphonates with placebo given in conjunction with standard treatment (either chemotherapy or hormonal treatment).[60–62] The first RCT (380 women with at least one lytic bone lesion who also received chemotherapy) found that intravenous pamidronate (90 mg as a 2 hour infusion every month for 12 cycles) significantly prolonged the median time to the first skeletal complication (13.1 months v 7.0 months, P = 0.005).[55] Significantly fewer women taking pamidronate developed skeletal complications (43% v 56%, P = 0.008), and there was significantly reduced requirement for radiotherapy to treat painful sites of bone disease (19% v 33%, P = 0.01). In an updated analysis in women who completed 2 years of treatment, those taking placebo were more than twice as likely to suffer a fracture than those taking pamidronate (OR 2.3, 95% CI 1.5 to 3.5).[63] The second RCT (173 women with bone metastases who may also have received either chemotherapy or hormonal treatment) found that the addition of oral clodronate 1600 mg daily significantly reduced the number of hypercalcaemic episodes (23% v 35%, P < 0.01) and the incidence of vertebral fractures (84 v 124 per 100 patient years, P < 0.025).[61] The third RCT (372 women with at least one lytic bone lesion who also received hormonal treatment) significantly prolonged the median time to the first skeletal complication (10.4 months v 6.9 months, P = 0.049).[62] Significantly fewer women taking pamidronate developed skeletal complications (2.4 v 3.8 events per year, P = 0.008), and there was significantly reduced requirement for radiotherapy to treat painful sites of bone disease (25% v 34%, P = 0.042). None of the three trials found an impact on overall survival. **Versus radiotherapy:** We found no RCTs.

Harms: In the first RCT, intravenous pamidronate was well tolerated, with no serious adverse events in those treated for up to 2 years.[63] One of the 185 women taking pamidronate developed symptomatic hypocalcaemia. Myalgia and arthralgia were more common in women taking pamidronate. Oral clodronate can be associated with minor gastrointestinal disturbance, but the RCT reported this in fewer than 5% of women.[61]

Comment: Large RCTs are in progress in the adjuvant setting to see whether these agents may delay or prevent the development of bone metastases.

OPTION   **RADIOTHERAPY**

Limited evidence from non-randomised studies suggests that persistent and localised bone pain can be successfully treated with radiotherapy in over 80% of cases. Longer courses and wide fields are rarely required, and adverse effects are minimal.

Benefits: We found no systematic review and no RCTs comparing radiotherapy versus no treatment or versus bisphosphonates (see comment). **Pain control:** Questionnaire studies found that control of pain was successful in over 80% of women who received radiotherapy for bone metastases, with concomitant use of appropriate analgesia according to the World Health Organization ladder,[64] which moves upwards from non-steroidal anti-inflammatory drugs and paracetamol to opiate containing analgesia (codeine based products) through to morphine and its derivatives (diamorphine, hydromorphone). **Cranial nerve compression:** In people with skull base metastases causing cranial nerve involvement, retrospective data suggest that radiotherapy leads to improvement in 50–80% of women, which is usually maintained.[65] **Different radiotherapy regimens:** We found two RCTs comparing different radiotherapy regimens. These found no significant differences between short courses (8 Gy as a single fraction) and longer courses (e.g. 20 Gy/5 fractions or 30 Gy/10 fractions).[66,67] Studies of accelerated fractionation schedules (e.g. twice daily treatments for 5 days) have failed to show any benefit over conventional regimens in the control of disease secondary to metastatic breast cancer.[68]

Harms: Adverse effects of radiotherapy for bone metastases include nausea and vomiting.[67] Higher dose fractions per day produce more toxic effects.

Comment: RCTs are notoriously difficult to perform in the field of palliative care. Randomised comparisons against no treatment or placebo would be considered unethical in palliative care, and even RCTs comparing one treatment versus another are difficult to undertake since it is reasonable to try many different options in order to make a patient comfortable. Rating of success of end of life care is difficult. Usual outcomes, such as response rates and survival duration, do not apply.[69] The prevention of nausea and vomiting caused by chemotherapy has been studied in one RCT (619 women). It compared placebo versus dexamethasone versus dexamethesone plus ondansetron following chemotherapy. In people who did not have acute nausea and vomiting with chemotherapy, dexamethasone alone was found to provide adequate protection against delayed nausea and vomiting.[70]

QUESTION **What are the effects of treatments for spinal cord, cerebral, and choroidal metastases?**

OPTION SPINAL CORD COMPRESSION

Spinal cord compression is an emergency. Retrospective studies suggest that early radiotherapy preserves function. One small RCT suggests that adding high dose steroids improves the chances of walking 6 months after radiotherapy for spinal cord compression.

Benefits: We found no systematic review. **Radiotherapy:** Retrospective analyses found an improvement with early radiotherapy, but that fewer than 10% of patients walked again if severe deterioration of motor function occurred before radiotherapy.[71] **Addition of high dose steroids:** One blinded RCT (n = 57) evaluated addition of high dose steroids to radiotherapy. It found that more people were walking 6 months after receiving intravenous dexamethasone 96 mg bolus followed by 96 mg orally for 3 days, compared with those who received no steroids (59% v 33%).[72]

Harms: In the RCT of high dose steroids,[72] significant adverse effects caused withdrawal from treatment in 11% of patients. Use of lower doses of glucocorticoids in the control of symptoms from cerebral metastases may result in short term agitation and the longer term development of Cushingoid facies.

Comment: See radiotherapy above.

OPTION | CEREBRAL METASTASES

Non-randomised evidence suggests that symptoms from cerebral metastases can be successfully controlled with radiotherapy.

Benefits: We found no systematic review and no RCTs comparing one form of treatment with another. **Radiotherapy:** Retrospective data suggest that whole brain radiation produces general improvement in neurological function in 40–70% of women with brain metastases secondary to breast cancer.[73] **Different radiotherapy regimens:** An RCT of 544 symptomatic people comparing two whole brain radiotherapy schedules (30 Gy/10 fractions v 12 Gy/2 fractions) found no evidence that the response rate or duration of response in people with multiple brain metastases were improved with higher doses of radiation compared with the shorter regimen.[68] **Surgical resection:** This is rarely indicated though may be beneficial in a small subgroup of people.[74] **Intrathecal chemotherapy:** We found no evidence that meningeal infiltration responds to intrathecal chemotherapy.

Harms: Adverse effects of radiotherapy in the treatment of cerebral metastases include hair loss and somnolence.[68] Higher dose fractions per day produce more toxic effects.

Comment: See radiotherapy, p 1012. Dexamethasone should be given immediately for raised intracranial pressure and anticonvulsants to control seizures if necessary.

OPTION | CHOROIDAL METASTASES

Non-randomised evidence suggests that symptoms from choroidal metastases can be successfully controlled with radiotherapy.

Benefits: We found no systematic review and no RCTs. Retrospective data suggest that radiotherapy benefits 70% of people.[75]

Harms: People with choroidal metastases who are treated with radiotherapy may lose the sight in that eye.

Comment: See radiotherapy, p 1012. People with deteriorating vision should be treated as an emergency.

GLOSSARY

Adjuvant treatment This usually refers to systemic chemotherapy or hormonal treatment or both, taken after removal of a primary tumour (in this case, surgery for early breast cancer), with the aim of killing any remaining micrometastatic tumour cells and thus preventing recurrence.

Aromatase inhibitors (anastrozole, letrozole, vorozole) Potent and highly selective non-steroidal inhibitors of the cytochrome P450 aromatase enzyme, which is responsible for peripheral conversion of androgens into oestrogens in postmenopausal women. These drugs cause oestrogen suppression in postmenopausal women.

Bisphosphonates (pamidronate, clodronate) Bone specific palliative drugs that inhibit osteoclast induced bone resorption associated with breast cancer metastases.

Combination chemotherapy regimens:

Classical CMF Cyclophosphamide (100 mg/m^2 orally days 1–14), methotrexate (40 mg/m^2 intravenously (iv) day 1 + 8), and 5-fluoruracil 600 mg/m^2 iv day 1 + 8, every 4 weeks for up to six cycles of treatment given dependency on response.

CAF Cyclophosphamide (500 mg/m^2 iv), doxorubicin (50 mg/m^2 iv), and 5-flurouracil (500 mg/m^2 iv), every 3 weeks for up to six cycles of treatment given dependency on response

FEC 5-flurouracil, epirubicin, and cyclophosphamide every 3 weeks for up to six cycles of treatment given dependency on response.

FAC 5-flurouracil, epirubicin, doxorubicin, and cyclophosphamide every 3 weeks for up to six cycles of treatment given dependency on response.

Complete response Disappearance of all known lesions on two separate measurements at least 4 weeks apart.

Disease free interval Time between surgery for early breast cancer (see below) and developing metastatic breast cancer.

Early breast cancer Operable disease, restricted to the breast and sometimes to local lymph nodes.

First line treatment Initial treatment for a particular condition that has previously not been treated. For example, first line treatment for metastatic breast cancer may include chemotherapy or hormonal treatment, or both.

Overall objective response rate The proportion of treated people in whom a complete (see above) or partial response (see below) is observed.

Partial response More than a 50% reduction in the size of lesions.

Progestins (medroxyprogesterone acetate, megestrol acetate) The antitumour effects of progestins may be mediated by a direct action on tumour cells, or an indirect effect on the pituitary–ovarian/adrenal axes.

Progression free survival (or time to progression) Interval between diagnosis of metastatic disease and diagnosis of progression (see below).

Progressive disease More than a 25% increase in the size of lesions or the appearance of new lesions.

Second line treatment Treatment given after relapse following first line treatment (see above).

Tamoxifen An oral, non-steroidal, competitive oestrogen receptor antagonist.

Substantive changes since last issue

Selective aromatase inhibitors in post-menopausal women Additional RCT; found that exemestane improved outcomes compared with progestins.[33–34]

First line chemotherapy Additional RCT comparing chemotherapy versus chemohormonal therapy for first line treatment; found similar response rates.[46]

Second line chemotherapy Additional RCT comparing doxorubicin plus vinorelbine v doxorubicin alone for first and second line treatment; found no significant difference in outcomes.[57]

REFERENCES

1. Pisani P, Parkin DM, Ferlay J. Estimates of the worldwide mortality from eighteen major cancers in 1985. Implications for prevention and projections of future burden. *Int J Cancer* 1993; 55:891–903.

2. Early Breast Cancer Trialists' Collaborative Group. Polychemotherapy for early breast cancer: an overview of the randomised trials. *Lancet* 1998; 352:30–42. Search date 1995; studies were identified using lists prepared by three international cancer research groups; by searching the international Cancer Research Data Bank, meeting abstracts, and references of published trials; and by consulting experts.

3. Slamon DJ, Clark GM, Wong SG, Levin WJ, Ullrich A, McGuire WL. Human breast cancer: correlation of relapse and survival with amplification of the HER-2/neu oncogene. *Science* 1987;235:177–182.

4. Rubens RD, Bajetta E, Bonneterre J, Kljin JGM, Lonning PE, Paridaens R. Treatment of relapse of breast cancer after adjuvant systemic therapy. *Eur J Cancer* 1994;30A:106–111.

5. Cold S, Jensen NV, Brincker H, et al. The influence of chemotherapy on survival after recurrence in breast cancer: a population based study of

patients treated in the 1950s, 1960s, and 1970s. *Eur J Cancer* 1993;29:1146–1152.

6. Jackson IM, Litherland S, Wakeling AE. Tamoxifen and other antioestrogens. In: Powels TJ, Smith IE ,eds. *Medical management of breast cancer*. London: Martin Dunitz, 1991:51–59.

7. Arafah BM, Pearson OH. Endocrine treatment of advanced breast cancer. In: Jordan VC, ed. *Estrogen/antiestrogen action and breast cancer therapy*. Madison: University of Wisconsin Press, 1986:417–429.

8. McGuire WL. Hormone receptors: their role in predicting prognosis and response to endocrine therapy. *Semin Oncol* 1978;5:428–443.

9. Kuss JT, Muss HB, Hoen H, Case LD. Tamoxifen as initial endocrine therapy for metastatic breast cancer: long term follow-up of two Piedmont Oncology Association (POA) trials. *Breast Cancer Res Treat* 1997;42:265–274.

10. Coates A, Gebski V, Signori D. Prognostic value of quality-of-life scores during chemotherapy for advanced breast cancer. *J Clin Oncol* 1992;10: 1833–1838.

11. European Organisation for Research and Treatment of Cancer (EORTC). A practical guide to EORTC studies. Brussels, Belgium: EORTC Data Center, 1996:126.

12. Miller AB, Hoogstraten B, Staquet M, Winkler A. Reporting results of cancer treatment. *Cancer* 1981;47:207–214.

13. Baum M, Priestman T, West RR, Jones EM. A comparison of subjective responses in a trial comparing endocrine with cytotoxic treatment in advanced carcinoma of the breast. In: Mouridsen HT, Palshof T, eds. *Breast cancer - experimental and clinical methods*. London: Pergamon Press, 1980:223–228.

14. Bernhard J, Thurlimann B, Schmitz SF, et al. Defining clinical benefit in postmenopausal patients with breast cancer under second-line endocrine treatment: Does quality of life matter? *J Clin Oncol* 1999;17:1672–1679.

15. Greenberg PA, Hortobagyi GN, Smith TL, Ziegler LD, Frye DK, Buzdar AU. Long-term follow-up of patients with complete remission following combination chemotherapy for metastatic breast cancer. *J Clin Oncol* 1997;14:2197–2205.

16. Geels P, Eisenhauer E, Bezjak A, et al. Palliative effect of chemotherapy: objective tumor response is associated with symptom improvement in patients with metastatic breast cancer. *J Clin Oncol* 2000;18:2395–2405.

17. Fossati R, Confalonieri C, Torri V, et al. Cytotoxic and hormonal treatment for metastatic breast cancer: a systematic review of published randomised trials involving 31 510 women. *J Clin Oncol* 1998;16:3439–3460. Search date 1997; primary sources Medline, Embase, and search of reference lists from retrieved articles and lists from relevant meetings.

18. Litherland S, Jackson IM. Antioestrogens in the management of hormone-dependent cancer. *Cancer Treat Rev* 1988;15:183–194.

19. Johnston SRD. Acquired tamoxifen resistance in human breast cancer – potential mechanisms and clinical implications. *Anti Cancer Drugs* 1997;8: 911–930.

20. Early Breast Cancer Trialists' Collaborative Group. Tamoxifen for early breast cancer: an overview of the randomised trials. *Lancet* 1998;351:1451–1467. Search date 1995; studies were identified using lists prepared by three international cancer research groups; by searching the international Cancer Research Data Bank, meeting abstracts, and references of published trials; and by consulting experts.

21. Hayes DF, Van Zyl JA, Goedhals L, et al.

Randomised comparison of tamoxifen and two separate doses of toremifine in postmenopausal patients with metastatic breast cancer. *J Clin Oncol* 1995;13:2556–2566.

22. Parazzini F, Colli E, Scatigna M, Tozzi L. Treatment with tamoxifen and progestins for metastatic breast cancer in postmenopausal women: a quantitative review of published randomised clinical trials. *Oncology* 1993;50:483–489. Search date 1991; primary sources Medline, handsearching, and reference lists of articles identified.

23. Pannuti F, Martoni A, Murari G, et al. Analgesic activity of medroxyprogesterone acetate in cancer patients: an anti-inflammatory mediated activity? *Int J Tissue React* 1985;7:505–508.

24. Muss HB, Case DL, Atkins JN, Bearden JD, Cooper MR, Cruz JM. Tamoxifen versus high-dose oral medroxyprogesterone acetate as initial endocrine therapy for patients with metastatic breast cancer: a Piedmont Oncology Association study. *J Clin Oncol* 1994;12:1630–1638.

25. Ingle JN, Ahmann DL, Green SJ. Randomised clinical trial of megesterol acetate versus tamoxifen in paramenopausal or castrated women with advanced breast cancer. *Am J Clin Oncol* 1982;5:155–160.

26. Panutti F, Martoni A, Zamagni C, Melotti B. Progestins. In: Powles TJ, Smith IE, eds. *Medical management of breast cancer*. London: Martin Dunitz, 1991:95–107.

27. Crump M, Sawka CA, DeBoer G, et al. An individual patient-based meta-analysis of tamoxifen versus ovarian ablation as first-line endocrine therapy for premenopausal women with metastatic breast cancer. *Breast Cancer Res Treat* 1997;44:201–210. Search date not stated; primary sources Medline, Cancerlit, hand searches of bibliographies of related publications, and personal contact with principal investigators of unpublished trials.

28. Sawka CA, Pritchard KI, Shelley W, et al. A randomised crossover trial of tamoxifen versus ovarian ablation for metastatic breast cancer in premenopausal women: a report of the National Cancer Institute of Canada clinical trials group trial MA1. *Breast Cancer Res Treat* 1997;44:211–215.

29. Taylor CW, Green S, Dalton WS, et al. Multicenter randomised clinical trial of goserelin versus surgical ovariectomy in premenopausal patients with receptor-positive metastatic breast cancer: an intergroup study. *J Clin Oncol* 1998;16:994–999.

30. Boccardo F, Rubagotti A, Perotta A, et al. Ovarian ablation versus goserelin with or without tamoxifen in pre-perimenopausal patients with advanced breast cancer: results of a multicentric Italian study. *Ann Oncol* 1994;5:337–342.

31. Buzdar A, Jonat W, Howell A, et al. Anastrozole, a potent and selective aromatase inhibitor, versus megesterol acetate in post-menopausal women with advanced breast cancer; results of overview analysis of two phase III trials. *J Clin Oncol* 1996; 14:2000–2011.

32. Buzdar A, Jonat W, Howell A, et al. Significant improved survival with Arimidex (anastrozole) versus megesterol acetate in postmenopausal advanced breast cancer; updated results of two randomised trials. *Proc Am Soc Clin Oncol* 1997; 16:A545.

33. Jones S, Vogel C, Arkhipov A, et al. Multicenter phase II trial of exemestane as third-line hormonal therapy of postmenopausal women with metastatic breast cancer. *J Clin Oncol* 1999;17: 3418–3425.

34. Kaufman M, Bajetta E, Dirix LY, et al. Exemestane is superior to megestrol acetate after tamoxifen

failure in postmenopausal women with advanced breast cancer: results of a phase III randomised double-blind trial. *J Clin Oncol* 2000;18:1399–1411.

35. Dombernowsky P, Smith IE, Falkson G, et al. Letrozole, a new oral aromatase inhibitor for advanced breast cancer: double-blind randomised trial showing a dose effect and improved efficacy and tolerability compared with megesterol acetate. *J Clin Oncol* 1998;16:453–461.

36. Gershanovich M, Chaudri HA, Campos D, et al. Letrozole, a new oral aromatase inhibitor: randomised trial comparing 2.5 mg daily, 0.5 mg daily and aminoglutethimide in postmenopausal women with advanced breast cancer. *Ann Oncol* 1998;9:639–645.

37. Goss PE, Winer EP, Tannock IF, Schwartz LH. Randomised phase III trial comparing the new potent and selective third-generation aromatase inhibitor vorozole with megestrol acetate in postmenopausal advanced breast cancer patients. *J Clin Oncol* 1999;17:52–63.

38. Engelsman E, Klijn JCM, Rubens RD, et al. "Classical" CMF versus a 3-weekly intravenous CMF schedule in postmenopausal patients with advanced breast cancer. *Eur J Cancer* 1991;27:966–970.

39. Tannock IF, Boyd NF, DeBoer G, et al. A randomised trial of two dose levels of cyclophosphamide, methotrexate and fluorouracil chemotherapy for patients with metastatic breast cancer. *J Clin Oncol* 1988;6:1377–1387.

40. A'Hern RP, Smith IE, Ebbs SR. Chemotherapy and survival in advanced breast cancer: the inclusion of doxorubicin in Cooper type regimens. *Br J Cancer* 1993;67:801–805. Search date not given; primary sources CancerLit, and communication with colleagues.

41. Cummings FJ, Gelman R, Horton J. Comparison of CAF versus CMFP in metastatic breast cancer: analysis of prognostic factors. *J Clin Oncol* 1985;3:932–940.

42. Smalley RV, Lefante J, Bartolucci A, Carpenter J, Vogel C, Krauss S. A comparison of cyclophosphamide, adriamicyn, and 5-fluorouracil (CAF) and cyclophosphamide, methotrexate, 5-fluorouracil, vincristine, and prednisolone (CMFVP) in patients with advanced breast cancer. *Breast Cancer Res Treat* 1983;3:209–220.

43. French Epirubicin Study Group. A prospective randomised phase III trial comparing combination chemotherapy with cyclophosphamide, fluorouracil, and either doxorubicin or epirubicin. *J Clin Oncol* 1988;6:679–688.

44. Italian Multicentre Breast Study with Epirubicin. Randomised phase III study of fluorouracil, doxorubicin, and cyclophosphamide in advanced breast cancer: an Italian multicentre trial. *J Clin Oncol* 1988;6:976–982.

45. Stewart DJ, Evans WK, Shepherd FA, et al. Cyclophosphamide and fluorouracil combined wish mitozanrone versus doxorubicin for breast cancer: superiority of doxorubicin. *J Clin Oncol* 1997;15:1897–1905.

46. Sledge GW, Hu P, Torney D, et al. Comparison of chemotherapy with chemohormonal therapy as first-line therapy for metastatic, hormone sensitive breast cancer. An Eastern Cooperative Oncology Group Study. *J Clin Oncol* 2000;18:262–66.

47. Ross MB, Buzdar AU, Smith TL, et al. Improved survival of patients with metastatic breast cancer receiving combination chemotherapy. *Cancer* 1985;55:341–346.

48. Goldhirsch A, Glick JH, Gelber RD, Senn H-J. International consensus panel on the treatment of primary breast cancer. *J Natl Cancer Inst* 1998;90:1601–1608.

49. Houston SJ, Richards MA, Bentley AE, Smith P, Rubens RD. The influence of adjuvant chemotherapy on outcome after relapse for patients with breast cancer. *Eur J Cancer* 1993;29A:1513–1518.

50. Stadtmauer E, O'Neill A, Goldstein L. Conventional-dose chemotherapy compared with high-dose chemotherapy plus autologous hematopoietic stem-cell transplantation for metastatic breast cancer. *N Engl J Med* 2000 (13 April) (http www/nejm.org/content/stadtmauer/1asp).

51. Hortobagyi GN, Bodey GP, Buzdar AU, Frye D, Legha SS, Malik R, et al. Evaluation of high-dose versus standard FAC chemotherapy for advanced breast cancer in protected environment units; a prospective randomised trial. *J Clin Oncol* 1987;5:354–364.

52. Bastholt L, Dalmark M, Gjedde S, Pfeiffer P, Pedersen D, Sandberg E, et al. Dose-response relationship of epirubicin in the treatment of post-menopausal patients with metastatic breast cancer: a randomised study of epirubicin at four different dose-levels performed by the Danish Breast Cancer Co-operative Group. *J Clin Oncol* 1996;14:1146–1155.

53. Vermoken JB, Ten Bokkel Huinick WW. Chemotherapy for advanced breast cancer: the place of active new drugs. *Breast* 1996;5:304–311.

54. Nabholtz JM, Senn HJ, Bezwoda WR, et al. Prospective randomised trial of docetaxel vs mitomycin plus vinblastine in patients with metastatic breast cancer progressing despite previous anthracycline-containing chemotherapy. *J Clin Oncol* 1999;17:1434–1424.

55. Sjorsom J, Blomqvist C, Mouridsen H, et al. Docetaxel compared with sequential methotrexate and 5-fluorouracil in patients with advanced breast cancer after anthracycline failure; a randomised phase III study with cross-over on progression by the Scandinavian Breast Group. *Eur J Cancer* 1999;35:1194–1201.

56. Chan S, Friedrichs K, Noel D, et al. Prospective randomised trial of docetaxel versus doxorubicin in patients with metastatic breast cancer. *J Clin Oncol* 1999;35:2341–2354.

57. Norris B, Pritchard KI, James K, et al. Phase III comparative study of vinorelbine combined with doxorubicin versus doxorubicin alone in disseminated metastatic/recurrent breast cancer: National Cancer Institute of Canada Clinical Trials Group Study MA8. *J Clin Oncol* 2000;18:2385–94.

58. Jones S, Winer E, Vogel C, Laufman L, et al. Randomised comparison of vinorelbine and melphalan in anthracycline-refractory advanced breast cancer. *J Clin Oncol* 1995;13:2567–2574.

59. Namer M, Soler-Michel P, Mefti F, et al. Is the combination FAC/FEC always the best regimen in advanced breast cancer? Utility of mitoxantrone and vinorelbine association as an alternative; results from a randomised trial [abstract]. *Breast Cancer Res Treat* 1997;46:94(A406).

60. Hortobagyi GN, Theriault RL, Porter L, et al. Efficacy of pamidronate in reducing skeletal complications in patients with breast cancer and lytic bone metastases. *N Engl J Med* 1996;335:1785–1791.

61. Paterson AHG, Powles TJ, Kanis JA, McCloskey E, Hanson J, Ashley S. Double-blind controlled trial of oral clodronate in patients with bone metastases from breast cancer. *J Clin Oncol* 1993;11:59–65.

62. Theriault RL, Lipton A, Hortobagyi GN. Pamidronate reduces skeletal morbidity in women

with advanced breast cancer and lytic bone lesions; a randomised placebo controlled trial. *J Clin Oncol* 1999;17:846–854.

63. Hortobagyi GN, Theriault RL, Lipton A, et al. Long-term prevention of skeletal complications of metastatic breast cancer with pamidronate. *J Clin Oncol* 1998;16:2038–2044.

64. World Health Organization. *Cancer pain relief.* Geneva: WHO, 1996.

65. Hall SM, Budzar AV, Blumenschein GR. Cranial nerve palsies in metastatic breast cancer due to osseous metastasis without intracranial involvement. *Cancer* 1983;52:180–184.

66. Bone Trial Working Party. 8 Gy single fraction radiotherapy for the treatment of metastatic skeletal pain: randomised comparison with a multifraction schedule over 12 months of patient follow-up. *Radiother Oncol* 1999;52:111–121.

67. Price P, Hoskin PJ, Easton D, Austin D, Palmer SG, Yarnold JR. Prospective randomised trial of single and multifraction radiotherapy schedules in treatment of painful bony metastases. *Radiother Oncol* 1986;6:247–255.

68. Priestman TJ, Dunn J, Brada M, Rampling R, Baker PG. Final results of the Royal College of Radiologists' trial comparing two different radiotherapy schedules in the treatment of brain metastases. *Clin Oncol* 1996;8:308–815.

69. Bretscher N. Care for dying patients: what is right? *J Clin Oncol* 2000;18:233–34.

70. The Italian Group for antiemetic research. Dexamethasone alone or in combination with ondansetron for the prevention of delayed nausea and vomiting induced by chemotherapy. *N Engl J Med* 2000;342:1554–1559.

71. Rades D, Blach M, Nerreter V, Bremer M, Karstens JH. Metastatic spinal cord compression. Influence of time between onset of motor deficits and start of irradiation on therapeutic effect. *Strahlenther Onkol* 1999;175:378–381.

72. Sorensen S, Helweg-Larsen S, Mouridsen H, Hansen HH. Effect of high-dose dexamethasone in carcinomatous metastatic spinal cord compression treated with radiotherapy: a randomised trial. *Eur J Cancer* 1994;30A:22–27.

73. Cancer Guidance Subgroup of the Clinical Outcomes Group. *Improving outcomes in breast cancer. The research evidence.* London: NHS Executive, 1996.

74. Diener-West M, Dobbins TW, Phillips TL, Nelson DF. Identification of an optimal subgroup for treatment evaluation of patients with brain metastases using RTOG study 7916. *Int J Radiat Oncol Biol Phys* 1989;16:669–673.

75. Ratanatharathorn V, Powers WE, Grimm J, Steverson N, Han I, Ahmad K. Eye metastasis from carcinoma of the breast: radiation treatment and results. *Cancer Treat Rev* 1991;18:261–276.

76. Hortobagyi GN. Treatment of breast cancer. *N Engl J Med* 1998;339:974–84.

Stephen Johnston
Senior Lecturer in Medical Oncology

Justin Stebbing
Specialist Registrar in Medical Oncology

The Royal Marsden NHS Trust
London
UK

Competing interests: None declared.

| TABLE 1 | Clinical factors that predict response to hormonal treatment in metastatic breast cancer, based on results of RCTs (see text, p 1002, p 1003, p 1007).[6–9,76] |

Factors predictive of good response to hormonal treatment

Postmenopausal status

Disease limited to soft tissue sites (skin, nodes)

Oestrogen receptor positive tumour

Long disease free interval since primary treatment for early breast cancer (> 18–24 months).

Factors making initial hormonal treatment less appropriate

Symptomatic visceral metasases (e.g. lymphangitis carcinomatosis or progressive liver metasatases)

Oestrogen receptor negative tumour

Short disease free interval (12–18 months)

Relapse on adjuvant tamoxifen (unless oestrogen receptor positive tumour and other features predictive of good response).

Breast cancer: non-metastatic

Updated this issue

J Michael Dixon, Alan Rodger and Stephen Johnston

INTERVENTIONS

DUCTAL CARCINOMA IN SITU
Likely to be beneficial

INVASIVE BREAST CANCER
Beneficial

Likely to be beneficial

Trade off between benefits and harms

Unknown effectiveness

Unlikely to be beneficial

To be covered in future issues of *Clinical Evidence*

Neoadjuvant (preoperative) systemic chemotherapy

Management of locally advanced breast cancer

Sentinel node biopsy

Covered elsewhere in this issue

Breast cancer: metastatic, p 1000

See glossary, p 1032

Key Messages

Ductal carcinoma in situ

- Two RCTs found that radiotherapy was associated with a reduced risk of local recurrence and invasive carcinoma, but with no evidence of a difference in survival.
- One RCT found that adjuvant tamoxifen reduced breast cancer events in women who had undergone wide excision and radiotherapy but with no evidence of an effect on survival.

Extent of surgery in operable breast cancer

- Systematic reviews of RCTs have found that, providing all local disease is excised, more extensive surgery is not associated with better outcomes in early invasive breast cancer. More extensive local resection in breast conserving surgery gives worse cosmetic results.

Radiotherapy in operable breast cancer

- One systematic review of RCTs has found that radiotherapy reduces the risk of isolated local recurrence and loss of a breast but does not increase 10 year survival compared with breast conserving surgery alone. Similar rates of survival and local recurrence are achieved with breast conserving surgery plus radiotherapy as with mastectomy.
- One systematic review of RCTs has found that radiotherapy to the chest wall after mastectomy reduces the risk of local recurrence by about two thirds and the risk of death from breast cancer at 10 years, but found no evidence of effect on overall 10 year survival.
- We found no direct evidence that radiotherapy to the internal mammary chain improves overall survival or breast cancer specific survival. Treatment may increase radiation induced cardiac morbidity.
- We found insufficient evidence to assess the impact on survival of irradiation of the ipsilateral supraclavicular fossa. RCTs suggest that radiotherapy is associated with reduced risk of supraclavicular fossa nodal recurrence. Morbidity associated with irradiation of the supraclavicular fossa is rare and where it occurs is mild and temporary.
- Three RCTs found that total nodal irradiation improved survival in high risk disease. Earlier RCTs found reduced locoregional recurrence but no evidence of improved survival.

Adjuvant systemic treatment in operable breast cancer

- One systematic review of RCTs has found that adjuvant chemotherapy reduces rates of recurrence and improves survival for women with early breast cancer. The benefit seems to be independent of nodal or menopausal status, although the absolute improvements are greater in those with node positive disease, and probably greater in younger women. The review found no evidence of a survival advantage from additional months of polychemotherapy (two or more drugs), nor did RCTs find survival advantage from increased or reduced dosages of polychemotherapy. Regimens containing anthracycline modestly improve survival compared with the standard cyclophosphamide, methotrexate, and 5-fluorouracil (CMF) regimen (see table 1, p 1036).
- One RCT found that adding combined chemotherapy to tamoxifen improved survival.
- One systematic review of RCTs has found that adjuvant tamoxifen taken for up to 5 years reduces the chance of recurrence and death in women with oestrogen receptor positive tumours irrespective of age, menopausal status,

nodal involvement, or the addition of chemotherapy. Tamoxifen slightly increases the risk of endometrial cancer, but we found no evidence of an overall adverse effect on non-breast cancer mortality.

- One systematic review of RCTs has found that ovarian ablation significantly improves long term survival in women aged under 50 years with early breast cancer.

Management of the axilla in operable breast cancer

- RCTs have found no evidence that axillary clearance is associated with improved survival compared with axillary node sampling, axillary radiotherapy, or sampling plus radiotherapy combined. One systematic review of mainly poor quality evidence found that the risk of arm lymphoedema was highest with axillary clearance plus radiotherapy, lower with axillary sampling plus radiotherapy and lowest with sampling alone.

DEFINITION	**Ductal carcinoma in situ (DCIS)** is a non-invasive tumour characterised by the presence of malignant cells in the breast ducts but with no evidence that they breach the basement membrane and invade into periductal connective tissues. **Invasive breast cancer** can be separated into three main groups: early or operable breast cancer, locally advanced disease, and metastatic breast cancer (see breast cancer: metastatic, p 1000). Women with early or operable breast cancer have disease that is apparently restricted to the breast and sometimes to local lymph nodes and can be surgically removed. Although these women do not have overt metastases at the time of staging, they remain at risk of local recurrence and of metastatic spread. They can be divided into those with tumours greater than 4 cm or multifocal cancers that can be treated by mastectomy, and those with tumours less than 4 cm or unifocal cancers that can be treated by breast conserving surgery (see glossary, p 1032). Locally advanced breast cancer is characterised by matted lymph nodes or involvement of the skin or chest wall. Management of locally advanced disease will be covered in a future issue of *Clinical Evidence*. The staging of breast cancer is based on the TNM system (see glossary, p 1033).[1]
INCIDENCE/ PREVALENCE	Breast cancer affects one in 12 women in the UK and causes about 21 000 deaths per year. Prevalence is about five times higher, with over 100 000 women living with breast cancer at any one time.
AETIOLOGY/ RISK FACTORS	The risk of breast cancer increases with age, doubling every 10 years up to the menopause. Risk factors include an early age at menarche, older age at menopause, older age at birth of first child, family history, atypical hyperplasia, alcohol, radiation exposure, oral contraceptive use, and postmenopausal hormone replacement therapy. Risk in different countries varies fivefold.
PROGNOSIS	Tumour size, axillary node status, histological grade, and oestrogen receptor status provide the most significant prognostic information. Seventy per cent of women with operable disease are alive 5 years after diagnosis and treatment. Risk of recurrence is highest during the first 5 years, but the risk remains even 15–20 years after surgery. Those with node positive disease have a 50–60% chance of recurrence within 5 years, compared with 30–35% for node nega-

tive disease. Adjuvant systemic drug treatment is given to most women in order to eliminate micrometastatic disease remaining after surgery.

AIMS

To improve survival; to prevent local or regional node recurrence; to obtain prognostic information on the type and extent of tumour and the status of the axillary lymph nodes; to optimise cosmetic results and minimise psychosocial impact; to minimise adverse effects of treatment; and to maximise quality of life.

OUTCOMES

Survival; rates of local and regional recurrence; rates of mastectomy after breast conserving treatment; rates of development of metastases; cosmetic outcomes; quality of life; incidence of adverse effects of treatment including upper limb lymphoedema.

METHODS

Clinical Evidence update search and appraisal May 2000. We appraised all identified systematic reviews and RCTs.

QUESTION | **What are the effects of interventions after breast conserving surgery for ductal carcinoma in situ (DCIS)?**

OPTION | RADIOTHERAPY

Two RCTs found that radiotherapy (see glossary, p 1033) was associated with a reduced risk of local recurrence and invasive carcinoma, but with no evidence of an effect on survival.

Benefits:
We found no systematic review. We found two RCTs comparing radiotherapy with no radiotherapy after surgery for DCIS. The first one (814 people) found no difference in survival at 8 years with radiotherapy, but a significant reduction in risk of local recurrence (survival 95% *v* 94%; local recurrence 12.1% *v* 26.8%, $P < 0.000005$; risk of recurrent DCIS 8.2% *v* 13.4%, $P = 0.007$; risk of invasive carcinoma 3.9% *v* 13.4%, $P < 0.0001$).[2] The second RCT (102 people) found, at median follow up of 4.25 years, significantly lower recurrence of DCIS in women given radiotherapy.[3] At 4 years, local relapse free survival was more likely with radiotherapy than with surgery alone (84% *v* 91%, $P = 0.005$, HR 0.62, 95% CI 0.44 to 0.87). More women were free of DCIS recurrence after 4 years with radiotherapy but the difference was not significant (92% *v* 95%, HR 0.65, 95% CI 0.43 to 1.03). There was a significant reduction in invasive recurrence (92% *v* 96%, HR 0.60, 95% CI 0.37 to 0.97).

Harms:
The second RCT found an increase in contralateral breast cancer associated with radiotherapy at year 4 (3% *v* 1%; HR 2.57, 95% CI 1.24 to 5.33).[3]

Comment:
Ongoing trials are evaluating radiotherapy in all grades of DCIS. Subset analyses may be required to identify subgroups of women who would benefit most after breast conserving surgery.

OPTION | TAMOXIFEN PLUS RADIOTHERAPY

One RCT found that adjuvant tamoxifen (see glossary, p 1033) reduced breast cancer events in women who had undergone wide excision and radiotherapy but no evidence of an effect on survival.

Benefits: We found no systematic review. We found one RCT in women with DCIS treated with wide excision and radiotherapy, which compared adjuvant tamoxifen 20 mg daily (902 people) with placebo (902 people) for 5 years.[4] At median follow up of 74 months, there were fewer breast cancer events with tamoxifen than placebo (OR 0.63, 95% CI 0.47 to 0.83), and fewer invasive ipsilateral or contralateral breast cancers (OR 0.57, 95% CI 0.38 to 0.85). However, there was no significant difference in overall survival (RR 0.88, 95% CI 0.33 to 2.28).

Harms: The trial found a non-significantly higher rate of endometrial cancers associated with tamoxifen (RR 3.4, 95% CI 0.6 to 33.4).[4]

Comment: There are ongoing RCTs of tamoxifen in DCIS (Dixon J, personal communication, 2000).

QUESTION	Is the extent of surgery related to outcome in early invasive breast cancer?

Systematic reviews of RCTs have found that more extensive surgery is not associated with better outcomes, providing that all local disease is excised. The more extensive the local resection in breast conserving surgery, the worse the cosmetic result.

Benefits: **Comparisons between supraradical, radical, and total mastectomy:** We found one systematic review (search date 1990) of five RCTs that compared supraradical with radical mastectomy, radical with total mastectomy (see glossary, p 1033), and supraradical with total mastectomy in 2090 women with operable breast cancer.[5] It found no significant difference in risk of death over 10 years (ARR of more extensive versus less extensive surgery 0.02, 95% CI −0.04 to +0.08). **Comparisons between radical, total, and simple mastectomy:** The same review included four RCTs comparing radical with simple mastectomy (three trials) and total with simple mastectomy (one trial) in 1296 women with operable breast cancer.[5] Meta-analysis found no significant difference in risk of death over 10 years (ARR for more extensive compared with less extensive surgery 2%, 95% CI −5% to +9%). **Mastectomy versus breast conservation:** We found two systematic reviews. One review (search date 1995) analysed data on 10 year survival from six RCTs comparing breast conservation with mastectomy.[6] Meta-analysis of data from five of the trials (3006 women) found no significant difference in the risk of death at 10 years (OR compared with mastectomy 0.91, 95% CI 0.78 to 1.05). The sixth trial used different protocols. Where more than half of node positive women in both mastectomy and breast conservation groups received adjuvant nodal radiotherapy, both groups had similar survival rates. Where fewer than half of node positive women in both groups received adjuvant nodal radiotherapy, survival was better with breast conservation (OR compared with mastectomy 0.69, 95% CI 0.49 to 0.97). The second review (search date 1990) identified nine RCTs in 4981 women potentially suitable for breast conserving surgery.[5] All participants received postoperative radiotherapy. Meta-analysis found no significant difference in risk of death over 10 years (RRR for breast conservation compared with mastectomy 0.02, 95% CI −0.05 to +0.09). It also found no significant difference in rates of local recurrence (six trials in 3107 women; RRR mastectomy v breast conservation 0.04, 95% CI –0.04 to +0.12). **Different extents of local excision in breast conservation:** We found no systematic review. We found one RCT (705 people) that compared lumpectomy (see glossary, p 1033) with quadrantectomy (see glossary, p 1033).[7] There were significantly more local recurrences with lumpectomy than with quadrantectomy (7% v 2%), but a major factor associated with local recurrence in the lumpectomy group was incomplete excision (see comment below).[8] We found no RCTs that compared wide local excision (complete excision microscopically) with quadrantectomy.

Harms: More extensive surgery results in greater mutilation and adverse psychosocial impact. Between 60–90% of women having breast conservation had an excellent or good cosmetic result (median 83%, 95% CI 67% to 87%).[7,9–17] The single most important factor influencing cosmetic outcome is the volume of tissue excised; the larger the amount of tissue excised the worse the cosmetic result.[7] The trial of different extents of local excision in breast conservation found that, in a subset of 148 women, there was a significantly higher rate of poor cosmetic outcome with quadrantectomy (RR compared with lumpectomy 3.11, 95% CI 1.2 to 8.1).[7] Only isolated small studies have shown no correlation between extent of surgical excision and cosmesis.[15]

Comment: The link between completeness of excision and local recurrence after breast conservation has been evaluated in 16 centres. In 13 of these, incomplete excision was associated with an increased relative risk of local recurrence compared with complete excision (estimated median RRI 3.4%, 95% CI 2.6% to 4.6%).[8] The three centres that did not report increased rates of local recurrence after incomplete excision gave much higher doses of local radiotherapy (65–72 Gy). Two centres also used re-excision, and women with involved margins had only focal margin involvement.

QUESTION What are the effects of different radiotherapy regimens in operable breast cancer?

OPTION RADIOTHERAPY AFTER BREAST CONSERVING SURGERY

One systematic review of RCTs has found that radiotherapy reduces the risk of isolated local recurrence and loss of a breast but does not increase 10 year survival compared with breast conserving surgery alone. Similar rates of survival and local recurrence are achieved with breast conserving surgery plus radiotherapy as with mastectomy.

Benefits: **Versus breast conserving surgery alone:** We found one systematic review (search date 1990), which identified four RCTs (381 to 1450 people) comparing surgery plus radiotherapy with surgery alone.[5] All four trials began before 1985 and used megavoltage X-rays. Pooled data from trials that reported sites of local recurrence (781 people) found that women with isolated local recurrence were less likely to have received radiotherapy (OR 0.25, 95% CI 0.16 to 0.34). Even a trial limited to "good prognosis disease" (tumour ≤ 2 cm, node negative, 381 people) found a significantly lower local relapse rate with radiotherapy at 5 and 10 years (5 years: relapse rate with radiotherapy 2.3%, 95% CI 1% to 4.3% versus no radiotherapy 18.4%, 95% CI 12.5% to 24.2%).[18] Ten year data found that radiotherapy was associated with lower local recurrence rates (8.5%, 95% CI 3.9% to 13.1% v 24%, 95% CI 17.6% to 30.4%, P = 0.0001) but no difference in overall survival (77.5% v 78%).[19] One subsequent RCT (585 people) also found that after 6 years the proportion of women free of locoregional disease and with breast conservation was higher with radiotherapy (93.8% v 81.3%).[20] Pooled data from all four trials found no significant difference in 10 year survival (80.1% v 78.9%). **Versus mastectomy:** The systematic review identified nine RCTs (4891 people) comparing breast radiotherapy after breast conserving surgery with simple or modified radical mastectomy in women with invasive breast cancer.[5] It found no difference in survival rates at 10 years (22.9% v 22.9%; no CIs available) or in local recurrence (6.2% v 5.9% from pooled data from six trials, 3107 people).[5]

Harms:
The RCTs and systematic review included in a consensus document published in 1998 (mainly of women undergoing breast conserving surgery or mastectomy with variation in radiotherapy techniques, doses, and fractionation) reported severe acute adverse effects of radiotherapy to be acute pneumonitis (0.7% to 7.0%) and pericarditis (0% to 0.3%), and long term adverse effects to be significant arm oedema (1% without axillary dissection), radionecrotic rib fracture (1.1% to 1.5%), and brachial plexopathy (0% to 1.8%).[21] The risk and severity of adverse effects increased with volume irradiated, total dose received, dose per fraction, previous surgery (e.g. axillary dissection), and radiotherapy techniques that caused overlap in irradiated tissues. The review found an increased risk of non-breast cancer death (OR 1.24, 95% CI 1.09 to 1.43).[3] One systematic review (search date not given) of 10 RCTs found that the excess of non-breast cancer deaths after chest wall radiotherapy was caused by cardiac deaths resulting from the radiotherapy, but recent trials with data beyond 10 years did not find an excess of cardiac deaths.[22–24] Studies assessing cosmetic results have mainly been retrospective using poorly validated outcomes. The effects of social, psychological, and financial disruptions from attending for 5–6 weeks of radiotherapy have not been clearly addressed. There is an extremely low reported incidence of radiation induced malignancy, usually soft tissue sarcomas, in the irradiated breast.

Comment:
The four trials comparing breast conserving surgery with and without radiotherapy, as well as retrospective case series, suggest that prognostic factors for local recurrence after breast conserving surgery include positive tumour margins, an extensive intraduct component, younger age, lymphovascular invasion, histological grade, and systemic treatment. The only consistent independent risk factor is avoiding radiotherapy.

OPTION   RADIOTHERAPY AFTER MASTECTOMY

RCTs have found that radiotherapy to the chest wall after mastectomy reduces the risk of local recurrence by about two thirds and reduces the risk of death from breast cancer at 10 years compared with mastectomy alone.

Benefits: We found one systematic review (search date 1995, 32 RCTs) comparing mastectomy with mastectomy followed by radiotherapy to the chest wall.[5] Five trials were of mastectomy alone (4541 people); four of mastectomy and axillary sampling (3286 people); and 23 of mastectomy and axillary clearance (6699 people). The review found that radiotherapy reduced local recurrence by two thirds and slightly reduced breast cancer mortality (OR 0.94, 95% CI 0.88 to 1.00), but found no significant difference in overall survival (OR 0.98, 95% CI 0.93 to 1.03).[5] Two subsequent trials in high risk women receiving adjuvant chemotherapy after mastectomy compared irradiation to the chest wall and peripheral lymphatics with no radiotherapy.[23,24] One found radiotherapy reduced relative locoregional relapse rates by 56% (RR 0.44, 95% CI 0.26 to 0.77) and the other by 76% (AR 58% v 14%).[23,24] One RCT found that survival at 10 years was higher with radiotherapy (54%, 95% CI 51% to 58% v 45%, 95% CI 42% to 48%).[24] The other, smaller trial found a 29% reduction in mortality at 15 years with radiotherapy (RR 0.71, CI 0.51 to 0.99), although when these results were pooled with the results of the review, no significant difference in overall mortality was detected (OR 0.96, 95% CI 0.91 to 1.01).[5,23,25,26] Another RCT in high risk postmenopausal women who underwent mastectomy and received tamoxifen 30 mg daily for 1 year, compared irradiation of the chest wall and peripheral lymphatics with no radiotherapy. It found that radiotherapy was associated with reduction in locoregional recurrence (as first site of recurrence) from 35% to 8%. Overall survival at 10 years was higher with radiotherapy (45%, 95% CI 41% to 49% v 36%, 95% CI 33% to 40%).[25] We found no evidence that reduction in relative risk of local recurrence was affected by age, nodal status, receptor status, tumour grade, or tumour size, nor that the effect of radiotherapy on mortality varied significantly with extent of surgery, type of radiotherapy (megavoltage or orthovoltage), years the trials commenced or completed recruitment, or whether systemic treatment was given.[26]

Harms: See radiotherapy after breast conserving surgery. Three recent trials of postmastectomy total nodal irradiation in high risk disease found no significant increase in cardiac mortality.[23–25]

Comment: The trials in the large systematic review were heterogeneous, in part because they began when trial methods were less developed.[5] They varied in randomisation processes, areas irradiated, use of systemic treatment, radiotherapy doses, fractionation, and treatment schedules. We found little strong evidence to identify which women should have postmastectomy radiotherapy to prevent local recurrence. One review of retrospective data found that extent of axillary node involvement, larger tumour size, higher histological grade, presence of lymphovascular invasion, and involvement of tumour margins reduced the chance of successful treatment.[26–29]

OPTION RADIOTHERAPY TO THE INTERNAL MAMMARY CHAIN

We found no direct evidence that radiotherapy to the internal mammary chain improves overall survival or breast cancer specific survival. Treatment may increase radiation induced cardiac morbidity.

Benefits: We found no systematic review. We found one RCT (270 women treated with breast conserving surgery and radiotherapy), which compared internal mammary chain irradiation with no internal mammary chain irradiation.[30] At median follow up of 2.7 years there was no significant difference in relapse or survival (figures not provided).

Harms: See harms under radiotherapy after breast conserving surgery, p 1024. Radiotherapy to the internal mammary chain is more likely to affect the heart compared with other types of radiotherapy.

Comment: The risk of internal mammary chain node involvement is related to the location and size of the primary tumour and, most importantly, histopathological axillary nodal status. Up to 30% of women with axillary involvement will also exhibit internal mammary chain nodal metastases. Central or medial breast cancers are more likely to metastasise to the internal mammary chain, as are larger tumours.[31,32] The risk of internal mammary chain recurrence is low, and after modified radical mastectomy alone is 2%.[33] Modern radiotherapy planning and delivery should involve an assessment of the position and depth of the internal mammary chain nodes to be treated (using CT or ultrasound) and computer assisted placement, arrangement, and determination of dose distribution, technologies unavailable at the time of most RCTs included in the reviews.[5,22] Recent indirect evidence from RCTs suggests improved survival from nodal irradiation (including radiation to the internal mammary chain) after modified radical mastectomy combined with systematic treatment.[23–25] Another trial of internal mammary chain irradiation has recently started (sponsored by the EORTC).

OPTION RADIOTHERAPY TO THE IPSILATERAL SUPRACLAVICULAR FOSSA

We found insufficient evidence to assess the impact on survival of irradiation of the ipsilateral supraclavicular fossa. RCTs suggest that radiotherapy is associated with reduced risk of supraclavicular fossa nodal recurrence. Morbidity associated with irradiation of the supraclavicular fossa is rare and where it occurs is mild and temporary.

Benefits: We found no systematic review or RCTs on radiotherapy to the ipsilateral supraclavicular fossa. One systematic review (search date 1990) found that postoperative radiotherapy was associated with reduced locoregional recurrence (see radiotherapy after breast conserving surgery, p 1023; radiotherapy after mastectomy, p 1025 and radiotherapy to internal mammary chain irradiation, p 1026).[5] RCTs have indicated that this includes reduced recurrence in the supraclavicular fossa. One trial in postmenopausal women at high risk of local recurrence who received tamoxifen after mastectomy found that radiotherapy was associated with lower recurrence in the supraclavicular fossa (37/686 [5.4%] v 9/689 [1.3%]) at median follow up of 123 months.[25]

Harms: The acute morbidity of irradiation to the supraclavicular fossa is mild and includes temporary upper oesophagitis in nearly all women. The risk of radiation pneumonitis increases with the volume of lung irradiated. Treatment irradiates the lung apex in addition to any lung included in the breast or chest wall fields. Possible late morbidity includes brachial plexopathy but this should not exceed 1.8% if attention is paid to limiting total dose to 50 Gy and the dose per fraction to 2 Gy or less and avoiding field junction overlaps.[21,34] Late apical lung fibrosis is common and usually of no clinical importance. Demyelination of the cervical cord is an extremely rare complication of supraclavicular fossa radiotherapy.

Comment: None.

OPTION TOTAL NODAL RADIOTHERAPY

Three RCTs found that total nodal irradiation (see glossary, p 1033) improved survival in high risk disease. Earlier RCTs found reduced locoregional recurrence but no evidence of improved survival.

Benefits: One systematic review (search date 1990) included RCTs of total regional nodal irradiation (to the internal mammary chain, supra-clavicular fossa, and axilla).[5] It found that postoperative radio-therapy was associated with reduced locoregional recurrence, but no evidence of improved 10 year survival.[4] However, three recent RCTs have found improved overall survival in women with high risk disease who underwent mastectomy, axillary dissection, and sys-temic adjuvant therapy, if total nodal postoperative radiotherapy was given.[23–25]

Harms: See radiotherapy to the internal mammary chain, p 1026, supra-clavicular fossa, p 1026, and axilla, p 1031. The three RCTs found no increase in cardiac mortality due to radiotherapy.[23–25]

Comment: None.

QUESTION What are the effects of adjuvant systemic treatment?

OPTION ADJUVANT COMBINATION CHEMOTHERAPY

One systematic review of RCTs has found that adjuvant chemotherapy reduces rates of recurrence and improves survival for women with early breast cancer. The benefit seems to be independent of nodal or menopausal status, although the absolute improvements are greater in those with node positive disease, and probably greater in younger women. The review found no evidence of a survival advantage from additional months of polychemotherapy (two or more drugs), nor did RCTs find survival advantage from increased or reduced dosages of polychemotherapy. Regimens containing anthracycline may modestly improve outcomes compared with the standard cyclophosphamide, methotrexate, and 5-fluorouracil (CMF) regimen (see table 1, p 1036).

Benefits: **Versus no chemotherapy:** We found one systematic review (search date 1995, 47 RCTs, 18 000 women) comparing prolonged combination chemotherapy (see glossary, p 1033) with no chemo-therapy.[35] Chemotherapy was associated with significantly lower rates of recurrence (women aged under 50 years, OR 0.65, 95% CI 0.61 to 0.69; women aged 50 to 69 years, OR 0.80, 95% 0.72 to 0.88) and death from all causes (women aged under 50 years, OR 0.73, 95% CI 0.68 to 0.78; women aged 50 to 69 years, OR 0.89, 95% CI 0.86 to 0.92). Rates of recurrence were similar for women with node negative and node positive disease. Ten year survival according to nodal and menopausal status is summarised in table (see table 1, p 1036). **Duration of treatment:** The same review identified 11 RCTs (6104 people) that compared longer regimens (doubling duration of chemotherapy from between 4 and 6 months to 8 to 12 months) with shorter regimens.[35] It found no additional benefit from longer treatment duration. **Different doses:** Several RCTs found no significant improvement from enhanced dose regimens, whereas others found little difference from untreated controls when suboptimal doses were used.[36,37] **Anthracycline regimens:** The systematic review identified 11 RCTs (5942 people) comparing regimens containing anthracycline (including the drugs doxorubicin or 4-epidoxorubicin) with standard CMF regimens.[35] It found a significant reduction in recurrence rates in those on anthracycline regimens (P = 0.006), and a modest but significant improvement in 5 year survival (69% v 72%; P = 0.02).

Harms:

Acute adverse effects: Adverse effects include nausea and vomiting, hair loss, bone marrow suppression, fatigue, and gastrointestinal disturbance. Prolonged chemotherapy is more likely to be associated with lethargy and haematological toxicity (anaemia and neutropenia), and anthracycline regimens cause complete hair loss. **Long term adverse effects:** Fertility and ovarian function may be permanently affected by chemotherapy, especially in women aged over 40 years, although for some women with hormone dependent cancer, reduced ovarian function may contribute to the benefit of adjuvant treatment (see glossary, p 1032). Other potential long term risks include induction of second cancers (especially haematological malignancies, although the risk is very low) and cardiac impairment with cumulative anthracycline dosages. Provided the cumulative dose of doxorubicin does not exceed 300–350 mg/m^2, the risk of congestive heart failure is less than 1%.

Comment:

The absolute benefits of these regimens need to be balanced against their toxicity for different women. Trials are under way of high dose chemotherapy with haematological support (bone marrow transplantation or peripheral stem cell support) in women with high risk disease (10 positive lymph nodes), although a recent RCT did not find survival advantage for high dose treatment.[38,39] New and highly active cytotoxic agents such as the taxanes are being examined with anthracyclines either in combination or sequence. Alternating sequences of cytotoxic agents may prove an effective way of circumventing acquired drug resistance and thus enhancing the efficacy of a regimen, such as the Milan regimen, of single agent anthracycline followed by standard CMF chemotherapy.[40]

OPTION   ADJUVANT TAMOXIFEN

One systematic review has found that adjuvant tamoxifen taken for up to 5 years reduces the chance of recurrence and death in postmenopausal

women, and in women with oestrogen receptor positive tumours irrespective of age, menopausal status, nodal involvement, or the addition of chemotherapy. Five years of treatment seems better than shorter durations, but available evidence does not find benefit associated with prolongation beyond 5 years. Tamoxifen carries a slightly increased risk of endometrial cancer, but we found no evidence of an overall adverse effect on non-breast cancer mortality (see table 2, p 1036).

Benefits: We found one systematic review (search date 1995, 55 RCTs, 37 000 women) that compared adjuvant tamoxifen with placebo.[41] It found that 5 years of adjuvant tamoxifen had similar effect on recurrence and long term survival in all age groups, irrespective of menopausal status or age. For women over 50 years old (usually postmenopausal), tamoxifen reduced the annual chance of recurrence by 29%, and of death from any cause by 20%. **Oestrogen receptor status:** Five years of tamoxifen treatment was associated with a greater reduction in the recurrence rate for women with oestrogen receptor positive rather than negative tumours (RRR 50% v 6%), and with a slightly greater reduction in the risk of 10 year recurrence in women with node positive compared with node negative disease (ARR 14.9% v 15.2%). **Duration of treatment:** The review found significantly greater reductions in recurrence with increasing duration of adjuvant tamoxifen (RRR 26% for 5 years of tamoxifen use v 12% for 1 year, P < 0.00001).[41] Table 2 presents findings on absolute improvement in 10 year survival from 5 years of tamoxifen (see table 2, p 1036). One RCT (3887 people) comparing 2 and 5 years of treatment found similar results.[42] The effects of prolonged treatment beyond 5 years are unclear. In the largest trial in the systematic review, 1153 women who had completed 5 years of tamoxifen were randomised to either placebo or 5 more years of tamoxifen.[41,43] Disease free survival after 4 years of further follow up was greater for those who switched to placebo rather than continued tamoxifen (92% v 86%, P = 0.003), although there was no significant difference in overall survival. Other studies found no detrimental effect or improvement in continuing tamoxifen beyond 5 years.[44]

Harms: The systematic review found an increased hazard ratio for endometrial cancer with tamoxifen (average HR 2.58, 95% CI 2.23 to 2.93).[41] For 5 years of tamoxifen treatment, this resulted in a cumulative risk over 10 years of two deaths (95% CI 0 to 4) per 1000 women. There was no evidence of an increased incidence of other cancers, nor of non-breast cancer related deaths (i.e. cardiac or vascular), although one extra death per 5000 women years of tamoxifen was attributed to pulmonary embolus. Bone loss was found in premenopausal women (1.4% bone loss per annum) but not in postmenopausal women, because of tamoxifen's partial agonist effects.[45] There were mixed effects on cardiovascular risk, with significant reductions in low density lipoprotein cholesterol associated with a reduced incidence of myocardial infarction in some studies, but an increased risk of thrombosis. Overall, no effect has been found on non-breast cancer mortality (HR 0.99 95% CI 0.88 to 1.16).[41]

Comment: The risk to benefit ratio may vary between women, with oestrogen receptor negative women deriving little benefit. Even in oestrogen receptor positive women, any benefit on breast cancer could be offset with prolonged treatment (beyond 5 years) by drug resistance and adverse effects on the endometrium. Two multicentre trials of tamoxifen duration are in progress (personal communication, Cancer Research Campaign, 2000), although because of concerns regarding long term toxicity with tamoxifen (see above) and in the absence of further definitive data, current practice outside the setting of a clinical trial has been to recommend tamoxifen for 5 years.[46] For women with completely oestrogen receptor negative disease, the overall benefit of adjuvant tamoxifen needs further research.

OPTION   COMBINED CHEMOTHERAPY PLUS TAMOXIFEN

One RCT found that adding combined chemotherapy to tamoxifen improved survival.

Benefits: We found no systematic review. We found one RCT of 2306 women with lymph node negative, oestrogen receptor positive early breast cancer that compared tamoxifen alone with tamoxifen plus CMF chemotherapy.[47] It found that adding chemotherapy to tamoxifen caused a further absolute improvement in disease free survival (at 5 years' follow up 90% v 85%, P = 0.006) and in overall survival (97% v 94%, P = 0.03).

Harms: Adding CMF chemotherapy to tamoxifen was associated with a greater incidence of grade three/four neutropenia (9% v 0%), greater than or equal to grade two nausea (35.2% v 3.7%), moderate/severe alopecia (35.6% v 0.4%), and thromboembolism/phlebitis (7.5% v 2.1%).[48]

Comment: None.

OPTION   OVARIAN ABLATION

One systematic review of RCTs has found that ovarian ablation (see glossary, p 1033) significantly improves long term survival in women aged under 50 years with early breast cancer.

Benefits: We found one systematic review (search date 1995, 12 RCTs with at least 15 years' follow up, 2102 premenopausal women) comparing ovarian ablation by irradiation or surgery with no ablation.[48] Significantly more women with ovarian ablation survived (52.4% v 46.1%, P = 0.001) and survived recurrence free (45% v 39%, P = 0.0007). Benefit was independent of nodal status.

Harms: We found no good evidence on long term adverse effects. Concerns exist about late sequelae of ovarian ablation, especially effects on bone mineral density and cardiovascular risk. Acute adverse effects are likely to be menopausal symptoms.

Comment: Five of the trials compared ovarian ablation plus chemotherapy with chemotherapy alone.[48] In these, the absolute benefit of ablation was smaller than in trials of ovarian ablation alone. It may be that cytotoxic chemotherapy itself suppresses ovarian function, making the effect of ablation difficult to detect in combined trials. When only pre-menopausal women were considered in the absence of chemotherapy, there was a 27% improvement in the odds of recurrence free survival. Trials are under way of reversible oophorectomy using gonadotrophin releasing hormone analogues, which would allow preservation of fertility in younger women with oestrogen receptor positive tumours.

QUESTION	What are the effects of axillary clearance, sampling, or radiotherapy in women with operable primary breast cancer?

RCTs have found no evidence that axillary clearance is associated with improved survival compared with axillary node sampling, axillary radiotherapy, or sampling plus radiotherapy (see glossary, p 1032) combined. One systematic review of mainly poor quality evidence found that the risk of arm lymphoedema was highest with axillary clearance plus radiotherapy, lower with axillary sampling plus radiotherapy, and lowest with sampling alone.

Benefits:
Versus axillary sampling: We found no systematic review. One RCT (466) in women undergoing breast conserving surgery found that sampling was associated with improved survival compared with axillary clearance, but the difference was not significant (estimated 5 year survival 88.6% v 82.1%).[49] Similar rates of node positivity were found in both groups. **Versus axillary radiotherapy:** We found one systematic review (search date 1990, 8 RCTs, 4370 women) comparing axillary clearance (level I, II, and III dissection) with axillary radiotherapy. It found no significant difference in mortality at 10 years (54.7% v 54.9%) nor in rates of recurrence (OR 1.01). Radiotherapy was associated with fewer isolated local recurrences (odds reduction 15%, 95% CI 7% to 22%).[5] **Versus sampling plus radiotherapy:** We found no systematic review. Two RCTs compared axillary clearance (level I, II, and III dissection) with sampling followed by radiotherapy in women with involved axillary nodes. They found no significant difference in local, axillary, or distant recurrence.[49,50] **Axillary clearance plus radiotherapy:** We found no evidence that radiotherapy in addition to axillary clearance (level I and II, or level I, II, and III dissection) improves regional control of disease.

Harms:
Axillary clearance: Adverse effects of axillary surgery include seroma formation, arm swelling, damage to the intercostobrachial nerve, and shoulder stiffness. We found one RCT that compared the morbidity of different axillary procedures.[49] It compared complete axillary clearance (levels I, II, and III dissection) with four node axillary sampling followed by radiotherapy if the nodes were involved. The rate of arm swelling was higher after clearance than after sampling whether or not women received postoperative radiotherapy (at 3 years, forearm girth was significantly greater, P = 0.005). After removal of axillary drains, between a quarter and a half of women who had undergone a level I and II or levels I, II, and III axillary dissection developed seromas requiring aspiration. **Axillary radiotherapy:** This usually includes irradiation of the supraclavicular fossa. Irradiation of this area incorporates some underlying lung that increases the risk of radiation pneumonitis. By increasing the volume of the lung irradiated compared with chest

wall or breast radiotherapy alone, the risk of acute pneumonitis is increased. The RCT comparing clearance with sampling plus radiotherapy for node positive disease found significantly reduced shoulder movement with radiotherapy, even though the shoulder joint was not irradiated.[49] At 6 months, both groups had significantly reduced shoulder movement compared with women receiving axillary sampling alone (P < 0.004).[49] However, by 3 years the axillary clearance group had improved and was not significantly different from the sampling group. **Arm lymphoedema:** One Australian systematic review of lymphoedema prevalence, risks, and management found that, although current information is of poor quality, the combination of axillary dissection (to or beyond level II) and axillary radiotherapy was associated with a risk of lymphoedema of between 12% and 60%, with most studies suggesting that at least one third of women are affected.[51] Studies of axillary sampling followed by irradiation found lower rates (between 6% and 32%), and for axillary sampling alone, lower still (between 0% and 21%). Studies of dissection beyond level I found rates between 0% to 42%, with most studies reporting a rate of 20–30% 1 year after operation.[51] In women who receive axillary radiotherapy without axillary surgery, the overall lymphoedema rate is about 8%.

Comment: **Axillary staging:** Both clearance and sampling provide important prognostic information on which decisions on local and systemic treatment can be based. Further RCTs of less invasive and potentially less morbid staging procedures such as sentinel node biopsy are under way. A decision on axillary management should be based on the risk of involvement of axillary nodes (which varies according to tumour size, grade, and the presence of vascular/lymphatic invasion) and potential treatment related morbidity. Two retrospective cohort studies found that level I dissection accurately assessed axillary lymph node status, providing that at least 10 nodes were removed.[52,53] One RCT found that a sample of four nodes provided sufficient information to categorise an axilla as histologically positive or negative.[54] Removal of nodes at level I and level II or removal of all nodes below the axillary vein (level I, II, and III) accurately stages the axilla.[52,53] Randomised trials comparing sentinel node biopsy with axillary node clearance and sampling are current under way and results of these will be incorporated in future issues (JM Dixon, personal communication, 2000).

GLOSSARY

Axillary clearance Clearance of level I, II and usually level III axillary lymph nodes. Level I nodes are lateral to the pectoralis minor muscle, level II nodes are under it, and level III nodes are medial to it at the apex of the axilla.

Axillary sampling Aims to remove the four largest, most easily palpable axillary lymph nodes, for histological examination.

Adjuvant treatment This usually refers to systemic chemotherapy or hormonal treatment, or both, taken by patients after removal of a primary tumour (in this case, surgery for early breast cancer), with the aim of killing any remaining micrometastatic tumour cells and thus preventing recurrence.

Breast conserving surgery Surgery that consists of lumpectomy (minimal free margins), wide local excision (wider free margins), or segmental or quadrant resection (usually with very wide free margins).

Combination chemotherapy Two or more cytotoxic drugs given intravenously every 3–4 weeks for 4–6 months.

Lumpectomy Gross tumour excision.

Ovarian ablation Surgical, medical, or radiation induced suppression of ovarian function in premenopausal women.

Quadrantectomy Tumour excised with at least 2 cm of normal surrounding breast tissue and with a segment of breast tissue from the periphery of the breast to the nipple.

Radical mastectomy Removal of breast and pectoralis major and minor muscles and axillary contents.

Radiotherapy Part of initial local and regional treatment. In early stage disease it may be an adjunct to surgery; in locally advanced disease (T4;N2) it may be the sole locoregional treatment. Radiotherapy may be delivered to the breast or postmastectomy chest wall, as well as to the lymphatic areas of the axilla, supraclavicular fossa or internal mammary node chain.

Staging of breast cancer A detailed description by tumour, nodal and metastatic parameters at a particular time (TNM).[1] These are amalgamated into broader categories called stages (0 to IV). Stages can be aggregated into even broader categories (non-invasive, early invasive and advanced breast cancer) (see table 3, p 1037). **Non-invasive breast cancer** (stage 0) is T_{is} (carcinoma in situ; intraductal carcinoma, lobular carcinoma in situ, or Paget's disease of the nipple with no associated tumor), and N_0 (no axillary nodal involvement) and M_0 (no metastases). **Early invasive breast cancer** (stage I or II) is M_0 with: T_1 or T_2 (tumour diameter 5 cm or less, no involvement of skin or chest wall) and N_0 or N_1 (mobile axillary nodes); or M_0 with T_3 (tumour diameter over 5 cm, no skin or chest wall involvement) but only N_0. **Advanced breast cancer** Locally advanced breast cancer (stage III) is M_0 with any combination of T and N not classified as non-invasive or early invasive breast cancer. Metastatic breast cancer (stage IV) is M1 (any supraclavicular fossa node involvement or distant metastases to bone, lung, liver etc) with any combination of tumour and node parameters.

Supraradical mastectomy Removal of breast, pectoralis major and minor muscles, axillary contents and internal mammary chain of nodes.

Tamoxifen A non-steroidal antioestrogen taken as daily oral tablets, usually for between 2–5 years.

Total mastectomy Removal of breast.

Total nodal irradiation Radiotherapy to the regional lymph nodes, including supraclavicular, infraclavicular, axillary nodes, and internal mammary nodes in the upper intercostal spaces.

REFERENCES

1. UICC International Union against Cancer. *TNM Classification of Malignant Tumours* 5th ed. Sobin LH, Wittekind Ch, eds. New York: Wiley–Liss Inc, 1997.

2. Fisher B, Dignam J, Wolmark N, et al. Lumpectomy and radiation therapy for the treatment of intraductal breast cancer: findings of the National Surgical Adjuvant Breast and Bowel Project B-17. *J Clin Oncol* 1998;16:441–452.

3. Julien J-P, Bijker N, Fentiman IS, Peterse JL, et al. Radiotherapy in breast-conserving treatment for ductal carcinoma in situ; first results of EORTC randomised phase III trial 10853. *Lancet* 2000; 355:528–533.

4. Fisher B, Dignam J, Wolmark N, et al. Tamoxifen in treatment of intraductal breast cancer: National Surgical Adjuvant Breast and Bowel Project B-24 randomised controlled trial. *Lancet* 1999;353: 1993–2000.

5. Early Breast Cancer Trialists' Collaborative Group. Effects of radiotherapy and surgery in early breast cancer: an overview of the randomised trials. *N Engl J Med* 1995;333:1444–1455. Search date not stated; the author sought information worldwide from investigators who conducted trials that began before 1985.

6. Morris AD, Morris RD, Wilson JF, et al. Breast conserving therapy versus mastectomy in early stage breast cancer: a meta-analysis of 10 year survival. *Cancer J Sci Am* 1997;3:6–12. Search date 1995, primary source Medline 1966 to 1995.

7. Sacchini V, Luini A, Tana S, et al. Quantitative and qualitative cosmetic evaluation after conservative treatment for breast cancer. *Eur J Cancer* 1991; 27:1395–1400.

8. Smitt NC, Nowels KW, Zdeblick MJ, et al. The importance of the lumpectomy surgical margin status in long-term results of breast conservation. *Cancer* 1995;76:259–267.

9. Wazer DE, DiPetrillo T, Schmidt-Ullrich R, et al. Factors influencing cosmetic outcome and complication risk after conservative surgery and radiotherapy for early-stage breast carcinoma. *J Clin Oncol* 1992;10:356–363.

10. Abner AL, Recht A, Vicini FA, et al. Cosmetic results after surgery, chemotherapy and radiation therapy for early breast cancer. *Int J Radiat Oncol Biol Phys* 1991;21:331–338.

11. Dewar JA, Benhamou S, Benhamou E, et al. Cosmetic results following lumpectomy axillary dissection and radiotherapy for small breast cancers. *Radiother Oncol* 1988;12:273–280.

12. Rochefordiere A, Abner A, Silver B, et al. Are cosmetic results following conservative surgery and radiation therapy for early breast cancer dependent on technique? *Int J Radiat Oncol Biol Phys* 1992;23:925–931.

13. Sneeuw KA, Aaronson N, Yarnold J, et al. Cosmetic and functional outcomes of breast conserving treatment for early stage breast cancer 1: comparison of patients' ratings, observers' ratings and objective assessments. *Radiother Oncol* 1992;25:153–159.

14. Ash DV, Benson EA, Sainsbury JR et al. Seven year follow-up on 334 patients treated by breast conserving surgery and short course radical postoperative radiotherapy: a report of the Yorkshire breast cancer group. *Clin Oncol* 1995;7:93–96.

15. Lindsey I, Serpell JW, Johnson WR, Rodger A. Cosmesis following complete local excision of breast cancer. *Aust N Z J Surg* 1997;67:428–432.

16. Touboul E, Belkacemi Y, Lefranc JP, et al. Early breast cancer: influence of type of boost (electrons or iridium-192 implant) on local control and cosmesis after conservative surgery and radiation therapy. *Radiother Oncol* 1995;34:105–113.

17. Halyard MY, Grado GL, Schomber PJ, et al. Conservative therapy of breast cancer: the Mayo Clinic experience. *Am J Clin Oncol* 1996;19:445–450.

18. Liljegren G, Holmberg L, Adami HO, Westman G, Graffman S, Bergh J for the Uppsala– rebro Breast Cancer Study Group. Sector resection with or without postoperative radiotherapy for stage I breast cancer: five year results of a randomised trial. *J Natl Cancer Inst* 1994;86:717–722.

19. Liljegren G, Holmberg J, Bergh, J, et al and the Uppsala– rebro Breast Cancer Study Group. 10-year results after sector resection with or without postoperative radiotherapy for stage I breast cancer: a randomized trial. *J Clin Oncol* 1999;17:2326–2333.

20. Forrest AP, Stewart HJ, Everington D, et al on behalf of the Scottish Cancer Trials Breast Group. Randomised controlled trial of conservation therapy in breast cancer: 6 year analysis of the Scottish trial. *Lancet* 1996;348:708–713.

21. Steering Committee on Clinical Practice Guidelines for the Care and Treatment of Breast Cancer. A Canadian consensus document. *Can Med Assoc J* 1998;158(suppl 3):S1–S84.

22. Cuzick J, Stewart H, Rutqvist L, et al. Cause-specific mortality in long term survivors of breast cancer who participated in trials of radiotherapy. *J Clin Oncol* 1994;12:447–453. Search date not given. Includes trials that started before 1975.

23. Ragaz J, Jackson SM, Le N, et al. Adjuvant radiotherapy and chemotherapy in node-positive premenopausal women with breast cancer. *N Engl J Med* 1997;337:956–962.

24. Overgaard M, Hansen PS, Overgaard J, et al. Postoperative radiotherapy in high-risk premenopausal women with breast cancer who receive adjuvant chemotherapy. *N Engl J Med* 1997;337:949–955.

25. Overgaard M, Jensen MB, Overgaard J, et al. Postoperative radiotherapy in high risk postmenopausal breast cancer patients given adjuvant tamoxifen: Danish Breast Cancer Cooperative Group DBCG 82c randomised trial. *Lancet* 1999;353:1641–1648.

26. Ghersi D, Simes J. Draft report of effectiveness of postmastectomy radiotherapy and risk factors for local recurrence in early breast cancer. Report to NHMRC National Breast Cancer Centre, Sydney, 1998.

27. O'Rourke S, Gaba MH, Morgan D, et al. Local recurrence after simple mastectomy. *Br J Surg* 1994;81:386–389.

28. Fowble B, Gray R, Gilchrist K, Goodman RL, Taylor S, Tormey D. Identification of a subset of patients with breast cancer and histologically positive nodes who may benefit from postoperative radiotherapy. *J Clin Oncol* 1988;6:1107–1117.

29. Houghton J, Baum M, Haybittle JL. Role of radiotherapy following total mastectomy in patients with early breast cancer: the closed trials working party of the CRC breast cancer trials group. *World J Surg* 1994;18:117–122.

30. Kaija H, Maunu P. Tangential breast irradiation with or without internal mammary chain irradiation: results of a randomised trial. *Radiother Oncol* 1995;36:172–176.

31. Handley R. Carcinoma of the breast. *Ann R Coll Surg Engl* 1975;57:59–66.

32. Veronesi U, Cascinelli NM, Bufalino R, et al. Risk of internal mammary lymph node metastases and its relevance on prognosis in breast cancer patients. *Ann Surg* 1983;198:681–684.

33. Veronesi U, Valagussa P. Inefficacy of internal mammary node dissection in breast cancer surgery. *Cancer* 1981;47:170–175.

34. Bates T, Evans RGB. Report of the Independent Review commissioned by The Royal College of Radiologists into Brachial Plexus Neuropathy following radiotherapy for breast cancer. London: Royal College of Radiologists, 1995.

35. Early Breast Cancer Trialists' Collaborative Group. Polychemotherapy for early breast cancer: an overview of the randomised trials. *Lancet* 1998; 352:930–942. Search date 1995; the authors sought information on each woman in any randomised trial that began before 1990.

36. Fisher B, Anderson S, Wickerham DL, et al. Increased intensification and total dose of cyclophosphamide in a doxorubicin-cyclophosphamide regimen for the treatment of primary breast cancer: findings from national surgical adjuvant breast and bowel project B-22. *J Clin Oncol* 1997;15:1858–1869.

37. Wood WC, Budman DR, Korzun AH. Dose and dose intensity of adjuvant chemotherapy for stage II, node-positive breast carcinoma. *N Engl J Med* 1994;330:1253–1259.

38. Peters WP, Ross M, Vredenburgh JJ, et al. High-dose chemotherapy and autologous bone marrow support as consolidation after standard-dose adjuvant chemotherapy for high-risk primary breast cancer. *J Clin Oncol* 1993;11:1132–1143.

39. Rodenhuis S, Richel DJ, van der Wall E, et al. Randomised trial of high-dose chemotherapy and haemopoietic progenitor-cell support in operable breast cancer with extensive axillary lymph-node involvement. *Lancet* 1998;352:515–521.

40. Bonadonna G, Zambeti M, Valagussa P. Sequential or alternating doxorubicin and CMF regimens in breast cancer with more than three positive nodes. *JAMA* 1995;273:542–547.

41. Early Breast Cancer Trialists' Collaborative Group. Tamoxifen for early breast cancer: an overview of

the randomised trials. *Lancet* 1998;351:1451–1467. Search date 1995, includes trials started before 1990. The authors sought data on each woman in any randomised trial that began before 1990.

42. Swedish Breast Cancer Cooperative Group. Randomised trial of two versus five years of adjuvant tamoxifen for post-menopausal early stage breast cancer. *J Natl Cancer Inst* 1996;88: 1543–1549.

43. Fisher B, Dignam J, Bryant J, et al. Five versus more than five years of tamoxifen therapy for breast cancer patients with negative lymph nodes and estrogen receptor-positive tumours. *J Natl Cancer Inst* 1996;88:1529–1542.

44. Stewart HJ, Forrest AP, Everington D, et al. Randomised comparison of 5 years of adjuvant tamoxifen with continuous therapy for operable breast cancer. *Br J Cancer* 1996;74:297–299.

45. Powles TJ, Hickish T, Kanis JA, Tidy A, Ashley S. Effect of tamoxifen on bone mineral density measured by dual-energy x-ray absorptiometry in healthy premenopausal and postmenopausal women. *J Clin Oncol* 1996;14:78–84.

46. Swain SM. Tamoxifen: the long and short of it. *J Natl Cancer Inst* 1996;88:1510–1512.

47. Fisher B, Dignam J, Wolmark N, et al. Tamoxifen and chemotherapy for lymph node-negative, estrogen receptor-positive breast cancer. *J Natl Cancer Inst* 1997;89:1673–1682.

48. Early Breast Cancer Trialists' Group. Ovarian ablation in early breast cancer: overview of the randomised trials. *Lancet* 1996;348:1189–1196. Search date 1995; the authors sought information

on each patient in any randomised trial that began before 1990.

49. Chetty U, Jack W, Prescott RJ, Tyler C, Rodger A. Management of the axilla in operable breast cancer treated by breast conservation: a randomised controlled trial. *Br J Surg* 2000;87: 163–169.

50. Stelle RJC, Forrest APM, Gibson R, Stuart HJ, Chetty U. The efficacy of lower axillary sampling in obtaining lymph node status in breast cancer: a controlled randomised trial. *Br J Surg* 1985;72: 368–369.

51. Browning C, Thomas and Associates; Redman S, Pillar C, Turner J, Boyle F. NHMRC National Breast Cancer Centre, Sydney 1998. Lymphoedema: prevalence risk factors and management: a review of research. Search date 1996; primary source Medline 1985 to 1996; and hand searches of article references and personal contact with key resources.

52. Axelsson CK, Mouridzsen HT, Zedeler K. Axillary dissection at level I and II lymph nodes is important in breast cancer classification. *Eur J Cancer* 1992;28A:1415–1418.

53. Kiricuta CI, Tausch J. A mathematical model of axillary lymph node involvement based on 1446 complete axillary dissections in patients with breast carcinoma. *Cancer* 1992;69:2496–2501.

54. Steele RJC, Forrest APM, Givson T, Stuart HJ, Chetty U. The efficacy of lower axillary sampling in obtaining lymph node status in breast cancer:a controlled randomised trial. *Br J Surg* 1985;72: 368–369.

J Michael Dixon
Honorary Senior Lecturer in Surgery
Western General Hospital
Edinburgh
UK

Alan Rodger
Professor of Radiation Oncology
William Buckland Radiotherapy Centre
The Alfred Hospital, Monash University
Melbourne
Australia

Stephen Johnston
Senior Lecturer in Medical Oncology
The Royal Marsden NHS Trust
London
UK

Competing interests: None declared.

TABLE 1 Ten year survival with combination chemotherapy versus placebo, according to nodal and age/menopausal status: results of a systematic review of RCTs (see text, p 1027).[35]

	Control (%)	Chemotherapy (%)	Absolute benefit (%)	SD (%)	Significance (two sided)
Age < 50 years					
Node +ve	41.4	53.8	+12.4	2.4	P < 0.00001
Node –ve	71.9	77.6	+5.7	2.1	P = 0.01
Age 50–69 years					
Node +ve	46.3	48.6	+2.3	1.3	P = 0.001
Node –ve	64.8	71.2	+6.4	2.3	P = 0.0025

SD, standard definition.

TABLE 2 Ten year survival in women treated with tamoxifen for 5 years compared with control treatment: results of a systematic review of RCTs (see text, p 1029).[41]

	Control (%)	Chemotherapy (%)	Absolute benefit (%)	SD (%)	Significance (two sided)
Node +ve	50.5	61.4	+10.9	2.5	P < 0.00001
Node –ve	73.3	78.9	+5.6	1.3	P < 0.00001

SD, standard definition.

TABLE 3	Staging of breast cancer (the individual terms are explained in the glossary, p 1032).[1]			
	Tumour	**Node**	**Metastases**	**Stage**
Non–invasive	T_{is}	N_0	M_0	0
Early invasive	T_{1-2}	N_{0-1}	M_0	I, II A or B
	T_3	N_0	M_0	II B
Advanced				
Locally advanced	T_{any}	N_2	M_0	III A
	T_3	N_{1-2}	M_0	III A
	T_4	N_{0-3}	M_0	III B
	T_{any}	N_3	M_0	III B
Metastatic	T_{any}	N_{any}	M_1	IV

SD, standard definition.

Breast pain

New topic

N Bundred

Key Messages

- We found limited evidence from RCTs suggesting that
  - A low fat, high carbohydrate diet reduces breast pain and tenderness.
  - Danazol reduces pain after 12 months but with increased adverse effects.
  - Tamoxifen is more effective than placebo. There is no significant difference between danazol and tamoxifen.
  - Bromocriptine relieves breast pain but with a high incidence of adverse effects.
  - Gestrinone reduces breast pain but with increased adverse effects. Tibolone is more effective than hormone replacement therapy (HRT).
- We found no good evidence from RCTs on the effects of evening primrose oil, luteinising hormone releasing hormone agonists, progestogen cream, pyridoxine, diuretics, antibiotics, or vitamin E.

DEFINITION	Breast pain can be differentiated into cyclical mastalgia (worse before a menstrual period) or non-cyclical mastalgia (unrelated to the menstrual cycle).[1,2] Cyclical pain is often bilateral, usually most severe in the upper outer quadrants of the breast, and may refer to the medial aspect of the upper arm.[1-3] Non-cyclical pain may caused by true breast pain or chest wall pain located over the costal cartilages.[1,2,4] Specific breast pathology and referred pain unrelated to the breasts are not included in this definition.
INCIDENCE/ PREVALENCE	Up to 70% of women develop breast pain in their lifetime.[1,2] Of 1171 American women attending a gynaecology clinic, 69% suffered regular discomfort, which was judged as severe in 11% of women, and 36% had consulted a doctor about breast pain.[2]
AETIOLOGY/ RISK FACTORS	The cause is multifactorial. Breast pain is more common in women aged 30 to 50 years.[1,2]
PROGNOSIS	Cyclical breast pain resolves spontaneously within 3 months of onset in 20–30% of women.[5] The pain tends to relapse and remit, and up to 60% of women develop recurrent symptoms 2 years after treatment.[1] Non-cyclical pain responds poorly to treatment but may resolve spontaneously in about 50% of women.[1]
AIMS	To reduce breast pain and improve quality of life.
OUTCOMES	Breast pain score based on the number of days of severe (score 2) or moderate (score 1) pain experienced in each menstrual cycle; visual analogue score of breast pain, heaviness or breast tenderness; questionnaires.
METHODS	We searched the Cochrane Library and Medline in April 2000 (key words: breast tenderness, discomfort, pain, mastalgia, mastodynia). Systematic reviews and subsequent RCTs that met *Clinical Evidence* quality criteria were included. Overall the evidence was poor and some studies with weaker methods were included when higher quality evidence was not found, as indicated in the text. Studies were included whatever the definition of breast pain, as indicated in the text.

QUESTION	What are the effects of treatments for breast pain?

OPTION	LOW FAT, HIGH CARBOHYDRATE DIET

One small RCT found that advice to follow a low fat, high carbohydrate diet reduced breast pain and tenderness more than general dietary advice.

Benefits: We found no systematic review. We found one RCT in 21 women with cyclical mastalgia for at least 5 years, which compared instruction to reduce fat content of the diet to 15% of total with general dietary advice for 6 months.[6] One woman in each group withdrew and was excluded from the analysis. Over 6 months the severity of self reported breast swelling (P = 0.04) and tenderness (P = 0.0001) was significantly reduced in women receiving low fat dietary advice compared with those receiving general dietary advice. However, no significant difference in breast swelling, tenderness, and nodularity was found on physical examination after 6

Breast pain

months (6/10 [60%] of women with diet, 2/9 [22%] of women with control; RR 2.7, 95% CI 0.75 to 4.13).

Harms: The small trial reported no ill effects.

Comment: Diets can be difficult to sustain in the long term.

OPTION EVENING PRIMROSE OIL

We found insufficient evidence on the effects of evening primrose oil.

Benefits: We found no systematic review and no good quality RCTs.

Harms: Poor quality RCTs found that adverse effects causing treatment discontinuation were similar with evening primrose oil and placebo (3%), and largely due to abdominal bloating.[5,7]

Comment: In one partially blinded RCT, 72 women received evening primrose oil or placebo for 3 months, followed by 3 months of evening primrose oil.[7] The RCT reported that pain, tenderness, and lumpiness improved in cyclical but not non-cyclical breast pain. However, the trial incorporated numerous methodological flaws, including post hoc revision of the inclusion criteria, subgroup analysis, exclusion of withdrawals, and the use of baseline comparisons (with the best response seen in women who were symptomatically worse at baseline). We found one survey of randomised and open studies, but data were reported as overall summary figures, making specific data extraction impossible.[6]

OPTION DANAZOL

One RCT found that danazol reduced cyclical breast pain compared with placebo after 12 months, but with increased adverse effects. It found no significant difference between danazol and tamoxifen.

Benefits: We found no systematic review. We found one good quality three arm outpatient based RCT in 93 women with severe cyclical mastalgia.[8] **Versus placebo:** It compared danazol 200 mg/day versus tamoxifen 10 mg/day versus placebo over 6 months. It found that more women achieved greater than 50% pain relief at the end of treatment with danazol than with placebo (pain relief AR 21/32 [66%] with danazol v 11/29 [38%] with placebo; RR 1.73, 95% CI 1.02 to 2.94; NNT 3, 95% CI 2 to 37). After 12 months of treatment the difference remained significant (pain relief AR 12/32 [38%] for danazol v 0/29 with placebo [0%]; RR 22, 95% CI 1.26 to 55).**Versus other drugs:** See tamoxifen, p 1042. The same RCT found no significant difference in pain relief after treatment with danazol compared with tamoxifen (AR 21/32 [66%] with danazol v 23/32 [72%] with tamoxifen; ARR 6%; RR 0.91, 95% CI 0.65 to 1.27).[8]

Harms: Adverse effects were reported in more women taking danazol than placebo.[8] These included weight gain (10 v 1), deepening of the voice (4 v 0), menorrhagia (4 v 0), and muscle cramps (3 v 0). The results were not assessed for significance.

Comment: Although we found no direct evidence, there is consensus that once a response is achieved, adverse effects can be avoided by reducing the dose of danazol to 100 mg daily, and confining treatment to the fortnight preceding menstruation.[8,9] Non-hormonal contraception is essential with danazol when given in 200 mg doses.[10]

OPTION   **BROMOCRIPTINE**

Two RCTs found limited evidence that bromocriptine relieves breast pain. One RCT found a high incidence of adverse effects.

Benefits: We found no systematic review but found two RCTs. The first outpatient based, European RCT, in 272 premenopausal women with diffuse fibrocystic disease of the breast, compared bromocriptine 2.5 mg twice daily with placebo. After 3 and 6 months it found that symptoms improved with bromocriptine compared with placebo on self assessed visual analogue scoring of breast pain, tenderness, and heaviness. Analysis did not use intention to treat, and 49 women (35%) withdrew on bromocriptine compared with 36 women (26%) on placebo.[11] The second RCT used a crossover design (n = 10), and also found that bromocriptine reduced pain compared with placebo (P < 0.02).[12]

Harms: The larger RCT found that with bromocriptine treatment 61/135 (45%) of women complained of adverse events compared with 41/137 (30%) on placebo (ARI 15%, 95% CI 3% to 28%; RR 1.51, 95% CI 1.11 to 1.92; NNH 7, 95% CI 4 to 29). Adverse effects caused 15/135 women (11%) to withdraw on active treatment compared with 8/137 women (6%) on placebo. The adverse reactions included nausea (32% v 13%), dizziness (12% v 7%), postural hypertension, and constipation.[11] The small RCT found that nausea and dizziness occurred in 8/10 women on bromocriptine compared with 0/10 on placebo.[12] Strokes and death have been reported after use of bromocriptine to inhibit lactation and the US Food and Drug Administration has withdrawn its license for this indication.[13]

Comment: Bromocriptine is now rarely used because frequent and intolerable adverse effects at the therapeutic dose outweigh the benefits for this indication.

OPTION   **HORMONE REPLACEMENT THERAPY IN BREAST PAIN**

One small RCT found that HRT reduced pain less than tibolone.

Benefits: We found no systematic review. **Versus placebo:** We found no RCTs (see tibolone under synthetic steroids, p 1043). **Versus tibolone:** One RCT in 44 postmenopausal woman compared tibolone 2.5 mg daily versus HRT (transdermal oestrogen patches 50μg, twice weekly for 3 weeks per month, plus progestogen 5 mg daily for 12 days/month per cycle), versus no treatment. After 1 year it found that breast pain was significantly increased in women on HRT compared with those on tibolone (total increase in breast pain was 53% v 5%, P < 0.02).[14]

Harms: The RCT did not report on adverse effects.[14] See harms of HRT under secondary prevention of ischaemic cardiac events, p 83.

Comment: Tibolone is a synthetic steroid reported to have oestrogenic, progestogenic, and weak androgenic, properties, which may be used as a form of HRT.[15]

Breast pain

OPTION	TAMOXIFEN

Two RCTs found limited evidence that tamoxifen is more effective than placebo. One RCT found no significant difference between tamoxifen and danazol.

Benefits:
We found no systematic review. **Versus placebo:** We found two RCTs. One double blind crossover RCT in 60 premenopausal women with cyclical breast pain compared tamoxifen with placebo.[15] It found that more women experienced pain relief (visual analogue scale over 3 months) with tamoxifen than placebo (71% v 38%; RR 1.87, 95% CI 1.20 to 1.87; NNT 3, 95% CI 2 to 13). The second RCT (n = 93) compared tamoxifen versus danazol versus placebo.[9] It found that significantly more women taking tamoxifen achieved a good outcome (greater than 50% reduction in mean pain score) at the end of treatment, 6 months later, and 12 months later, compared with placebo (pain relief after treatment AR 23/32 [72%] v 11/29 [38%] with placebo; ARI 0.34; RR 1.89, 95 CI 1.13 to 2.37). **Dose response:** One RCT in 301 women with cyclical breast pain for more than 6 months compared 10 mg with 20 mg of tamoxifen daily from days 15–25 in the menstrual cycle for 3 months. It found no significant difference in pain relief or nodularity (pain relief 127/155 [82%] v 107/142 [75%]; ARR 7%, 95% CI −3% to +13%; RR 1.09, 95% CI 0.96 to 1.18; nodularity 41/155 [26%] v 52/142 [36%]; ARR −9%, 95% CI −18.6% to +0.4%; RR 0.72, 95% CI 0.49 to 1.01).[16] Another RCT (n = 60) compared 10 mg with 20 mg daily doses of tamoxifen for 3 and 6 months in cyclical and non-cyclical mastalgia.[17] Three month response rates were similar (12/14 [86%] had pain relief with 10 mg [86%] v 14/15 [93%] with 20 mg; ARR 8%, 95% CI 5% to 61%; RR 0.92, 95% CI 0.35 to 1.06). **Versus other treatments:** One RCT found no significant difference between tamoxifen and danazol[9] (see versus other drugs in benefits section of danazol, p 1040).

Harms:
One RCT found more women experienced hot flushes (26% v 10%; ARI 16%; RRI 1.49; 95% CI −0.34 to +3.33) and vaginal discharge (16% v 7%; ARI 9.2%; RRI 1.34; 95% CI −0.97 to +3.64) in women taking tamoxifen compared with placebo.[16] Two RCTs found that fewer adverse effects occurred with a daily dose of 10 mg than 20 mg.[16,17] The largest RCT found that adverse effects were reported in 66% of women taking 20 mg daily compared with 52% on 10 mg daily (ARI 15%, 95% CI 3% to 26%; RR 0.78, 95% CI 0.60 to 0.95).[15] The adverse effects primarily consisted of hot flushes (AR 54/142 [38%] with 20 mg dose of tamoxifen v 33/155 [21%] with the 10 mg dose; RR 1.79, 95% CI 1.24 to 2.58; NNH 6, 95% CI 3 to 16) and gastrointestinal disturbances (AR 54/142 [38%] with 20 mg v 30/155 [19%] with 10 mg tamoxifen; RR 1.97, 95% CI 1.34 to 2.88; NNH 6, 95% CI 4 to 12). See adverse effects of tamoxifen in the treatment of breast cancer, p 1018.

Comment:
Tamoxifen is not licensed for mastalgia in the UK or the USA. There is consensus that it should not be used for more than 6 months at a time. Due to the high incidence of adverse effects it should be used only under expert supervision and with appropriate non-hormonal contraception. Tamoxifen is contraindicated in pregnancy because of potential teratogenicity.[18]

OPTION	LUTEINISING HORMONE RELEASING HORMONE AGONISTS

We found no good evidence on the effects of luteinising hormone releasing hormone agonists (e.g. goserelin) in women with breast pain.

Benefits: We found no systematic review or good quality RCTs.

Harms: Adverse effects of goserelin may include hot flushes, headaches, nausea, depression, loss of libido, and amenorrhoea.

Comment: None.

OPTION	SYNTHETIC STEROIDS (GESTRINONE, TIBOLONE)

One RCT found that gestrinone relieved breast pain more than placebo. One small RCT found that tibolone reduced breast pain more than HRT.

Benefits: We found no systematic review. **Gestrinone:** We found one double blinded outpatient based RCT in 145 premenopausal women with cyclical breast pain comparing gestrinone 2.4 mg twice weekly with placebo.[19] It found that gestrinone reduced breast pain more than placebo after 3 months (using visual analogue score 0 to 100 where 0 = no pain, 100 = worst pain: pain score reduced from 59.5 to 11.0 with gestrinone compared with 58.2 to 36.7 with placebo, $P < 0.0001$) (see HRT versus tibolone, p 1041).[14]

Harms: The first RCT found that 41% of women on gestrinone had androgenic effects, including greasy skin, hirsutism, acne, reduction in breast size, headache, and depression compared with 14% on placebo (ARI 0.27; RR 2.96, 95% CI 1.70 to 4.40).[19] The second RCT did not report on adverse effects.[15]

Comment: Gestrinone is a synthetic steroid, reported to have androgenic, anti-oestrogenic and anti-progestogenic properties, which may be used for the treatment of endometriosis.[20]

OPTION	PROGESTOGENS

We found no good evidence on the effects of progestogens in women with breast pain.

Benefits: We found no systematic review or good quality RCTs.

Harms: We found no evidence from RCTs.

Comment: None.

OPTION	OTHER AGENTS

We found no evidence that pyridoxine, diuretics, antibiotics, or vitamin E, are effective compared with placebo for the treatment of breast pain.

Benefits: We found no systematic review or good quality RCTs.

Harms: We found no good evidence.

Comment: None.

REFERENCES

1. Gateley CA, Mansel RE. Management of the painful and nodular breast. *Br Med Bull* 1991; 47,702:284–294.
2. Ader DN, Shriver CD. Cyclical mastalgia: prevalence and impact in an outpatient breast clinic sample. *J Am Coll Surg* 1997;185:466–470.
3. Harding C, Osundeko O, Tetlow L, Faragher EB, Howell A, Bundred NJ. Hormonally-regulated proteins in breast secretions are markers of target organ sensitivity. *Br J Cancer* 2000;2:354–360
4. Maddox PR, Harrison BJ, Mansel RE, Hughes LE. Non-cyclical mastalgia: improved classification and treatment. *Br J Surg* 1989;76:901–904.
5. Kumar S, Mansel RE, Scanlon MF, et al. Altered responses of prolactin, luteinizing hormone and follicle stimulating hormone secretion to thyrotrophin releasing hormone/gonadotrophin releasing hormone stimulation in cyclical mastalgia. *Br J Surg* 1984;71:870–873.
6. Boyd NF, McGuire V, Shannon P, et al. Effect of a low-fat high-carbohydrate diet on symptoms of cyclical mastopathy. *Lancet* 1988;2:128–32.
7. Preece PE, Hanslip JI, Gilbert L, et al. Evening primrose oil (Efamol) for mastalgia. In: Horrobin D, ed. *Clinical uses of essential fatty acids.* Montreal: Eden Press Inc, 1982:147–154.
8. Kontostolis E, Stefanidis K, Navrozoglou I, Lolis D. Comparison of tamoxifen with danazol for treatment of cyclical mastalgia. *Gynecol Endocrinol* 1997;11:393–397.
9. Maddox PR, Harrison BJ, Mansel RE. Low-dose danazol for mastalgia. *Br J Clin Pract* 1989;68: 43–47.
10. Anonymous. Danazol. In: *The ABPI Compendium of Data Sheets and Summaries of Product Characteristics.* London: Datapharm Publications Ltd, 1999–2000:1395.
11. Mansel RE, Dogliotti L. European multicentre trial of bromocriptine in cyclical mastalgia. *Lancet* 1990;335:190–193.
12. Blichert-Toft M, Anderson AN, Henrikson OB, Mygind T. Treatment of mastalgia with bromocriptine: a double blind crossover study. *BMJ* 1979;1:237.
13. Arrowsmith-Lowe T. Bromocriptine indications withdrawn. *FDA Med Bull* 1994;24:2
14. Colacurci N, Mele D, De Franciscis P, Costa V, Fortunato N, De Seta L. Effects of tibolone on the breast. *Eur J Obs Gynae and Rep Bio* 1998;80: 235–238.
15. Fentiman IS, Caleffi M, Brame K, Choudary A, Hayward JL. Double blind controlled trial of Tamoxifen therapy for mastalgia. *Lancet* 1986;1: 287–288.
16. GEMB Group. Tamoxifen therapy for cyclical mastalgia: dose randomised trial. *Breast* 1997;5: 212–213.
17. Fentiman IS, Hamed H, Caleffi M, Choudary MA. Dosage and duration of Tamoxifen treatment for mastalgia: a controlled trial. *Br J Surg* 1988;845–846.
18. Anonymous. Nolvadex. In: *The ABPI Compendium of Data Sheets and Summaries of Product Characteristics.* London: Datapharm Publications Ltd, 1999–2000:1799.
19. Peters F. Multicentre study of gestinone in cyclical breast pain. *Lancet* 1992;339:205–208.
20. Kathleen Parfitt, ed. *Martindale. The complete drug reference,* 32nd ed. London: Pharmaceutical Press, 1999:1447–1448.

N Bundred

Reader in Surgical Oncology and
Consultant Surgeon
University of Manchester
Department of Surgery and
South Manchester University Hospital
Manchester
UK

Competing interests: NB has received reimbursement by AstraZeneca, the maker of Tamoxifen, for attending several conferences and running education programmes. NB has also received support by Serle Pharmaceuticals for attending and speaking at Symposia.

INTERVENTIONS

Key Messages

- One systematic review of RCTs has found that aspirin is more effective for pain relief than placebo but less effective than naproxen and ibuprofen. One RCT found limited evidence that paracetamol/dextropropoxyphene (DPH) is more effective than placebo.

- One systematic review of RCTs found strong evidence that naproxen, ibuprofen, and mefenamic acid are more effective than placebo for pain relief. The review found some evidence of increased adverse effects with naproxen.

- Three small RCTs found insufficient evidence that oral contraceptives are effective for pain relief.

- One small RCT found limited evidence suggesting that laparoscopic uterine nerve ablation (LUNA) was more effective than diagnostic laparoscopy. A second RCT compared LUNA and laparoscopic presacral neurectomy (LPSN) and found no significant difference in pain relief in the short term. However, LPSN was significantly more effective in the long term.

- Small RCTs found that high frequency transcutaneous electrical nerve stimulation and acupuncture achieved more effective pain relief than placebo.

- We found insufficient evidence to determine the effectiveness of behavioural interventions, spinal manipulation, or herbal remedies.

- One large RCT found that vitamin B_1 was more effective than placebo. RCTs evaluating other dietary interventions were too small to provide adequate evidence of effectiveness.

DEFINITION Dysmenorrhoea comprises painful menstrual cramps of uterine origin. It is commonly divided into primary dysmenorrhoea (pain without organic pathology) and secondary dysmenorrhoea (pelvic pain associated with an identifiable pathological condition, such as endometriosis or ovarian cysts). The initial onset of primary dysmenorrhoea is usually shortly after menarche (6–12 months) when ovulatory cycles are established. The pain duration is commonly 8–72 hours and is usually associated with the onset of the menstrual flow. Secondary dysmenorrhoea may arise as a new symptom during a woman's fourth and fifth decades.[1]

INCIDENCE/ PREVALENCE Variations in the definition of dysmenorrhoea make it difficult to determine the precise prevalence. Various types of studies nonetheless consistently demonstrate a high prevalence in women of different ages and nationalities. A recent systematic review of the prevalence of chronic pelvic pain summarising both community and hospital surveys (search date December 1996) estimated the prevalence at 45–95%.[2] Reports focus on adolescent girls and generally include only primary dysmenorrhoea, although this is not always specified. Studies of prevalence are summarised in table 1, p 1056.

AETIOLOGY/ RISK FACTORS A longitudinal study of a representative sample of women born in 1962 found that severity of dysmenorrhoea was significantly associated with duration of menstrual flow (average duration of menstrual flow was 5 days for women with no dysmenorrhoea and 5.8 days for women with severe dysmenorrhoea, $P < 0.001$, WMD −0.8, 95% CI −1.36 to −0.24); younger average menarcheal age (13.1 in women without dysmenorrhoea v 12.6 in women with severe dysmenorrhoea, $P < 0.01$, WMD 0.5, 95% CI 0.09 to 0.91); and cigarette smoking (41% of smokers and 26% of non-smokers experienced moderate or severe dysmenorrhoea).[9]

PROGNOSIS Primary dysmenorrhoea is a chronic recurring condition that affects most young women. Studies of the natural history of this condition are sparse. One longitudinal study in Scandinavia found that primary dysmenorrhoea often improves in the third decade of a woman's reproductive life, and is also reduced following childbirth.[9]

AIMS To relieve pain from dysmenorrhoea, with minimal adverse effects.

OUTCOMES Pain relief, measured either by visual analogue scale, other pain scales, or as a dichotomous outcome (pain relief achieved yes/no); overall improvement in dysmenorrhoea measured by change in dysmenorrhoeic symptoms either self-reported or observed, quality of life scales, or other similar measures such as the Menstrual Distress or Menstrual Symptom questionnaire; adverse effects of treatment (incidence and type of adverse effects); proportion of women requiring analgesics in addition to their assigned treatment; proportion of women reporting activity restriction or absences from work or school, and hours or days of absence as a more selective measure.

METHODS *Clinical Evidence* search and appraisal March 2000.

OPTION   ASPIRIN, PARACETAMOL, AND COMPOUND ANALGESICS

One systematic review of RCTs has found that aspirin is more effective for pain relief than placebo but less effective than naproxen and ibuprofen. One RCT found limited evidence that paracetamol/ dextropropoxyphene (DPH) is more effective than placebo.

Benefits:
We found one systematic review (see table 2, p 1057) of the effects of analgesics in primary dysmenorrhoea (search date 1997, 13 RCTs), which compared analgesics with placebo, each other, or common non-steroidal anti-inflammatory drugs (NSAIDs).[10] **Aspirin versus placebo:** The review identified eight RCTs comparing aspirin with placebo (n = 486, 650 mg four times daily). For the outcome of pain relief, aspirin was significantly better than placebo (5 RCTs, RR 1.60, 95% CI 1.12 to 2.29). There was no significant difference between aspirin and placebo in the need for additional medication (3 RCTs, RR 0.79, 95% CI 0.58 to 1.08), or restriction of daily activity and absence from work (3 RCTs, RR 0.82, 95% CI 0.64 to 1.04; 1 RCT, RR 1.28, 95% CI 0.24 to 6.76). Overall, 10 women need to be treated with aspirin to achieve pain relief in one additional women (NNT 10, 95% CI 5 to 50). **Paracetamol versus placebo:** One RCT comparing paracetamol 500 mg four times daily with placebo found no significant difference in pain relief (n = 35, RR 1.00, 95% CI 0.28 to 3.63). **Paracetamol/DPH versus placebo:** The review identified one placebo controlled RCT, which found that paracetamol/DPH was significantly more effective in achieving marked or moderate pain relief than placebo (n = 72, 650 mg/65 mg four times daily, RR 3.72, 95% CI 2.13 to 6.52). **Paracetamol versus aspirin:** One RCT comparing aspirin and paracetamol (n = 35) found that pain relief from paracetamol was not significantly different from aspirin (using visual analogue scale, the median change from baseline was 1.6, 95% CI 0.4 to 3.3 with paracetamol v 1.2, 95% CI 0 to 2.7 with aspirin). **Aspirin or paracetamol versus NSAIDs:** There were six comparisons of aspirin or paracetamol versus NSAIDs (n = 313). Aspirin 650 mg four times daily was found to be less effective for pain relief than both naproxen 275 mg four times daily (one RCT, RR 2.29, 95% CI 1.16 to 4.29) and ibuprofen 400 mg four times daily (one RCT, RR 1.9, 95% CI 1.13 to 2.78). One RCT found no significant difference in pain relief (defined as at least moderate relief) between paracetamol 1000 mg three times daily and ibuprofen 400 mg three times daily (one RCT, RR 0.86, 95% CI 0.68 to 1.10). **Paracetamol/DPH versus NSAIDs:** The review identified one RCT that compared paracetamol/DPH 650 mg/65 mg three times daily with mefenamic acid 500 mg three times daily. The RCT found that mefenamic acid was significantly better for relief of all dysmenorrhoea related symptoms (P < 0.01). The need for additional medication was also lower in the mefenamic acid group (a mean of 2.6 v 6.8, no P value reported). There was no significant difference between treatments in terms of absence from work or school. Two RCTs (n = 98) compared paracetamol/DPH with naproxen 275 mg three times daily. Neither found a significant difference in pain

severity (P > 0.05), but naproxen achieved better pain control on some of the days measured (P < 0.05).

Harms: The most commonly experienced adverse effects were nausea or abdominal discomfort, headaches, and dizziness. Adverse effects occurred in 7–17% of women taking aspirin and 3–17% of those taking placebo. Aspirin and paracetamol were not significantly different from placebo in terms of adverse effects (RR 1.31, 95% CI 0.79 to 2.17; RR 1.00, 95% CI 0.36 to 2.75). More women taking paracetamol/DPH experienced adverse effects than those taking naproxen (23–58% v 15–25%; RR 1.94, 95% CI 1.11 to 3.41).[10]

Comment: Most RCTs included in the systematic review were short (usually only one menstrual cycle on each treatment), small, and used a crossover design without a washout period. All of the RCTs, except one of paracetamol/DPH versus naproxen, used double blinding. All the RCTs used oral administration of treatment in the form of tablets or capsules.

OPTION   **NON-STEROIDAL ANTI-INFLAMMATORY DRUGS**

One systematic review of RCTs has found strong evidence that naproxen, ibuprofen, and mefenamic acid are all more effective than placebo for pain relief. The RCT found some evidence of increased adverse effects with naproxen.

Benefits: We found one recent systematic review of the effects of NSAIDs in primary dysmenorrhoea (search date March 1997), which included 23 RCTs of naproxen (n = 1728), 18 of ibuprofen (n = 748) and five of mefenamic acid (n = 257).[10] **NSAIDs versus placebo:** The systematic review found that all three NSAIDs provided significant pain relief compared with placebo (naproxen: 13 RCTs, RR 3.17, 95% CI 2.72 to 3.67, NNT 2.6, 95% CI 2 to 3.4; ibuprofen: 9 RCTs, RR 2.41, 95% CI 1.58 to 3.68, NNT 2.4, 95% CI 1.7 to 3.8; mefenamic acid: 3 RCTs, RR 2.03, 95% CI 1.65 to 2.48, NNT 2.4, 95% CI 1.6 to 4.5). The need for additional analgesics was significantly reduced for all NSAIDs when compared with placebo. Women taking naproxen were 60% less likely to require additional analgesics (10 RCTs; RR 0.4, 95% CI 0.3 to 0.4); those taking ibuprofen were 70% less likely (2 RCTs; RR 0.2, 95% CI 0.1 to 0.4); and those on mefenamic acid were 35% less likely (1 RCT; RR 0.7, 95% CI 0.5 to 0.8). Restriction of daily life was significantly less for naproxen (7 RCTs; RR 0.71, 95% CI 0.60 to 0.85) and ibuprofen (3 RCTs; RR 0.82, 95% CI 0.64 to 1.04). Absence from work or school was reduced significantly with naproxen (7 RCTs; RR 0.29, 95% CI 0.13 to 0.66) but not with ibuprofen (1 RCT; RR 0.14, 95% CI 0.02 to 1.10). **Comparison of NSAIDs:** The review identified five comparative RCTs. Three found no significant difference in pain relief between naproxen and ibuprofen (RR 1.1, 95% CI 0.8 to 1.5). One RCT found that naproxen provided more pain relief than mefenamic acid (RR 2.4, 95% CI 1.4 to 4.1), and a comparison of ibuprofen and mefenamic acid found no significant difference between the two treatments (no RR or P values reported).

Harms: The most commonly reported adverse effects were nausea, dizziness, and headaches. Naproxen caused significantly more adverse effects than placebo (RR 1.45, 95% CI 1.03 to 2.04). There was no significant difference in adverse effects with ibuprofen and mefenamic acid compared with placebo (RR 1.12, 95% CI 0.85 to 1.47; RR 0.59, 95% CI 0.28 to 1.23).[10]

Comment: All the RCTs used oral treatment. NSAIDs can be administered as suppositories, which have been shown to have a similar effect on overall pain relief but are less effective than tablets for spasmodic pain (P < 0.05).[11] The majority of the RCTs included in this systematic review used a crossover design without a washout period and were of short duration, usually only one menstrual cycle on each treatment. Nine of the included trials were only single blind. Many of the trials on NSAIDs were sponsored by industry. Pain relief figures used above refer to RCTs that include women with primary dysmenorrhoea only. However, some of the other figures regarding use of additional medication included data from women with undefined dysmenorrhoea. A systematic review with stricter inclusion criteria and methodological quality assessment is in progress (ML Wilson, personal communication, 2000).

OPTION	COMBINED ORAL CONTRACEPTIVES

Three small RCTs found insufficient evidence that oral contraceptives are effective for pain relief.

Benefits: We found no systematic review. We found three placebo controlled RCTs evaluating high dose oestrogen combined oral contraceptives for treatment of primary dysmenorrhoea.[12–14] The first double blind RCT evaluated Norinyl (norethisterone 2 mg and mestranol 0.1 mg). Primary dysmenorrhoea was diagnosed by physical examination and 35/44 women completed the study. Complete or partial pain relief was achieved in 14/17 (82%) receiving treatment compared with 3/18 (17%) on placebo.[12] The second RCT evaluated Sequens (mestranol 0.08 mg taken from day 5 to day 25, and chlormadinone acetate 2 mg added for the last 5 days). Only 29 women completed the trial. Pain relief was significantly higher with treatment compared with placebo (P < 0.02; further data extraction was not possible as the data were presented in graphic form).[13] The third RCT (n = 28) evaluated an oral contraceptive pill (OCP) comprising 0.05 mg ethinyl oestradiol and 0.5 mg norgestrel taken from day 5 to day 25 of the cycle, for 3–6 months. This RCT found pain relief was much better in the OCP group when the number of menstrual cycles with relief across the entire trial was compared (22/44 treated menstrual cycles with complete pain relief versus 1/31 placebo treated menstrual cycles, P < 0.05).[13] However, if the average number of women with pain relief was reported, there was no significant difference due to the small number of women in the trial (5/11 v 0/7; OR 12.69, 95% CI 0.58 to 27).

Harms: No adverse effects were reported, although in the third trial 2/18 women receiving the OCP reported breakthrough bleeding.[13]

Comment: All three RCTs evaluated oral contraceptives that are either banned or no longer commonly prescribed. All the RCTs were of poor methodological quality. A Cochrane systematic review is currently in progress (ML Wilson, personal communication, 2000).

QUESTION What are the effects of surgical treatments?

One small RCT found limited evidence suggesting that laparoscopic uterine nerve ablation (LUNA) was more effective than diagnostic laparoscopy. A second RCT compared LUNA and laparoscopic presacral neurectomy (LPSN) and found no significant difference in pain relief in the short term. However, LPSN was significantly more effective in the long term.

Benefits: We found one systematic review of surgical pelvic nerve interruption for primary and secondary dysmenorrhoea (6 RCTs, search date December 1998).[15] Only two of the six RCTs included women with primary dysmenorrhoea. Meta-analysis was not possible because of trial heterogeneity. One trial (21 women) compared LUNA with diagnostic laparoscopy as a control. There was a significant difference in pain relief in favour of LUNA at 3 months (OR 15.5, 95% CI 2.91 to 82.7) and at 12 months (OR 10.9, 95% CI 1.5 to 77.4). The other trial (68 women) compared LUNA with LPSN. There was no significant difference in pain relief between the two treatments at 3 months follow up (OR 0.7, 95% CI 0.2 to 2.7). However, at 12 months follow up, the LPSN group had significantly better pain relief scores (OR 0.26, 95% CI 0.10 to 0.71).

Harms: Adverse effects were more common with LPSN than with LUNA. Constipation occurred in 94% of women receiving LPSN compared with 0% receiving LUNA (OR 0.02, 95% CI 0.01 to 0.06).

Comment: Two larger trials of LUNA are currently in progress, and data will be included in an update of the systematic review. We found a second relevant systematic review, but have not included it in this chapter because it includes lower levels of evidence, such as case studies.[16]

QUESTION What are the effects of complementary treatments?

OPTION TRANSCUTANEOUS ELECTRICAL NERVE STIMULATION

Two small RCTs found that high frequency transcutaneous electrical nerve stimulation (TENS) (see glossary, p 1054) was more effective than placebo for pain relief.

Benefits: We found no systematic review but found three small RCTs with a total of 71 participants.[17–19] **High frequency TENS versus placebo:** For pain relief, high frequency TENS was found to be more effective than placebo in two RCTs.[18,19] In one double blind trial, 14/32 women experienced at least moderate pain relief in the TENS group compared with 1/32 in the placebo group (OR 24, 95% CI 2.9 to 199). A single blind trial had nine women in each group: the mean decrease in pain was 72% with treatment and 26% with placebo (WMD 45, 95% CI 23 to 67). **Low frequency TENS versus placebo:** The third RCT (n = 18) found no significant benefit from low frequency TENS compared with placebo (WMD 24, 95% CI –2.9 to +51).[18] **High frequency TENS versus low frequency TENS:** One RCT found no significant difference between high frequency and low frequency TENS for pain relief (WMD 21, 95% CI

4.4 to 46).[18] **High frequency TENS versus NSAIDs:** One unblinded RCT found that high frequency TENS was less effective than ibuprofen, with 14/32 women experiencing pain relief compared with 24/32 using ibuprofen (OR 0.26, 95% CI 0.09 to 0.75)[17]. Naproxen and high frequency/high intensity TENS were both shown to significantly reduce pain in a unblinded crossover trial of 12 women (P < 0.001), but were not significantly different from each other (data were presented in graphic form but no OR or P values were reported).[19]

Harms:
Adverse effects of muscle vibrations, tightness, headaches, and slight burning or redness after use were experienced by four women on treatment and none on placebo (OR 10, 95% CI 0.5 to 199, P = 0.12).[17] In the unblinded crossover trial, 10/12 women considered TENS to be temporarily painful but were prepared to accept this effect for the pain relief achieved. None of the 12 women reported any adverse effects during treatment with naproxen.[19]

Comment:
A systematic review is currently underway (ML Wilson, personal communication, 2000).

OPTION ACUPUNCTURE

One small RCT found that acupuncture achieved more effective pain relief than placebo.

Benefits:
We found no systematic review. We found one RCT (n = 48) comparing acupuncture, placebo acupuncture (see glossary, p 1054), and two no-treatment control groups, one of which had extra visits with a physician.[20] Treatment was for 30–40 minutes once a week for 3 weeks a month, for a total of 3 months. The proportion of women showing improvement in pain was significantly higher in the acupuncture group compared with all other groups ($\chi^2 = 13.6$, P < 0.001). Acupuncture was significantly more effective than placebo acupuncture in achieving pain relief (OR 17.5, 95% CI 1.6 to 192).

Harms:
The trial did not report on adverse effects.

Comment:
A systematic review is currently underway (ML Wilson, personal communication, 2000).

OPTION BEHAVIOURAL INTERVENTIONS

We found insufficient evidence of the effectiveness of behavioural interventions (see glossary, p 1054).

Benefits:
We found no systematic review. We found two small RCTs on behaviour therapy. One involved relaxation and imagery,[21] the other aerobic exercise.[22] **Relaxation therapy:** The first trial included 69 women divided into three groups. The treatment group used muscle relaxation combined with positive imagery regarding menstruation. A pseudo treatment group included self-directed group discussion about menstruation, and the third group was a waiting list control group. The groups were also divided into women with spasmodic or congestive dysmenorrhoea using the Menstrual Symptom Questionnaire. Spasmodic dysmenorrhoea was defined as spasms of

pain mainly around the abdomen, and congestive dysmenorrhoea was defined as a dull aching pain in the lower abdomen and other areas of the body. The muscle relaxation group had significantly more pain and symptom relief than the waiting list controls ($P < 0.01$). However, only the women with spasmodic dysmenorrhoea had significantly more relief with relaxation than with all treatments ($P < 0.001$).[21] **Aerobic exercise:** The second trial had a training group that participated in 30 minutes of exercise 3 days a week and a sedentary control group. Results for the 26 women who completed the study showed that during the menstrual phase, the training group had significantly lower Menstrual Distress Questionnaire scores than controls ($P < 0.05$). Data were presented in a graph, making further data extraction impossible.

Harms: The trials did not report on adverse effects.

Comment: Both RCTs were small and of poor methodological quality. The classification of dysmenorrhoea into spasmodic and congestive categories is no longer commonly used and has little meaning. A systematic review is in progress (ML Wilson, personal communication, 2000).

OPTION   SPINAL MANIPULATION

One RCT found no evidence that spinal manipulation was effective in pain relief.

Benefits: We found no systematic review. We found one RCT in 138 women randomised either to spinal manipulative therapy or a low-force mimic manoeuvre used as a control.[23] The RCT found no significant differences in visual analogue pain scores between the two groups after two treatment cycles. The mean change in pain score from baseline in treatment group was 10.1 (95% CI 6.5 to 13.7) v 8.01 (95% CI 4.17 to 11.85) in the control group. There was also no significant difference between pre- and post-intervention pain scores after four treatment cycles ($P = 0.29$).

Harms: Soreness in the lower back region within 48 hours of the intervention occurred in 2/69 women in the control group and 3/69 in the treatment group. Soreness resolved within 24 hours. No other adverse effects were reported.

Comment: The RCT's overall methodological quality was good; low withdrawal rate (2%), adequate randomisation method, blinding of the outcome assessor, and potential blinding of the participants as the control procedure was very similar to the treatment.

OPTION   HERBAL REMEDIES

We found insufficient evidence to determine the effectiveness of herbal remedies.

Benefits: We found no systematic review. We found one trial (n = 40) comparing the Japanese herbal remedy toki-shakuyaku-san (taken three times daily for 6 months) versus a placebo remedy.[24] Pain relief using a visual analogue scale was significantly better in the treatment group ($P < 0.005$). The requirement for additional medication (diclofenac sodium) was also significantly less in the treatment group (P < 0.01). The data were presented in a graph, making further data extraction impossible.

Harms: The trials did not report on adverse affects.

Comment: Toki-shakuyaku-san is a mixture of six herbs, including angelica and peony root.

| OPTION | DIETARY SUPPLEMENTS |

One large RCT found vitamin B$_1$ to be more effective than placebo. RCTs of other dietary remedies were too small to provide evidence of effectiveness.

Benefits: We found no systematic review. We found four RCTs on four different treatments: magnesium, vitamin B$_1$, vitamin E/ibuprofen, and fish oil (an omega-3 fatty acid comprised of vitamin E, eicosapentaenoic acid, and docosapantaenoic acid). **Magnesium versus placebo:** One RCT (n = 50) evaluated magnesium aspartate taken three times daily.[25] After 6 months magnesium was significantly better than placebo in achieving pain relief (no pain in 21/25 on magnesium v no pain in 7/25 on placebo, RR 3.0, 95% CI 1.6 to 5.8, NNT 1.8). **Vitamin B versus placebo:** One RCT (n = 556) evaluated thiamine hydrochloride 100 mg daily for 3 months.[26] After 60 days, prior to crossover, the treatment group had significantly more pain relief than the placebo group (no pain in 142/277 on treatment v no pain in 0/279 on placebo; RR 287, CI 95% 18 to 4589; NNT 2). After completion of the trial, 87% of all participants experienced no pain. **Vitamin E plus ibuprofen versus ibuprofen:** One crossover RCT in 50 women evaluated vitamin E 100 mg daily for 20 days prior to menses, then ibuprofen 400 mg at the outset of painful menstruation. The comparison was ibuprofen 400 mg at the onset of pain.[27] Women were treated over two cycles, with treatments crossed over after one cycle. Pain relief was more effective with combined vitamin E/ibuprofen, but the confidence intervals were wide (cycle 1: no pain in 23/26 women on combined treatment v 17/24 on ibuprofen alone, OR 3.2, 95% CI 0.7 to 14; cycle 2: no pain in 17/20 women on combined treatment v 16/22 women on ibuprofen alone, OR 2.1, 95% CI 0.5 to 10). **Fish oil versus placebo:** One RCT in 42 women compared taking fish oil capsules twice daily versus placebo for 1 month.[28] Menstrual symptom scores were significantly lower with fish oil than placebo (44 v 70, P < 0.001). Less additional medication (ibuprofen 200 mg) was consumed in the fish oil group (mean 4.7 tablets with treatment v 10.1 with placebo, P = 0.015).

Harms: Circulation problems and intestinal discomfort were experienced by 5/25 women taking magnesium compared with 0/25 taking placebo, although relief of these symptoms occurred when the dose was reduced from three to two tablets daily. In the fish oil group, 2/42 women reported nausea and 1/42 participants reported acne.

Comment: The trial of vitamin B$_1$ used double blinding and was of good methodological quality.

Women's health

GLOSSARY

Behavioural interventions Treatments that attempt modification of thought and beliefs (cognition) about symptoms and pain and/or modification of behavioural or physiological responses to symptoms and pain.

Placebo acupuncture Also known as sham acupuncture, a commonly used control intervention involving the use of acupuncture needles to stimulate non-acupuncture points not located on Chinese meridians. These points can be identified by a point detector as areas of the skin that do not have skin electrical activity similar to acupuncture points. There is some disagreement over correct needle placement, as placement of a needle in any position may elicit some biological response that can complicate interpretation of results.

Transcutaneous electrical nerve stimulation Electrodes are placed on the skin and different electrical pulse rates and intensities are used to stimulate the areas. Low frequency TENS (also referred to as acupuncture-like TENS) usually consists of pulses delivered at 1–4 Hz at high intensity so they evoke visible muscle fibre contractions. High frequency TENS (conventional TENS) usually consists of pulses delivered at 50–120 Hz at a low intensity, so there are no muscle contractions.

REFERENCES

1. Fraser I. Prostaglandins, prostaglandin inhibitors and their roles in gynaecological disorders. *Bailliere's Clinical Obstet Gynaecol* 1992;6:829–857.
2. Zondervan KT, Yudkin PL, Vessey MP, et al. The prevalence of chronic pelvic pain in the United Kingdom: a systematic review. *Br J Obstet Gynaecol* 1998;105:93–99. Search date December 1996; primary sources Medline from 1966, Embase from 1980, Psychlit from 1974.
3. Harlow SD, Park M. A longitudinal study of risk factors for the occurrence, duration and severity of menstrual cramps in a cohort of college women. *Br J Obstet Gynaecol* 1996;103:1134–1142.
4. Campbell MA, McGrath PJ. Use of medication by adolescents for the management of menstrual discomfort. *Arch Pediatr Adolesc Med* 1997;151:905–913.
5. Robinson JC, Plichta S, Weisman CS, et al. Dysmenorrhoea and the use of oral contraceptives in adolescent women attending a family planning clinic. *Am J Obstet Gynecol* 1992;166:578–583.
6. Andersch B, Milsom I. An epidemiologic study of young women with dysmenorrhea. *Am J Obstet Gynecol* 1982;144:655–660.
7. Pedron Neuvo N, Gonzalez-Unzaga LN, De Celis-Carrillo R, et al. Incidence of dysmenorrhea and associated symptoms in women aged 12–24 years. *Ginecologia y Obstetrica de Mexico* 1998;66:492–494.
8. Klein JR, Litt IF. Epidemiology of adolescent dysmenorrhea. *Pediatrics* 1981;68(5):661–664.
9. Sundell G, Milsom I, Andersch B. Factors influencing the prevalence and severity of dysmenorrhoea in young women. *Br J Obstet Gynaecol* 1990;97:588–594.
10. Zhang WY, LiWanPo A. Efficacy of minor analgesics in primary dysmenorrhoea: a systematic review. *Br J Obstet Gynaecol* 1998;105:780–789. Search date March 1997; primary sources Medline, Embase and Science Citation Index 1966–1997.
11. Ylikorkala O, Puolakka J, Kauppila A. Comparison between naproxen tablets and suppositories in primary dysmenorrhea. *Prostaglandins* 1980;20:463–438.
12. Kremser E, Mitchell GM. Treatment of primary dysmenorrhoea with a combined type oral contraceptive — a double blind study. *J Am Coll Health* 1971;19:195–196.
13. Nakano R, Takemura H. Treatment of function

dysmenorrhoea: a double-blind study. *Acta Obstet Gynaecol Jpn* 1971;18:41–44.
14. Matthews AE, Clarke JE. Double-blind trial of a sequential oral contraceptive (Sequens) in the treatment of dysmenorrhoea. *J Obstet Gynaecol Br Commonw* 1968;75:1117–1122.
15. Wilson ML, Farquhar CM, Sinclair OJ, et al. Surgical interruption of pelvic nerve pathways for primary and secondary dysmenorrhoea. In: The Cochrane Library, Issue 1, 2000. Oxford: Update Software. Search date December 1998; primary sources Medline 1966–December 1998, Embase 1980–December 1998, Cochrane Controlled Trials Register 1966–December 1998, hand-searched citation lists and conference proceedings.
16. Khan KS, Khan SF, Nwosu CR, et al. Laparoscopic uterosacral nerve ablation in chronic pelvic pain: an overview. *Gynaecol Endosc* 1999;8:257–265. Search date 1997; primary sources Medline 1966–1997; Embase 1980–1997, Science Citation Index.
17. Dawood MY, Ramos J. Transcutaneous electrical nerve stimulation (TENS) for the treatment of primary dysmenorrhea: a randomized crossover comparison with placebo TENS and ibuprofen. *Obstet Gynecol* 1990;75:656–660.
18. Mannheimer JS, Whalen EC. The efficacy of transcutaneous electrical nerve stimulation in dysmenorrhea. *Clin J Pain* 1985;1:75–83.
19. Hedner N, Milsom I, Eliasson T, et al. Tens bra vid smatsam mens. [TENS is effective in painful menstruation.] *Lakartidningen* 1996;93:1219–1222 (in Swedish).
20. Helms JM. Acupuncture for the management of primary dysmenorrhea. *Obstet Gynecol* 1987;69:51–56.
21. Chesney MA, Tasto DL. The effectiveness of behavior modification with spasmodic and congestive dysmenorrhea. *Behav Res Ther* 1975;13:245–253.
22. Israel RG, Sutton M, O'Brien KF. Effects of aerobic training on primary dysmenorrhea symptomatology in college females. *J Am Coll Health* 1985;33:241–244.
23. Hondras MA, Long CR, Brennan PC. Spinal manipulation therapy versus a low force mimic maneuver for women with primary dysmenorrhea: a randomized, observer-blinded clinical trial. *Pain* 1999;81:105–114.
24. Kotani N, Oyama T, Sakai I, et al. Analgesic effect

of a herbal medicine for treatment of primary dysmenorrhea — a double-blind study. *Am J Chin Med* 1997;25s:205–212.

25. Seifert B, Wagler P, Dartsch S, et al. Magnesium — a new therapeutic alternative in primary dysmenorrhea. *Zentralbl Gynakol* 1989;111: 755–60 (in German).

26. Gokhale LB. Curative treatment of primary (spasmodic) dysmenorrhoea. *Indian J Med Res* 1996;103:227–231.

27. De Roldan MES, Ruiz-Castro S. Primary dysmenorrhea treatment with ibuprofen and vitamin E. *Rev Obstet Ginecol Venez* 1993;53: 35–37 (in Spanish).

28. Harel Z, Biro FM, Kottenhahn RK, et ak. Supplementation with omega-3 polyunsaturated fatty acids in the management of dysmenorrhea in adolescents. *Am J Obstet Gynecol* 1996;174(4): 1335–1338.

Michelle Wilson

Cynthia Farquhar
Associate Professor

School of Medicine
University of Auckland
Auckland
New Zealand

Competing interests: None declared.

TABLE 1 Prevalence of dysmenorrhoea: results of community and hospital surveys (see text, p 1046).[3-8]

Study population	Population size	Location	Year	Prevalence
College students aged 17–19 years[3]	165	USA	1996	72% (13% severe)
High school students aged 14–21 years[4]	291	Canada	1997	93% (5% severe)
Adolescents attending an inner city family planning clinic[5]	308	USA	1992	80% (18% severe)
Women from an urban population aged 19 years[6]	596	Sweden	1982	73% (15% severe)
Students aged 12–24 years[7]	1066	Mexico	1998	52–64%
Adolescents aged 12–17 years[8]	2699	USA	1981	60% (14% severe)

TABLE 2   Effects of aspirin, paracetamol, and compound analgesics for dysmenorrhoea: results of a systematic review of RCTs (see text).[10]

Comparison	Usual dosage	Number of RCTs	Number of women	Pain relief	Adverse effects	Conclusion
Aspirin v placebo	650 mg four times daily	8	486	RR 1.60 (95% CI 1.12 to 2.29)	More frequent on aspirin (7–17% v 3–17% on placebo, RR 1.3, 95% CI 0.79 to 2.17)	Aspirin more effective than placebo (NNT 10, 95% CI 5 to 50)
Aspirin v paracetamol	650 mg v 500 mg four times daily	1	35	Median pain relief: paracetamol 1.6 (95% CI 0.4 to 3.3), aspirin 1.2 (95% CI 0 to 2.7)		No significant difference
Aspirin v naproxen	650 mg v 275 mg four times daily	1	32	RR 2.29 (95% CI 1.16 to 4.29)		Naproxen more effective than aspirin
Aspirin v ibuprofen	650 mg v 400 mg four times daily	1	56	RR 1.9 (95% CI 1.13 to 2.78)		Ibuprofen more effective than placebo
Paracetamol v placebo	500 mg four times daily	1	35	RR 1.00 (95% CI 0.28 to 3.63)	No significant difference (RR 1.00, 95% CI 0.36 to 2.75)	No significant difference
Paracetamol v ibuprofen	1000 mg v 400 mg three times daily	1	67	RR 0.86 (95% CI 0.68 to 1.10)		No significant difference
Paracetamol/DPH v placebo	650 mg/65 mg four times daily	1	72	RR 3.72 (95% CI 2.13 to 6.52)		Paracetamol/DPH more effective than placebo
Paracetamol/DPH v naproxen	650 mg/65 mg v 275 mg three times daily	2	98	P > 0.05 (no other data could be obtained from the report)	More frequent on paracetamol/DPH (23–58% v 15–25% on naproxen, RR 1.94, 95% CI 1.11 to 3.41)	No significant difference
Paracetamol/DPH v mefenamic acid	650 mg/65 mg v 500 mg three times daily	1	30	P < 0.01 (no other evidence can be obtained from the trial)		Mefenamic acid more effective than paracetamol/DPH

DPH; dextropropoxyphene.

Women's health

Updated this issue

Cynthia Farquhar

Key Messages

Hormonal treatment at diagnosis

■ Four small systematic reviews found that all hormonal treatments, except dydrogesterone, reduced pain attributed to endometriosis compared with placebo, and were equally effective. One systematic review of small RCTs found no evidence that hormonal treatments improved fertility. Adverse effects of hormonal treatment were common.

Surgical treatment

■ We found insufficient evidence on the effects of laparoscopic uterine nerve ablation (LUNA) in women with pain attributed to endometriosis.

■ We found insufficient evidence on the effects of laparoscopic ablation of deposits on its own. One RCT found that combined treatment with ablation of deposits plus LUNA reduced pain more than diagnostic laparoscopy at 6 months. One RCT found that laparoscopic surgery increased fertility compared with diagnostic laparoscopy, a subsequent smaller RCT found no significant difference.

- We found no RCTs comparing medical and surgical treatments.

Postoperative hormonal treatment

- RCTs found that 6 months' postoperative hormonal treatment significantly reduced pain and delayed the recurrence of pain compared with placebo; treatment for 3 months did not seem to be effective. RCTs found no evidence of an effect of postoperative hormonal treatment on fertility. Adverse effects of hormonal treatment were common.

Preoperative treatment

- One RCT found no evidence that preoperative treatment with GnRH analogues facilitated surgery.

Endometrioma

- One RCT found that pain and subfertility caused by ovarian endometrioma were improved more by cystectomy than drainage. Complication rates were similar.

DEFINITION	Endometriosis is characterised by ectopic endometrial tissue, which can cause dysmenorrhoea, dyspareunia, non-cyclical pelvic pain, and subfertility. Diagnosis is made by laparoscopy. Most endometrial deposits are found in the pelvis (ovaries, peritoneum, uterosacral ligaments, pouch of Douglas, and rectovaginal septum). Extrapelvic deposits, including those in the umbilicus and diaphragm, are rare. Severity of endometriosis is defined by the American Fertility Society: this review uses the terms mild (stage I and II), moderate (stage III), and severe (stage IV).[1] Endometriomas are cysts of endometriosis within the ovary.
INCIDENCE/ PREVALENCE	In asymptomatic women, the prevalence of endometriosis ranges from 2–22%, depending on the diagnostic criteria used and the populations studied.[2–5] In women with dysmenorrhoea, the incidence of endometriosis ranges from 40–60%, and in women with subfertility from 20–30%.[3,6,7] The severity of symptoms and the probability of diagnosis increase with age.[8] Incidence peaks at about age 40.[9] Symptoms and laparoscopic appearance do not always correlate.[10]
AETIOLOGY/ RISK FACTORS	The cause of endometriosis is unknown. Risk factors include early menarche and late menopause. Embryonic cells may give rise to deposits in the umbilicus, whereas retrograde menstruation may deposit endometrial cells in the diaphragm.[11,12] Use of oral contraceptives reduces the risk of endometriosis, and this protective effect persists for up to one year after their discontinuation.[9]
PROGNOSIS	We found one small RCT in which laparoscopy was repeated in the women treated with placebo. Over 12 months, endometrial deposits resolved spontaneously in one quarter, deteriorated in nearly half, and were unchanged in the remainder.[13]
AIMS	To relieve pain (dysmenorrhoea, dyspareunia, and other pelvic pain) and to improve fertility, with minimal adverse effects.

OUTCOMES American Fertility Society scores for size and number of deposits;[1] recurrence rates; time between stopping treatment and recurrence; rate of adverse effects of treatment. **In women with pain:** relief of pain, assessed by visual analogue scale ranging from 0–10, and subjective improvement. **In women with subfertility:** cumulative pregnancy rate, live birth rate. **In women undergoing surgery:** ease of surgical intervention (rated as easy, average, difficult, or very difficult).[14]

METHODS *Clinical Evidence* update search and appraisal for systematic reviews May 2000. We sought RCTs by electronic searching of databases, hand searching of 30 key journals, searching the reference lists of other RCTs, and identifying unpublished studies from abstracts, proceedings, and pharmaceutical companies. We used the search strategy and database of the Cochrane Menstrual Disorders and Subfertility Group to identify RCTs on Medline and Embase. We included RCTs that used adequate diagnostic criteria for inclusion of participants (endometriosis diagnosed either by laparoscopy or laparotomy in association with dysmenorrhoea, dyspareunia, other pelvic pain, or infertility) and clinical outcomes (see outcomes above). Studies of assisted reproductive technologies were not included. Trials comparing different hormonal treatments of the same class were not included.

QUESTION What are the effects of hormonal treatments at diagnosis?

Four small systematic reviews found that all hormonal treatments except dydrogesterone reduced pain attributed to endometriosis compared with placebo, and were equally effective. One systematic review of small RCTs found no evidence that hormonal treatments improved fertility. Adverse effects of hormonal treatments were common.

Benefits: **In women with pain attributed to endometriosis:** We found four systematic reviews (search dates 1998, 1996, 1997, 1997) evaluating 6 months' continuous ovulation suppression using danazol, gestrinone, depot medroxyprogesterone acetate (DMPA), dydrogesterone, oral contraceptives, or GnRH analogues.[15–18] The systematic reviews found that all treatments were equally effective at reducing severe and moderate pain at 6 months, except dydrogesterone which, given at two different dosages in the luteal phase, showed no evidence of effect. The first systematic review (search date 1998) of seven RCTs comparing danazol with GnRH analogues (nearly 400 women) found no significant difference in reduction of pain or in resolution of endometrial deposits after 6 months' treatment.[15] The second systematic review[16] included one RCT (269 women) that compared danazol (200 mg a day) with gestrinone (2.5 mg twice a week). It found no difference in pain reduction.[19] The first systematic review[15] included one RCT (49 women) that compared combined oral contraceptives (COC) with GnRH analogues.[20] It found no significant differences in rate of relief for all types of pain except menstrual pain, for which oral contraceptives were better. A subsequent RCT (102 women) compared 12 months of COC versus 4 months of COC, *versus* 8 months of GnRH analogues. At 12 months, no difference was found in pain reduction (either menstrual or non menstrual).[21] The second systematic review included two RCTs of DMPA (140 women).[16] The larger RCT (80 women) compared DMPA (150 mg every 3 months) with COC plus danazol (50 mg a day). It found DMPA was more effective at reducing dysmenorrhoea but not for any other outcomes. **In women with subfertility attributed to endometriosis:** We found one systematic review (search date 1996, 4 RCTs), in 244 women with "visually diagnosed" endometriosis attempting conception for more than 12 months.[22] The trials evaluated 6 months' treatment with danazol, medroxyprogesterone, or GnRH analogues versus placebo. They found no evidence of an effect on the likelihood with danazol of pregnancy (OR for pregnancy compared with placebo RR 0.90, 95% CI 0.66 to 1.21).

Harms: **GnRH analogues:** The first systematic review found that GnRH analogues were associated with more hot flushes than placebo (approximately 80% v 30%).[15] Headaches were also more frequent with GnRH analogues compared with placebo (33% v 10%). GnRH analogues are associated with hypo-oestrogenic symptoms, such as hot flushes and vaginal dryness. RCTs have found that adding oestrogen, progesterone, or tibolone significantly relieves hot flushes caused by GnRH analogues (reducing symptom scores by 50% or more).[14,23,24] **Danazol:** In one trial of 6 months' postoperative danazol, (100 mg a day) versus no treatment, more adverse effects were associated with danazol; spotting (12% v 7%), bloating (16% v 9%), headache (21% v 13%), and weight gain (22% v 14%) (see postoperative hormonal treatment, p 1062).[25] **Gestrinone:** One trial found a significantly higher frequency of hot flushes versus GnRH analogues; other trials found greater frequency of greasy skin and hirsutism compared with danazol, but less reduction in breast size, muscle cramps, and hunger.[16] **Medroxyprogesterone:** The trials gave no information on adverse effects of medroxyprogesterone. One trial found more adverse events with DMPA versus danazol plus COC; amennorrhoea (20% v 0%); breakthrough bleeding (15% v 0%); spotting (65% v 10%); bloating (63% v 28%); and weight gain (53% v 30%).[26]

Comment: The trials were mainly small with no long term follow up. No summary statistics could be calculated because the trials compared different drugs versus placebo or no treatment. Trials comparing different hormonal treatments of the same class were not included.

QUESTION What are the effects of surgical treatments?

OPTION LAPAROSCOPIC UTERINE NERVE ABLATION (LUNA)

We found insufficient evidence on the effects of LUNA in women with pain attributed to endometriosis.

Benefits: We found one systematic review (search date 1998, 2 RCTs) in 132 women with endometriosis, stages I–III, age range 18–40 years.[27] It found no significant difference in pain relief between women treated with LUNA and those who were not. The largest trial (81 women) found that satisfaction with treatment was high in both groups (73% v 68%).

Harms: The trials gave no information on adverse effects. Potential harms include denervation of pelvic structures and uterine prolapse.[27]

Comment: The trials may have been too small to exclude a significant effect.[27]

OPTION LAPAROSCOPIC ABLATION OF ENDOMETRIAL DEPOSITS

We found insufficient evidence on the effects of laparoscopic ablation of deposits alone. One RCT found that combined treatment with ablation of deposits plus LUNA reduced pain more than diagnostic laparoscopy at 6 months. One RCT found that laparoscopic surgery increased fertility compared with diagnostic laparoscopy, another smaller RCT found no significant difference.

Benefits: We found no systematic review. **In women with pain attributed to endometriosis:** We found no RCTs evaluating laparoscopic ablation of deposits alone. We found one RCT (63 women with mild to moderate endometriosis) comparing ablation of deposits plus LUNA versus diagnostic laparoscopy.[28,29] It found that ablation plus LUNA reduced pain at 6 months (median decrease in pain score 2.85 for ablation v 0.05 for diagnostic laparoscopy; P = 0.01). **In women with subfertility attributed to endometriosis:** We found two RCTs in women with subfertility attributed to mild or moderate endometriosis of laparoscopic ablation/excision of mild to moderate endometriotic deposits versus diagnostic laparoscopy.[30,31] In the larger study (341 women) laparoscopic surgery increased cumulative pregnancy rates (RR of pregnancy after 36 weeks 1.7, 95% CI 1.2 to 2.6; NNT 8). A more recent RCT[30] (101 women) did not find a significant difference in pregnancy rates at the end of 12 months follow up (OR 0.75, 95% CI 0.31 to 1.88). When the results of the studies were combined, the difference was not significant (OR 1.56, 95% CI 1.01 to 2.43), but the studies did have different lengths of follow up.[31] **Laser versus diathermy ablation:** We found no RCTs.

Harms: The trials gave no information on adverse effects.[28–31] Potential harms include adhesions, reduced fertility, and damage to other pelvic structures.

Comment: Further RCTs of ablation alone versus ablation plus LUNA are under way, (Sutton C, Dover R, personal communication, 1998). A systematic review of laser versus diathermy ablation is planned, (C Farquhar, N Johnson, personal communication, 1999).

QUESTION What are the effects of postoperative hormonal treatment?

RCTs found that 6 months' postoperative hormonal treatment significantly reduced pain and delayed the recurrence of pain compared with placebo; treatment for 3 months did not seem to be effective. RCTs found no evidence of an effect of postoperative hormonal treatment on fertility. Adverse effects of hormonal treatment were common.

Benefits: We found no systematic review. We found six placebo controlled RCTs of medical treatment in 443 women who had undergone surgery for endometriosis (GnRH analogues in 3 trials; danazol in 2 trials; and 1 trial comparing danazol versus DMPA versus expectant management).[22,30-32] **Pain relief:** One RCT (77 women) compared danazol (600 mg a day) for 3 months with placebo after surgery in moderate to severe endometriosis. It found no significant difference in pain relief 6 months after finishing treatment.[33] A second RCT compared danazol (100 mg a day) for 6 months with expectant management in 28 women with moderate endometriosis who had undergone conservative surgery followed by monthly injections of decapeptyl for 6 months.[25] Danazol significantly reduced pain at both 12 months ($P < 0.01$) and 24 months ($P < 0.05$). Overall recurrence at 24 months was 44% with danazol versus 67% with expectant management. A third RCT in 60 women with mild to severe endometriosis found that postoperative danazol (600 mg a day) or medroxyprogesterone (100 mg a day) for 180 days reduced pain more than placebo at 6 months.[34] Three trials assessed GnRH analogues. The smallest of these (75 women with endometriosis stages I and II) evaluated 3 months' treatment and found no difference in pain relief at follow up;[32] the two larger trials (109 women and 269 women with mild to moderate symptomatic endometriosis) evaluated 6 months' treatment and found that GnRH analogues significantly reduced pain scores ($P = 0.008$) and delayed the recurrence of pain by more than 12 months.[35,36] **Fertility:** Three of the trials (28, 75, and 269 women, all stages of endometriosis) looked at effects of postoperative hormonal treatment on fertility and found no difference in pregnancy rates or time to conception compared with placebo.[25,32,36]

Harms: See harms of hormonal treatments, p 1061.

Comment: The trials were mainly small with no long term follow up. No summary statistics could be calculated because the trials compared different drugs with placebo or no treatment.

QUESTION   **What are the effects of preoperative hormonal treatment?**

One RCT found no evidence that preoperative treatment with GnRH analogues facilitated surgery.

Benefits: We found no systematic review. We found one RCT in 75 women with moderate or severe endometriosis comparing 3 months' preoperative treatment with a GnRH analogue versus no treatment.[37] It found no significant difference in ease of surgery between the two groups, although more women with preoperative hormonal treatment were appraised as easy to treat by the surgeon (56% v 36%).

Harms: See harms of hormonal treatments, p 1061.

Comment: The trial may have been too small to exclude a clinically significant effect.

Endometriosis

QUESTION	What are the effects of treatments for ovarian endometrioma?

OPTION	LAPAROSCOPIC DRAINAGE VERSUS LAPAROSCOPIC CYSTECTOMY

One RCT found that pain and fertility improved more with cystectomy versus drainage; there was no evidence of a difference in complication rates.

Benefits:
We found no systematic review. We found one RCT (64 women) comparing laparoscopic cystectomy versus laparoscopic drainage.[38] **In women with pain attributed to endometrioma:** Cystectomy versus drainage reduced recurrence of pain at 2 years (OR 0.2, 95% CI 0.05 to 0.77) and increased the pain free interval after operation (median interval 19 months v 9.5 months, P < 0.05). **In women with subfertility attributed to endometrioma:** Compared with drainage, cystectomy increased the pregnancy rate (67% v 24%; OR 8.25, 95% CI 1.15 to 59).

Harms:
The trial reported no intraoperative or postoperative complications in either group.

Comment:
None.

Substantive changes since last issue

Hormonal treatments at diagnosis New RCT comparing COC versus GnRH; conclusion unchanged.
Laparoscopic ablation of deposits New RCT; conclusion unchanged.

REFERENCES

1. American Fertility Society. Revised American Fertility Society (RAFS) classification of endometriosis. *Fertil Steril* 1985;43:351–352.
2. Mahmood TA, Templeton A. Prevalence and genesis of endometriosis. *Hum Reprod* 1991;6: 544–549.
3. Gruppo Italiano per lo studio dell'endometriosi. Prevalence and anatomical distribution of endometriosis in women with selected gynaecological conditions: results from a multicentric Italian study. *Hum Reprod* 1994;9: 1158–1162.
4. Moen MH, Schei B. Epidemiology of endometriosis in a Norwegian County. *Acta Obstet Gynecol Scand* 1997;76:559–562.
5. Eskenazi B, Warner ML. Epidemiology of endometriosis. *Obstet Gynecol Clin North Am* 1997;24:235–258.
6. Ajossa S, Mais V, Guerriero S, et al. The prevalence of endometriosis in premenopausal women undergoing gynecological surgery. *Clin Exp Obstet Gynecol* 1994;21:195–197.
7. Waller KG, Lindsay P, Curtis P, et al. The prevalence of endometriosis in women with infertile partners. *Eur J Obstet Gynecol Reprod Biol* 1993;48:135–139.
8. Berube S, Marcoux S, Maheux R. Characteristics related to the prevalence of minimal or mild endometriosis in infertile women. Canadian Collaborative Group on Endometriosis. *Epidemiology* 1998;9:504–510.
9. Vessey MP, Villard-Mackintosh L, Painter R. Epidemiology of endometriosis in women

attending family planning clinics. *BMJ* 1993;306: 182–184.
10. Vercellini P, Trespidi L, DeGiorgi O, et al. Endometriosis and pelvic pain: relation to disease stage and localization. *Fertil Steril* 1996;65:299–304.
11. Rock JA, Markham SM. Pathogenesis of endometriosis. *Lancet* 1992;340:1264–1267.
12. McLaren J, Prentice A. New aspects of pathogenesis of endometriosis. *Curr Obstet Gynecol* 1996;6:85–91.
13. Cooke ID, Thomas EJ. The medical treatment of mild endometriosis. *Acta Obstet Gynecol Scand Suppl* 1989;150:27–30.
14. Compston JE, Yamaguchi K, Croucher PI, et al. The effects of gonadotrophin-releasing hormone agonists on iliac crest cancellous bone structure in women with endometriosis. *Bone* 1995;16:261–267.
15. Prentice A, Deary AJ, Goldbeck-Wood S, et al. Gonadotrophin releasing hormone analogues (GnRHAs) for painful symptoms associated with endometriosis. In: Cochrane Library, Issue 3, 2000. Oxford: Update Software. Search date December 1998; primary sources Medline 1966 to August 1998; Embase 1987 to August 1998; Cochrane Controlled Trials Register 1966 to August 1999; plus unpublished trials by UK distributors of GnRHAs.
16. Prentice A, Deary AJ, Goldbeck-Wood S, et al. Progestogens and antiprogestogens for painful symptoms associated with symptomatic endometriosis. In: Cochrane Library, Issue 2, 2000. Oxford: Update Software. Search date

January 2000; primary sources Medline 1966 to September 1996; Embase 1987 to September 1996; Cochrane Controlled Trials Register 1966 to September 1996.

17. Selak V, Farquhar C, Prentice A, et al. Danazol versus placebo for the treatment of endometriosis. Cochrane Library. Issue 3, 2000. Oxford: Update Software. Search date February 1997; primary sources Medline 1966 to February 1997; Embase 1987 to February 1997; Cochrane Controlled Trials Register 1966 to February 1997; and hand searched journals and conference proceedings.

18. Moore J, Kennedy S, Prentice A. Modern combined oral contraceptives for the treatment of painful symptoms associated with endometriosis. In: Cochrane Library, Issue 3, 2000. Oxford: Update Software. Search date August 1997; primary sources Medline 1966 to August 1997; Embase 1987 to August 1997; Cochrane Controlled Trials Register 1966 to August 1997.

19. Bromham DR, Bookere MW, Rose R, et al. Updating the clinical experience in endometriosis – The European perspective. B J Obstet Gynaecol 1995(suppl);102:12–16.

20. Vercellini P, Trespidi L, Colombo A, et al. A gonadotropin-releasing hormone agonist versus a low-dose oral contraceptive for pelvic pain associated with endometriosis. Fertil Steril 1993; 60:75–79.

21. Parazzini F, Di Cintio E, Chatenoud L, et al. Estroprogestin vs. gonadotrophin agonists plus estroprogestin in the treatment of endometriosis-related pelvic pain: a randomized trial. Gruppo Italiano per lo Studio dell'Endometriosis. Eur J Obstet, Gynecol Repro Biol 2000;88:11–14.

22. Hughes E, Fedorkow D, Collins J, et al. Ovulation suppression versus placebo in the treatment of endometriosis. In: Cochrane Library, Issue 4, 1999. Oxford: Update Software. Search date February 1996; primary sources Medline 1966 to February 1996; Embase 1987 to February 1996; Cochrane Controlled Trials Register 1966 to February 1996; and hand searched journals and conference proceedings.

23. Gregoriou O, Konidaris S, Vitoratos N, et al. Gonadotropin-releasing hormone analogue plus hormone replacement therapy for the treatment of endometriosis: a randomized controlled trial. Int J Fertil Womens Med 1997;42:406–411.

24. Taskin O, Yalcinoglu AI, Kucuk S. Effectiveness of tibolone on hypoestrogenic symptoms induced by goserelin treatment in patients with endometriosis. Fertil Steril 1997;67:40–45.

25. Morgante G. Low-dose danazol after combined surgical and medical therapy reduces the incidence of pelvic pain in women with moderate and severe endometriosis. Human Reprod 1999; 14:2371–2374.

26. Vercellini P, De-Giorgi O. Depot medroxyprogesterone acetate versus an oral contraceptive combined with very-low-dose danazol for long-term treatment of pelvic pain associated with endometriosis. Am J Obstet

Gynecol 1996;175:396–401.

27. Wilson M, Farquhar CM, Sinclair O, et al. Surgical interruption of pelvic nerve pathways for primary and secondary dysmenorrhoea. In: Cochrane Library, Issue 4, 1999. Oxford: Update Software. Search date 1998; primary sources Medline 1966 to 1998; Embase 1974 to 1998; Cochrane Controlled Trials Register 1966 to 1998, and hand searched journals, conference proceedings and references.

28. Sutton CJG, Ewen SP, Whitelaw N, et al. A prospective, randomised, double-blind, controlled trial of laser laparoscopy in the treatment of pelvic pain associated with minimal, mild and moderate endometriosis. Fertil Steril l994;62:696–700.

29. Sutton CJG, Pooley AS, Ewen SP. Follow-up report on a randomised, controlled trial of laser laparoscopy in the treatment of pelvic pain associated with minimal to moderate endometriosis. Fertil Steril 1997;68:170–174.

30. Marcoux S, Maheux R, Berube S, et al. Laparoscopic surgery in infertile women with minimal or mild endometriosis. Canadian Collaborative Group on Endometriosis. N Engl J Med 1997;337:217–222.

31. Parazzini F. Ablation of lesions or no treatment in minimal-mild endometriosis in infertile women: a randomized trial. Gruppo Italiano per lo Studio dell'Endometriosis. Hum Reprod 1999;14:1332–1334.

32. Parazzini F, Fedele L, Busacca M, et al. Postsurgical medical treatment of advanced endometriosis: results of a randomized clinical trial. Am J Obstet Gynecol 1994;171:1205–1207.

33. Bianchi S, Busacca M, Agnoli B, et al. Effects of 3 month therapy with danazol after laparoscopic surgery for stage III/IV endometriosis: a randomized study. Hum Reprod 1999;14:1335–1337.

34. Telimaa S, Ronnberg L, Kauppila A. Placebo-controlled comparison of danazol and high-dose medroxyprogesterone acetate in the treatment of endometriosis after conservative surgery. Gynecol Endocrinol 1987;1:363–371.

35. Hornstein MD, Hemmings R, Yuzpe AA, et al. Use of nafarelin versus placebo after reductive laparoscopic surgery for endometriosis. Fertil Steril 1997;68:860–864.

36. Vercellini P, Crosignani PG, Fadini R, et al. A gonadotrophin-releasing hormone agonist compared with expectant management after conservative surgery for symptomatic endometriosis. Br J Obstet Gynaecol 1999;106: 672–677.

37. Audebert A, Descampes P, Marret H, et al. Pre or post operative medical treatment with nafarelin in Stage III-IV endometriosis: a French Multicentered Study. Eur J Obstet Gynecol Reprod Biol 1998;79: 145–148.

38. Beretta P, Franchi M, Ghezzi F, et al. Randomised clinical trial of two laparoscopic treatments of endometriomas: cystectomy versus drainage and coagulation. Fertil Steril 1998;709:1176–1180.

Cynthia Farquhar
Associate Professor
School of Medicine
University of Auckland
Auckland
New Zealand

Competing interests: None declared.

Essential vulvodynia (vulval pain)

Updated this issue

Earlando Thomas, Damian Murphy and Charles Redman

QUESTIONS
Effects of treatments. 1067

INTERVENTIONS

Unknown effectiveness
Amitriptyline 1067
Pudendal nerve
   decompression 1067

To be covered in future issues of
Clinical Evidence
Topical steroids

Key Messages

- We found no randomised evidence on the effects of amitriptyline or pudendal nerve decompression in women with essential vulvodynia.

DEFINITION	Essential vulvodynia is characterised by a diffuse, unremitting burning of the vulva, which may extend to the perineum, thigh or buttock, and is often associated with urethral or rectal discomfort. Hyperaesthesia over a wide area is usually the only abnormal finding on physical examination. It is found primarily in postmenopausal women.
INCIDENCE/ PREVALENCE	We found no data on the prevalence of essential vulvodynia.
AETIOLOGY/ RISK FACTORS	The cause is unknown. Similar symptoms may be caused by pudendal nerve damage.[1-3]
PROGNOSIS	Without treatment, the unremitting symptoms of essential vulvodynia may reduce the quality of life. Frequency of micturition, stress incontinence, and chronic constipation may also rarely develop.[1-3]
AIMS	To control symptoms and improve quality of life with minimal adverse effects.
OUTCOMES	Symptom scores for itching, burning, pain, and dyspareunia; range from 0–3 (3 represents the most severe).
METHODS	*Clinical Evidence* update search and appraisal May 2000. Where we found no good RCTs, we used the best available observational studies.

QUESTION   What are the effects of treatments?

OPTION   AMITRIPTYLINE

We found no randomised evidence on the effects of amitriptyline in women with essential vulvodynia.

Benefits: We found no systematic review or RCTs.

Harms: In one retrospective cohort study, adverse effects, mostly drowsiness and dry mouth, occurred in 45% (9/20) of women. Weight gain occurred in 10–15%. Tinnitus and palpitation were each reported by one women.[3]

Comment: None.

OPTION   PUDENDAL NERVE DECOMPRESSION

We found no randomised evidence on the effects of pudendal nerve decompression in women with essential vulvodynia.

Benefits: We found no systematic review or RCTs.

Harms: No adverse effects were found during follow up.

Comment: Pudendal nerve decompression may be technically challenging. Experience suggests that success depends on selection of suitable patients for surgical or medical management.

Women's health

REFERENCES

1. Turner MLC, Marinoff SC. Pudendal neuralgia. *Am J Obstet Gynecol* 1991;165:1233–1236.
2. Shafik A. Pudendal canal syndrome as a cause of vulvodynia and its treatment by pudendal nerve decompression. *Eur J Obstet Gynecol* 1998;80: 215–220.
3. McKay M. Dysesthetic ("essential") vulvodynia. Treatment with amitriptyline. *J Reprod Med* 1993; 38:9–13.

Earlando Thomas
Senior Specialist Registrar
Department of Obstetrics and
Gynecology
Rochester General Hospital
Rochester, NY
USA

Damian Murphy
Consultant Obstetrician and
Gynaecologist
Department of Obstetrics and
Gynaecology
New Cross Hospital
Wolverhampton
UK

Charles Redman
Consultant Obstetrician and
Gynaecologist
Department of Obstetrics and
Gynaecology
City General Hospital
Stoke-on-Trent
UK
Competing interests: None declared.

Updated this issue

Kirsten Duckitt

INTERVENTIONS

To be covered in future issues of Clinical Evidence
Counselling
Adoption

Covered elsewhere in this issue
See erectile dysfunction, p 468
See endometriosis, p 1058
See pelvic inflammatory disease,
    p 934

See glossary, p 1085

Key Messages

In women with infertility caused by ovulation disorders

- One systematic review of randomised crossover trials has found that clomiphene increases the chances of becoming pregnant. We found no trials that compared clomiphene with other interventions in women with ovulation disorders. RCTs have compared follicle stimulating hormone, human menopausal gonadotrophin, and laparoscopic ovarian drilling. They found no difference in pregnancy rates. None of these interventions has been directly compared with placebo in women with ovulation disorders.

In women with tubal infertility

- We found no adequate RCTs of the main interventions (selective salpingography and tubal catheterisation, tubal surgery, and in vitro fertilisation (IVF).
- One systematic review found insufficient evidence to support the routine use of hydrotubation or second look laparoscopy following tubal surgery.

In women with infertility caused by endometriosis

- Systematic reviews of cohort studies have found that pregnancy rates are higher with surgical than medical treatment. IVF has not been adequately evaluated in this context.

In couples with male factor infertility

- One systematic review of RCTs has found that intrauterine insemination achieves higher pregnancy rates than intracervical insemination or natural intercourse.
- We found insufficient evidence on intracytoplasmic sperm injection plus IVF.
- Donor insemination achieves live birth rates of about 10% in women with no evidence of reduced fertility or in whom problems with fertility have been corrected.

In couples with unexplained infertility

- We found no evidence to support the use of clomiphene.
- Three systematic reviews of RCTs have found that intrauterine insemination achieves higher pregnancy rates than timed intercourse, especially when ovarian stimulation with gonadotrophins is also used.
- We found no RCTs of gamete intrafallopian transfer in couples with unexplained infertility. Limited data from RCTs found no difference in pregnancy rates between ovarian hyperstimulation and IVF.

Interventions involving ovarian stimulation

- These carry the risk of multiple pregnancy and ovarian hyperstimulation syndrome. The risk of each varies with the type of ovarian stimulation used. Moderate to severe ovarian hyperstimulation complicates 4% of ovulation induction cycles and up to 10% of all IVF cycles. Multiple pregnancy occurs in 29% of women with polycystic ovaries when conventional (as opposed to low dose) regimens of gonadotrophins are used.

DEFINITION   Normal fertility has been defined as achieving a pregnancy within 2 years by regular sexual intercourse.[1] Many, however, define infertility as the failure to conceive after 1 year of unprotected intercourse. Infertility can be primary, in couples who have never conceived, or secondary, in couples who have previously conceived. Infertile couples include those who are sterile (who will never achieve a natural pregnancy) and those who are subfertile (who should eventually achieve a pregnancy).

INCIDENCE/ PREVALENCE	Although there is no evidence of a major change in prevalence of infertility, many more couples are seeking help than previously. Currently, about one in seven couples in industrialised countries will seek medical advice for infertility.[2] Rates of primary infertility vary widely between countries, ranging from 10% in Africa to about 6% in North America and Europe.[1] Reported rates of secondary infertility are less reliable.
AETIOLOGY/ RISK FACTORS	In the UK nearly a third of cases of infertility are unexplained. The rest are caused by ovulatory failure (27%), low sperm count or quality (19%), tubal damage (14%), endometriosis (5%), and other causes (5%).[3]
PROGNOSIS	In developed countries, 80–90% of couples attempting to conceive are successful after 1 year, and 95% after 2 years.[3] The chances of becoming pregnant vary with the cause and duration of infertility, the woman's age, the couple's previous pregnancy history, and the availability of different treatment options.[4,5] For the first 2–3 years of unexplained infertility, cumulative conception rates remain high (27–46%) but decrease with increasing age of the woman and duration of infertility. The background rates of spontaneous pregnancy in infertile couples can be calculated from longitudinal studies of infertile couples who have been observed without treatment.[4]
AIMS	To achieve the delivery of one healthy baby; to reduce the distress associated with infertility; to help people come to terms with childlessness if treatments fail or are unavailable.
OUTCOMES	Rates of pregnancy, live birth, miscarriage, and multiple pregnancy; incidence of ovarian hyperstimulation syndrome; satisfaction with services and treatments; acceptance of childlessness if treatment is unsuccessful. Ovulation is an intermediate outcome. Pregnancy rate is an intermediate outcome but one that is important in itself to many people. A large number of pregnancies in infertile couples will occur spontaneously without treatment.[4] Effectiveness of treatments for infertility should be assessed on the basis of pregnancy rates over and above the spontaneous pregnancy rates. Otherwise the impacts of treatments will be overestimated.
METHODS	*Clinical Evidence* update search and appraisal May 2000. **Crossover design:** For infertility, RCTs with a crossover design may overestimate the treatment effect, because pregnancies occurring in the first half of the trial will remove couples from the second half.[6] Crossover trials were included in some systematic reviews where no or very few RCTs using a parallel group design were available. Ideally, only data from the first half of the trial, before crossover, should be used. However, a study that used a computer model to compare the results of crossover and parallel designed trials suggests that any overestimation may be clinically irrelevant.[7]

QUESTION What are the effects of treatments for infertility caused by ovulation disorders?

OPTION CLOMIPHENE

One systematic review of RCTs found that clomiphene increases the likelihood of pregnancy in women who ovulate infrequently. We found insufficient evidence that prolonged use of clomiphene increases the risk of ovarian cancer. The incidence of multiple pregnancy (mostly with twins) is increased. Clomiphene has not been adequately compared with other treatments for ovulation disorders.

Benefits:
Versus placebo: See table 1, p 1090. One systematic review (updated in 1996) identified three double blind, crossover RCTs comparing clomiphene 50–200 mg versus placebo in 217 cycles in women who ovulate infrequently.[8] Pregnancy was over three times more likely per treatment cycle with clomiphene than placebo (OR 3.41, 95% CI 1.23 to 9.48). **Versus tamoxifen:** We found no systematic review. We found three studies comparing clomiphene versus tamoxifen in 102 anovulatory or infrequently ovulating women. One RCT used a parallel group design, one used alternate cycles design, and one was an observational study.[9–11] Two small studies based estimates of pregnancy rates on fewer than 30 pregnancies.[9,11]

Harms:
Ovarian cancer: Eleven women with ovarian cancer were detected in a cohort of 3837 infertile women.[12] One nested case control study found a sevenfold increase in risk of ovarian cancer in women using clomiphene citrate for 12 or more cycles (RR 7.2, 95% CI 1.2 to 43.9), which increased to 11-fold when adjusted for gravidity at enrolment (RR 11.1, 95% CI 1.5 to 82.3). The association was present for both gravid and nulligravid women and for infertile women both with ovulatory disorders and with infertility from other causes. No subsequent studies have found an association between clomiphene and ovarian cancer.[13–16] **Multiple pregnancy:** Multiple pregnancy occurs in 2–13% of women with all causes of infertility taking clomiphene, compared with a spontaneous multiple pregnancy rate of about 1–2% of women in North American and European populations.[17,18] In a 1 year survey in the UK, 25 of the 44 triplet pregnancies reported were attributable to clomiphene.[19] Clomiphene was also implicated in two of the eight sets of quads and quins reported. **Ovarian hyperstimulation syndrome:** Clomiphene tends to cause only mild ovarian hyperstimulation that does not require treatment.

Comment:
Clomiphene was first introduced in the 1960s and all the trials took place in the 1970s, before more recent quality standards for RCTs were established.

OPTION GONADOTROPHINS

One systematic review of RCTs found no evidence of a difference in pregnancy rates between human menopausal gonadotrophin and urinary follicle stimulating hormone (FSH) or laparoscopic ovarian drilling. However, compared with FSH, human menopausal gonadotrophin carried

greater risk of ovarian hyperstimulation syndrome. Gonadotrophins have not been compared with placebo or with clomiphene. We found insufficient evidence of an increased risk of ovarian cancer from using gonadotrophins.

Benefits: **Versus placebo:** We found no RCTs. **Versus clomiphene:** We found no RCTs. **Human menopausal gonadotrophin versus FSH:** One systematic review (updated in 1996) identified six RCTs, three of which used crossover designs. The RCTs compared human menopausal gonadotrophin versus purified urinary FSH in 182 women with clomiphene resistant polycystic ovary syndrome (see table 1, p 1090).[20] There was no significant difference in pregnancy rates (37% v 27%; OR for pregnancy v FSH 0.66, 95% CI 0.35 to 1.24). **Urinary versus recombinant FSH:** We found no systematic review. We found two RCTs comparing recombinant versus urinary FSH in 223 women with clomiphene resistant, normogonadotrophic anovulation.[21,22] No significant differences in pregnancy rates were found between either group in either trial. However, in one trial, a significantly lower total dose and shorter duration of recombinant FSH achieved ovulation.[21] One recent systematic review (published in 1999) identified 12 RCTs that compared recombinant FSH versus urinary FSH in cycles using either IVF or intracytoplasmic sperm injection (ICSI) cycles.[23] There was a 20% increase in clinical pregnancy rates per started cycle when recombinant FSH was used compared with baseline (OR 1.20, 95% CI 1.02 to 1.42). The risk difference represented an increase in clinical pregnancy rate per cycle started with recombinant FSH rather than urinary FSH of 3.7% (95% CI 0.5% to 6.9%). **Versus laparoscopic ovarian drilling:** See option, p 1074.

Harms: **Ovarian cancer:** One case control study of 200 women with ovarian cancer and 408 area matched controls found that women with non-invasive ovarian tumours were over three times more likely to have been exposed to any ovulation induction agents (adjusted OR 3.52, 95% CI 1.23 to 10.1), particularly to human menopausal gonadotrophin (adjusted OR 9.38, 95% CI 1.66 to 52.1).[15] Women with invasive ovarian tumours were no more likely to have been exposed to any ovulation induction agents. **Multiple pregnancy:** Multiple pregnancy occurs in 29% of women with polycystic ovaries when conventional regimens of gonadotrophins are used to induce ovulation.[24] **Ovarian hyperstimulation:** The risk of moderate to severe ovarian hyperstimulation was lower with FSH than with human menopausal gonadotrophin (OR versus human menopausal gonadotrophin 0.20, 95% CI 0.09 to 0.46).[20] **Urinary versus recombinant FSH:** One large RCT found no significant difference in the risk of multiple pregnancy or ovarian hyperstimulation syndrome.[21]

Comment: Despite not being placebo controlled, trials of gonadotrophins often included women who were not ovulating, and therefore provide some evidence that treatment is effective. The avoidance of gonadotrophins may reduce the risk of multiple pregnancy and ovarian hyperstimulation syndrome. Recombinant FSH is not derived from human tissues.

Women's health

One systematic review of RCTs has found no evidence of a significant difference in pregnancy rates between laparoscopic ovarian drilling and gonadotrophins.

Benefits: We found one systematic review (updated in 1998), which identified two RCTs (one using a crossover design) in 112 women with anovulatory, clomiphene resistant polycystic ovary syndrome, comparing laparoscopic ovarian drilling (see glossary, p 1085) versus gonadotrophins (see table 1, p 1090).[25] They found no significant difference in pregnancy rates (OR 0.72, 95% CI 0.29 to 1.78).

Harms: Laparoscopic drilling incurs the risks and morbidity of the laparoscopy under general anaesthetic and postoperative adhesion formation. We found no evidence to support the suggestion that laparoscopic drilling increases the long term risk of premature ovarian failure. However, it carried no increased risk of multiple pregnancy.

Comment: The trials of laparoscopic drilling included women who were not ovulating and therefore provide some evidence that treatment is effective despite the lack of placebo controls. Two more RCTs are in progress (N Bayran and C Farquhar, personal communication, 2000).

We found that pulsatile gonadotrophin releasing hormone (GnRH) has not yet been adequately evaluated in women with infertility caused by ovulation disorders.

Benefits: We found one systematic review (published in 1999), which identified three RCTs and one non-randomised comparative trial comparing pulsatile GnRH versus another treatment to induce ovulation in subfertile women with clomiphene resistant polycystic ovary syndrome.[26] The trials described four different comparisons, were small (each reporting between one and four pregnancies), and of short duration (1–3 cycles), and so provided insufficient evidence to assess the value of pulsatile GnRH in polycystic ovary syndrome. Case series in 256 anovulatory women with hypogonadotrophic hypogonadism undergoing 1043 treatment cycles found cumulative pregnancy rates of 59–73% at 6 months and 81–92% at 12 months.[27–29] Only one series reported the live birth rate; this was 65% after 12 treatment cycles.[27]

Harms: One retrospective analysis in 229 cycles in 71 women compared pulsatile GnRH versus gonadotrophins alone, and found no significant difference in multiple pregnancy rates after six cycles.[30] However, 75% of the multiple pregnancies in the gonadotrophin group were triplets or higher order multiple pregnancies, whereas all multiple pregnancies in the GnRH group were twins.

Comment: Pulsatile GnRH is used in women with anovulation caused by low serum gonadotrophins and oestrogen concentrations. It is a well defined condition so the evidence, although only from case series, should be generalisable to all women with hypogonadotrophic hypogonadism.

OPTION   SELECTIVE SALPINGOGRAPHY/TUBAL CATHETERISATION

We found no RCTs of selective salpingography and tubal catheterisation. Non-randomised studies found that, if used in isolated proximal tubal obstruction, these procedures reduced the need for tubal surgery or IVF in some women.

Benefits: We found no RCTs. One recent systematic review (published in 1999) combined the raw data from 10 cohort and other observational studies of selective salpingography and tubal cannulation (482 women), and four studies from hysteroscopic cannulation for proximal tubal blockage (133 women).[31] The ongoing pregnancy rate (> 20 weeks' gestation) for the radiographic series was 23% versus 49% for the hysteroscopic series. One prospective cohort study followed 43 women with bilateral proximal tubal obstruction and 33 control women undergoing reversal of tubal sterilisation.[32] Those in whom tubal catheterisation was unsuccessful went on to have microsurgical resection and anastomosis. Cumulative pregnancy rates at 12 months were 68% with successful tubal catheterisation, 56% with microsurgery, and 29% in the control group.

Harms: Tubal perforation, which does not seem to be clinically important, occurred in 2% and ectopic pregnancy in 3–9.4% of women undergoing selective salpingography and tubal catheterisation.[31,33]

Comment: None of the published studies included an untreated group, so it is not possible to give the treatment related pregnancy rate over and above the spontaneous pregnancy rate. Tubal patency and pregnancy without treatment have been reported in women diagnosed with bilateral proximal tube obstruction.[34]

OPTION   TUBAL SURGERY

We found limited evidence that surgical division of tubal adhesions improves pregnancy rates, and that laparoscopic techniques offer no benefit over open microsurgical techniques. We found no RCTs comparing tubal surgery with IVF. One systematic review found insufficient evidence to support the routine use of hydrotubation or second look laparoscopy following tubal surgery.

Benefits: **Versus IVF:** We found no systematic review or RCTs. Case series of tubal surgery have been compared with large databases of couples undergoing IVF. These found that tubal surgery was as effective as IVF in women with filmy adhesions, mild distal tubal occlusion, or proximal obstruction.[35–40] Success rates with tubal surgery depend on the severity and site of disease. The best figures from surgery in women with distal tubal occlusion are live birth rates of 20%–30% with rates of up to 60% reported for the less common proximal occlusion.[35,41–44] **Different types of tubal surgery:** We found two systematic reviews.[45,46] The first (updated in 1998) identified eight RCTs and 14 non-randomised trials looking at all aspects of infertility surgery.[45] It found that pregnancy rates were higher with microsurgery for adhesiolysis plus salpingostomy than with macrosurgery (full term rates 36.8% v 20.0%; RR 1.94, 95% CI 1.15 to 3.29). Pregnancy rates were higher with adhesiolysis compared with no treatment. Pregnancy rates were no different with laparoscopic than with open microsurgical adhesiolysis (total pregnancy rates 85.2% v 75.0%; RR 1.14, 95% CI 0.79 to 1.63). The review found no difference in pregnancy rates between carbon dioxide laser for adhesiolysis, salpingostomy, or reversal of sterilisation than with standard techniques. Total and intrauterine pregnancy rates were lower with laparoscopic than with open microsurgical salpingostomy. However, the last conclusion was based on four trials reported between 1987 and 1991. The second systematic review (updated in 1999) of five RCTs concluded that all the studies were either poor quality or underpowered. It found insufficient evidence to support the routine practice of hydrotubation or second look laparoscopy following tubal surgery.[46] **Proximal tubal blockage:** We found no RCTs. One recent systematic review (published in 1999) evaluated the raw data from five cohort and other observational studies (175 women) that used microsurgical techniques for proximal tubal blockage, and from two studies (104 women) that used macrosurgical techniques.[31] The overall pregnancy rate after microsurgery was 59%, with ongoing pregnancy rates of 47% and an ectopic rate of 7.4%. For macrosurgery the overall pregnancy rate was 42%, the ongoing pregnancy rate was 16%, and the ectopic rate was 16%. Ongoing pregnancy rates after microsurgery were significantly higher than those after macrosurgery (RR 2.2, 95% CI 1.5 to 3.2).

Harms:　　Tubal surgery involves general anaesthesia and admission to hospital, although the laparoscopic approach reduces hospital stay and recovery time. There is a risk of ectopic pregnancy caused by pre-existing tubal damage; rates of 7–9% have been reported compared with 1–3% with IVF.[47,48] IVF carries the risk of multiple pregnancy and ovarian hyperstimulation syndrome (see harms of IVF, p 1077).

Comment:　　These data precede recent improvements in case selection and laparoscopic training. RCTs of current practice are needed. If successful, tubal surgery allows women to have more pregnancies without further medical intervention and without the risks associated with IVF.[49]

| OPTION | IN VITRO FERTILISATION |

Two RCTs found improved pregnancy and live birth rates with immediate compared with delayed IVF. Data from IVF databases suggest higher pregnancy rates compared with expected spontaneous pregnancy rates without treatment.

Benefits:　　We found no systematic review. We found two RCTs comparing immediate versus delayed IVF in 598 infertile couples with all causes of infertility.[50,51] The delayed group served as untreated controls for at least 6 months. One RCT found increased rates of live birth in the immediate compared with the delayed group (11.6% v 4.9%; RR of live birth 2.36, 95% CI 1.03 to 5.66).[50] The other RCT found an increase in crude and cumulative pregnancy rates in the immediate compared with the delayed group, but the effect was significant only in women with severe bilateral tubal disease.[51] **Versus tubal surgery:** See option, p 1078. In all causes of infertility, IVF produced live birth rates per cycle of 15% in the UK and 20% in the USA.[5] If 3–5 cycles of IVF were possible, 59–77% of women with tubal infertility became pregnant, better than the best outcomes from tubal surgery.[52] **Versus IVF plus intracytoplasmic sperm injection (ICSI):** One RCT found no evidence of a benefit from adding ICSI to IVF for tubal infertility if the semen analysis is normal (see option, p 1080).[53]

Harms: **Multiple pregnancy:** Multiple pregnancy rates were not reported in the RCTs mentioned above. However, of the 5538 live births following IVF in the UK in 1995–1996, 32% were multiple, including 230 (4.2%) sets of triplets and five sets of quads.[54] In the UK, the number of embryos that can be replaced is restricted to three. In the USA, where there are no such restrictions, 7939 deliveries included 36.6% multiple births, 7% of which were triplets and above. **Ovarian hyperstimulation syndrome:** Severe ovarian hyperstimulation syndrome occurs in 0.5–2% of all IVF cycles.[55] Ovarian hyperstimulation syndrome rates were not reported in the RCTs above.

Comment: Similar clinics, ostensibly using the same methods, report different success rates. In the UK, the live birth rates per cycle vary from 0–28% with an average of 15%.[54] The equivalent average figure in the USA is nearly 20%, but again results vary widely.[56,57] In the UK, larger centres (200 or more cycles per year) report slightly higher live birth rates than smaller centres (15.7% per cycle started compared with 12.7%).[5] Such a difference has not been consistently reported in the USA. The success of IVF is influenced by age, duration of infertility, and previous pregnancy history. Pregnancy rates are highest between the ages of 25 and 35 years and decline steeply after 35.[5] A systematic review of nine retrospective comparative series and five abstracts found that the presence of a hydrosalpinx during an IVF cycle reduced pregnancy, implantation, and live birth rates and increased rates of early pregnancy loss.[58] However, RCTs are needed to establish whether routine salpingectomy in these women would be beneficial prior to IVF.

QUESTION **What are the effects of treatment for infertility associated with endometriosis?**

OPTION **DRUG-INDUCED OVARIAN SUPPRESSION**

One systematic review of RCTs found no evidence of a significant difference in pregnancy rates between drugs that induce ovarian suppression and either placebo or danazol in women with endometriosis. Ovarian suppression is less effective than surgical treatment.

Benefits: We found one systematic review (updated in 1996), which identified 13 RCTs.[59] **Versus placebo:** Five RCTs compared ovulation suppression agents (medroxyprogesterone acetate, gestrinone, combined oral contraceptive pills, and GnRH analogues) versus placebo in 244 women with visually diagnosed endometriosis who had been attempting conception for over 12 months. Ovulation suppression agents versus placebo did not significantly increase the pregnancy rate (OR 0.83, 95% CI 0.50 to 1.39). **Versus danazol:** Eight RCTs compared ovulation suppression versus danazol in 658 similar women. They found no significant difference in pregnancy rates (OR compared with danazol 1.20, 95% CI 0.85 to 1.68). **Versus surgery:** See option below.

Harms: Drugs that suppress ovulation had important adverse effects that included weight gain, hot flushes, and osteoporosis.[60] Adverse effects of danazol were dose related. An average weight gain of 2–4 kg was common with 3 months of treatment. Other adverse effects included androgenic effects such as acne, seborrhoea, hirsutism, voice changes, and general complaints, including irritability, musculoskeletal pains, and tiredness. Hot flushes and breast atrophy were sometimes observed. Most of these adverse effects were reversible on stopping treatment.[61]

Comment: None of the RCTs in the systematic review used a crossover design. Combination of clomiphene with other infertility drugs was used in three of the trials. Treatment using ovulation suppression could waste valuable time for women who are trying to get pregnant, as the opportunity for spontaneous conceptions is lost during treatment.[60]

OPTION   **SURGICAL TREATMENT**

Systematic reviews of cohort studies have found that surgery is more effective than ovarian suppression in women with infertility related to endometriosis, and that there is no significant difference in pregnancy rates between open and laparoscopic surgery. We found no RCTs that compared surgery with IVF in women with endometriosis.

Benefits: **Versus placebo or ovarian suppression:** We found one systematic review (published in 1993) and one non-systemic review (published in 1994), which together identified 21 cohort studies and one quasi randomised trial in a total of 3879 women with all stages of endometriosis.[62,63] Interventions were laparoscopic or open surgery versus medical treatment or no treatment. Surgical treatment produced a two fifths increase in pregnancy rate compared with medical treatment or no treatment (RR 1.38, 95% CI 1.28 to 1.48), but there was no significant difference between laparoscopic and open surgery (RR 0.93, 95% CI 0.84 to 1.02).[63] In women with mild or minimal endometriosis, analysis of pooled data found that laparoscopic surgery achieved higher pregnancy rates than danazol or no treatment (OR 2.7, 95% CI 2.1 to 3.5).[62] **Versus diagnostic laparoscopy:** We found two RCTs with conflicting results published since the reviews.[64,65] Both compared laparoscopic surgery (ablation or resection of endometriosis) versus diagnostic laparoscopy in a total of 452 infertile women with minimal or mild endometriosis. In the larger trial (n = 341), the women undergoing laparoscopic surgery had a 13% absolute increase in the probability of a pregnancy occurring within 36 weeks and lasting longer than 20 weeks (RR 1.7, 95% CI 1.2 to 2.6; NNT 8).[64] However, the smaller trial (which was powered to detect a

2.5-fold difference in pregnancy rates between the groups) found no difference between the groups either in conception rates (24% v 29%) or birth rates at 1 year (20% v 22%).[65]

Harms: The risks and morbidity of surgery under general anaesthesia, and of postoperative adhesion formation, have to be balanced against the adverse effects of treatments involving ovarian suppression or stimulation. One multicentre series of 29 966 diagnostic and operative gynaecological laparoscopies found a mortality of 3.33 per 100 000 laparoscopies, and a complication rate of 3.20 per 1000.[66]

Comment: In the RCT described above, 14% of the women who received surgery for their endometriosis also had periadnexal adhesions lysed, which may have affected their fecundity.[64]

OPTION   IN VITRO FERTILISATION

Retrospective studies suggest that IVF achieves similar rates of pregnancy in women with endometriosis as in those with other causes of infertility. We found no evidence comparing IVF with drug induced ovarian suppression or with surgery for women with moderate or severe endometriosis.

Benefits: We found no systematic review or RCTs. We found two retrospective cohort studies of women undergoing IVF.[67,68] They compared pregnancy rates in those with endometriosis and those with other causes of infertility. There were no significant differences in pregnancy rates for different stages of endometriosis or for endometriosis compared with other causes of infertility.

Harms: See harms of IVF for tubal fertility, p 1077.

Comment: There is a need for properly controlled prospective studies that present their results for different stages of endometriosis using a validated classification system. Comparisons with assisted reproductive techniques are also required.

QUESTION   What are the effects of treatments for male infertility?

OPTION   INTRAUTERINE INSEMINATION

One systematic review of RCTs has found that intrauterine insemination more than doubles the chance of pregnancy compared with intracervical insemination or natural intercourse in couples with male infertility.

Benefits: We found two systematic reviews, published in 1997 and 1999.[69,70] The earlier review identified 10 RCTs (2082 treatment cycles) comparing intrauterine insemination versus intracervical insemination or natural intercourse.[69] In couples reported as having male infertility, intrauterine insemination more than doubled the pregnancy rate compared with intracervical insemination or timed natural intercourse (OR 2.20, 95% CI 1.43 to 3.39). Pregnancy rate per cycle was 6.5% with intrauterine insemination versus 3.1% with intracervical insemination or timed natural intercourse. The more recent review identified 17 RCTs (3662 completed treatment cycles) comparing intrauterine insemination with timed intercourse in either natural or stimulated cycles in couples with male subfertility.[70] Intrauterine insemination more than doubled the pregnancy rate compared with timed intercourse, both in natural cycles (OR 2.43, 95% CI 1.54 to 3.83) and in cycles where controlled ovarian hyperstimulation was also used (OR 2.14, 95% CI 1.30 to 3.51). Intrauterine insemination in cycles with controlled ovarian hyperstimulation improved the probability of conception compared with intrauterine insemination in natural cycles, but did not reach significance (OR 1.79, 95% CI 0.98 to 3.25). When intrauterine insemination in controlled ovarian hyperstimulation cycles was compared with timed intercourse in natural cycles, the probability of conception was significantly increased (OR 6.2, 95% CI 2.35 to 16.5).

Harms: Apart from the risks of ovarian hyperstimulation syndrome and multiple pregnancy associated with ovarian stimulation, intrauterine insemination may increase the likelihood of infection and may be associated with some discomfort.[71] However, data from RCTs are scarce.

Comment: We found three RCTs that addressed the optimum number of inseminations in controlled ovarian stimulation cycles. Two trials found that two inseminations performed in the pre-ovulatory and peri-ovulatory periods produced significantly higher pregnancy rates than one peri-ovulatory insemination.[72,73] The other trial found a non-significant increase in pregnancy rates with two similarly timed inseminations.[74] One small crossover RCT addressed the timing of insemination in clomiphene stimulated cycles. It found similar pregnancy rates per cycle whether insemination was timed with a urinary luteinising hormone (LH) kit or whether ultrasound monitoring with human chorionic gonadotrophin (hCG) induction of ovulation was used.[75]

OPTION | INTRACYTOPLASMIC SPERM INJECTION PLUS IVF

The combination of intracytoplasmic sperm injection (ICSI) plus IVF has not been rigorously tested in RCTs compared with no treatment.

Benefits: **Versus IVF alone:** We found one systematic review[76] and one subsequent RCT.[53] The systematic review (published in 1999) identified 10 RCTs (total 437 couples) comparing ICSI plus IVF versus IVF alone (eight compared ICSI with conventional IVF, one compared ICSI with subzonal sperm injection, and one compared ICSI with additional IVF).[76] For couples with normal semen, no evidence of a difference was found in fertilisation rates per retrieved oocyte or pregnancy rates between IVF alone and ICSI. However, there seemed to be a slight benefit of ICSI over IVF alone if fertilisation rate per inseminated oocytes was considered (combined OR 1.42, 95% CI 1.17 to 1.72). For couples with borderline semen (concentration 10–20 million/ml, motility 30–50%, morphology 4–14% normal forms), ICSI resulted in higher fertilisation rates compared with conventional IVF both for fertilisations per oocyte retrieved (OR 3.79, 95% CI 2.97 to 4.85) and for fertilisations per oocyte inseminated (OR 3.90, 95% CI 2.96 to 5.15). For couples with very poor semen (concentration < 10 million/ml, motility < 30%, morphology < 4% normal forms) two RCTs found better fertilisation outcomes with ICSI than with subzonal sperm injection or additional IVF. The subsequent RCT randomised 76 couples with tubal factor infertility but normal semen analysis to either ICSI plus IVF or IVF alone. No significant difference was found in clinical pregnancy rates per cycle (21.0% v 21.1%) or take home baby rates (18.4% v 15.8%).[53]

Harms: We found conflicting reports of congenital abnormality in children born after intracytoplasmic sperm injection. Some found no increase over background rates of abnormality. Others found that major birth defects may be twice as likely and minor defects 50% more likely.[77,78] There has also been a suggestion that sex chromosomal defects may be more likely in children born as a result of ICSI.[79,80]

Comment: Many couples have a strong preference for a child genetically related to both partners.[81] The data on congenital and chromosome abnormalities with intracytoplasmic sperm injection are constantly being revised as experience increases.

OPTION **IVF VERSUS GAMETE INTRAFALLOPIAN TRANSFER**

We found insufficient evidence to compare IVF and gamete intrafallopian transfer in male infertility.

Benefits: We found no systematic review. We found one RCT in 14 couples with male infertility.[82] This found no evidence of a difference in pregnancy rates.

Harms: See harms of IVF, p 1077.

Comment: None.

OPTION **DONOR INSEMINATION**

Analysis of data from large databases has found live birth rates of about 10% with donor insemination in women without evidence of reduced fertility or in whom problems with fertility have been corrected. No RCTs have compared donor insemination with other treatments for male infertility. One systematic review found that intrauterine insemination of frozen donor sperm led to higher pregnancy rates than intracervical insemination (ICI) in centres where pregnancy rates per cycle for ICI were under 6%.

Benefits: **Versus no treatment:** We found no systematic reviews or RCTs that compared donor insemination with no treatment or other interventions for male infertility. **Type of insemination:** One systematic review (12 RCTs, 2215 treatment cycles) found that intrauterine insemination of frozen donor sperm led to higher pregnancy rates than intracervical insemination (ICI) in centres where pregnancy rates per cycle for ICI were under 6%.[83]

Harms: Few adverse effects are reported if ovarian stimulation is not used. The fact that the child is not the man's genetic offspring may be difficult for couples to come to terms with.

Comment: Data are available from large databases, but it is sometimes unclear whether ovarian stimulation was also used. The live birth rate per cycle in the UK Human Fertilisation and Embryology Authority database (based on 7136 women) was 9%.[54] Similar rates are reported from the French donor insemination database (23 700 women over 4 years), with a mean pregnancy rate of 10.3% per cycle, and the Sheffield database (343 women, 980 treatment cycles), with an 11.3% overall live birth rate.[84,85] Comparisons of donor insemination versus no treatment or other interventions may be inappropriate as, for many couples, donor insemination is not an acceptable option. RCTs have tended to concentrate on comparisons between different techniques of donor insemination.

QUESTION   What are the effects of treatment for unexplained infertility?

OPTION   CLOMIPHENE

Systematic reviews of RCTs have found no evidence of benefit from the use of clomiphene in couples with unexplained infertility.

Benefits: We found two systematic reviews[86,87] and one additional RCT[88] of clomiphene versus placebo in couples with unexplained infertility. The first systematic review (updated in 1996) identified five placebo controlled RCTs, four using crossover designs, in women with unexplained infertility (458 cycles).[86] It found that clomiphene versus placebo significantly increased the chance of pregnancy per cycle (OR 2.5, 95% CI 1.35 to 4.62). When only cycles before crossover were included (which was only possible with the data from three of these trials), the positive effect increased (OR 5.0, 95% CI 1.75 to 14.3). A subsequent RCT using a parallel group design in 33 women with unexplained infertility found significantly higher pregnancy rates in spontaneous cycles compared with clomiphene cycles.[88] When added to the review, the combined odds ratio for pregnancy compared with placebo/no treatment fell to 1.4 and was no longer significant, showing no evidence of benefit from clomiphene in women with unexplained infertility (J Collins, personal communication, 1998). The other systematic review (published in 1997) identified 22 RCTs in couples with all causes of infertility. It found no independent effect of clomiphene compared with no ovarian stimulation.[87]

Harms: See harms of clomiphene, p 1072.

Comment: The RCTs were generally of poor quality, and it is possible that, if one further medium sized RCT was performed, the direction of the overall effect found with meta-analysis could change again. The review highlighted important differences between the trials: two RCTs included women with surgically treated endometriosis, one included only couples with primary infertility, and one included couples with a short duration of infertility (median of 28 months). Three of the trials included co-intervention with intrauterine insemination or cervicovaginal insemination. The trials also differed in their design (four were crossover trials) and in the quality of randomisation (only one used properly concealed randomisation). The additional RCT also lacked a secure method of randomisation.[88] One large double blind RCT without co-interventions in a well defined group of couples with unexplained infertility is needed to clarify the role of clomiphene in unexplained infertility.

OPTION   INTRAUTERINE INSEMINATION

Systematic reviews have found that, in couples with unexplained infertility receiving FSH, intrauterine insemination increases the rate of pregnancy compared with timed intercourse. Two reviews found that intrauterine insemination doubles the rate of pregnancy, although a third found that the apparent benefit disappears when intrauterine insemination is compared with intercourse timed favourably rather than late.

Benefits: We found three systematic reviews.[69,87,89] The first (published in 1997) identified eight RCTs (number of treatment cycles not stated) comparing intrauterine insemination versus timed intercourse in couples with unexplained infertility receiving FSH.[87] In stimulated cycles, intrauterine insemination more than doubled the likelihood of pregnancy compared with timed intercourse (OR 2.37, 95% CI 1.43 to 3.90). The review also assessed the independent effects of FSH, clomiphene, and intrauterine insemination across 22 trials in couples with all causes of infertility. The likelihood of pregnancy was more than doubled with FSH (OR 2.35, 95% CI 1.87 to 2.94), and nearly trebled with intrauterine insemination (OR 2.82, 95% CI 2.18 to 3.66). Clomiphene did not increase the chances of pregnancy compared with no ovarian stimulation. The second review (published in 1998) identified seven RCTs (980 treatment cycles) comparing intrauterine insemination versus timed intercourse in couples with unexplained infertility (both interventions in addition to ovarian stimulation with gonadotrophins).[89] In stimulated cycles, intrauterine insemination achieved nearly twice the rate of pregnancy (20%) compared with timed intercourse (11.4%; OR 1.84, 95% CI 1.30 to 2.62). The third systematic review (published in 1997) identified seven RCTs comparing intrauterine insemination versus timed intercourse or intracervical insemination in couples with unexplained infertility (934 treatment cycles).[69] Four RCTs used gonadotrophins, two used clomiphene, and three used no ovarian stimulation. There was no significant difference in pregnancy rates with intrauterine insemination versus intracervical insemination or timed intercourse (OR 1.47, 95% CI 0.98 to 2.21). The addition of ovarian stimulation with gonadotrophins to any of the three interventions increased the overall pregnancy rates from 9.0% to 19.3% (NNT 10). One RCT (932 couples with unexplained infertility) published after the reviews compared intracervical insemination, intrauterine insemination, ovarian stimulation plus intracervical insemination, and ovarian stimulation plus intrauterine stimulation for four cycles or until pregnancy was achieved. It found pregnancy rates of 10% with intracervical insemination, 18% with intrauterine insemination, 19% with ovarian stimulation plus intracervical insemination, and 33% with ovarian stimulation plus intrauterine insemination.[90] Women treated with ovarian stimulation and intrauterine insemination were more likely to become pregnant than those in the intracervical insemination group (OR 3.2, 95% CI 2.0 to

5.3) and more likely than those in the intrauterine insemination group (OR 1.7, 95% CI 1.2 to 2.6). One underpowered crossover RCT (58 women, 174 cycles) suggests ovarian stimulation with clomiphene (50–100 mg day 3–7 of cycle) was at least as effective as ovarian stimulation with human menopausal gonadotrophin (150 IU days 4, 6, 8, and 9) before intrauterine insemination for either unexplained, male factor or female factor infertility in terms of clinical pregnancy rate and live birth rate.[91] **Versus fallopian tube sperm perfusion:** Fallopian tube sperm perfusion is based on a pressure injection of 4 ml sperm suspension with an attempt to seal the cervix to prevent semen reflux. It ensures a sperm flushing of the fallopian tubes and an overflowing of the inseminate into the pouch of Douglas. We found one RCT (with a review and meta-analysis of previous trials), which identified five RCTs comparing fallopian tube sperm perfusion versus intrauterine insemination in couples with unexplained infertility.[92] All five studies used gonadotrophins or gonadotrophins in combination with clomiphene citrate. In total, 293 cycles of intrauterine insemination and 317 cycles of fallopian sperm perfusion were evaluated. Fallopian sperm perfusion almost doubled the pregnancy rate when compared with intrauterine insemination (22% v 13%; OR 1.9, 95% CI 1.2 to 3.0). **Versus gamete intrafallopian transfer:** See option, p 1085. **Versus IVF:** One RCT randomised 258 couples with either unexplained infertility or male subfertility to six cycles of intrauterine insemination in natural cycles, to intrauterine insemination in stimulated cycles or to IVF. Pregnancy rates per started treatment cycle were similar in all groups (7.4%, 8.7%, and 12.2%, respectively) with no differences between the different diagnostic groups. More couples in the IVF group failed to complete their six cycles of treatment, and cumulative pregnancy rates after six cycles did not differ significantly between treatment groups. Multiple pregnancy rates were 4%, 29%, and 21%, respectively. Mild ovarian hyperstimulation syndrome occurred in two women in the stimulated intrauterine insemination group, and severe ovarian hyperstimulation syndrome occurred in three women in the IVF group.[93]

Harms: Apart from the risks of ovarian hyperstimulation syndrome and multiple pregnancy associated with the ovarian stimulation (see harms of gonadotrophins, p 1073), intrauterine insemination may increase the likelihood of infection and may be associated with some discomfort. However, data from RCTs are scarce. A recent RCT compared low dose, step up FSH versus a conventional FSH regimen combined with intrauterine insemination in 97 couples with unexplained infertility.[94] There was no significant difference in pregnancy rates (14.3 % v 14.6%), but the low dose group had significantly reduced incidence of ovarian hyperstimulation syndrome (8.3% v 27.1%) and ovarian hyperstimulation syndrome requiring hospitalisation (0% v 16.7%). However, the low dose regimen did not completely prevent multiple pregnancies.

Comment: Only three of the RCTs were common to all three systematic reviews. One of the reviews scored the included studies for validity.[89] They scored from 49–70% when 100% was taken as the ideal study. The evidence from RCTs for timing and the optimum number of inseminations per cycle is conflicting (see intrauterine insemination, p 1079).

| OPTION | GAMETE INTRAFALLOPIAN TRANSFER |

We found weak evidence suggesting that gamete intrafallopian transfer is more effective than no treatment in couples with unexplained infertility. RCTs comparing it with other treatments (intrauterine insemination, timed intercourse, and IVF) found no evidence of a difference.

Benefits: **Versus no treatment:** We found no systematic review or RCTs. One prospective cohort study (99 treatment cycles, 53 couples) reported pregnancy rates in couples with unexplained infertility before and after gamete intrafallopian transfer. It found that treatment with gamete intrafallopian transfer resulted in more pregnancies compared with no treatment.[95] **Versus intrauterine insemination or timed intercourse:** We found no systematic review. We found three RCTs in 283 couples with unexplained infertility. The first compared gamete intrafallopian transfer versus ovarian stimulation plus either timed intercourse or timed cervical donor insemination.[96] It found no significant difference. Of the other two RCTs, one found higher pregnancy rates with gamete intrafallopian transfer than with ovarian stimulation plus intrauterine insemination, and the other found no significant difference.[97,98] **Versus IVF:** See option below.

Harms: Potential harms include the risks attributable to general anaesthesia and laparoscopy. Multiple pregnancy rates vary with the number of oocytes transferred.

Comment: Gamete intrafallopian transfer, unlike IVF, gives no diagnostic information regarding fertilisation, and involves a laparoscopy and general anaesthetic, both of which are usually avoided with IVF. Success rates decrease with increasing age.[99,100]

| OPTION | IN VITRO FERTILISATION |

Limited data provide no evidence of a difference in pregnancy rates between IVF and gamete intrafallopian transfer in unexplained infertility.

Benefits: We found no systematic review. We found two RCTs in 155 couples with unexplained infertility.[82,101] Neither found a significant difference between gamete intrafallopian transfer and IVF.

Harms: See harms of IVF, p 1077.

Comment: The RCTs were too small to rule out a beneficial effect.

GLOSSARY

Laparoscopic ovarian drilling Ovarian drilling can be performed laparoscopically by either cautery or laser vaporisation (using CO_2, argon or Nd:YAG lasers), which are used to create multiple perforations (approximately 10 holes/ovary) of the ovarian surface and stroma (inner area of the ovary). This is thought to cause ovulation by restoring the intraovarian hormonal environment to normal, which in turn beneficially affects the hypothalamic–pituitary–ovarian axis.

Substantive changes since last issue

RCTs with crossover design A computer model comparing crossover and parallel designed trials suggested that any overestimation of effect may be clinically irrelevant.[7]

Hydrotubation or second look laparoscopy One new systematic review found insufficient evidence to support their routine use following tubal surgery.[46]

IVF alone versus IVF plus intracytoplasmic sperm injection (ICSI) One RCT found no evidence of a benefit from adding ICSI to IVF for tubal infertility where the semen analysis is normal.[53]

Intrauterine insemination for male infertility One RCT found similar pregnancy rates whether insemination was timed with a urinary LH kit or whether ultrasound monitoring with hCG induction of ovulation was used.[75]

Donor insemination for male infertility One systematic review found that intrauterine insemination of frozen donor sperm led to higher pregnancy rates than intracervical insemination (ICI) in centres where pregnancy rates per cycle for ICI were under 6%.[83]

Intrauterine insemination for unexplained infertility One underpowered crossover RCT suggests ovarian stimulation with clomiphene is at least as effective as ovarian stimulation with human menopausal gonadotrophin before intrauterine insemination for either unexplained, male factor or female factor infertility in terms of clinical pregnancy rate and live birth rate.[91]

Intrauterine insemination for unexplained infertility versus IVF One RCT found no differences between pregnancy rates in couples, with either unexplained infertility or male subfertility, randomised to six cycles of intrauterine insemination in natural cycles, intrauterine insemination in stimulated cycles or IVF.[93]

REFERENCES

1. European Society for Human Reproduction and Embryology. Guidelines to the prevalence, diagnosis, treatment and management of infertility, 1996. *Hum Reprod* 1996;11:1775–1807.

2. Schmidt L, Munster K. Infertility, involuntary infecundity, and the seeking of medical advice in industrialized countries 1970–1992: a review of concepts, measurements and results. *Hum Reprod* 1995;10:1407–1418.

3. Effective Health Care. The management of subfertility. *Effective Health Care Bulletin* 1992;3:13. Search date and primary sources not stated.

4. Collins JA, Burrows EA, Willan AR. The prognosis for live birth among untreated infertile couples. *Fertil Steril* 1995;64:22–28.

5. Templeton A, Morris JK. IVF — factors affecting outcome. In: Templeton A, Cooke ID, O'Brien PMS, eds. *35th RCOG study group evidence-based fertility treatment*. London: RCOG Press, 1998.

6. Khan KS, Daya S, Collins JA, Walter SD. Empirical evidence of bias in infertility research: overestimation of treatment effect in crossover trials using pregnancy as the outcome measure. *Fertil Steril* 1996;65:939–945.

7. Cohlen BJ, te Velde ER, Looman CW, Eijckemans R, Habbema JD. Crossover or parallel design in infertility trials? The discussion continues. *Fertil Steril* 1998;70:40–45.

8. Hughes E, Collins J, Vandekerckhove P. Clomiphene citrate vs placebo for ovulation induction in oligo-amenorrhoiec women. In: The Cochrane Library, Issue 4, 1999. Search date not stated; primary source Cochrane Subfertility Group Register of Controlled Trials.

9. Buvat J, Buvat-Herbaut M, Marcolin G, Ardaens-Boulier K. Antiestrogens as treatment of female and male infertilities. *Horm Res* 1987;28:219–229.

10. Messinis IE, Nillius SJ. Comparison between tamoxifen and clomiphene for induction of ovulation. *Acta Obstet Gynecol Scand* 1982;61:377–379.

11. Gerhard I, Runnebaum B. Comparison between tamoxifen and clomiphene therapy in women with anovulation. *Arch Gynecol* 1979;227:279–288.

12. Rossing MA, Daling JR, Weiss NS, Moore DE, Self SG. Ovarian tumours in a cohort of infertile women. *N Engl J Med* 1994;331:771–776.

13. Parazzini F, Negri E, La Vecchia C, Moroni S, Franceschi S, Crosignani PG. Treatment for infertility and risk of invasive epithelial ovarian cancer. *Hum Reprod* 1997;12:2159–2161.

14. Mosgaard BJ, Lidegaard O, Kjaer SK, Schou G, Andersen AN. Infertility, fertility drugs, and invasive ovarian cancer: a case-control study. *Fertil Steril* 1997;67:1005–1012.

15. Shushan A, Paltiel O, Iscovich J, Elchalal U, Peretz T, Schenker JG. Human menopausal gonadotrophin and the risk of epithelial ovarian cancer. *Fertil Steril* 1996;65:13–18.

16. Venn A, Watson L, Lumley J, Giles G, King C, Healy D. Breast and ovarian cancer incidence after infertility and IVF. *Lancet* 1995;346:995–1000.

17. Dunn A, Macfarlane A. Recent trends in the incidence of multiple births and associated mortality in England and Wales. *Arch Dis Child Fetal Neonatal Ed* 1996;75:F10–19.

18. State-specific variation in rates of twin births — United States, 1992–1994. *MMWR Morb Mortal Wkly Rep* 1997;46:121–125.

19. Levene MI, Wild J, Steer P. Higher multiple births and the modern management of infertility in Britain. *Br J Obstet Gynaecol* 1992;99:607–613.

20. Hughes E, Collins J, Vandekerckhove P. Ovulation induction with urinary follicle stimulating hormone vs human menopausal gonadotrophin for clomiphene-resistant polycystic ovary syndrome. In: The Cochrane Library, Issue 4, 1999. Oxford: Update Software. Search date not stated; primary source Cochrane Subfertility Group Register of Controlled Trials.

21. Coelingh-Bennink HJ, Fauser BC, Out HJ. Recombinant follicle-stimulating hormone (FSH; Puregon) is more efficient than urinary follicle

stimulating hormone (Metrodin) in women with clomiphene-resistant, normogonadotropic, chronic anovulation: a prospective, multicenter, assessor-blind, randomized, clinical trial. European Puregon collaborative anovulation study group. *Fertil Steril* 1998;69:19–25.

22. Yarali H, Bukulmez O, Gurgan T. Urinary follicle stimulating hormone (FSH) versus recombinant FSH in clomiphene citrate resistant normogonadotropic, chronic anovulation: a prospective randomised study. *Fertil Steril* 1999; 72:276–281.

23. Daya S, Gunby J. Recombinant versus urinary follicle stimulating hormone for ovarian stimulation in assisted reproduction. *Hum Reprod* 1999;14: 2207–2215. Search date 1999; primary sources Medline, Excerpta Medica Fertility Database, and hand searches of article bibliographies and meeting abstracts.

24. Wang CF, Gemzell C. The use of human gonadotrophins for the induction of ovulation in women with polycystic ovarian disease. *Fertil Steril* 1980;33:479–486.

25. Farquhar C, Vandekerckhove P, Arnot M, Lilford R. Polycystic ovary syndrome: laparoscopic "drilling" by diathermy or laser for ovulation induction in patients with anovulatory polycystic ovarian syndrome. In: The Cochrane Library, Issue 4, 1999. Oxford: Update Software. Search date not stated; primary source Cochrane Menstrual Disorders and Subfertility Group Register of Controlled Trials.

26. Bayram N, van Wely M, Vandekerckhove P, Lilford R, van der Veen F. Pulsatile luteinising hormone releasing hormone for ovulation induction in subfertility associated with polycystic ovary syndrome. In: The Cochrane Library, Issue 4, 1999. Oxford: Update Software. Search date not stated; primary sources Cochrane Menstrual Disorders and Subfertility Group Register of Controlled Trials, and hand searches of reference lists of included trials.

27. Balen AH, Braat DD, West C, Patel A, Jacobs HS. Cumulative conception and live birth rates after the treatment of anovulatory infertility: safety and efficacy of ovulation induction in 200 patients. *Hum Reprod* 1994;9:1563–1570.

28. Braat DD, Schoemaker R, Schoemaker J. Life table analysis of fecundity in intravenously gonadotropin-releasing hormone-treated patients with normogonadotropic and hypogonadotropic amenorrhea. *Fertil Steril* 1991;55:266–271.

29. Filicori M, Flamigni C, Dellai P, et al. Treatment of anovulation with pulsatile gonadotropin-releasing hormone: prognostic factors and clinical results in 600 cycles. *J Clin Endocrinol Metab* 1994;79: 1215–1220.

30. Martin KA, Hall JE, Adams JM, Crowley WF, Jr. Comparison of exogenous gonadotropins and pulsatile gonadotropin-releasing hormone for induction of ovulation in hypogonadotropic amenorrhea. *J Clin Endocrinol Metab* 1993;77: 125–129.

31. Honore GM, Holden AE, Schenken RS. Pathophysiology and management of proximal tubal blockage. *Fertil Steril* 1999;71:785–795. Search date not stated; primary sources Medline, Science Citation Index.

32. Ransom MX, Garcia AJ. Surgical management of cornual-isthmic tubal obstruction. *Fertil Steril* 1997;68:887–891.

33. Thurmond AS. Pregnancies after selective salpingography and tubal recanalization. *Radiology* 1994;190:11–13.

34. Marana R. Proximal tubal obstruction: are we overdiagnosing and overtreating? *Gynaecol Endoscopy* 1992;1:99–101.

35. Winston RM, Margara RA. Microsurgical salpingostomy is not an obsolete procedure. *Br J Obstet Gynaecol* 1991;98:637–642.

36. Filippini F, Darai E, Benifla JL, et al. Distal tubal surgery: a critical review of 104 laparoscopic distal tuboplasties. *J Gynecol Obstet Biol Reprod* 1996; 25:471–478.

37. Donnez J, Casanas-Roux F. Prognostic factors of fimbrial microsurgery. *Fertil Steril* 1986;46:200–204.

38. Tomazevic T, Ribic-Pucelj M, Omahen A, Colja B. Microsurgery and in vitro fertilization and embryo transfer for infertility resulting from pathological proximal tubal blockage. *Hum Reprod* 1996;11: 2613–2617.

39. Wu CH, Gocial B. A pelvic scoring system for infertility surgery. *Int J Fertil* 1988;33:341–346.

40. Oelsner G, Sivan E, Goldenberg M, Carp HJ, Admon D, Mashiach S. Should lysis of adhesions be performed when in vitro fertilization and embryo transfer are available? *Hum Reprod* 1994;9: 2339–2341.

41. Singhal V, Li TC, Cooke ID. An analysis of factors influencing the outcome of 232 consecutive tubal microsurgery cases. *Br J Obstet Gynaecol* 1991; 98:628–636.

42. Marana R, Quagliarello J. Distal tubal occlusion: microsurgery versus in vitro fertilization: a review. *Int J Fertil* 1988;33:107–115.

43. Marana R, Quagliarello J. Proximal tubal occlusion: microsurgery versus IVF: a review. *Int J Fertil* 1988;33:338–340.

44. Patton PE, Williams TJ, Coulam CB. Results of microsurgical reconstruction in patients with combined proximal and distal occlusion: double obstruction. *Fertil Steril* 1987;47:670–674.

45. Watson A, Vandekerchove P, Lilford R. Techniques for tubal surgery. In: The Cochrane Library, Issue 4, 1999. Oxford: Update Software. Search date not stated; primary source Cochrane Menstrual Disorders and Subfertility Group Register of Controlled Trials.

46. Johnson NP, Watson A. Postoperative procedures for improving fertility following pelvic reproductive surgery. In: The Cochrane Library, Issue 1, 2000. Oxford: Update Software. Search date not stated; primary source Cochrane Menstrual Disorders and Subfertility Group Register of Controlled trials.

47. Holst N, Maltau JM, Forsdahl F, Hansen LJ. Handling of tubal infertility after introduction of in vitro fertilization: changes and consequences. *Fertil Steril* 1991;55:140–143.

48. Vilos GA, Verhoest CR, Martin JS, Botz C. Economic evaluation of in vitro fertilization-embryo transfer and neosalpingostomy for bilateral tubal obstruction. *J Soc Obstet Gynecol Can* 1998;20: 139–147.

49. Gillett WR, Clarke RH, Herbison GP. First and subsequent pregnancies after tubal surgery: evaluation of the fertility index. *Fertil Steril* 1998; 68:1033–1042.

50. Jarrell J, Labelle R, Goeree R, Milner R, Collins J. In vitro fertilization and embryo transfer: a randomized controlled trial. *Online J Curr Clin Trials* 1993;2:Doc 73

51. Soliman S, Daya S, Collins J, Jarrell J. A randomized trial of in vitro fertilization versus conventional treatment for infertility. *Fertil Steril* 1993;59:1239–1244.

52. Benadiva CA, Kligman I, Davis O, Rosenwaks Z. In vitro fertilization versus tubal surgery: is pelvic reconstructive surgery obsolete? *Fertil Steril* 1995; 64:1051–1061.

53. Bukulmez O, Yarali H, Yucel A, Sari T, Gurgan T. Intracytoplasmic sperm injection versus in vitro fertilization for patients with a tubal factor as their sole cause of infertility: a prospective, randomized

trial. *Fertil Steril* 2000;73:38–42.

54. Human Fertilisation and Embryology Authority. Sixth Annual Report 1997. London: HFEA, 1998.

55. Brinsden PR, Wada I, Tan SL, Balen A, Jacobs HS. Diagnosis, prevention and management of ovarian hyperstimulation syndrome. *Br J Obstet Gynaecol* 1995;102:767–772.

56. Centers for Disease Control and Prevention. US Department of Health and Human Services. 1995 Assisted Reproductive Technology Success Rates. National Summary and Fertility Clinic Reports 1997;1–23.

57. Chapko KM, Weaver MR, Chapko MK, Pasta D, Adamson GD. Stability of in vitro fertilization-embryo transfer success rates from the 1989,1990, and 1991 clinic-specific outcome assessments. *Fertil Steril* 1995;64:757–763.

58. Camus E, Poncelet C, Goffinet F, et al. Pregnancy rates after in vitro fertilization in cases of tubal infertility with and without hydrosalpinx: a meta-analysis of published comparative studies. *Hum Reprod* 1999;14:1243–1249. Search date not stated; primary sources Medline and Cochrane Database of Systematic Reviews.

59. Hughes E, Fedorkow DM, Collins J, Vandekerckhove P. Ovulation suppression versus placebo in the treatment of endometriosis. In: The Cochrane Library, Issue 4, 1999. Oxford: Update Software. Search date not stated; primary source Cochrane Subfertility Group Register of Controlled Trials.

60. Hughes E, Fedorkow D, Collins J, Vandekerckhove P. Ovulation suppression for endometriosis. In: The Cochrane Library, Issue 3, 2000. Oxford: Update Software. Search date not stated; primary source Cochrane Subfertility Group Register of Controlled Trials.

61. Dockeray CJ, Sheppard BL, Bonnar J. Comparison between mefenamic acid and danazol in the treatment of established menorrhagia. *Br J Obstet Gynaecol* 1989;96:840–844.

62. Hughes EG, Fedorkow DM, Collins J. A quantitative overview of controlled trials in endometriosis-associated infertility. *Fertil Steril* 1993;59:963–970. Search date not stated; primary sources Medline 1966 to 1992; Science Citation Index January 1986 to December 1989; abstracts from scientific meetings 1986 to 1992, and hand searches of relevant trials and personal contacts.

63. Adamson GD, Pasta DJ. Surgical treatment of endometriosis-associated infertility: meta-analysis compared with survival analysis. *Am J Obstet Gynecol* 1994;171:1488–1504.

64. Marcoux S, Maheux R, Berube S. Laparoscopic surgery in infertile women with minimal or mild endometriosis. *N Engl J Med* 1997;337:217–222.

65. Parazzini, F. Ablation of lesions or no treatment in minimal-mild endometriosis in infertile women: a randomized trial. Gruppo Italiano per lo Studio dell'Endometriosi. *Hum Reprod* 1999;14:1332–1334.

66. Chapron C, Querleu D, Bruhat M, et al. Surgical complications of diagnostic and operative gynaecological laparoscopy: a series of 29 966 cases. *Hum Reprod* 1998;13:867–872.

67. Olivennes F, Feldberg D, Liu H-C, Cohen J, Moy F, Rosenwaks Z. Endometriosis: a stage by stage analysis — the role of in vitro fertilization. *Fertil Steril* 1995;64:392–398.

68. Geber S, Paraschos T, Atkinson G, Margara M, Winston RML. Results of IVF in patients with endometriosis: the severity of the disease does not affect outcome or the incidence of miscarriage. *Hum Reprod* 1995;10:1507–1511.

69. Ford WCL, Mathur RS, Hull MGR. Intrauterine insemination: is it an effective treatment for male factor infertility? *Balliere Clin Obstet Gynecol* 1997;11:691–710. Search date not stated; primary sources Medline, BIDS, and manual scanning of leading reproductive journals.

70. Cohlen BJ, Vandekerckhove P, te Velde ER, Habbema JDF. Timed intercourse versus intra-uterine insemination with or without ovarian hyperstimulation for subfertility in men. In: The Cochrane Library, Issue 4, 1999. Oxford: Update Software. Search date 1996/7; primary sources Medline, Embase, DDFU, Biosis, SciSearch, handsearching, and conference abstracts.

71. O'Brien P, Vandekerckhove P. Intra-uterine versus cervical insemination of donor sperm for subfertility. In: The Cochrane Library, Issue 3, 2000. Oxford: Update Software. Search date not stated; primary source Cochrane Subfertility Group Specialist Register of Controlled Trials.

72. Ragni G, Maggioni P, Guermandi E, et al. Efficacy of double intrauterine insemination in controlled ovarian hyperstimulation cycles. *Fertil Steril* 1999; 72:619–622.

73. Silverberg KM, Johnson JV, Olive DL, Burns WN, Schenken RS. A prospective, randomized trial comparing two different intrauterine insemination regimens in controlled ovarian hyperstimulation cycles. *Fertil Steril* 1992;576:357–361.

74. Ransom MX, Blotner MB, Bohrer M, Corsan G, Kemmann E. Does increasing frequency of intrauterine insemination improve pregnancy rates significantly during superovulation cycles? *Fertil Steril* 1994;61:303–307.

75. Zreik TG, Garcia-Velasco JA, Habboosh MS, Olive DL, Arici A. Prospective, randomized, crossover study to evaluate the benefit of human chorionic gonadotrophin-timed versus urinary luteinising hormone-timed intrauterine inseminations in clomiphene citrate-stimulated treatment cycles. *Fertil Steril* 1998;71:1070–1074.

76. van Rumste MME, Evers JLH, Farquhar CM, Blake DA. Intra-cytoplasmic sperm injection versus partial zona dissection, subzonal insemination and conventional techniques for oocyte insemination during IVF. In: The Cochrane Library, Issue 4, 1999. Oxford: Update Software. Search date not stated; primary source Cochrane Menstrual Disorders and Subfertility Group Specialised Register of Controlled Trials.

77. Bonduelle M, Legein J, Buyesse A, Van Assche E, Wisanto A, Devroey P. Prospective follow-up study of 423 children born after intracytoplasmic sperm injection. *Hum Reprod* 1996;11:1558–1564.

78. Kurinczuk J, Bower C. Birth defects in infants conceived by intracytoplasmic sperm injection: an alternative interpretation. *BMJ* 1997;315:1260–1265.

79. Bonduelle M, Legein J, Derde M, et al. Comparative follow-up study of 130 children born after ICSI and 130 children born after IVF. *Hum Reprod* 1995;10:3327–3331.

80. Velde E, van Baar A, van Kooije R. Concerns about assisted reproduction. *Lancet* 1998;351: 1524–1525.

81. de Wert G. Ethics of intracytoplasmic sperm injection: proceed with care. *Hum Reprod* 1998; 13(suppl 1):219–227.

82. Leeton J, Healy D, Rogers P. A controlled study between the use gamete intrafallopian transfer (GIFT) and in vitro fertilization and embryo transfer in the management of idiopathic and male infertility. *Fertil Steril* 1987;48:605–607.

83. O'Brien P, Vandekerckhove P. Intra-uterine versus cervical insemination of donor sperm for subfertility. In: The Cochrane Library, Issue 4, 1999. Oxford: Update Software. Search date not stated; primary source Cochrane subfertility group's specialised register of controlled trials.

84. Le Lannou D, Lansac J. Artificial procreation with frozen donor sperm: the French experience of CECOS. In: Barratt CLR, Cooke ID, eds. *Donor insemination*. Cambridge: Cambridge University Press, 1993;152–169.

85. Cooke ID. Donor insemination – timing and insemination method. In: Templeton A, Cooke ID, O'Brien PMS, eds. *35th RCOG Study Group evidence-based fertility treatment*. London: RCOG Press, 1998.

86. Hughes E, Collins J, Vandekerckhove P. Clomiphene citrate vs placebo or no treatment in unexplained subfertility. In: The Cochrane Library, Issue 4, 1999. Oxford: Update Software. Search date not stated; primary source Cochrane menstrual disorders and subfertility group's register of controlled trials.

87. Hughes EG. The effectiveness of ovulation induction and intrauterine insemination in the treatment of persistent infertility: a meta-analysis. *Hum Reprod* 1997;12:1865–1872. Search date not stated; primary source Cochrane menstrual disorders and subfertility group's register of controlled trials.

88. Fujii S, Fukui A, Fukushi Y, Kagiya A, Saito Y. The effects of clomiphene citrate on normally ovulatory women. *Fertil Steril* 1997;68:997–999.

89. Zeyneloglu HB, Arici A, Olive DL, Duleba AJ. Comparison of intrauterine insemination with timed intercourse in superovulated cycles with gonadotrophins: a meta-analysis. *Fertil Steril* 1998;69:486–491. Search date 1997; primary sources Medline and hand searches of bibliographies of relevant publications and review articles.

90. Guzick DS, Carson SA, Coutifaris C, et al. Efficacy of superovulation and intrauterine insemination in the treatment of infertility. National Cooperative Reproductive Medicine Network. *N Engl J Med* 1999;340:177–183.

91. Ecochard R, Mathieu C, Royere D, Blache G, Rabilloud M, Czyba JC. A randomized prospective study comparing pregnancy rates after clomiphene citrate and human menopausal gonadotrophin before intrauterine insemination. *Fertil Steril* 2000;73:90–93.

92. Trout SW, Kemmann E. Fallopian sperm perfusion versus intrauterine insemination: a randomized controlled trial and metaanalysis of the literature. *Fertil Steril* 1999;71:881–885. Search date not stated; primary source Medline.

93. Goverde AJ, McDonnell J, Vermeiden JPW, Schats R, Rutten FFH, Schoemaker J. Intrauterine insemination or in vitro fertilisation in idiopathic subfertility and male subfertility: a randomised trial and cost-effectiveness analysis. *Lancet* 2000; 355:13–18.

94. Sengoku K, Tamate K, Takaoka Y, et al. The clinical efficacy of low-dose step-up follicle stimulating hormone administration for treatment of unexplained infertility. *Hum Reprod* 1999;14:349–353.

95. Murdoch AP, Harris M, Mahroo M, Williams M, Dunlop W. Is GIFT (gamete intrafallopian transfer) the best treatment for unexplained infertility. *Br J Obstet Gynaecol* 1991;98:643–647.

96. Hogerzeil HV, Spiekerman JCM, de Vries JWA, de Schepper G. A randomized trial between GIFT and ovarian stimulation for the treatment of unexplained infertility and failed artificial insemination by donor. *Hum Reprod* 1992;7:1235–1239.

97. Murdoch AP, Harris M, Mahroo M, Williams M, Dunlop W. Gamete intrafallopian transfer (GIFT) compared with intrauterine insemination in the treatment of unexplained infertility. *Br J Obstet Gynaecol* 1991;98:1107–1111.

98. Wessels PHX, Cronje HS, Oosthuizen AP, Trumpelmann MD, Grobler S, Hamlett DK. Cost-effectiveness of gamete intrafallopian transfer in comparison with induction of ovulation with gonadotrophins in the treatment of female infertility: a clinical trial. *Fertil Steril* 1992;57:163–167.

99. Rombauts L, Dear M, Breheny S, Healy DL. Cumulative pregnancy rates and live birth rates after gamete intra-fallopian transfer. *Hum Reprod* 1997;12:1338–1342.

100. Society for Assisted Reproductive Technology and the American Society for Reproductive Medicine. Assisted reproductive technology in the United States and Canada: 1995 results generated from the American Society for Reproductive Medicine/Society for Assisted Reproductive Technology Registry. *Fertil Steril* 1998;69:389–398.

101. Ranieri M, Beckett VA, Marchant S, Kinis A, Serhal P. Gamete intra-fallopian transfer or in vitro fertilization after failed ovarian stimulation and intrauterine insemination in unexplained infertility. *Hum Reprod* 1995;10:2023–2026.

102. Meirow D, Schenker JG, Appraisal of Gift: *Eur J Obstet Gynecol Reprod* 1995;58:59–65.

103. RCOG Infertility Giudeline Group. *The management of infertility in secondary care*. London: RCOG, 1998. Primary Sources Medline, Embase, Cochrane Library, hand searching major journals.

104. Wahab M, Li TC, Cooke ID. Reversal of sterilization versus IVF. *J Obst Gynaecol* 1997; 17:180–185.

Kirsten Duckitt
Former Research Fellow
Royal College of Obstetricians and
Gynaecologists
London
UK

Competing interests: None declared.

TABLE 1 Comparative success rates of treatments for infertility: evidence from RCTs and analysis of database data (see text, pp 1072–1074.)

Treatment	Live birth rates	Pregnancy rates	Adverse effects
All causes of infertility			
IVF (per treated cycle)	UK 15%; US 20%[5]	59–77% (with 3–5 treatment cycles)[52]	Ectopic pregnancy: 1–3%[47,48]
GIFT (per cycle) (not including tubal infertility)	23%[102]	–	23%[78]
Infertility caused by ovulation disorders			
Clomiphene to induce ovulation in amenorrhoeic women (cumulative rate after 11 cycles of treatment)		90% 33 times more likely than with placebo[8]	Risk of ovarian cancer, unproved. MP: 2–13%, mostly twins.[16] OHSS: infrequent and mild
Gonadotrophins to induce ovulation in clomiphene resistant PCOS (cumulative rate after four months of treatment)		27–40%[3,20]	Risk of ovarian cancer, unproved. MP: 29%[24] OHSS: 4%
Laparoscopic drilling (cumulative rate 1–2 years after treatment)		FSH 27%[20] 48%[25,103]	Risks of laparoscopy, general anaesthesia, and adhesions. Risk of premature ovarian failure unproved
Tubal infertility			
Tubal surgery for distal occlusion (cumulative rate 2 years after surgery)	20–30%[35,41,42]		Risks of general anaesthesia. Ectopic pregnancy: 7–9%[47,48]
Tubal surgery for proximal occlusion (cumulative rate)	40–60%[43,44]		
Reversal of female sterilisation (cumulative live birth rate 1–2 years after surgery)	50–90%[104] depending on method used for sterilisation		
Infertility associated with endometriosis			
Surgery (per cycle)		13–38%†[62-64]	Risks of surgery and general anaesthesia (for laparoscopic surgery. Mortality 3.33/100 000; complication rate 3.2/1000)[66]
Male infertility			
IUI ± ovarian stimulation (per cycle)	20%[5]	6.5%[69]	
ICSI plus IVF (per cycle)	9–12%[54,84,85]		
Donor insemination* (per cycle)		9–12% without stimulation; 19–20% with stimulation[69,89]	No adverse effects if no ovarian stimulation is given, but child is not male partner's genetic offspring
Unexplained infertility			
IUI ± ovarian stimulation (per cycle)			

*Using frozen donor sperm in women without female factor or with corrected female factor infertility; †Over spontaneous rate; MP, multiple pregnancy; OHSS, ovarian hyperstimulsyndrome; IUI, intrauterine insemination; IVF, in vitro fertilisation; ICSI, intracytoplasmic sperm injection; GIFT, gamete intrafallopian transfer; PCOS, polycystic ovary syndrome.

Updated this issue

Janice Rymer and Edward Morris

Women's health

QUESTIONS

INTERVENTIONS

Key Messages

- Systematic reviews of RCTs have found that oestrogen relieves symptoms of urogenital atrophy and vasomotor symptoms. RCTs have found that oestrogen improves quality of life in the short term.

- Pooled estimates from observational studies have found that long term use of oestrogen is associated with an increased risk of thromboembolic disease, and endometrial and breast cancers.

- RCTs have found that:
  - Progestogens relieve vasomotor symptoms when used in high doses.
  - Tibolone relieves vasomotor symptoms and improves sexual symptoms.
  - Clonidine reduces hot flushes.

- Limited evidence from small RCTs suggests that soy flour, which contains phyto-oestrogens, may relieve vasomotor menopausal symptoms.

- We found insufficient evidence on the effects of testosterone and antidepressants on menopausal symptoms.

Menopausal symptoms

DEFINITION	Menopause begins 1 year after the last menstrual period. Symptoms often begin in the perimenopausal years.
INCIDENCE/ PREVALENCE	In the UK, the mean age for the start of the menopause is 50 years and 9 months. The median onset of the perimenopause is between 45.5 and 47.5 years. One Scottish survey (6096 women aged 45–54 years) found that 84% had experienced at least one of the classic menopausal symptoms, with 45% finding one or more symptoms a problem.[1]
AETIOLOGY/ RISK FACTORS	Urogenital symptoms of menopause are caused by decreased oestrogen concentrations, but the cause of vasomotor symptoms and psychological effects is complex and remains unclear.
PROGNOSIS	Menopause is a physiological event. Its timing may be determined genetically. Although endocrine changes are permanent, menopausal symptoms such as hot flushes, which are experienced by about 70% of women, usually resolve with time.[2] However, some symptoms may remain the same or worsen, for example genital atrophy.
AIMS	To reduce or prevent menopausal symptoms; and to improve quality of life, with minimum adverse effects.
OUTCOMES	Frequency and severity of vasomotor, urogenital, and psychological symptoms; quality of life.
METHODS	*Clinical Evidence* update search and appraisal May 2000. We included only RCTs and systematic reviews that met *Clinical Evidence* quality criteria.

QUESTION What are the effects of medical treatments?

OPTION OESTROGENS

Over 40 RCTs have found that oestrogen improves vasomotor symptoms. Systematic reviews of RCTs have found that oestrogen improves urogenital symptoms and depressed mood. Important adverse effects include venous thromboembolic disease, breast cancer, and endometrial cancer.

Benefits: **Vasomotor symptoms:** We found no systematic review. We found over 40 RCTs comparing oestrogen versus placebo and versus each another. Most found that oestrogen reduced vasomotor symptoms (data from one RCT in 875 women: OR 0.53, 95% CI 0.31 to 0.93).[3] Two RCTs found that transdermal oestrogen at a low dose of 25 μg daily reduced severity of vasomotor symptoms compared with placebo.[4,5] **Urogenital system:** We found one systematic review (search date 1995) and three subsequent RCTs.[6] The review pooled data from six RCTs. It found that oestrogen improved urogenital symptoms regardless of the route of administration (no figures available). One subsequent RCT (n = 136) found that low dose transdermal oestrogen (25 μg daily) combined with norethisterone acetate significantly reduced vaginal dryness and dyspareunia compared with placebo over 6 months.[4] Two other RCTs (n = 192) found that local administration of oestrogen using a silicone oestradiol releasing vaginal ring over 24–36 weeks improved vaginal oestrogenisation and pH compared with placebo.[7,8] One of these trials also found a significant reduction in incidence of urinary tract infection in treated women (P = 0.008).[7] **Psychological symptoms:** We found one systematic review (search date 1995, 14 RCTs, 12 cohort studies), which found that oestrogen reduced depressed mood among menopausal women.[9] Duration of treatment ranged from 1 month to 2 years. Data pooling for oestrogen versus placebo (10 studies) found that oestrogen reduced depressive symptoms (no figures available). We found no RCTs of oestrogen treatment in women with clinically proven depression. We found one systematic review (search date 1996, 10 controlled trials and nine observational studies) of the effects of oestrogen on cognitive function in postmenopausal women and women with Alzheimer's disease.[10] Studies were too weak to allow reliable conclusions. An additional crossover RCT (n = 62) found a beneficial effect of oestrogen on sleep quality compared with placebo over 7 months.[11] **Quality of life:** We found no systematic review. We found four RCTs (639 women, three placebo controlled RCTs, three versus progestogen), which found significant improvement in quality of life in women treated with oestrogen compared with baseline or placebo.[12–15] The largest RCT (242 women) found that oestrogen improved quality of life (P = 0.0003) and wellbeing (P = 0.003) compared with placebo over 12 weeks.[12]

Harms: Many RCTs have found that oestrogen causes weight gain and breast tenderness in the short term. Although many women report an increase in weight when starting oestrogen, we found no evidence from RCTs that oestrogen causes significant weight gain in the long term. One recent systematic review (search date 1998) of 22 studies has found no effect of either unopposed or combined hormone replacement therapy (HRT) on body weight.[16] The most important long term adverse effects are increased risk of venous thromboembolic disease, endometrial cancer, and breast cancer (see HRT under prevention of ischaemic cardiac events, p 83.[17,18] The relationship between oestrogen (as HRT) and breast cancer was reviewed in a reanalysis of 51 studies of more than 160 000 women.[19] The review found that the risk of breast cancer increased by 2.3% (95% CI 1.1% to 3.6%) each year in women using HRT. Five or more years after stopping HRT, there was no significant excess of breast cancer.[19]

Comment: Many studies used selected populations such as women attending hospital clinics, who may be different in their behaviour, personality, and symptom profile to women of the same age seen in primary care or those who do not seek medical advice.

OPTION   PROGESTOGENS

We found good evidence from RCTs that progestogens reduce vasomotor symptoms. We found no good quality evidence on other outcomes, including quality of life.

Benefits: We found no systematic review. **Vasomotor symptoms:** We found five RCTs (257 women, all trials less than a year long), which found that women taking progestogens experienced a significant reduction in vasomotor symptoms compared with placebo.[20-24] An RCT comparing oestrogen alone versus progesterone (150 mg of depot medroxyprogesterone for 25 days a month) found that over 3 months, 18% of women taking oestrogens and 33% taking progestogen reported no vasomotor symptoms.[21] One RCT (n = 102) found that transdermal progesterone cream 20 mg daily improved vasomotor symptoms compared with placebo (P < 0.001), but had no beneficial effect on bone density.[25] **Urogenital system:** We found no RCTs evaluating the effects of progestogens alone on urinary incontinence, the lower genital tract, or sex life. **Psychological symptoms:** We found no RCTs. **Quality of life:** One RCT of cyclical progestogen plus oestrogen for 6 months found no evidence of an effect on quality of life.[26] We found no studies of progestogen alone on quality of life.

Harms: We found two RCTs that evaluated harms of progestogens. The first compared continuous progestogen (norgestrel) versus placebo in 321 women who had undergone hysterectomy and were already taking conjugated oestrogen. The study found no difference in symptoms (including weight gain and bloating).[27] The second RCT (875 women) compared various oestrogen/progestogen combinations over 3 years.[3] It found that additional progestogen increased breast discomfort (OR 1.92, 95% CI 1.16 to 3.09). Neither trial found evidence of an effect on cardiovascular events.

Comment: Progestogen is seldom given alone, which makes it hard to isolate its effects. When given without oestrogen, doses of progestogens were high, the lowest dose being 20 mg medroxyprogesterone acetate per day.

OPTION   TIBOLONE

RCTs found that tibolone significantly improved vasomotor symptoms, libido, and vaginal lubrication.

Benefits: We found no systematic review. **Vasomotor symptoms:** We found three RCTs, two of tibolone versus continuous combined oestrogen/progestogen treatment over 48 and 52 weeks (672 women with menopausal symptoms)[28,29] and one versus placebo over 16 weeks (82 women with menopausal symptoms).[30] The first RCT found that the combined regimen versus tibolone reduced hot flushes over 48 weeks (P = 0.01). The second trial found a significant reduction in vasomotor symptoms from baseline in both groups (67/72 women on HRT and 58/68 women on tibolone, P < 0.001) but no significant difference between groups. The third trial found tibolone reduced vasomotor symptoms by 39% compared with placebo (P = 0.001). **Urogenital system:** We found two RCTs.[28,31] The first RCT found no significant difference between tibolone and combined hormonal treatment in terms of subjective reports of vaginal lubrication; both interventions improved lubrication compared with baseline.[28] The second RCT (437 women) found that tibolone improved sexual satisfaction compared with oestradiol plus norethisterone (P < 0.05).[31] We found no RCTs examining effects on urinary incontinence. **Psychological symptoms:** We found no RCTs. **Quality of life:** We found no RCTs.

Bone density: We found nine RCTs, which found that tibolone increased bone density over periods from 6 to 36 months compared with baseline or placebo.[32]

Harms: We found no evidence on adverse effects from RCTs. One non-randomised controlled trial found that the main adverse effect of tibolone was breakthrough bleeding, which occurred in about 10% of users.[33] We found no good evidence of androgenic adverse effects, such as hair growth and greasiness of the skin. Two RCTs of short term use found a 33% reduction in plasma high density lipoproteins with tibolone,[34,35] although the long term effects on cardiovascular disease are unknown.

Comment: None.

| OPTION | PHYTO-OESTROGENS |

Limited evidence from small RCTs suggests that soy flour, which contains phyto-oestrogens, may relieve vasomotor menopausal symptoms.

Benefits: We found no systematic review. **Vasomotor symptoms:** We found four placebo controlled RCTs. Two double blind RCTs evaluated soy supplements (which contain phyto-oestrogen); the other, which was not blinded, evaluated isoflavone. The first RCT (58 postmeno-pausal women) compared soy flour with wheat flour for 12 weeks. Hot flushes, though significantly reduced compared with baseline in both groups, were not reduced significantly more with soy flour than with wheat (40% reduction with soy *v* 25% with wheat).[36] The second RCT used a crossover design to evaluate 6 weeks' admin-istration of soy protein 34 mg daily. The trial found reduced severity but not frequency of vasomotor symptoms.[37] The third crossover RCT (n = 51) compared isoflavone 40 mg daily versus placebo. It found benefit from placebo compared with baseline, but not with isoflavone.[38] The fourth RCT (n = 39) found that soy flour reduced flushes more than placebo (45% reduction with soy *v* 25% with placebo, P < 0.01).[39] **Urogenital system:** We found no RCTs. **Psychological symptoms:** We found no RCTs. **Beneficial effects of treatment on quality of life:** We found no RCTs.

Harms: We found no evidence of significant adverse effects.

Comment: None.

| OPTION | CLONIDINE |

Two RCTs found that clonidine reduced vasomotor symptoms.

Benefits: We found no systematic review. **Vasomotor symptoms:** We found two RCTs.[40,41] One crossover RCT (66 women) found that clonidine reduced the mean number of flushing attacks in the 14 days after crossover compared with placebo (56.8 *v* 64.3, P < 0.05).[30] The second RCT (30 women) found that more women taking clonidine reported reduced flushes at 8 weeks (12/15 *v* 5/14, P < 0.04).[41] **Psychological symptoms:** We found no RCTs. **Quality of life:** We found no RCTs.

Harms: The two RCTs found no significant difference in the incidence of unwanted effects between placebo and active treatment groups.[40,41]

Comment: None.

OPTION TESTOSTERONE

We found evidence from RCTs that testosterone improves sexual enjoyment and libido. We found no studies evaluating effects on other commonly experienced menopausal symptoms.

Benefits: We found no systematic review. **Vasomotor symptoms:** We found no RCTs evaluating testosterone alone in women with menopausal symptoms. We found one RCT (93 postmenopausal women) comparing oestrogen alone versus oestrogen plus methyltestosterone. It found that the addition of a small dose of methyltestosterone reduced the dose of oestrogen needed to control menopausal symptoms.[42] **Urogenital system:** We found two RCTs, one in 40 women and one crossover study in 53 women. Both found benefit from exogenous testosterone on self-reported sexual enjoyment, desire, and arousal.[43,44] **Psychological symptoms:** We found no RCTs. **Beneficial effects of treatment on quality of life:** We found no RCTs.

Harms: We found no evidence from RCTs or other controlled studies on the incidence of androgenic adverse effects with testosterone.

Comment: None.

OPTION ANTIDEPRESSANTS

We found insufficient evidence on the effects of antidepressants on menopausal symptoms.

Benefits: We found no systematic review or RCTs that specifically addressed the effects of antidepressants on menopausal symptoms or quality of life in menopausal women.

Harms: We found no evidence on adverse effects in postmenopausal women. Antidepressants as a group can cause many central nervous system adverse effects, including sedation and agitation, as well as urinary and vision problems, liver dysfunction, and cardiac dysrhythmias (see antidepressants under depressive disorders, p 520).

Comment: None.

Substantive changes since last issue

Phyto-oestrogens Additional RCT; no change to conclusions.[39]

REFERENCES

1. Porter M, Penney G, Russell D, Russell E, Templeton A. A population based survey of women's experience of the menopause. *Br J Obstet Gynaecol* 1996;103:1025–1028.
2. Hagsta TA, Janson PO. The epidemiology of climacteric symptoms. *Acta Obstet Gynecol Scand* 1986;134(suppl):59.
3. Greendale GA, Reboussin BA, Hogan P, et al.

Symptom relief and side effects of postmenopausal hormones: results from the postmenopausal estrogen/progestin interventions trial. *Obstet Gynecol* 1998;92:982–988.
4. Mattsson L-A. Clinical experience with continuous combined transdermal hormone replacement therapy. *J Menopause* 1999;6:25–29.
5. Utian WH, Burry KA, Archer DF, et al. Efficacy and

safety of low, standard, and high dosages of an estradiol transdermal system (Esclim) compared with placebo on vasomotor symptoms in highly symptomatic menopausal patients. The Esclim Study Group. *Am J Obstet Gynecol* 1999;181:71–79.

6. Cardozo L, Bachmann G, McClish D, Fonda D. Meta-analysis of estrogen therapy in the management of urogenital atrophy in postmenopausal women: second report of the hormones and urogenital therapy committee. *Obstet Gynecol* 1998;2:722–727. Search date April 1995; primary sources Medline, Excerpta Medica, Biosis, and hand searched journals.

7. Eriksen B. A randomized, open, parallel-group study on the preventive effect of an estradiol-releasing vaginal ring (Estring) on recurrent urinary tract infections in postmenopausal women. *Am J Obstet Gynecol* 1999;180:1072–1079.

8. Casper F, Petri E. Local treatment of urogenital atrophy with an estradiol-releasing vaginal ring: a comparative and a placebo-controlled multicenter study. Vaginal Ring Study Group. *Int Urogynecol J Pelvic Floor Dysfunct* 1999;10:171–176.

9. Zweifel JE, O'Brien WH. A meta-analysis of the effect of HRT upon depressed mood. *Psychoneuroendocrinology* 1997;22:189–212.

10. Haskell SG, Richardson ED, Horwitz RI. The effect of ORT on cognitive function in women: a critical review of the literature. *J Clin Epidemiol* 1997;50:1249–1264.

11. Polo-Kantola P, Erkkola R, Irjala K, Pullinen S, Virtanen I, Polo O. Effect of short-term transdermal estrogen replacement therapy on sleep: a randomized, double-blind crossover trial in postmenopausal women. *Fertil Steril* 1999;71:873–880.

12. Wiklund I, Karlberg J, Mattsson L. Quality of life of postmenopausal women on a regimen of transdermal estradiol therapy: a double-blind placebo-controlled study. *Am J Obstet Gynecol* 1993;168:824–830.

13. Karlberg J, Mattsson L, Wiklund I. A quality of life perspective on who benefits from estradiol replacement therapy. *Acta Obstet Gynecol Scand* 1995;74:367–372.

14. Derman RJ, Dawood MY, Stone S. Quality of life during sequential hormone replacement therapy – a placebo-controlled study. *Int J Fertil Menopausal Stud* 1995;40:73–78.

15. Hilditch JR, Lewis J, Ross AH, et al. A comparison of the effects of oral conjugated equine estrogen and transdermal estradiol-17 beta combined with an oral progestin on quality of life in postmenopausal women. *Maturitas* 1996;24:177–184.

16. Norman RJ, Flight IHK, Rees MCP. Oestrogen and progestogen hormone replacement therapy for peri-menopausal and post-menopausal women: weight and body fat distribution. In: The Cochrane Library, Issue 1, 2000. Search date 1998; primary sources Medline, Embase, Current Contents, Biological Abstracts and Cinahl, citation lists, and contact with authors of eligible trails retrieved.

17. Grady D, Sawaya G. Postmenopausal hormone therapy increases risk of deep vein thrombosis and pulmonary embolism. *Am J Med* 1998;105:41–43.

18. Barrett-Connor E. Fortnightly review: hormone replacement therapy. *BMJ* 1998;317:457–461.

19. Collaborative Group on Hormonal Factors in Breast Cancer. Breast cancer and hormone replacement therapy: collaborative reanalysis of data from 51 epidemiological studies of 52 705 women with breast cancer and 108 411 women without breast cancer. *Lancet* 1997;350:1047–1059.

20. Loprinzi CL, Michalak JC, Quella SK, et al.

Megestrol acetate for the prevention of hot flashes. *N Engl J Med* 1994;331:347–352.

21. Lobo RA, McCormick W, Singer F, Roy S. DMPA compared with conjugated oestrogens for the treatment of postmenopausal women. *Obstet Gynecol* 1984;63:1–5.

22. Aslaksen K, Frankendal B. Effect of oral MPA on menopausal symptoms on patients with endometrial carcinoma. *Acta Obstet Gynecol Scand* 1982;61:423–428.

23. Schiff I, Tulchinsky D, Cramer D, Ryan KJ. Oral MPA in the treatment of postmenopausal symptoms. *JAMA* 1980;244:1443–1445.

24. Bullock JL, Massey FM, Gambrell RD. Use of MPA to prevent menopausal symptoms. *Obstet Gynecol* 1975;46:165–168.

25. Leonetti HB, Longo S, Anasti JN. Transdermal progesterone cream for vasomotor symptoms and postmenopausal bone loss. *Obstet Gynecol* 1999;94:225–228.

26. Reginster JY, Zartarian M, Colau JC. Influence of nomogestrel acetate on the improvement of the quality of life induced by estrogen therapy in menopausal women. *Contracept Fertil Sex* 1996;24:847–851.

27. Medical Research Council's General Practice Research Framework. Randomised comparison of oestrogen versus oestrogen plus progestagen hormone replacement therapy in women with hysterectomy. *BMJ* 1996;312:473–478.

28. Hammar M, Christau S, Nathorst-Boos J, Rud T, Garre K. A double-blind, randomised trial comparing the effects of tibolone and continuous combined hormone replacement therapy in postmenopausal women with menopausal symptoms. *Br J Obstet Gynaecol* 1998;105:904–911.

29. Al Azzawi F, Wahab M, Habiba M, Akkad A, Mason T. Continuous combined hormone replacement therapy compared with tibolone. *Obstet Gynecol* 1999;93:258–264.

30. Kicovic PM, Cortes-Prieto J, Luisi M, Milojevic S, Franchi F. Placebo-controlled cross-over study of effects of Org OD14 in menopausal women. *Reproduccion* 1982;6:81–91.

31. Nathorst-Boos J, Hammar M. Effect on sexual life – a comparison between tibolone and a continuous estradiol-norethisterone acetate regimen. *Maturitas* 1997;26:15–20.

32. Moore RA. Livial: a review of clinical studies. *Br J Obstet Gynaecol* 1999:106(suppl 19):1–21.

33. Morris EP, Wilson POG, Robinson J, Rymer JM. Long term effects of tibolone on the genital tract in postmenopausal women. *Br J Obstet Gynaecol* 1999;106:954–959.

34. Benedek-Jaszmann LJ. Long-term placebo-controlled efficacy and safety study of Org OD14 in climacteric women. *Maturitas* 1987;1:25–33.

35. Walker ID, Davidson JF, Richards A, Yates R, McEwan HP. The effect of the synthetic steroid Org OD14 on fibrinolysis and blood lipids in postmenopausal women. *Thromb Haemost* 1985;53:303–305.

36. Murkies AL, Lombard C, Stauss BJ, Wilcox G, Burger HG, Morton MS. Dietary flour supplementation decreases postmenopausal hot flushes: effect of soy and wheat. *Maturitas* 1995;21:189–195.

37. Washburn S, Burke GL, Morgan T, Anthony M. Effect of soy protein supplementation on serum lipoproteins, blood pressure, and menopausal symptoms in perimenopausal women. *Menopause* 1999;6:7–13.

38. Baber RJ, Templeman C, Morton T, Kelly GE, West L. Randomized placebo-controlled trial of an isoflavone supplement and menopausal symptoms in women. *Climacteric* 1999;2:85–92.

39. Scambia G, Mango D, Signorile PG, et al. Clinical effects of a standardized soy extract in postmenopausal women: a pilot study. *Menopause* 2000;7:105–111.

40. Edington RF, Chagnon JP. Clonidine (Dixarit) for menopausal flushing. *Can Med Assoc J* 1980; 123:23–26.

41. Nagamani M, Kelver ME, Smith ER. Treatment of menopausal hot flashes with transdermal administration of clonidine. *Am J Obstet Gynecol* 1987;156:561–565.

42. Simon J, Klaiber E, Wiita B, Bowen A, Yang HM. Differential effects of estrogen-androgen and estrogen-only therapy on vasomotor symptoms, gonadotropin secretion, and endogenous androgen bioavailability in postmenopausal women. *Menopause* 1999;6:138–146.

43. Dow MG, Hart DM, Forrest CA. Hormonal treatments of sexual unresponsiveness in postmenopausal women: a comparative study. *Br J Obstet Gynaecol* 1983;90:361–366.

44. Sherwin BB, Gelfand MM, Brender W. Androgen enhances sexual motivation in females: a prospective crossover study of sex steroid administration in the surgical menopause. *Psychosom Med* 1985;47:339–351.

Janice Rymer
Senior Lecturer/Consultant in Obstetrics
and Gynaecology
Guys, Kings, and St Thomas'
Medical School
London
UK

Edward Morris
Senior Registrar/Honorary Lecturer
HRT Research Unit, Guys Hospital
London
UK

Competing interests: JR has been sponsored to attend conferences by Organon, Solvay Healthcare Ltd, Wyeth, Novo Nordisk, and Janssen-Cilag. JR has also received research funding from Organon, and consultancy fees from Organon, Wyeth, and Janssen-Cilag. EM, none declared.

Updated this issue

Kirsten Duckitt

INTERVENTIONS

Key Messages

Medical treatments

- Systematic reviews of RCTs have found that non-steroidal anti-inflammatory drugs (NSAIDs) and tranexamic acid reduce menstrual blood loss. NSAIDs also alleviate dysmenorrhoea. Systematic reviews of RCTs have found danazol to be effective, but unacceptable adverse effects occur in two fifths of women.
- One systematic review of RCTs on ethamsylate has found conflicting results that suggest at most a small reduction in menstrual blood flow.
- We found no placebo controlled RCTs of oral or intrauterine progestogens. Two systematic reviews of comparative RCTs have found little benefit from oral progestogens given in the luteal phase, although oral progestogen treatment for 21 days of the cycle significantly reduces menstrual blood loss from baseline. We found one systematic review of the levonorgestrel releasing intrauterine device (IUD), which identified four small RCTs. It found no evidence of a difference compared with norethisterone and found it less effective than endometrial resection.
- We found no good evidence on the effects of oral contraceptives or gonadotrophin releasing hormone (GnRH) analogues in women with menorrhagia.

Surgical treatments

- Hysterectomy and endometrial destruction are suitable only for women who have completed childbearing. One systematic review of RCTs has found high levels of patient satisfaction after both procedures but significantly higher levels after hysterectomy. It found that 30–90% of women who had undergone endometrial destruction experienced continued bleeding, although in most cases this was light.

- One prospective cohort study found that hysterectomy caused major and minor complications in about one third of women. One RCT found that by 4 years, 38% of women who had undergone endometrial destruction required repeat surgery.
- RCTs have found no evidence of a difference in effectiveness between different methods of endometrial destruction.
- We found no good quality evidence on the effects of dilatation and curettage or myomectomy in women with menorrhagia.
- RCTs comparing resection versus medical treatments found conflicting results.
- One systematic review of RCTs has found that medical treatment to thin the endometrium before hysteroscopic surgery facilitates and reduces the duration of surgery and increases the rate of postoperative amenorrhoea.

DEFINITION	Menorrhagia is defined as heavy but regular menstrual bleeding. Idiopathic ovulatory menorrhagia is regular heavy bleeding in the absence of recognisable pelvic pathology or a general bleeding disorder. Objective menorrhagia is taken to be a total menstrual blood loss of 80 ml or more each menstruation.[1] Subjectively, menorrhagia may be defined as a complaint of regular excessive menstrual blood loss occurring over several consecutive cycles in a woman of reproductive years.
INCIDENCE/ PREVALENCE	In the UK, 5% of women, aged 30–49 years, consult their general practitioner each year with menorrhagia.[2]
AETIOLOGY/ RISK FACTORS	Idiopathic ovulatory menorrhagia is thought to be caused by disordered prostaglandin production within the endometrium.[3] Prostaglandins may also be implicated in menorrhagia associated with uterine fibroids, adenomyosis, or the presence of an IUD. Fibroids have been reported in 10% of women with menorrhagia (80–100 ml/cycle) and 40% of those with severe menorrhagia ($\geq$ 200 ml/cycle).[4]
PROGNOSIS	Menorrhagia limits normal activities and causes iron deficiency anaemia in two thirds of women proved to have objective menorrhagia.[1,5,6] One in five women in the UK and one in three women in the USA will have a hysterectomy before the age of 60 years; menorrhagia is the main presenting problem in at least half of these women.[7–9] About half of the women who have a hysterectomy for menorrhagia have a normal uterus removed.[10]
AIMS	To reduce menstrual bleeding, improve quality of life, and prevent or correct iron deficiency anaemia with minimum adverse effects.
OUTCOMES	Menstrual blood flow (assessed objectively [ml/cycle] or subjectively), haemoglobin concentration, quality of life, patient satisfaction, incidence of adverse drug effects, and incidence of postoperative complications. Whether a particular percentage reduction in menstrual blood loss is considered clinically important will depend on pretreatment menstrual loss and the individual woman's perception of acceptable menstrual loss.
METHODS	*Clinical Evidence* update search and appraisal May 2000. We also hand searched reference lists of non-systematic reviews and stud-

ies obtained from the initial search, and recent issues of key journals. We did not systematically search the "grey literature" (conference abstracts, theses, unpublished trials).

| QUESTION | What are the effects of medical treatments? |

| OPTION | NON-STEROIDAL ANTI-INFLAMMATORY DRUGS |

One systematic review of RCTs has found that NSAIDs, with the exception of ibuprofen, significantly reduce menstrual blood loss compared with placebo. Another systematic review of RCTs found no evidence of a difference in effectiveness between mefenamic acid and naproxen. One systematic review of a few small RCTs found no evidence of a difference between NSAIDs and other medical treatments. NSAIDs have the additional advantage of relieving dysmenorrhoea in three quarters of women.

Benefits: **Versus placebo:** We found one systematic review comparing NSAIDs (mefenamic acid, naproxen, meclofenamic acid, ibuprofen, and diclofenac) versus placebo (search date 1996, 12 RCTs, n = 313).[11] All the NSAIDs tested, except ibuprofen, reduced menstrual blood loss compared with placebo. Treatment was taken only during menstruation, but doses varied depending on the specific drug. The mean reduction in menstrual blood loss compared with placebo ranged from 23 ml (mefenamic acid) to 74 ml (diclofenac). When all the NSAIDs were combined, the difference compared with placebo was a reduced blood loss of 35 ml (WMD −35 ml, 95% CI −43 ml to −27 ml). **Versus other NSAIDs and other drugs:** We found one systematic review comparing different NSAIDs, and NSAIDs versus other drugs (search date not given, 16 RCTs).[12] It found no important difference between mefenamic acid and naproxen. In the few small studies suitable for evaluation it also found no important difference between NSAIDs and oral progestogens given in the luteal phase, the combined oral contraceptive, or a progesterone releasing IUD.

Harms: Commonly reported adverse effects were headaches and gastrointestinal disturbances, including indigestion, nausea, vomiting, and diarrhoea. These occurred in at least half of women taking NSAIDs in the RCTs that reported data on adverse effects, but similar levels of adverse effects were found in placebo cycles.[11,12]

Comment: NSAIDs have the additional benefit of relieving dysmenorrhoea. One systematic review (search date 1983, 51 RCTs) found that three quarters of women with dysmenorrhoea reported significant pain relief with NSAIDs.[13] A more recent systematic review (search date 1997, 56 RCTs) found that naproxen, ibuprofen, and mefenamic acid were all significantly better than placebo in relieving dysmenorrhoea (RR for relief of dysmenorrhoea versus placebo: 3.17, 95% CI 2.72 to 3.65 with naproxen; 2.41, 95% CI 1.58 to 3.68 with ibuprofen; and 2.03, 95% CI 1.65 to 2.48 with mefanamic acid).[14]

OPTION · TRANEXAMIC ACID

Two systematic reviews of RCTs have found that tranexamic acid significantly reduces menstrual blood loss compared with placebo. One of these reviews has also found that tranexamic acid significantly reduces menstrual blood loss compared with luteal phase oral progestogens, mefenamic acid, and ethamsylate. Small individual RCTs found that tranexamic acid was significantly more effective than mefenamic acid, ethamsylate, flurbiprofen, diclofenac, and norethisterone. Leg cramps occurred in one third of women. Long term follow up studies have found no evidence to confirm the possibility of an increased risk of thromboembolism.

Benefits: **Versus placebo:** We found two systematic reviews. The first review (search date 1996, 5 RCTs, n = 153) found a significant reduction in mean menstrual blood loss with tranexamic acid (250–500 mg 4 times a day during menstruation) compared with placebo (WMD −52 ml, graph in published report shows significant difference).[11] Few studies measured patient satisfaction. The second systematic review (search date 1997, 7 RCTs) identified two RCTs that compared tranexamic acid (1 g 4 times a day) or a pro-drug of tranexamic acid (Kabi 2161, 1.2 g twice a day) versus placebo.[15] It found a significant reduction in mean blood loss compared with placebo (WMD −94 ml, 95% CI −151 ml to −37 ml). **Versus other drugs:** We found two systematic reviews.[11,15] One review (search date 1997) found a significant reduction in mean menstrual blood loss compared with luteal phase oral progestogens (WMD −111 ml, 95% CI −179 ml to −44 ml) and mefenamic acid (WMD −73 ml, 95% CI −123 ml to −23 ml).[15] The other review (search date 1996) identified but did not pool data from several RCTs comparing tranexamic acid versus other drugs.[11] The trials consistently found that tranexamic acid was significantly more effective than mefenamic acid, ethamsylate, flurbiprofen, diclofenac, and norethisterone. One of the RCTs that looked at quality of life (n = 46) found that tranexamic acid reduced limitations on social activities and sex life significantly more than norethisterone.[16]

Harms: Nausea and leg cramps occur in a third of women taking tranexamic acid. One systematic review (search date not given) found no increase in gastrointestinal adverse effects compared with either placebo or other drugs.[15] Isolated case reports have suggested a risk of thromboembolism, but a large population based study over 19 years found no evidence that this was higher than expected in the normal population.[17]

Comment: Unlike NSAIDs, tranexamic acid has no effect on dysmenorrhoea.

OPTION · ETHAMSYLATE

One systematic review of RCTs has found a small reduction in menstrual blood loss compared with baseline, with minimal adverse effects. We found limited evidence from RCTs suggesting that ethamsylate is less effective than tranexamic acid, mefenamic acid, and aminocaproic acid.

Benefits: We found one systematic review (search date not given, 4 RCTs) comparing ethamsylate versus placebo (one trial), mefenamic acid (one trial), aminocaproic acid (one trial), and mefenamic acid plus tranexamic acid (one trial).[18] Most results were presented as comparison with baseline. The review concluded that ethamsylate achieved an overall reduction in menstrual blood loss compared with baseline of 13.1% (95% CI 10.9% to 15.3%), which may not be clinically significant. The individual trials reported conflicting results. One RCT (n = 23) found a 7% reduction in blood loss with ethamsylate and a 56% reduction with aminocaproic acid. A second RCT (n = 34) found a 20% reduction in blood loss with ethamsylate and a 24% reduction with mefenamic acid. A third RCT (n = 82) was the only one of the four to give direct comparative results rather than comparison with baseline.[19] It found that both tranexamic acid and mefenamic acid were significantly more effective than ethamsylate (WMD tranexamic acid v ethamsylate –97 ml, 95% CI –140 ml to –54 ml, and mefenamic acid v ethamsylate –51 ml, 95% CI –96 ml to –6 ml). The only placebo controlled trial (n = 22) found that ethamsylate reduced menstrual blood loss by 50% compared with baseline in women with "primary menorrhagia" and by 19% in women who were using IUDs.

Harms: The review found no significant difference between different regimens, in the rate of adverse effects such as nausea, headaches, and dizziness, and these seldom caused women to withdraw from studies.[18]

Comment: The individual trials differed in their methods. Two included women who were using IUDs as well as women with "idiopathic" menorrhagia and did not require a menstrual blood loss of more than 80 ml before entry. The other two studies looked only at women with a pretreatment menstrual blood loss greater than 80 ml. The placebo controlled trial may not be comparable with the other trials because it did not use the normally accepted alkaline haematin method to determine menstrual blood loss, and the women started ethamsylate 5 days before the expected start of their period instead of on day one as in the other trials.[18]

OPTION   DANAZOL

One systematic review of RCTs has found that danazol reduces menstrual blood flow more than placebo. Individual RCTs found that danazol was as or more effective than luteal phase oral progestogens, mefenamic acid, naproxen, or oral contraceptives. Unacceptable adverse effects occurred in 40% of women.

Benefits: **Versus placebo:** We found one systematic review comparing danazol (200 mg/day continuously for 2–3 months) versus placebo (search date 1996, 3 RCTs, n = 127).[11] It found a significant reduction in menstrual blood loss compared with placebo (WMD –108 ml, 95% CIs presented graphically). **Versus other drugs:** Several RCTs have found no difference or greater effectiveness with danazol compared with luteal phase oral progestogens, mefenamic acid, naproxen, and oral contraceptives.[20–23]

Harms: In one RCT (n = 40) adverse effects occurred in three quarters of those given danazol (200 mg daily) compared with one third of those given mefenamic acid; 40% of these adverse effects were deemed unacceptable.[20] An average weight gain of 2–4 kg occured in about a quarter of women after 3 months' treatment. Other adverse effects, which together occur in about half of women, include androgenic effects such as acne, seborrhoea, hirsutism, voice changes, and general complaints, including irritability, musculoskeletal pains, and tiredness. Hot flushes and breast atrophy can sometimes occur. Most of these adverse effects are reversible on cessation of treatment.

Comment: Women must be advised to use barrier methods of contraception because of potential virilisation of the fetus if pregnancy occurs during treatment.

OPTION   COMBINED ORAL CONTRACEPTIVES

We found insufficient evidence on the effects of oral contraceptives in the treatment of menorrhagia.

Benefits: We found one systematic review (search date 1997), which identified one small RCT (n = 38) comparing the combined oral contraceptive versus danazol, mefenamic acid, or naproxen.[24] It found no significant difference between any of the interventions but was too small to rule out a clinically important difference.

Harms: Minor adverse effects are common and include nausea, headache, breast tenderness, changes in body weight, hypertension, changes in libido, and depression.

Comment: One non-randomised controlled trial (n = 164) found that a 50 mg oral contraceptive pill led to a 53% reduction in menstrual blood loss compared with baseline. Aminocaproic acid (n = 85) led to a 54% reduction, and tranexamic acid (n = 172) led to a 47% reduction.[25] Two longitudinal case control studies found that women taking the pill were less likely than those not taking the pill to experience heavy menstrual bleeding or anaemia.[26,27] The oral contraceptive has the advantage of reducing symptoms of dysmenorrhoea and providing effective contraception. See oral contraceptives under dysmenorrhoea, p 1045.

OPTION   ORAL PROGESTOGENS

We found no placebo controlled RCTs. Two systematic reviews of comparative RCTs have found little benefit from oral progestogens given in the luteal phase, although oral progestogen treatment for 21 days of the cycle significantly reduces menstrual blood loss from baseline.

Benefits: **Versus placebo:** We found no placebo controlled RCTs. **Versus other drugs:** We found two systematic reviews (search dates not given).[18,28] The earlier systematic review identified four comparative RCTs.[18] Results were presented as comparison with baseline. The review found that norethisterone (taken on days 15–26 or 19–26) was associated with a small significant increase in menstrual loss from baseline (WMD in percentage reduction –3.6%, 95% CI –6.1% to –1.1%). Only two of the RCTs gave direct comparative data. One found a 16% reduction in blood loss with norethisterone (n = 15) and a 34% reduction with mefenamic acid (n = 17). The other found a 4% increase in blood flow with nore-thisterone (n = 18) and a 40% reduction with danazol (n = 19). The later systematic review identified seven comparative RCTs, including three RCTs not in the earlier review.[28] Mean menstrual blood loss was significantly greater with luteal progestogen than with danazol (WMD −56 ml, 95% CI −96 ml to −15 ml), tranexamic acid (WMD −111 ml, 95% CI −179 ml to −43.5 ml), and the progesterone releasing IUD (WMD −51 ml, 95% CI −84 ml to −18 ml). Luteal progestogens were associated with a significantly greater self assessed blood loss than danazol (OR 4.2, 95% CI 1.5 to 12.0). **Longer treatment cycle:** One RCT included in the review evaluated a longer regimen of progestogen (21 days/cycle) in 48 women.[28] It found no significant difference in the reduction in menstrual blood loss between norethisterone and the levonorgestrel releasing IUD (94 ml v 104 ml). There was a large and significant reduction from baseline with both treatments (P < 0.001), but a higher proportion of women who were using the levonorgestrel releasing IUD had menstruation reduced to "normal" (< 80 ml/cycle) compared with women taking oral progestogens.

Harms: Adverse effects were reported in one third to half of the women but were not usually serious. They consisted mainly of headache, breast tenderness, premenstrual symptoms, and gastrointestinal distur-bances.[18,28] In the trial of the longer treatment cycle, only 44% of women said they liked the treatment "well" or "very well", and only 22% elected to continue with treatment after the 3 months of the study.

Comment: The large number of withdrawals (27%) from the norethisterone group of one RCT may make the findings less valid.

| OPTION | INTRAUTERINE PROGESTOGENS |

We found one systematic review evaluating the levonorgestrel releasing IUD, which identified four small RCTs. It found no evidence of a difference compared with norethisterone and found the IUD less effective than endometrial resection.

Benefits: We found one systematic review of progesterone/progestogen releasing IUDs in menorrhagia (search date not given).[29] **Progest-erone releasing IUD:** The systematic review found one RCT that examined effects of a progesterone releasing IUD (65 µg/day), danazol, mefenamic acid, or norethisterone in women with menor-rhagia.[29] The review found that all treatments reduced menstrual blood loss from baseline, but did not compare treatments. **Levonorgestrel releasing IUD:** The review found four RCTs that examined effects of levonorgestrel releasing IUDs (20µg/day).[29] Two trials (n = 60 and n = 70) compared levonorgestrel releasing IUDs versus transcervical endometrial resection (see glossary, p 1111), using the pictorial blood loss assessment chart. A system-atic review of these trials found that at 1 year follow up, resection reduced blood loss from baseline more than levonorgestrel releas-ing IUDs (WMD for reduction in blood loss, resection v IUD 27, 95% CI 17 to 38).[29] However, mean blood loss and satisfaction rates were not significantly different between groups (WMD for mean blood loss, resection v IUD 12.2, 95% CI −1.9 to +26.3; satisfaction rate 85% with IUD, 94% with resection, P = NS).[29] The third RCT (n = 44) found no significant difference in reduction of blood loss or rates of satisfaction between norethisterone (15 ml/day, day 5 to day 26 of cycle) and levonorgestrel releasing IUDs (median reduction from baseline for norethisterone 6 ml/cycle v 20 ml/cycle for levonorgestrel; satisfaction data not given).[29] The fourth RCT (n = 56) found that levonorgestrel releasing IUDs improved all the quality of life scores that were assessed when compared with medical treatment (details of medical treatment and results not given). After 6 months of treatment, women using levonorgestrel releasing IUDs were more likely to cancel their hysterectomy than women using medical treatment (levonorgestrel releasing IUDs, AR of cancellation 64%, 95% CI 44% to 81%, v medical treatment, 14%, 95% CI 4% to 33%).[29]

Harms: Progesterone releasing IUDs were withdrawn in the UK because of concerns about increased rates of ectopic pregnancy. We found no evidence of this adverse effect. The systematic review found that most adverse effects in women using a levonorgestrel releasing IUD were typical of progestogens (bloating, weight gain, breast tenderness). One included trial found that 56% of women had at least one adverse event with the IUD, compared with 26% for transcervical endometrial resection (RR 2.17, 95% CI 1.2 to 3.0).[30] One further trial found that a greater proportion of women were amenorrhoeic after 3 months of treatment with levonorgestrel releasing IUDs compared with norethisterone (32% v 0%).[31] The other main adverse effect was irregular (although not usually heavy) menstrual bleeding. RCTs looking at the contraceptive effect of levonorgestrel releasing IUDs in younger women found that during the first few months of use, the total number of bleeding days (including menstrual bleeding, intermenstrual bleeding, and spotting) increased in most women.[32] However, by 12 months most women bled lightly for only 1 day a month and about 15% were amenorrhoeic.[33]

Comment: None of the trials included in the systematic review compared progestogen-releasing IUDs versus placebo.[29] Long term follow up on women with menorrhagia is required to assess continuation rates, satisfaction, and whether surgical treatment is avoided or just postponed. The trials that considered long term bleeding patterns were mainly in women aged under 40. It is not yet known whether these data can be extrapolated to older women with menorrhagia.

OPTION **GONADOTROPHIN RELEASING HORMONE (GNRH) ANALOGUES**

We found insufficient evidence on the effects of GnRH analogues in women with menorrhagia.

Benefits: We found no systematic review or RCTs. A few small non-randomised studies have looked at GnRH analogues in menorrhagia. Others have looked at their effects in women with fibroids or on thinning the endometrium before ablation or resection.

Harms: Adverse effects are mainly caused by reduced oestrogens. Hormone replacement to counteract hypo-oestrogenism has been tried with limited success to reduce hot flushes.[34] Bone demineralisation occurs in most women after 6 months of treatment but is reversible after treatment is stopped.[35]

Comment: Contraception is not guaranteed.[36]

QUESTION If medical treatments fail, what are the effects of surgical treatments?

OPTION DILATATION AND CURETTAGE

We found insufficient evidence on the effects of dilatation and curettage in women with menorrhagia.

Benefits: We found no systematic review or RCTs.

Harms: The procedure has small risks of serious morbidity, including uterine perforation and cervical laceration as well as the usual risks of general anaesthesia.[37]

Comment: Dilatation and curettage still plays a part in the investigation of menorrhagia. We found one uncontrolled cohort study (n = 50) that measured blood loss before and after dilatation and curettage. It found a reduction in menstrual blood loss immediately after the procedure, but losses returned to previous levels or higher by the second menstrual period.[38]

OPTION HYSTERECTOMY

Hysterectomy is the only certain way to stop all menstrual loss. One systematic review of RCTs has found that patient satisfaction is significantly higher after hysterectomy than after endometrial destruction. One large cohort study reported major and minor complications in about a third of women.

Benefits: **Versus endometrial resection or laser ablation:** We found two systematic reviews (search dates 1996 and not stated).[11,39] Both identified the same five RCTs (708 premenopausal women) comparing either transcervical endometrial resection or laser ablation (see glossary, p 1111) versus hysterectomy. Two of the authors were common to both reviews, and the conclusions were essentially the same. Follow up ranged from 1–4 years. The five RCTs consistently found a significantly greater reduction in menstrual blood loss with hysterectomy. Fewer women experienced reduction in blood loss with endometrial destruction compared with hysterectomy (RR for improvement 0.87, 95% CI 0.82 to 0.91). After longer follow up, the differences in improvement in blood loss between the groups seemed to narrow, possibly because of retreatment in the endometrial ablation group or women reaching the menopause. The reviews found that between 30–90% of women continued bleeding after endometrial destruction, although blood loss was usually light. The proportion of women who were very or moderately satisfied was significantly lower after endometrial ablation, both at 1 and 2 years (1 year: RR 0.93, 95% CI 0.89 to 0.99; 2 years: RR 0.87, 95% CI 0.81 to 0.94).[11,39] Two studies included in the review found no significant difference between satisfaction rates at longer follow up

(3 and 4 years). However, the duration of surgery, hospital stay, and time to return to work were all significantly shorter with endometrial destruction than with hysterectomy (reduced by a mean of 23 minutes, 5 days, and 4.5 weeks, respectively). Risk of repeat surgery was significantly higher at all follow up periods after endometrial destruction than after hysterectomy (first year: OR 7.3, 95% CI 4.2 to 12.9; second year: OR 7.5, 95% CI 4.2 to 13.4; third year: OR 4.5, 95% CI 1.8 to 11.2; fourth year: OR 9.8, 95% CI 4.9 to 19.7). One RCT found that by 4 years, 38% of women who had undergone endometrial destruction required repeat surgery for menstrual problems compared with 1% of those who had undergone hysterectomy.[40] **Different techniques:** We found no systematic review. A few small RCTs (total 334 women) compared abdominal, vaginal, or laparoscopic hysterectomy.[41–45] They found no evidence of a difference in effectiveness or complication rates. However, operating and recovery times varied.

Harms: Large population based analyses stratified by age have found a mortality after hysterectomy for non-malignant conditions of 1/2000 women aged under 50.[46] When compared with endometrial destruction, hysterectomy had a greater risk of sepsis, blood transfusion, urinary retention, anaemia, pyrexia, vault and wound haematoma, and cautery of hypergranulation before hospital discharge. One large, prospective cohort study of hysterectomy for non-malignant conditions found combined major and minor complication rates (mainly fever) of 25% for vaginal hysterectomy and 43% for abdominal hysterectomy.[47]

Comment: None.

| OPTION | ENDOMETRIAL DESTRUCTION (RESECTION OR ABLATION) |

One systematic review of RCTs has found that, although patient satisfaction is high after endometrial destruction, it is significantly lower than after hysterectomy. Endometrial destruction has several short term advantages over hysterectomy: shorter operating time, fewer complications, faster recovery, and less need for analgesia. Between 30–90% of women treated with endometrial destruction will experience continued bleeding, although in most cases this is light. One RCT found that about 40% of women required repeat surgery within 4 years. RCTs have found no evidence of a difference in effectiveness between different methods of endometrial destruction. RCTs comparing medical treatment and endometrial destruction found conflicting results.

Benefits: **Endometrial destruction versus hysterectomy:** See hysterectomy, p 1107. **Resection versus laser ablation:** We found no systematic review. We found one RCT (n = 372) comparing transcervical endometrial resection versus laser ablation.[48] It found no significant differences in operative complications (23% v 19.5%), satisfaction rates (90.3% v 89%), or need for further treatment (20% v 16%). It also found no significant difference in recovery times or symptom relief. **Rollerball ablation versus electrosurgical ablation:** We found no systematic review. One recent RCT (n = 276) comparing rollerball ablation (see glossary, p 1111) versus electrosurgical ablation (see glossary, p 1111) found no significant difference in reduction of blood loss assessed at 12 months by pictorial blood loss assessment charts (91% v 94%), and no significant difference in the proportion of women reporting amenorrhoea (39.6% v 31.8%).[49] **Resection versus microwave ablation:** We found no systematic review. One RCT (n = 263) comparing transcervical endometrial resection with microwave endometrial ablation (see glossary, p 1112) found no significant difference in patient satisfaction at 12 months, the same rates of amenorrhoea at 6 months, and a similar proportion of both groups requiring further surgery at 12 months. Satisfaction rates 75% with resection v 77% with microwave ablation. Rates of amenorrhoea in both groups 40%. Proportion requiring further surgery 7.8% with ablation v 9.7% with resection.[49] The mean operating time was significantly shorter for ablation compared with resection (11.4 minutes v 15 minutes).[50] **Rollerball ablation versus thermal balloon therapy:** We found no systematic review. One multicentre RCT (n = 255) comparing thermal uterine balloon therapy (see glossary, p 1111) versus hysteroscopic rollerball ablation, found no significant difference in mean menstrual blood loss at 12 months (85.5% v 91.7%).[51] Significantly more women were amenorrhoeic after rollerball ablation than after thermal balloon therapy (27.2% v 15.2%). However, 85.6% of women after balloon therapy and 86.7% of women after rollerball ablation were highly satisfied with the results 12 months after their ablative procedure (measured by quality of life questionnaires). **Resection versus medical treatment:** We found no systematic review. We found two RCTs, which reported conflicting results.[52] One RCT (n = 70) found no significant difference in menstrual blood loss or patient satisfaction between a levonorgestrel releasing IUD and transcervical endometrial resection. The other RCT (n = 197) found that satisfaction was significantly lower among women treated with one of a variety of medical treatments (not including a levonorgestrel releasing IUD) other than with transcervical endometrial resection (27% v 76%).[52] However, the women in this trial had already found no benefit from medical management and may differ from women newly presenting with menorrhagia. A 2 year follow up study on these women has recently been published.[51] It found increased average satisfaction for all women but higher satisfaction with transcervical endometrial resection than medical management. Satisfaction after resection was 79% compared with 55% after medical management (95% CI for the difference 9% to 36%). Bleeding and pain had also improved with medical management at 2 years and were comparable to levels in women who had undergone resection. These results could have arisen because 59% of women in the medical group had gone on to either transcervical endometrial resection or hysterectomy. However, 20% of women continued to take medical treatment and 41% of women avoided surgery.

Harms: Intraoperative complications include uterine perforation, haemorrhage, and fluid overload from the distension medium. Immediate postoperative complications include infection, haemorrhage and, rarely, bowel injury. Complication rates in the five RCTs described above ranged from 0–15%.[48–51,53] One large prospective survey of 10 686 women undergoing endometrial destructive procedures in the UK found an immediate complication rate of 4.4%.[54] Intraoperative emergency procedures were performed in 1.26%, and two procedure related deaths occurred. Newer methods of endometrial destruction, such as thermal balloon therapy have been evaluated only in small numbers of women and, although complications in the RCTs seem minimal, safety data for routine use are awaited.

Comment: These were good quality RCTs with results that should be widely generalisable. The prospective survey gave a good indication of what happened when the procedure was used in clinical practice.[54] RCTs of other methods of endometrial destruction are in progress.

OPTION   MYOMECTOMY

We found insufficient evidence on the effects of myomectomy in women with menorrhagia.

Benefits: We found no systematic review. **Open versus laparoscopic myomectomy:** We found no RCTs or other studies in women with menorrhagia that measured menstrual blood loss. **Hysteroscopic myomectomy:** We found no RCTs. One uncontrolled study (15 women, 10 with additional symptoms) reported objective measures of menstrual blood loss.[55] Mean menstrual blood loss, assessed preoperatively and at 3 and 6 months postoperatively, was significantly reduced (261 ml at baseline; 76 ml at 3 months, and 57 ml at 6 months). The study found a significant reduction in pain scores and menstrual duration, despite the fibroids removed measuring only 1–4 cm.

Harms: Intraoperative complications for hysteroscopic myomectomy are similar to those with endometrial destructive procedures that use a hysteroscope. The main complication of open myomectomy is haemorrhage, making a hysterectomy necessary.

Comment: RCTs are needed that use objective assessment of menstrual blood loss. This is especially important in the evaluation of surgical procedures because of the greater difficulty in blinding.

QUESTION   What are the effects of endometrial thinning before hysteroscopic surgery?

OPTION   ENDOMETRIAL THINNING BEFORE SURGERY

One systematic review of RCTs has found that use of GnRH analogues to thin the endometrium before hysteroscopic surgery facilitates and reduces the duration of surgery, and increases the rate of postoperative amenorrhoea. The review found that danazol was also effective but less so than GnRH analogues. There was insufficient evidence on the use of progestogens in this context.

Benefits: We found one systematic review evaluating medical treatment to thin the endometrium before hysteroscopic surgery for menorrhagia (search date not given, 8 RCTs, n = 946).[56] **GnRH analogues:** Four RCTs (n = 566) compared the GnRH analogue goserelin versus placebo or no treatment, with 6–12 months' follow up. Goserelin was associated with significant reductions in endometrial thickness on ultrasound (n = 358, 1.61 mm v 3.53 mm); weight of endometrium removed (n = 60, 2.4 g v 7.8 g, P < 0.01); duration of surgery (time difference ranging from 2–14 minutes, WMD –4.7 minutes, 95% CI –6.1 minutes to –3.2 minutes); volume of distension medium absorbed (no statistical analysis given); and operative difficulty (RR of encountering difficulty during procedure compared with placebo or no treatment 0.32, 95% CI 0.22 to 0.46). Goserelin was also associated with a significant increase in the rate of postoperative amenorrhoea (RR compared with placebo or no treatment 1.73, 95% CI 0.13 to 0.25, NNT for one additional case of postoperative amenorrhoea 5.3), and lighter menstrual periods (RR of continuing to have moderate or heavy periods 0.74, 95% CI 0.59 to 0.92). The data did not suggest any major difference in intraoperative complications, (uterine perforations were reported in 2/266 on goserelin and in 1/275 on no treatment or placebo), patient satisfaction, or the likelihood of undergoing further surgery. **GnRH analogue versus danazol:** Three RCTs (n = 340) compared danazol versus GnRH analogues (goserelin or decapeptyl). GnRH analogues were associated with significant reductions in endometrial thickness, greater uterine atrophy (RR of atrophic or inactive glands compared with danazol 1.42, 95% CI 1.11 to 1.82), and a significant increase in the rate of postoperative amenorrhoea (RR 1.57, 95% CI 1.06 to 2.33, NNT for 2 months 5.9). However, there was no significant difference in operative difficulty (RR 0.68, 95% CI 0.31 to 1.51). On the basis of data from two RCTs, duration of surgery seemed to be less with GnRH analogues (WMD –3.9 minutes, 95% CI –6.1 minutes to –1.7 minutes). None of the trials reported any intraoperative complications. **Progestogens:** One RCT (n = 40) compared progestogens versus GnRH analogues versus danazol versus no treatment. The trial was too small to allow firm conclusions to be drawn.

Harms: Hot flushes, reduced libido, depression, and vaginal dryness were significantly more common with goserelin than danazol. Oily skin, hirsutism, and weight gain were significantly more common with danazol. Withdrawals from trials because of adverse effects occurred in 1/566 women receiving goserelin (headache) and 11/139 receiving danazol.

Comment: None of the trials used objective measures of postoperative menstrual blood loss. One used allocation concealment and one used intention to treat analysis. Rates of withdrawal or loss to follow up were low in all studies.

GLOSSARY

Transcervical endometrial resection A hysteroscopic procedure in which endometrium is removed under direct vision by using an electrosurgical loop.

Electrosurgical ablation A procedure in which an inflatable device with electrodes on the outside is inserted into the uterine cavity via the cervix. The electrodes make contact with the endometrium and cause necrosis.

Thermal uterine balloon therapy A procedure in which a balloon catheter is passed through the cervix into the uterine cavity. The balloon is then filled with fluid which is heated to about 87°C, and left for 8 minutes. This causes necrosis of the endometrium.

Rollerball ablation A hysteroscopic procedure in which endometrium is destroyed under direct vision by the use of diathermy applied by a rollerball.

Menorrhagia

Microwave endometrial ablation A procedure in which a microwave probe is passed through the cervix into the uterine cavity. When activated it is moved slowly from side to side over the whole surface of the uterine cavity in order to destroy the endometrium.

Laser ablation A hysteroscopic procedure in which endometrium is destroyed under direct vision by a laser beam.

Substantive changes since last issue

Intrauterine progestogens: New systematic review.[29] Found no evidence of a difference compared with norethisterone and found intrauterine progestogens less effective than endometrial resection. One included trial found that treatment with levonorgestrel releasing IUDs was more likely than norethisterone to result in amenorrhoea.

Endometrial destruction: New RCT.[47] Found no evidence of a difference in outcome between microwave endometrial ablation and transcervical endometrial resection.

REFERENCES

1. Hallberg L, Hogdahl A, Nilsson L, et al. Menstrual blood loss – a population study: variation at different ages and attempts to define normality. *Acta Obstet Gynecol Scand* 1966;45:320–351.
2. Vessey MP, Villard-Mackintosh L, McPherson K, et al. The epidemiology of hysterectomy: findings in a large cohort study. *Br J Obstet Gynaecol* 1992;99: 402–407.
3. Smith SK, Abel MH, Kelly RW, et al. A role for prostacyclin (PGI$_2$) in excessive menstrual bleeding. *Lancet* 1981;i:522–524.
4. Rybo G, Leman J, Tibblin R. Epidemiology of menstrual blood loss. In: Baird DT, Michie EA, eds. *Mechanisms of menstrual bleeding*. New York: Raven Press, 1985:181–193.
5. Alexander DA, Naji AA, Pinion SB, et al. Randomised trial comparing hysterectomy with endometrial ablation for dysfunctional uterine bleeding: psychiatric and psychosocial aspects. *BMJ* 1996;312:280–284.
6. Coulter A, Peto V, Jenkinson C. Quality of life and patient satisfaction following treatment for menorrhagia. *Fam Pract* 1994;11:394–401.
7. Coulter A, McPherson K, Vessey M. Do British women undergo too many or too few hysterectomies? *Soc Sci Med* 1988;27:987–994.
8. Pokras R, Hufnagel VG. *Hysterectomy in the United States, 1965–84*. Washington, DC: Public Health Service, 1987:87–1753.
9. Coulter A, Kelland J, Long A. The management of menorrhagia. *Effective Health Care Bull* 1995;9: 1–14.
10. Clarke A, Black N, Rowe P, et al. Indications for and outcome of total abdominal hysterectomy for benign disease: a prospective cohort study. *Br J Obstet Gynaecol* 1995;102:611–620.
11. Working Party of the National Health Committee New Zealand. *Guidelines for the management of heavy menstrual bleeding*. Wellington: Ministry of Health, 1998. (Available from The Ministry of Health, 133 Molesworth Street, PO Box 5013, Wellington, New Zealand.) Search date 1996; primary sources Medline, Embase, Current Contents, Biological Abstracts, Social Sciences Index, Psychlit, Cinahl.
12. Lethaby A, Augood C, Duckitt K. Nonsteroidal anti-inflammatory drugs vs either placebo or any other medical treatment for heavy menstrual bleeding (menorrhagia). In: The Cochrane Library, Issue 2, 2000. Oxford: Update Software. Search date not given; primary sources Cochrane Menstrual Disorders and Subfertility Group trials register,

Medline, Embase, Psychlit, Current Contents, Biological Abstracts, Social Sciences Index, Cinahl, reference lists and drug companies.
13. Owen PR. Prostaglandin synthetase inhibitors in the treatment of primary dysmenorrhoea. *Am J Obstet Gynecol* 1984;148:96–103. Search date January 1982; primary sources Medline 1974–1982.
14. Zhang WY, Li Wan Po A. Efficacy of minor analgesics in primary dysmenorrhoea: a systematic review. *Br J Obstet Gynaecol* 1998; 105:780–789. Search date 1997; primary sources Medline, Embase, Science Citation Index, reference lists of retrieved RCTs, review articles, communication with the manufacturers.
15. Cooke I, Lethaby A, Farquhar C. Antifibrinolytics for heavy menstrual bleeding. In: The Cochrane Library, Issue 2, 2000. Oxford: Update Software. Search date 1997; primary sources Cochrane Menstrual Disorders and Subfertility Group trials register, Medline, Embase and hand searches of reference lists from experts and drug companies.
16. Preston JT, Cameron IT, Adams EJ, et al. Comparative study of tranexamic acid and norethisterone in the treatment of ovulatory menorrhagia. *Br J Obstet Gynaecol* 1995;102: 401–406.
17. Rybo G. Tranexamic acid therapy is effective treatment in heavy menstrual bleeding: clinical update on safety. *Ther Adv* 1991;4:1–8.
18. Coulter A, Kelland J, Peto V, et al. Treating menorrhagia in primary care. An overview of drug trials and a survey of prescribing practice. *Int J Technol Assess Health Care* 1995;11:456–471. Search date not given; primary sources Medline, Embase.
19. Bonnar J, Sheppard BL. Treatment of menorrhagia during menstruation: randomised controlled trial of ethamsylate, mefenamic acid, and tranexamic acid. *BMJ* 1996;313:579–582.
20. Dockeray CJ, Sheppard BL, Bonnar J. Comparison between mefenamic acid and danazol in the treatment of established menorrhagia. *Br J Obstet Gynaecol* 1989;96:840–844.
21. Higham JM, Shaw RW. A comparative study of danazol, a regimen of decreasing doses of danazol, and norethindrone in the treatment of objectively proven unexplained menorrhagia. *Am J Obstet Gynecol* 1993;169:1134–1139.
22. Fraser IS, McCarron G. Randomized trial of 2 hormonal and 2 prostaglandin-inhibiting agents in women with a complaint of menorrhagia. *Aust NZ*

J Obstet Gynaecol 1991;31:66–70.

23. Dunphy BC, Goerzen J, Greene CA, et al. A double-blind randomised study comparing danazol and medroxyprogesterone acetate in the management of menorrhagia. *J Obstet Gynaecol* 1998;18:553–555.

24. Iyer V, Farquhar C, Jepson R. The effectiveness of oral contraceptive pills versus placebo or any other medical treatment for menorrhagia. In: The Cochrane Library, Issue 2, 2000. Oxford: Update Software. Search date 1997; primary sources Cochrane Register of Controlled Trials.

25. Nilsson L, Rybo G. Treatment of menorrhagia. *Am J Obstet Gynecol* 1971;5:713–720.

26. Ramcharan S, Pellegrin FA, Ray MR, et al. The Walnut Creek contraceptive drug study – a prospective study of the side effects of oral contraceptives. Vol III. An interim report: a comparison of disease occurrence leading to hospitalization or death in users and nonusers of oral contraceptives. *J Reprod Med* 1980;25:345–372.

27. Royal College of General Practitioners. *Oral contraceptives and health*. London: Pitman Medical, 1974.

28. Lethaby A, Irvine G, Cameron I. Cyclical progestogens for heavy menstrual bleeding. In: The Cochrane Library, Issue 2, 2000. Oxford: Update Software. Search date not given; primary sources Cochrane Menstrual Disorders and Subfertility Group trials register, Medline, Embase, Psychlit, Current Contents, Biological Abstracts, Social Sciences Index, Cinahl, reference lists.

29. Lethaby AE, Cooke I, Rees M. Progesterone/progestogen releasing intrauterine systems versus either placebo or any other medication for heavy menstrual bleeding. In: The Cochrane Library, Issue 2, 2000. Oxford: Update Software. Search date 1999; primary sources Medline, Embase, Cochrane Library, and experts contacted.

30. Crosignani PG, Vercellini P, Mosconi P, et al. Levonorgestrel-releasing intrauterine device versus hysteroscopic endometrial resection in the treatment of dysfunctional uterine bleeding. *Obstet Gynecol* 1997;90:257–263.

31. Irvine GA, Campbell-Brown MB, Lumsden MA, et al. Randomised comparative study of the levonorgestrel intrauterine system and norethisterone for the treatment of idiopathic menorrhagia. *Br J Obstet Gynaecol* 1998;105:592–598.

32. Long-acting progestogen-only contraception. *Drug Ther Bull* 1996;34:93–96.

33. Luukkainen T. The levonorgestrel-releasing IUD. *Br J Fam Plann* 1993;19:221–224.

34. Thomas EJ, Okuda KJ, Thomas NM. The combination of a depot gonadotrophin releasing hormone agonist and cyclical hormone replacement therapy for dysfunctional uterine bleeding. *Br J Obstet Gynaecol* 1991;98:1155–1159.

35. Eldred JM, Haynes PJ, Thomas EJ. A randomized double blind placebo controlled trial of the effects on bone metabolism of the combination of nafarelin acetate and norethisterone. *Clin Endocrinol* 1992;37:354–359.

36. Pickersgill A, Kingsland CR, Garden AS, et al. Multiple gestation following gonadotrophin releasing hormone therapy for the treatment of minimal endometriosis. *Br J Obstet Gynaecol* 1998;101:260–262.

37. Smith JJ, Schulman H. Current dilatation and curettage practice: a need for revision. *Obstet Gynecol* 1985;65:516–518.

38. Haynes PJ, Hodgson H, Anderson AB, et al. Measurement of menstrual blood loss in patients complaining of menorrhagia. *Br J Obstet Gynaecol* 1977;84:763–768.

39. Lethaby A, Shepperd S, Cooke I, et al. Endometrial resection and ablation versus hysterectomy for heavy menstrual bleeding. In: The Cochrane Library, Issue 2, 2000. Oxford: Update Software. Search date not stated; primary sources Cochrane Menstrual Disorders and Subfertility Group Register of Trials, Medline, Embase, Psychlit, Current Contents, Biological Abstracts, Social Sciences Index, and Cinahl.

40. Aberdeen Endometrial Ablation Trials Group. A randomised trial of endometrial ablation versus hysterectomy for the treatment of dysfunction uterine bleeding: outcome at four years. *Br J Obstet Gynaecol* 1999;106:360–366.

41. Phipps JH, John M, Nayak S. Comparison of laparoscopically assisted vaginal hysterectomy and bilateral salpingo-oophorectomy with conventional abdominal hysterectomy and bilateral salpingo-oophorectomy. *Br J Obstet Gynaecol* 1993;100:698–700.

42. Raju KS, Auld BJ. A randomised prospective study of laparoscopic vaginal hysterectomy versus abdominal hysterectomy each with bilateral salpingo-oophorectomy. *Br J Obstet Gynaecol* 1994;101:1068–1071.

43. Richardson RE, Bournas N, Magos AL. Is laparoscopic hysterectomy a waste of time? *Lancet* 1995;345:36–41.

44. Summitt RL Jr, Stovall TG, Lipscomb GH, et al. Randomized comparison of laparoscopy-assisted vaginal hysterectomy with standard vaginal hysterectomy in an outpatient setting. *Obstet Gynecol* 1992;80:895–901.

45. Langebrekke A, Eraker R, Nesheim B, et al. Abdominal hysterectomy should not be considered as primary method for uterine removal. *Acta Obstet Gynecol Scand* 1996;75:404–407.

46. Carlson KJ. Outcomes of hysterectomy. *Clin Obstet Gynecol* 1997;40:939–946.

47. Dicker RC, Greenspan JR, Strauss LT, et al. Complications of abdominal and vaginal hysterectomy among women of reproductive age in the United States—the Collaborative Review of Sterilization. *Am J Obstet Gynecol* 1982;144:841–848.

48. Bhattacharya S, Cameron IM, Parkin DE, et al. A pragmatic randomised comparison of transcervical resection of the endometrium with endometrial laser ablation for the treatment of menorrhagia. *Br J Obstet Gynaecol* 1997;104:601–607.

49. Corson SL, Brill AI, Brooks PG, et al. Interim results of the American Vesta trial of endometrial ablation. *J Am Assoc Gynecol Laparosc* 1999;6:45–49.

50. B. Cooper KG, Bain C, Parkin DE. Comparison of microwave endometrial ablation and transcervical resection of the endometrium for treatment of heavy menstrual bleeding: a randomised trial. *Lancet* 1999;354:1859–1863.

51. Meyer WR, Walsh BW, Grainger DA, et al. Thermal balloon and rollerball ablation to treat menorrhagia: a multicenter comparison. *Obstet Gynecol* 1998;92:98–103.

52. Cooper KG, Parkin DE, Garratt AM, et al. A randomised comparison of medical versus hysteroscopic management in women consulting a gynaecologist for treatment of heavy menstrual loss. *Br J Obstet Gynaecol* 1997;104:1360–1366.

53. Cooper KG, Parkin DE, Garratt AM, et al. Two-year follow up of women randomised to medical management or transcervical resection of the endometrium for heavy menstrual loss: clinical and quality of life outcomes. *Br J Obstet Gynaecol* 1999;106:258–265.

54. Overton C, Hargreaves J, Maresh M. A national survey of the complications of endometrial destruction for menstrual disorders: the MISTLETOE study. Minimally invasive surgical techniques — laser, endothermal or endoresection. *Br J Obstet Gynaecol* 1997;104: 1351–1359.

55. Broadbent JAM, Magos AL. Menstrual blood loss after hysteroscopic myomectomy. *Gynaecol Endoscop* 1995;4:41–44.

56. Sowter MC, Singla AA, Lethaby A. Pre-operative endometrial thinning agents before hysteroscopic surgery for heavy menstrual bleeding. In: The Cochrane Library, Issue 2, 2000. Oxford: Update Software. Search date not stated; primary sources Medline, Embase, Psychlit, Cinahl, biological abstracts, reference lists, authors of conference abstracts, Zeneca Pharmaceuticals and Sanofi Winthrop.

Kirsten Duckitt
Clinical Lecturer
John Radcliffe Hospital
Oxford
UK

Competing interests: None declared.

Updated this issue

Earlando Thomas, Damian Murphy and Charles Redman

QUESTIONS

Effects of treatments for lichen sclerosus 1116
Effects of treatments for vulval intraepithelial neoplasia (VIN) 1118

INTERVENTIONS

LICHEN SCLEROSUS

Likely to be beneficial
Topical clobetasol propionate
(0.05%) 1116

Trade off between benefits and harms
Oral retinoids (acitretin) 1117
Surgery (vulvectomy, cryosurgery,
laser) 1118

Likely to be ineffective or harmful
Topical testosterone 1116

VULVAL INTRAEPITHELIAL NEOPLASIA

Unknown effectiveness
Surgical treatments 1118
Topical α interferon 1119

To be covered in future issues of *Clinical Evidence*
Lichen sclerosus: effects of topical
lignocaine
VIN: effects of 5-fluorouracil
Petroleum jelly

See glossary, p 1119

Key Messages

Lichen sclerosus

- Limited evidence from three small RCTs suggests that topical clobetasol propionate is the most effective treatment for lichen sclerosus. Good quality prospective observational studies reported minimal adverse effects when clobetasol was used as required for maintenance treatment.

- Small RCTs found no evidence that testosterone was more effective than petroleum jelly, either as initial treatment or as maintenance treatment after treatment with clobetasol propionate. Testosterone is associated with virilisation.

- One small RCT found acitretin significantly reduced symptoms compared with placebo, but was associated with hair loss and severe skin peeling.

- We found insufficient evidence on the effects of surgery in women with lichen sclerosus.

Vulval intraepithelial neoplasia

- We found insufficient evidence on the effects of surgical or topical treatments in women with vulval intraepithelial neoplasia (VIN).

DEFINITION There are two recognised premalignant conditions of the vulva. **Lichen sclerosus** is characterised by epithelial thinning, inflammation, and distinctive histological changes in the dermis. It affects all age groups but is typically found in the anogenital region in post-menopausal women. The most common presentation is severe intractable itching (pruritus vulvae) and vaginal soreness with dyspareunia. **Vulval intraepithelial neoplasia (VIN)** is dysplasia of the vulval epithelium, categorised as mild (VIN I), moderate (VIN II), or severe (VIN III). The vulval lesions are often multifocal and are usually associated with itching and pain.

INCIDENCE/ PREVALENCE We found no data on the prevalence of lichen sclerosus. The true incidence of VIN is unknown, but it is being diagnosed with increased frequency in the UK and the USA. This may be because of increased recognition of the disease or a true increase in incidence.[1–3]

AETIOLOGY/ RISK FACTORS The cause is unknown. VIN is associated with human papilloma virus 16.[1]

PROGNOSIS There is currently no cure for lichen sclerosus, but the risk of progression to vulval carcinoma ranges from 0% to 9%.[4] People with concomitant squamous cell hyperplasia are at increased risk of malignancy.[5] Malignant transformation appears to be low in women with VIN I and II, but has been reported in 2–4% of women with VIN III.[2,6] About 30% of vulval carcinomas are associated with VIN.[1]

AIMS To control symptoms, to reduce the risk of malignant transformation, and to improve quality of life, with minimal adverse effects.

OUTCOMES Scores for symptoms (itching, burning, pain, and dyspareunia), gross appearance (relating to severity of lesions and extent of vulval involvement), and histological stage. Scores range from 0 to 3, where 3 represents the most severe. Other outcomes are rates of histological regression, recurrence, malignant transformation, and adverse effects of treatment.

METHODS *Clinical Evidence* update search and appraisal May 2000. We included all RCTs that were appropriately randomised and double-blinded with follow up of 80% or more participants, and with a minimum of 15 people in each study arm. Where confidence intervals were not reported but adequate information was provided, we calculated them using the software Statsdirect.[7] Where we found no good RCTs, we used the best available observational studies.

QUESTION What are the effects of treatments for lichen sclerosus?

OPTION TOPICAL CORTICOSTEROIDS AND TOPICAL TESTOSTERONE

We found limited evidence from three small RCTs suggesting that topical clobetasol propionate is more effective than topical testosterone propionate or petroleum jelly. We found no evidence that topical testosterone is more effective than petroleum jelly. Testosterone is associated with virilisation and pain.

Benefits: We found no systematic review. **Short term treatment:** We found two placebo- or vehicle- (petroleum jelly) controlled RCTs. One RCT compared clobetasol propionate 0.05% (n = 20), testosterone propionate (n = 20), and petroleum jelly (n = 19) for 3 months, with follow up of 3 months.[8] Clobetasol propionate was associated with significantly higher rates of symptom control and reversal of histological changes (AR for symptom control 75% on clobetasol, 20% on testosterone, and 10.5% on petroleum jelly). A significant difference in both gross and histological changes occurred only in the clobetasol group.[8] A second RCT compared testosterone propionate in petroleum jelly (n = 30) versus petroleum jelly alone (n = 28) for 12 months with at least 12 months' follow up. There was no significant difference in response rates (75% v 66.6%; AR difference 8.3%, 95% CI –31.1% to +15.5%, calculated from data reported).[9] **Maintenance treatment:** Recurrence of symptoms on maintenance treatment was more common with topical testosterone than with petroleum jelly (AR 9/16 [56%] with testosterone, 3/16 [19%] with petroleum jelly; ARI [38%], 95% CI 2% to 67%; NNH 3, 95% CI 1 to 53). There was no significant difference in control of gross features between testosterone and petroleum jelly.[10]

Harms: One RCT found no evidence that topical clobetasol propionate was associated with adverse effects,[8] and good prospective observational studies reported minimal adverse effects when clobetasol propionate was used as required for maintenance treatment for 1–3 years (see glossary, p 1119).[11,12] Topical testosterone was associated with virilisation (4/20 women),[8] hypertrichosis (1/30),[9] pruritus and pain (3/30),[9] and burning (4/16).[10] No harmful effects were reported with petroleum jelly.[8–10,13]

Comment: None of the RCTs was double-blinded and none included a power calculation to justify sample size. All had follow up rates of > 80% for assessment of treatment efficacy. The high response rate to petroleum jelly may have been more than a placebo effect: petroleum jelly has a soothing effect on the vulvar skin.

| OPTION | ORAL RETINOIDS (ACITRETIN) |

One small RCT found that acitretin was more effective than placebo. Acitretin is associated with severe peeling of palms and soles, and with hair loss.

Benefits: We found no systematic review. We found one RCT comparing acitretin versus placebo for 12–16 weeks with 4–6 weeks' follow up in 46 eligible patients.[13] Compared to placebo, acitretin reduced the incidence of pruritus, atrophic features, hyperkeratosis, burning, and large lesions (8/22 v 18/24; ARR: 38.6%, 95% CI 9.8% to 61.1%; NNT 3, 95% CI 2 to 10).

Harms: Adverse effects were reported in 100% of people taking acitretin and 56% of those taking placebo.[13] Acitretin was associated with severe peeling of the palms and soles (11/39 people) and increased rates of hair loss (23/39 v 2/39 on placebo).[13] Acitretin was associated with congenital abnormalities in women exposed during the first trimester of pregnancy,[14,15] and is therefore contraindicated in pregnancy. Contraception has been recommended for use during treatment and for 2 years afterwards.[16]

Comment: The RCT was double-blinded. Follow up rates were > 80% for assessment of treatment efficacy.

OPTION SURGICAL TREATMENTS

We found insufficient evidence on the effects of surgery in lichen sclerosus.

Benefits: We found no systematic review, RCTs, or good quality observational studies.

Harms: Three cohort studies reported reoperation rates after vulvectomy (33%, 23%, and 50%). The reasons for reoperating were recurrence, progression to vulval cancer, and constricted vaginal outlet.[4]

Comment: We found one non-systematic review, which identified uncontrolled cohort studies of vulvectomy, cryosurgery and laser treatment.[4] **Vulvectomy:** Five studies were reviewed. Four evaluated simple, partial, or complete vulvectomy (44–120 women, follow up 3–23 years, recurrence rates 39–59%). One study evaluated skinning vulvectomy (see glossary, p 1119) and skin graft (n = 4, follow up 4–8 years, recurrence rate 50%). **Cryosurgery:** One study was reviewed (n = 12, follow up 3 years, two women lost to follow up, rate of recurrence/failed treatment 42%). Complete healing took up to 3 months. **Laser treatment:** Four studies were reviewed. The largest (n = 62, follow up 0.3–7years) found a 16% recurrence rate. The other studies were small (5–7 women, follow up 1–6 years, recurrence rates 0–14%). Complete healing took up to 6 weeks.

QUESTION What are the effects of treatments for vulval intraepithelial neoplasia?

OPTION SURGICAL TREATMENTS

We found insufficient evidence on the effects of surgical treatments in women with vulval intraepithelial neoplasia (VIN).

Benefits: We found no systematic review or RCTs.

Harms: Laser skinning vulvectomy may be associated with labial fusion (14%), and in 5% of cases laser treatment of perianal lesions caused an incomplete anal sphincter. Moderate to severe postoperative pain is also common after laser vaporisation.[3,17] Vaporisation using carbon dioxide produces a plume containing carcinogenic substances, and the radiant energy can cause thermal burns, fires, and eye injuries in the operator. The risk of aerosol produced during ultrasound surgical aspiration is unclear, and precautions to protect surgeons from patients' body fluids may be required.[18,19] Cryosurgery may be associated with oedema, pain, and ulceration. Difficulties with precision and control may also result in vulval scarring and distortion.[18]

Comment: A minimum of 5 years' follow up would be necessary to assess properly the effects of treatment on rates of recurrence and malignant transformation in women with VIN. One retrospective cohort study in women with VIN I, II, or III reported on rates of recurrence or persistence, at a mean of 31 months, after local excision (n = 61, recurrence 25%), primary surgery including local excision, simple vulvectomy, and knife skinning vulvectomy with grafting (n = 103, recurrence 39%) and laser vaporisation (n = 30, recurrence 67%). The difference between laser vaporisation and local excision was significant (P ≤ 0.001). By 10 years, histological recurrence was seen in 79% of women treated with laser compared with 36% treated with local excision. Progression to malignant disease occurred after surgical intervention in nine women (7%).[2] A smaller cohort study found recurrence or persistence in 21% of women after simple vulvectomy (n = 9, median follow up 74 months), 44% after local excision (n = 14, median follow up 74 months), and 52% after laser skinning vulvectomy (n = 21, median follow up 38 months).[3] Other small, uncontrolled studies found recurrence rates of 8.6% with laser vaporisation (n = 35, follow up 12–36 months),[17] 22% with ultrasound surgical aspiration (n = 9, median follow up 12 months),[20] and 90% with cryosurgery (n = 10, mean follow up 12 months).[6]

| OPTION | TOPICAL α INTERFERON |

We found insufficient evidence on the effects of topical α interferon in women with VIN.

Benefits: We found no systematic review and no placebo controlled or comparative RCTs. We found one small blinded crossover RCT (n = 18) evaluating topical α interferon with and without 1% nonoxinol-9. Outcomes were symptom control (itching, burning, and pain), reversal of histological changes, and adverse effects of treatment. Overall, 14/18 (67%) of participants had some response to α interferon (no P values or CIs reported). The addition of 1% nonoxinol-9 made no significant difference to the number of complete responders (complete response occurred in 3/10 treatment episodes with 1% nonoxinol-9 and 6/14 without).[21]

Harms: Topical α interferon was associated with transitory adverse effects, including fever (8%), mild discomfort, and mild pruritus (17%).[21]

Comment: None.

GLOSSARY

Skinning vulvectomy The epidermis and the underlying dermis of the vulva are removed by knife or laser. Split thickness skin graft is usually employed to cover the defect following knife excision.

REFERENCES

1. Crum CP, McLachlin CM, Tate JE, Mutter GL. Pathobiology of vulvar squamous neoplasia. *Curr Opin Obstet Gynecol* 1997;9:63–69.

2. Herod JJO, Shafi MI, Rollason TP, et al. Vulvar intraepithelial neoplasia: long term follow up treated and untreated. *Br J Obstet Gynaecol* 1996;103:446–452.

3. Shafi MI, Luesley DM, Byrne P, et al. Vulval

intraepithelial neoplasia – management and outcome. *Br J Obstet Gynaecol* 1989;96:1339–1344.

4. Abramov Y, Elchalal U, Abramov D, Goldfarb A, Schenker JG. Surgical treatment of vulvar lichen sclerosus: a review. *Obstet Gynecol Surv* 1996;51:193–199.

5. Elchalal U, Gilead L, Vardy DA, et al. Treatment of

vulvar lichen sclerosus in the elderly: an update. *Obstet Gynecol Surv* 1995;50:155–162.

6. Marren P, Dawber R, Wojnarowska F, et al. Failure of cryosurgery to eradicate vulval intraepithelial neoplasia: a pilot study. *J Eur Acad Dermatol Venereol* 1993;2:247–252.

7. Buchan IE. Statsdirect http://www.statsdirect.com. Cambridge (England) CamCode 2000.

8. Bracco GL, Carli P, Sonni L, et al. Clinical and histologic effects of topical treatments of vulval lichen sclerosus. *J Reproductive Med* 1993;38: 37–40.

9. Sideri M, Origoni L, Spinaci L, Ferrari A. Topical testosterone in the treatment of vulvar lichen sclerosus. *Int J Gynaecol Obstet* 1994;46:53–56.

10. Cattaneo A, Carli P, De Marco A, et al. Testosterone maintenance therapy. Effects on vulval lichen sclerosus treated with clobetasol propionate. *J Reprod Med* 1996;41:99–102.

11. Dalziel KL, Wojnarowska F. Long-term control of vulval lichen sclerosus after treatment with a potent topical steroid cream. *J Reprod Med* 1993; 38:25–27.

12. Bornstein J, Heifetz S, Kellner Y, et al. Clobetasol dipropionate 0.05% versus testosterone propionate 2% topical application for severe vulval lichen sclerosus. *Am J Obstet Gynecol* 1998;178: 80–84.

13. Bousema MT, Romppanen U, Geiger J-M, et al. Acitretin in the treatment of severe lichen sclerosus ou atrophicus of the vulva: a double-blind, placebo-controlled study. *J Am Acad Dermatol* 1994;30:225–231.

14. De Die-Smulders CE, Sturkenboom MC, Veraart J, van Katwijk C, Sastrowijoto P, van der Linden E. Severe limb defects and craniofacial anomalies in a fetus conceived during acitretin therapy. *Teratology* 1995;52:215–219.

15. Geiger JM, Baudin M, Saurat JH. Teratogenic risk with etretinate and acitretin treatment. *Dermatology* 1994;89:109–116.

16. *British National Formulary*. London: British Medical Association/Royal Pharmaceutical Society of Great Britain, September 1999;38:504.

17. Baggish MS, Dorsey JH. CO2 laser for the treatment of vulvar carcinoma in situ. *Obstet Gynecol* 1981;57:371–374.

18. Townsend DE, Levine RU, Richart RM, et al. Management of vulvar intraepithelial neoplasia by carbon dioxide laser. *Obstet Gynecol* 1982;60:49–51.

19. Adelson MD. Ultrasonic surgical aspiration in the treatment of vulvar disease. *Obstet Gynecol* 1991; 78:477–479.

20. Rader JS, Leake JF, Dillon MB, et al. Ultrasound surgical aspiration in the treatment of vulvar disease. *Obstet Gynecol* 1991;77:573–576.

21. Spirtos NM, Smith LH, Teng NNH. Prospective randomised trial of α-interferon (α-interferon gels) for the treatment of vulvar intraepithelial neoplasia III. *Gynecol Oncol* 1990;37:34–38.

Earlando Thomas
Senior Specialist Registrar
Department of Obstetrics and Gynecology
Rochester, New York
USA

Damian Murphy
Consultant Obstetrician and Gynaecologist
Department of Obstetrics and Gynaecology
New Cross Hospital
Wolverhampton
UK

Charles Redman
Consultant Obstetrician and Gynaecologist
Department of Obstetrics and Gynaecology
City General Hospital
Stoke on Trent
UK

Competing interests: None declared.

Updated this issue

Katrina Wyatt, Paul Dimmock and PMS O'Brien

QUESTIONS

INTERVENTIONS

Key Messages

- RCTs have found that selective serotonin reuptake inhibitors (SSRI) and prostaglandin inhibitors relieve premenstrual symptoms. Antidepressants and ovulation suppression with danazol and gonadotrophin releasing hormone (GnRH) analogues are also effective but have significant adverse effects, including the masculinising effects of danazol and the "menopausal" effects of GnRH analogues.

- We found limited evidence suggesting that oestrogen, tibolone, vitamin B6, evening primrose oil, exercise, and chiropractic therapy may also be beneficial.

- RCTs have found that bromocriptine is effective for breast symptoms and that diuretics are effective for bloatedness and swelling. Both treatments can have adverse effects.

© *Clinical Evidence* 2000;4:1121–1133.

Premenstrual syndrome

- We found no good evidence on the effects of progesterone or oral contraceptives.
- Few treatments have been adequately evaluated in RCTs.

DEFINITION	A woman has premenstrual syndrome (PMS) if she complains of recurrent psychological or somatic symptoms (or both), occurring specifically during the luteal phase of the menstrual cycle and resolving by the end of menstruation (see table 1, p 1133).[1]
INCIDENCE/ PREVALENCE	Premenstrual symptoms occur in 95% of all women of reproductive age; severe, debilitating symptoms (premenstrual syndrome) occur in about 5% of those women.[1]
AETIOLOGY/ RISK FACTORS	The aetiology is unknown, but hormonal and other (possibly neuroendocrine) factors probably contribute.[2,3] There may be enhanced sensitivity to progesterone, possibly caused by a deficiency of serotonin.[3]
PROGNOSIS	Except after oophorectomy, symptoms usually recur when treatment is stopped.
AIMS	To improve or eliminate physical and psychological symptoms; to minimise the impact on normal functioning, interpersonal relationships, and quality of life; to minimise adverse effects of treatment.
OUTCOMES	Symptom severity. There is no consensus on how this should be assessed. One review of PMS outcomes found 65 different questionnaires or scales, measuring 199 different symptoms or signs.[4]
METHODS	We used the search strategy of the Cochrane Collaboration's Menstrual Disorders and Subfertility Group.[5] A *Clinical Evidence* update search and appraisal was performed in May 2000. A well controlled trial should show the existence of PMS before treatment by prospectively administered, validated scales; should include a pre-randomisation placebo cycle to exclude women who have a non-specific response; and should contain sufficient cycles to allow for symptom variability between cycles. Few trials fulfilled these criteria. The wide range of diagnostic scales, outcome criteria, and dosing regimens made comparison between trials difficult. Detailed numerical analysis for each intervention awaits systematic review and possible meta-analysis.

QUESTION   What are the effects of drug treatments?

OPTION   PROGESTERONE

One systematic review of progesterone versus control treatments found no improvement in overall premenstrual symptoms.

Benefits: We found one systematic review (search date July 2000, 14 RCTs, 609 women with previously diagnosed premenstrual syndrome). It found no improvement in overall premenstrual symptoms for women taking progesterone compared with control treatments (WMD −0.003, 95% CI −0.010 to +0.015; OR 1.005, 95% CI 0.98 to 1.03). Three trials (138 people) used oral progesterone and 11 trials (471 people) used progesterone suppositories.[6]

Harms: Some RCTs reported adverse effects such as abdominal pain, nausea, headache, vaginal pruritus, dizziness, drowsiness, excessive bleeding, and dysmenorrhoea.[6]

Comment: We found no direct evidence to support the theory that PMS may by caused by progesterone deficiency, nor to support the use of progesterone to treat PMS.

OPTION   **PROGESTOGENS (SYNTHETIC PROGESTERONE-LIKE DRUGS)**

We found conflicting evidence from RCTs.

Benefits: We found no systematic review. We identified seven RCTs comparing dydrogesterone with placebo.[7–13] Three trials found improvement with dydrogesterone for some premenstrual symptoms.[9,11,13] The remaining four found no therapeutic effect.[7,8,10,12] Three trials compared medroxyprogesterone acetate with placebo.[14–16] Two of these found an improvement in women taking the drug while the third found no difference.

Harms: The most common adverse effects were nausea, breast discomfort, headache, and menstrual irregularity.

Comment: The most commonly used progestogen for PMS is dydrogesterone. Medroxyprogesterone acetate is occasionally used to suppress ovulation. Paradoxically, progestogens may induce PMS symptoms during hormone replacement therapy.

OPTION   **OESTROGEN**

Limited evidence from RCTs suggests benefit from oestradiol.

Benefits: We found no systematic review. We found three RCTs that compared oestrogen with placebo. One (using oral conjugated equine oestrogens) found no difference in premenstrual symptoms.[17] Oestradiol (given as a transdermal patch or subcutaneous implant) improved overall premenstrual symptoms.[18,19] One trial found oestradiol gel was effective for premenstrual migraine.[19]

Harms: Adverse effects included mastalgia, nausea, weight gain, headache, and skin pigmentation (in the patch trial).[18]

Comment: The studies suggest that oestrogenic ovarian suppression may eliminate PMS. To avoid endometrial hyperplasia and adenocarcinoma, a 12 day progestogen course is needed every 28 days. Progestogen may induce PMS symptoms. To avoid this systemic effect, progestogen may be given locally (using a levonorgestrel intrauterine device or progesterone gel). We found no RCTs evaluating this approach.

OPTION   **TIBOLONE**

We found limited evidence of benefit from two small RCTs.

Benefits: We found no systematic review. We found two RCTs. One RCT compared tibolone with placebo and the other compared tibolone with a multivitamin supplement.[20,21] Both found a significant improvement with tibolone for all premenstrual symptoms.

Harms: No significant adverse effects were reported.

Comment: Both trials included very small numbers of women on active treatment.

OPTION   DANAZOL

RCTs have found danazol to be of some benefit, but with notable adverse effects and long term risks associated with masculinisation.

Benefits: We found no systematic review. Of the seven RCTs identified, five found that danazol given continuously was significantly better than placebo.[22–28] **Luteal phase danazol:** In two trials where danazol was given in the luteal phase only, one found it to be better than placebo for overall symptoms, whereas the other, larger trial found it to be better for premenstrual breast pain only.[26,28]

Harms: Danazol has important adverse effects and there are long term risks with continued use. Osteoporosis seems not to be a risk, but masculinising effects can be notable. These include effects on the voice, hirsutism, and weight gain, and possibly effects on plasma lipids and hence cardiovascular risk. **Luteal phase danazol:** The two trials did not find a significantly higher rate of adverse effects than placebo. However, long term adverse effects were not assessed.[26–28]

Comment: Danazol is used in PMS because it suppresses the ovarian cycle in most women.

OPTION   GNRH ANALOGUES

RCTs have found benefit from GnRH analogues. Treatment with GnRH analogues for more than 6 months carries significant risk of osteoporosis, limiting their usefulness for long term treatment. It may be possible to extend treatment when "add back" hormonal treatment is included.

Benefits: We found no systematic review. We found 10 RCTs that compared GnRH analogues with placebo.[29–38] Nine found an improvement with the drug over placebo. The other found no significant difference between drug and placebo.[31] In three of these trials, "add back" treatment with oestrogen and medroxyprogesterone or norethisterone was also given.[33,34,37] Two found the treatment better than placebo, and one found no improvement over placebo.[37] The most recent trial used low dose GnRH analogues to avoid the need for add back treatment. This trial found an improvement in premenstrual depression and irritability.[38]

Harms: Adverse effects of GnRH analogues, other than osteoporosis, include hot flushes, night sweats, decreased libido, pruritus, nausea, and bronchospasm.[30,32]

Comment: A true double blind controlled trial of GnRH analogues would be hard to conduct because women receiving these agents experience amenorrhoea.

OPTION BROMOCRIPTINE

RCTs have found that bromocriptine relieves breast tenderness, although adverse effects are common.

Benefits: We found no systematic review. One survey of 14 trials found no evidence that bromocriptine was effective for PMS, although it found limited evidence of effectiveness for premenstrual mastalgia.[39]

Harms: Bromocriptine has a high incidence of adverse effects, including nausea, dizziness, headache, weight increase, and swelling.[40–42] The survey did not include any mention of adverse effects, which on analysis of individual trials are well documented.[39] There have been very rare case reports of stroke and death following bromocriptine treatment to prevent lactation.[43]

Comment: None.

OPTION ORAL CONTRACEPTIVES

We found limited and conflicting evidence from RCTs on the effects of oral contraceptives in PMS.

Benefits: We found no systematic review. Four RCTs compared oral contraceptives with placebo. Three found no improvement over placebo, and one found improvement in premenstrual breast pain and bloating.[44–47]

Harms: Some women develop PMS-like symptoms for the first time when taking the oral contraceptive pill. Few adverse effects were mentioned in the trials.

Comment: Anecdotal evidence suggests that oral contraceptives may be beneficial in PMS. Continuous combined regimens (those without a 1 week break) should, in theory, suppress ovulation and provide symptom relief, but we found no published trials.

OPTION DIURETICS

RCTs have found that diuretics improve breast tenderness and bloating.

Benefits: We found no systematic review. Six RCTs used spironolactone.[14,48–52] Five found an improvement in premenstrual symptoms compared with placebo (particularly those associated with bloating and breast tenderness) and one found no difference between drug and placebo. Metolazone was significantly more effective than placebo for physical and somatic symptoms.[53] Ammonium chloride plus caffeine significantly reduced premenstrual weight gain compared with placebo.[54] There was no significant difference between placebo and chlorthalidone.[55]

Harms: Adverse effects included nausea, dizziness, palpitations, excess diuresis, and weakness.[14,50,52,53]

Comment: Diuretics are widely used, in the belief that many symptoms of PMS are the direct consequence of fluid retention, although there is little evidence of water retention in most women with PMS.

OPTION PROSTAGLANDIN INHIBITORS

RCTs have found benefit from prostaglandin inhibitors for a range of premenstrual symptoms but not for premenstrual breast pain.

Benefits: We found no systematic review. **Mefenamic acid:** We found five placebo controlled RCTs.[56–60] All found an improvement with mefenamic acid compared with placebo for many premenstrual symptoms but not for breast pain. **Naproxen sodium:** Two trials used naproxen sodium. One found it more effective than placebo for physical symptoms, whereas the other reported a significant improvement in mood change and headache for naproxen sodium over placebo.[61,62]

Harms: Adverse effects included nausea, gastrointestinal disturbances, and rashes.[56–58]

Comment: None.

OPTION ANXIOLYTICS/NON-SSRI ANTIDEPRESSANTS

RCTs have found benefit for one or more symptoms of PMS, but a proportion of women stop treatment because of adverse effects.

Benefits: We found no systematic review. We found 18 adequately controlled trials of antidepressants/anxiolytic drugs for PMS. Most (14/18) reported some positive effects for one or more symptoms. Six trials used antidepressants (bupropion, clomipramine, nortriptyline, and desipramine) and eight trials used anxiolytics (alprazolam and buspirone).[63–76] Three trials used β blockers (atenolol and propanolol), two with some positive effects.[74,76–78] Lithium was assessed in two trials, which found no significant difference compared with placebo.[55,79] Methylscopolamine was compared with desipramine in one trial, which found that both treatments were associated with some symptom relief.[68]

Harms: Adverse effects such as drowsiness, nausea, anxiety, and headache led to problems with adherence to treatment in most of the trials.[61,65,66,73]

Comment: Although there may be some benefit from the use of antidepressants/anxiolytics in PMS, this must be weighed carefully against the adverse effects.

OPTION SELECTIVE SEROTONIN REUPTAKE INHIBITORS

One systematic review of RCTs has found major improvement in overall symptoms.

Benefits: We found one preliminary systematic review and two subsequent RCTs. The review (search date July 2000, 15 RCTs, 882 women with PMS) found significant improvement in overall symptoms on SSRIs compared with placebo (WMD −1.07, 95% CI −1.38 to −0.75; OR for symptom relief 6.9, 95% CI 3.9 to 12.2, in favour of SSRIs).[80] SSRIs used in the trials were fluoxetine (7 trials), sertraline (5 trials), citalopram (1 trial), fluvoxamine (1 trial) and paroxetine (1 trial).

Harms: Common adverse effects were headache, nervousness, insomnia, drowsiness/fatigue, sexual dysfunction, and gastrointestinal disturbances.[80]

Comment: Secondary analysis found that SSRIs were effective in treating physical as well as behavioural symptoms.[80]

QUESTION   **What are the effects of nutritional supplements?**

OPTION   VITAMIN B6

A systematic review of poor quality RCTs found benefit with vitamin B6 for overall symptoms. Three RCTs found conflicting evidence of the benefits of vitamin B6.

Benefits: We found one systematic review and three additional RCTs.[81–84] The review (search date July 1998, 9 RCTs, 940 women with PMS) found no high quality RCTs comparing vitamin B6 (either as a single supplement or as part of a multivitamin supplement) with placebo.[81] The pooled odds ratio for relief of overall PMS symptoms was 2.32 (95% CI 1.95 to 2.54) in favour of vitamin B6. There was no dose related response. One additional RCT compared vitamin B6 with *Vitex agnus castus*; an improvement over placebo was found with both treatments.[82] Another RCT with weak methods found no improvement over placebo whilst the third additional RCT found a significant improvement.[73,83]

Harms: High doses (> 200 mg/day) have been associated with a reversible peripheral neuropathy.[81]

Comment: None of these trials met established criteria for inclusion in a systematic review.[81]

OPTION   EVENING PRIMROSE OIL

Limited evidence from one systematic review of small RCTs suggests that evening primrose oil may have a small beneficial effect.

Benefits: We found one systematic review (search date July 1993), which identified eight placebo controlled RCTs.[84] Although the trials found a small beneficial effect, patient numbers were low. The authors concluded that there was insufficient evidence for evening primrose oil in PMS.

Harms: Few adverse effects have been reported. There are rare reports of evening primrose oil causing seizures in people with epilepsy.

Comment: Evening primrose oil is one of the most popular "self help" remedies for PMS, although in the UK it is licensed only for the treatment of premenstrual mastalgia.

| OPTION | DIETARY SUPPLEMENTS |

We found insufficient evidence on the effects of dietary supplements in PMS.

Benefits: We found no systematic review. Three RCTs used magnesium as a supplement for relieving PMS symptoms.[85–87] One trial found an improvement in overall PMS symptoms compared with placebo, but another found no effect.[85,86] The third trial found that magnesium supplements improved symptoms of bloating.[87] Two RCTs looked at the effect of calcium.[88,89] One found it effective for water retention and pain (breast tenderness and swelling, headaches, and abdominal cramps).[88] The other found it effective for overall symptoms.[89] A further controlled study investigated the effect of dietary calcium plus manganese, and found a reduction in physical and behavioural symptoms for women taking the recommended daily allowance of both supplements.[90]

Harms: None reported.

Comment: One RCT found benefit from high dose (6 g/day) L-tryptophan, but this was not presented as a potential treatment option.[91] A low fat vegetarian diet was found to reduce both dysmenorrhoea and premenstrual symptoms, but the patients were not randomised on their PMS symptoms.[92]

| QUESTION | What are the effects of non-drug treatments? |

| OPTION | COGNITIVE BEHAVIOURAL TREATMENT |

We found conflicting evidence from RCTs.

Benefits: We found no systematic review. Five trials compared cognitive behavioural treatment with a dummy treatment or placebo.[93–97] One trial (dydrogesterone v cognitive behavioural treatment v relaxation) found cognitive behavioural treatment more effective than the other interventions.[93] Two trials found cognitive behavioural treatments to be better than remaining on a waiting list.[94,95] Two other trials found no benefit over placebo.[96,97]

Harms: None reported.

Comment: None.

| OPTION | EXERCISE AND PHYSICAL THERAPY |

RCTs have found that both exercise and physical therapy improve symptoms of PMS.

Benefits: We found no systematic review. Three controlled trials found that moderate aerobic exercise improved symptoms.[98–100] One placebo controlled crossover RCT compared chiropractic therapy with a placebo therapy.[101] Active treatment was associated with a significant decrease in PMS scores, but women who received placebo first did not experience any additional improvement when they were switched to chiropractic therapy.

Harms: None reported.

Comment: None.

OPTION   RELAXATION TREATMENT

We found insufficient evidence on the effects of relaxation treatment in PMS.

Benefits: We found no systematic review. Two controlled trials (relaxation treatment alone v keeping a daily symptoms chart v reading leisure material plus keeping a daily symptoms chart) found conflicting results.[97,102] One trial found relaxation treatment effective for physical and emotional symptoms but the other found no overall benefit.

Harms: None mentioned.

Comment: Most studies of relaxation techniques have used them as an adjunct to other treatment.

QUESTION   What are the effects of surgical treatments?

OPTION   HYSTERECTOMY WITH OR WITHOUT OOPHORECTOMY

RCTs have found that hysterectomy plus bilateral oophorectomy is curative. Hysterectomy alone may reduce symptoms, but evidence is limited because of the difficulty in providing controls. The risks are those of major surgery. Infertility is an irreversible consequence of bilateral oophorectomy.

Benefits: We found no systematic review. We found two trials in which hysterectomy alone relieved PMS symptoms, and two trials in which hysterectomy with bilateral oophorectomy relieved PMS symptoms.[103–106]

Harms: Potential risks include those associated with major surgery.[107]

Comment: Surgery is rarely used but may be indicated if there are coexisting gynaecological problems.

OPTION   LAPAROSCOPIC BILATERAL OOPHORECTOMY

We found insufficient evidence for this treatment in PMS.

Benefits: We found no systematic review or RCTs.

Harms: Insufficient evidence.

Comment: After oophorectomy, oestrogen replacement and hence cyclical progesterone are needed to prevent endometrial hyperplasia and carcinoma. Progesterone may restimulate PMS.

OPTION   ENDOMETRIAL ABLATION

We found insufficient evidence for endometrial ablation in PMS.

Benefits: We found no systematic review or RCTs.

Harms: Insufficient evidence.

Comment: Studies claiming that endometrial ablation may relieve symptoms of PMS have been in the context of menorrhagia, and thus women were not randomised on the basis of PMS.

Substantive changes since last issue

Progesterone New systematic review of progesterone versus placebo found no improvement in overall premenstral symptoms. Progesterone was moved from unknown effectiveness to likely to be ineffective or harmful after re-evaluation of the evidence.

REFERENCES

1. O'Brien PMS. *Premenstrual syndrome*. London: Blackwell Science, 1987.
2. O'Brien PMS. Helping women with premenstrual syndrome. *BMJ* 1993;307:1471–1475.
3. Rapkin AJ, Morgan M, Goldman L, Brann DW, Simone D, Mahesh VB. Progesterone metabolite allopregnanolone in women with premenstrual syndrome. *Obstet Gynecol* 1997;90:709–714.
4. Budeiri DJ, Li WP, Dorman JC. Clinical trials of treatments of premenstrual syndrome: entry criteria and scales for measuring treatment outcomes. *Br J Obstet Gynaecol* 1994;101:689–695.
5. Cochrane Menstrual Disorders and Subfertility Group. Search strategy for specialist registrar (Collaborative Review Groups) In: The Cochrane Library, Issue 4. Oxford: Update software, 1999.
6. Wyatt KM, Dimmock PW, Jones PW, O'Bryen PMS. Progesterone therapy; a systematic review of its efficacy in the premenstrual syndrome. *Neuropsychopharmacology* 23;S2:2000.
7. Sampson GA, Heathcote PR, Wordsworth J, Prescott P, Hodgson A. A premenstrual syndrome. A double-blind cross-over study of treatment with dydrogesterone and placebo. *Br J Psychiatry* 1988;153:232–235.
8. Dennerstein L, Morse C, Gotts G, et al. Treatment of premenstrual syndrome: a double-blind trial of dydrogesterone. *J Affect Disord* 1986;11:199–205.
9. Kerr GD, Day JB, Munday MR, Brush MG, Watson M, Taylor RW. Dydrogesterone in the treatment of the premenstrual syndrome. *Practitioner* 1980;224:852–855.
10. Hoffmann V, Pedersen PA, Philip J, Fly P, Pedersen C. The effect of dydrogesterone on premenstrual symptoms: a double-blind, randomized, placebo-controlled study in general practice. *Scand J Prim Health Care* 1988;6:179–183.
11. Haspels AA. A double blind, placebo controlled multi-centre study of the efficacy of dydrogesterone (Duphaston). In: Van Keep PA, Utian WH, eds. *The premenstrual syndrome*. Lancaster, UK: MTP Press, 1980:81–92.
12. Williams JGC, Martin AJ, Hulkenberg-Tromp A. PMS in 4 European countries: part 2. a double blind controlled study of dydrogesterone. *Br J Sex Med* 1983;10:8–18.
13. Coppen AJ, Milne HB, Outram DH, Weber JCP. Dytide, norethisterone and placebo in the premenstrual syndrome. *Clin Trials J* 1969;6:33–35.
14. Hellberg D, Claesson B, Nilsson S. Premenstrual tension: a placebo-controlled efficacy study with spironolactone and medroxyprogesterone acetate. *Int J Gynaecol Obstet* 1991;34:243–248.
15. Jordheim O. The premenstrual syndrome: clinical trials of treatment with a progestogen combined with a diuretic compared with both a progestogen alone and with a placebo. *Acta Obstet Gynecol Scand* 1972;51:77–80.
16. West CP. Inhibition of ovulation with oral progestins: effectiveness in premenstrual syndrome. *Eur J Obstet Gynecol Reprod Biol* 1990;34:119–128.
17. Dhar V, Murphy BE. Double-blind randomized crossover trial of luteal phase estrogens (Premarin) in the premenstrual syndrome (PMS). *Psychoneuroendocrinology* 1990;15:489–493.
18. Watson NR, Studd JW, Savvas M, Garnett T, Baber RJ. Treatment of severe premenstrual syndrome with oestradiol patches and cyclical oral norethisterone. *Lancet* 1989;2:730–732.
19. de Lignieres B, Vincens M, Mauvais-Jarvis P, et al. Prevention of menstrual migraine by percutaneous oestradiol. *BMJ* 1986;293:1540.
20. Taskin O, Goekdeniz R, Yalcinoglu A, et al. Placebo controlled crossover study of effects of tibolone on premenstrual symptoms and peripheral endorphin concentrations in premenstrual syndrome. *Hum Reprod* 1998;13:242–245.
21. Taskin O, Gokdeniz R, Yalcinoglu A, Buhur A, Burak F, Atmaca R, Ozekici. Placebo-controlled cross-over study of effects of tibolone on premenstrual symptoms and peripheral beta-endorphin concentrations in premenstrual syndrome. *Hum Reprod* 1998;13:2402–2405.
22. Gilmore DH, Hawthorn RJ, Hart DM. Danol for premenstrual syndrome: a preliminary report of a placebo-controlled double-blind study. *J Int Med Res* 1985;13:129–130.
23. Halbreich U, Rojansky N, Palter S. Elimination of ovulation and menstrual cyclicity (with danazol) improves dysphoric premenstrual syndromes. *Fertil Steril* 1991;56:1066–1069.
24. Watts JF, Butt WR, Logan ER. A clinical trial using danazol for the treatment of premenstrual tension. *Br J Obstet Gynaecol* 1987;94:30–34.
25. Deeny M, Hawthorn R, McKay HD. Low dose danazol in the treatment of the premenstrual syndrome. *Postgrad Med J* 1991;67:450–454.
26. Sarno APJ, Miller EJJ, Lundblad EG. Premenstrual syndrome: beneficial effects of periodic, low-dose danazol. *Obstet Gynecol* 1987;70:33–36.
27. Hahn PM, Van Vugt DA, Reid RL. A randomized, placebo-controlled, crossover trial of danazol for the treatment of premenstrual syndrome. *Psychoneuroendocrinology* 1995;20:193–209.
28. O'Brien PMS, Abukhalil IEH. Randomised controlled trial of the management of premenstrual syndrome and premenstrual mastalgia using luteal phase only danazol. *Am J Obstet Gynecol* 1999;180:18–23.
29. Freeman EW, Sondheimer SJ, Rickels K. Gonadotropin-releasing hormone agonist in the treatment of premenstrual symptoms with and without ongoing dysphoria: a controlled study. *Psychopharmacol Bull* 1997;33:303–309.
30. Brown CS, Ling FW, Andersen RN, Farmer RG,

Arheart KL. Efficacy of depot leuprolide in premenstrual syndrome: effect of symptom severity and type in a controlled trial. *Obstet Gynecol* 1994;84:779–786.

31. Helvacioglu A, Yeoman RR, Hazelton JM, Aksel S. Premenstrual syndrome and related hormonal changes. Long-acting gonadotrophin releasing hormone agonist treatment. *J Reprod Med* 1993; 38:864–870.

32. Muse KN, Cetel NS, Futterman LA, Yen SC. The premenstrual syndrome. Effects of "medical ovariectomy". *N Engl J Med* 1984;311:1345–1349.

33. Mortola JF, Girton L, Fischer U. Successful treatment of severe premenstrual syndrome by combined use of gonadotrophin-releasing hormone agonist and estrogen/progestin. *J Clin Endocrinol Metab* 1991;72:252A–252F.

34. Mezrow G, Shoupe D, Spicer D, Lobo R, Leung B, Pike M. Depot leuprolide acetate with estrogen and progestin add-back for long-term treatment of premenstrual syndrome. *Fertil Steril* 1994;62: 932–937.

35. Hammarback S, Backstrom T. Induced anovulation as treatment of premenstrual tension syndrome: a double-blind cross-over study with GnRH-agonist versus placebo. *Acta Obstet Gynecol Scand* 1988; 67:159–166.

36. West CP, Hillier H. Ovarian suppression with the gonadotrophin-releasing hormone agonist goserelin (Zoladex) in management of the premenstrual tension syndrome. *Hum Reprod* 1994;9:1058–1063.

37. Leather AT, Studd JWW, Watson NR, Holland EFN. The treatment of severe premenstrual syndrome with goserelin with and without 'add-back' estrogen therapy: a placebo-controlled study. *Gynecol Endocrinol* 1999;13:48–55.

38. Sundstrom I, Nyberg S, Bixo M, Hammarback S, Backstrom T. Treatment of premenstrual syndrome with gonadotrophin-releasing hormone agonist in a low dose regimen. *Acta Obstet Gynecol Scand* 1999;78:891–899.

39. Andersch B. Bromocriptine and premenstrual symptoms: a survey of double blind trials. *Obstet Gynecol Surv* 1983;38:643–646.

40. Ylostalo P, Kauppila A, Puolakka J, Ronnberg L, Janne O. Bromocriptine and norethisterone in the treatment of premenstrual syndrome. *Obstet Gynecol* 1982;59:292–298.

41. Graham JJ, Harding PE, Wise PH, Berriman H. Prolactin suppression in the treatment of premenstrual syndrome. *Med J Aust* 1978;2:18–20.

42. Kullander S, Svanberg L. Bromocriptine treatment of the premenstrual syndrome. *Acta Obstet Gynecol Scand* 1979;58:375–378.

43. Arrowsmith-Lowe T. Bromocriptine indications withdrawn. *FDA Med Bull* 1994;24:2.

44. Cullberg J. Mood changes and menstrual symptoms with different gestagen/estrogen combinations: a double blind comparison with a placebo. *Acta Psychiatr Scand Suppl* 1972; 236: 1–86.

45. Morris NM, Udry JR. Contraceptive pills and day-by-day feelings of well-being. *Am J Obstet Gynecol* 1972;113:763–765.

46. Graham CA, Sherwin BB. A prospective treatment study of premenstrual symptoms using a triphasic oral contraceptive. *J Psychosom Res* 1992;36: 257–266.

47. Silbergeld S, Brast N, Noble EP. The menstrual cycle: a double blind study of symptoms, mood and behaviour and biochemical variables using Enovid and placebo. *Psychosom Med* 1971;33: 411–428.

48. Smith SL. Mood and the menstrual cycle. In: Sachar EJ, ed. *Topics in psychoendocrinology*. New York: Grune and Stratton, 1975:19–58.

49. Wang M, Hammarback S, Lindhe BA, Backstrom T. Treatment of premenstrual syndrome by spironolactone: a double-blind, placebo-controlled study. *Acta Obstet Gynecol Scand* 1995;74:803–808.

50. Burnet RB, Radden HS, Easterbrook EG, McKinnon RA. Premenstrual syndrome and spironolactone. *Aust N Z J Obstet Gynaecol* 1991; 31:366–368.

51. Vellacott ID, Shroff NE, Pearce MY, Stratford ME, Akbar FA. A double-blind, placebo-controlled evaluation of spironolactone in the premenstrual syndrome. *Curr Med Res Opin* 1987;10:450–456.

52. O'Brien PM, Craven D, Selby C, Symonds EM. Treatment of premenstrual syndrome by spironolactone. *Br J Obstet Gynaecol* 1979;86: 142–147.

53. Werch A, Kane RE. Treatment of premenstrual tension with metolazone: a double-blind evaluation of a new diuretic. *Curr Ther Res Clin Exp* 1976;19:565–572.

54. Hoffman JJ A double blind crossover clinical trial of an OTC diuretic in the treatment of premenstrual tension and weight gain. *Curr Ther Res* 1979;26: 575–580.

55. Mattsson B, von Schoultz B. A comparison between lithium, placebo and a diuretic in premenstrual tension. *Acta Psychiatr Scand Suppl* 1974;255:75–84.

56. Mira M, McNeil D, Fraser IS, Vizzard J, Abraham S. Mefenamic acid in the treatment of premenstrual syndrome. *Obstet Gynecol* 1986;68: 395–398.

57. Jakubowicz DL, Godard E, Dewhurst J. The treatment of premenstrual tension with mefenamic acid: analysis of prostaglandin concentrations. *Br J Obstet Gynaecol* 1984;91: 78–84.

58. Wood C, Jakubowicz D. The treatment of premenstrual symptoms with mefenamic acid. *Br J Obstet Gynaecol* 1980;87:627–630.

59. Gunston KD. Premenstrual syndrome in Cape Town. Part II: a double-blind placebo-controlled study of the efficacy of mefenamic acid. *S Afr Med J* 1986;70:159–160.

60. Budoff PW. *No more menstrual cramps and other good news*. New York: GP Putman and Sons, 1980.

61. Facchinetti F, Fioroni L, Sances G, Romano G, Nappi G, Genazzani AR. Naproxen sodium in the treatment of premenstrual symptoms: a placebo-controlled study. *Gynecol Obstet Invest* 1989;28: 205–208.

62. Budoff PW. Use of prostaglandin inhibitors in the treatment of PMS. *Clin Obstet Gynecol* 1987: 30(2);453–464.

63. Pearlstein TB, Stone AB, Lund SA, Scheft H, Zlotnik C, Brown WA. Comparison of fluoxetine, buproprion, and placebo in the treatment of premenstrual dysphoric disorder. *J Clin Psychopharmacol* 1997;17:261–266.

64. Sundblad C, Hedberg MA, Eriksson E. Clomipramine administered during the luteal phase reduces the symptoms of premenstrual syndrome: a placebo-controlled trial. *Neuropsychopharmacology* 1993;9:133–145.

65. Sundblad C, Modigh K, Andersch B, Eriksson E. Clomipramine effectively reduces premenstrual irritability and dysphoria: a placebo-controlled trial. *Acta Psychiatr Scand* 1992;85:39–47.

66. Harrison WM, Endicott J, Nee J. Treatment of premenstrual depression with nortriptyline: a pilot study. *J Clin Psychiatry* 1989;50:136–139.

67. Freeman EW, Rickels K, Sandheimer SJ, Polansky

M. Differential response to antidepressants in women with premenstrual syndrome/premenstrual dysphoric disorder. *Arch Gen Psychiatry* 1999;56; 932–939.

68. Taghavi E, Menkes DB, Howard RC, Mason PA, Shaw JP, Spears GFS. Premenstrual syndrome: a double blind controlled trial of desipramine and methylscopolamine. *Int Clin Psychopharmacol* 1995;10:119–122.

69. Freeman EW, Rickels K, Sondheimer SJ, Polansky M. A double-blind trial of oral progesterone, alprazolam, and placebo in treatment of severe premenstrual syndrome. *JAMA* 1995;274:51–57.

70. Schmidt PJ, Grover GN, Rubinow DR. Alprazolam in the treatment of premenstrual syndrome: a double-blind, placebo-controlled trial. *Arch Gen Psychiatry* 1993;50:467–473.

71. Harrison WM, Endicott J, Rabkin JG, Nee JC, Sandberg D. Treatment of premenstrual dysphoria with alprazolam and placebo. *Psychopharmacol Bull* 1987;23:150–153.

72. Smith S, Rinehart JS, Ruddock VE, Schiff I. Treatment of premenstrual syndrome with alprazolam: results of a double- blind, placebo-controlled, randomized crossover clinical trial. *Obstet Gynecol* 1987;70:37–43.

73. Harrison WM, Endicott J, Nee J. Treatment of premenstrual dysphoria with alprazolam: a controlled study. *Arch Gen Psychiatry* 1990;47: 270–275.

74. Diegoli MSC, DaFonseca AM, Diegoli CA, Pinotti JA. A double-blind trial of four medications to treat severe premenstrual syndrome. *Int J Gynecol Obstet* 1998;62:63–67.

75. Evans SM, Haney M, Levin FR, Foltin RW Fischman MW. Mood and performance changes in women with premenstrual dysphoric disorder: acute effects of alprazolam. *Neuropsychopharmacology* 1998;19:499–516.

76. Rickels K, Freeman E, Sondheimer S. Buspirone in treatment of premenstrual syndrome. *Lancet* 1989;1:777.

77. Rausch JL, Janowsky DS, Golshan S, Kuhn K, Risch SC. Atenolol treatment of late luteal phase dysphoric disorder. *J Affect Disord* 1988;15:141–147.

78. Parry BL, Rosebthal NE, James SP, Wehr TA. Atenolol in premenstrual syndrome: A test of the melatonin hypothesis. *Psychiatry Res* 1991;37: 131–138.

79. Singer K, Cheng R, Schou M. A controlled evaluation of lithium in the premenstrual tension syndrome. *Br J Psychiatry* 1974;124:50–51.

80. Dimmock PW, Wyatt KM, Jones PW, O'Brien PMS. Efficacy of selective serotonin–reuptake inhibitors in premenstrual syndrome: A systematic. *Lancet* 2000;356:1131–1136.

81. Wyatt KM, Dimmock PW, O'Brien PMS. Vitamin B6 therapy: a systematic review of its efficacy in premenstrual syndrome. *BMJ* 1999;318:1375–1381. Search date 1998 (before July); primary sources Medline 1966 to May 1998; Psychlit 1974 to 1996; Cinahl 1982 to May 1998.

82. Lauritzen CH, Reuter HD, Repges R, Bohnert KJ, Schmidt U. Treatment of premenstrual tension syndrome with vitex agnus castus, controlled double blind study vs pyridoxine. *Phytomedicine* 1994;4(3):183–189.

83. Lauritzen C. Die behandling des premenstreullen syndoms. Doppelblind studie mi hochdosertem vitamin B6 gegen placebo. *Z Allg Med* 1988;64: 275–278.

84. Budeiri D, Li WP, Dornan JC. Is evening primrose oil of value in the treatment of premenstrual syndrome? *Control Clin Trials* 1996;17:60–68. Search date July 1993; primary sources Science Citation Index 1987 to July 1993; Medline 1966

to July 1993; Dissertation Abstracts 1964 to July 1992; companies who marketed evening primrose oil were approached for any published or unpublished trials.

85. Facchinetti F, Borella P, Sances G, Fioroni L, Nappi RE, Genazzani AR. Oral magnesium successfully relieves premenstrual mood changes. *Obstet Gynecol* 1991;78:177–181.

86. De Souza MC, Walker AF, Bolland KM, Robinson PA. A synergistic effect of magnesium and vitamin B6 supplementation for the relief of symptoms of the premenstrual syndrome (PMS). *Proc Nutr Soc* 996;56:75a.

87. Walker AF, De Souza MC, Vickers MF, Abeyasekera S, Collins ML, Trinca LA. Magnesium supplementation alleviates premenstrual symptoms of fluid retention. *J Womens Health* 1998;7:1157–1165.

88. Thys-Jacobs S, Ceccarelli S, Bierman A, Weisman H, Cohen MA, Alvir J. Calcium supplementation in premenstrual syndrome: a randomized crossover trial. *J Gen Intern Med* 1989;4:183–189.

89. Thys-Jacobs S, Starkey P, Bernstein D, Tian J. Calcium carbonate and the premenstrual syndrome: effects on premenstrual and menstrual symptoms. Premenstrual Syndrome Study Group. *Am J Obstet Gynecol* 1998;179:444–452.

90. Penland JG, Johnson PE. Dietary calcium and manganese effects on menstrual cycle symptoms [see comments]. *Am J Obstet Gynecol* 1993; 168(5):1417–1423.

91. Steinberg S, Annable L, Young SN, Liyanage N. A placebo-controlled clinical trial of L-tryptophan in premenstrual dysphoria. *Biol Psychiatry* 1999;45: 313–320.

92. Barnard ND, Scialli AR, Hurlock D, Bertron P. Diet and sex-hormone binding globulin, dysmenorrhea, and premenstrual symptoms. *Obstet Gynecol* 2000;95(2):245–250.

93. Morse C, Dennerstein L, Farrell E. A comparison of hormone therapy, coping skills training and relaxation for the relief of premenstrual syndrome. *J Behav Med* 1991;14:469–489.

94. Kirkby RJ. Changes in premenstrual symptoms and irrational thinking following cognitive - behavioural coping skills training. *J Consult Clin Psychol* 1994; 62:1026–1032.

95. Blake F, Salkovskis P, Gath D, Day A, Garrod A. Cognitive therapy for premenstrual syndrome: a controlled trial. *J Psychosom Res* 1998;45:307–318.

96. Corney RH, Stanton R, Newell R. Comparison of progesterone, placebo and behavioural psychotherapy in the treatment of premenstrual syndrome. *J Psychosom Obstet Gynaecol* 1990; 11:211–220.

97. Christensen AP, Oei TPS. The efficacy of cognitive behaviour therapy in treating premenstrual dysphoric changes. *J Affect Disord* 1995;33:57–63.

98. Prior JC, Vigna Y, Alojada N. Conditioning exercise decreases premenstrual symptoms. A prospective controlled three month trial. *Eur J Appl Physiol* 1986;55:349–355.

99. Lemos D. The effects of aerobic training on women who suffer from premenstrual syndrome. *Dissert Abstracts Int* 1991;52:563.

100. Bibi KW. The effects of aerobic exercise on premenstrual syndrome symptoms. *Dissert Abstracts Int* 1995;56:6678.

101. Walsh MJ, Polus BI. A randomised, placebo-controlled clinical trial on the efficacy of chiropractic therapy on PMS. *J Manipulative Physiol Ther* 1999;22;582–585.

102. Goodale IL, Domar AD, Benson H. Alleviation of premenstrual syndrome symptoms with the

relaxation response. *Obstet Gynecol* 1990;75: 649–655.

103. Metcalf MG, Braiden V, Livesey JH, Wells JE. The premenstrual syndrome: amelioration of symptoms after hysterectomy. *J Psychosom Res* 1992;36:569–584.

104. Osborn M, Gath D. Psychological and physical determinants of premenstrual symptoms before and after hysterectomy. *Psychol Med* 1990;20: 565–572.

105. Casper RF, Hearn MT. The effect of hysterectomy and bilateral oophorectomy in women with severe premenstrual syndrome. *Am J Obstet Gynecol* 1990;162:105–109.

106. Casson P, Hahn PM, Van Vugt DA, Reid RL. Lasting response to ovariectomy in severe intractable premenstrual syndrome. *Am J Obstet Gynecol* 1990;162:99–105.

107. Shaw RW, Soutter WP, Stanton SL. *Gynaecology*. New York: Churchill Livingstone, 1997.

Katrina Wyatt
Non-clinical Lecturer in Reproductive
Endocrinology

Paul Dimmock
Research Scholar

PMS O'Brien
Professor and Head of Department

North Staffordshire NHS Trust, and
School of Postgraduate Medicine
Keele University
Stoke on Trent
UK

Competing interests: PMS O'Brien has been reimbursed for lectures and conferences by the following companies: Hoechst Marion Roussel Ltd., Shire Pharmaceuticals, SmithKline Beecham, Eli Lilly, Searle, Sanofi Winthrop, Zeneca, Solvay Pharmaceuticals, and Novo Nordisk. He has also received funds for research personnel from Searle, SmithKline Beecham, Eli Lilly, and Sanofi Winthrop. He is married to a member of the research department of Zeneca Pharmaceuticals. KMW and PWD, none declared.

TABLE 1	Commonly reported symptoms in women with PMS (see text, p 1122).[4]
Psychological symptoms	Irritability, depression, crying/tearfulness, anxiety, tension, mood swings, lack of concentration, confusion, forgetfulness, unsociableness, restlessness, temper outbursts/anger, sadness/blues, loneliness.
Behavioural symptoms	Fatigue, dizziness, sleep/insomnia, decreased efficiency, accident prone, sexual interest changes, increased energy, tiredness.
Physical symptoms: pain	Headache/migraine, breast tenderness/soreness/pain/swelling (collectively known as premenstrual mastalgia), back pain, abdominal cramps, general pain.
Physical symptoms: bloatedness and swelling	Weight gain, abdominal bloating or swelling, oedema of arms and legs, water retention.
Appetite symptoms	Increased appetite, food cravings, nausea.

Pyelonephritis in non-pregnant women

Updated this issue

Bruce Cooper and Ruth Jepson

INTERVENTIONS

Beneficial
Oral antibiotics for women with
   uncomplicated infection . . .1135
Intravenous antibiotics in women
   admitted to hospital with
   uncomplicated infection . . .1137

Unknown effectiveness
Inpatient versus outpatient
   management. 1137

Key Messages

- RCTs have consistently found that oral antibiotic treatment with trimethoprim–sulfamethoxazole (TMP-SMZ), amoxycillin–clavulanic acid, or a fluoroquinolone (ciprofloxacin, norfloxacin, levofloxacin, or lomefloxacin) is effective in women outpatients with uncomplicated infection.

- We found limited evidence suggesting that intravenous antibiotics are effective in women admitted to hospital with uncomplicated infection, and that ampicillin should not be used alone to treat infection with *Escherichia coli* because of antimicrobial resistance.

- We found no well designed trials comparing newer intravenous antibiotics with older, standard regimens.

- We found no direct evidence comparing the inpatient and outpatient management of acute uncomplicated pyelonephritis in non-pregnant women. One RCT found no significant difference between oral and intravenous antibiotics in the duration of fever or symptoms.

DEFINITION	Acute pyelonephritis, or upper urinary tract infection, is an infection of the kidney, characterised by dysuria, fever, flank pain, nausea, and vomiting. Pyuria is almost always present, and occasionally white blood cell casts are seen on urine microscopy. Uncomplicated infection occurs in an otherwise healthy person without underlying comorbidity. Complicated infection occurs in people with structural or functional urinary tract abnormalities or comorbid diseases. People with acute pyelonephritis can be divided into those able to take oral antibiotics and without signs of sepsis who may be managed at home, and those requiring parenteral treatment in hospital.
INCIDENCE/ PREVALENCE	In the USA, there are 250 000 cases of acute pyelonephritis per year.[1] Worldwide prevalence and incidence are unknown.
AETIOLOGY/ RISK FACTORS	Pyelonephritis is most commonly caused when bacteria in the bladder ascend the ureters and invade the renal parenchyma. In some cases, this results in bacteraemia.
PROGNOSIS	With prompt diagnosis and treatment, the prognosis is good. Complications include sepsis, metastatic infection, renal impairment, and renal abscess. Comorbidity such as renal disease, diabetes mellitus, and immunosuppression may worsen prognosis, with a potential increase in risk of sepsis and death, but we found no good long term data for such people.
AIMS	To reduce the duration and severity of symptoms; to prevent or minimise potential complications, with minimum adverse effects.
OUTCOMES	Urine culture after treatment, signs and symptoms of infection, rates of complications of infection, and adverse effects of treatment.
METHODS	*Clinical Evidence* update search and appraisal May 2000, using the MeSH terms pyelonephritis, upper urinary tract infection, hospitalisation, outpatient therapy, and oral antibiotics. We included RCTs and systematic reviews that focused on the inpatient and outpatient management of acute uncomplicated pyelonephritis in non-pregnant women. We excluded studies that were primarily in men, pregnant women, and people with complicated infections.

QUESTION **What are the effects of treatments for acute pyelonephritis?**

OPTION **ORAL ANTIBIOTICS**

One systematic review of RCTs has found that oral antibiotic treatment with trimethoprim–sulfamethoxazole (TMP-SMZ), amoxycillin–clavulanic acid, or a fluoroquinolone (ciprofloxacin, norfloxacin, levofloxacin, and lomefloxacin) is effective in healthy, non-pregnant women with acute pyelonephritis who are able to take oral treatment and lack signs of sepsis.

Benefits: We found one systematic review (search date 1991) and two subsequent RCTs. The review identified nine RCTs comparing different oral antibiotics with one another in 470 men and non-pregnant women with acute pyelonephritis (see table 1, p 1139).[2] Five trials were conducted with people outside hospital and four in people admitted to hospital. The studies were conducted in the USA, Europe, and Peru. All included more women than men. Most studies excluded people with complicating factors such as structural abnormalities of the urinary tract, comorbid illnesses, pregnancy, or signs of possible sepsis. All except one found no significant difference in rates of early cure (negative urine culture within 7–10 days), and six of the nine studies found no significant difference in rates of late cure (negative urine culture 2–4 weeks or more after stopping treatment). However, several of the individual studies were too small to rule out a difference between antibiotic regimens. Of the subsequent RCTs, the first, a multicentre RCT in 47 people with acute uncomplicated pyelonephritis who were admitted to hospital, compared oral lomefloxacin 400 mg daily versus oral TMP-SMZ 160 mg/800 mg twice daily, both for 14 days.[3] At 5–9 days, there was a significantly higher rate of bacteriological eradication on lomefloxacin compared with TMP-SMZ (100% v 88.9%, P = 0.05) but no significant difference in clinical cure rates. At 4–6 weeks, there were no significant differences. The other RCT compared 10 days of levofloxacin 250 mg daily versus 10 days of ciprofloxacin 500 mg twice daily or 14 days of lomefloxacin 400 mg daily in 186 outpatients (87% women) with acute uncomplicated pyelonephritis.[4] There was no significant difference in rates of early cure (defined as a negative urine culture 5–9 days after treatment, which occurred in 94% of people on each of the three drugs) or microbiologic relapse at long term follow up.

Harms: Adverse effects were reported in 12% of people taking lomefloxacin and 17% taking TMP-SMZ.[3] The most frequent adverse effects were skin reactions. Three people taking TMP-SMZ withdrew from treatment, one because of dermatitis and one because of hepatocellular damage. There were no withdrawals because of adverse events in people taking lomefloxacin.[3] Adverse effects were reported in 2% of people on levofloxacin, 8% on ciprofloxacin, and 5% on lomefloxacin.[4] Gastrointestinal symptoms were common with both ciprofloxacin and levofloxacin, whereas rash was the most common adverse effect with lomefloxacin. One of the 186 people discontinued treatment (lomefloxacin) because of adverse effects.[4]

Comment: Calculated cure rates from the systematic review are likely to overestimate rates that would be achieved in clinical practice because many patients were excluded, including those who experienced adverse effects, had growth of a resistant bacteria on initial culture, or did not adhere to treatment. The high rate of ampicillin resistance found in laboratory tests has led to a consensus view that ampicillin and amoxicillin are not recommended in pyelonephritis. We found no direct evidence to confirm or refute this view. Ampicillin and amoxycillin were found in the trials to have cure rates comparable with other antibiotics, but the studies were too small to exclude a clinically important difference.

OPTION INTRAVENOUS ANTIBIOTICS

One RCT found that intravenous TMP-SMZ or ampicillin plus gentamicin were effective and well tolerated in non-pregnant women admitted to hospital with acute uncomplicated pyelonephritis. We found no well designed trials comparing newer intravenous antibiotics with these standard regimens.

Benefits: We found no systematic review. We found one RCT in 85 women admitted to hospital for acute uncomplicated pyelonephritis. This compared intravenous ampicillin 1 g every 6 hours versus intravenous TMP-SMZ 160 mg/800 mg every 12 hours, initiated before culture results were known.[5] Both regimens were combined with gentamicin and followed by oral treatment with either ampicillin or TMP-SMZ. *E coli* was the sole microorganism isolated from the urine in 91% of women. Fourteen of the 42 women (32%) treated with ampicillin and gentamicin were infected with ampicillin resistant isolates and were withdrawn from the study. No women allocated to TMP-SMZ required a change of treatment, and there were no other treatment failures in either group. **New versus standard regimens:** We found no adequately designed RCTs comparing quinolones, cephalosporins, and broad spectrum β lactams with standard treatment. **Versus oral antibiotics:** See inpatient versus outpatient management below.

Harms: Adverse effects varied by agent. In the RCT,[5] adverse effects that may have been a result of treatment were reported equally in the two groups (33% ampicillin, 32% TMP-SMZ) but the nature of these adverse effects was not reported. One person from each group discontinued treatment because of adverse effects.[5] Common adverse effects with ampicillin include rash, diarrhoea, and vaginitis, and with TMP-SMZ include nausea, vomiting, and vaginitis.

Comment: There is a consensus view that the choice of empirical antibiotics should take into account the setting, medical history of the patient, Gram stain of the urine, previous infecting organism, and local antibiotic sensitivities.

OPTION INPATIENT VERSUS OUTPATIENT MANAGEMENT

We found no direct evidence comparing inpatient and outpatient management of acute, uncomplicated pyelonephritis in non-pregnant women. One RCT found no significant difference between oral or intravenous antibiotics in the duration of fever or symptoms.

Benefits: We found no systematic review and no RCTs comparing outpatient with inpatient management of acute uncomplicated pyelonephritis in non-pregnant women. **Intravenous versus oral antibiotics:** We found one Swiss based multicentre RCT in 163 people admitted to hospital with pyelonephritis or complicated UTI (infection associated with a structural or functional abnormality of the urinary tract or nosocomially acquired), which compared oral ciprofloxacin 500 mg every 12 hours versus intravenous ciprofloxacin 200 mg every 12 hours. The analysis included 83 non-pregnant women. It found no significant difference between oral and intravenous ciprofloxacin in the duration of symptoms (1.7 days, 95% CI 1.5 to 1.9 with oral *v*

1.9 days, 95% CI 1.7 to 2.2 with intravenous, P = 0.15) or fever (1.8 days, 95% CI 1.4 to 2.2 v 1.8 days, 95% CI 1.4 to 2.2, P = 0.85), the number of people with persistent infection after 3–5 days of treatment (2 v 1, P = 0.95), or the median duration of hospitalisation (7 days, 95% CI 2 to 35 v 8 days, 95% CI 2 to 32, P = 0.15). There were no infection related deaths.[6]

Harms: In the RCT, one person on oral ciprofloxacin discontinued treatment because of the development of mental confusion. Another person on intravenous ciprofloxacin developed pruritus, but treatment was continued until completed. No other adverse affects were reported.[6]

Comment: The results of the RCT suggest that oral ciprofloxacin is as effective as intravenous ciprofloxacin in people with either community or hospital acquired pyelonephritis, even in those with underlying structural or functional urinary abnormalities. Whether this can be generalised to treatment outside hospital is not clear, as both groups in this study received close monitoring and supervision in an inpatient setting.

REFERENCES

1. Stamm WE, Hooton TM, Johnson JR. Urinary tract infection: from pathogenesis to treatment. *J Infect Dis* 1989;15:400–406.
2. Pinson AG, Philbrick JT, Lindbeck GH, et al. Oral antibiotic therapy for acute pyelonephritis: a methodologic review of the literature. *J Gen Intern Med* 1992;7:544–553. Search date 1991; primary sources Medline 1965 to 1990, Current Contents 1990 to 1991.
3. Mouton Y, Ajana F, Chidiac C, et al. A multicenter study of lomefloxacin and trimethoprim/sulfamethoxazole in the treatment of uncomplicated acute pyelonephritis. *Am J Med* 1992;92 (suppl):87–90.
4. Richard GA, Klimberg IN, Fowler CL, et al. Levofloxacin versus ciprofloxacin versus lomefloxacin in acute pyelonephritis. *Urology* 1998;52:51–55.
5. Johnson JR, Lyons MF, Pearce W, et al. Therapy for women hospitalized with acute pyelonephritis: a randomized trial of ampicillin versus trimethoprim-sulfamethoxazole for 14 days. *J Infect Dis* 1991; 163:325–330.
6. Mombelli G, Pezzoli R, Pinoja-Lutz G, et al. Oral vs intravenous ciprofloxacin in the initial empirical management of severe pyelonephritis or complicated urinary tract infections: a prospective randomized clinical trial. *Arch Intern Med* 1999; 159:53–58.

Bruce Cooper
Renal Research Fellow
University of Sydney, Royal North Shore
Hospital, St Leonards
Sydney
Australia

Ruth Jepson
Research Fellow
NHS Centre for Reviews and
Dissemination
York
UK

Competing interests: None declared.

TABLE 1   Oral antibiotic treatment for acute pyelonephritis: results of RCTs (see text, p 1135).[2]

Study number	Oral antibiotic regimens	Total number of patients	Early cure* rates %	Late cure* rates %	P value
1	Amoxycillin 500 mg three times daily for 14 days	16	–	94	NS
	TMP-SMZ (160 mg/800 mg) twice daily for 14 days	12	–	92	
2	Norfloxacin 400 mg twice daily for 10 days	14	100	86	NS
	TMP-SMZ (160 mg/800 mg) twice daily for 10 days	10	100	90	
3	Ampicillin 500 mg four times daily for 10 days	8	88	–	NS
	Cefaclor 250 mg twice daily for 10 days	6	67	–	
4	Norfloxacin 400 mg twice daily for 7 days or longer	3	67	–	NS
	TMP-SMZ (160 mg/800 mg) twice daily for 7 days or longer	12	92	–	
5	Amoxycillin-clavulanic acid 250 mg/125 mg three times daily for 10 days	54	94	85	P = 0.02 for late cure; NS for early cure
	TMP-SMZ (160 mg/800 mg) twice daily for 10 days	50	82	64	
6	Ampicillin 500 mg four times daily for 2 or 6 weeks	17	100	47	P = 0.004 for late cure; NS for early cure
7	TMP-SMZ (160 mg/800 mg) twice daily for 2 or 6 weeks	22	100	91	NS
	Amoxycillin 2000 mg one time dose then 1000 mg twice daily for 9 days	22	100	100	
8	Amoxycillin 750 mg three times daily for 12 days	23	96	87	NS
	Cefetamet 2000 mg daily or 1000 mg twice daily for 10–15 days	28	93	79	
	Cefadroxil 1000 mg twice daily for 10–15 days	22	73	52	
9	Norfloxacin 400 mg twice daily for 14 days	76	91	82	P < 0.0001 for both early and late cures
	Cefadroxil 1000 mg twice daily for 14 days	75	59	44	

Table adapted with permission.[2] NS, not significant. *Early cure: negative urine culture within 7–10 days of starting treatment; late cure: negative urine culture 2–4 weeks or more after stopping treatment.

Recurrent cystitis in non-pregnant women

Updated this issue

Bruce Cooper and Ruth Jepson

QUESTIONS
How to prevent further recurrence 1141
Who to investigate for urinary tract abnormalities 1144

INTERVENTIONS

Beneficial
Continuous antibiotic
  prophylaxis 1141
Postcoital antibiotic
  prophylaxis 1142

Likely to be beneficial
Self treatment with
  antibiotics 1143
Long term antibiotic
  prophylaxis 1143

Unknown effectiveness
Cranberry juice and cranberry
  products 1143

Unlikely to be beneficial
Routine investigation of the urinary
  tract in women with
  uncomplicated recurrent
  infection 1144

To be covered in future issues of
Clinical Evidence
Advice to pass urine after
  intercourse

Key Messages

- Consistent evidence from RCTs has found that antibiotic prophylaxis (either continuous or postcoital), using nitrofurantoin, a quinolone, trimethoprim, or trimethoprim-sulfamethoxazole (also known as co-trimoxazole or TMP-SMZ) reduces infection rates in women with high rates of recurrent urinary tract infections (at least two per year).

- One RCT has found that intermittent, single dose, self administered treatment taken at the onset of symptoms is an effective alternative management strategy to continuous antibiotic prophylaxis in women with high rates of recurrent infection.

- A cohort study has found that long term prophylaxis is likely to benefit women with a baseline rate of more than two infections per year over many years. However, long term treatment has not yet been evaluated in RCTs.

- The effects of cranberry juice and other cranberry products have not been adequately assessed.

- In women who experience recurrent, uncomplicated urinary tract infections, we found no good evidence to support routine investigation of the urinary tract with excretory urography, ultrasonography, cystoscopy, or voiding cystourethrography. No subgroups of women who would clearly benefit from investigation have yet been adequately defined.

© *Clinical Evidence* 2000;4:1140–1147.

DEFINITION	Cystitis is an infection of the lower urinary tract causing dysuria, frequency, urgency, haematuria, or suprapubic pain. Pyuria and bacteriuria are almost always present. The presence of fever, flank pain, nausea, or vomiting suggests pyelonephritis (see pyelonephritis in non-pregnant women, p 1134). Recurrent cystitis may be either a reinfection (after successful eradication of infection) or a relapse after inadequate treatment.
INCIDENCE/ PREVALENCE	The incidence of cystitis among premenopausal sexually active women is 0.5–0.7 infections per person year,[1] and 20–40% of women will experience cystitis during their lifetime. Of those, 20% will develop recurrence, almost always (90% of cases) because of reinfection rather than relapse. Rates of infection fall during the winter months.[2]
AETIOLOGY/ RISK FACTORS	Cystitis is caused by uropathogenic bacteria in the faecal flora that colonise the vaginal and periurethral introitus and ascend the urethra into the bladder. Prior infection, sexual intercourse, and exposure to vaginal spermicide are risk factors for developing cystitis.[3,4]
PROGNOSIS	We found little evidence on the long term effects of untreated cystitis. One study found that progression to upper urinary tract infection was infrequent, and that most cases of cystitis regressed spontaneously, although symptoms sometimes persisted for several months.[5] Women with a baseline rate of more than two infections per year, over many years, are likely to continue to suffer from recurrent infections.[6]
AIMS	To prevent recurrent infection in women predisposed to frequent infections, with minimal adverse effects.
OUTCOMES	Rate of infection based on urine culture and symptoms.
METHODS	*Clinical Evidence* update search and appraisal May 2000. We reviewed all systematic reviews and RCTs comparing different forms of prophylaxis or comparing prophylaxis versus placebo in non-pregnant women with a history of recurrent urinary tract infection. We excluded studies in populations consisting mainly of men or pregnant women.

QUESTION **Which interventions prevent further recurrence in women experiencing at least two infections per year?**

OPTION CONTINUOUS ANTIBIOTIC PROPHYLAXIS

RCTs have found that continuous antibiotic prophylaxis using trimethoprim, TMP-SMZ, nitrofurantoin, cefaclor, or a quinolone reduces rates of recurrent urinary tract infection in non-pregnant women. We found no good evidence of any difference between different continuous regimens, nor between continuous and postcoital regimens.

Benefits:	We found no systematic review. We found seven RCTs comparing different regimens for continuous antibiotic prophylaxis lasting 6–12 months in women with high rates of recurrent urinary tract infection (at least two episodes per year) (see table 1, p 1146).[7–13] Three of the RCTs included a placebo or no treatment arm.[7–9] All

found significantly lower rates of infection with active treatment (nitrofurantoin, ciprofloxacin, norfloxacin, or TMP-SMZ), but confidence intervals were not given. **Versus each other:** Five RCTs compared different antibiotic regimens.[7,10–13] One study of 72 patients found significantly fewer infections (P < 0.05) in women taking a nocturnal dose of nitrofurantoin compared with those using a nocturnal dose of trimethoprim.[10] In the other larger studies comparing different regimens over 6–12 months, no significant differences were found.[7,11–13] Most of the reported rates of infection in these studies were much less than 0.6 per patient year, suggesting that they were all as effective in reducing the rate of infection in patients with a history of recurrent cystitis. However, these studies were not powered to exclude a clinically important difference between treatments. **Versus postcoital prophylaxis:** One RCT compared daily versus postcoital treatment with ciprofloxacin in 135 women. It found no significant difference in rates of infection, but no confidence interval was given.[8]

Harms: Rates of adverse effects in these studies ranged from 7–40% for trimethoprim; 0–40% for nitrofurantoin; 5% for cefaclor; 7–21% for norfloxacin; and 13% for ciprofloxacin.[7–9,11–13] The most common adverse effects for all agents were gastrointestinal symptoms, rash, and yeast vaginitis.

Comment: Many of the studies were not placebo controlled or blinded, and had small study populations. Despite the small study sizes, however, infection rates were significantly less in women using continuous prophylactic antibiotics compared to those without antibiotics. Adjustments were not made for confounding factors such as frequency of sexual intercourse.

OPTION   POSTCOITAL ANTIBIOTIC PROPHYLAXIS

RCTs have found that taking nitrofurantoin, a quinolone, trimethoprim, or TMP-SMZ within 2 hours after sexual intercourse significantly reduces the rates of infection in women with recurrent urinary tract infection. One RCT found no evidence of any difference between postcoital and continuous daily antibiotic regimens.

Benefits: We found no systematic review. We found four RCTs of postcoital antibiotic regimens (treatment taken within 2 hours of sexual intercourse), evaluated over 6–14 months, in women with high rates of recurrent urinary tract infection (at least two episodes per year) (see table 2, p 1147).[8,14–16] **Versus placebo or no treatment:** All trials found a significant reduction in rates of infection with active treatment (TMP-SMZ, nitrofurantoin or a quinolone). **Versus continuous daily prophylaxis:** One RCT compared continuous daily versus postcoital treatment with ciprofloxacin in 135 women.[8] It found no evidence of a significant difference in rates of infection.

Harms: Rates of adverse effects were as follows: TMP-SMZ 18%; ciprofloxacin 6%; and nitrofurantoin less than 1%.[8,14–16] The most common adverse effects for all agents were gastrointestinal symptoms, rash, and yeast vaginitis.

Comment: Only one of the studies was placebo controlled and blinded.[14] Adjustments were not made for confounding factors such as frequency of sexual intercourse.

OPTION   SELF TREATMENT WITH ANTIBIOTICS

Limited evidence from one small RCT suggests that self treatment with a single dose of TMP-SMZ is an effective alternative management strategy to continuous antibiotic prophylaxis in women with high rates of infection.

Benefits: We found no systematic review. We found one RCT using a cross-over design in 38 non-pregnant women with two or more culture documented urinary tract infections in the previous 12 months.[17] This compared continuous antibiotic prophylaxis with TMP-SMZ (40 mg/200 mg) versus a self administered single dose of TMP-SMZ (40 mg/200 mg) to be taken at the onset of symptoms of cystitis. The self treatment group was given enough tablets for four single treatments. Although infection rates were higher in the self treatment group (2.2 per patient year compared with 0.22 per patient year with continuous prophylaxis; P < 0.001, see comment below), 85% of infections responded to a single dose. We found no evidence relating to effects on quality of life.

Harms: The trial found no evidence of significant differences in adverse effects between continuous antibiotic prophylaxis and self administered treatment.

Comment: The trial found that the women were almost always able to diagnose their own infections from symptoms (positive predictive value 92%).[17] The higher rate of infections in the self treatment group is to be expected since self treatment was only administered after the onset of symptoms.

OPTION   LONG TERM ANTIBIOTIC PROPHYLAXIS

Long term antibiotic prophylaxis (longer than 12 months) has not yet been adequately evaluated in RCTs.

Benefits: We found no systematic review or RCTs. One cohort study followed 51 non-pregnant women treated for over 112 person years with continuous trimethoprim, TMP-SMZ, or nitrofurantoin, and found that this intervention was effective in preventing cystitis and pyelo-nephritis.[2]

Harms: The cohort study reported no significant adverse effects, even when treatment continued for as long as 5 years. The development of bacterial resistance from continuous antibiotic prophylaxis was rare. However, the number of TMP-SMZ resistant organisms increased during the latter part of the study.[2]

Comment: None.

OPTION   CRANBERRY JUICE AND CRANBERRY PRODUCTS

A systematic review has found no reliable evidence on the effects of cranberry juice and other cranberry products.

Benefits: We found one systematic review (search date 1998) assessing the effectiveness of cranberry juice and other cranberry products in the prevention of urinary tract infections in susceptible populations.[18] It identified two RCTs in women. One was a crossover trial comparing cranberry capsules versus placebo in women with recurrent infections (n = 19, withdrawal rate 47%). This reported 21 infections among the 10 remaining women, of which six infections occurred while taking cranberry capsules. The other trial compared cranberry juice versus placebo in elderly women (n = 192, withdrawal rate 20%), and found that cranberry juice significantly reduced the rate of infection (defined as ≥ 100 000 organisms per ml plus pyuria) compared with placebo (OR 0.42, P = 0.004).

Harms: No data on adverse effects were reported.

Comment: These studies were small, with high withdrawal rates, and the lack of intention to treat analyses in either trial may mean that they overestimated the effectiveness of cranberry juice and products. High withdrawal rates suggest that long term adherence may be difficult to achieve.

| QUESTION | Which women with recurrent infections should undergo investigation for urinary tract abnormalities? |

We found limited evidence suggesting that routine investigation is unlikely to be beneficial. Subgroups of women who would clearly benefit from investigation have not yet been adequately defined.

Benefits: We found no systematic review or RCTs.

Harms: We found two cross-sectional studies[19–20] and one prospective study[21] of routine excretory urography (see comment below). The studies had insufficient power to report on harms. Excretory urography with iodinated dye can cause anaphylactoid reactions and renal dysfunction. Cystoscopy can cause bleeding and other complications depending upon the type of procedure and anaesthesia used. Ultrasonography has no known adverse effects.

Comment: Two older, cross sectional studies[19,20] and one prospective study[21] examined the yield of routine excretory urography in women with recurrent urinary tract infections. Among the 421 women studied, urography was normal in 88%, showed anatomic variants in about 6%, and was abnormal in about 5%. None of the abnormalities detected were correctable or thought to be causally related to infection. Two of the studies found no evidence that cystoscopy detected clinically important abnormalities.[20,21] In a more recent cross sectional study, 186 women were non-randomly selected from a larger group of 475 women with recurrent urinary tract infections because the referring physician suspected an underlying problem.[22] Of these, 21% had an abnormality reported on cystoscopy, excretory urography, ultrasonography, or voiding cystourethrography. The reported rates of detection of abnormalities in these observational stuides [19–21] are likely to be overestimates because the studies took place in specialist urology units. Results from the more recent cross sectional study are difficult to interpret because there was no standard protocol for evaluation and results were collected retrospectively.[22]

REFERENCES

1. Hooton TM, Scholes D, Hughes JP, et al. A prospective study of risk factors for symptomatic urinary tract infection in young women. *N Engl J Med* 1996;335:468–474.
2. Stamm WE, McKevitt M, Roberts PL, White NJ. Natural history of recurrent urinary tract infections in women. *Rev Infect Dis* 1991;13:77–84.
3. Fihn SD, Latham RH, Roberts P, Running K, Stamm WE. Association between diaphragm use and urinary tract infection. *JAMA* 1985;254:240–245.
4. Fihn SD, Boyko EJ, Normand EH, et al. Association between use of spermicide-coated condoms and *Escherichia coli* urinary tract infection in young women. *Am J Epidemiol* 1996; 144:512–520.
5. Mabeck CE. Treatment of uncomplicated urinary tract infection in non-pregnant women. *Postgrad Med J* 1972;48:69–75.
6. Stamm WE, Counts GW, McKevitt M, Turck M, Holmes KK. Urinary prophylaxis with trimethoprim and trimethoprim-sulfamethoxazole: efficacy, influence on the natural history of recurrent bacteriuria and cost control. *Rev Infect Dis* 1982; 4:450–455.
7. Stamm WE, Counts GW, Wagner KF, et al. Antimicrobial prophylaxis of recurrent urinary tract infections: a double-blind placebo-controlled trial. *Ann Intern Med* 1980;92:770–775.
8. Melekos MD, Asbach HW, Gerharz E, Zarakovitis IE, Weingaertner K, Naber KG. Post-intercourse versus daily ciprofloxacin prophylaxis for recurrent urinary tract infections in premenopausal women. *J Urol* 1997;157:935–939.
9. Nicolle LE, Harding GKM, Thompson M, Kennedy J, Urias B, Ronald AR. Prospective, randomized, placebo-controlled trial of norfloxacin for the prophylaxis of recurrent urinary tract infection in women. *Antimicrob Agents Chemother* 1989;33:1032–1035.
10. Brumfitt W, Smith GW, Hamilton-Miller JMT, Gargan RA. A clinical comparison between macrodantin and trimethoprim for prophylaxis in women with recurrent urinary infection. *J Antimicrob Chemother* 1985;16:111–120.
11. Raz R, Boger S. Long-term prophylaxis with norfloxacin versus nitrofurantoin in women with recurrent urinary tract infection. *Antimicrob Agents Chemother* 1991;35:1241–1242.
12. Brumfitt W, Hamilton-Miller JMT, Smith GW, Al-Wali W. Comparative trial of norfloxacin and macrocrystalline nitrofurantoin (Macrodantin) in the prophylaxis of recurrent urinary tract infection in women. *Q J Med* 1991;81:811–820.
13. Brumfitt W, Hamilton-Miller JMT. A comparative trial of low-dose cefaclor and macrocrystalline nitrofurantoin in the prevention of recurrent urinary tract infection. *Infection* 1995;23:98–102.
14. Stapleton A, Latham RH, Johnson C, Stamm WE. Postcoital antimicrobial prophylaxis for recurrent urinary tract infection: a randomized, double-blind placebo-controlled trial. *JAMA* 1990;264:703–706.
15. Pfau A, Sacks TG. Effective postcoital quinolone prophylaxis of recurrent urinary tract infection in women. *J Urol* 1994;152:136–138.
16. Pfau A, Sacks T, Englestein D. Recurrent urinary tract infections in premenopausal women: prophylaxis based on an understanding of the pathogenesis. *J Urol* 1983;129:1153–1156.
17. Wong ES, McKevitt M, Running K, Counts GW, Turck M, Stamm WE. Management of recurrent urinary tract infections with patient-administered single-dose therapy. *Ann Intern Med* 1985;102:302–307.
18. Jepson RG, Mihaljevic L, Craig J. Cranberries for preventing urinary tract infections. In: The Cochrane Library. Issue 1, 2000. Oxford: Update Software. Search date 1998; primary sources Medline; Embase; Psychlit; LILACS; Cinahl; Biological Abstracts; Current Contents; Cochrane Controlled Trials Register; Cochrane Renal Group; The Internet; Conference Proceedings, and hand searched references.
19. Fair WR, McClennan BL, Jost RG. Are excretory urograms necessary in evaluating women with urinary tract infection? *J Urol* 1979;121:313–315.
20. Engle G, Schaeffer AJ, Grayhack JT, Wendel EF. The role of excretory urography and cystoscopy in the evaluation and management of women with recurrent urinary tract infection. *J Urol* 1980;123:190–191.
21. Fowler JE Jr, Pulaski ET. Excretory urography, cystography, and cystoscopy in the evaluation of women with urinary tract infection: a prospective study. *N Engl J Med* 1981;304:462–465.
22. Nickel JC, Wilson, J, Morales A, Heaton J. Value of urologic investigation in a targeted group of women with recurrent urinary tract infections. *Can J Surg* 1991;34:591–594.

Bruce Cooper
Renal Research Fellow
University of Sydney Royal North
Shore Hospital
St Leonards
Australia

Ruth Jepson
Research Fellow
NHS Centre for Reviews and
Dissemination University of York
York
UK
Competing interests: None declared.

| TABLE 1 | Continuous antimicrobial prophylactic regimens for recurrent urinary tract infections: results of RCTs (see text, p 1141).[1] |

Study	Total number of participants	Regimen	Duration of prophylaxis (months)	Infections per patient year	P value (placebo v drug treatment)
Stamm, et al[7] (placebo controlled RCT) 1980	60	Placebo	6	2.80	< 0.001
		TMP-SMZ (40 mg/200 mg) at bedtime		0.15	
		Nitrofurantoin 100 mg at bedtime		0.14	
		Nitrofurantoin 100 mg at bedtime		0	
Melekos, et al[8] (open RCT) 1997	135	Without prophylaxis	12	3.62–3.66	< 0.001
		Ciprofloxacin 125 mg postcoital		0.043	
		Ciprofloxacin 125 mg daily		0.031	
Nicolle, et al[9] (placebo controlled RCT) 1989	30	Placebo	12	1.6	< 0.001
		Norfloxacin 200 mg at bedtime		0	
Brumfitt, et al[10] (open RCT) 1985	72	Trimethoprim 100 mg at bedtime	12	1.00	< 0.05
		Nitrofurantoin 100 mg bedtime		0.17	
Raz, et al[11] (open RCT) 1991	94	Norfloxacin 200 mg at bedtime	6	0.04	= 0.05
		Nitrofurantoin 50 mg at bedtime		0.60	
Brumfitt, et al[12] (open RCT) 1991	88	Norfloxacin 200 mg at bedtime	12	0.002	Not reported
		Nitrofurantoin 100 mg at bedtime		0.003	
Brumfitt, et al[13] (open RCT) 1995	97	Cefaclor 250 mg at bedtime	12	0.006	Not reported
		Nitrofurantoin 50 mg at bedtime		0.006	

TMP-SMZ = trimethoprim-sulphamethoxazole.

TABLE 2   Postcoital regimens for recurrent urinary tract infections: results of RCTs (see text, p 1142).

Study	Total number of participants	Regimen	Duration of prophylaxis (months)	Infections per patient year	P value
Stapleton, et al[14] (placebo controlled RCT) 1990	27	Placebo	6	3.6	= 0.0001
		Postcoital TMP-SMZ (40 mg/20 mg)		0.3	
Pfau, et al[15] (open RCT) 1994	33	Without prophylaxis	14	6.13	= 0.0000
		Postcoital prophylaxis with either ofloxacin 100 mg, Norfloxacin 200 mg or ciprofloxacin 125 mg		0.02	
Melekos, et al[8] (open RCT) 1997	135	Without prophylaxis	12	3.62–3.66	< 0.0001
		Ciprofloxacin 125 mg daily		0.031	
		Ciprofloxacin 125 mg postcoital		0.043	
Pfau, et al[16] (open RCT) 1983	56	Without prophylaxis	12	4.6	< 0.001
		Postcoital prophylaxis with either TMP-SMZ 80 mg/400 mg		0	
		Nitrofurantoin 50–100 mg		0.1	

TMP-SMZ, trimethoprim-sulphamethoxazole.

Stress incontinence

Updated and expanded this issue

Jason Coop and Ash Monga

Women's health

INTERVENTIONS

Key Messages

- One RCT has found that postpartum pelvic floor muscle exercises reduce the risk of developing stress incontinence in the short term. The effect of antenatal exercises in preventing stress incontinence has not been assessed in good quality RCTs.

- One systematic review of RCTs has found that pelvic floor muscle exercises and electrical stimulation of the pelvic floor improve objective measures of stress incontinence.

- Meta-analysis of a systematic review of RCTs has found that biofeedback is associated with a higher cure rate compared with pelvic floor exercises. The difference was not quite significant.

- RCTs found no evidence of benefit from oestrogen in postmenopausal women.
- One RCT found no evidence of a difference between pelvic floor muscle exercises and α adrenergic agonists.
- RCTs comparing different surgical procedures found that colposuspension and slings were the most effective approach, both in the short and long term.
- We found limited evidence suggesting that endoscopic procedures are currently less effective than open procedures.

DEFINITION   Urinary incontinence is defined as involuntary loss of urine that is objectively demonstrable and is a social or hygienic problem.[1] There are two main types of urinary incontinence: stress incontinence (see glossary, p 1156) and detrusor instability (see glossary, p 1156), which together account for more than 80% of all cases of urinary incontinence. Urinary incontinence is eight times more common in women than in men. This review deals specifically with stress incontinence.

INCIDENCE/   Prevalence is increasing as the population ages. In 1990, the
PREVALENCE number of women in the UK suffering from urinary incontinence was estimated at 2.5 million (see table 1, p 1158).[2,3] A community based study in the USA found that the self reported, age adjusted prevalence of female urinary incontinence was 48% (95% CI 45% to 52%).[4] A questionnaire based study in Sweden estimated the prevalence of urinary incontinence to be 3% in women aged 20–29 years old, increasing to 32% in women > 80 years old.[5]

AETIOLOGY/   Stress incontinence is made more likely with some genetic alter-
RISK FACTORS ations in connective tissue, pregnancy and childbirth, menopause, aging, obesity, some races, chronic constipation, other causes of chronic raised intra-abdominal pressure, and pelvic surgery.[6] Psychological factors, bladder neck surgery, caffeine, and smoking may aggravate the condition. Other causes of urinary incontinence include urinary tract infection, immobility, loss of physical function and dexterity, dementia, and other conditions causing impaired mental state.

PROGNOSIS   Urinary incontinence affects physical, psychological, and social wellbeing, and impairs quality of life. We found no good studies of its natural history. Prognosis after treatment is probably better for stress incontinence than for most other forms of urinary incontinence.

AIMS   To improve or cure urinary incontinence, and to restore normal social functioning and confidence, with minimal adverse effects.

OUTCOMES   Objective demonstration of urinary loss by urodynamic investigation; subjective improvement in urinary loss; improvement in quality of life indicators; adverse effects of drug treatment; complications of surgical treatment.

METHODS   *Clinical Evidence* update search and appraisal May 2000.

OPTION   PELVIC FLOOR MUSCLE EXERCISES

We found no evidence of sufficient quality on the effectiveness of antenatal pelvic floor exercises in the prevention of postpartum stress incontinence. One RCT has found that postnatal pelvic floor exercises significantly reduce stress incontinence in the short term.

Benefits: We found no systematic review. **Antenatal pelvic floor exercises:** We found one RCT (72 primigravidas) which found pelvic floor exercise training starting at 20 weeks gestation versus routine care reduced urinary incontinence symptoms during late pregnancy and up to 6 months postpartum. The RCT had methodological problems (see comment below).[7] **Postnatal pelvic floor exercises:** We found one RCT published in abstract form, which compared instructed pelvic floor exercises plus bladder retraining versus routine postnatal exercises. Nearly 8000 women responded to a questionnaire survey 3 months after delivery. Of these, 749 who reported incontinence were randomised. At 12 months postpartum, the intervention group showed a significant reduction in stress incontinence (rates of stress incontinence 58% v 68%, P = 0.02).[8]

Harms: None reported.

Comment: The RCT of pelvic muscle exercises versus normal care[7] recruited 72 people but reported results for only 46 (63%) of them; dropouts were due to conceiving the second child within 1 year of the first birth (5 women), no data collection (eight women), and partial data collection (7 women). Overall, 13 of the 72 women had caesarean deliveries; more women had caesarean deliveries in the treatment group than in the control group. A subgroup analysis of 37 women who had vaginal delivery found no significant effect of training for pelvic floor exercises versus control treatment.

QUESTION   What are the effects of non-surgical treatments?

OPTION   PELVIC FLOOR MUSCLE EXERCISES

One systematic review and additional RCTs have found that pelvic floor muscle exercises reduce symptoms of stress incontinence, and that high intensity exercise is more effective than low intensity. RCTs have found that pelvic floor muscle exercises are more effective than electrical stimulation of the pelvic floor or vaginal cones. Meta-analysis of three RCTs found biofeedback to be significantly more effective than pelvic floor muscle exercises.

Benefits: We found one systematic review (search date 1997), which identi-fied 11 RCTs of conservative treatments for stress incontinence in women.[9] Included trials had at least 50 participants in each group, appropriate randomisation and blinding, less than 10% withdrawal rate, and relevant baseline and outcome measurements. **Versus no treatment:** The review identified two RCTs comparing pelvic floor muscle exercises versus no treatment. One found that women in the pelvic floor muscle exercise group were more likely to be dry or mildly incontinent than the no treatment group (61% v 3%). After 3 months, the mean weekly frequency of incontinent episodes fell from 17.3 to 4.8 in the treatment group, whereas in the controls it increased from 23.1 to 25.3. The second RCT found major decreases in frequency of incontinence episodes in the pelvic floor muscle exercise group, with no significant change in the control group (reduction in frequency 54% v 6%).[9] **High versus low intensity exercises:** The review identified one RCT comparing high and low intensity home based pelvic floor muscle exercise programmes and found a greater rate of "cure or almost cure" for high intensity exercise (60% v 17%). It also found improved social and urodynamic parameters.[9] **Plus intravaginal resistance devices or biofeedback:** The systematic review[9] identified three RCTs of sufficient quality comparing pelvic floor muscle exercises alone and in combination with an intravaginal resistance device (one RCT) or biofeedback (two RCTs). These found no significant difference in the frequency of incontinent episodes per week. **Versus biofeedback:** The systematic review identified five RCTs comparing biofeedback versus pelvic floor muscle exercises.[9] One trial found a significant difference in favour of biofeedback and four trials found no significant difference. Meta-analysis of the three trials with a common outcome measure (published separately) found no significant increase in the proportion of women cured after biofeedback (OR 2.1, 95% CI 0.99 to 4.4).[10] **Versus electrical stimulation or vaginal cones:** One RCT (107 women) compared pelvic floor muscle exercises versus electrical stimulation, vaginal cones, or no treatment.[11] It found no significant difference between electrical stimulation, resistance devices, and no treatment. However, pelvic floor muscle exercises versus other interventions or no treatment increased muscle strength and social activity index, and decreased leakage over 3 days (P < 0.01). Significantly more women reported being continent or almost continent in the exercise group than in other groups (control 1/30, exercise 12/25, electrical stimulation 3/25, cones 5/27; P < 0.001 for exercise compared with other groups). **Versus or combined with bladder training:** One RCT (145 women) compared pelvic floor muscle training versus bladder training or the two treatments combined.[12] Combined treatment was associated with greater satisfaction immediately after treatment began, but at 3 months, there were no significant differences between groups. Reduction of incontinence episodes by 50% or more was reported 59% with combination treatment, 56% with pelvic muscle exercises alone, and 41% with bladder training alone.

Harms: None reported.

Comment: The RCT that compared pelvic floor muscle training versus bladder training or the two treatments combined found that outcomes improved with increased contact between women in the trial and the intervention team.[12] The authors speculated that specific treatment may not be as important as having a structured intervention programme with education, counselling, and frequent patient contact.

Stress incontinence

OPTION **ELECTRICAL PELVIC FLOOR STIMULATION**

Two systematic reviews of RCTs have found conflicting evidence on the effects of electrical stimulation of the pelvic floor in women with stress incontinence. RCTs have found it to be less effective than pelvic floor muscle exercises.

Benefits: We found two systematic reviews. The first review (search date 1997) identified two RCTs of sufficient quality comparing electrical and sham stimulation of the pelvic floor in women with stress incontinence.[9] Electrical stimulation was associated with improvements in daily and weekly leakage episodes, pelvic floor muscle strength, and pad tests. In the first RCT (35 women), voiding diaries indicated a 50% or greater improvement in 48% of participants in the active group compared with 13% in the sham group. The second RCT, in 14 women, also compared active versus sham electrical stimulation, but all participants were also treated with pelvic floor muscle exercises. It found improvements in pelvic floor muscle strength and endurance and significantly reduced episodes of incontinence in the women receiving electrical stimulation. None of the women receiving electrical stimulation required further treatment, compared with a third of those receiving sham treatment. The second review (search date 1996) identified two additional RCTs and excluded the smaller of the two RCTs identified in the first review.[13] Neither of the two additional RCTs found significant benefit compared with controls. **Versus pelvic floor muscle exercises:** See pelvic floor muscle exercises, p 1150. **Versus pelvic floor muscle exercises plus biofeedback:** One RCT (70 people) compared electrical stimulation versus pelvic floor muscle exercises plus biofeedback. There was no significant difference in outcomes between groups.[14]

Harms: Adverse effects included vaginal irritation and infection, pain, and urinary tract infection.

Comment: There were considerable variations in the methods used for delivering the electrical stimulation. Further trials are needed that compare electrical stimulation alone versus no treatment, using adequate sample sizes and sufficiently long treatment periods.

OPTION **OESTROGEN SUPPLEMENTATION IN POSTMENOPAUSAL WOMEN**

RCTs have found no evidence that oestrogen supplementation improves stress incontinence. The combination of oestrogen plus an α adrenergic agonist may improve objective measures.

Benefits: **Oestrogen alone:** We found one systematic review (published in 1994, 6 RCTs: 1 vaginal oestrogen, 5 oral oestrogen), and 17 uncontrolled trials of oestrogen on the treatment of urinary incontinence in women.[15] It concluded that, although the uncontrolled trials (5 vaginal, 9 oral, 3 intramuscular oestrogen found there was subjective improvement in symptoms of incontinence, 3 RCTs (84 women with genuine stress incontinence) found no objective improvement assessed from various measures of urine loss. The two subsequent RCTs (135 postmenopausal women with genuine stress incontinence) found no significant difference between treated and placebo groups in the number of incontinent episodes at 3–6 months follow up.[16–17] **Combined with an α adrenergic agonist:** See benefits of α adrenergic agonists below.

Harms: Adverse effects of long term hormone replacement therapy include increased risk of breast cancer and thromboembolic disease.

Comment: The studies included clinically heterogeneous groups, and used a range of diagnostic criteria, therapeutic interventions, and outcome assessments.

OPTION α ADRENERGIC AGONISTS (PHENYLPROPANOLAMINE)

One RCT found no evidence of a difference in effectiveness between phenylpropanolamine and pelvic floor muscle exercises. Limited evidence suggests that combination of phenylpropanolamine with oestrogen in postmenopausal women improves objective measures of urinary incontinence more than oestrogen alone.

Benefits: **Versus placebo:** We found no RCTs. **Versus pelvic floor muscle exercises:** We found one systematic review,[9] which identified one RCT of sufficient quality. The RCT found no significant difference between pelvic floor muscle exercises and phenylpropanolamine (77% v 84% improvement from baseline). **Combined with oestrogen:** A non-systematic review of combined oestrogen and phenylpropanolamine (published in 1995) reviewed two trials of combination therapy in 84 postmenopausal women, and concluded that frequency and nocturia improved more with combined treatment than with oestrogen alone.[18] Levels of significance were not given in the review. Stress incontinence improved subjectively in all groups but objectively only in the combined group.

Harms: We found no evidence from RCTs.

Comment: Limited data are available, which limits generaliseability. A consensus view exists that α adrenergic agonists should be used with care or not at all in women with hypertension, hyperthyroidism, or coronary heart disease, or in those taking monoamine oxidase inhibitors.

OPTION OTHER CONSERVATIVE INTERVENTIONS

One RCT found that vaginal cones were less effective than pelvic floor muscle exercises but not significantly different compared with electrical stimulation of the pelvic floor or no treatment. We found insufficient evidence on the effects of regulation of fluid intake and weight loss in women with stress incontinence.

Benefits: **Vaginal cones versus pelvic floor muscle exercises or electrical stimulation:** See pelvic floor muscle exercises, p 1150. **Fluid intake and weight loss:** We found no systematic review or adequate RCTs.

Harms: Insufficient data.

Comment: None.

| QUESTION | How do the main surgical treatments for stress incontinence compare? |

| OPTION | COLPOSUSPENSION, ANTERIOR COLPORRHAPHY, NEEDLE SUSPENSION, SLINGS, AND IMPLANTABLE DEVICES |

From limited data, colposuspension seems to be the most successful surgical procedures for stress incontinence. We found limited and conflicting evidence that sling procedures (see glossary, p 1156) may have a similar cure rate as colposuspension. We found no evidence to support the use of anterior colporrhaphy or needle suspension. Newer treatments such as injectable devices and artificial slings (see glossary, p 1156) have not been adequately evaluated in RCTs. One RCT found that tension free vaginal tape had similar effectiveness as colposuspension at 6 months follow up. One small RCT found that the Marshall-Marchetti-Krantz urethropexy (see glossary, p 1156) compared with colposuspension increases the 1 year subjective cure rate. We found no good comparative data on the harms of different procedures.

Benefits: We found two systematic reviews of surgery for stress incontinence in women (first review published in 1996; 11 RCTs, 20 non-randomised trials/prospective cohort studies, and 45 retrospective cohort studies).[19] The second review will be appraised in the next issue.[20] **Colposuspension versus anterior colporrhaphy:** The review identified four RCTs and 11 non-randomised prospective studies. The studies were small and most were not able to exclude a clinically important effect. Overall, they found that colposuspension cured or improved stress incontinence after 1 year more than anterior colporrhaphy (see table 2, p 1158). The benefits of colposuspension were sustained for at least 5 years whereas those of anterior colporrhaphy seemed to diminish rapidly.[19] Three RCTs published since the review compared open colposuspension versus anterior colporrhaphy. One (35 woman) found significantly greater improvement 1 year after surgery with colposuspension than with colporrhaphy (16/18 v 5/16; RR 0.15, 95% CI 0.04 to 0.59).[21] The second RCT (81 women) found no difference at 2 months, but significantly greater cure rate with colposuspension at 3 years' follow up (88% v 57%; P < 0.001).[22] The third RCT (68 women) found that 14 years after surgery colposuspension versus anterior colporrhaphy improved both the objective cure rate (26/35 [74%] v 14/33 [42%]; OR 3.9, 95% CI 1.3 to 12.5) and the subjective cure rate (30/35 [86%] v 17/33 [52%]; OR 5.6, 95% CI 1.6 to 21.6).[23] **Colposuspension versus needle suspension:** The review identified three RCTs and 10 non-randomised studies comparing colposuspension versus needle suspension procedures.[19] Two RCTs and two non-randomised studies found a higher success rate with colposuspension, whereas one RCT and eight non-randomised studies found no significant difference. **Colposuspension versus slings:** The review[19] identified no RCTs and we found two subsequent small RCTs.[24,25] The first RCT found that colposuspension versus paravaginal repair increased the number of women with subjective cure at follow up of 1 to 3 years (18/18 [100%] v 13/18 [72%], P = 0.02).[24] The second RCT (36 women) found a similar cure rate 3 months after both colposuspension and suburethral sling.[25] **Colposuspension versus tension free vaginal tape:** One RCT (344 women) found that colposuspension versus tension free vaginal tape had no significant effect on subjective cure rates after 6 months (71% v 66%) or on objective cure rate (66% v 68%).[26] **Colposuspension versus Marshall-Marchetti-Krantz urethropexy:** One RCT in 30 women found that more were subjectively cured at 1 year after Marshall-Marchetti-Krantz urethropexy versus colposuspension (subjective cure rate 100% v 66%; P = 0.02).[27] **Anterior colporrhaphy versus needle suspension:** The review identified three RCTs and five non-randomised prospective studies, which found no difference in the effectiveness of anterior colporrhaphy and needle suspension procedures.[19] **Implantable devices and artificial sphincters:** We found no RCTs.

Harms: Reported complications of surgery include urinary retention, frequency, and urgency. However, we found no good data on the frequency of complications.

Comment: A review published in 1997 identified 282 articles with acceptable outcome data (as determined by an expert panel, rejection encompassing such points as being published only in abstract form, lack of original data, or inadequate follow up).[28] Combined data from the 282 included articles gave cure rates of 84% for retropubic suspensions, 65–79% for transvaginal suspensions, 61–85% for anterior repairs, and 82–83% for paravaginal sling procedures. The authors concluded that at 48 months' follow up, retropubic suspensions (colposuspension) and slings were more effective than anterior colporrhaphy or needle suspension. No differentiation was made between primary and secondary procedures. Studies suffered from lack of standardisation on definition, severity, and diagnosis of stress incontinence. Information on detrusor instability, prior surgery, quality of life measurements, surgical technique, length of follow up, and external validity were often not available. One cohort study of 259 women who underwent the Stamey endoscopic bladder neck suspension found a 6% success rate at 10 year follow up.

QUESTION **How do endoscopic and open colposuspension compare?**

We found limited evidence suggesting that open colposuspension procedures are currently superior to endoscopic colposuspension.

Benefits: We found one systematic review (search date 1996)[29] and one subsequent RCT.[30] The review identified one RCT (60 women), comparing open versus laparoscopic colposuspension. At both 1 year and in a follow up study at 3 years, open colposuspension was significantly more effective as judged by visual analogue scores and pad tests (P = 0.03).[31,32] The subsequent RCT (minimum follow up 1 year, 92 women) also found that open colposuspension was significantly more effective than laparoscopic. Based on objective outcome measures, success rate for the open procedure was 96% (95% CI 90% to 100%) compared with 80% (95% CI 69% to 92%) for laparoscopic.[30]

Harms: The review also identified four non-randomised comparisons and 10 case series.[29] Rates of postoperative complication in these studies were low. Other studies have reported postoperative complications including bladder injuries, postoperative urinary retention, haematuria, urinary tract infection, ureteric injury, and detrusor instability.[33] We also found two reported cases of transmural bladder sutures.[34] The subsequent RCT found that rates of postoperative complication were higher with open than with laparoscopic colposuspension.[30]

Comment: None.

GLOSSARY

Detrusor instability Diagnosed when the detrusor muscle contracts, spontaneously or on provocation, during the filling phase, while the woman is attempting to inhibit micturition.[1]

Stress incontinence Diagnosed when, in the absence of a detrusor contraction, the pressure inside the bladder exceeds the pressure in the urethra.

Sling procedure Typically a piece of fascia placed under the bladder neck and then secured to either bone, abdominal wall, or ligament. This sling then support the urethra where it connects to the bladder and may restore the valve mechanism at the bladder neck. It is performed through the vagina or the abdomen.

Artificial sling There are many different types of sling procedure that differ in the type of material, sutures, and points of anchoring. Many artificial materials have been used in the construction of slings (e.g. polyester, polytetrafluoroethylene [Gore-Tex]).

Marshall-Marchetti-Krantz urethropexy A surgical procedure through an incision in the lower abdomen in which the bladder neck and urethra are elevated by suturing tissues around the urethra and bladder to the periosteum on the rear of the symphysis pubis. The aim is to create a valve mechanism at the bladder neck. The procedure has been modified in various ways (e.g. Burch colposuspension, Stamey urethropexy, Pereyra procedure, paravaginal repair).

Substantive changes since last issue

Antenatal pelvic floor exercises One new RCT; conclusion unchanged.[7]

Colposuspension versus anterior colporrhaphy One new RCT; conclusion unchanged.[23]

Colposuspension versus slings One new RCT; conclusion unchanged.[25]

Colposuspension versus tension free vaginal tape One new RCT; conclusion unchanged. Found no difference in subjective or objective cure rate after 6 months.[25]

Colposuspension versus Marshall-Marchetti-Krantz Urethropexy New subheading. One new RCT found that more women were subjectively cured at 1 year after urethrotherapy versus colposuspension.[27]

REFERENCES

1. Abrams P, Blaivas JG, Stanton SL, et al. Standardisation of terminology of lower urinary tract function. *Scand J Urol Nephrol* 1988; 114(suppl):5–19.
2. MORI Health Survey Questionnaire 1990. London: Market and Opinion Research International (MORI).
3. Royal College of Physicians. *Incontinence: causes, management and provision of services. Report of a working party.* London: Royal College of Physicians, 1995.
4. Roberts RO, Jacobsen SA, Reilly WT, et al. Prevalence of combined fecal and urinary incontinence: A community–based study. *J Am Geriatr Soc* 1999;47:837–841.
5. Simeonova Z, Milsom I, Kullendorff A-E, et al. The prevalence of urinary incontinence and its influence on the quality of life in women from an urban Swedish population. *Acta Obstet Gynecol Scand* 1999;78:546–551.
6. Handa VL, Harris TA, Ostergard DR. Protecting the pelvic floor: obstetric management to prevent incontinence and pelvic organ prolapse. *Obstet Gynecol* 1996;88:470–478.
7. Sampselle CM, Miller JM, Mims BL, et al. Effect on pelvic muscle exercise on transient incontinence during pregnancy and after birth. *Obstet Gynecol* 1998;91:406–412.
8. Gladzener CMA, Lang G, Wilson PD, et al. Postnatal incontinence: a multicentre randomised controlled trial of conservative treatment. *Br J Obstet Gynaecol* 1998;105(suppl 117):47.

9. Berghmans LCM, Hendriks HJM, Bo K, et al. Conservative treatment of stress urinary incontinence in women: a systematic review of randomised controlled trials. *Br J Urol* 1998;82: 181–191. Search date 1997; primary sources Medline, Excerpta Medica, Cochrane Field in Therapies and Rehabilitation database, Dutch National Institute of Allied Professions database.

10. Weatherall M. Biofeedback or pelvic floor muscle exercises for female genuine stress incontinence: a meta-analysis of trials identified in a systematic review. *BJU Int* 1999;83:1015–1016.

11. Bo K, Talseth T, Holme I. Single blind randomised controlled trial of pelvic floor exercises, electronical stimulation, vaginal cones, and no treatment in management of genuine stress incontinence. *BMJ* 1999;318:487–493.

12. Wyman JF, Fantl JA, McClish DK, et al. Comparative efficacy of behavioural interventions in the management of female urinary incontinence. *Am J Obstet Gynecol* 1998;179: 999–1007.

13. Bo K, Effect of electronic stimulation on stress and urge incontinence. *Acta Obstet Gynaecol Scand* 1998;77(suppl 168):3–11. Search date 1996; primary source Medline and hand searches of relevant journals.

14. Knight S, Laycock J, Naylor D. Evaluation of neuromuscular electronical stimulation in the treatment of genuine stress incontinence. *Physiotherapy* 1998;84:61–71.

15. Fantl JA, Cardozo LD, Ekberg J, et al. Estrogen therapy in the management of urinary incontinence in post-menopausal women: a meta-analysis. *Obstet Gynecol* 1994;83:12–18. Search date 1992; primary sources English language articles found in Excerpta Medica, Biosis and Medline.

16. Fantl JA, Bump RC, Robinson D, et al. and the Continence Program for Women Research Group. Efficacy of oestrogen supplementation in the treatment of urinary incontinence. *Obstet Gynecol* 1996;88:745–749.

17. Jackson S, Shepherd A, Brookes S, et al. The effect of oestrogen supplementation on post-menopausal urinary stress incontinence: A double blind placebo controlled trial. *Br J Obstet Gynaecol* 1999; 106:711–718.

18. Cardozo LD, Kelleher CJ. Sex hormones, the menopause and urinary problems. *Gynecol Endocrinol* 1995;9:75–84.

19. Black NA, Downs SH. The effectiveness of surgery for stress incontinence in women: a systematic review. *Br J Urol* 1996;78:497–510. Search dates and primary sources: English and non-English articles found in Medline (1966 to June 1995), Embase (1980 to June 1995), Science Citation Index (1980 to June 1995), British Library Information Index (1995), together with information from experts.

20. Anterior vaginal repair for unrinary incontinence in women. In: The Cochrane Library. Issue 1, 2000. Oxford: Update software. Search date 1999; primary sources Cochrane Incontinence Group's trials register and reference lists of relevant articles.

21. Kammerer-Doak DN, Dorin MH, Rogers RG, et al. A randomised trial of Burch retropubic urethropexy and anterior colporrhaphy for stress urinary incontinence. *Obstet Gynecol* 1999;93:75–78.

22. Liapis A, Pyrgiotis E, Kontoravdis A, et al. Genuine stress incontinence: prospective randomised comparison of two operative methods. *Eur J Obstet Gynaecol Reprod Biol* 1996;64:69–72.

23. Colombo M, Vitobello D, Proietti F, et al. Randomized comparison of Burch colposuspension versus anterior colporrhaphy in women with stress urinary incontinence and anterior vaginal wall prolapse. *Br J Obstet Gynaecol* 2000;107:544–551.

24. Colombo M, Milani R, Vitobello P, et al. A randomised comparison of Burch colposuspension and abdominal paravaginal defect repair for female stress urinary incontinence. *Am J Obstet Gynecol* 1996;175:78–84.

25. Sand PK, Winkler H, Blackhurst DW, et al. A prospective randomized study comparing modified Burch retropubic urethropexy and suburethral sling for treatment of genuine stress incontinence. *Am J Obstet Gynecol* 2000;182:30–34.

26. Ward KL, Hilton P, Browning J. A randomised trial of colposuspension and tension free vaginal tape for primary genuine stress incontinence (abstract) Neurourol Urodynam 2000;19:386–388.

27. Quadri G, Magatti F, Belloni C, et al. Marshall-Marchetti-Krantz urethropexy and Burch colposuspension for stress urinary incontinence in women with low pressure and hypermobility of the urethra: early results of a prospective randomized clinical trial. *Am J Obstet Gynecol* 1999; 181:12–18.

28. Leach GE, Dmochowski RR, Appell RA, et al. Female stress urinary incontinence clinical guidelines panel summary report on surgical management of female stress urinary incontinence. *J Urol* 1997;158:875–880.

29. Lose G. Laparoscopic Burch colposuspension. *Acta Obstet Gynaecol Scand* 1998;88(suppl 168):29–33. Search date 1991–1996, primary sources Medline search of English language articles, and search of references cited in all identified studies.

30. Su T-H, Wang D-G, Hsu C-Y, et al. Prospective comparison of laparoscopic and traditional colposuspensions in the treatment of genuine stress incontinence. *Acta Obstet Gynecol Scand* 1997;76:576–582.

31. Burton GA. A randomised comparison of laparoscopic and open colposuspension. *Neurol Urodyn* 1994;88:29–33.

32. Burton G. A three year prospective randomised urodynamic study comparing open and laparoscopic colposuspension. Neurourol Urodyn 1997;16:353–354.

33. Aslan P, Woo HH. Ureteric injury following laparoscopic colposuspension. *Br J Obstet Gynecol* 1997;104:266–68.

34. Flax S. The gasless laparoscopic Burch bladderneck suspension; early experience. *J Urol* 1996;156:1105–1107.

Jason Cooper
Consultant Gynaecologist
City General Hospital
Stoke on Trent
UK

Ash Monga
Consultant Urogynaecologist
Princess Anne Hospital
Southampton
UK

Competing interests: None declared.

TABLE 1	Proportion of women in the UK of different ages and in different settings suffering urinary incontinence (see text, p 1149).[3]

Women living at home	%
15–44 years	5–7
45–64 years	8–15
> 65 years	10–20
Institutionalised women	
Residential homes	25
Nursing homes	40
Hospitals: long stay care	50–70

TABLE 2	Results of RCTs in the systematic review comparing colposuspension versus anterior colporrhaphy and needle suspension (see text, p 1154).[19]

Study	Follow up (years)	Anterior colporrhaphy		Colposuspension	
		cured	total (%)	cured	total (%)
34	1	88/101	87	70/99	70
35	1	5/19	25	0/15	0
36	1	34/38	89	23/35	65
37	5	27/33	82	11/30	37

Study	Follow up (years)	Anterior colporrhaphy		Needle suspension	
		cured	total (%)	cured	total (%)
34	1	88/101	87	66/98	67
35	1–3.7	17/24	71	15/26	58
37	5	27/33	82	13/30	43

*In some cases the numbers of people cured has been calculated from the information provided in the papers.

Updated this issue

Nicky Cullum, E Andrea Nelson and Jane Nixon

QUESTIONS

Effects of preventive interventions. 1161
Effects of treatments 1163

INTERVENTIONS

PREVENTION

Beneficial
Foam alternatives (compared with
  standard foam mattresses) .1161
Pressure relieving overlays on
  operating tables. 1161

Likely to be beneficial
Low air loss beds in intensive care
  (compared with standard
  beds) 1161

Unknown effectiveness
Relative effectiveness of different
  seat cushions 1161
Constant low pressure
  supports 1161
Alternating pressure surfaces .1161
Low air loss hydrotherapy
  beds. 1161
Repositioning 1162
Sheepskin 1162
Topical lotions and dressings .1162

Likely to be ineffective or harmful
Air filled vinyl boots with foot
  cradle. 1162

TREATMENT

Likely to be beneficial
Low air loss beds 1163

Beneficial
Air fluidised supports (compared
  with standard care) 1163

Unknown effectiveness
Seat cushions. 1163
Hydrocolloid dressings (compared
  with gauze soaked in saline or
  hypochlorite) 1163
Debridement 1163
Surgery 1163
Nutritional supplements. 1163
Electrotherapy. 1163
Ultrasound 1163
Becaplermin (recombinant human
  platelet derived growth factor
  (rh-PDGF BB) 1163
Low level laser therapy New .1163

See glossary, p 1165

Key Messages

Prevention

- One systematic review of RCTs has found that foam alternatives to the standard hospital foam mattress reduce the incidence of pressure sores in people at high risk.

- The relative merits of alternating and constant low pressure, and of the different alternating pressure devices, are unclear.

- One systematic review of RCTs has found that pressure relieving overlays on operating tables reduce the incidence of pressure sores.

- We found insufficient evidence on the effects of seat cushions, constant low pressure devices, regular repositioning ("turning"), sheepskins, topical lotions, or dressings.

- One RCT found that air filled vinyl boots with foot cradles were associated with more rapid development of pressure sores.

Treatment

- Systematic reviews of RCTs have found that air fluidised support and low air loss beds may improve healing rates.
- We found insufficient evidence on the effects of other types of beds and mattresses, seat cushions, becaplermin, dressings, debridement, surgery, nutritional supplementation, electrotherapy, ultrasound, or low level laser therapy on healing rates of pressure sores.

DEFINITION	Pressure sores (also known as pressure ulcers, bed sores, and decubitus ulcers) may present as persistently hyperaemic, blistered, broken, or necrotic skin, and may extend to underlying structures, including muscle and bone. Whether blanching and non-blanching erythema constitute pressure sores remains controversial.
INCIDENCE/ PREVALENCE	The most comprehensive data on prevalence and incidence come from hospital populations. Studies have found prevalences of 6.6–10.1% in NHS hospitals in the UK[1] and 8.7% in a teaching hospital in the USA.[2]
AETIOLOGY/ RISK FACTORS	Pressure sores are caused by unrelieved pressure, shear, or friction, and are most common below the waist and at bony prominences such as the sacrum, heels, and hips. They occur in all healthcare settings. Increased age, reduced mobility, and impaired nutrition emerge consistently as risk factors. However, the relative importance of these and other factors is uncertain.[3]
PROGNOSIS	The presence of pressure sores has been associated with a two- to fourfold increased risk of death in elderly people in intensive care.[4,5] However, pressure sores are a marker for underlying disease severity and other comorbidities rather than an independent predictor of mortality.[4] Pressure sores vary considerably in size and severity.
AIMS	To prevent pressure sore formation, to heal existing pressure sores, to improve quality of life.
OUTCOMES	Incidence and severity of pressure sores, rate of change of area and volume, and time to heal. Interface pressure recorded at various anatomical sites is a surrogate outcome sometimes used in studies of preventive interventions; it has not yet been linked to clinical outcomes.
METHODS	We searched the Specialist Trials Register of the Cochrane Wounds Group in June 2000. The register is compiled by searching 19 electronic databases, including Medline (1966 to December 1999), Cinahl, BIDS, and Embase, and hand searching journals and conference proceedings. We reviewed all RCTs that used objective clinical outcome measures. For many trials, we could not be sure that pressure sore size was evenly distributed between groups at baseline. Unequal distribution of wound size at baseline will impact on all measures of wound healing. Ideally, studies of treatment should stratify randomisation by initial wound area and be of sufficient size to ensure even distribution of baseline wound size. Many of the studies performed by manufacturers were in

healthy people who are not representative of clinical subjects, and these studies have been excluded.

QUESTION   **What are the effects of preventive interventions?**

OPTION   PRESSURE RELIEVING SURFACES

One systematic review of RCTs has found that foam alternatives to the standard hospital foam mattress reduce the incidence of pressure sores in people at high risk. There is no obvious "best" foam alternative. The relative merits of alternating and constant low pressure, and of the different devices used in alternating pressure therapy, are unclear. We found insufficient evidence on the effects of seat cushions and low tech constant low pressure supports. The systematic review has found that the use of pressure relieving overlays on operating tables reduces the incidence of pressure sores.

Benefits: We found one systematic review (search date February 1999)[6] and three subsequent RCTs.[7–9] **Foam alternatives versus standard hospital mattress:** The systematic review identified four RCTs.[6] The RCTs found that using various foam alternatives to the standard hospital mattress reduced the risk of sores (RRR 71%, 95% CI 57% to 81%; NNT for 10–14 days treatment to prevent one additional sore 4, 95% CI 3 to 6). **Different foam alternatives:** The systematic review identified four RCTs comparing different foam alternatives.[6] One reported a reduction in the risk of pressure sores associated with using a five section foam and fibre replacement compared with a 4 inch (10 cm) thick dimpled foam overlay (RRR 58%, 95% CI 10% to 82%; NNT for 10–21 days treatment 3, 95% CI 2 to 25). The other studies were too small to distinguish between the foam alternatives. **Cushions:** The systematic review identified two RCTs in 194 people comparing different types of seat cushion for preventing pressure sores.[6] They found no significant difference. **Low tech constant low pressure supports:** See glossary, p 1165. The systematic review identified eight RCTs.[6] Most were too small or flawed to allow conclusions. **Low air loss beds:** See glossary, p 1165. The systematic review identified one RCT in 98 people in intensive care (ICU), and one more has subsequently been published.[6,9] The ICU trial found a reduction in the risk of developing a new sore on low air loss beds compared with a standard intensive care unit bed (RRR 76%, 95% CI 45% to 91%; NNT 3, 95% CI 2 to 5).[6] The second trial in incontinent people admitted to acute and long stay hospital wards found a non-significant increased risk of developing a sore in the low air loss hydrotherapy bed (RRI 167%, 95% CI –8.7% to +690%) compared with a range of support surfaces.[9] **Alternating pressure therapy:** See glossary, p 1165. The systematic review identified eight comparisons of standard foam or constant low pressure with alternating pressure devices in the prevention of pressure sores,[6] and one has been published subsequently.[8] Most studies were too small to rule out a clinically important difference. One trial reported a significant reduction in the incidence of pressure sores in people on an alternating pressure device versus a standard foam mattress (RRR 68%, 95% CI 28% to 86%; NNT for 10 days treatment 11, 95% CI

6 to 34). Another trial compared a range of constant low pressure supports with a range of alternating pressure devices and reported that the incidence of pressure sores was significantly reduced with alternating pressure. The other seven comparisons found no significant difference between alternating pressure devices and constant low pressure supports. The relative merits of the different alternating pressure devices are unclear. **Pressure relieving overlays on the operating table:** The systematic review identified three RCTs.[6] The first compared a viscoelastic polymer pad versus a standard table in people undergoing elective major general, gynaecological, or vascular surgery. It found a significant reduction in the incidence of postoperative pressure sores with the polymer pad (RRR 48%, 95% CI 17% to 68%; NNT 11, 95% CI 6 to 36). The other two RCTs compared an alternating system used both during and after surgery versus a gel pad during surgery and a standard mattress after surgery for 7 days. Meta-analysis of these two trials gave a significant reduction in the incidence of pressure sores with the alternating system (RRR 80%, 95% CI 35% to 94%; NNT 16, 95% CI 9 to 48).

Harms: Hypothermia has been reported in a small number of people using low air loss hydrotherapy beds.[9]

Comment: Studies have tended to be small, of poor quality, and few comparisons have been undertaken more than once. Foam alternatives use foam of varying densities, often within the same mattress, and are sometimes sculptured.

| OPTION | OTHER PREVENTIVE INTERVENTIONS |

We found no good evidence that regular repositioning ("turning"), sheepskins, topical lotions, or dressings are effective. This may, however, represent a lack of evidence rather than a lack of benefit from these interventions. One RCT found that air filled vinyl boots with foot cradles were associated with more rapid development of pressure sores.

Benefits: We found one systematic review (search date February 1999)[10] and one subsequent RCT.[7] **Repositioning/turning:** The systematic review identified three RCTs of regular manual repositioning.[10] These were small and found no significant difference between experimental and control groups. We found no RCTs that evaluated the impact of positioning patients in different ways. **Sheepskin:** The systematic review identified one small trial of sheepskin overlays.[10] This was inconclusive and of poor quality. **Topical lotions and dressings:** We found one RCT, which compared a lotion containing hexachlorophene versus one containing cetrimide in 120 participants and found no significant difference in skin condition.[11] **Air filled vinyl boot with foot cradle:** We identified one small RCT comparing hospital pillows versus a vinyl, air filled boot with a built in foot cradle for the prevention of heel pressure sores in hospitalised people.[7] Sores developed significantly more quickly in the people wearing the boot (mean time to skin breakdown 10 days v 13 days; P < 0.036 log rank test).

Harms: We found no direct or indirect evidence of harm arising from repositioning, sheepskins, topical applications, or dressings.

Comment: The RCTs were small, of poor quality, and few comparisons have been undertaken more than once.

OPTION PRESSURE RELIEVING SURFACES

One systematic review of RCTs has found that air fluidised supports improve healing rates. We found insufficient evidence on the effects of seat cushions or other types of bed or mattress.

Benefits: We found one systematic review (search date February 1999)[6] and two further RCTs.[12,13] **Constant low pressure supports:** See glossary, p 1165. One trial found no difference in healing rates between a layered foam replacement mattress and a water mattress in elderly people in a nursing home who had existing pressure sores.[12] **Air fluidised support:** See glossary, p 1165. The systematic review identified four RCTs comparing air fluidised support versus standard care.[6] In two trials of people in hospital, standard care involved use of pressure relieving surfaces such as alternating pressure mattresses, regular changes of position, sheepskin or gel pads, and limb protectors. Both trials found that air fluidised support was more effective in healing established sores. A third RCT in 97 people being cared for at home found no significant difference. However, this trial had a high withdrawal rate. The fourth RCT was small and involved people who had undergone plastic surgery to repair pressure sores. It found no significant difference between air fluidised support and dry flotation. **Low air loss beds:** See glossary, p 1165. The systematic review identified one RCT comparing low air loss with foam beds and one has been identified subsequently.[6,13] There was no significant difference in the number of sores healed in these trials. We found no RCTs comparing low air loss beds versus alternating pressure or air fluidised supports. **Seat cushions:** The systematic review identified one RCT in 25 people.[6] This found no significant difference between seat cushions using dry flotation compared with alternating pressure.

Harms: Hypothermia has been reported in a small number of people using low air loss hydrotherapy beds.[9]

Comment: **Air fluidised support:** People are unable to move into and out of bed independently while using an air fluidised bed, and this limits the type of people for whom it is suitable. Air fluidised support has been evaluated in a range of settings, including surgical and medical wards and home care. Thus, the evidence could be viewed as generally applicable to people with pressure sores. The trials were of varying quality. **Low air loss beds:** These have been evaluated in a range of acute and elderly care settings.

OPTION OTHER TREATMENTS

Evidence on the effects of dressings is unclear. A meta-analysis of trials comparing hydrocolloids and gauze dressings found no significant difference. We found no good evidence on the effects of other types of

dressings, debridement, surgery, nutritional supplementation, electrotherapy, therapeutic ultrasound, or low level laser therapy on healing rates of pressure sores.

Benefits: **Hydrocolloid and gauze dressings:** We found one systematic review (28 RCTs)[14] and one subsequent RCT.[15] Most trials were small, of poor quality, and did not find significant results. Both the meta-analysis within the review and the subsequent RCT found a significant effect. However, a subsequent meta-analysis (personal communication from the authors) using preferred statistical techniques found no significant difference (RR 1.63, 95% CI 0.97 to 2.75).[15-20] The wide confidence intervals only just crossing the line of no effect suggests this may represent a lack of evidence of benefit rather than evidence of no benefit. **Other dressings:** Twelve of the RCTs identified in the systematic review compared hydrocolloid versus other dressings, 11 trials compared other dressing types such as foam and alginate, and two (one using hydrocolloid versus saline-gauze dressings and the other using becaplermin gel versus placebo) have been published subsequently.[21,22] All were too small and most were too flawed to allow conclusions to be drawn. **Debridement:** One systematic review (search date October 1998) found no RCTs comparing debridement versus no debridement.[23] It identified 32 RCTs comparing different debriding agents, but these were small, included a range of wounds, and few comparisons were undertaken more than once. The authors concluded that there was insufficient evidence to promote the use of any particular debriding agent over another. **Surgery:** We found no RCTs evaluating surgical treatments for pressure sores. **Nutritional supplements:** We found two RCTs of ascorbic acid supplementation for healing pressure sores. One small trial in people undergoing surgery who had pressure sores found that ascorbic acid supplementation (500 mg twice daily versus placebo) improved healing rates.[24] A larger trial (n = 88) found no significant difference in healing rates between those receiving ascorbic acid 500 mg twice daily and those receiving 10 mg twice daily.[25] We found no RCTs of the effects of parenteral nutrition or hyperalimentation on wound healing. **Electrotherapy:** See glossary, p 1165. We found four RCTs comparing electrotherapy versus sham treatment.[26-29] The trials were of varying quality. Overall, they suggested that electrotherapy improved healing of pressure sores, but confirmatory studies are needed. **Ultrasound:** We found three RCTs comparing ultrasound versus sham or standard treatment.[30-32] All found no difference, but they were too small to rule out a beneficial effect. **Low level laser therapy:** We found one systematic review (search date 1998, 1 RCT, n = 18) of low level laser therapy in pressure sores. It found no evidence of benefit in this trial.[33]

Harms: We found no reports of harms with these treatments.

Comment: Overall, the evidence relating to these treatments is poor.

GLOSSARY

Air fluidised support A membrane covering a layer of particles, which are fluidised by having air forced through them. The air flow can be turned off, making the surface solid again, to allow the person to be moved. It is difficult for people to get in and out of these beds independently; therefore they are usually reserved for people who spend most of the day in bed.

Alternating pressure therapy Mattresses or overlays made of one or two layers of parallel air sacs. Alternate sacs are inflated and deflated, providing alternating pressure and then release for each area of skin.

Constant low pressure supports Mattresses, overlays, and cushions made of high density or contoured foam, or filled with fibre, gel, water, beads, or air. They increase the area of contact between the person and the support surface and therefore reduce the interface pressure.

Electrotherapy The application of electrical fields by placing electrodes near a wound. Treatments include pulsed electromagnetic therapy, low intensity direct current, negative polarity and positive polarity electrotherapy, and alternating polarity electrotherapy.

Therapeutic ultrasound The application of ultrasound to a wound, using a transducer and a water based gel. The power of ultrasound waves used in wound healing is low in order to avoid heating the tissues.

Low air loss beds A mattress comprising inflatable upright sacs made of semi-permeable fabric. Inflating the sacs increases the area of contact between the individual and the support surface and reduces the pressure on the skin. It is difficult for people to get in and out of these beds independently; therefore they are usually reserved for people who spend most of the day in bed.

Substantive changes since last issue

Low level laser therapy One systematic review found no evidence of benefit.[33]

REFERENCES

1. O'Dea K. Prevalence of pressure damage in hospital patients in the UK. *J Wound Care* 1993; 2:221–225.
2. Granick MS, Solomon MP, Wind S, Goldberg M. Wound management and wound care. *Adv Plastic Reconstruct Surg* 1996;12:99–121.
3. Allman RM. Pressure ulcer prevalence, incidence, risk factors, and impact. *Clin Geriatr Med* 1997; 13:421–436.
4. Thomas DR, Goode PS, Tarquine PH, Allman RM. Hospital acquired pressure ulcers and risk of death. *J Am Geriatr Soc* 1996;44:1435–1440.
5. Clough NP. The cost of pressure area management in an intensive care unit. *J Wound Care* 1994;3: 33–35.
6. Cullum N, Deeks J, Sheldon TA, Song F, Fletcher AW. Beds, mattresses and cushions for pressure sore prevention and treatment. In: The Cochrane Library, Issue 4, 1999. Oxford. Update Software. Primary sources Medline (1966 to February 1999); Cinahl (to February 1999).
7. Tymec AC, Pieper B, Vollman K. A comparison of two pressure relieving devices in the prevention of heel pressure ulcers. *Adv Wound Care* 1997;10: 39–44.
8. Price P, Bale S, Newcombe R, Harding K. Challenging the pressure sore paradigm. *J Wound Care* 1999;8:187–190.
9. Bennett RG, Baran PJ, DeVone L, et al. Low airloss hydrotherapy versus standard care for incontinent hospitalized patients. *J Am Geriatr Soc* 1998;46:569–576.
10. Cullum N, Deeks JJ, Fletcher AW, Sheldon TA, Song F. Preventing and treating pressure sores. *Qual Health Care* 1995;4:289–297. Primary

sources Medline (1966 to February 1999); Cinahl (February 1995); hand searching of five journals.
11. Van der Cammen TJ, O'Callaghan U, Whitefield M. Prevention of pressure sores. A comparison of new and old pressure sore treatments. *Br J Clin Pract* 1987;41:1009–1011.
12. Groen HW, Groenier KH, Schuling J. Comparative study of a foam mattress and a water mattress. *J Wound Care* 1999;8:333–335.
13. Mulder GD, Taro N, Seeley JE, Andrews K. A study of pressure sore response to low air loss beds versus conventional treatment. *J Geriatr Dermatol* 1994;2:87–91.
14. Bradley M, Cullum N, Nelson EA, Petticrew M, Sheldon T, Torgerson D. Systematic reviews of wound care management: (2) Dressings and topical agents used in the healing of chronic wounds. *Health Technol Assess* 1999;3(17 pt 2) Search date 1997; primary source Medline.
15. Matzen S, Peschardt A, Alsbjørn B. A new amorphous hydrocolloid for the treatment of pressure sores: a randomised controlled study. *Scand J Plast ReconstrSurg Hand Surg* 1999;33: 13–15.
16. Barrois B. Comparison of Granuflex and medicated paraffin gauze in pressure sores. *Proceedings of the 2nd European Conference on Advances in Wound Management*. London: Macmillan, 1993: 209.
17. Alm A, Hornmark AM, Fall PA, et al. Care of pressure sores: a controlled study of the use of a hydrocolloid dressing compared with wet saline gauze compresses. *Acta Derm Venereol Suppl (Stockh)* 1989;149:1–10.
18. Colwell JC, Foreman MD, Trotter JP. A comparison

of the efficacy and cost-effectiveness of two methods of managing pressure ulcers. *Decubitus* 1993;6:28–36.

19. Xakellis GC, Chrischilles EA. Hydrocolloid versus saline-gauze dressings in treating pressure ulcers: a cost-effectiveness analysis. *Arch Phys Med Rehabil* 1992;73:463–469.

20. Gorse GJ, Messner RL. Improved pressure sore healing with hydrocolloid dressings. *Arch Dermatol* 1987;123:766–771.

21. Thomas DR, Goode PS, LaMaster K, Tennyson T. Acemann hydrogel dressing versus saline dressing for pressure ulcers. A randomized, controlled trial. *Adv Wound Care* 1998;11:273–276.

22. Rees RS, Robson MC, Smiell JM, et al. Becaplermin gel in the treatment of pressure ulcers: a phase II randomized, double-blind, placebo controlled study. *Wound Repair Regen* 1999;7:141–147.

23. Bradley M, Cullum N, Sheldon T. The debridement of chronic wounds: a systematic review. *Health Technol Assess* 1999;3(17 pt 1). Search undertaken of 19 electronic databases, including Medline and Embase up until June 1998.

24. Taylor TV, Rimmer S, Day B, Butcher J, Dymock IW. Ascorbic acid supplementation in the treatment of pressure sores. *Lancet* 1974;2:544–546.

25. Ter Riet G, Kessels AG, Knipschild PG. Randomized clinical trial of ascorbic acid in the treatment of pressure ulcers. *J Clin Epidemiol* 1995;48:1453–1460.

26. Salzberg CA, Cooper Vastola SA, Perez F, Viehbeck MG, Byrne DW. The effects of non-thermal pulsed electromagnetic energy on wound healing of pressure ulcers in spinal cord-injured patients: a randomized, double-blind study. *Ostomy Wound Manage* 1995;41:42–48.

27. Wood JM, Evans PE 3rd, Schallreuter KU, et al. A multicenter study on the use of pulsed low-intensity direct current for healing chronic stage II and stage III decubitus ulcers. *Arch Dermatol* 1993;129:999–1009.

28. El-Zeky F. Efficacy of high voltage pulsed current for healing of pressure ulcers in patients with spinal cord injury. *Phys Ther* 1991;71:433–442.

29. Kloth LC, Feedar JA. Acceleration of wound healing with high voltage, monophasic, pulsed current. *Phys Ther* 1988;68:503–508.

30. McDiarmid T. Ultrasound in the treatment of pressure sores. *Physiotherapy* 1985;February:66–70.

31. Ter Riet G, Kessels AG, Knipschild P. Randomised clinical trial of ultrasound treatment for pressure ulcers. *BMJ* 1995;310:1040–1041.

32. Nussbaum EL, Biemann I, Mustard B. Comparison of ultrasound/ultraviolet-C and laser for treatment of pressure ulcers in patients with spinal cord injury. *Phys Ther* 1994;74:812–823.

33. Lucas C, Stanborough RW, Freeman CL, De Haan RJ. Efficacy of low level laser therapy on wound healing in human subjects. A systematic review. *Lasers Med Sci* 2000; 15:84–93.

Nicky Cullum
Reader

E Andrea Nelson
Research Fellow

Centre for Evidence Based Nursing
Department of Health Studies
University of York
York
UK

Jane Nixon
Research Fellow
Centre for Evidence Based Nursing
Department of Health Studies
University of York
York
UK

Competing interests: EAN has been reimbursed for attending symposia by Smith and Nephew, Huntleigh Healthcare Ltd, and Convatec. JN has received lecture fees and expenses from Central Medical Supplies, UK, Huntleigh Healthcare Ltd, and Hill Rom.

INTERVENTIONS

Key Messages

- RCTs have found that compression heals venous leg ulcers more effectively than no compression and that oral oxpentifylline increases the proportion of ulcers that heal completely.

- One systematic review found that, in the presence of compression, hydrocolloid dressings do not heal venous leg ulcers more effectively than simple, non-adherent dressings.

- We found insufficient evidence to determine whether any particular occlusive or non-occlusive dressing increases healing or reduces the pain of venous leg ulcers.

- Limited evidence suggests that human skin equivalent or peri-ulcer injection of granulocyte–macrophage colony stimulating factor may accelerate healing.

- Limited evidence suggests that flavonoids may accelerate healing, but we found no evidence that either stanozolol or rutoside decrease recurrence rates.

- We found no good evidence on the effects of aspirin, intermittent pneumatic compression, oral zinc supplements, ultrasound, low level laser therapy, skin grafting, or vein surgery.

- We found limited evidence that compression prevents recurrence of venous leg ulcers.

DEFINITION	Definitions of leg ulcers vary, but the following is widely used: loss of skin on the leg or foot that takes more than 6 weeks to heal. Some definitions exclude ulcers confined to the foot, whereas others include ulcers on the whole of the lower limb. This review deals with ulcers of venous origin in people without concurrent diabetes mellitus, arterial insufficiency, or rheumatoid arthritis.
INCIDENCE/ PREVALENCE	Between 1.5 and 3 people per 1000 have active leg ulcers. Prevalence increases with age to around 20 per 1000 in people aged over 80 years.[1]
AETIOLOGY/ RISK FACTORS	Leg ulceration is strongly associated with venous disease. However, about a fifth of people with leg ulceration have arterial disease, either alone or in combination with venous problems, which may require specialist referral.[1] Venous ulcers (also known as varicose or stasis ulcers) are caused by venous reflux or obstruction, both of which lead to poor venous return and venous hypertension.
PROGNOSIS	People with leg ulcers have a poorer quality of life than age matched controls because of pain, odour, and reduced mobility.[2] In the UK, audits have found wide variation in the types of care (hospital inpatient care, hospital clinics, outpatient clinics, home visits), in the treatments used (topical agents, dressings, bandages, stockings), in healing rates, and in recurrence rates (26–69% in 1 year).[3,4]
AIMS	To promote healing; to reduce recurrence; to improve quality of life, with minimal adverse effects.
OUTCOMES	Ulcer area, number of ulcers healed, number of ulcer free limbs, recurrence rates, number of new ulcer episodes, number of ulcer free weeks or months, number of people who are ulcer free, frequency of dressing/bandage changes, quality of life, adverse effects of treatment.
METHODS	We used the search strategy for the Cochrane Wounds Group: search date June 2000, primary sources Cochrane Library, Medline, Embase, and Cinahl. *Clinical Evidence* update search and appraisal May 2000. We included RCTs with clinically important and objective outcomes: proportion of wounds healed, healing rates, incidence of new or recurring wounds, infection, and quality of life.

QUESTION What are the effects of treatments?

OPTION COMPRESSION

One systematic review of RCTs has found that compression heals venous leg ulcers more effectively than no compression. Elastomeric multilayer, high compression bandages, Unna's boot, high compression hosiery, and European short stretch bandages are all effective. We found insufficient evidence to compare different methods of compression.

Benefits: **Compression versus no compression:** We found one recent systematic review (search date May 2000, 6 RCTs, n = 260), comparing compression versus no compression.[5] The review found that compression (e.g. short stretch bandages, double layer bandage, and Unna's boot — see glossary, p 1175) healed venous leg ulcers more effectively than no compression (e.g. dressing alone). The trials were heterogeneous, using different forms of compression in different settings and patient populations. The results were not pooled. The results of individual RCTs consistently favoured compression. **Elastomeric versus non-elastomeric multilayer compression:** See glossary, p 1175. The systematic review identified three RCTs (n = 273) comparing elastomeric multilayer high compression bandages versus non-elastomeric multilayer compression.[5] Meta-analysis found an increase in the proportion of people whose ulcers healed with 12–15 weeks of high compression treatment versus controls (RRI for healing 54%, 95% CI 19% to 100%; NNT 5, 95% CI 3 to 12) (see table 1, p 1177).[5] **Multilayer high compression versus short stretch regimens:** The systematic review identified four small RCTs (n = 164), which found no difference between multilayer high compression and short stretch regimens (RRI for healing 10%, 95% CI –22% to +55%).[5] The lack of power in these small studies means that a clinically important difference cannot be excluded. **Multilayer high compression versus single layer bandage:** The systematic review identified four RCTs (n = 280) comparing multilayer high compression versus a single layer of bandage.[5] Meta-analysis found an increase in the proportion of ulcers healing with multilayered compression versus controls (RRI 41%, 95% CI 11% to 80%; NNT 6, 95% CI 4 to 18) (see table 1, p 1177).

Harms: High levels of compression applied to limbs with insufficient arterial supply, or inexpert application of bandages, can lead to tissue damage and, at worst, amputation.[10] Complication rates were rarely reported in trials.

Comment: People suitable for high compression were those with clinical signs of venous disease (ulcer in the gaiter region, from the upper margin of the malleolus to the bulge of the gastrocnemius; peri-ulcer staining; or eczema); no concurrent diabetes mellitus or rheumatoid arthritis; and adequate arterial supply to the foot as determined by ankle/brachial pressure index. The precise ankle/brachial pressure index below which compression is contraindicated is often quoted as 0.8; however, many trials used the higher cut off of 0.9.[5] Effectiveness is likely to be influenced by the ability of those applying the bandage to generate safe levels of compression. Bandages may be applied by the person with the leg ulcer, their carer, nurse, or doctor. We found no comparisons of healing rates between specialist and non-specialist application of compression. Training improves bandaging technique among nurses.[11] Bandages containing elastomeric fibres can be applied weekly as they maintain their tension over time. Bandages made of wool or cotton, or both, such as short stretch bandages, may need to be reapplied more frequently as they do not maintain their tension.

| OPTION | INTERMITTENT PNEUMATIC COMPRESSION |

Three small RCTs have found no evidence of a significant effect on healing with intermittent pneumatic compression in conjunction with compression bandages.

Benefits: We found one systematic review (search date April 1997, 2 RCTs, n = 67) comparing intermittent pneumatic compression (see glossary, p 1175) in conjunction with compression (bandages or hosiery) versus compression alone.[9] We found one subsequent RCT (n = 53).[12] These trials were all different in design. Pooling of results, using a random effects model, found no difference in healing rates.

Harms: No harmful effects have been reported.

Comment: Availability may vary widely between healthcare settings. Treatment can be delivered in the home, in outpatient clinics, or in the hospital ward. Clinical trials have evaluated the use of intermittent pneumatic pressure for 1 hour twice a week and 3–4 hours a day. Treatment requires resting for 1–4 hours daily, which may reduce quality of life.

| OPTION | DRESSINGS AND TOPICAL AGENTS | New |

We found no strong evidence on the effects of occlusive and non-occlusive dressings, topical agents, or antimicrobial agents compared with simple primary dressings such as gauze. Given that the trials were small and have not been replicated, they provide no evidence of benefit rather than firm evidence of no benefit.

Benefits: **Simple low adherent dressings versus occlusive or semi-occlusive dressings:** We found one systematic review (search date October 1997, 16 RCTs) comparing occlusive (hydrocolloids) or semi-occlusive dressings (foam, film, alginates) versus simple dressings (such as paraffin-tulle, knitted viscose dressings).[13] Nine of the trials compared hydrocolloid dressings versus simple dressings, in the presence of compression. A pooled analysis of seven RCTs (n = 714) found no evidence of benefit. Two comparisons of foam dressings versus simple dressings; two of film dressings versus simple dressings; and one comparing an alginate versus a simple dressing failed to find evidence of benefit. The trials, however, were too small (10–132 participants, median 60) to detect anything but a very large difference in effectiveness. **Topical agents versus inert comparators:** The same systematic review identified 16 RCTs comparing topical agents (such as growth factors, cell suspensions, oxygen free-radical scavengers) versus either placebo preparations or standard care in the treatment of venous leg ulcers.[13] There was insufficient evidence to recommend any topical agent. The studies were small (9–233 participants, median 45) and heterogeneous, and therefore could not be pooled. Four RCTs of topical agents have been published since the systematic review search. One RCT (n = 66) of calcitonin gene related peptide and vasoactive intestinal polypeptide administered by iontophoresis (see glossary, p 1175) versus electrical stimulation, found no evidence of benefit.[14] One RCT (n = 60) comparing a 13 week course of peri-ulcer injections of granulocyte–macrophage colony stimulating factor (GM-CSF) 400 µg versus placebo found a benefit for the treatment (RRI for the proportion of ulcers completely healed 236%, 95% CI 13% to 1134%; NNT 2, 95% CI 1 to 19) (see table 1, p 1177).[7] One RCT (n = 293) comparing a cultured allogenic bilayer skin (see glossary, p 1175) replacement that contained both epidermal and dermal components with a non-adherent dressing, found a greater proportion of ulcers healed completely in 6 months with the skin replacement (RRI for the proportion of ulcers healed 29%, 95% CI 4% to 61%; NNT 7, 95% CI 4 to 41) (see table 1, p 1177)[8] One RCT (n = 40) of topically applied mesoglycan, a profibrinolytic agent, found no evidence of benefit.[15] **Antimicrobial agents versus placebo or standard care:** We found one systematic review (search date October 1997, 14 RCTs) comparing antimicrobial agents versus either placebo agents or standard care.[16] The trials were small (25–153 participants, median 56), of poor quality, and no firm conclusions could be drawn.

Harms: It is unlikely that low adherent primary wound dressings would cause harm, although dressings containing iodine may affect thyroid function if used over large surface areas for extended periods.[17] People with venous leg ulcers exhibit a high rate (50–85%) of contact sensitivity to preservatives, perfumes, and dyes; therefore, simple products should be used where possible.[18]

Comment: Simple primary dressings maintain a moist environment beneath compression bandages by preventing loss of moisture from the wound.[19]

| OPTION | THERAPEUTIC ULTRASOUND |

We found insufficient evidence of the effects of therapeutic ultrasound in the treatment of venous leg ulcers.

Benefits: We found one systematic review (search date December 1999, 7 RCTs, n = 470) comparing therapeutic ultrasound (see glossary, p 1175) versus no ultrasound or sham ultrasound for venous leg ulcers.[20] Results for all studies tended to favour ultrasound, but a significant difference in ulcer healing was found in only four out of seven individual RCTs.

Harms: Mild erythema, local pain, and small areas of bleeding have been reported in some trials.

Comment: None.

| OPTION | DRUG TREATMENTS |

One systematic review found good evidence that oral oxpentifylline accelerates the healing of venous leg ulcers. We found limited evidence suggesting that sulodexide or flavonoids accelerate the healing of venous leg ulcers. We found no good evidence on the effects of aspirin or oral zinc supplements.

Benefits: **Oxpentifylline:** We found one systematic review (search date August 1999, 9 RCTs).[6] Eight RCTs compared oxpentifylline (1200 mg or 2400 mg a day) versus placebo in venous leg ulcers. The review pooled results from five RCTs, in which compression was standard therapy, and found that more ulcers healed with oxpentifylline than placebo (RRI for healing 30%, 95% CI 10% to 54%; NNT for 6 months' treatment 6, 95% CI 4 to 14). One trial found no evidence of benefit for oxpentifylline compared with defibrotide (see table 1, p 1177). **Flavonoids:** We found one RCT (n = 91) comparing a flavonoid versus placebo in venous leg ulcers. This trial found that 1000 mg (900 mg diosmin and 100 mg hesperidin) increased the rate of complete healing of ulcers that were initially less than 10 cm in diameter (relative increase in proportion of ulcers healed 150%, 95% CI 9% to 485%; NNT for 2 months' treatment 5, 95% CI 3 to 50) (see table 1, p 1177).[21] **Thromboxane α2 antagonists:** We found one RCT (n = 165) comparing an oral thromboxane α_2 antagonist versus placebo in venous leg ulcers. There was no significant difference in the proportion of ulcers healing in the two groups (54% v 55%).[22] **Oral zinc:** We found one systematic review (search date December 1997, 5 RCTs, n = 151) comparing daily doses of 440–600 mg oral zinc sulphate with placebo. The review found no evidence of benefit for oral zinc.[23] **Aspirin:** We found one small RCT of aspirin (300 mg a day, enteric coated) versus placebo. This reported that more ulcers healed with aspirin (38% v 0%), but the trial had several weaknesses.[24] **Sulodexide:** We found one RCT (n = 94), which compared the addition of a profibrinolytic agent, sulodexide, to compression therapy. Sulodexide was administered by daily intramuscular injection for 30 days and then orally for 30 days. More ulcers healed in the sulodexide group than the control group (35% v 58%; RRI 61%, 95% CI 3.5% to 163%; NNT 4, 95% CI 2 to 64, for 60 days treatment).[25]

Harms: The systematic review found that more adverse effects were reported in the oxpentifylline group, although this was not significant (for adverse effects with oxpentifylline RR 1.25, 95% CI 0.87 to 1.80). Nearly half of the adverse effects reported were gastrointestinal, such as dyspepsia, vomiting, and diarrhoea.[20] Adverse effects of flavonoids, such as gastrointestinal disturbances, were reported in 10% of people.

Comment: Sulodexide is not widely available and daily injections may be unacceptable to some people.

OPTION VEIN SURGERY

We found insufficient evidence of the effects of vein surgery on ulcer healing.

Benefits: We found no systematic review. We found one RCT (n = 47) comparing vein surgery (perforator ligation) versus no surgery or surgery plus skin grafting.[26] There was no difference in the proportion of ulcers healed after 1 year or the rate of ulcer healing. The trial was too small to rule out a beneficial effect.

Harms: Vein surgery carries the usual risks of surgery and anaesthesia.

Comment: Several operative approaches are commonly used, including perforator ligation, saphenous vein stripping, and a combination of both procedures.

OPTION SKIN GRAFTING   New

We found insufficient evidence of the effects of skin grafting on ulcer healing.

Benefits:	We found one systematic review (search date October 1999, 6 RCTs, n = 197) of skin grafts (autografts or allografts) for venous leg ulcers. In five trials people also received compression bandaging; two trials (n = 98) evaluated split thickness autografts; three trials (n = 92) evaluated cultured keratinocyte allografts; and one (n = 7, 13 ulcers) compared tissue engineered skin (artificial skin) with a split thickness skin graft. There was insufficient evidence to determine whether skin grafting increased the healing of venous ulcers.[27]
Harms:	Grafts harvested from the patient will leave an additional wound that requires management and may cause pain. We found no evidence of harm from tissue engineered skin.
Comment:	None.

OPTION LOW LEVEL LASER THERAPY New

We found insufficient evidence of the effects of low level laser therapy on ulcer healing.

Benefits:	We found two systematic reviews.[28,29] The larger review (search date 1998, 4 RCTs) of laser therapy for venous leg ulcers included the only two RCTs identified by the smaller review. Two RCTs compared low level laser therapy (see glossary, p 1175) with sham; one RCT compared laser with ultraviolet therapy; and one RCT with non-coherent, unpolarised red light. Neither of the two RCTs comparing laser with sham found a significant difference in healing rates. There was no significant difference in healing rates with laser when the trials were pooled. A three arm study (n = 30) compared laser therapy with laser therapy plus infrared light and with non-coherent, unpolarised red light. Significantly more ulcers healed completely in the group receiving a combination of laser and infrared light compared with non-coherent, unpolarised red light (RRI 140%, 95% CI 22% to 442%; NNT 2, 95% CI 1 to 9, for 9 months' treatment). A fourth trial compared laser and ultraviolet light and found no difference.[28]
Harms:	Eye protection is required when using some types of laser as the high energy beam may lead to damage of the retina.
Comment:	The laser power, wavelength, frequency, duration and follow up of treatment were different for all the studies.

QUESTION What are the effects of interventions to prevent recurrence?

OPTION COMPRESSION

We found limited evidence that compression reduces recurrence rates but non-compliance with compression is a risk factor for recurrence.

Benefits:	We found one systematic review (search date April 1997), which identified no RCTs comparing compression hosiery versus no compression.[9] The review identified two RCTs comparing different types of compression. One trial (n = 166) compared two brands of UK

Class 2 stockings (see comment below) and found no difference in recurrence rates. The larger trial (n = 300) compared recurrence rates using Class 2 and Class 3 stockings (see table 1, p 1177 and comment below). With an intention to treat analysis, the trial found no significant reduction in recurrence at 5 years' follow up associated with high compression hosiery (UK Class 3) compared with moderate compression hosiery (UK Class 2). This analysis may underestimate the effectiveness of the Class 3 hosiery because a significant proportion of people changed from Class 3 to Class 2. Both trials found that non-compliance with compression hosiery was associated with recurrence.

Harms: The application of high compression to limbs with reduced arterial supply may result in ischaemic tissue damage and, at worst, amputation.[10]

Comment: Compression hosiery is classified according to the magnitude of pressure exerted at the ankle; the UK classification states that Class 2 hosiery is capable of applying 18–24 mm Hg pressure, and Class 3 is capable of applying 25–35 mm Hg pressure at the ankle. Other countries use different classification systems. Hosiery reduces venous reflux by locally increasing venous pressure in the legs relative to the rest of the body. This effect only takes place while hosiery is worn. The association between non-compliance with compression and recurrence of venous ulceration provides some indirect evidence of the benefit of compression in prevention. People are advised to wear compression hosiery for life. It is considered good practice to reassess arterial supply regularly as patients might develop arterial disease and hence risk pressure necrosis caused by their compression hosiery. Other measures designed to reduce leg oedema, such as resting with the leg elevated, may be useful.

| OPTION | SYSTEMIC DRUGS |

We found insufficient evidence on the effects of systemic drugs on ulcer recurrence.

Benefits: We found one systematic review (search date April 1997, 2 RCTs, n = 198) of drugs in the prevention of leg ulcer recurrence.[9] The review concluded that there was no evidence that stanozolol or rutoside decreased recurrence rates. One trial (n = 60), of stanozolol versus placebo, found no significant difference in recurrence rates (17% v 20%). The other trial (n = 139), of rutoside versus placebo, found no significant difference in recurrence rates (32% v 34%).

Harms: Stanozolol is an anabolic steroid; adverse effects included acne, hirsutism, amenorrhoea, oedema, headache, dyspepsia, rash, hair loss, depression, jaundice, and changes in liver enzymes. Tolerance of rutoside was reported to be good; adverse effects included headache, flushing, rashes, and mild gastrointestinal disturbances.[30]

Comment: None.

| OPTION | VEIN SURGERY |

We found insufficient evidence on the effects of vein surgery on ulcer recurrence.

Benefits: We found one systematic review (search date April 1997, 1 RCT, n = 30).[9] The identified trial, which was poorly controlled, compared surgery plus compression hosiery versus compression hosiery alone for prevention of recurrence. The trial found a reduced rate of recurrence when surgery was carried out in addition to the use of elastic stockings (5% v 24%; RRR 0.79, 95% CI 0.20 to 0.97).

Harms: Vein surgery has the usual risks of surgery and anaesthesia.

Comment: The results of this small, poorly controlled trial should be interpreted with caution.

GLOSSARY

Cultured allogenic bilayer skin equivalent Also called human skin equivalent. This is made of a lower (dermal) layer of bovine collagen containing living human dermal fibroblasts, and an upper (epidermal) layer of living human keratinocytes.

Elastomeric multilayer high compression bandages Generally a layer of padding material followed by 1–3 additional layers of elastomeric bandages.

Intermittent pneumatic compression External compression applied by inflatable leggings or boots either over, or instead of, compression hosiery or bandages. A pump successively inflates and deflates the boots to promote the return of blood from the tissues. Newer systems have separate compartments in the boots so that the foot is inflated before the ankle, which is inflated before the calf.

Iontophoresis The delivery of an ionic substance by application of an electrical current.

Short stretch bandages Minimally extensible bandages usually made of cotton with few or no elastomeric fibres. They are applied at near full extension to form a semi-rigid bandage.

Therapeutic ultrasound Application of ultrasound to a wound, using a transducer and a water based gel. Prolonged application can lead to heating of the tissues, but when used in wound healing the power used is low, and the transducer is constantly moved by the therapist, so that the tissue is not significantly heated.

Unna's boot An inner layer of zinc oxide impregnated bandage, which hardens as it dries to form a semi-rigid layer against which the calf muscle can contract. It is usually covered in an elastomeric bandage.

Low level laser therapy Application of treatment energy ($< 10J/cm^2$) using lasers of 50 mW or less.

Substantive changes since last issue

Topical agents One RCT of topical mesoglycan found no evidence of benefit.[14]

Ultrasound One new systematic review found insufficient evidence of the effects of therapeutic ultrasound in the treatment of venous leg ulcers.[19]

Oral oxpentifylline One new systematic review found that oral oxpentifylline increases the healing of venous leg ulcers; no change in conclusion.[20]

Drug treatments: Aspirin New component in the option; one RCT.[24]

Drug treatments: Sulodexide New component in the option; one RCT.[25]

REFERENCES

1. Callam MJ, Ruckley CV, Harper DR, et al. Chronic ulceration of the leg: extent of the problem and provision of care. *BMJ* 1985;290:1855–1856.
2. Roe B, Cullum N, Hamer C. Patients' perceptions of chronic leg ulceration. In: Cullum N, Roe B, eds. *Leg ulcers: nursing management*. Harrow: Scutari, 1995:125–134.
3. Roe B, Cullum N. The management of leg ulcers: current nursing practice. In: Cullum N, Roe B, eds. *Leg ulcers: nursing management*. Harrow: Scutari, 1995:113–124.
4. Vowden KR, Barker A, Vowden P. Leg ulcer management in a nurse-led, hospital-based clinic. *J Wound Care* 1997;6:233–236.
5. Cullum N, Nelson EA, Fletcher AW, et al. Compression bandages and stockings in the treatment of venous leg ulcers. In: The Cochrane Library, Issue 3, 2000. Oxford: Update Software. Search date May 2000; primary sources 19 electronic databases, hand searches and personal contacts.
6. Jull AB, Waters J, Arroll B. Oral oxpentifylline for treatment of venous leg ulcers. In: The Cochrane Library, Issue 3, 2000. Oxford: Update Software. Search date 1999; primary sources Cochrane Peripheral Vascular Diseases and Wounds Group, specialised registers, hand searches of reference lists, relevant journals and conference proceedings, personal contact with Hoechst, manufacturers of pentoxifylline, and experts in the field.
7. Da Costa RM, Ribeiro Jesus FM, Aniceto C, et al. Randomized, double-blind, placebo-controlled, dose-ranging study of granulocyte–macrophage colony stimulating factor in patients with chronic venous leg ulcers. *Wound Repair Regen* 1999;7:17–25.
8. Falanga V, Margolis D, Alvarez O, et al. Rapid healing of venous ulcers and lack of clinical rejection with an allogeneic cultured human skin equivalent. Human Skin Equivalent Investigators Group. *Arch Dermatol* 1998;134:293–300.
9. Cullum N, Fletcher A, Semlyen A, et al. Compression therapy for venous leg ulcers. *Qual Health Care* 1997;6:226–231. Search date April 1997; primary sources 18 databases, including Medline, Embase and Cinahl with no restriction on date, hand search of relevant journals, conference proceedings, and correspondence with experts to obtain unpublished papers.
10. Callam MJ, Ruckley CV, Dale JJ, et al. Hazards of compression treatment of the leg: an estimate from Scottish surgeons. *BMJ* 1987;295:1382.
11. Nelson EA, Ruckley CV, Barbenel J. Improvements in bandaging technique following training. *J Wound Care* 1995;4:181–184.
12. Schuler JJ, Maibenco T, Megerman J, et al. Treatment of chronic venous leg ulcers using sequential gradient intermittent pneumatic compression. *Phlebology* 1996;11:111–116.
13. Bradley M, Nelson EA, Cullum N, et al. Dressings and topical agents for healing of chronic wounds: a systematic review. NHS Health Technology Assessment Report 1999;3(17pt2). Search date October 1997; primary sources Cochrane Library, Medline, Embase, Cinahl.
14. Gherardini G, Gurlek A, Evans GRD, et al. Venous ulcers: improved healing by iontophoretic administration of calcitonin gene-related peptide and vasoactive intestinal polypeptide. *Plast Reconstr Surg* 1998;101:90–93.
15. La Marc G, Pumilia G, Martino A. Effectiveness of mesoglycan topical treatment of leg ulcers in subjects with chronic venous insufficiency. *Minerva Cardioangiol* 1999;47:315–319.
16. O'Meara S, Cullum N, Majid M, et al. A systematic review of systemic and topical antimicrobial agents used in the treatment of chronic wounds. NHS Health Technology Assessment Report 1999; 3(17pt2). Search date October 1997; primary sources Cochrane Library, Medline, Embase, Cinahl.
17. Thomas S. *Wound management and dressings*. London: Pharmaceutical Press, 1990.
18. Cameron J, Wilson C, Powell S, et al. Contact dermatitis in leg ulcer patients. *Ostomy Wound Manage* 1992;38:10–11.
19. Wu P, Nelson EA, Reid WH, et al. Water vapour transmission rates in burns and chronic leg ulcers: influence of wound dressings and comparison with in vitro evaluation. *Biomaterials* 1996;17:1373–1377.
20. Flemming K, Cullum N. Therapeutic ultrasound for venous leg ulcers (Protocol for a Cochrane Review). In: The Cochrane Library, Issue 3, 2000. Oxford: Update Software.
21. Guilhou JJ, Dereure O, Marzin L, et al. Efficacy of Daflon 500 mg in venous leg ulcer healing: a double-blind, randomized, controlled versus placebo trial in 107 patients. *Angiology* 1997;48:77–85.
22. Lyon RT, Veith FJ, Bolton L, et al. Clinical benchmark for healing of chronic venous ulcers. Venous Ulcer Study Collaborators. *Am J Surgery* 1998;176:172–175.
23. Wilkinson EAJ, Hawke CI. Does oral zinc aid the healing of chronic leg ulcers? A systematic literature review. *Arch Dermatol* 1998;134:1556–1560. Search date 1997; primary sources Medline, Embase, Cinahl, Science Citation Index, Biosis, British Diabetic Association Database, Ciscom, Cochrane Controlled Register of Clinical Trials, Dissertation Abstracts, Royal College of Nursing Database, electronic databases of ongoing research, hand searches of wound care journals and conference proceedings, and contact with manufacturer of zinc sulphate tablets.
24. Layton AM, Ibbotson SH, Davies JA, et al. Randomised trial of oral aspirin for chronic venous leg ulcers. *Lancet* 1994;344:164–165.
25. Scondotto G, Aloisi D, Ferrari P, et al . Treatment of venous leg ulcers with sulodexide. *Angiology* 99;50:883–889.
26. Warburg FE, Danielsen L, Madsen SM, et al. Vein surgery with or without skin grafting versus conservative treatment for leg ulcers. *Acta Dermatol Vereol* 1994;74:307–309.
27. Jones JE, Nelson EA. Skin grafting for venous leg ulcers. In: The Cochrane Library, Issue 3, 2000. Oxford: Update Software. Search date 1999; primary sources Cochrane Wounds Group Specialised Register, hand searches of reference lists, relevant journals, conference proceedings, and personal contact with experts in the field.
28. Flemming K, Cullum N. Laser therapy for venous leg ulcers. In: The Cochrane Library, Issue 3, 2000. Oxford: Update Software. Search date 1998; primary sources 19 databases, hand searches of journals, conference proceedings, and bibliographies.
29. Lucas C, Stanborough RW, Freeman CL, et al. Efficacy of low level laser therapy on wound healing in human subjects: a systematic review. *Lasers Med Sci* 2000;15:84–93. Search date 1998; primary sources Medline, Embase, Cinahl, Cochrane Rehabilitation, and Related Therapies Register of Trials.
30. Taylor HM, Rose KE, Twycross RG. A double-blind clinical trial of hydroxyethylrutosides in obstructive arm lymphoedema. *Phlebology* 1993;8(suppl 1):22–28.

E Nelson
Research Fellow

Nicky Cullum
Reader

Centre for Evidence Based Nursing
University of York
York
UK

June Jones
Clinical Nurse Specialist
North Sefton and West Lancashire
Community Services NHS Trust
Southport
UK

Competing interests: AN has been reimbursed for attending symposia by Smith and Nephew, Huntleigh Healthcare, and Convatec; JJ has been reimbursed for attending symposia by 3M and Convatec.

TABLE 1 NNTs for interventions (see text, p 1169).

Intervention	NNT (95% CI)
Elastomeric multilayer compression v non-elastomeric multilayer compression bandages	5 (3 to 12)[5]
Multilayer high compression v single layer compression bandages	6 (4 to 18)[5]
Oxpentifylline 400 mg three times a day v placebo (concurrent use of compression)	6 (4 to 14)[6]
Peri-ulcer injection of GM-CSF* (400 µg) v placebo	2 (1 to 19)[7]
Cultured allogenic bilayer skin equivalent v non-adherent dressing	7 (4 to 41)[8]
Class 3 v class 2 compression hosiery for prevention of recurrence	9 (5 to 236)[9]

*GM–CSF, granulocyte–macrophage colony stimulating factor.

Estimating cardiovascular risk and treatment benefit

Adapted from the New Zealand guidelines on management of dyslipidaemia[1] and raised blood pressure [2] by Rod Jackson

How to use these colour charts

The charts help the estimation of a person's absolute risk of a cardiovascular event and the likely benefit of drug treatment to lower cholesterol or blood pressure. For these charts cardiovascular events include: new angina, myocardial infarction, coronary death, stroke or transient ischaemic attack (TIA), onset of congestive cardiac failure or peripheral vascular syndrome.

There is a group of patients in whom risk can be assumed to be high (>20% in 5 years) without using the charts. They include those with symptomatic cardiovascular disease (angina, myocardial infarction, congestive heart failure, stroke, TIA, and peripheral vascular disease), or left ventricular hypertrophy on ECG.

To estimate a person's absolute five-year risk:
■ Find the table relating to their sex, diabetic status (on insulin, oral hypoglycaemics or fasting blood glucose over 8 mmol/l), smoking status and age. The age shown in the charts is the mean for that category, i.e. age 60 = 55 to 65 years.
■ Within the table find the cell nearest to the person's blood pressure and total cholesterol : HDL ratio. For risk assessment it is enough to use a mean blood pressure based on two readings on each of two occasions, and cholesterol measurements based on one laboratory or two non-fasting Reflotron measurements. More readings are needed to establish the pre-treatment baseline.
■ The colour of the box indicates the person's five-year cardiovascular disease risk (see below).

Notes: (1) People with a strong history of CVD (first degree male relatives with CVD before 55 years, female relatives before 65 years) or obesity (body mass index above 30 kg/m^2) are likely to be at greater risk than the tables indicate. The magnitude of the independent predictive value of these risk factors remains unclear—their presence should influence treatment decisions for patients at borderline treatment levels. (2) If total cholesterol or total cholesterol:HDL ratio is greater than 8 then the risk is at least 15%. (3) Nearly all people aged 75 years or over also have an absolute cardiovascular risk over 15%.

Charts reproduced with permission from The National Heart Foundation of New Zealand. Also available on http://www.nzgg.org.nz/library/gl_complete/bloodpressure/chart1.htm

REFERENCES

1. Dyslipidaemia Advisory Group. 1996 National Heart Foundation clinical guidelines for the assessment and management of dyslipidaemia. *NZ Med J* 1996;109:224–232.
2. National Health Committee. Guidelines for the management of mildly raised blood pressure in New Zealand: Ministry of Health National Health Committee Report, Wellington, 1995.

	RISK LEVEL Five-year CVD risk (non-fatal and fatal)	BENEFIT (1) CVD events prevented per 100 treated for five years*	BENEFIT (2) Number needed to treat for five years to prevent one event*
Very High	>30%	>10 per 100	<10
Very High	25–30%	9 per 100	11
Very High	20–25%	7.5 per 100	13
High	15–20%	6 per 100	16
Moderate	10–15%	4 per 100	25
Mild	5–10%	2.5 per 100	40
Mild	2.5–5%	1.25 per 100	80
Mild	<2.5%	<0.8 per 100	>120

*Based on a 20% reduction in total cholesterol or a reduction in blood pressure of 10–15 mmHg systolic or 5–10 mmHg diastolic, which is estimated to reduce CVD risk by about one third over 5 years.

RISK LEVEL: MEN

DIABETES

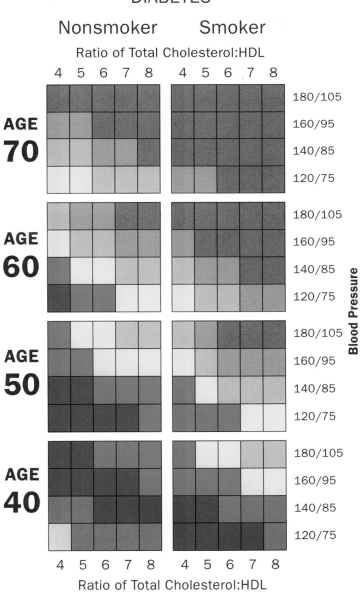

Nonsmoker   Smoker

Ratio of Total Cholesterol:HDL

Appendix 1

RISK LEVEL: WOMEN

NO DIABETES

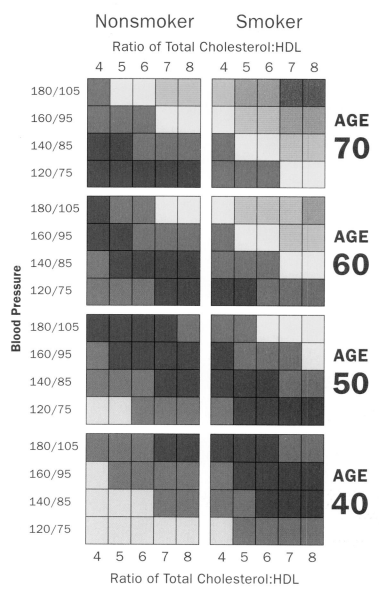

Nonsmoker   Smoker

Ratio of Total Cholesterol:HDL

Blood Pressure

AGE 70
AGE 60
AGE 50
AGE 40

Ratio of Total Cholesterol:HDL

Estimating cardiovascular risk and treatment benefit

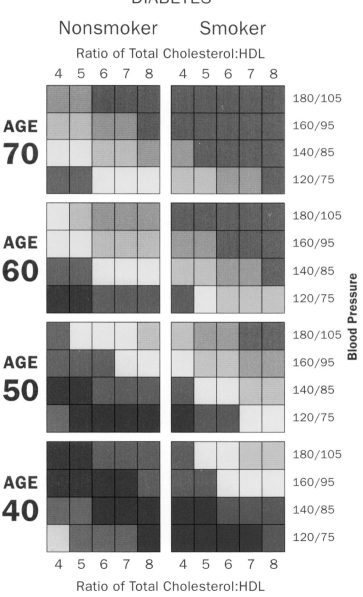

DIABETES

Nonsmoker   Smoker

Ratio of Total Cholesterol:HDL

Ratio of Total Cholesterol:HDL

Blood Pressure

The number needed to treat: adjusting for baseline risk

Adapted with permission from Chatellier et al, 1996[1]

BACKGROUND

The number needed to treat (NNT) to avoid a single additional adverse outcome is a meaningful way of expressing the benefit of an active treatment over a control. It can be used both to summarise the results of a therapeutic trial or series of trials and to help medical decision making about an individual patient.

If the absolute risk of adverse outcomes in a therapeutic trial is ARC in the control group and ART in the treatment group, then the absolute risk reduction (ARR) is defined as (ARC − ART). The NNT is defined as the inverse of the ARR:

$$NNT = 1/(ARC - ART)$$

Since the Relative Risk Reduction (RRR) is defined as (ARC − ART)/ARC, it follows that NNT, RRR and ARC are related by their definitions in the following way:

$$NNT \times RRR \times ARC = 1$$

This relationship can be used to estimate the likely benefits of a treatment in populations with different levels of baseline risk (that is different levels of ARC). This allows extrapolation of the results of a trial or meta-analysis to people with different baseline risks. Ideally, there should be experimental evidence of the RRR in each population. However in many trials, subgroup analyses show that the RRR is approximately constant in groups of patients with different characteristics. Cook and Sackett therefore proposed that decisions about individual patients could be made by using the NNT calculated from the RRR measured in trials and the baseline risk in the absence of treatment estimated for the individual patient.[2]

The method may not apply to periods of time different to that studied in the original trials.

USING THE NOMOGRAM

The nomogram shown on the next page allows the NNT to be found directly without any calculation: a straight line should be drawn from the point corresponding to the estimated absolute risk for the patient on the left hand scale to the point corresponding to the relative risk reduction stated in a trial or meta-analysis on the central scale. The intercept of this line with the right hand scale gives the NNT. By taking the upper and lower limits of the confidence interval of the RRR, the upper and lower limits of the NNT can be estimated.

REFERENCES

1. Chatellier G, Zapletal E, Lemaitre D, Menard J, Degoulet P. The number needed to treat: a clinically useful nomogram in its proper context. *BMJ* 1996;321:426–429.
2. Cook RJ, Sackett DL. The number needed to treat: a clinically useful measure of treatment effect. *BMJ* 1995;310:452–454.

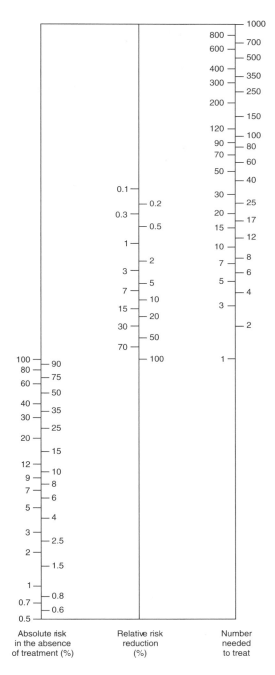

Abbreviations

AR	Absolute risk	**NS**	Not significant
ARR	Absolute risk reduction	**OR**	Odds ratio
ARI	Absolute risk increase	**P**	P value
CI	Confidence interval	**RCT**	Randomised controlled trial
CCT	Controlled clinical trial	**RR**	Relative risk
HR	Hazard ratio	**RRI**	Relative risk increase
NNH	Number needed to harm	**RRR**	Relative risk reduction
NNT	Number needed to treat	**WMD**	Weighted mean difference

How to calculate risk

AR = # events (good or bad) in treated or control groups/ # people in that group

ARC = AR of events in the control group

ART = AR of events in the treatment group

ARR = ARC − ART

RR = ART/ARC = 1 − RRR

RRR = (ARC − ART)/ARC = 1 − RR

NNT = 1/ARR

To express decimals as percentages, multiply by 100.

If:

the RR (or OR) = 1, or the CI includes 1, there is no significant difference between treatment and control groups

the RR > 1 and the CI does not include 1, events are significantly more likely in the treatment than the control group

the RR < 1 and the CI does not include 1, events are significantly less likely in the treatment than the control group

RR of 0.8 means a RRR of 20% (meaning a 20% reduction in the relative risk of the specified outcome in the treatment group compared with the control group).

RRR is usually constant across a range of absolute risks. But the ARR is higher and the NNT lower in people with higher absolute risks.

Example: If a person's AR of stroke, estimated from his age and other risk factors (see appendix 1), is 0.25 without treatment but falls to 0.20 with treatment, the ARR is 25% −20% = 5%; the RRR is (25% −20%)/25% = 20%; and the NNT is 1/0.05 = 20. In a person with an AR of stroke of only 0.025 without treatment, the same treatment will still produce a 20% RRR, but treatment will reduce her AR of stroke to 0.2, giving a much smaller ARR of 2.5% −2% = 0.5%, and a NNT of 200.

Note

When looking up a class of drug, the reader is advised to also look up specific examples of that class of drug where additional entries may be found. The reverse situation also applies. Abbreviations used: CVD, cardiovascular disease; HRT, hormone replacement therapy; HSV, herpes simplex virus; IVF, in vitro fertilisation; MI, myocardial infarction; PMS, premenstrual syndrome; NSAIDs, non- steroidal anti-inflammatory drugs; STD, sexually transmitted disease; TIA, transient ischaemic attack.

INDEX